Trust Carol J. Buck and Elsevier
to take you through the levels of coding success

Step 4:
Professional Resources

Step 3:
Certify

With the resources you need for every level of coding success, Carol J. Buck and Elsevier are with you every step of your coding career. From beginning to advanced, from the classroom to the workplace, from application to certification, the Step Series products are your guides to greater opportunities and successful career advancement.

Step 2:
Practice

Step 1:
Learn

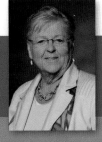

Keep climbing with the most trusted name in medical coding.

Author and Educator
Carol J. Buck, MS, CPC, COC, CCS-P

B-00

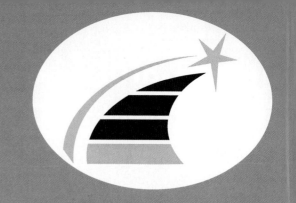
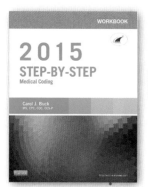
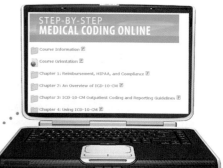
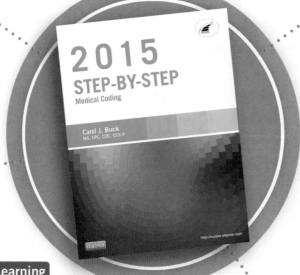
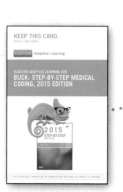

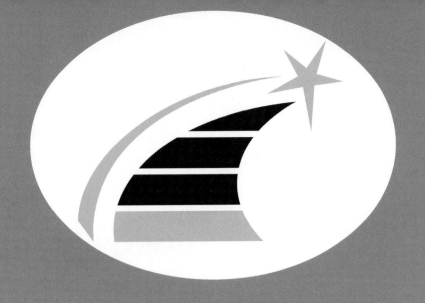

Step 1: Learn

"A journey of a thousand miles begins with a single step."

— Lao-tzu

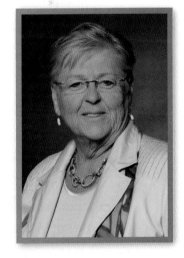

Congratulations! You are embarking on an exciting and rewarding career, and you have taken a great first step. Coding is a career that gives you a chance to pursue excellence at a variety of levels, and I am happy that you have chosen to start with my *Step* line of products. As a lifelong coder and educator, I am dedicated to giving you the tools you need to succeed. ***So, get out there and code!***

— Carol J. Buck, MS, CPC, COC, CCS-P

Track your progress!

**See the checklist in the back of this book
to learn more about your next step toward coding success!**

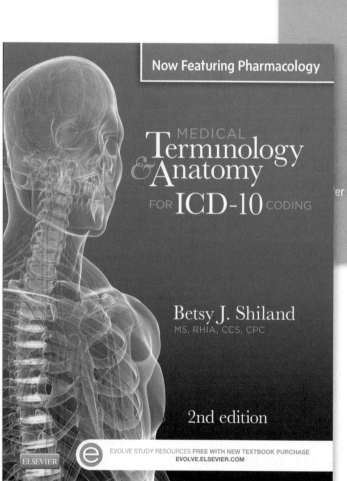
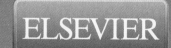

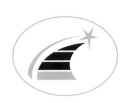

2015
STEP-BY-STEP
Medical Coding

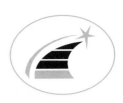

2015
STEP-BY-STEP
Medical Coding

Carol J. Buck
MS, CPC, COC, CCS-P

Former Program Director
Medical Secretary Programs
Northwest Technical College
East Grand Forks, Minnesota

ELSEVIER

http://evolve.elsevier.com

SAUNDERS

3251 Riverport Lane
St. Louis, Missouri 63043

STEP-BY-STEP MEDICAL CODING, 2015 EDITION

ISBN: 978-0-323-27981-9
ISSN: 2210-6529

International Standard Book Number: 978-0-323-27981-9

Director, Private Sector Education & Professional/Reference: Jeanne R. Olson
Content Development Manager: Luke Held
Senior Content Development Specialist: Joshua S. Rapplean
Publishing Services Manager: Pat Joiner
Project Manager: Lisa A. P. Bushey
Senior Designer: Amy Buxton

Printed in Canada

Last digit is the print number: 9 8 7 6 5 4 3 2

Dedication

To the students, whose drive and determination to learn serve as my endless source of inspiration and enrichment.

To teachers, whose contributions are immense and workloads daunting. May this work make your preparation for class a little easier.

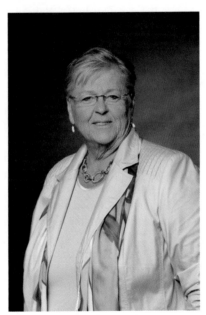

Carol J. Buck

Acknowledgments

This book was developed in collaboration with educators and employers in an attempt to meet the needs of students preparing for careers in the medical coding allied health profession. Obtaining employers' input about the knowledge, skills, and abilities desired of entry-level coding employees benefits educators tremendously. This text is an endeavor to use this information to better prepare our students.

There are several other people who deserve special thanks for their efforts in making this text possible.

Jacqueline Grass, Lead Technical Collaborator, for her technical knowledge, interest in student learning, and long hours of dedicated service to developing education materials.

Patricia Cordy Henricksen, Query Manager, who graciously lends her amazing knowledge and attention to detail to the query process. Her dedication to excellence consistently improves this work.

Nancy Maguire, for her dedication to superior education and her lifetime of devotion to the coding career.

Jeanne R. Olson, Director, Private Sector Education & Professional/Reference, who managed to maintain an excellent sense of humor while jumping into the fray and who is a valued member of the team. **Josh Rapplean,** Senior Content Development Specialist, who manages the developmental duties of this text with calm, confidence, and tremendous efficiency. **Kelly Boutross,** Production Editor, Graphic World, who has assumed responsibility for many projects while maintaining a high degree of professionalism.

The publisher would also like to acknowledge and thank the following people for their enthusiasm and dedication to the coding profession and tremendous contributions to this work:

Patricia Champion
Beverly Comsa
Maria Coslett
Ellen Dooley
Robert H. Ekvall
Christopher P. Galeziewski
Patricia Cordy Henricksen
Belinda D. Inabinet
Lori Koetje

Lynda Kross
Stephanie A. Lewis
Karla R. Lovaasen
Nancy Maguire
Debbi Miller
Tom Mobley
Regine Monfette
Genieve R. Nottage
John R. Nuemann III
Sharon J. Oliver
Zarrina Ostowari

Barbara Oviatt
Christine A. Patterson
Letitia Patterson
Damaris Ramirez
Keith Russell
Patricia Sommerfeld
Martha Tracy
Jane A. Tuttle
Joan E. Wolfgang

Preface

Thank you for purchasing *Step-by-Step Medical Coding*, the leading textbook for medical coding education. This 2015 edition has been carefully reviewed and updated with the latest content, making it the most current textbook for your class. The author and publisher have made every effort to equip you with skills and tools you will need to succeed on the job. To this end, *Step-by-Step Medical Coding* presents essential information for all major health care coding systems and covers the skills needed to be a successful medical coder. No other text on the market brings together such thorough coverage of the coding systems in one source.

ORGANIZATION OF THIS TEXTBOOK

Developed in collaboration with employers and educators, *Step-by-Step Medical Coding, 2015 Edition*, takes a practical approach to training for a successful career in medical coding. The text is divided into five units covering Reimbursement, ICD-10-CM, ICD-9-CM, CPT and HCPCS, and Inpatient Coding.

Unit 1, Reimbursement, is a chapter that introduces the reimbursement, HIPAA, and compliance processes, noting the connections between coding and reimbursement.

Unit 2, ICD-10-CM, provides an overview of the ICD-10-CM codes and their use in medical coding. A highlight of this unit is the inclusion of the *ICD-10-CM Official Guidelines for Coding and Reporting* within the chapter text, as they apply to the content.

Unit 3, ICD-9-CM, provides an overview of the ICD-9-CM codes and their use in medical coding. A highlight of this unit is the inclusion of the *ICD-9-CM Official Guidelines for Coding and Reporting* within the chapter text, as they apply to the content.

Unit 4, CPT and HCPCS, begins with an introduction to the CPT manual, followed by an in-depth explanation of the sections found in the code set. Organized by body systems to follow the CPT codes, the chapters include important information about anatomy, terminology, and various procedures, as well as demonstrations and examples of how to code each service.

Unit 5, Inpatient Coding, provides an overview of reporting facility services provided to patients in acute inpatient facilities and the reporting of these services with ICD-10-PCS and ICD-9-CM, Volume 3, procedures codes.

Some of the CPT code descriptions for physician services include physician extender services. Physician extenders, such as nurse practitioners, physician assistants, and nurse anesthetists, etc., provide medical services typically performed by a physician. Within this educational material the term "physician" may include "and other qualified health care professionals" depending on the code. Refer to the official CPT® code descriptions and guidelines to determine codes that are appropriate to report services provided by non-physician practitioners.

DISTINCTIVE FEATURES OF OUR APPROACH

This book was designed to be the first step in your coding career, and it has many unique features to help you along the way.

- The repetition of skills in each chapter reinforces the material and creates a logical progression for learning and applying each skill—a truly "step-by-step" approach!
- In-text exercises further reinforce important concepts and allow you to check your comprehension as you read (answers are located in Appendix B).
- The format for exercise and review answers guides you in the development of your coding ability by including three response variations:

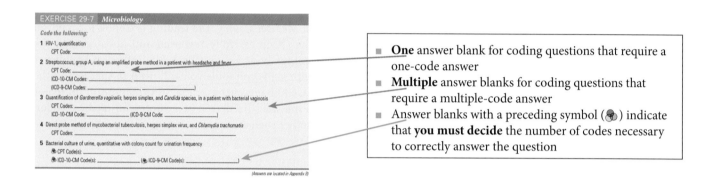

- **One** answer blank for coding questions that require a one-code answer
- **Multiple** answer blanks for coding questions that require a multiple-code answer
- Answer blanks with a preceding symbol (⊛) indicate that **you must decide** the number of codes necessary to correctly answer the question

- *Quick Checks* are located throughout the chapters, providing short follow-up questions after a key concept has been covered to immediately assess learning (answers are located in Appendix C).

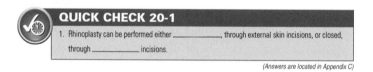

QUICK CHECK 20-1

1. Rhinoplasty can be performed either _____, through external skin incisions, or closed, through _____ incisions.

(Answers are located in Appendix C)

- A full-color design brings a fresh look to the material, visually reinforcing new concepts and examples.
- Medical procedures or conditions are illustrated and discussed in the text to help you understand the services being coded.

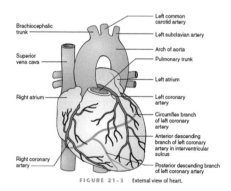

FIGURE 21-3   External view of heart.

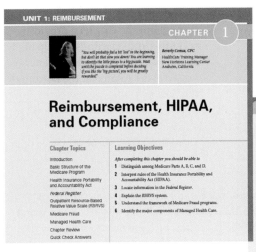

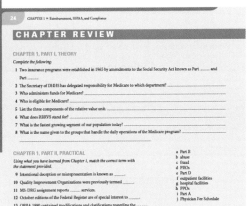

- Chapter learning objectives and end-of-chapter review questions help readers focus on essential chapter content (answers are available only in the TEACH Instructor Resources on Evolve).

- Concrete "real-life" examples illustrate the application of important coding principles and practices.

Example
A lesion was excised and determined to be malignant. The patient was returned to the operating room a few days later for a re-excision of the malignancy. Report the re-excision with modifier -58 because the second procedure was performed within the global period of the first procedure and related to the first procedure.

ICD-10 OFFICIAL GUIDELINES FOR CODING AND REPORTING

SECTION I.B.
6. Conditions that are not an integral part of a disease process
Additional signs and symptoms that may not be associated routinely with a disease process should be coded when present.

- *ICD-10-CM Official Guidelines for Coding and Reporting* boxes in Chapters 2-7 contain excerpts of the actual guidelines, presenting the official wording alongside in-text discussions.
- *ICD-9-CM Official Guidelines for Coding and Reporting* boxes in Chapters 8-12 contain excerpts of the actual guidelines, presenting the official wording alongside in-text discussions.

- *From the Trenches* boxes highlight a different real-life medical coding practitioner in each chapter, with photographs throughout the chapter alongside quotes that offer practical advice or motivational comments.

From the Trenches

"Don't be afraid to write in your coding books! As you study and read, highlight important rules. Write instructions 'in your own words' so you will understand when you go back to look at it again."
BEVERLY

- *Coding Shots* contain tips for the new coder.

 CODING SHOT

Included in the Biopsy codes are codes for biopsies of mucous membranes. A mucous membrane is tissue that covers a variety of body parts, such as the tongue and the nasal cavities.

- *CMS RULES* boxes highlight correct coding methods as required for Medicare claims.

CMS RULES

When a covered colonoscopy is attempted but cannot be completed due to extenuating circumstances (e.g., the inability to extend beyond the splenic flexure), Medicare will usually pay for the interrupted colonoscopy at the rate of a flexible sigmoidoscopy.

TOOLBOX

Susan recently graduated as a medical coder and has been employed at Island Clinic for three months. While coding last Monday, she encountered a superbill for a Medicare patient for an office visit for $62, but there was no supporting documentation in the patient's medical record. Susan questioned the physician and he said that he just forgot to do the paperwork and asked her to send the claim to Medicare with a promise to complete the paperwork later.

QUESTIONS

Susan should do which of the following:
a. Complete the claim and send it in, and write a reminder to the physician to complete the documentation.
b. Wait until the physician completes the documentation.
c. Inform the physician that she cannot submit a claim without appropriate documentation in the medical record.

▼ ANSWERS

c. Never submit a claim for any patient, at any time, for any reason without appropriate documentation in the medical record that supports the claim.

■ *Toolbox* features are located throughout the chapters, providing scenarios and questions to help apply chapter content to realistic scenarios (answers are located at the bottom of the *Toolbox*).

STOP *You were just presented with some very important information about the use of certain codes in the CPT manual. The plus (+) symbol next to any CPT code—not just next to Qualifying Circumstances codes—indicates that that code cannot be used alone. Throughout the remaining sections of the CPT manual, the plus symbol will appear to caution you to use the code only as an adjunct code (with other codes).*

■ *Stop* notes halt you for a reality check, offering a brief summary of material that was just covered and providing a transition into the next topic.

CAUTION *Unlisted codes are assigned only after thorough research fails to reveal a more specific code.*

■ *Caution!* notes warn you about common coding mistakes and reinforce the concept of coding as an exact science.

CHECK THIS OUT! The American Medical Association (AMA) has a website located at www.ama-assn.org.

■ *Check This Out!* boxes offer notes about accessing reference information related to coding, primarily via the Internet.

V45.01:   309t, 891, 901
V72.5:   263

ICD-10-CM CODES

A00.0:   31, 54, 54b
A00.1:   31
A00-A99:   98
A00-B99:   31, 40, 97, 104–105

■ A *Coder's Index* is located in the back of the book, providing easy reference when looking for specific codes.

EXTENSIVE SUPPLEMENTAL RESOURCES

Considering the broad range of students, programs, and institutions in which this textbook is used, we have developed an extensive package of supplements designed to complement *Step-by-Step Medical Coding*. Each of these comprehensive supplements has been developed with the needs of both students and instructors in mind.

Student Online Activities

The online activities supplement the text with 47 chapter activities and 25 coding cases. The variety of activity styles include multiple choice, fill in the blank, matching, and coding exercises. These activities will reinforce material learned in the text and offer students another study tool. Answers are available only in the TEACH Instructor Resources on Evolve.

Activity 20-2, Match the Terms
Directions: Match the term with the correct definition by dragging the term to the definition.

A. lavage   B. pleurectomy   C. cordectomy

D. intramural   E. thoracotomy

1. within the organ wall
2. surgical incision into the chest wall
3. surgical excision of the pleura
4. surgical removal of the vocal cord(s)
5. washing out of an organ

Exit   Main Menu   Print Activity   Reset Activity   Back   Next

Student Workbook

The fully updated workbook supplements the text with more than 1500 questions and terminology exercises, as well as over 90 original source documents to familiarize the user with documents he or she will encounter in practice. (Odd-numbered answers are located in Appendix B, and the full answer key is available only in the TEACH Instructor Resources on Evolve.) Reports are included in a variety of areas, including arthroscopy, muscle repair, thoracentesis, tubal ligation, and endarterectomy. The workbook questions also follow the same answer format of the main text, improving coding skills and promoting critical thinking.

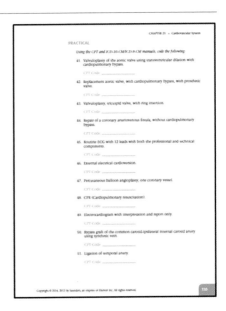

TEACH Instructor Resources on Evolve

No matter what your level of teaching experience, this total-teaching solution will help you plan your lessons with ease, and the author has developed all the curriculum materials necessary to use *Step-by-Step Medical Coding* in the classroom. Instructors can download:

- All answers to the textbook, online activities, and workbook exercises.
- Extra coding cases with answers.
- Course calendar and syllabus.
- Curriculum with TEACH lesson plans.
- Multiple curriculum outline options.
- Ready-made tests for easy assessment.
- Test bank in ExamView. The ExamView test generator will help you quickly and easily prepare quizzes and exams, and the test banks can be customized to your specific teaching methods.
- Comprehensive PowerPoint collection that can be easily customized to support your lectures, formatted with PowerPoint as overhead transparencies, or formatted as handouts for student note-taking.
- Interactive PowerPoint slides.

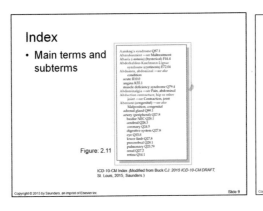

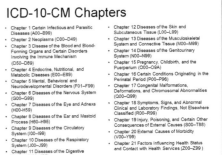

Evolve Learning Resources

The Evolve Learning Resources offer helpful material that will extend your studies beyond the classroom. Encoder practice exercises provide added practice and help you understand how to utilize an Encoder product.

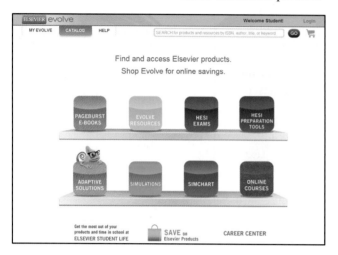

Official Guidelines for Coding and Reporting, Code Updates, and Chapter WebLinks offer you the opportunity to expand your knowledge base and stay current with this ever-changing field. Extra Coding Cases, ICD GEMs files, and Coding Tips are also available to check your understanding.

A Course Management System is also available free to instructors who adopt this textbook. This web-based platform gives instructors yet another resource to facilitate learning and to make medical coding content accessible to students. In addition to the Evolve Learning Resources available to both faculty and students, there is an entire suite of tools available that allows for communication between instructors and students.

To access this comprehensive online resource, simply go to the Evolve home page at http://evolve.elsevier.com and enter the user name and password provided by your instructor. If your instructor has not set up a Course Management System, you can still access the free Evolve Learning Resources at http://evolve.elsevier.com/Buck/step/.

Step-by-Step Medical Coding Online

Designed to accommodate diverse learning styles and environments, *Step-by-Step Medical Coding Online* is an online course supplement that works in conjunction with the textbook to provide you with a wide range of visual, auditory, and interactive learning materials. The course amplifies course content, synthesizes concepts, reinforces learning, and demonstrates practical applications in a dynamic and exciting way. As you move through the course, interactive exercises, quizzes, and activities allow you to check your comprehension and learn from immediate feedback while still allowing you to use your textbook as a resource. Because of its design, this course offers students a unique and innovative learning experience.

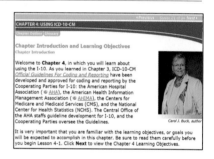

ELSEVIER   pageburst·

Spend less time searching and more time learning with electronic access to *Step-by-Step Medical Coding, 2015 Edition.* With easy access from virtually any device with an Internet connection, you can search across all of your Elsevier e-textbooks, paste important text and images from multiple sources into a focused, custom document, make notes and highlights, and more. Please contact an Elsevier customer service representative for more information, or visit pageburst.elsevier.com.

Development of This Edition

This book would not have been possible without a team of educators and professionals, including practicing coders and technical consultants. The combined efforts of the team members have made this text an incredible learning tool.

LEAD TECHNICAL COLLABORATOR

Jacqueline Klitz Grass, MA, CPC
Coding and Reimbursement Specialist
Grand Forks, North Dakota

QUERY MANAGER

Patricia Cordy Henricksen, MS, CHCA, CPC-I, CPC, CCP-P, ACS-PM
AAPC/AHIMA Approved ICD-10-CM Trainer
Auditing, Coding, and Education Specialist
Soterion Medical Services/Merrick Management
Lexington, Kentucky

SENIOR COLLABORATOR AND ICD-10-CM CONSULTANT

Nancy Maguire, ACS, CRT, PCS, FCS, HCS-D, APC, AFC
Physician Consultant for Auditing and Education
Winchester, Virginia

ICD-10-CM CONSULTANT

Kathy Buchda, CPC, CPMA
Revenue Recognition
New Richmond, Wisconsin

EDITORIAL REVIEW BOARD

To ensure the accuracy of the material presented in this textbook, many reviewers have provided feedback over several editions of this text. We are deeply grateful to the numerous people who have shared their suggestions and comments. Reviewing a book or supplement takes an incredible amount of energy and attention, and we are glad so many colleagues were able to take the time to give us their feedback on the material. It takes a village of coders to keep this work relevant. If you have input, suggestions, or criticisms regarding this material, or if you are interested in reviewing this book, please contact us at BuckStep@elsevier.com. Any updates, including corrections, will be posted to the Evolve site and included in the next edition.

Julie Alles, MSCTE, RHIA
Assistant Professor/Program Director
Allendale, Michigan

Kelly M. Anastasio, CPC, COC, CPC-I, CPC-P
Associate Director
Yale University, Yale Center for Clinical Investigation
New Haven, Connecticut

Garry Argro-Marino, BSN, RMA
Instructor
Drake College of Business
Elizabeth, New Jersey

Kathleen G. Bailey, CPA, MBA, CPC, CPMA, CPC-I, CCS-P
AAPC Approved ICD-10-CM & Licensed PMCC Instructor
Healthcare Management Consultant & Educator
Practice Management Solutions
Tampa, Florida

Janice L. Barker, MS, CMOM
Instructor/Program Coordinator, Office Information Systems
Bay de Noc Community College
Escanaba, Michigan

Katherine Barnes, CMBS
Academic Advisor
Laguna Hills, California

Brenda Parks Brown, HCA, MHS, CCS
Instructor
Roanoke, Virginia

Angela R. Campbell, RHIA
AHIMA Approved ICD-10-CM/PCS Trainer
Medical Insurance Manager
Eastern Illinois University
Charleston, Illinois;
Health Information Technology Faculty
Northwestern College
Chicago, Illinois;
Health Information Technology Faculty
Ultimate Medical Academy
Tampa, Florida

Charlene A. Crump, CPC, AHI, CMAS
Financial Counselor
Healthspan
Cleveland, Ohio

Brenda J. Dombkowski, RMA, CPC, CPMA, CIMC
Compliance Auditor and Educator
New Haven, Connecticut

Ann S. Faigin, BS, CPC, CPC-I, CGSC
Academic Coach/Medical Billing and Coding Tutor
Ultimate Medical Academy
Tampa, Florida

Mona F. Falcon, CPC, CMBS, CMAA
Academic Advisor
Laguna Hills, California

Yakima Fleming-Thomas, MSNM, RHIA, CPC
Healthcare Consultant
Chicago, Illinois

Johnna L. Floyd, CPMA, CPCO, CPC, CPC-P
Director of Auditing and Provider Education
All Care Health Networks
Tampa, Florida

Julia E. Huston, BS, CPC, COC, CCS
Adjunct Faculty
Phoenix College;
Consultant
AAPC Chapter: Glendale Coders
Phoenix, Arizona

Robin M. Moore, CPC
Northwest Surgical Specialists
Maumee, Ohio;
Owner, Robin Moore Coding & Billing
Toledo, Ohio

Kathy O'Brien, MBA-HM, CPC, COC
Allied Health Instructor
Brown Mackie College
Fenton, Missouri

Yvette Pawlowski, M.Ed, RHIT, CMT
Professor
Central Texas College
Killeen, Texas

Kathleen M. Skolnick, CPC, COC, CPCO, CPB, CPMA, CPPM, CPC-I
Certified ICD-10-CM Instructor
Medical Coding for Professionals, LLC
Linden, New Jersey

Mary Lynn Taylor, MA-HIM, CMS, CPC, CPC-I
CEO
Professional Coding Services
Fairbanks, Alaska

Diana G. Wilson, MA, CPC, CPMA, CPC-I
Medical Coding Training and Instruction
Ultimate Medical Academy Online Division
Tampa, Florida

Introduction

The number of people seeking health care services has increased as a result of an aging population, technologic advances, and better access to health care. At the same time, there is an increase in the use of outpatient facilities. This increase is due in part to the government's tighter controls over patient services. The government continues to increase its involvement in and control over health care through reimbursement of services for Medicare and Medicaid patients. Other insurance companies are following the government's lead and adopting reimbursement systems that have proved effective in reducing third-party payer costs but place further pressure on the health care system.

Health care in America has undergone tremendous change in the recent past, and more changes are promised for the future. These changes have resulted in an ever-increasing demand for qualified medical coders. The Bureau of Labor Statistics states that employment of medical records and health information technicians "is projected to grow 22 percent from 2012 to 2022, much faster than the average for all occupations. The demand for health services is expected to increase as the population ages."[1]

There is also an increase in the number of medical tests, treatments, and procedures, as well as an increase in claims review by third-party payers. Credentialed coders are on average paid more than the non-credentialed coder. According to the 2013 AAPC Salary Survey (which was the latest available upon publication of this text) the overall average salary for a coder is $46,847![2] Figure 1 illustrates the earnings by region; Figure 2 shows salary by job responsibility; and Figure 3 charts salary by workplace. The COC™, the hospital outpatient certification, pays more ($56,284) than the CPC®, the physician outpatient certification ($48,593)[2]. Coders working in a solo practice and small group practices earn on the lower end at $42,202, while coders working in health systems earn on the higher end at $48,789.[2] Further information can be obtained about the AAPC and the certifications offered by the organization at www.aapc.com.

CHECK THIS OUT ! Be sure to check your free Evolve student resources for updated salary figures. Go to the *Course Documents* section, click *Resources,* then click *Content Updates – Student.*

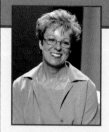

From the Trenches

"Coding can really open doors to a variety of things. You're not tied into one job—there are many roads you can take and many things you can do with a coding background."

MARIA

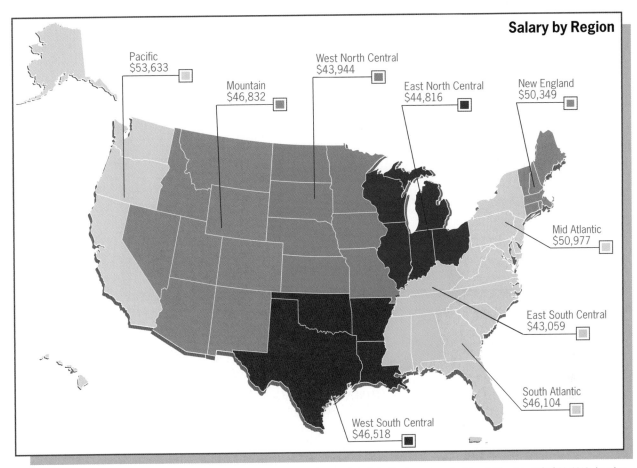

Salary by Region

Pacific
$53,633

Mountain
$46,832

West North Central
$43,944

East North Central
$44,816

New England
$50,349

Mid Atlantic
$50,977

East South Central
$43,059

South Atlantic
$46,104

West South Central
$46,518

FIGURE 1 Average Salaries by Region. (Modified from Blackmer D: Salary Survey 2013: Coder Employment on the Rise, *Cutting Edge* 24[10]:39, 2013, American Academy of Professional Coders.)

Salary by Job Responsibility

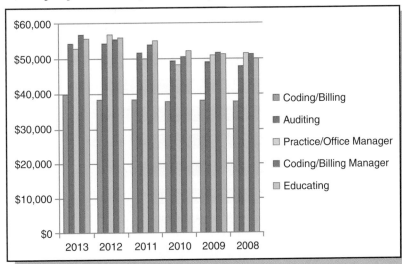

- Coding/Billing
- Auditing
- Practice/Office Manager
- Coding/Billing Manager
- Educating

FIGURE 2 Salary by Job Responsibility. (Modified from Blackmer D: Salary Survey 2013: Coder Employment on the Rise, *Cutting Edge* 24[10]:39, 2013, American Academy of Professional Coders.)

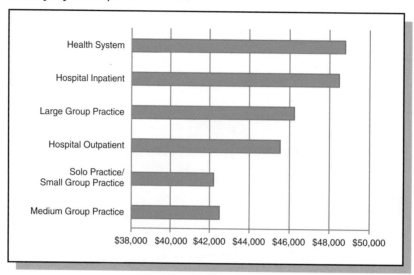

FIGURE 3   Salary by Workplace. (Modified from Blackmer D: Salary Survey 2013: Coder Employment on the Rise, *Cutting Edge* 24[10]:39, 2013, American Academy of Professional Coders.)

The American Health Information Management Association (AHIMA) is a health care organization that offers the Certified Coding Specialist—Physician-based (CCS-P) certification. The AHIMA 2012 Salary Study (which was the latest available upon publication of this text) indicated "The overall 2012-year ending average salary across all AHIMA Salary Survey respondents . . . came in at approximately $65,963."[3] Figure 4 illustrates the average salary by work setting. Figure 5 illustrates the average salary by job level. Figure 6 illustrates the average salary for coders by credential. Further information about AHIMA and the certifications offered can be accessed at the organization's website, www.ahima.org.

Medical coding is far more than assigning numbers to services and diagnoses. Coders abstract information from the patient record and combine that information with their

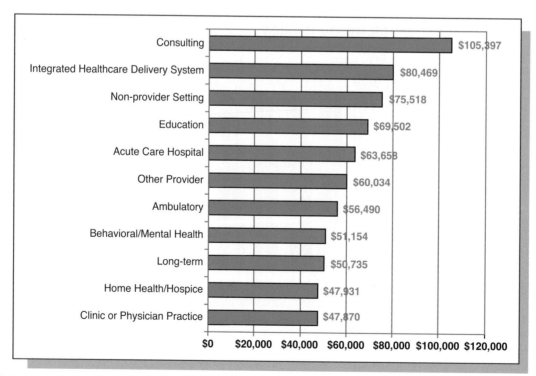

FIGURE 4   Average Salary by Work Setting. (AHIMA 2012 Salary Survey, Courtesy of the American Health Information Management Association)

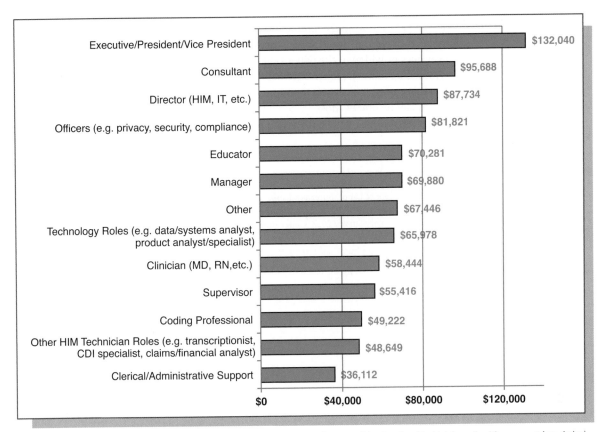

FIGURE 5 Average Salary by Job Level. (AHIMA 2012 Salary Survey, Courtesy of the American Health Information Management Association)

CHECK THIS OUT ☞ Be sure to check your free Evolve student resources for updated salary figures. Go to the *Course Documents* section, click *Resources,* then click *Content Updates – Student.*

AHIMA Credential	Coding Professional		
	2010 Avg	2012 Avg	% Change
RHIT	$44,807	$49,446	10.4%
RHIA	$50,494	$56,807	12.5%
CCA	$37,428	$40,930	9.4%
CCS	$50,244	$53,862	7.2%
CCS-P	$46,859	$48,740	4.0%

FIGURE 6 Average Salary by Credential. (AHIMA 2012 Salary Survey, Courtesy of the American Health Information Management Association)

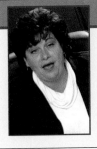

From the Trenches

"You need to be committed. . . . Be prepared to spend some time and effort to study and work hard. Do whatever you have to do to get your foot in the door."

BARBARA

knowledge of reimbursement and coding guidelines to optimize physician payment. Coders have been called the "fraud squad" because they optimize but never maximize and code only for services provided to the patient that are documented in the medical record.

According to the October 2013 Salary Survey in *Cutting Edge,* "Almost half the respondents stated that coding/billing was their long-term career goal."[2] There is a demand for skilled coders, and you can be one of those in demand. Put your best efforts into building the foundation of your career, and you will be rewarded for a lifetime.

References

1. U.S. Department of Labor, Bureau of Labor Statistics, Employment Projections. www.bls.gov/ooh/healthcare/medical-records-and-health-information-technicians.htm.
2. Blackmer D: Salary Survey 2013: Coder Employment on the Rise, *Cutting Edge* 24[10]:36–38, 2013, American Academy of Professional Coders.
3. AHIMA 2012 Salary Survey, Courtesy of the American Health Information Management Association.

Contents

UNIT 3
ICD-9-CM

UNIT 5
Inpatient Coding

CHAPTER 1

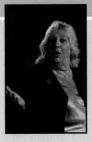

"You will probably feel a bit 'lost' in the beginning, but don't let that slow you down! You are learning to identify the little pieces to a big puzzle. Wait until the puzzle is completed before deciding if you like the 'big picture'; you will be greatly rewarded."

Beverly Comsa, CPC

HealthCare Training Manager
New Horizons Learning Center
Anaheim, California

Reimbursement, HIPAA, and Compliance

Chapter Topics

Introduction

Basic Structure of the Medicare Program

Health Insurance Portability and Accountability Act

Federal Register

Outpatient Resource-Based Relative Value Scale (RBRVS)

Medicare Fraud

Managed Health Care

Chapter Review

Learning Objectives

After completing this chapter you should be able to

1 Distinguish among Medicare Parts A, B, C, and D.

2 Interpret rules of the Health Insurance Portability and Accountability Act (HIPAA).

3 Locate information in the *Federal Register*.

4 Explain the RBRVS system.

5 Understand the framework of Medicare Fraud programs.

6 Identify the major components of Managed Health Care.

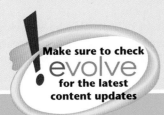

Make sure to check
evolve
for the latest
content updates

NOTE: *The 2015 ICD-10-CM DRAFT and 2015 ICD-10-PCS DRAFT were used in preparing this text.*

INTRODUCTION

Coding systems are used in the outpatient and inpatient health care settings. Each of the coding systems plays a role in the reimbursement of patient health care services. As a medical coder, it is your responsibility to ensure that you code accurately and completely to optimize reimbursement for services provided. To accomplish this, you not only need to know the coding systems but also the environment in which the modern medical office functions.

Medical advances allow people to live longer and healthier lives than ever before. In 2010, the Administration on Aging (AOA) of the Department of Health and Human Services published a population survey that indicated in 1900 persons 65 and older were only 4.1% of the population of the United States. In 2010 that same group had grown to 13%. By 2050, the elderly will be over 20% of the population.[1] The elderly compose the fastest growing segment of our population, and this growth will place additional demands on health care providers and facilities.

In 2014 the Administration for Community Living (ACL) reports in its *Justification of Estimates for Appropriations Committees,* "The U.S. population over age 60 is projected to increase by 26 percent between 2012 and 2020, from 61 million to 77 million. Over the same period, the number of seniors age 65 and older with severe disabilities—defined as 3 or more limitations in activities of daily living—who are at greatest risk of nursing home admission, is projected to increase by nearly 30 percent. The US Census Bureau also estimates that 37 million people have a disability, representing 12.1 percent of the civilian noninstitutionalized population."[2]

According to the National Health Expenditure (NHE) Projections 2010-2020 report, "Over the projection period (2010-2020), average annual health spending growth (5.8 percent) is anticipated to outpace average annual growth in the overall economy by 1.1 percentage points (4.7 percent). By 2020, national health spending is expected to reach $4.6 trillion and comprise 19.8 percent of GDP."[3] The number of persons enrolled in government health programs will increase as the enrollment in private health programs will decrease as the aging population enrolls in Medicare and as the government expands its ever increasing control over the national health care sector.

Increasing numbers of elderly people, technologic advances, and improved access to health care have increased consumer use of health care services. As more people utilize health care services, coding becomes even more important to appropriate reimbursement and cost control.

As a coder, it is your responsibility to ensure that the data reported are as accurate as possible, not only for classification and study purposes but also to obtain appropriate reimbursement. Ethical issues will arise and will require attention by coding personnel. Guidelines must always be followed in the assignment of codes. Instruction from internal and external sources (e.g., administration, review organizations, third-party payers) that may increase reimbursement but conflict with coding guidelines must be discussed and resolved.

Reimbursement usually comes from third-party payers. By far, the largest third-party payer is the government through the Medicare program. Because the Medicare program plays such an important role in reimbursement, the rules and regulations that govern Medicare reimbursement will be the first topic of study.

BASIC STRUCTURE OF THE MEDICARE PROGRAM

The Medicare program was established in 1965 with the passage of the Social Security Act. The Medicare program dramatically increased the involvement of the government in health care and consists of **Part A** (Hospital Insurance) and **Part B** (Supplemental Medical Insurance). Part A pays for the cost of hospital/facility care, and Part B pays for physician services and durable medical equipment not paid for under Part A. Part A insurance also helps to cover hospice care and some care services that are rendered in the home.

Medicare was originally designed for people 65 and over. In 1972 people who were eligible for disability benefits from Social Security were also covered under the Medicare program, along with those patients experiencing end-stage renal disease. Individuals covered under Medicare are termed **beneficiaries**.

The Secretary of the Department of Health and Human Services (DHHS) is responsible for the administration of the Federal Medicare program. Within the Department, the operation of Medicare is delegated to the Centers for Medicare and Medicaid Services (CMS), formerly the Health Care Financing Administration (HCFA). The funds to run Medicare are generated from payroll taxes paid by employers and employees. The Social Security Administration is responsible for collecting and handling the funds. CMS's function is to promote the general welfare of the public, and its stated mission and vision are:

CMS's mission is to serve Medicare & Medicaid beneficiaries.

The CMS vision is to become the most energized, efficient, customer friendly Agency in the government. CMS will strengthen the health care services & information available to Medicare & Medicaid beneficiaries & the health care providers who serve them.[4]

CMS handles the daily operation of the Medicare program through the use of Medicare Administrative Contractors (MACs) (formerly Fiscal Intermediaries, FIs). The MACs do the paperwork for Medicare and are usually insurance companies that bid for a contract with CMS to handle the Medicare program in a specific area. The monies for Medicare flow from the Social Security Administration through the CMS to the MACs and, finally, are paid to beneficiaries and providers.

In 2003, the Medicare Prescription Drug Improvement and Modernization Act passed and allowed CMS to reduce the administrative structure from 48 FIs to 19 MACs. Originally, there were 15 Part A and B MACs (Fig. 1-1)[5] and 4 Durable Medical Equipment (DME) MACs (Fig. 1-2).[6] CMS now believes that the efficiency and effectiveness of its contracted Medicare claims operations can be further increased by consolidating some of the smaller A/B MAC

Part A and B MAC Jurisdictions

Original Jurisdiction	New Jurisdiction	States Included in Jurisdiction
1	E	American Samoa, California, Guam, Hawaii, Nevada, and Northern Mariana Islands
2	F	Alaska, Idaho, Oregon, and Washington
3	F	Arizona, Montana, North Dakota, South Dakota, Utah, and Wyoming
4	H	Colorado, New Mexico, Oklahoma, and Texas
5	G	Iowa, Kansas, Missouri, and Nebraska
6	G	Illinois, Minnesota, and Wisconsin
7	H	Arkansas, Louisiana, and Mississippi
8	I	Indiana and Michigan
9	N	Florida, Puerto Rico, and U.S. Virgin Islands
10	J	Alabama, Georgia, and Tennessee
11	M	North Carolina, South Carolina, Virginia, and West Virginia
12	L	Delaware, District of Columbia, Maryland, New Jersey, and Pennsylvania
13	K	Connecticut and New York
14	K	Maine, Massachusetts, New Hampshire, Rhode Island, and Vermont
15	I	Kentucky and Ohio

FIGURE 1 – 1   Part A and B MAC Jurisdictions.

Durable Medical Equipment (DME) MAC Jurisdictions

Jurisdiction	States Included in Jurisdiction
A	Connecticut, Delaware, District of Columbia, Maine, Maryland, Massachusetts, New Hampshire, New Jersey, New York, Pennsylvania, Rhode Island, and Vermont
B	Illinois, Indiana, Kentucky, Michigan, Minnesota, Ohio, and Wisconsin
C	Alabama, Arkansas, Colorado, Florida, Georgia, Louisiana, Mississippi, New Mexico, North Carolina, Oklahoma, Puerto Rico, South Carolina, Tennessee, Texas, U.S. Virgin Islands, Virginia, and West Virginia
D	Alaska, American Samoa, Arizona, California, Guam, Hawaii, Idaho, Iowa, Kansas, Missouri, Montana, Nebraska, Nevada, North Dakota, Northern Mariana Islands, Oregon, South Dakota, Utah, Washington, and Wyoming

FIGURE 1-2 Durable Medical Equipment (DME) Jurisdictions.

workloads to form larger A/B MAC jurisdictions, further reducing the size range among the A/B MACs. CMS believes that reducing the number of A/B MAC contracts to ten will improve the efficiency and effectiveness of CMS's internal MAC procurement and contract administration process. This will be done over the next several years. The jurisdictions will have their names changed from numbers (Jurisdiction 1) to letters (Jurisdiction E) as shown in Fig. 1-1. CMS will consolidate the following ten A/B MAC workloads, comprising five pairings, to form five consolidated A/B MAC contracts.[5]

- A/B MAC Jurisdictions 2 and 3 (Alaska, Washington, Oregon, Idaho, North Dakota, South Dakota, Montana, Wyoming, Utah, and Arizona)
- A/B MAC Jurisdictions 4 and 7 (Louisiana, Arkansas, Mississippi, Texas, Oklahoma, Colorado, and New Mexico)
- A/B MAC Jurisdiction 5 and 6 (Minnesota, Wisconsin, Illinois, Kansas, Nebraska, Iowa, and Missouri)
- A/B MAC Jurisdictions 8 and 15 (Kentucky, Ohio, Michigan, and Indiana)
- A/B MAC Jurisdictions 13 and 14 (New York, Connecticut, Massachusetts, Rhode Island, Vermont, Maine, and New Hampshire)

CMS intends to re-compete five A/B MAC contracts/jurisdictions based on their present area boundaries, which will not be increased or reduced in size by CMS's consolidation strategy.

- A/B MAC Jurisdiction 1 (California, Hawaii, Nevada, Pacific Islands)
- A/B MAC Jurisdiction 9 (Florida, Puerto Rico, U.S. Virgin Islands)
- A/B MAC Jurisdiction 10 (Alabama, Georgia, Tennessee)
- A/B MAC Jurisdiction 11 (North Carolina, South Carolina, Virginia, West Virginia)
- A/B MAC Jurisdiction 12 (Delaware, Maryland, Pennsylvania, New Jersey, Washington DC)

Physicians, hospitals, and other suppliers that furnish care or supplies to Medicare patients are called **providers**. Providers must be licensed by local and state health agencies to be eligible to provide services or supplies to Medicare patients. Providers must also meet various additional Medicare requirements before being eligible for payments.

Medicare pays for 80% of allowable charges, and the beneficiary pays the remaining 20% for office visits to a health care provider. The beneficiary pays deductibles, premiums, and coinsurance payments. (The 2014 deductible for Part A is $1216 per hospital stay of 1-60 days and for Part B, $147.)[7] The **coinsurance** is the 20% that Medicare does not pay. Often, beneficiaries have additional insurance to cover out-of-pocket expenses or non-covered services.

Beneficiary Pays: Deductible, premiums, coinsurance (20%), 100% of non-covered services

Medicare Pays: Covered services (80%)

As of January 2011, the Affordable Care Act waived the Part B deductible and the 20 percent coinsurance for a grade A (strongly recommended) or grade B (recommended) preventative services or the annual wellness examination.

The maximum out-of-pocket amounts are set each year according to formulas established by Congress and published in the *Federal Register*. New amounts usually take effect each January 1.

Quality Improvement Organizations (QIOs)

Claims sent in by the providers of services are processed by MACs according to Medicare guidelines. QIOs providers were previously termed PROs (Peer Review Organizations). Under the direction of CMS, the Quality Improvement Organizations program consists of a national network of QIOs, responsible for each state, territory, and the District of Columbia. QIOs work with consumers and physicians, hospitals, and other caregivers to refine care delivery systems to make sure patients get the right care at the right time, particularly patients from underserved populations. Providers can sign a Quality Improvement Organizations (QIOs) agreement with a MAC to accept assignment on all claims submitted to Medicare. When a provider accepts assignment, the provider agrees to accept the Medicare allowable for services provided. The provider also agrees not to bill the patient for the difference between what the service costs and what Medicare allows. For example, a QIO provider renders a service that costs $100 and bills Medicare for the service; Medicare allows $58, and the provider accepts the Medicare payment as payment in full. Now, you are probably asking yourself why anyone would agree to this. The patient does not pay the $42 difference, nor does Medicare. The amount is written off by the provider as if the service really cost only $58. This is a good deal for Medicare and the patient, but what about the provider? Why would a provider agree to decreased payments? Incentives have been established to encourage providers to become QIO providers. Congress has mandated the following incentives:

FOR QIO PROVIDERS:

- Direct payment is made to the provider on all claims.
- A 5% higher fee schedule than that for non-QIO providers.
- Faster processing of claims.
- The provider's name is listed in the QIO directory, which is made available to each Medicare patient, along with identification as a QIO provider who accepts assignment on all claims.
- Hospital referrals for outpatient care must provide the patient with the name and address of at least one QIO provider.

FOR NON-QIO PROVIDERS:

- Payment goes to the patient on all claims.
- A 5% lower fee schedule than that for QIO providers.
- Slower processing of claims is the norm.
- A statement on the Medicare Summary Notice (MSN) sent to the patient reminds the patient that the use of a participating physician will lower out-of-pocket expenses.

FOR QIO:

- A bonus is offered for each recruited and enrolled QIO provider.

There are incentives for providers to participate in the Medicare program! These incentives are backed by Congress. Currently, more than half of all physicians in the nation are participating providers.

Part A: Hospital Insurance

Hospitals report Part A services by using diagnosis codes and procedure codes that together determine Medical Severity-Diagnosis Related Groups (MS-DRG) assignment. You will be learning more about MS-DRGs in Chapter 31 of this text.

Beneficiaries are automatically eligible for Part A, hospital insurance, when they are eligible for Medicare benefits.

During a hospital inpatient stay, Part A pays for a semiprivate room (two to four beds), meals and special diet, plus all other medically necessary services except personal-convenience items and private-duty nurses. Also covered are general nursing, drugs as part of the inpatient treatment, and other hospital services and supplies. Part A can also help pay for inpatient care in a Medicare-certified skilled nursing facility if the patient's condition requires daily skilled nursing or rehabilitation services that can be provided only in a skilled nursing facility. Skilled nursing care means care that can be performed only by or under the supervision of licensed nursing personnel. Skilled rehabilitation services may include such services as physical therapy performed by or under the supervision of a professional therapist. The skilled nursing care and skilled rehabilitation services received must be based on a physician's orders. Part A pays for a semiprivate room in the skilled nursing facility, plus meals, nursing services, and drugs.

Part A can pay for covered home health care visits from a participating home health agency. The visits can include part-time skilled nursing care and physical therapy or speech therapy when the services are approved by a physician.

Hospice provides relief (palliative) care and support care to terminally ill patients. Part A also pays for hospice care for terminally ill patients when a physician has certified that the patient is terminally ill and is expected to live 6 months or less if the disease runs its normal course. Further, the patient has elected to receive care from a hospice rather than the standard Medicare benefits, and the hospice is Medicare-certified. Items covered include nursing services, physician services, services of a home health care aide, homemaker services, medical supplies, counseling, and any other item or service, which is specified in the plan and for which payment may otherwise be made under this title.[8]

Part B: Supplementary Insurance

Part B is not automatically provided to beneficiaries when they become eligible for Medicare. Instead, beneficiaries must purchase the benefits with a monthly premium. Part B helps pay for medically necessary professional services, outpatient hospital services, home health care, and a number of other medical services and supplies that are not covered by Part A. Beneficiaries pay a premium each month. There are circumstances in which the premium may vary. If Medicare recipients do not sign up for Medicare when they become eligible, they will be penalized. The cost of enrolling in Medicare will increase by 10% each year that they could have obtained coverage, unless they qualify under a special case. The penalty will be in effect as long as they retain coverage. These Part B services are reported using diagnosis codes, CPT codes for the procedure (service), and HCPCS codes (National Level II codes) for the additional supplies and services.

Part C: Medicare Advantage Organizations

Medicare Part C is also known as Medicare Advantage Organizations (formerly Medicare + Choice) and is a set of health care options from which Medicare beneficiaries can choose their health care providers. The options available under Part C are:

- Health Maintenance Organization (HMO)
- Preferred Provider Organization (PPO)
- Private Fee-for-Service Plan (PFFS)
- Special Needs Plan (SNP)
- Medical Savings Account (MSA)
- HMO Point of Service (HMOPOS)

Medicare Advantage Plans may offer the option to purchase additional benefits, such as vision, hearing, dental, and/or health and wellness programs, and prescription drug coverage that the original Medicare does not offer. The managed plan, such as an HMO, has a contract to deliver Medicare services under the plan and provides the same services to all beneficiaries enrolled under Part C. The beneficiary is still under the coverage of Medicare but has opted to utilize a different way of receiving services.

Part D: Prescription Drugs

The Medicare Prescription Drug, Improvement, and Modernization Act of 2003 (MMA) (Pub. L. 108–173, enacted December 8, 2003) established a prescription drug benefit under

Part D of the Medicare program. On January 1, 2006, Medicare beneficiaries could enroll in the Medicare prescription drug plan (Part D) and choose between several plans that offered drug coverage. Medicare beneficiaries are charged a premium each month to be a member of these plans and receive the Medicare Part D drug benefit, pay a deductible, and a copayment.

QUICK CHECK 1-1

Match the Medicare part(s) with the correct phrase(s) below.

a. Part A   b. Part B   c. Part C   d. Part D

1. Automatic coverage under Social Security _____
2. Optional coverage under Social Security _____
3. Hospice care coverage _____
4. Prescription drug coverage _____
5. Physician visit coverage _____
6. Beneficiary pays premium for coverage _____
7. Codes assigned for payment using diagnoses; CPT; and HCPCS _____

(Answers are located in Appendix C)

EXERCISE 1-1 *Medicare*

Using the information presented in this chapter, complete the following:

1 The major third-party payer in the United States is the _____.

2 The Medicare program was established in what year? _____

3 Hospital Insurance is Medicare, Part _____.

4 Supplemental Medical Insurance is Medicare, Part _____.

(Answers are located in Appendix B)

CHECK THIS OUT ☞ The CMS website is located at www.cms.gov and contains information about the Medicare program. Through it, you can link to useful information concerning Medicare providers.

HEALTH INSURANCE PORTABILITY AND ACCOUNTABILITY ACT[9]

HIPAA stands for the Health Insurance Portability and Accountability Act of 1996 (also known as the Kennedy-Kassebaum Law) and includes provisions for governing:

- Health coverage portability
- Health information privacy
- Administrative simplification
- Medical savings accounts
- Long-term care insurance

The section of the Act that has resulted in the most major change to the health care industry is the administrative simplification portion of which there are four parts:

- Electronic transactions and code sets standard requirements
- Privacy requirements
- Security requirements
- National identifier requirements

Electronic Transactions

Uniformity is one goal of the change that took place by adopting transaction standards for several types of electronic health information transactions. Third-party payers (insurers) could no longer have unique requirements for processing claims. Providers and payers covered by HIPAA are required to provide the same information using standard formats for processing claims and payments, as well as for the maintenance and transmission of electronic health care information and data. With HIPAA there is now only one way to process electronic claims.

Transactions are activities involving the transfer of health care information. **Transmission** is the movement of electronic data between two entities and the technology that supports the transfer. For example, if you send claims electronically to a payer, you utilize Electronic Data Interchange **(EDI)** technology. HIPAA identified 10 standard transactions for EDI transmission:

1. Claims or equivalent encounter information
2. Payment and remittance advice
3. Claim status inquiry and response
4. Eligibility inquiry and response
5. Referral certification and authorization inquiry and response
6. Enrollment and disenrollment in a health plan
7. Health plan premium payments
8. Coordination of benefits
9. Claims attachments
10. First report of injury

Providers must complete a Standard Electronic Data Interchange (EDI) Enrollment Form before submitting electronic media claims (EMC) or other EDI transactions. The software that supports the electronic transmissions must be compatible with the HIPAA transaction standard **Version 5010** and the National Council for Prescription Drug Programs (NCPDP) version **D.0.**

CODING SHOT

Years ago, each payer had different requirements for codes and forms in medical insurance billing. The federal government determined that in addition to providing an employee the opportunity to continue coverage during a job change or loss, and limiting coverage exclusion for pre-existing conditions, health care would benefit if every payer and provider used the same standardized forms and codes, and if everyone stored and transmitted medical insurance data electronically. But electronic information has the potential for unauthorized access, so legislation was needed to protect the public while at the same time streamlining medical reporting. HIPAA was created to govern health care portability, privacy of information, simplification of reporting by standardizing code sets, billing forms, and rules. Today, more than 99 percent of Part A and 96 percent of Part B claims are filed electronically.[10]

Code Sets

Code sets are composed of numbers and/or letters that identify specific diagnosis and clinical procedures on claims and encounter forms. The CPT, ICD-10-CM, ICD-10-PCS, and ICD-9-CM codes are examples of code sets for procedure and diagnosis coding. Other code sets adopted under the administrative simplification provisions of HIPAA include those for claims involving:

Groups	Code Sets
1. Physician services/other health services	HCPCS and CPT
2. Medical supplies, orthotics, and DME (durable medical equipment)	HCPCS (A-V codes)
3. Diagnosis codes	ICD-10-CM, ICD-9-CM, Vols 1, 2
4. Inpatient hospital procedures	ICD-10-PCS, ICD-9-CM, Vol 3
5. Dental services	Dental codes (HCPCS, D codes)
6. Drugs/biologics	National Drug Classifications (NDC)

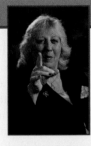

From the Trenches

"Don't be afraid to write in your coding books! As you study and read, highlight important rules. Write instructions 'in your own words' so you will understand when you go back to look at it again."

BEVERLY

Privacy Requirements

HIPAA also has privacy requirements that govern disclosure of patient protected health information (PHI) placed in the medical record by physicians, nurses, and other health care providers. This includes conversations with nurses and other staff about the patient's health care or treatment. All PHI is included in the privacy requirements.

Security Requirements

There are security regulations that address the administrative, technical, and physical safeguards required to prevent unauthorized access to protected health care information. There are significant penalties for those who breach the security of the medical record or PHI. Do not access any medical documentation that you are not authorized to access. You are only to access information that you have a work-related reason to access.

Facilities must train their employees in their privacy procedures and designate an individual to be responsible for ensuring the procedures are followed. If an employee fails to follow the established procedures, the facility is required by law to take appropriate disciplinary action.

Security has become a significant concern since computers are being used to store patient information. The two major terms used to describe the format of the electronic health record are:

- Electronic medical record (**EMR**)—a computerized health record limited to one practice
- Electronic health record (**EHR**)—the entire health record compiled from multiple sources

National Provider Identification

HIPAA also requires health care providers, health plans, and employers to have National Provider Identification (NPI) numbers that are unique identification on transactions. The NPI is entered onto the claim forms to identify the provider(s) of the services.

Further information about HIPAA is located on the CMS website: www.cms.gov/HIPAAGenInfo.

FEDERAL REGISTER

The *Federal Register* is the official publication for all "Presidential Documents," "Rules and Regulations," "Proposed Rules," and "Notices." When the government institutes national changes, those changes are published in the *Federal Register*. You must be aware of the changes listed in the *Federal Register* that relate to reimbursement of Medicare so as to submit Medicare charges correctly.

Most of the information in this chapter is about rules that the government developed and introduced through the *Federal Register*. You might wonder why so much time is to be spent on learning how to follow the guidelines set by the government for reimbursement when it is only one third-party payer. The answer is simple: Because the government is the largest third-party payer in the nation and even a slight change in the rules governing reimbursement to providers can have major consequences. For example, there was a 45% decrease in the number of inpatient hospital beds between 1975 and 1996,[11] directly related to a government-implemented inpatient reimbursement system that you will learn about in Chapter 31, the MS-DRGs. Often, more than half of the patients in a hospital are Medicare patients. Because the government is such an important payer in the health care system, you must know how to interpret the government's directives published in the *Federal Register*. In addition, most commercial insurers have adopted Medicare payment philosophies for their own reimbursement policies. The government has changed health care reimbursement through the Medicare program, and even more changes are promised for the future.

If you have the *Federal Register* available to you through a library or via the Internet, locating and reviewing some of the issues would be an excellent educational activity for you.

CHECK THIS OUT ☞ You can access the *Federal Register* at www.gpo.gov/fdsys/, the Federal digital system.

The October editions of the *Federal Register* are of special interest to **hospital** facilities because the hospital updates are released in that edition. **Outpatient** facilities are especially interested in the November or December edition of the *Federal Register* because Medicare reimbursements for outpatient services are usually published in one of those editions. Each year, when changes to the various payment systems are proposed, those proposed changes are published early in the year, and a period of several months is offered to interested parties to comment and make suggestions on the proposed changes. The final rules are usually published in the fall editions and implemented in the following calendar year. Some addendums are particularly helpful to the coder because they list the active codes, noncovered codes, bundled codes, etc.

Fig. 1-3 shows a copy of a portion of the *Federal Register;* it is marked to indicate the location of the following details[12]:

1. The regulation's issuing office
2. The subject of the notice
3. The agency
4. The action

5. A summary
6. The dates
7. Contacts for further information
8. Supplementary information

Items 1 through 8 are always placed before the Final Rule, which is the official statement of the entire rule.

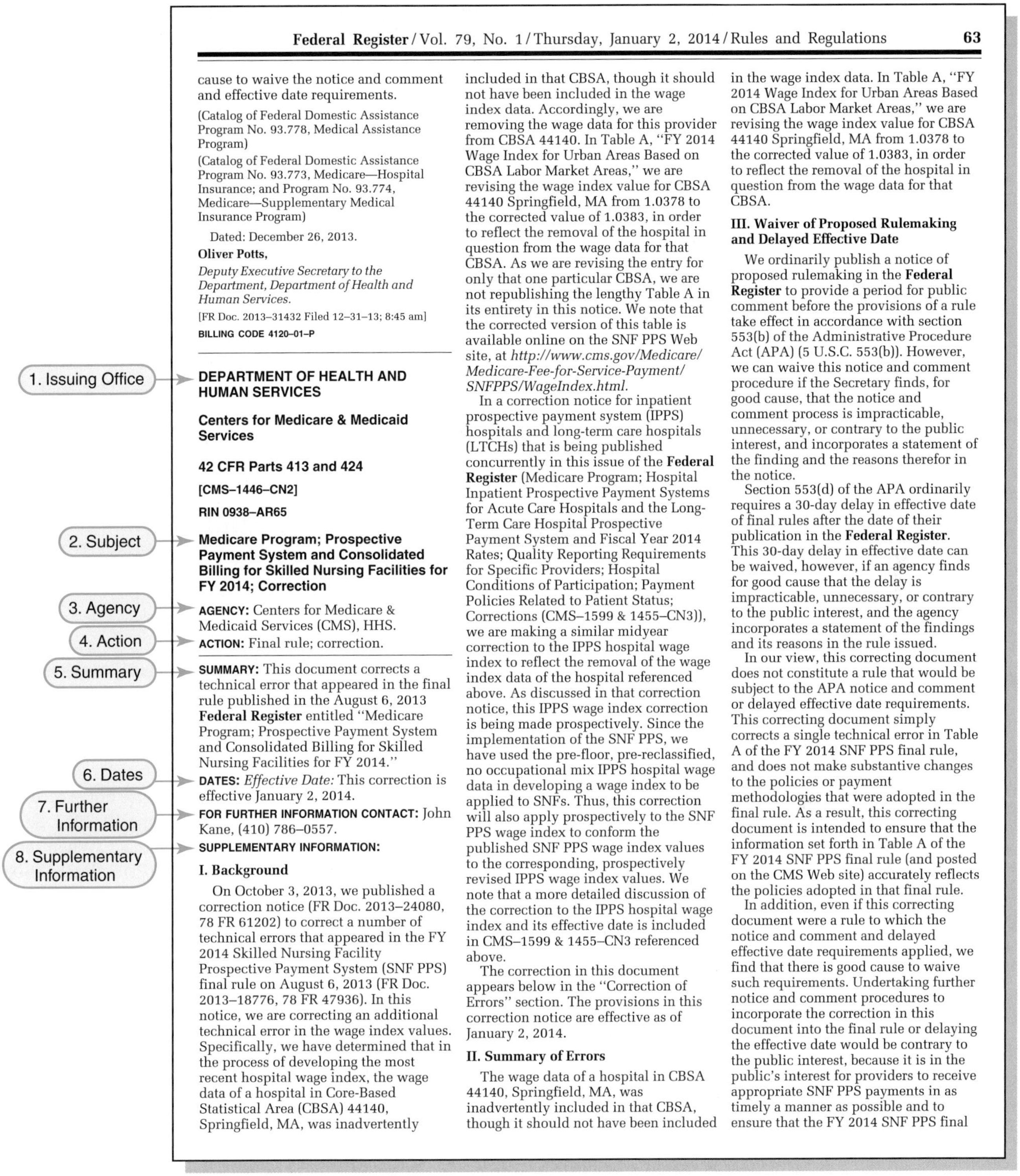

cause to waive the notice and comment and effective date requirements.

(Catalog of Federal Domestic Assistance Program No. 93.778, Medical Assistance Program)

(Catalog of Federal Domestic Assistance Program No. 93.773, Medicare—Hospital Insurance; and Program No. 93.774, Medicare—Supplementary Medical Insurance Program)

Dated: December 26, 2013.

Oliver Potts,

Deputy Executive Secretary to the Department, Department of Health and Human Services.

[FR Doc. 2013–31432 Filed 12–31–13; 8:45 am]

BILLING CODE 4120–01–P

1. Issuing Office →

DEPARTMENT OF HEALTH AND HUMAN SERVICES

Centers for Medicare & Medicaid Services

42 CFR Parts 413 and 424

[CMS–1446–CN2]

RIN 0938–AR65

2. Subject →

Medicare Program; Prospective Payment System and Consolidated Billing for Skilled Nursing Facilities for FY 2014; Correction

3. Agency →

AGENCY: Centers for Medicare & Medicaid Services (CMS), HHS.

4. Action →

ACTION: Final rule; correction.

5. Summary →

SUMMARY: This document corrects a technical error that appeared in the final rule published in the August 6, 2013 **Federal Register** entitled "Medicare Program; Prospective Payment System and Consolidated Billing for Skilled Nursing Facilities for FY 2014."

6. Dates →

DATES: *Effective Date:* This correction is effective January 2, 2014.

7. Further Information →

FOR FURTHER INFORMATION CONTACT: John Kane, (410) 786–0557.

8. Supplementary Information →

SUPPLEMENTARY INFORMATION:

I. Background

On October 3, 2013, we published a correction notice (FR Doc. 2013–24080, 78 FR 61202) to correct a number of technical errors that appeared in the FY 2014 Skilled Nursing Facility Prospective Payment System (SNF PPS) final rule on August 6, 2013 (FR Doc. 2013–18776, 78 FR 47936). In this notice, we are correcting an additional technical error in the wage index values. Specifically, we have determined that in the process of developing the most recent hospital wage index, the wage data of a hospital in Core-Based Statistical Area (CBSA) 44140, Springfield, MA, was inadvertently

included in that CBSA, though it should not have been included in the wage index data. Accordingly, we are removing the wage data for this provider from CBSA 44140. In Table A, "FY 2014 Wage Index for Urban Areas Based on CBSA Labor Market Areas," we are revising the wage index value for CBSA 44140 Springfield, MA from 1.0378 to the corrected value of 1.0383, in order to reflect the removal of the hospital in question from the wage data for that CBSA. As we are revising the entry for only that one particular CBSA, we are not republishing the lengthy Table A in its entirety in this notice. We note that the corrected version of this table is available online on the SNF PPS Web site, at *http://www.cms.gov/Medicare/ Medicare-Fee-for-Service-Payment/ SNFPPS/WageIndex.html.*

In a correction notice for inpatient prospective payment system (IPPS) hospitals and long-term care hospitals (LTCHs) that is being published concurrently in this issue of the **Federal Register** (Medicare Program; Hospital Inpatient Prospective Payment Systems for Acute Care Hospitals and the Long-Term Care Hospital Prospective Payment System and Fiscal Year 2014 Rates; Quality Reporting Requirements for Specific Providers; Hospital Conditions of Participation; Payment Policies Related to Patient Status; Corrections (CMS–1599 & 1455–CN3)), we are making a similar midyear correction to the IPPS hospital wage index to reflect the removal of the wage index data of the hospital referenced above. As discussed in that correction notice, this IPPS wage index correction is being made prospectively. Since the implementation of the SNF PPS, we have used the pre-floor, pre-reclassified, no occupational mix IPPS hospital wage data in developing a wage index to be applied to SNFs. Thus, this correction will also apply prospectively to the SNF PPS wage index to conform the published SNF PPS wage index values to the corresponding, prospectively revised IPPS wage index values. We note that a more detailed discussion of the correction to the IPPS hospital wage index and its effective date is included in CMS–1599 & 1455–CN3 referenced above.

The correction in this document appears below in the "Correction of Errors" section. The provisions in this correction notice are effective as of January 2, 2014.

II. Summary of Errors

The wage data of a hospital in CBSA 44140, Springfield, MA, was inadvertently included in that CBSA, though it should not have been included

in the wage index data. In Table A, "FY 2014 Wage Index for Urban Areas Based on CBSA Labor Market Areas," we are revising the wage index value for CBSA 44140 Springfield, MA from 1.0378 to the corrected value of 1.0383, in order to reflect the removal of the hospital in question from the wage data for that CBSA.

III. Waiver of Proposed Rulemaking and Delayed Effective Date

We ordinarily publish a notice of proposed rulemaking in the **Federal Register** to provide a period for public comment before the provisions of a rule take effect in accordance with section 553(b) of the Administrative Procedure Act (APA) (5 U.S.C. 553(b)). However, we can waive this notice and comment procedure if the Secretary finds, for good cause, that the notice and comment process is impracticable, unnecessary, or contrary to the public interest, and incorporates a statement of the finding and the reasons therefor in the notice.

Section 553(d) of the APA ordinarily requires a 30-day delay in effective date of final rules after the date of their publication in the **Federal Register**. This 30-day delay in effective date can be waived, however, if an agency finds for good cause that the delay is impracticable, unnecessary, or contrary to the public interest, and the agency incorporates a statement of the findings and its reasons in the rule issued.

In our view, this correcting document does not constitute a rule that would be subject to the APA notice and comment or delayed effective date requirements. This correcting document simply corrects a single technical error in Table A of the FY 2014 SNF PPS final rule, and does not make substantive changes to the policies or payment methodologies that were adopted in the final rule. As a result, this correcting document is intended to ensure that the information set forth in Table A of the FY 2014 SNF PPS final rule (and posted on the CMS Web site) accurately reflects the policies adopted in that final rule.

In addition, even if this correcting document were a rule to which the notice and comment and delayed effective date requirements applied, we find that there is good cause to waive such requirements. Undertaking further notice and comment procedures to incorporate the correction in this document into the final rule or delaying the effective date would be contrary to the public interest, because it is in the public's interest for providers to receive appropriate SNF PPS payments in as timely a manner as possible and to ensure that the FY 2014 SNF PPS final

FIGURE 1–3   Example of page from *Federal Register.*

EXERCISE 1-2   *Federal Register*

Answer the following questions:

1 Which edition of the *Federal Register* is of special interest to hospital facilities? _____

2 Which edition of the *Federal Register* is of special interest to outpatient facilities? _____

Using Fig. 1-3, answer the following questions:

3 What is the issuing office? _____

4 What is the Effective Date? _____

5 According to the Summary section in Fig. 1-3, what does the document correct? _____

6 According to the "For Further Information Contact" section in Fig. 1-3, who could give you further information related to the issue addressed in this *Federal Register*? _____

(Answers are located in Appendix B)

OUTPATIENT RESOURCE-BASED RELATIVE VALUE SCALE (RBRVS)

Physician payment reform was implemented to:
1. Decrease Medicare expenditures
2. Redistribute physicians' payments more equitably
3. Ensure quality health care at a reasonable rate

Before January 1, 1992, payment under Medicare Part B for physicians' services was based on a reasonable charge that, under the Social Security Act, could not exceed the lowest of (1) the physician's actual charge for the service, (2) the physician's customary charge for the service, or (3) the prevailing charges of physicians for similar services in the locality.

The act also required that the local prevailing charge for a physician's service not exceed the level in effect for that service in the locality for the fiscal year ending on June 30, 1973. Some provision was made for changes in the level on the basis of economic changes. When there were economic changes in the country, the Medicare Economic Index (MEI) reflected these changes. Until 1992, the MEI tied increases in the Medicare prevailing charges to increases in the costs of physicians' practice and general wage rates throughout the economy as compared with the index base year. The MEI was first published in the *Federal Register* on June 16, 1975, and has been recalculated annually since then.

Congress mandated the MEI as part of the 1972 Amendment to the Social Security Act. The 1972 Amendment to the Act did not specify the particular type of index to be used; however, the present form of the MEI follows the recommendations outlined by the Senate Finance Committee in its report accompanying the legislation. The MEI attempts to present an equitable measure for changes in the costs of physicians' time and operating expenses.

A major change took place in Medicare in 1989 with the enactment of the Omnibus Budget Reconciliation Act of 1989 (OBRA), Public Law 101-239. Section 6102 of PL 101-239 amended Title XVIII of the Social Security Act by adding Section 1848, Payment for Physician Services. The new section contained three major elements:
1. Establishment of standard rates of increase of expenditures for physicians' services
2. Replacement of the reasonable charge payment mechanism by a fee schedule for physicians' services
3. Replacement of the maximum actual allowable charge (MAAC), which limits the total amount non-QIO physicians could charge

Revisions were made and a new Omnibus Budget Reconciliation Act of 1990 was passed. OBRA 1990 contained several modifications and clarifications of the provisions establishing the physician fee schedule. This final rule required that before January 1 of each year, beginning with 1992, the Secretary establish, by regulation, fee schedules that determine payment amounts for all physicians' services furnished in all fee schedule areas for the year.

The physician fee schedule is updated each April 15 and is composed of three basic elements:
1. The relative value units (RVUs) for each service
2. A geographic adjustment factor to adjust for regional variations in the cost of operating a health care facility
3. A national conversion factor

CHECK THIS OUT ☞ The CMS Physician Fee Schedule Search can be accessed at www.cms.gov/apps/physician-fee-schedule/search/search-criteria.aspx.

Medicare volume performance standards have been developed to be used as a tool to monitor annual increases in Part B expenditures for physicians' services and, when appropriate, to adjust payment levels to reflect the success or failure in meeting the performance standards. Various financial protections have been designed and instituted on behalf of the Medicare beneficiary.

Relative Value Unit

Nationally, unit values are assigned for each service and are determined on the basis of the resources necessary to the physician's performance of the service. By analyzing a service, a Harvard team was able to identify its separate parts and assign each part a relative value unit (RVU). These parts or components are as follows:
1. **Work.** The work component is identified as the amount of time, the intensity of effort, and the technical expertise required for the physician to provide the service.
2. **Overhead.** The overhead component or **practice expense** is identified as the allocation of costs associated with the physician's practice (e.g., rent, staffing, supplies) that must be expended in order to provide a service.
3. **Malpractice.** The malpractice component is identified as the cost of the medical malpractice insurance coverage/risk associated with providing the service.

The sum of the units established for each component of the service equals the total RVUs of a service.

A relative value was established for a midlevel, established-patient office visit (99213) and all other services are valued at, above, or below this service relative to the work, overhead, and malpractice expenses associated with the service.

Geographic Practice Cost Index

The Urban Institute developed scales that measure cost differences in various areas. The Geographic Practice Cost Indices (GPCIs) have been established for each of the prevailing charge localities. An entire state may be considered a locality for purposes of physician payment reform. The GPCIs reflect the relative costs of practice in a given locality compared with the national average. A separate GPCI has been established and is applied to each component of a service.

Conversion Factor

The conversion factor (CF) is a national dollar amount that is applied to all services paid on the basis of the Medicare Fee Schedule. Congress provided a CF to be used to convert RVUs to dollars. Updated annually on the basis of the data sources, the CF indicates:
- Percent changes to the Medicare Economic Index (MEI)
- Percent changes in physician expenditures
- Relationship of expenditures to volume performance standards
- Change in access and quality

The CF varies according to the type of service provided (e.g., medical, surgical, nonsurgical).

CHECK THIS OUT 🖎 The Physician Fee Schedule (PFS) is located at www.cms.gov/ PhysicianFeeSched/PFSRVF/list.asp.

Medicare Volume Performance Standards

The Medicare Volume Performance Standards (MVPS) are best thought of as an object. "It" represents the government's estimate of how much growth is appropriate for nationwide physician expenditures paid by the Part B Medicare program. The purpose of MVPS is to guide Congress in its consideration of the appropriate annual payment update.

The Secretary of Health and Human Services must make MVPS recommendations to Congress by April 15 for the upcoming fiscal year, and by May 15, the Physician Payment Review Commission (PPRC) must make its recommendations for the fiscal year. Congress has until October 15 to establish the MVPS by either accepting or modifying the two proposed MVPS recommendations.

If Congress does not react by October 15, the MVPS rate is established by using a default mechanism. If the default mechanism is used, the Secretary is then required to publish a notice in the *Federal Register* that provides the formula for deriving the MVPS.

Variations in health care usage by Medicare patients occur every year. Because Medicare strives for a balanced budget, if CMS agrees to pay for additional services not previously paid for or increases the weights of CPT codes, thus increasing reimbursement, then discounts are taken across the board so that more money than authorized is not spent and the budget remains balanced.

Beneficiary Protection

Several provisions in the Physician Payment Reform were designed to protect Medicare beneficiaries.

1. As of September 1, 1990, all providers must file claims for their Medicare patients (free of charge). In addition, claims must be submitted according to timely filing guidelines. As of January 1, 2010, the Patient Protection and Affordable Care Act requires physicians and suppliers to submit claims within 12 months of the service date. Assigned claims submitted more than 12 months after the date of service will be denied payment.
2. The Omnibus Budget Reconciliation Act of 1989 requires participating physicians to accept the amount paid for eligible Medicaid services (mandatory assignment) as payment in full.
3. Effective January 1, 1991, the Maximum Actual Allowable Charge (MAAC) limitations that applied to nonparticipating physician charges were replaced by new limits called limiting charges. The provisions of the new limitations state that nonparticipating physicians and suppliers cannot charge more than the stated limiting charge.

Limiting Charge

In 1991 and 1992, the limiting charge was specific to each physician. Beginning in 1993, the limiting charge for a service has been the same for all physicians within a locality, regardless of specialty.

The limiting charge applies to every service listed in the Medicare Physicians' Fee Schedule that is performed by a nonparticipating physician. This includes global, professional, and technical services performed by a physician. When a nonphysician provider (e.g., portable x-ray supplier, laboratory technician) performs the technical component of a service that is on the fee schedule, the limiting charge does not apply. CPT codes are assigned many different prices. The amount is determined by multiplying the RVU weight by the geographic index and the conversion factor for the fee schedule amount. If a physician is participating, he or she receives the fee schedule amount. If the physician is not participating, the fee schedule amount or the allowable payment is slightly less than the participating physician's payment.

The limiting charge is a percentage over the allowable (e.g., 115% times the allowable amount). The limiting charge is important because that is the maximum amount a Medicare patient can be billed for a service. For covered services, Medicare usually pays 80% of the allowable amount for participating physicians. The beneficiary is then balance-billed, which means that the patient is billed the difference between what Medicare pays and the limiting charge.

Example

Limiting charge is	$115	(Maximum charge)
Allowable is	$100	
Medicare pays	$80	(Medicare pays 80%)
Patient is billed	$35	($20, 20% of $100, and $15, the remainder of the limiting charge maximum)

Physicians may round the limiting charge to the nearest dollar if they do this consistently for all services.

Uniformity Provision

Equitable use of the Medicare fee schedule requires a payment system with uniform policies and procedures. Because the relative value of the work component of a service is the same nationwide (except for a geographic practice cost adjustment), it is important that when physicians across the country are paid for a service, they be paid the same amount, or "package." For example, the preoperative and postoperative periods included in the payment must be the same. To prevent variation in interpretation, standard definitions of services are required.

Adjustments

Whenever an adjustment of the full fee schedule amount is made to a service, the limiting charge for that service must also be adjusted. These adjustments are identified on the physician disclosure, which is provided to all physicians during the participating enrollment period each year.

Adjustments to the limiting charge must be manually calculated before submitting claims for all services in which a fee schedule limitation applies.

Payments to nonparticipating physicians do not exceed 95% of the physician fee schedule for a service.

Site-of-Service Limitations

Services that are performed primarily in office settings are subject to a payment discount if they are performed in an outpatient hospital department. There is a national list of procedures that are performed 50% of the time in the office setting. These procedures are subject to site-of-service limitations for which a discount is taken on any service that is performed in a setting other than a clinic setting. For instance, an arthrocentesis is normally performed in the office. If a physician provides this service in a hospital outpatient setting, the limiting charge will be less than that for the office setting. This is because the hospital will also be billing Medicare for the use of the room and the supplies. Medicare has a built-in practice expense, or overhead, for the clinic setting (the RVU weight for practice expense), and Medicare doesn't want to pay twice for the overhead; therefore, part of the overhead is reduced from the physician's payment to offset the hospital payment. For these procedures, the practice expense RVU is reduced by 50%. Payment is the lower of the actual charge or the reduced fee schedule amount.

There are many rules and regulations when reporting Medicare services, and these rules and regulations become "adjustments" to the final payments providers receive. As an example, review the following rules regarding the assignment of just a few modifiers.

Surgical Modifier Circumstances

Multiple Surgeries

General. If a surgeon performs more than one procedure on the same patient on the same day, discounts are made on all subsequent procedures, excluding add-on codes. Medicare will pay 100% of the fee for the highest value procedure, 50% for the second most expensive procedure, and 50% for the third, fourth, and fifth procedures. Each procedure after the fifth procedure requires documentation and special review to determine the payment amount. Discounting is why the order of the codes and the use of modifiers are so important! These discount amounts are subject to review every year by the CMS.

Third-party payers often follow different discount limits rules from those of Medicare. It is necessary to keep abreast of payer discounting rules.

Endoscopic Procedures. In the case of multiple endoscopic procedures, in the same indented category of the CPT, Medicare allows the full value of the highest valued endoscopy, plus the difference between the next highest endoscopy and the highest valued endoscopy. As in all other reimbursement issues, some non-Medicare carriers follow this pricing method, whereas others follow their own multiple-procedure discounting policies.

Dermatologic Surgery. For certain dermatology services, there are CPT codes that indicate that multiple surgical procedures have been performed. When a CPT code description states "additional," the general multiple-procedure rules do not apply. For example, code 11001, which is an indented code under 11000, states "each additional" in the code description, and the general multiple-procedure rules do not apply because of this statement in the code description.

Providers Furnishing Part of the Global Fee Package.
Under the fee schedule, Medicare pays the same amount for surgical services furnished by several physicians as it pays if only one physician furnished all of the services in the global package.

Medicare pays each physician for his or her part of the global surgical services. The policy is written with the assumption that the surgeon always furnishes the usual and necessary preoperative and intraoperative services and also, with a few exceptions, in-hospital postoperative services. In most cases, the surgeon also furnishes the postoperative office services necessary to ensure normal recovery from the surgery. Recognizing that there are cases in which the surgeon turns over the out-of-hospital recovery care to another physician, Medicare has determined percentages of payment if the postoperative care is furnished by someone other than the surgeon. These are weighted percentages based on the percentage of total global surgical work.

For example:
- Preoperative care   15%
- Intraoperative service   70%
- Postoperative care   15%

Again, become familiar with individual third-party payer policies, because some may not split their global payments in this manner.

Physicians Who Assist at Surgery.
Physicians assisting the primary physician in a procedure receive a set percentage of the total fee for the service. Medicare sets the payment level for assistants-at-surgery at 16% of the fee schedule amount for the global surgical service. Non-Medicare payers may set this percentage at 20% or more. CPT modifiers -80 (Assistant Surgeon), -81 (Minimum Assistant Surgeon), and -82 (Assistant Surgeon, when qualified resident surgeon not available) and HCPCS modifier -AS (Assistant at Surgery) would be appended to the code to indicate the type of assistant.

Two Surgeons and Surgical Team.
When two primary surgeons (usually of different specialties) perform a procedure, each is paid an equal percentage of the global fee. For co-surgeons, Medicare pays 125% of the global fee, dividing the payment equally between the two surgeons (each will receive the lesser of the actual charge or 62.5% of the

global fee). No payment is made for an assistant-at-surgery when co-surgeons perform the procedure.

For team surgery, a medical director determines the payment amounts on an individual basis. Modifiers -62 (Two Surgeons) or -66 (Surgical Team) would be appended to the procedure code.

Purchased Diagnostic Services. For physicians who bill for a diagnostic test performed by an outside supplier, the fee schedule amount is limited to the lower of the billing physician's fee schedule amount or the price paid for the service.

Reoperations. The amount paid by Medicare for a return to the operating room for treatment of a complication is limited to the intraoperative portion of the code that best describes the treatment of the complications.

When an unlisted procedure is reported because no other code exists to describe the treatment, payment is usually based on a maximum of 50% of the value of the intraoperative services originally performed.

Modifiers -78 (Return to Operating/Procedure Room for a Related Procedure During the Postoperative Period) or -79 (Unrelated Procedure or Service by the Same Physician or Other Qualified Health Care Professional During the Postoperative Period) would be appended to the code to more specifically identify that the service was a reoperation.

Third-party payers have their own guidelines. Many do not apply discounts for these subsequent surgical procedures.

CHECK THIS OUT ☞ CMS publishes the RVUs on their website (www.cms.gov/ PhysicianFeeSched/PFSRVF/list.asp). In your job in the medical office, you may be responsible for downloading the new RVUs when they are posted, usually in October of each year. So, it is a good idea to know where to locate this information!

EXERCISE 1-3 *RBRVS*

Fill in the blanks with the correct words:

1 What does RBRVS stand for?

_____

2 The Medicare Economic Index is published in what publication?

_____

3 In 1989, a major change took place in Medicare with the enactment of

_____.

(Answers are located in Appendix B)

MEDICARE FRAUD

Fraud Defined

The Medicare program is subject to fraud, as is any third-party payer program. But because Medicare is the largest third-party payer, it has the most comprehensive anti-fraud program. You must understand the specifics of this program because you will be submitting Medicare claims. CMS is responsible for establishing the regulations that monitor the Medicare program for fraud. CMS publishes fraud guidelines for professionals (www.cms.gov/FraudAbuseforProfs/) that contain links to the latest fraud and abuse information.

Fraud is the intentional deception or misrepresentation that an individual knows to be false or does not believe to be true and makes it knowing that the deception could result in some unauthorized benefit to himself/herself or some other person. Fraud involves both deliberate intention to deceive and an expectation of an unauthorized benefit. By this definition, it is fraud if a claim is filed for a service rendered to a Medicare patient when that service was not actually provided. How could this type of fraud happen? The fact is that most Medicare patients sign a standing approval, which assigns benefits to the provider and is kept on file in the medical office. Having a standing approval is convenient for the patient and for the coding staff. After the patient has received a service, the Medicare claim is filed automatically, without the patient's actual signature. But a standing approval also makes it easy for unscrupulous persons to submit charges for services never provided. This circumstance also makes it possible for extra services to be submitted in addition to services that were provided (upcoding). Suppose, for example, a patient came in for an office visit and a claim was submitted for an in-office surgical procedure that was not performed. That's also fraud.

> 🖐 **CAUTION**   *The most common kind of fraud arises from a false statement or misrepresentation made, or caused to be made, that results in additional payment by the Medicare program.*

Who Are the Violators?   The violator may be a physician or other practitioner, a hospital or other institutional provider, a clinical laboratory or other supplier, an employee of any provider, a billing service, a beneficiary, a Medicare employee, or any person in a position to file a claim for Medicare benefits. You will be the person filing Medicare claims so you have to be careful about the claims you submit. It is important to validate that the service was provided by consulting the medical record or the physician.

Medicare Learning Network (MLN), the CMS educational Center on the Web, contains publications and computer-based training (CBT) modules on fraud and abuse (www.cms.gov/Outreach-and-Education/Medicare-Learning-Network-MLN/MLNProducts/WebBasedTraining.html). The heading labeled "Related Links Inside CMS" has a link to "Web Based Training (WBT) Modules" that directs you to a list of courses, and one of them is "Medicare Fraud and Abuse."

Fraud schemes range from those committed by individuals acting alone to broad-based activities perpetrated by institutions or groups of individuals, sometimes employing sophisticated telemarketing and other promotional techniques to lure consumers into serving as unwitting tools in the schemes. Seldom do such perpetrators target just one insurer; nor do they focus exclusively on either the public or the private sector. Rather, most are found to be defrauding several private- and public-sector victims such as Medicare simultaneously.

What Forms Does Fraud Take?   The most common forms of Medicare fraud are:

■ Billing for services not furnished
■ Misrepresenting a diagnosis to justify a payment
■ Soliciting, offering, or receiving a kickback
■ Unbundling, or "exploding," charges
■ Falsifying certificates of medical necessity, plans of treatment, and medical records to justify payment
■ Billing for additional services not furnished as billed-up coding
■ Routine waiver of copayment

Who Says What Is Fraudulent?   CMS administers the Medicare program. CMS's responsibilities include managing claims payment, overseeing fiscal audit and/or overpayment prevention and recovery, and developing and monitoring the payment safeguards necessary to detect and respond to payment errors or abusive patterns of service delivery. Within CMS's Bureau of Program Operations is the Office of Benefits Integrity (OBI), which oversees Medicare's payment safeguard program related to fraud, audit, medical review, the collection of overpayments, and the imposition of civil monetary penalties (CMPs) for certain violations of Medicare law.

The Office of the Inspector General (OIG), Department of Health and Human Services, is responsible for developing an annual work plan that outlines the ways in which the Medicare program is monitored to identify fraud and abuse. The plan is a published public document that provides the evaluation methods and approaches that will be taken the following year to monitor the Medicare program. For example, in the 2014 Work Plan, the following was listed as an item for review during 2014:

NEBULIZER MACHINES AND RELATED DRUGS—SUPPLIER COMPLIANCE WITH PAYMENT REQUIREMENTS (NEW)

Billing and Payments. We will review Medicare Part B payments for nebulizer machines and related drugs to determine whether medical equipment suppliers' claims are for nebulizers and related drugs that are medically necessary and are supported in accordance with Medicare requirements. Context—Prior OIG work found that suppliers were overpaid approximately $46 million for inhalation drugs used with nebulizer machines. Medicare requires that such items be "reasonable and necessary." (Social Security Act § 1862(a)(1)(A).) Further, the local coverage determinations (LCD) issued by the four Medicare contractors that process medical equipment and supply claims contain utilization guidelines and documentation requirements. (OAS; W-00-14-35465; expected issue date: FY 2015; new start)[13]

This excerpt from the OIG Work Plan identifies a specific area that was monitored in 2014. The OIG charges the MACs with doing the actual monitoring. The OIG Work Plan sets the broad boundaries for monitoring the Medicare program for fraud and abuse.

CHECK THIS OUT 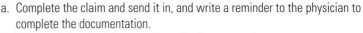 The site http://oig.hhs.gov/reports-and-publications/archives/workplan/2014/Work-Plan-2014.pdf contains the OIG work plan for 2014.

TOOLBOX

Susan recently graduated as a medical coder and has been employed at Island Clinic for three months. While coding last Monday, she encountered a superbill for a Medicare patient for an office visit for $62, but there was no supporting documentation in the patient's medical record. Susan questioned the physician and he said that he just forgot to do the paperwork and asked her to send the claim to Medicare with a promise to complete the paperwork later.

QUESTIONS

Susan should do which of the following:

a. Complete the claim and send it in, and write a reminder to the physician to complete the documentation.

b. Wait until the physician completes the documentation.

c. Inform the physician that she cannot submit a claim without appropriate documentation in the medical record.

▼ **ANSWER**

c. Never submit a claim for any patient, at any time, for any reason without appropriate documentation in the medical record that supports the claim.

Specific Regulations Are in the IOMs

CMS establishes the specific regulations in the *Internet-Only Manuals (IOMs)* for the providers and carriers to follow. You will deal with regulations as you report Medicare services in order to know what is allowable and what fraud and abuse are.

CHECK THIS OUT The IOMs are located at www.cms.gov/Manuals/IOM/list.asp and publication 100-08, Medicare Program Integrity Manual presents principles and values to protect the Medicare program from fraud and abuse.

Attempts to defraud the Medicare program may take a variety of forms. The following are some more examples of how fraud may be perpetrated:

■ Billing for services or supplies not provided;

■ Deliberately applying for duplicate payment (e.g., billing both Medicare and the beneficiary for the same service or billing both Medicare and another insurer in an attempt to get paid twice);

- Soliciting, offering, or receiving a kickback, bribe, or rebate (e.g., paying for a referral of patients in exchange for the ordering of diagnostic tests and other services or medical equipment);
- Unbundling or "exploding" charges (e.g., the billing of a multichannel set of lab tests to appear as if the individual tests had been performed);
- Completing Certificates of Medical Necessity (CMN) for patients not personally and professionally known by the provider;
- Misrepresenting the services rendered (up coding or the use of procedure codes not appropriate for the item or service actually furnished), amounts charged for services rendered, identity of the person receiving the services, dates of services, etc.;
- Billing for noncovered services (e.g., routine foot care billed as a more involved form of foot care to obtain payment);
- Participating in schemes that involve collusion between a provider and a beneficiary, or between a supplier and a provider, and result in higher costs or charges to the Medicare program;
- Using another person's Medicare card to obtain medical care;
- Utilizing split billing schemes (e.g., billing procedures over a period of days when all treatment occurred during one visit);
- Participating in schemes that involve collusion between a provider and a carrier employee where the claim is assigned (e.g., the provider deliberately overbills for services, and the carrier employee then generates adjustments with little or no awareness on the part of the beneficiary);
- Billing based on "gang visits" (e.g., a physician visits a nursing home and bills for 20 nursing home visits without furnishing any specific service to, or on behalf of, individual patients).

How to Protect Yourself. As you can see from the preceding information about Medicare fraud, CMS is very serious about identifying those who try to take advantage of the program. As the person submitting the Medicare claims, you are one of those whom CMS holds responsible for submitting truthful and accurate claims. If you are unsure about a charge or a request, check with the physician or other supervisory personnel to ensure that you are submitting the correct charges for each patient. In this way, you protect the Medicare program, your facility, and yourself.

CHECK THIS OUT ☞ CMS Fraud and Abuse Web-Based Training Module is available at www.cms.gov/Outreach-and-Education/Medicare-Learning-Network-MLN/MLNProducts/WebBasedTraining.html.

MANAGED HEALTH CARE

People come from all over the world to the United States of America to access the health care that U.S. residents take for granted. Physicians and health care have traditionally been held in high esteem by U.S. citizens. Whatever it took to provide access to high-quality health care is what these citizens demanded. Historically, the government responded to these demands by funding the research, facilities, and services necessary to keep the U.S. health system on the cutting edge of medical advances. But the research, facilities, and services are extremely expensive, and many U.S. citizens are also demanding a balanced federal budget.

Health care services in the United States are undergoing rapid change. The U.S. health care system has been financed through traditional health insurance systems, which paid providers on a fee-for-service basis and allowed beneficiaries relative freedom in their selection of health care providers. Health insurance has become an important benefit of employment. Employers became the primary purchasers of health insurance, and the rising cost of health care is reflected in the premiums employers pay and the subsequent decrease in employer-sponsored coverage. Private purchasers of health insurance have also seen a steady increase in their health insurance premiums, while fewer people now have health insurance coverage as a benefit of their employment. One way of containing health care costs that has widespread popularity is managed health care.

The term "managed health care" refers to the concept of establishing networks of health care providers that offer an array of health care services under the umbrella of a single organization. A managed health care organization may be a group of physicians, hospitals, and health plans responsible for the health services for an enrolled individual or group. The organization coordinates the total health care services required by its enrollees. The purpose of managed health care is to provide cost-effectiveness of services and theoretically to improve the health care services provided to the enrollee by ensuring access to all required health services.

Many models are used to deliver managed health care: Health Maintenance Organization (HMO), Individual Practice Association (IPA), Group Practice, Multiple Option Plan, Medicare Risk HMO, Preferred Provider Organization (PPO), and the Staff model. Each of these models delivers managed health care using a different structure.

The use of the managed health care approach varies widely with geography. There continues to be a rise in the percentage of employers opting for a managed care health plan for their employees; this indicates the employers' search for cost containment while offering the benefit of health coverage to employees.

The pressure on the government to cut expenses and balance the budget guarantees the continued increases in market share for managed care. The government mandated the use of managed care within the Medicaid program, and the number of Medicaid beneficiaries enrolled in managed care continues to increase.

The managed care industry has evolved from small, regional nonprofit plans to large, national, for-profit companies. In the early stages of development, the managed care market included networks that allowed the enrollees a broad choice of providers. As the market segments for managed care expanded, choice for the enrollees decreased.

Types of HMOs

A **Managed Care Organization (MCO)** is a group that is responsible for the health care services offered to an enrolled group or person. The organization coordinates or manages the care of the enrollee. The MCO contains costs by negotiating with various health care entities—hospitals, clinics, laboratories, and so forth—for a discounted rate for services provided to its enrollees. Providers of the health care services must receive prior approval from the MCO before services are rendered. For example, a physician may want to conduct a certain high-cost diagnostic test, but before the test can be conducted, the MCO must give the physician approval. The MCO uses a gatekeeper, usually the primary care physician of the patient, who can authorize the patient's need to seek health care services outside of the established organization. For example, a certain specialist may not be available within the MCO, and the primary care physician may recommend that the enrollee be referred to such a specialist. If the enrollee were to see the specialist without the recommendation of the primary care physician and the approval of the MCO, the enrollee would be responsible for charges incurred. MCOs develop practice guidelines that evaluate the appropriateness and medical necessity of medical care provided to the enrollee by the physicians, which gives the MCO control over what care is provided to the enrollee.

A **Preferred Provider Organization (PPO)** is a group of providers who form a network and who have agreed to provide services to enrollees at a discounted rate. Enrollees are usually responsible for paying a portion of the costs (cost sharing) when using a PPO provider. Enrollees who seek health care outside of the PPO providers pay an additional out-of-pocket cost. The out-of-pocket costs are established by the PPO to discourage the use of outside providers. The PPOs do not use a gatekeeper, but they do have strict guidelines that denote approved expenses and how much the enrollee will pay.

A **Health Maintenance Organization (HMO)** is a delivery system that allows the enrollee access to all health care services. The HMO is the "total package" approach to health care organizations, and the out-of-pocket expenses are minimal. However, the enrollee is assigned a primary care physician who manages all the health care needs of the enrollee and acts as the gatekeeper for the enrollee. Services are prepaid by the HMO. For example, the HMO pays a laboratory to provide services at a negotiated price and the services are prepaid by the HMO. The gatekeeper has authority to allow the enrollee access to the services available or authorize services outside of those the HMO has available.

The gatekeeper has strong incentives to contain costs for the HMO by controlling and managing the health care services provided to the enrollee. The HMO can directly employ the physician in the Staff Model HMO or contract the physician through the **Individual Practice Associations (IPA)** model in which the physician provides services for a set fee. Either way, the physician has an incentive to service the cost containment needs of the HMO.

An **Exclusive Provider Organization (EPO)** has many of the same features as an HMO except that the providers of the services are not prepaid. Instead, the providers are paid on a fee-for-service basis. The **Group Practice Model (GPM)** is a form of HMO in which an organization of physicians contracts with the HMO to provide services to the enrollees of the HMO. A payment is negotiated, the HMO pays the group, and then the group pays the individual physicians.

Medicare Advantage (formerly Medicare + Choice) is a Medicare-funded alternative to the standard Medicare supplemental coverage. Medicare Advantage is an HMO; however, it is provided to Medicare beneficiaries rather than the traditional fee-for-service model historically used by Medicare. The enrollees pay out of pocket if they choose to go outside the network of providers. **Point-of-Service (POS)** benefits allow enrollees to receive services outside of the HMO's health care network, but at increased cost in copayments, in coinsurance, or in a deductible. The POS benefit is one that the HMO may choose to offer, but it is not required, and CMS does not provide any additional funding for this benefit. However, the HMO that offers this option is more attractive to a potential enrollee, because the lack of access to providers outside of a predefined network is the one reason people do not join a managed health care organization. The POS benefit option is also referred to as an **open-ended HMO** or a **self-referral option**. The POS benefit is attractive not only to Medicare enrollees who wish to be treated by providers not available in their plan's network but also to those who travel and would like access to routine medical care while temporarily (fewer than 90 days) out of their plan's service area.

Program for All-Inclusive Care for the Elderly (PACE) is a program developed to address the needs of long-term care clients, providers, and payers. The program provides a comprehensive package of services that permits the clients to continue to live in their homes while receiving services rather than being placed in an institution.

Managed health care is now part of the fabric of the U.S. health care system. The "richer" plans of traditional insurance companies are often no longer an option to a great segment of the population.

Drawbacks of the HMO. There are some significant drawbacks to the HMO concept in terms of access to health care. Consider that providers (physicians in particular) have an incentive to keep treatment costs to a minimum. Traditionally, a physician's primary concern was what was in the best interest of the patient, not what was in the best interest of cost containment. This fundamental change transformed physicians into gatekeepers for third-party payers and transformed third-party payers into developers of guidelines that ultimately control the services patients can and do receive. The patient-physician relationship has shifted to include a physician/third-party-payer relationship, which leaves the patient at the mercy of the third-party payer. Many lawsuits have been brought by patients who allege that lack of treatment caused harm and sometimes death. Cost-containment issues, and hence HMOs, raise many ethical and legal issues that will continue to involve patients, providers, and third-party payers.

In March 2010, the President signed into law the Affordable Care Act. The law puts into place comprehensive health insurance reforms by 2015 with the hope that insurance companies would be more accountable, lower health care costs, guarantee more health care choices, and enhance the quality of health care.[14]

CHECK THIS OUT 🖘 For more information about the key features of the Affordable Care Act, go to www.hhs.gov/healthcare/facts/timeline/index.html.

EXERCISE 1-4 *Medicare Fraud/Abuse and Managed Health Care*

Fill in the blanks for the following questions:

1 This term is the intentional deception or misrepresentation that an individual knows to be false or does not believe to be true and makes knowing that the deception could result in some unauthorized benefit. _____

2 This organization develops a work plan to identify areas of the Medicare program that will be monitored. _____

3 The physician responsible for controlling and managing the health care of an HMO enrollee is the _____.

4 What does the abbreviation PACE stand for? _____

(Answers are located in Appendix B)

CHAPTER REVIEW

CHAPTER 1, PART I, THEORY

Complete the following:

1 Two insurance programs were established in 1965 by amendments to the Social Security Act known as Part _____ and Part _____.

2 The Secretary of DHHS has delegated responsibility for Medicare to which department? _____

3 Who administers funds for Medicare? _____

4 Who is eligible for Medicare? _____

5 List the three components of the relative value unit: _____

6 What does RBRVS stand for? _____

7 What is the fastest growing segment of our population today? _____

8 What is the name given to the groups that handle the daily operations of the Medicare program? _____
_____

CHAPTER 1, PART II, PRACTICAL

Using what you have learned from Chapter 1, match the correct term with the statement provided.

9 Intentional deception or misrepresentation is known as _____.

10 Quality Improvement Organizations were previously termed _____.

11 MS-DRG assignment reports _____ services.

12 October editions of the Federal Register are of special interest to _____.

13 OBRA 1990 contained modifications and clarifications regarding the _____.

a Part B
b abuse
c fraud
d PROs
e Part D
f outpatient facilities
g hospital facilities
h PPOs
i Part A
j Physician Fee Schedule

Chapter Review answers are only available in the TEACH Instructor Resources on Evolve

REFERENCES

1. Administration on Aging (AOA): *Projected Future Growth of the Older Population,* www.aoa.gov/AoARoot/Aging_Statistics/future_growth/future_growth.aspx

2. Administration for Community Living (ACL): *Justification of Estimates for Appropriations Committees,* http://acl.gov/About_ACL/Budget/docs/FY2014_ACL_CJ.pdf

3. Centers for Medicare and Medicaid Services: *National Health Expenditure Projections 2010-2020,* www.cms.gov/NationalHealthExpendData/Downloads/proj2010.pdf

4. Centers for Medicare and Medicaid Services: *CMS Mission, Vision, & Goals,* http://surveyortraining.cms.hhs.gov/bhfs/m1/M1S1_180.aspx

5. Centers for Medicare and Medicaid Services: A/B MAC Jurisdictions, www.cms.gov/Medicare/Medicare-Contracting/Medicare-Administrative-Contractors/A-B_MAC_Jurisdictions.html

6. Centers for Medicare and Medicaid Services: *DME MAC Jurisdictions,* www.cms.gov/Medicare/Medicare-Contracting/Medicare-Administrative-Contractors/DME-MAC-Jurisdictions.html

7. Centers for Medicare and Medicaid Services: *Medicare & You 2014,* www.medicare.gov/Pubs/pdf/10050.pdf

8. Centers for Medicare and Medicaid Services: *Hospice,* www.cms.gov/Hospice/

9. Centers for Medicare and Medicaid Services: *HIPAA Electronic Transactions and Code Sets, HIPAA Information Series,* www.cms.gov/EducationMaterials/Downloads/HIPAA101-1.pdf

10. Centers for Medicare and Medicaid Services: New Health Care Electronic Transactions Standards Versions 5010, D.0, and 3.0, www.cms.gov/ICD10/Downloads/w5010BasicsFctSht.pdf

11. 1996 HCFA Statistics. Bureau of Data Management, HCFA Pub. No. 03394, Sept. 1996.

12. *Federal Register,* 79(1), January 2, 2014, p. 63.

13. Office of Inspector General: *Work Plan for Fiscal Year 2014,* http://oig.hhs.gov/reports-and-publications/archives/workplan/2014/Work-Plan-2014.pdf

14. Key features of the Affordable Care Act: www.hhs.gov/healthcare/facts/timeline/index.html

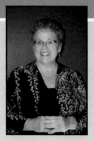

"What an exciting time to be a coder! The implementation of ICD-10 will bring so many changes, coders will be more important than ever before. It's a great time to begin a career in coding."

Sheri Poe Bernard, CPC, COC, CPC-I
Coding Education Specialist
Salt Lake City, Utah

An Overview of ICD-10-CM

Chapter Topics

The ICD-10-CM

ICD-10-CM Replaces the ICD-9-CM, Volumes 1 and 2

Improvements in the ICD-10-CM

Structure of the System

Mapping

ICD-10-CM Format

Index

Tabular

Official Instructional Notations in the ICD-10-CM

Chapter Review

Learning Objectives

After completing this chapter you should be able to

1 Explain the development of the ICD-10-CM.

2 Describe how the ICD-10-CM replaces the ICD-9-CM, Volumes 1 and 2.

3 Identify the improvements in the ICD-10-CM.

4 List the official instructional notations in ICD-10-CM.

5 Describe the format of ICD-10-CM.

NOTE: The 2015 ICD-10-CM DRAFT and 2015 ICD-10-PCS DRAFT were used in preparing this text.

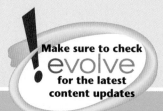

Make sure to check **evolve** for the latest content updates

Note: In this text **ICD-10** is the WHO's code system and **I-10** refers to the ICD-10-CM. The ICD-9-CM is referred to as **I-9**.

THE ICD-10-CM

The International Classification of Diseases, 10th Revision, Clinical Modification (ICD-10-CM) is designed for the classification of patient morbidity (sickness) and mortality (death) information for statistical purposes and for the indexing of health records by disease and operations, data storage and retrieval.

The 10th revision of the *International Classification of Diseases* (ICD-10) was issued in 1993 by the World Health Organization (WHO), and WHO is responsible for maintaining it. The ICD-10, the WHO version, does not include a procedure classification. Each world government is responsible for adapting the ICD-10 to suit its own country's needs. For example, Australia uses the ICD-10-AM, that is, the ICD-10-Australian Modification. Each government is responsible for ensuring that its modification conforms with the WHO's conventions in the ICD-10. In the United States, the Centers for Medicare and Medicaid Services is responsible for developing the procedure classification entitled the ICD-10-PCS (Procedure Coding System). The National Center for Health Statistics (NCHS) is responsible for the disease classification system entitled ICD-10-CM (CM stands for Clinical Modification).

The ICD-10 is already widely used in Europe, but conversion to the new edition in the United States has taken a great deal of time to implement. One reason for the additional time needed for conversion is that the I-9 is the basis for the hospital inpatient billing system in the United States. I-10 was set for implementation on October 1, 2014; however, the Senate passed a bill in March of 2014 which again delayed the I-10 implementation date. I-10 is now scheduled to replace I-9 on October 1, 2015.

The material in this text is based on the 2015 DRAFT version of the I-10. Guidance for the use of I-10 is available at www.cms.gov/ICD10.

Through the years, the use of diagnostic coding has grown. The Medicare Catastrophic Coverage Act of 1988 (P.L. 100-360) required the submission of the appropriate diagnosis codes, with charges submitted to Medicare Part B (outpatient services). The law was later repealed, but the coding requirement still stands.

Although coding was originally designed to provide access to medical records through retrieval for medical research, education, and administration, today codes are used to:
1. Facilitate payment of health services
2. Evaluate patients' use of health care facilities (utilization patterns)
3. Study health care costs
4. Research the quality of health care
5. Predict health care trends
6. Plan for future health care needs

The use and results of coding are widespread and evident in our everyday lives. Many people hear the results of coding on a regular basis and don't even know it. Anytime you listen to the news and hear the newscaster refer to a specific number of AIDS cases in the United States or read a news article about an epidemic of measles, you are seeing the results of diagnostic coding. The I-10 classification system is totally compatible with its parent system (ICD-10), thus meeting the need for comparability of morbidity and mortality statistics at the international level. A classification system means that each condition or disease can be coded to only one code as much as possible to ensure the validity and reliability of data; this classification system is used to track morbidity and mortality.

Coding must be performed correctly and consistently to produce meaningful statistics. (Refer to Fig. 2-1 for the AAPC Code of Ethics.) To code accurately, it is necessary to have an in-depth knowledge of medical terminology, anatomy and physiology, disease conditions, and pharmacology, along with an understanding of the I-10 coding guidelines, format, and conventions.

Transforming verbal or narrative descriptions of diseases, injuries, conditions, and procedures into alphanumeric designations is a complex activity and should not be undertaken without proper training. Learning to use the I-10 codes will be a valuable tool to you in any health care career.

AAPC Code of Ethics

Commitment to ethical professional conduct is expected of every AAPC member. The specification of a Code of Ethics enables AAPC to clarify to current and future members, and to those served by members, the nature of the ethical responsibilities held in common by its members. This document establishes principles that define the ethical behavior of AAPC members. All AAPC members are required to adhere to the Code of Ethics and the Code of Ethics will serve as the basis for processing ethical complaints initiated against AAPC members.

AAPC members shall:

- Maintain and enhance the dignity, status, integrity, competence, and standards of our profession.
- Respect the privacy of others and honor confidentiality
- Strive to achieve the highest quality, effectiveness and dignity in both the process and products of professional work.
- Advance the profession through continued professional development and education by acquiring and maintaining professional competence.
- Know and respect existing federal, state and local laws, regulations, certifications and licensing requirements applicable to professional work.
- Use only legal and ethical principles that reflect the profession's core values and report activity that is perceived to violate this Code of Ethics to the AAPC Ethics Committee.
- Accurately represent the credential(s) earned and the status of AAPC membership.
- Avoid actions and circumstances that may appear to compromise good business judgment or create a conflict between personal and professional interests.

Adherence to these standards assures public confidence in the integrity and service of medical coding, auditing, compliance and practice management professionals who are AAPC members.

Failure to adhere to these standards, as determined by AAPC's Ethics Committee, may result in the loss of credentials and membership with AAPC.

FIGURE 2–1   AAPC Code of Ethics. (From American Academy of Professional Coders: AAPC Code of Ethics [website]: www.aapc.com/aboutus/code-of-ethics.aspx. Accessed July 7, 2014.)

EXERCISE 2-1   *The ICD-10-CM*

Without the use of reference material, answer the following:

1 The I-10 was originally issued in 1993 by _____.

   a CMS

   b AHIMA

   c AHA

   d WHO

2 This country currently uses the ICD-10-AM: _____.

   a Argentina

   b Africa

   c Australia

   d Austria

3 The I-10 is designed for the classification of patient _____ or _____.

4 The CM in ICD-10-CM stands for _____.

5 List four of the six reasons why diagnosis codes are used today.

_____

_____.

6 The I-10 is used to translate what descriptive information into alphanumeric codes?

_____ **or** _____.

Continued

7 I-10 is scheduled for full implementation in America on this date: _____

   a November 1, 2015

   b October 1, 2016

   c October 30, 2015

   d October 1, 2015

(Answers are located in Appendix B)

ICD-10-CM REPLACES THE ICD-9-CM, VOLUMES 1 AND 2

The I-10 was developed by the National Center for Health Statistics (NCHS) and will replace I-9, Volumes 1 and 2 on October 1, 2015. Prior to the implementation of the new edition, extensive consultation and review must take place with physician groups, clinical coders, and others. The NCHS established a 20-member Technical Advisory Panel of representatives of the health care and coding communities to provide input during the development of the 10th revision.

IMPROVEMENTS IN THE ICD-10-CM

Notable improvements in the content and format of the I-10 include the following:

1. Addition of information relevant to ambulatory and managed care encounters

Example

Y92.53 **Ambulatory health services establishments as the place of occurrence of the external cause**

    Y92.530 **Ambulatory surgery center as the place of occurrence of the external cause**

        Outpatient surgery center, including that connected with a hospital as the place of occurrence of the external cause

        Same day surgery center, including that connected with a hospital as the place of occurrence of the external cause

2. Expansion of injury codes

Example

Y93 **Activity codes**

    Y93.4 **Activities involving dancing and other rhythmic movement**

        EXCLUDES1:   activity, martial arts (Y93.75)

        Y93.41 **Activity, dancing**

        Y93.42 **Activity, yoga**

        Y93.43 **Activity, gymnastics**

            Activity, rhythmic gymnastics

            EXCLUDES1:   activity, trampolining (Y93.44)

        Y93.44 **Activity, trampolining**

        Y93.45 **Activity, cheerleading**

3. Extensive expansion of the injury codes, allowing for greater specificity

Example

S50.351 is the code for superficial foreign body of right elbow. The 7th character designates the encounter: A - Initial encounter, D - subsequent encounter, S - sequela.

4. Creation of combination diagnosis/symptom codes to reduce the number of codes needed to fully describe a condition

Example

I25.110 is the code for atherosclerotic heart disease of native coronary artery with unstable angina pectoris. Only one code is required in ICD-10-CM.

5. The addition of a sixth character

Example

S06.336 is the code to report unspecified contusion and laceration of the cerebrum, with loss of consciousness greater than 24 hours without return to pre-existing conscious level with the patient surviving (requires a 7th character to describe the encounter (A, D, or S).

6. The incorporation of common fourth- and fifth-character subclassifications

Example

F10.14 is the five-character code to report alcohol abuse with alcohol-induced mood disorder.

7. Updating and greater specificity of diabetes mellitus codes

Example

E11.21 reports Type 2 diabetes mellitus with diabetic nephropathy.

8. Facilitation of providing greater specificity when assigning codes

CHECK THIS OUT ☞ Third-party companies typically employ **Clinical Documentation Improvement (CDI)** specialists, who are then hired by medical providers to advise and implement programs that improve documentation practices. The use of CDI is especially important to ensure documentation is specific enough to support the level of detail required from ICD-10-CM/ICD-10-PCS. Ultimately, it's the coders' responsibility to follow up with the provider in order to ensure proper documentation that meets the quality of coding, medical necessity, and denial standards of ICD-10-CM/ICD-10-PCS.

QUICK CHECK 2-1

1. According to the previous information on injury codes, what code would you reference for an activity code for an injury on a trampoline? _____

(Answers are located in Appendix C)

STRUCTURE OF THE SYSTEM

Chapter titles in the I-10 remain similar to those in the I-9 with the presence of two new chapters: Chapter 7, Diseases of the Eye and Adnexa, and Chapter 8, Diseases of the Ear and Mastoid Process.

Chapter 1 Certain Infectious and Parasitic Diseases (A00-B99)

Chapter 2 Neoplasms (C00-D49)

Chapter 3 Diseases of the Blood and Blood-Forming Organs and Certain Disorders Involving the Immune Mechanism (D50-D89)

Chapter 4 Endocrine, Nutritional, and Metabolic Diseases (E00-E89)

Chapter 5 Mental, Behavioral and Neurodevelopmental Disorders (F01-F99)

Chapter 6 Diseases of the Nervous System (G00-G99)

Chapter 7 Diseases of the Eye and Adnexa (H00-H59)

Chapter 8 Diseases of the Ear and Mastoid Process (H60-H95)

Chapter 9 Diseases of the Circulatory System (I00-I99)

Chapter 10 Diseases of the Respiratory System (J00-J99)

Chapter 11 Diseases of the Digestive System (K00-K95)

Chapter 12 Diseases of the Skin and Subcutaneous Tissue (L00-L99)

Chapter 13 Diseases of the Musculoskeletal System and Connective Tissue (M00-M99)

Chapter 14 Diseases of the Genitourinary System (N00-N99)

Chapter 15 Pregnancy, Childbirth, and the Puerperium (O00-O9A)

Chapter 16 Certain Conditions Originating in the Perinatal Period (P00-P96)

Chapter 17 Congenital Malformations, Deformations and Chromosomal Abnormalities (Q00-Q99)

Chapter 18 Symptoms, Signs, and Abnormal Clinical and Laboratory Findings, Not Elsewhere Classified (R00-R99)

Chapter 19 Injury, Poisoning and Certain Other Consequences of External Causes (S00-T88)

Chapter 20 External Causes of Morbidity (V00-Y99)

Chapter 21 Factors Influencing Health Status and Contact with Health Services (Z00-Z99)

MAPPING

As a part of the conversion, two sets of diagnosis code General Equivalence Mappings (GEMs) have been developed. This mapping is a type of crosswalk to find corresponding diagnosis codes between the two code sets. The two GEMs files are:

1. I-9 to I-10, which is forward mapping
2. I-10 to I-9, which is backward mapping

Fig. 2-2 displays GEMs mapping files for codes from I-9 to I-10. Note that the GEMs files do not contain decimal points. For example, in the GEMs file for I-9, code 001.0 is 0010 and code 001.1 is 0011. For I-10 codes, A00.0 is A000 and A00.1 is A001. In Fig. 2-2, column 1 displays the I-9 codes and column 2 displays the I-10 codes. Fig. 2-3 displays the mapping for codes from the I-10 code system to the I-9 code system. In Fig. 2-3, column 1 displays the I-10 code and column 2 displays the equivalent I-9 code. Column 3 in both figures is the "Flag" designation, which will be reviewed next.

Flags

There are three different types of flag designations:

- Approximate
- No Map
- Combination

Approximate

Approximate, Flag 0. The Approximate, Flag 0, means there is a direct match between the two coding systems, and the GEMs file directs the coder to a **single** entry. The conversion between the two code sets is straightforward: the I-10 code A02.21 maps to 003.21 in the I-9 code system.

Example

003.21 (Salmonella meningitis)
A02.21 (Salmonella meningitis)

I-9	I-10	Flag
0010	A000	00000
0011	A001	00000
0019	A009	00000
0020	A0100	10000
0021	A011	00000
0022	A012	00000
0023	A013	00000
0029	A014	00000
0030	A020	00000
0031	A021	10000
00320	A0220	00000
00321	A0221	00000
00322	A0222	00000
00323	A0223	00000
00324	A0224	00000

FIGURE 2–2 GEMs mapping files I-9 to I-10.

I-10	I-9	Flag
A000	0010	00000
A001	0011	00000
A009	0019	00000
A0100	0020	10000
A0101	0020	10000
A0102	0020	10000
A0103	0020	10000
A0104	0020	10000
A0105	0020	10000
A0109	0020	10000
A011	0021	00000
A012	0022	00000
A013	0023	00000
A014	0029	00000
A020	0030	00000
A021	0031	10111
A021	99591	10112
A0220	00320	00000
A0221	00321	00000
A0222	00322	00000
A0223	00323	00000
A0224	00324	00000

FIGURE 2–3 GEMs mapping files I-10 to I-9.

Example

I-10	I-9	Flag
A0221	00321	00000

Approximate, Flag 1. The I-10 code set has a more consistent level of detail, such as a more extensive vocabulary of clinical concepts, body part specificity, and patient encounter information. There are five times more codes in the I-10 (69,000+) than in the I-9 (14,000+), so the I-9 code is often linked to more than one I-10 code. The Approximate, Flag 1, assists in the process of conversion by identifying those times when more than one code in the I-10 is available to replace an I-9 code. For example, stress fractures in the I-9 are reported with codes in the 733.93-733.98 range, and although some of the codes are for specific bones (e.g., fibula, metatarsals, femur), a code such as 733.95 reports "other" bones. Code 733.95 is reported when there is not a specific code to report the stress fracture stated in the diagnosis. As such, 733.95 becomes an umbrella code that is assigned to a wide variety of stress fracture diagnoses. The I-10 code set expands the stress fracture codes (M84.3) to be more specific. For example, Fig. 2-4 illustrates the specificity of code M84.31, Stress fracture, shoulder.

Note that M84.311 reports the right shoulder and M84.312 reports the left shoulder. This **laterality** is utilized throughout I-10.

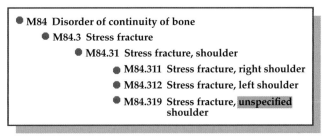

FIGURE 2-4   Specificity of M84.31, Stress fracture, shoulder.

Note that in addition to the specific anatomical location and laterality (right, left) of M84.31, a 7th character is also reported to indicate the episode of care, as illustrated in Fig. 2-5. This greater detail in the I-10 results in one I-10 code reporting what would have taken several I-9 codes to report.

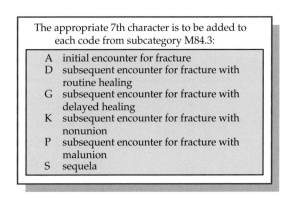

FIGURE 2-5   M84.3 7th character assigned to increase specificity.

The Approximate, Flag 1, assists the coder in choosing the correct code to reference by listing all of the possible choices. For example, the I-9 to I-10 GEMs file maps 16 possible I-10 codes for 733.95, Stress fracture of other bone, based on the specific location of

I-9	I-10	Flag	I-10 Tabular Code Description
73395	M84373A	10000	**M84.373A** Stress fracture, unspecified ankle, initial encounter for fracture
73395	M84343A	10000	**M84.343A** Stress fracture, unspecified hand, initial encounter for fracture
73395	M84339A	10000	**M84.339A** Stress fracture, unspecified ulna and radius initial encounter for fracture
73395	M84329A	10000	**M84.329A** Stress fracture, unspecified humerus, initial encounter for fracture
73395	M84319A	10000	**M84.319A** Stress fracture, unspecified shoulder, initial encounter for fracture
73395	M8430XA	10000	**M84.30XA** Stress fracture, unspecified site, initial encounter for fracture
A			B

FIGURE 2–6 **A**, I-9 to I-10 GEMs file entries for code 733.95. **B**, I-10 Tabular code descriptions.

🖐 **CAUTION** *The medical documentation must be reviewed to determine the exact location of the stress fracture for correct I-10 code assignment.*

the fracture. Some of the GEMs file entries for 733.95 are displayed in Fig. 2-6 along with the I-10 Tabular entries for the codes.

Entire chapters of the I-10, such as obstetrics, have been reorganized, and the conversion from I-9 to I-10 is more complex. For example, spotting complicating pregnancy in the I-9 is based on **episode of care** and in the I-10 these codes are based on the **trimester**.

Example

ICD-9

649.50	Spotting complicating pregnancy, **unspecified as to episode of care or not applicable**
649.51	Spotting complicating pregnancy, **delivered with or without mention of antepartum condition**
649.53	Spotting complicating pregnancy, **antepartum condition or complication**

ICD-10

O26.851 Spotting complicating pregnancy, **first trimester**
O26.852 Spotting complicating pregnancy, **second trimester**
O26.853 Spotting complicating pregnancy, **third trimester**
O26.859 Spotting complicating pregnancy, **unspecified trimester**

Example

In the I-9 to I-10 GEMs file, the entry for 649.50-649.53 indicates that the choice of correct code would be based on the new information of trimester:

I-9	I-10	Flag
64950	O26859	10000
64951	O26851	10000
64951	O26852	10000
64951	O26853	10000
64953	O26852	10000
64953	O26853	10000
64953	O26851	10000

Example

In the I-10 to I-9 GEMs file, the entry for O26.851-O26.859 is:

I-10	I-9	Flag
O26851	64951	10000
O26851	64953	10000
O26852	64953	10000
O26852	64951	10000
O26853	64951	10000
O26853	64953	10000

The 10000 flag indicates that although there is a one-to-one code mapping, the codes may not be exactly the same because the choice of code depends on the trimester. The majority of the flags in the GEMs files are Flag 1 with either a 1 or 0.

No Map. **No Map** means that there is no similar code from one coding system to the other. When this occurs, there will be a 1 as the second character in Flag 2. For example, the I-10 code, T36.6X6A, Poisoning by, adverse effect of and underdosing of rifampicins, initial encounter, has no match in I-9. In the I-9 column, "NoDx" appears and there is a 1 in the Flag 2 position.

Example

I-10	I-9	Flag
T366X6A	NoDx	11000

Combination. The **Combination** Flag 3 (third character in the flag) contains a 1 when a code from the source system must be linked to more than one code in the target system to be valid. For example, in the I-10 system, R65.21, Severe sepsis with septic shock, would require two I-9 codes (995.92, Severe sepsis, and 785.52, Septic shock) to fully report. The I-10 GEMs file displays this requirement with a 1 in the third field, as illustrated in Fig. 2-7.

Scenario and Choice List. The fourth field is the **Scenario** field and the fifth field is the **Choice List**. These two numbers appear after the three flags and indicate a further subdivision of the flags. The Scenario is the number of variations of diagnosis combinations included in the source system code. As illustrated in Fig. 2-8, in R65.21, the fourth character is 1, indicating that there is only one valid combination of I-9 codes (995.92 and 785.52).

The Choice List indicates the possible target system codes that when combined are one valid scenario. For example, in Fig. 2-8 the 2 in the Choice List position (5th place) for 995.92 indicates that the code is the second of two codes that when combined with the Choice List 1 makes a valid scenario.

I-10	I-9	Flag
R6521	99592	10112
R6521	78552	10111

FIGURE 2-7 I-10 mapping files for combination code R65.21.

I-10	I-9	Flag
R6521	99592	10112
R6521	78552	10111

1 in the **Scenario** field (4th field) indicates there is only ONE combination.

1 in the **Choice List** field (5th field) indicates the first code in the combination and the 2 indicates the second code in the combination.

FIGURE 2–8 Scenario and Choice List fields.

There are times when the fourth field (Scenario) is a number other than a 0 or 1. For example, in the I-9, there is a code for poisoning by succinimides (966.2) and a code for poisoning by oxazolidine derivatives (oxazolidinediones) (966.0). Either of these codes could be combined with E855.8 (Other specified drugs acting on central and autonomic nervous systems) to report how the poisoning occurred. However, in the I-10 coding system the two substances are combined in one code: T42.2X1A, Poisoning by succinimides and oxazolidinediones, accidental (unintentional), initial encounter. This means that both 996.2 and E855.8 are reported with the one I-10 code T42.2X1A and both 996.0/E855.8 are also reported with T42.2X1A. The GEMs file illustrates that E855.8 can be used in multiple combinations by placing a 2 in the fourth field (Fig. 2-9).

I-10	I-9	Flag
T422X1A	9662	10111
T422X1A	E8558	10112
T422X1A	9660	10121
T422X1A	E8558	10122

The 2 in the Scenario field indicates this combination is a second combination possibility.

FIGURE 2–9 GEMs file for E8558.

EXERCISE 2-2 GEMs Files and Activity Codes

To access the GEMs files, start by logging into your Evolve Learning Resources (or registering for FREE at http://evolve.elsevier.com/Buck/step). Access your "Step-by-Step Medical Coding 2015 Edition" course, then:

- Click "Course Documents"
- Click "Resources"
- Click "Coding Updates, Tips, and Links"
- Click "GEMs files (2015)"
- Select the appropriate GEMs Files

With the use of the two GEMs files, answer the following:

Using the I-9 to I-10 GEMs file, map the following codes:

1 005.89 _____   a C15.3

2 016.01 _____   b T07

3 150.0 _____   c A05.8

4 919.8 _____   d Z39.1

5 E841.3 _____   e A18.11

6 V24.1 _____   f V95.8XXA

Continued

According to the I-10 to I-9 GEMs file, map the following codes:

7 S06.1X8A _____

8 T38.903S _____

9 D75.81 _____

10 A02.29 _____

11 M35.09 _____

12 R65.20 _____

a 003.29

b 289.83

c 854.05 and 348.5

d 995.92

e 710.2

f 909.0 and E969

According to the examples previously presented in the text or in the I-10 Tabular, match the activity code description to the correct I-10 code:

13 Y93.01 _____

14 Y93.11 _____

15 Y93.34 _____

a bungee jumping

b walking, marching, and hiking

c swimming

16 When 00000 is displayed in the Flag field, the following is true about the target coding system: _____

a there are multiple entries available

b there is only a single entry available

c there is no code available

d any of the above may be true

17 The third character in the Flag field is this type of flag: _____

a combination

b approximate

c scenario

d choice list

(Answers are located in Appendix B)

ICD-10-CM FORMAT

The I-10 Alphabetic Index and Tabular are used in outpatient settings to substantiate the reason for receiving medical services (medical necessity) by assigning diagnosis codes. ICD-10-PCS is used for coding surgical, therapeutic, and diagnostic procedures and is used primarily by hospitals. Today, more than 95 percent of claims are filed electronically using the 5010 claim format required under HIPAA. Examples of the 5010 format can be seen in Figs. D-1 through D-8 (located in Appendix D). I-10 codes can also be reported on the CMS-1500 insurance claim form (Fig. 2-10). Government and private insurers require diagnostic codes to be submitted to show the medical necessity of services provided. Several publishing companies produce versions of the I-10 manual. All versions are based on the official government version of the I-10.

There are four groups whose function it is to deal with in-depth coding principles and practices: Centers for Medicare and Medicaid Services (CMS), which was formerly known as the Health Care Financing Administration (HCFA); National Center for Health Statistics (NCHS); American Health Information Management Association (AHIMA); and American Hospital Association (AHA).

HEALTH INSURANCE CLAIM FORM

APPROVED BY NATIONAL UNIFORM CLAIM COMMITTEE (NUCC) 02/12

☐☐ PICA   PICA ☐☐

| 1. MEDICARE ☐ (Medicare#) | MEDICAID ☐ (Medicaid#) | TRICARE ☐ (ID#DoD#) | CHAMPVA ☐ (Member ID#) | GROUP HEALTH PLAN ☐ (ID#) | FECA BLK LUNG ☐ (ID#) | OTHER ☐ | 1a. INSURED'S I.D. NUMBER | (For Program in Item 1) |

2. PATIENT'S NAME (Last Name, First Name, Middle Initial)

3. PATIENT'S BIRTH DATE MM | DD | YY   SEX   M ☐   F ☐

4. INSURED'S NAME (Last Name, First Name, Middle Initial)

5. PATIENT'S ADDRESS (No., Street)

6. PATIENT RELATIONSHIP TO INSURED   Self ☐ Spouse ☐ Child ☐ Other ☐

7. INSURED'S ADDRESS (No., Street)

CITY   STATE

8. RESERVED FOR NUCC USE

CITY   STATE

ZIP CODE   TELEPHONE (Include Area Code) ( )

ZIP CODE   TELEPHONE (Include Area Code) ( )

9. OTHER INSURED'S NAME (Last Name, First Name, Middle Initial)

10. IS PATIENT'S CONDITION RELATED TO:

11. INSURED'S POLICY GROUP OR FECA NUMBER

a. OTHER INSURED'S POLICY OR GROUP NUMBER

a. EMPLOYMENT? (Current or Previous)   YES ☐   NO ☐

a. INSURED'S DATE OF BIRTH MM | DD | YY   SEX   M ☐   F ☐

b. RESERVED FOR NUCC USE

b. AUTO ACCIDENT?   PLACE (State)   YES ☐   NO ☐

b. OTHER CLAIM ID (Designated by NUCC)

c. RESERVED FOR NUCC USE

c. OTHER ACCIDENT?   YES ☐   NO ☐

c. INSURANCE PLAN NAME OR PROGRAM NAME

d. INSURANCE PLAN NAME OR PROGRAM NAME

10d. CLAIM CODES (Designated by NUCC)

d. IS THERE ANOTHER HEALTH BENEFIT PLAN?   YES ☐   NO ☐   *If yes,* complete items 9, 9a, and 9d.

READ BACK OF FORM BEFORE COMPLETING & SIGNING THIS FORM.
12. PATIENT'S OR AUTHORIZED PERSON'S SIGNATURE I authorize the release of any medical or other information necessary to process this claim. I also request payment of government benefits either to myself or to the party who accepts assignment below.

SIGNED _____   DATE _____

13. INSURED'S OR AUTHORIZED PERSON'S SIGNATURE I authorize payment of medical benefits to the undersigned physician or supplier for services described below.

SIGNED _____

14. DATE OF CURRENT ILLNESS, INJURY, or PREGNANCY(LMP) MM | DD | YY   QUAL.

15. OTHER DATE QUAL. | MM | DD | YY

16. DATES PATIENT UNABLE TO WORK IN CURRENT OCCUPATION MM | DD | YY FROM   TO MM | DD | YY

17. NAME OF REFERRING PROVIDER OR OTHER SOURCE

17a.
17b. NPI

18. HOSPITALIZATION DATES RELATED TO CURRENT SERVICES MM | DD | YY FROM   TO MM | DD | YY

19. ADDITIONAL CLAIM INFORMATION (Designated by NUCC)

20. OUTSIDE LAB?   YES ☐   NO ☐ $ CHARGES

21. DIAGNOSIS OR NATURE OF ILLNESS OR INJURY Relate A-L to service line below (24E)   ICD Ind. |

A. |_____   B. |_____   C. |_____   D. |_____
E. |_____   F. |_____   G. |_____   H. |_____
I. |_____   J. |_____   K. |_____   L. |_____

22. RESUBMISSION CODE   ORIGINAL REF. NO.

23. PRIOR AUTHORIZATION NUMBER

24. A. DATE(S) OF SERVICE						B. PLACE OF SERVICE	C. EMG	D. PROCEDURES, SERVICES, OR SUPPLIES (Explain Unusual Circumstances) CPT/HCPCS	MODIFIER	E. DIAGNOSIS POINTER	F. $ CHARGES	G. DAYS OR UNITS	H. EPSDT Family Plan	I. ID. QUAL.	J. RENDERING PROVIDER ID. #
From MM	DD	YY	To MM	DD	YY										
1														NPI	
2														NPI	
3														NPI	
4														NPI	
5														NPI	
6														NPI	

25. FEDERAL TAX I.D. NUMBER   SSN ☐ EIN ☐

26. PATIENT'S ACCOUNT NO.

27. ACCEPT ASSIGNMENT? (For govt. claims, see back)   YES ☐   NO ☐

28. TOTAL CHARGE $

29. AMOUNT PAID $

30. Rsvd for NUCC Use $

31. SIGNATURE OF PHYSICIAN OR SUPPLIER INCLUDING DEGREES OR CREDENTIALS (I certify that the statements on the reverse apply to this bill and are made a part thereof.)

SIGNED _____   DATE _____

32. SERVICE FACILITY LOCATION INFORMATION

a. NPI   b.

33. BILLING PROVIDER INFO & PH # ( )

a. NPI   b.

NUCC Instruction Manual available at: www.nucc.org   *PLEASE PRINT OR TYPE*   APPROVED OMB-0938-1197 FORM 1500 (02-12)

FIGURE 2–10 CMS–1500 Health Insurance Claim Form

INDEX

The I-10 Index is alphabetic, as illustrated in Fig. 2-11. As in the I-9, the I-10 index presents the main terms in bold type, and subterms indented under the main term. After the index entry, a code is provided. Sometimes, only the first four characters of the code are listed. To ensure that you have chosen the correct code and/or to obtain the remaining characters, you must always reference the Tabular.

Aarskog's syndrome Q87.1
Abandonment —*see* Maltreatment
Abasia (-astasia) (hysterical) F44.4
Abderhalden-Kaufmann-Lignac
    syndrome (cystinosis) E72.04
Abdomen, abdominal —*see also*
    condition
    acute R10.0
    angina K55.1
    muscle deficiency syndrome Q79.4
Abdominalgia —*see* Pain, abdominal
Abduction contracture, hip or other
    joint —*see* Contraction, joint
Aberrant (congenital) —*see also*
    Malposition, congenital
    adrenal gland Q89.1
    artery (peripheral) Q27.8
        basilar NEC Q28.1
        cerebral Q28.3
        coronary Q24.5
        digestive system Q27.8
        eye Q15.8
        lower limb Q27.8
        precerebral Q28.1
        pulmonary Q25.79
        renal Q27.2
        retina Q14.1

FIGURE 2–11 ICD-10-CM Index.

QUICK CHECK 2-2

According to Fig. 2-11, what is the code you would reference in the Tabular for:
1. aberrant basilar artery? _____
2. acute abdomen? _____

(Answers are located in Appendix C)

TABULAR

The 21 chapters of the Tabular are arranged in numeric order after the first letter assigned to the chapter. The chapters are as follows:

Chapter 1 Certain Infectious and Parasitic Diseases (A00-B99)
Chapter 2 Neoplasms (C00-D49)
Chapter 3 Diseases of the Blood and Blood-Forming Organs and Certain Disorders Involving the Immune Mechanism (D50-D89)
Chapter 4 Endocrine, Nutritional, and Metabolic Diseases (E00-E89)
Chapter 5 Mental, Behavioral and Neurodevelopmental Disorders (F01-F99)
Chapter 6 Diseases of the Nervous System (G00-G99)
Chapter 7 Diseases of the Eye and Adnexa (H00-H59)
Chapter 8 Diseases of the Ear and Mastoid Process (H60-H95)
Chapter 9 Diseases of the Circulatory System (I00-I99)
Chapter 10 Diseases of the Respiratory System (J00-J99)
Chapter 11 Diseases of the Digestive System (K00-K95)
Chapter 12 Diseases of the Skin and Subcutaneous Tissue (L00-L99)
Chapter 13 Diseases of the Musculoskeletal System and Connective Tissue (M00-M99)
Chapter 14 Diseases of the Genitourinary System (N00-N99)
Chapter 15 Pregnancy, Childbirth, and the Puerperium (O00-O9A)
Chapter 16 Certain Conditions Originating in the Perinatal Period (P00-P96)
Chapter 17 Congenital Malformations, Deformations and Chromosomal Abnormalities (Q00-Q99)
Chapter 18 Symptoms, Signs, and Abnormal Clinical and Laboratory Findings, Not Elsewhere Classified (R00-R99)
Chapter 19 Injury, Poisoning and Certain Other Consequences of External Causes (S00-T88)
Chapter 20 External Causes of Morbidity (V00-Y99)
Chapter 21 Factors Influencing Health Status and Contact with Health Services (Z00-Z99)

If you compare the chapters in ICD-10-CM to those in ICD-9-CM, you will see that the flow is very similar. That is because the World Health Organization used ICD-9 as the foundation to create the ICD-10. To increase the capacity of the system, WHO replaced the first numerals 0-9 with letters A-Z. The results are sometimes a parallel, for example:

ICD-9-CM		ICD-10-CM	
021	Tularemia	A21	Tularemia
021.0	Ulceroglandular tularemia	A21.0	Ulceroglandular tularemia
021.1	Enteric tularemia	A21.1	Oculoglandular tularemia
021.2	Pulmonary tularemia	A21.2	Pulmonary tularemia
021.3	Oculoglandular tularemia	A21.3	Gastrointestinal tularemia
		A21.7	Generalized tularemia
021.8	Other specified tularemia	A21.8	Other forms of tularemia
021.9	Unspecified tularemia	A21.9	Tularemia, unspecified

As you can see, the classifications are nearly identical. In ICD-9-CM, generalized tularemia is reported with 021.9 unspecified tularemia, so the creation of A21.7 in the ICD-10-CM adds additional specificity to the reporting of generalized tularemia. (Tularemia is an infectious disease caused by bacterium.)

The ICD-9-CM classification begins with 0 and continues through 9. ICD-10-CM begins with A and continues through Z. Due to the complexity of some chapters in ICD-10-CM, a chapter may use more than one letter (example: Neoplasms are all of the letter C and half of the letter D), or only part of one letter (example: Eye and Adnexa are half of the letter H). Although there is no significance to the letters assigned to each chapter other than alphabetic order, there are numerous chapter code sets that start with letters that seem intuitive. For example, Chapter 15 Pregnancy, Childbirth and the Puerperium, uses only the letter O. If you think "obstetrics," you will instantly know which letter pregnancy codes begin with. This trick is called a mnemonic (new-MON-ick) device, and there are many for remembering ICD-10 chapters:

Neoplasms (C00-D49)	"C for cancer"
Endocrine, Nutritional, and Metabolic Diseases (E00-E89)	"E for endocrine"
Nervous System (G00-G99)	"G for ganglia"
Ear and Mastoid Process (H60-H95)	"H for hearing"
Circulatory System (I00-I99)	"I for infarct"
Musculoskeletal System and Connective Tissue (M00-M99)	"M for musculoskeletal"
Genitourinary System (N00-N99)	"N for nephrology"
Certain Conditions Originating in the Perinatal Period (P00-P96)	"P for perinatal"

Think of your own mnemonic devices for the other chapters, as they are very helpful when beginning to work with a new coding system.

Fig. 2-12 illustrates a portion of the chapter concerning symptoms. Note that in the Index (see Fig. 2-11) the main entry is Abdomen, abdominal, and the first subterm is "acute," directing the coder to the Tabular location, R10.0. Now, note in the Tabular (see Fig. 2-12) the location of R10.0 as Acute abdomen.

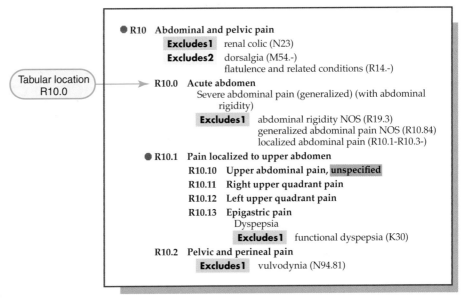

FIGURE 2-12 ICD-10-CM Tabular, R codes.

EXERCISE 2-3   *ICD-10-CM Index and Tabular*

Using the information previously presented, answer the following:

1 The code range for Mental, Behavioral and Neurodevelopmental Disorders is _____.

   a V00-Y99

   b O00-O9A

   c F01-F99

   d N00-N99

2 The code range for Certain Conditions Originating in the Perinatal Period is _____.

   a P00-P96

   b Z00-Z99

   c I00-I99

   d G00-G99

3 According to Fig. 2-11, when referencing "Aberrant (congenital), artery, eye" in the Index of the I-10, the coder is directed to reference this code in the Tabular. _____.

   a Q98.0

   b Q15.8

   c R15

   d Z49.31

4 In the Index of the I-10, the main term is identified in this typeface. _____.

   a italic

   b red

   c underlined

   d bold

(Answers are located in Appendix B)

OFFICIAL INSTRUCTIONAL NOTATIONS IN THE ICD-10-CM

The I-10 has instructional notations to provide guidance to the coder. Although publishers will enhance their I-10s with various notations and symbols, all publishers present the notations that are part of the official version of the coding system. Let's review these official instructional notations.

Includes

The word "Includes" appears under certain categories to further define or give examples of the content of the category. For example, Fig. 2-13 illustrates an "Includes" in Chapter 1 of the I-10.

CHAPTER 1

CERTAIN INFECTIOUS AND PARASITIC DISEASES (A00-B99)

   Includes   diseases generally recognized as communicable or transmissible

---

FIGURE 2-13   Includes notation in I-10.

Excludes

The I-10 has two types of Excludes notes. Each note has a different meaning.

Excludes1. An Excludes1 note is a pure excludes. It means "NOT CODED HERE!" and indicates that the code excluded should **not be assigned** at the same time as the code above the Excludes1 note. In Fig. 2-14 codes in Chapter 1 are not to be reported with certain localized infections (the first Excludes1).

An Excludes1 is used when two conditions cannot occur together, such as a congenital form versus an acquired form of the same condition.

CHAPTER 1

CERTAIN INFECTIOUS AND PARASITIC DISEASES (A00-B99)

Includes   diseases generally recognized as communicable or transmissible

Use additional code to identify resistance to antimicrobial drugs (Z16.-)

Excludes1   certain localized infections - see body system-related chapters

FIGURE 2–14 Excludes1 notation in I-10.

Excludes2. An Excludes2 note represents "Not included here." An Excludes2 note indicates that the condition excluded is not part of the condition it is excluded from and a patient may have both conditions at the same time. When an Excludes2 note appears under a code, it is acceptable to use both the code and the Excludes2 code together. For example, the first Exludes2 note in Chapter 1 indicates that the infectious and parasitic disease does not include a carrier or suspected carrier of infectious disease as shown in Fig. 2-15 and it is possible for the patient to have both conditions.

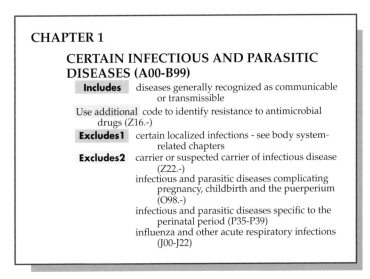

CHAPTER 1

CERTAIN INFECTIOUS AND PARASITIC DISEASES (A00-B99)

Includes   diseases generally recognized as communicable or transmissible

Use additional code to identify resistance to antimicrobial drugs (Z16.-)

Excludes1   certain localized infections - see body system-related chapters

Excludes2   carrier or suspected carrier of infectious disease (Z22.-)

infectious and parasitic diseases complicating pregnancy, childbirth and the puerperium (O98.-)

infectious and parasitic diseases specific to the perinatal period (P35-P39)

influenza and other acute respiratory infections (J00-J22)

FIGURE 2–15 Excludes2 notation in I-10.

QUICK CHECK 2-3

According to Fig. 2-15, Chapter 1 Excludes 2, what is the code you reference when reporting
1. infectious and parasitic diseases complicating pregnancy, childbirth and the puerperium?

_____

2. influenza and other acute respiratory infections? _____

(Answers are located in Appendix C)

Code First/Use Additional Code

The "Code first" and "Use additional code" notations indicate etiology/manifestation paired codes. Certain conditions have both an underlying etiology and multiple body system manifestations. For such conditions, the I-10 has a coding convention that requires the underlying condition be sequenced first followed by the manifestation. Wherever such a combination exists there is a "Use additional code" note at the **etiology** code, and a "Code first" note at the **manifestation** code. These instructional notes indicate the proper sequencing order of the codes—etiology followed by manifestation. For example, as illustrated in Fig. 2-16, the Code first notation at code A40 directs the coder to report certain conditions first.

In most cases the manifestation codes will have in the code title, "in diseases classified elsewhere." Codes with this title are a component of the etiology/manifestation convention. The code title "in diseases classified elsewhere" indicates that the code is a manifestation code. "In diseases classified elsewhere" codes are never first-listed codes. Rather, these codes must be used in conjunction with an underlying condition code and must follow the underlying condition code. For example, the Code first notation at D77 directs the coder to first report the underlying disease, such as illustrated in Fig. 2-17. The black dot to the left of D77 in Fig. 2-17 indicates an "Unacceptable First-Listed Diagnosis." (The black dot is an enhancement placed by the publisher and is not part of the official code set.)

Code Also

A "Code also" note instructs that two codes may be required to fully describe a condition but the sequencing of the two codes is discretionary, depending on the severity of the conditions and the reason for the encounter. For example, at D61.82, the coder is directed to also code an underlying disorder, if one is present, as shown in Fig. 2-18.

● **A40   Streptococcal sepsis**

Code first
   postprocedural streptococcal sepsis (T81.4)
   streptococcal sepsis during labor (O75.3)
   streptococcal sepsis following abortion or ectopic or
      molar pregnancy (O03-O07, O08.0)
   streptococcal sepsis following immunization (T88.0)
   streptococcal sepsis following infusion, transfusion or
      therapeutic injection (T80.2-)

FIGURE 2–16 I-10 Tabular, Code first notation.

▶ **D77 Other disorders of blood and blood-forming organs in diseases classified elsewhere**

Code first underlying disease, such as:
amyloidosis (E85.-)
congenital early syphilis (A50.0)
echinococcosis (B67.0-B67.9)
malaria (B50.0-B54)
schistosomiasis [bilharziasis] (B65.0-B65.9)
vitamin C deficiency (E54)

FIGURE 2-17 ICD-10-CM Tabular, Code first underlying disease notation.

D61.82 Myelophthisis
Leukoerythroblastic anemia
Myelophthisic anemia
Panmyelophthisis
Code also the underlying disorder, such as:
malignant neoplasm of breast (C50.-)
tuberculosis (A15.-)

FIGURE 2-18 I-10 Tabular, Code also notation.

7th Characters and Placeholder X

For codes less than 6 characters that require a 7th character a placeholder X is assigned for all characters less than 6.

For the initial encounter of a sprain of an unspecified acromioclavicular joint, the correct code, as shown in Fig. 2-19, is S43.50. Following the instructions under Category S43, a 7th character A is required. In order for the A to be a 7th character, an X is added as a 6th character to S43.50. The correct code is S43.50XA. In other cases, the classification itself presents an X to identify a placeholder that may be expanded in the future. For example, see Fig. 2-20. In this case, the classification may in the future be divided into individual disorders of the patella for more specific coding. The 7th character now and in the future will identify whether the disorder is of the right or left knee.

● **S43 Dislocation and sprain of joints and ligaments of shoulder girdle**

The appropriate 7th character is to be added to each code from category S43

A initial encounter
D subsequent encounter
S sequela

● **S43.5 Sprain of acromioclavicular joint**
Sprain of acromioclavicular ligament
X ● **S43.50 Sprain of unspecified acromioclavicular joint**
X ● **S43.51 Sprain of right acromioclavicular joint**
X ● **S43.52 Sprain of left acromioclavicular joint**

FIGURE 2-19 Determining X as the placeholder.

● **M22.8 Other disorders of patella**
    ● **M22.8X Other disorders of patella**
            M22.8X1 Other disorders of patella, right knee
            M22.8X2 Other disorders of patella, left knee

FIGURE 2–20   X as the placeholder.

EXERCISE 2-4   *Official Instructional I-10 Notations*

With the use of the information previously presented, match the following notation with the correct description:

1 Includes _____

2 Excludes1 _____

3 Excludes2 _____

4 Code First _____

5 Code Also _____

a. two codes may be required to fully describe the condition but the sequencing of the two codes is discretionary

b. pure excludes

c. indicates a manifestation due to underlying etiology

d. not included here

e. gives further definition or examples of content

(Answers are located in Appendix B)

CHAPTER REVIEW

CHAPTER 2, PART I, THEORY

Without the use of reference material, answer the following:

1 I-10 codes are alphanumeric.

   True   False

2 I-10 is indexed in a similar manner to ICD-9-CM.

   True   False

3 Like I-9, I-10 contains 17 chapters.

   True   False

4 All versions of the ICD-10-CM are based on the official government version.

   True   False

5 I-10 was issued in 1993 by _____.
   a CMS
   b AHIMA
   c AHA
   d WHO

6 The acronym used in the United States for the I-10 system that reports inpatient procedures is the _____.
   a PDQ
   b PCS
   c PHI
   d none of the above

7 Implementation of the I-10 system is scheduled for this date in America: _____
   a November 1, 2015
   b October 1, 2016
   c October 30, 2015
   d October 1, 2015

8 The expansion of the injury codes in the I-10 has been done with _____ codes.
   a sport
   b ambulatory
   c activity
   d dynamic

9 The mapping files that crosswalk I-9 to I-10 and I-10 to I-9 are known as _____.
   a ACTs
   b GEMs
   c HIMs
   d PQIs

10 A code that reports more than one diagnosis with one code is a _____ code.
   a multiple
   b compound
   c complex
   d combination

Chapter Review answers are only available in the TEACH Instructor Resources on Evolve

CHAPTER 2, PART II, PRACTICAL

GEMs FILES REQUIRED. *Using the I-9 to I-10 GEMs file, map the following codes. The I-9 codes may have more than one correct I-10 code.*

11 004.0 _____

12 456.1 _____

13 803. 81 _____

14 290.40 _____

15 530.0 _____
   a K22.0
   b I85.00
   c S06.360A
   d A03.0
   e F01.50
   f S0291XB

GEMs FILES REQUIRED. *Using the I-10 to I-9 GEMs file, map the following codes and drag and drop the I-9 code or codes to the correct I-10 code.*

16 R56.9 _____

17 S52.513S _____

18 Z99.89 _____

19 W16.832S _____

20 V04.99XS _____
   a 905.2
   b E929.0
   c V46.8
   d E929.3
   e 780.39

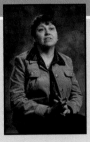

"The implementation of ICD-10-CM will require a shift for providers in their documentation habits. More specific information will be required to accurately report conditions. I think it would be beneficial for coders to be proactive in working with their providers now to coach them in more thorough documentation."

Joan E. Wolfgang, MEd, RHIT, CPC, COC, CPC-I, CCA

Faculty
Milwaukee Area Technical College
Milwaukee, Wisconsin

ICD-10-CM Outpatient Coding and Reporting Guidelines

Chapter Topics

First-Listed Diagnosis

Unconfirmed Diagnosis

Outpatient Surgery

Additional Diagnoses

Z Codes

Observation Stay

First-Listed Diagnosis and Coexisting Conditions

Uncertain Diagnosis

Chronic Diseases

Documented Conditions

Diagnostic Services

Therapeutic Services

Preoperative Evaluation

Prenatal Visits

Chapter Review

Learning Objectives

After completing this chapter you should be able to

1 Identify a first-listed diagnosis.

2 Define assignment of codes for unconfirmed diagnosis.

3 Describe code assignment for outpatient surgery.

4 Outline assignment of additional diagnoses.

5 Describe Z code reporting.

6 Define observation stay.

7 Delineate the differences between first-listed and coexisting conditions.

8 Explain uncertain diagnosis.

9 Understand assignment of codes for chronic diseases.

10 Recognize diagnostic services.

11 Recognize therapeutic services.

12 Illustrate reporting of preoperative evaluations.

13 Explain prenatal visits.

14 Apply the *Official Guidelines for Coding and Reporting.*

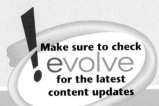

Make sure to check
evolve
for the latest
content updates

NOTE: *The 2015 ICD-10-CM DRAFT and 2015 ICD-10-PCS DRAFT were used in preparing this text.*

FIRST-LISTED DIAGNOSIS

The majority of the services that a physician will provide are outpatient services, so this chapter will start with assigning I-10 diagnosis codes for outpatient services in accordance with the I-10 *Official Guidelines for Coding and Reporting*, Section IV.

ICD-10 OFFICIAL GUIDELINES FOR CODING AND REPORTING

SECTION IV. Diagnostic Coding and Reporting Guidelines for Outpatient Services

These coding guidelines for outpatient diagnoses have been approved for use by hospitals/providers in coding and reporting hospital-based outpatient services and provider-based office visits.

Information about the use of certain abbreviations, punctuation, symbols, and other conventions used in the ICD-10-CM Tabular List (code numbers and titles), can be found in Section IA of these guidelines, under "Conventions Used in the Tabular List." **Section I. B. contains general guidelines that apply to the entire classification. Section I. C. contains chapter-specific guidelines that correspond to the chapters as they are arranged in the classification.** Information about the correct sequence to use in finding a code is also described in Section I.

The terms encounter and visit are often used interchangeably in describing outpatient service contacts and, therefore, appear together in these guidelines without distinguishing one from the other.

Though the conventions and general guidelines apply to all settings, coding guidelines for outpatient and provider reporting of diagnoses will vary in a number of instances from those for inpatient diagnoses, recognizing that:

> The Uniform Hospital Discharge Data Set (UHDDS) definition of principal diagnosis applies only to inpatients in acute, short-term, long-term care, and psychiatric hospitals.

> Coding guidelines for inconclusive diagnoses (probable, suspected, rule out, etc.) were developed for inpatient reporting and do not apply to outpatients.

A. Selection of first-listed condition

> In the outpatient setting, the term first-listed diagnosis is used in lieu of principal diagnosis.

> In determining the first-listed diagnosis the coding conventions of ICD-10-CM, as well as the general and disease specific guidelines take precedence over the outpatient guidelines.

> Diagnoses often are not established at the time of the initial encounter/visit. It may take two or more visits before the diagnosis is confirmed.

> The most critical rule involves beginning the search for the correct code assignment through the Alphabetic Index. Never begin searching initially in the Tabular List as this will lead to coding errors.

Examples

Select the First-Listed Diagnosis

Established 50-year-old patient was seen in the clinic for acute bronchitis. Patient also received a prescription for a refill of medication for hypertension. The first-listed diagnosis is acute bronchitis.

Initial office visit for a 36-year-old female complaining of irregular menses. Review of systems identified unexplained weight loss. The first-listed diagnosis is irregular menses.

Established patient is a 75-year-old male complaining of substernal chest pain, which is relieved with rest. Patient has hypertension and blood pressure is above baseline on this visit. The first-listed diagnosis is substernal chest pain.

Most physicians will document the "chief complaint" of the patient for each encounter in the medical record. The chief complaint (CC) is the reason the patient presents for the medical visit. The CC is one of the keys to determining the first-listed diagnosis. The chief complaint is the reason for the visit from the patient's perspective. For example, a patient consumed a soup that contained shellfish. The patient is allergic to shellfish, and develops hives. The chief complaint and the first-listed diagnosis is allergic hives, due to allergy to shellfish:

L50.0	**Allergic urticaria**
Z91.013	**Allergy to seafood**

Other times, the patient's complaint is a symptom of a more complex diagnosis. For example, a patient presents with a chief complaint of a backache, and after examination, the physician determines the patient has an acute kidney infection due to *Escherichia coli*. The chief complaint is a backache, but the first-listed diagnosis is an acute kidney infection due to *E. coli*. The backache was a symptom of the acute kidney infection.

N10	**Acute tubulo-interstitial nephritis**
B96.2	**Escherichia coli [E. coli] as the cause of diseases classified elsewhere**

The patient may also schedule a visit without a chief complaint. As examples, the patient requests a physical to qualify for insurance or may be an expectant parent seeking to establish a pediatrician. The reason for these visits can be reported as first-listed codes using codes from Chapter 21:

Z02.6	**Encounter for examination for insurance purposes**
Z76.81	**Expectant parent(s) prebirth pediatrician visit**

EXERCISE 3-1   *First-Listed Diagnosis*

Identify the first-listed diagnosis in the following encounters or visits:

1 Established patient complaining of painful urination and frequency. Patient is a type 2 diabetic. Lab work revealed a urinary tract infection and blood glucose was within normal limits.

First-listed Diagnosis: _____

2 Established patient presented to clinic with exacerbation of Crohn's disease. Patient's rheumatoid arthritis is stable and no medication changes were made.

First-listed Diagnosis: _____

3 Initial office visit for sprained left knee. Patient has a history of hypertension and asthma, both stable at this time.

First-listed Diagnosis: _____

4 Initial office visit for patient requiring equal management of COPD and CHF.

First-listed Diagnosis: _____

5 Established patient seen for cough, fever, and shortness of breath. Chest x-ray confirmed physician's diagnosis of pneumonia and patient was sent home on antibiotics.

First-listed Diagnosis: _____

(Answers are located in Appendix B)

UNCONFIRMED DIAGNOSIS

Often, it may take several encounters before the diagnosis is confirmed. In these instances, report the symptoms or signs that occasioned the encounter.

Examples

Two or More Visits Before A Diagnosis is Confirmed

1. Initial office visit, 30-year-old woman complains of fatigue, abnormal weight gain, and constipation. Lab studies including thyroid function test were ordered. Patient will return in two weeks.

   In this case the only reportable diagnoses are symptom codes as no specific diagnosis has been confirmed during this visit.

   Codes: R53.83 fatigue, R63.5 abnormal weight gain, and K59.00 constipation.

2. Follow-up office visit, 30-year-old woman with continued complaints of fatigue, weight gain, and constipation. Lab results confirm that patient has hypothyroidism and she was started on Synthroid. She will have repeat thyroid function studies on her next visit.

   Code: E03.9 hypothyroidism. The patient was told that she has hypothyroidism and the fatigue, weight gain, and constipation are common symptoms and would likely improve with treatment of her hypothyroidism. No additional treatment was directed at the patient's symptoms.

3. Follow-up office visit, 30-year-old woman is seen following her repeat thyroid function studies and her hypothyroidism has responded to the Synthroid. She will be maintained on her current dose.

   Code: E03.9 hypothyroidism is the reason for the visit.

EXERCISE 3-2 *Unconfirmed Diagnosis*

Using reference material, assign codes to the following:

1 Initial office visit for a 28-year-old male with persistent abdominal pain and bloody diarrhea. Patient was scheduled for small-bowel x-rays and colonoscopy and will be seen in the office following those outpatient procedures.

Codes: _____, _____

2 Follow-up office visit for a 28-year-old male with recent colonoscopy with biopsy and small bowel x-rays. The biopsy and small bowel x-rays confirmed that the patient had ulcerative colitis and the patient was started on sulfasalazine.

Code: _____

3 Initial office visit for 55-year-old male with fatigue and jaundice. Laboratory tests were ordered and patient will return in 1 week for the results.

Codes: _____, _____

4 Follow-up office visit for 55-year-old male with jaundice and fatigue. Diagnostic tests confirm that the patient has hepatitis C. He will be treated with interferon therapy.

Code: _____

(Answers are located in Appendix B)

OUTPATIENT SURGERY

ICD-10 OFFICIAL GUIDELINES FOR CODING AND REPORTING

SECTION IV.A.

1. Outpatient Surgery

When a patient presents for outpatient surgery (same day surgery), code the reason for the surgery as the first-listed diagnosis (reason for the encounter), even if the surgery is not performed due to a contraindication.

Examples

Outpatient Surgery

Patient with a history of asthma presents for an outpatient T&A due to chronic tonsillitis.

First-listed diagnosis: J35.01 Chronic tonsillitis.

Outpatient Surgery That has been Canceled

Patient presented for a right inguinal hernia repair. Following assessment of the patient by the nurse, it was discovered that the patient had breakfast and the surgery was canceled and will be rescheduled for next week.

First-listed diagnosis: K40.90 Inguinal hernia, followed by Z53.09 (procedure not carried out due to other contraindication).

EXERCISE 3-3 | *Outpatient Surgery*

Identify the first-listed diagnoses in the following:

1 A female patient was admitted as an outpatient for elective bilateral tubal ligation. The patient was noted to be wheezing during the nurse's assessment. She was seen by her physician and her surgery was canceled because of an exacerbation of her asthma.

First-listed Diagnosis: _____

2 A male patient was admitted as an outpatient for transurethral prostatic resection for symptomatic benign prostatic hypertrophy.

First-listed Diagnosis: _____

3 A patient was admitted as an outpatient for a cystoscopy for hematuria. The procedure was performed without complications. No abnormality or explanation for the hematuria was found.

First-listed Diagnosis: _____

(Answers are located in Appendix B)

ADDITIONAL DIAGNOSES

In the preceding guidelines and exercises, we were concerned primarily with the identification of the first-listed diagnosis. In some cases, additional diagnoses would be reported to describe complications, reasons for canceled procedures, and other coexisting conditions.

ICD-10 OFFICIAL GUIDELINES FOR CODING AND REPORTING

SECTION IV.B. Codes from A00.0 through T88.9, Z00-Z99

The appropriate code(s) from A00.0 through T88.9, Z00-Z99 must be used to identify diagnoses, symptoms, conditions, problems, complaints, or other reason(s) for the encounter/visit.

The Guidelines state that it is acceptable to use any of the codes throughout the entire Tabular List to identify the reason(s) for an outpatient visit including the use of Z codes. Z codes are used more frequently in the outpatient setting.

This guideline assures data integrity by promoting accurate I-10 diagnosis codes that are supported by documentation in the health record. It is important to code all the conditions or problems that are being managed during an encounter.

ICD-10 OFFICIAL GUIDELINES FOR CODING AND REPORTING

SECTION IV.C. Accurate reporting of ICD-10-CM diagnosis codes

For accurate reporting of ICD-10-CM diagnosis codes, the documentation should describe the patient's condition, using terminology which includes specific diagnoses as well as symptoms, problems, or reasons for the encounter. There are ICD-10-CM codes to describe all of these.

According to Guideline D, it is acceptable for symptoms and signs to be reported if no definitive diagnosis has been established by the provider. Chapter 18 of the I-10 contains codes (R00-R99) for most of these symptom or sign codes, but there are other such codes throughout the I-10.

ICD-10 OFFICIAL GUIDELINES FOR CODING AND REPORTING

SECTION IV.D. Codes that describe symptoms and signs

Codes that describe symptoms and signs, as opposed to diagnoses, are acceptable for reporting purposes when a diagnosis has not been established (confirmed) by the provider. Chapter 18 of ICD-10-CM, Symptoms, Signs, and Abnormal Clinical and Laboratory Findings Not Elsewhere Classified (codes R00-R99) contain many, but not all codes for symptoms.

Z CODES

There are 21 chapters in Volume 1, Tabular List, of the I-10. Each of the chapters represents a different organ system or type of disease. You will review each of the chapters, but first, there are some special codes that you need to know about—Z codes (located in Chapter 21 of the I-10).

When abstracting information from the medical record as the basis for code assignment, the intent is to communicate the story of the patient encounter. Sometimes, important information contributing to the care of the patient is not an illness. As you read through the medical record, always ask yourself, "Is this information pertinent to the care provided?" For example, the patient may have a history of cancer, but the cancer has been surgically removed. As another example, a patient lives in difficult circumstances at his home and these circumstances are affecting the patient's health or are affecting the physician's ability to treat the patient's primary condition, putting the patient at risk. There are also circumstances in which patients need counseling or may have been exposed to a disease that they may or may not have contracted. The Z codes are assigned to report these types of encounters and capture the story accurately. Sometimes the Z code will be the first-listed code, and sometimes the Z code will be a supplemental code.

Examples

1. The patient complains to her family practitioner of blood in her sputum. An x-ray shows a coin lesion in the right lung. The patient is seven years post-mastectomy for breast cancer.

   The history of breast cancer is pertinent to the patient's chief complaint. Although the patient has been symptom-free for seven years, her history of breast cancer will contribute to the diagnostic path the physician chooses. Report:

R04.2	**Hemoptysis**
R91.1	**Other coin lesion lung**
Z85.3	**Personal history of malignant neoplasm of breast**

2. John went camping last month in the Rockies with several friends who now have been diagnosed with Giardia from drinking from the mountain stream. John also drank from the stream but has no symptoms. He presents to the office today to be tested for Giardia. The laboratory results indicate that he has been infected with *Giardia lamblia* and is prescribed a 10-day course of Flagyl.

   John did not have a chief complaint and had no symptoms. He presented for a screening test and laboratory results indicated an infection. Report:

Z11.0	**Encounter for screening for intestinal Infectious diseases**
A07.1	**Giardiasis [lambliasis]**

Read the following Guidelines about assignment of codes in the Z00-Z99 range:

ICD-10 OFFICIAL GUIDELINES FOR CODING AND REPORTING

SECTION IV.E. Encounters for circumstances other than a disease or injury

ICD-10-CM provides codes to deal with encounters for circumstances other than a disease or injury. The Factors Influencing Health Status and Contact with Health Services codes (Z00-Z99) are provided to deal with occasions when circumstances other than a disease or injury are recorded as diagnosis or problems.

See Section I.C.21. Factors influencing health status and contact with health services.

SECTION IV.Q. Encounters for routine health screenings

See Section I.C.21. Factors influencing health status and contact with health services, Screening

SECTION I.C.21. Chapter 21: Factors influencing health status and contact with health services (Z00-Z99)

Note: The chapter specific guidelines provide additional information about the use of Z codes for specified encounters.

a. Use of Z codes in any healthcare setting

Z codes are for use in any healthcare setting. Z codes may be used as either a first-listed (principal diagnosis code in the inpatient setting) or secondary code, depending on the circumstances of the encounter. Certain Z codes may only be used as first-listed or principal diagnosis.

b. Z Codes indicate a reason for an encounter

Z codes are not procedure codes. A corresponding procedure code must accompany a Z code to describe any procedure performed.

c. Categories of Z Codes

1) Contact/Exposure

Category Z20 indicates contact with, and suspected exposure to, communicable diseases. These codes are for patients who do not show any sign or symptom of a

Continued

disease but are suspected to have been exposed to it by close personal contact with an infected individual or are in an area where a disease is epidemic.

Category Z77, Other contact with and (suspected) exposures hazardous to health.

Contact/exposure codes may be used as a first-listed code to explain an encounter for testing, or, more commonly, as a secondary code to identify a potential risk.

2) Inoculations and vaccinations

Code Z23 is for encounters for inoculations and vaccinations. It indicates that a patient is being seen to receive a prophylactic inoculation against a disease. Procedure codes are required to identify the actual administration of the injection and the type(s) of immunizations given. Code Z23 may be used as a secondary code if the inoculation is given as a routine part of preventive health care, such as a well-baby visit.

QUICK CHECK 3-1

1. According to the Guidelines, which category code would you reference to report inoculations and vaccinations? _____

2. According to the Guidelines, this category is referenced when reporting suspected exposure to a communicable disease: _____

3. Can Z codes only be used in the outpatient setting?
   Yes   No

(Answers are located in Appendix C)

Status Code

A status code is assigned to indicate that a patient has a sequelae or residual of a past disease or condition or is a current carrier of a disease. There are codes and categories of Z codes assigned to report a status.

ICD-10 OFFICIAL GUIDELINES FOR CODING AND REPORTING

SECTION I.C.21.
3) Status

Status codes indicate that a patient is either a carrier of a disease or has the sequelae or residual of a past disease or condition. This includes such things as the presence of prosthetic or mechanical devices resulting from past treatment. A status code is informative, because the status may affect the course of treatment and its outcome. A status code is distinct from a history code. The history code indicates that the patient no longer has the condition.

A status code should not be used with a diagnosis code from one of the body system chapters, if the diagnosis code includes the information provided by the status code. For example, code Z94.1, Heart transplant status, should not be used with a code from subcategory T86.2, Complications of heart transplant. The status code does not provide additional information. The complication code indicates that the patient is a heart transplant patient.

For encounters for weaning from a mechanical ventilator, assign a code from subcategory J96.1, Chronic respiratory failure, followed by code Z99.11, Dependence on respirator [ventilator] status.

The status Z codes/categories are:

Z14   Genetic carrier
                 Genetic carrier status indicates that a person carries a gene, associated with
                 a particular disease, which may be passed to offspring who may develop that
                 disease. The person does not have the disease and is not at risk of developing
                 the disease.

Continued

Z15	Genetic susceptibility to disease

Genetic susceptibility indicates that a person has a gene that increases the risk of that person developing the disease.

Codes from category Z15 should not be used as principal or first-listed codes. If the patient has the condition to which he/she is susceptible, and that condition is the reason for the encounter, the code for the current condition should be sequenced first. If the patient is being seen for follow-up after completed treatment for this condition, and the condition no longer exists, a follow-up code should be sequenced first, followed by the appropriate personal history and genetic susceptibility codes. If the purpose of the encounter is genetic counseling associated with procreative management, code Z31.5, Encounter for genetic counseling, should be assigned as the first-listed code, followed by a code from category Z15. Additional codes should be assigned for any applicable family or personal history.

Z16	Resistance to antimicrobial drugs

This code indicates that a patient has a condition that is resistant to antimicrobial drug treatment. Sequence the infection code first.

Z17	Estrogen receptor status
Z18	Retained foreign body fragments
Z21	Asymptomatic HIV infection status

This code indicates that a patient has tested positive for HIV but has manifested no signs or symptoms of the disease.

Z22	Carrier of infectious disease

Carrier status indicates that a person harbors the specific organisms of a disease without manifest symptoms and is capable of transmitting the infection.

Z28.3	Underimmunization status
Z33.1	Pregnant state, incidental

This code is a secondary code only for use when the pregnancy is in no way complicating the reason for visit. Otherwise, a code from the obstetric chapter is required.

Z66	Do not resuscitate

This code may be used when it is documented by the provider that a patient is on do not resuscitate status at any time during the stay.

Z67	Blood type
Z68	Body mass index (BMI)
Z74.01	Bed confinement status
Z76.82	Awaiting organ transplant status
Z78	Other specified health status

Code Z78.1, Physical restraint status, may be used when it is documented by the provider that a patient has been put in restraints during the current encounter. Please note that this code should not be reported when it is documented by the provider that a patient is temporarily restrained during a procedure.

Z79	Long-term (current) drug therapy

Codes from this category indicate a patient's continuous use of a prescribed drug (including such things as aspirin therapy) for the long-term treatment of a condition or for prophylactic use. It is not for use for patients who have addictions to drugs. This subcategory is not for use of medications for detoxification or maintenance programs to prevent withdrawal symptoms in patients with drug dependence (e.g., methadone maintenance for opiate dependence). Assign the appropriate code for the drug dependence instead.

Continued

	Assign a code from Z79 if the patient is receiving a medication for an extended period as a prophylactic measure (such as for the prevention of deep vein thrombosis) or as treatment of a chronic condition (such as arthritis) or a disease requiring a lengthy course of treatment (such as cancer). Do not assign a code from category Z79 for medication being administered for a brief period of time to treat an acute illness or injury (such as a course of antibiotics to treat acute bronchitis).
Z88	Allergy status to drugs, medicaments and biological substances
	Except: Z88.9, Allergy status to unspecified drugs, medicaments and biological substances status
Z89	Acquired absence of limb
Z90	Acquired absence of organs, not elsewhere classified
Z91.0-	Allergy status, other than to drugs and biological substances
Z92.82	Status post administration of tPA (rtPA) in a different facility within the last 24 hours prior to admission to current facility
	Assign code Z92.82, Status post administration of tPA (rtPA) in a different facility within the last 24 hours prior to admission to current facility, as a secondary diagnosis when a patient is received by transfer into a facility and documentation indicates they were administered tissue plasminogen activator (tPA) within the last 24 hours prior to admission to the current facility.
	This guideline applies even if the patient is still receiving the tPA at the time they are received into the current facility.
	The appropriate code for the condition for which the tPA was administered (such as cerebrovascular disease or myocardial infarction) should be assigned first.
	Code Z92.82 is only applicable to the receiving facility record and not to the transferring facility record.
Z93	Artificial opening status
Z94	Transplanted organ and tissue status
Z95	Presence of cardiac and vascular implants and grafts
Z96	Presence of other functional implants
Z97	Presence of other devices
Z98	Other postprocedural states
	Assign code Z98.85, Transplanted organ removal status, to indicate that a transplanted organ has been previously removed. This code should not be assigned for the encounter in which the transplanted organ is removed. The complication necessitating removal of the transplant organ should be assigned for that encounter.
	See section I.C19. for information on the coding of organ transplant complications.
Z99	Dependence on enabling machines and devices, not elsewhere classified
	Note: Categories Z89-Z90 and Z93-Z99 are for use only if there are no complications or malfunctions of the organ or tissue replaced, the amputation site or the equipment on which the patient is dependent.

External Cause Index

Chapter 20 in the I-10 classifies External Causes. The External Cause Index is located after the Table of Drugs and Chemicals in the I-10. The index classifies environmental events (tornadoes, floods), circumstances, and other conditions as the cause of injury and other adverse effects alphabetically. **The External Cause codes are never reported as a first-listed diagnosis.** Rather these codes are reported to clarify injury or adverse effects.

> **Assault** (homicidal) (by) (in) Y09
>   arson X97
>   bite (of human being) Y04.1
>   bodily force Y04.8
>   bite Y04.1
>   bumping into Y04.2
>   sexual —*see* subcategories T74.0,
>   T76.0
>   unarmed fight Y04.0
>   bomb X96.9
>   antipersonnel X96.0
>   fertilizer X96.3
>   gasoline X96.1
>   letter X96.2
>   petrol X96.1
>   pipe X96.3
>   specified NEC X96.8
>   brawl (hand) (fists) (foot) (unarmed)
>   Y04.0

FIGURE 3-1 External Cause Index of the I-10.

The code terms describe the external circumstances under which an accident, injury, or act of violence occurred. The main terms in the code index usually represent the type of accident or violence (e.g., assault, collision), with the specific agent or other circumstance listed below the main term. "Assault" in Fig. 3-1 illustrates a main term and indented subterms that further define how the assault occurred. You will not find these codes in the Index to Disease of the I-10; rather you must reference the External Cause Index.

External cause codes have their own index, and the external cause codes are not listed in the Index to Diseases. When an external cause code is reported, it is reported **in addition** to an injury code from the Tabular List of the I-10. The external cause codes are codes that provide greater detail. Most groups of codes have Includes or Excludes notes that provide further detail about assigning the codes.

Index Locations

The Z codes are located at the end of the Tabular. If you have an I-10 manual available, locate the Z codes in the Tabular now. Z codes can be located in the Index like any other code. Often, the most difficult thing about the Z code is locating the Z code term in the Index. To help you become familiar with how to locate Z codes in the Index, review Fig. 3-2 for the most common Index terms for locating Z codes.

Admission	Examination	Replacement
Aftercare	Fitting (and adjustment) (of)	Screening
Attention (to)	Healthy	Status
Care (of)	History	Supervision (of)
Carrier	Maintenance	Test
Checking	Maladjustment	Transplant
Contraception	Observation	Unavailability (of)
Counseling	Problem	Vaccination
Dialysis	Procedure (surgical)	
Donor	Prophylactic	

FIGURE 3-2 Most common Index terms for locating Z codes.

EXERCISE 3-4   *External Cause Codes*

Using the I-10 manual, locate the correct External Cause code indicated for each of the following:

1 Railway accident involving derailment without antecedent collision, injuring a porter

   Place of occurrence code: _____

2 Motor vehicle traffic accident due to tire blowout; driver of the car was injured, initial encounter

   Injured person code: _____

3 Driver of an ATV (off-road vehicle) is injured when he collides with a fence

   Injured person code: _____

4 Horse being ridden, rider injured, and non-motor vehicle collision, initial encounter

   Injured person code: _____

5 Accident to watercraft causing other injury; occupant of small powered boat injured due to collision, initial encounter

   External cause code: _____

(Answers are located in Appendix B)

Circumstances to Assign Z Codes

Z codes are most often assigned in the outpatient settings, that is, ambulatory care centers, physicians' offices, and outpatient departments of hospitals.

1. When a person who is currently not sick encounters the health services for some specific purpose, such as to act as donor of an organ or tissue, to receive a preventive vaccination, or to discuss a problem that is in itself not a disease or injury. Occurrences such as these are more common among outpatients at health clinics.

Example

The patient is donating a kidney.

Code: Z52.4 indicates a donor of a kidney; the donor is not sick but encounters health care
You would first locate "Donor, kidney," in the Index, and then verify code Z52.4 in the Z codes of the Tabular List.

Example

A student seeks health care to discuss a problem with school maladjustment with classmates.

Z55	**Problems related to education and literacy**
	Z55.4 Educational maladjustment and discord with teachers and classmates

Z55 is the category code and Z55.4 is the subcategory code.

Code: Z55.4 indicates a patient who is not ill but encounters health care for a psychosocial circumstance. The Index location is "Dissatisfaction with, school environment."

2. A patient with a known disease or injury receives health services for specific treatment of the disease or injury.

Example

A female patient with breast cancer reports to the outpatient department of the hospital for a chemotherapy session. The patient receives health care services for treatment of cancer.

Index:	**Chemotherapy,** neoplasm Z51.11
Tabular:	**Z51 Encounter for other aftercare**
	Z51.1 Encounter for antineoplastic chemotherapy and immunotherapy
	Z51.11 Encounter for antineoplastic chemotherapy
Code:	Z51.11 Chemotherapy treatment

The breast cancer (C50.919) would also be reported, but you will learn about the details of that later; for now, concentrate on the use of the Z codes. Also, Z codes should not be mistaken for procedure codes.

---

3. A circumstance or problem is present and influences a patient's health status but is not in itself a current illness or injury. (In these situations the Z code should be used only as a supplementary or secondary code.)

Example

A patient who is allergic to penicillin is admitted to the hospital for treatment of pneumonia using intravenous antibiotics. The patient receives treatment for the pneumonia, but the patient's allergy to penicillin is a special consideration in the treatment received.

Index:	**History,** personal (of), allergy to, penicillin Z88.0
Tabular:	**Z88 Allergy status to drugs, medicaments and biological substances**
	Z88.0 Allergy status to penicillin
Code:	Z88.0, History of allergy to penicillin

Additionally, the pneumonia (J18.9) would be reported as the first-listed diagnosis, but you are focusing only on the use of Z codes right now.

---

4. To indicate the birth status and outcome of the delivery of a newborn.

Example

A live, healthy newborn infant is the result of a vaginal delivery in the hospital.

Index:	**Infant(s),** liveborn (singleton), born in hospital Z38.00
Tabular:	**Z38.00 Single liveborn, delivered vaginally**

The first "0" in Z38.00 reports born in hospital, and the last "0" reports a vaginal delivery.

Code:	Z38.00 Vaginal delivery of a single, live-born newborn in the hospital

History of

Often, the patient record states that there is a "history of" a disease: for example, "history of diabetes type 2 mellitus without complications." This does not mean that the patient no longer has diabetes mellitus but that the patient's medical history includes diabetes mellitus. You would not assign a Z code to indicate a previous history of diabetes mellitus but instead would assign the code for the current disease of diabetes mellitus (E11.9). If there is any question regarding the current status of the disease, check with the physician. You may also want to offer some physician education regarding the documentation of past history of diseases.

EXERCISE 3-5 | *Z Codes*

Locate the Z codes in the I-10 manual in Volume 2, Alphabetic Index, and then in Volume 1, Tabular List. Code the following:

1 A person who has been in contact with smallpox

Index location: _____

Code: _____

2 Prophylactic vaccination against smallpox

Index location: _____

Code: _____

3 Personal history of malignant neoplasm of the lip

Index location: _____

Code: _____

Assign the Z code for the following:

4 Admission for cardiac pacemaker adjustment

Code: _____

5 Initial prescription and insertion of subdermal implantable contraceptive

Code: _____

6 Personal history of cancer of the prostate

Code: _____

7 Baby in for MMR (measles, mumps, rubella) vaccination

Code: _____

8 Screening mammogram

Code: _____

9 Clinic visit for pre-employment physical examination

Code: _____

(Answers are located in Appendix B)

OBSERVATION STAY

ICD-10 OFFICIAL GUIDELINES FOR CODING AND REPORTING

SECTION IV.A.
2. Observation Stay

When a patient is admitted for observation for a medical condition, assign a code for the medical condition as the first-listed diagnosis.

When a patient presents for outpatient surgery and develops complications requiring admission to observation, code the reason for the surgery as the first reported diagnosis (reason for the encounter), followed by codes for the complications as secondary diagnoses.

The two categories of Z codes that report observation are **Z03** and **Z04**. These observation codes are reported only as the first-listed diagnosis for medical observation for suspected conditions and conditions ruled out. Other codes may be reported in addition to the observation codes but only when that condition or conditions are unrelated to the reason for the observation. For example, a patient admitted for observation for suspected exposure to anthrax (Z03.810) demonstrates no signs or symptoms but is admitted to observation to determine if the exposure will result in the patient developing anthrax. If the patient also has primary hypertension (I10), the hypertension may be reported as it is unrelated to the anthrax exposure and observation.

QUICK CHECK 3-2

1. The I-10 code to report observation for suspected exposure to anthrax, ruled out, is
   _____.

2. When reporting the diagnosis for a patient admitted to observation status for a medical condition, assign a code for the _____ condition as the first-listed diagnosis.

(Answers are located in Appendix C)

Example

Observation for a Medical Condition
A patient was admitted for observation due to chest pain. The patient has chronic obstructive pulmonary disease (COPD). After testing, no evidence of cardiac cause was found. The patient was discharged home. Discharge Diagnosis: Noncardiac chest pain.

First-listed diagnosis: R07.89 Noncardiac chest pain.

Codes P00-P04 report observation and evaluation of newborns for suspected conditions that are not found. These codes are only reported when a healthy newborn is evaluated for a condition that is suspected, but after a study has determined the condition not to be present. If the newborn has signs or symptoms of a suspected problem, you would report the signs or symptoms and not a code from the P00-P04 observation codes.

EXERCISE 3-6   *Observation Stay*

Answer the following:

1 The patient fell off his motorcycle when turning too sharply and hit his head on the sidewalk. The patient was wearing a helmet. The examination reveals no outward apparent head injury. The only injury noted on examination is abrasion of the right upper arm. The patient is admitted overnight to the observation unit to rule out head injury. No head injury was found.

   a Hospital observation is located in the Index under the main term "Observation." Listed under the main term are the reasons for observation. The subterm is "accident NEC" and subterm "transport." Check the code in the Tabular. What is the Z code?

      Code: _____

   b The second code is for the abrasion to the right upper arm. When you locate "Abrasion" and subterm "arm (upper)," you are directed to S40.81- (the "-" indicates that the Tabular is to be referenced for the additional character[s]). What is the code for the abrasion?

      Code: _____

2 An adult patient is admitted for observation and further evaluation following an alleged rape, ruled out.

   a There is only one code for this case. What is that Z code?

      Code: _____

3 A 35-year-old female patient was admitted to observation for severe nausea and vomiting following diagnostic laparoscopy for pelvic pain.

    First-listed diagnosis: _____

4 A male patient was admitted to observation following an endoscopic retrograde cholangiopancreatography (ERCP) for acute pancreatitis. Patient has a biliary duct stricture.

    First-listed diagnosis: _____

5 Patient was admitted for observation because of urinary retention following a Dilation and Curettage (D&C) for post-menopausal bleeding.

    First-listed diagnosis: _____

(Answers are located in Appendix B)

FIRST-LISTED DIAGNOSIS AND COEXISTING CONDITIONS

You have already had practice at selecting the first-listed diagnoses and you know that it is possible for the first-listed diagnosis to be a symptom. The important information in this Guideline is that additional codes should be assigned for any coexisting conditions that are present or treated during that visit or encounter. Sometimes there is more than one symptom that is present.

ICD-10 OFFICIAL GUIDELINES FOR CODING AND REPORTING

SECTION IV.G. ICD-10-CM code for the diagnosis, condition, problem, or other reason for encounter/visit

List first the ICD-10-CM code for the diagnosis, condition, problem, or other reason for encounter/ visit shown in the medical record to be chiefly responsible for the services provided. List additional codes that describe any coexisting conditions. In some cases the first-listed diagnosis may be a symptom when a diagnosis has not been established (confirmed) by the physician.

Examples

Coexisting Conditions

An established patient was seen in the clinic for dyspnea on exertion. The patient has hypertension and Graves' disease. No etiology for the dyspnea was determined. The patient's medication prescriptions for hypertension and Graves' disease were refilled.

> Codes: R06.00 dyspnea, I10 hypertension, E05.00 Graves' disease.

An initial office visit for a 55-year-old male with jaundice and fatigue. Laboratory tests were ordered and patient will return in 1 week for the results.

> Codes: R17 jaundice, R53.83 fatigue (either of these diagnoses could be the first-listed diagnosis).

EXERCISE 3-7 │ *First-Listed Diagnosis and Coexisting Conditions*

Identify the first-listed diagnosis and any coexisting conditions. Assign the I-10 codes.

1 Patient was seen in the office for a consultation for palpitations. Patient also has rheumatoid arthritis. Medications that the patient takes for the arthritis were reviewed to see if they could be the cause of the palpitations.

    First-listed diagnosis: _____

    Code: _____

    Other diagnosis: _____

    Code: _____

2 Patient is an established patient with memory loss. Patient also has a long-term (current) use of insulin for diabetes type 2.

    First-listed diagnosis: _____

    Code: _____

    Other diagnoses: _____ and _____

    Codes: _____ and _____

3 Patient is a new patient who was seen for flank pain and diagnosed with a urinary tract infection, and antibiotics were prescribed. Patient has psoriasis, which is stable at this time.

    First-listed diagnosis: _____

    Code: _____

    Other diagnosis: _____

    Code: _____

(Answers are located in Appendix B)

UNCERTAIN DIAGNOSES

In an inpatient setting, uncertain diagnoses are reported, but in the outpatient setting these uncertain diagnoses are not reported as explained in the Section IV.H of the Guidelines.

ICD-10 OFFICIAL GUIDELINES FOR CODING AND REPORTING

SECTION IV.H. Uncertain diagnosis

Do not code diagnoses documented as "probable", "suspected," "questionable," "rule out," or "working diagnosis" or other similar terms indicating uncertainty. Rather, code the condition(s) to the highest degree of certainty for that encounter/visit, such as symptoms, signs, abnormal test results, or other reason for the visit.

Please note: This differs from the coding practices used by short-term, acute care, long-term care and psychiatric hospitals.

Examples

Uncertain Diagnosis

A chest x-ray is ordered to rule out pneumonia. Patient has cough and fever. The x-ray is normal.

> Codes: R05 cough, R50.9 fever. The pneumonia cannot be coded as it is documented as a rule out and has not been confirmed.

A 55-year-old male was seen with loss of appetite and jaundice. Further diagnostic studies are needed for suspected cancer of the pancreas.

> Codes: R17 jaundice, R63.0 loss of appetite. No code can be assigned for cancer of the pancreas because it is "suspected" and not yet confirmed.

EXERCISE 3-8 | *Uncertain Diagnoses*

Identify the diagnoses and I-10 codes that should be assigned:

1 Patient is seen in the office for pain and stiffness of the right knee. X-rays to rule out osteoarthritis were performed.

Reported diagnosis and code: _____

Reported diagnosis and code: _____

Diagnosis not reported: _____

2 Office visit for established patient with left wrist pain and numbness of fingertips. Studies ordered for probable carpal tunnel syndrome.

Reported diagnosis and code: _____

Reported diagnosis and code: _____

Diagnosis not reported: _____

3 Office consultation for a new patient with amenorrhea and galactorrhea. Studies to rule out pituitary tumor were ordered.

Reported diagnosis and code: _____

Reported diagnosis and code: _____

Diagnosis not reported: _____

4 Initial visit for a patient with a breast lump. Working diagnosis is breast cancer. Diagnostic workup has been scheduled.

Reported diagnosis and code: _____

Diagnosis not reported: _____

(Answers are located in Appendix B)

CHRONIC DISEASES

If a patient has a chronic condition that is treated on an ongoing basis, you can report the condition as many times as the patient receives care or treatment for the condition.

ICD-10 OFFICIAL GUIDELINES FOR CODING AND REPORTING

SECTION IV.I. Chronic diseases

Chronic diseases treated on an ongoing basis may be coded and reported as many times as the patient receives treatment and care for the condition(s).

Examples

Chronic Diseases
An established patient is seen for equal management of mild, intermittent, uncomplicated asthma and type 2 diabetes.

> Codes: J45.20 Asthma, E11.9 Diabetes, type 2 (either code could be the first-listed)

An established patient is seen for continued management of systemic lupus erythematosus.

> Code: M32.9 Systemic lupus erythematosus

DOCUMENTED CONDITIONS

Code conditions that coexist at the time of the encounter and for which the physician provides care, treatment, or management.

ICD-10 OFFICIAL GUIDELINES FOR CODING AND REPORTING

SECTION IV.J. Code all documented conditions that coexist

Code all documented conditions that coexist at the time of the encounter/visit, and require or affect patient care treatment or management. Do not code conditions that were previously treated and no longer exist. However, history codes (categories Z80-Z87) may be used as secondary codes if the historical condition or family history has an impact on current care or influences treatment.

Examples

Coexisting Conditions
An established patient is seen in follow-up for coronary artery disease of a native artery. The patient is also a diabetic on oral medications. The patient had a coronary artery bypass graft 6 months ago. Labs were reviewed and prescriptions for diabetic medications were renewed.

> Codes: I25.10 coronary artery disease, E11.9 diabetes, type 2 (chronic coexisting conditions that were managed during this visit), Z95.1 history of CABG (acceptable to report as this is important in a patient with coronary artery disease).

An established patient is seen for management of hypertension and congestive heart failure. Patient has a family history of colonic polyps.

> Codes: I10 hypertension, I50.9 congestive heart failure (either could be first-listed diagnosis). No Z code is necessary to identify the family history of colonic polyps as it has no bearing on the treatment of hypertension and congestive heart failure.

EXERCISE 3-9   *Chronic Diseases*

Identify the I-10 codes that should be assigned:

1 Harry Drew, a patient with chronic obstructive pulmonary disease, presents for a one-week follow-up for bronchitis. He continues to smoke 1 package of cigarettes per day, against repeated medical advice.

Codes: _____, _____

2 Harry Drew presents 10 days later for repeated follow-up regarding his bronchitis and to ensure that the infection had responded to the antibiotic prescribed 10 days previously. The physician determined that the bronchitis had responded well and no further bronchitis was identified. The patient's COPD continues to inhibit his activities. He continues to smoke 1 package of cigarettes per day and since his bronchitis has improved, he says he is smoking "a bit more."

Codes: _____, _____

(Answers are located in Appendix B)

DIAGNOSTIC SERVICES

When a diagnostic service is provided to a patient during an encounter, the reason for the service is the diagnosis stated in the medical record, or when no diagnostic statement is available, report the primary reason the patient presented for the service.

ICD-10 OFFICIAL GUIDELINES FOR CODING AND REPORTING

SECTION IV.K. Patients receiving diagnostic services only

For patients receiving diagnostic services only during an encounter/visit, sequence first the diagnosis, condition, problem, or other reason for encounter/visit shown in the medical record to be chiefly responsible for the outpatient services provided during the encounter/visit. Codes for other diagnoses (e.g., chronic conditions) may be sequenced as additional diagnoses.

For encounters for routine laboratory/radiology testing in the absence of any signs, symptoms, or associated diagnosis, assign Z01.89, Encounter for other specified special examinations. If routine testing is performed during the same encounter as a test to evaluate a sign, symptom, or diagnosis, it is appropriate to assign both the **Z** code and the code describing the reason for the non-routine test.

For outpatient encounters for diagnostic tests that have been interpreted by a physician, and the final report is available at the time of coding, code any confirmed or definitive diagnosis(es) documented in the interpretation. Do not code related signs and symptoms as additional diagnoses.

Please note: This differs from the coding practice in the hospital inpatient setting regarding abnormal findings on test results.

Examples

Diagnostic Services Only

Patient encounter for blood typing prior to outpatient surgery tomorrow.

> Z01.83 encounter for blood typing.

Patient is having an MRI of the head to monitor the progression of brain tumor.

> D49.6 brain tumor.

Patient without any symptoms had a CBC (complete blood count).

> Z01.89 laboratory examination without any sign or symptom documented.

Patient was seen for shortness of breath and fever with a negative x-ray. Patient returned the next day for a CT of chest, which confirmed the presence of pneumonia.

> J18.9 pneumonia.

EXERCISE 3-10　*Diagnostic Services*

Identify the diagnoses and I-10 codes that should be assigned:

1 David presents for blood typing for his surgery in two days.

Code: _____

2 Chris, a 43-year-old male patient, presents for his annual examination.

Code: _____

(Answers are located in Appendix B)

THERAPEUTIC SERVICES

Report the diagnosis, condition, problem, or other reason for the encounter when a patient presents for a therapeutic service.

ICD-10 OFFICIAL GUIDELINES FOR CODING AND REPORTING

SECTION IV.L. Patients receiving therapeutic services only

For patients receiving therapeutic services only during an encounter/visit, sequence first the diagnosis, condition, problem, or other reason for encounter/visit shown in the medical record to be chiefly responsible for the outpatient services provided during the encounter/visit. Codes for other diagnoses (e.g., chronic conditions) may be sequenced as additional diagnoses.

The only exception to this rule is that when the primary reason for the admission/encounter is chemotherapy or radiation therapy, the appropriate Z code for the service is listed first, and the diagnosis or problem for which the service is being performed listed second.

Examples

Therapeutic Services Only

Patient had an outpatient phlebotomy performed for polycythemia vera.

> D45 polycythemia vera.

Female patient received outpatient chemotherapy for breast cancer with metastasis to the axillary lymph nodes.

> Z51.11 encounter for chemotherapy, C50.919 breast cancer, and C77.3 metastasis to axillary lymph nodes.

Patient had monthly B12 shot for pernicious anemia.

> D51.0 pernicious anemia, congenital.

EXERCISE 3-11   *Therapeutic Services*

Identify the I-10 codes that should be assigned.

1 The patient presents for a chemotherapy treatment due to primary, malignant ovarian cancer of the left ovary.

Codes: _____, _____

2 A patient with dietary folate deficiency anemia presents for a folate injection.

Code: _____

3 A patient presents for allergy testing.

Code: _____

(Answers are located in Appendix B)

PREOPERATIVE EVALUATION

ICD-10 OFFICIAL GUIDELINES FOR CODING AND REPORTING

SECTION IV.M. Patients receiving preoperative evaluations only

For patients receiving preoperative evaluations only, sequence first a code from subcategory Z01.81, Encounter for pre-procedural examinations, to describe the pre-op consultations. Assign a code for the condition to describe the reason for the surgery as an additional diagnosis. Code also any findings related to the pre-op evaluation.

Usually, a surgeon will want a preoperative clearance performed by the patient's primary care provider, often due to a chronic or pre-existing condition. When the primary care provider reports the diagnosis for this visit, the first-listed diagnosis will be the appropriate Z code to indicate the encounter is for preop clearance; then the reason for the upcoming surgery is reported followed by the condition requiring the clearance. The Z code will be one of the following:

Z01.810 Preoperative cardiovascular examination

Z01.811 Preoperative respiratory examination

Z01.812 Preoperative laboratory examination

> Blood and urine tests prior to treatment or procedure

Z01.818 Other preprocedural examination

TOOLBOX

Sam is a 7-year-old male patient who is brought to Dr. Well's office for a pre-procedural consultation for a mass on his left lung. Dr. Well reviews the patient's x-rays and MRI taken the previous week and sent from Dr. Grossman, Sam's pediatrician.

QUESTIONS
1. What Z code would you report for the pre-procedural consultation? _____
2. In addition to the Z code, you would report what diagnosis? _____
3. Would the Z code or diagnosis code be first-listed? _____

▼ **ANSWERS**

1. Z01.811, 2. lung mass, 3. Z code

EXERCISE 3-12 *Preoperative Evaluations*

Match the following code descriptions to the correct codes:

1 Z01.810 _____ **a** Preoperative cardiovascular examination

2 Z01.811 _____ **b** Preoperative respiratory examination

3 Z01.818 _____ **c** Preoperative examination

(Answers are located in Appendix B)

Preoperative Evaluations Only

When the only service is a preoperative examination, report the appropriate Z code along with any codes that indicate significant conditions.

Examples

Preoperative Examinations
Patient is seen by cardiologist for surgical clearance for upcoming cataract surgery. The patient has coronary artery disease (CAD) and has a history of angioplasty and cardiac stent. Patient's medical condition from a cardiac standpoint is stable. Patient can proceed with cataract removal.

Z01.810 preoperative cardiovascular examination, H26.9 cataract, I25.10 coronary artery disease, Z95.5 history of cardiac angioplasty with stent placement.

Patient is seen by internist for medical clearance for inguinal hernia repair. The patient has a number of chronic medical conditions, including hypertension, diabetes type 2, and chronic atrial fibrillation.

Z01.818 other specified preoperative examination, K40.90 inguinal hernia, I10 hypertension, E11.9 diabetes type 2, I48.92 chronic atrial fibrillation.

ICD-10 OFFICIAL GUIDELINES FOR CODING REPORTING

SECTION IV.N. Ambulatory surgery

For ambulatory surgery, code the diagnosis for which the surgery was performed. If the postoperative diagnosis is known to be different from the preoperative diagnosis at the time the diagnosis is confirmed, select the postoperative diagnosis for coding, since it is the most definitive.

Examples

Pre and Postoperative Diagnoses are the Same
The patient has an EGD for upper gastrointestinal bleeding. The postoperative diagnosis is upper gastrointestinal bleeding, etiology undetermined, K92.2.

Pre and Postoperative Diagnoses are Different
The patient has an EGD for upper gastrointestinal bleeding. The postoperative diagnosis is gastrointestinal bleeding due to gastric ulcer, K25.4.

PRENATAL VISITS

There are specific rules for reporting routine prenatal visits that are provided in an outpatient setting. Read the Guidelines to learn the details regarding this assignment.

ICD-10 OFFICIAL GUIDELINES FOR CODING AND REPORTING

SECTION IV.O. Routine outpatient prenatal visits
See Section I.C.15. Routine outpatient prenatal visits.
SECTION I.C.
15.b. Selection of OB Principal or First-listed Diagnosis

1) Routine outpatient prenatal visits

For routine outpatient prenatal visits when no complications are present, a code from category Z34, Encounter for supervision of normal pregnancy, should be used as the first-listed diagnosis. These codes should not be used in conjunction with chapter 15 codes.

2) Prenatal outpatient visits for high-risk patients

For routine prenatal outpatient visits for patients with high-risk pregnancies, a code from category O09, Supervision of high-risk pregnancy, should be used as the first-listed diagnosis. Secondary chapter 15 codes may be used in conjunction with these codes if appropriate.

Examples

First Pregnancy Without Complication

A 25-year-old female presents for initial prenatal visit. This is her first pregnancy. No problems were identified. Z34.00

Second Pregnancy Without Complication

A 25-year-old female presents for initial prenatal visit. Patient had an uncomplicated vaginal delivery of a term female infant 3 years ago. No problems were identified. Z34.80

Prenatal Visit with Complication (Code from Chapter 15)

A 25-year-old female is seen for a routine prenatal visit in second trimester. Her laboratory results indicate that she has a urinary tract infection. She is given a prescription for antibiotics and will return in 1 week for repeat urinalysis. O23.92

CHAPTER REVIEW

CHAPTER 3, PART I, THEORY

Answer the following questions about the Diagnostic Coding and Reporting Guidelines for Outpatient Services:

1 When a patient is to have outpatient surgery and the surgery is not performed due to contraindication, the reason that the surgery was not performed is the first-listed diagnosis.

   True   False

2 It is appropriate to code the postoperative diagnosis as it is the most definitive diagnosis for ambulatory surgery.

   True   False

3 Chronic diseases that are treated on an ongoing basis should be coded and reported as often as the patient receives treatment and care for the chronic conditions.

   True   False

4 In the physician office it is acceptable to report Z codes as a first-listed diagnosis.

   True   False

5 In the outpatient setting it is unacceptable to have a sign or symptom as the first-listed diagnosis.

   True   False

6 When coding an encounter for preoperative evaluation, the reason that the patient is having the surgery or procedure performed is the first-listed diagnosis.

   True   False

7 In the outpatient setting, diagnoses that are documented as "probable," "suspected," "rule out," or "questionable" are reported to the highest degree of certainty.

   True   False

8 The first-listed diagnosis is defined as the diagnosis that is the most serious.

   True   False

9 It is acceptable to report a code from Chapter 15 in conjunction with Z34.00 or Z34.80.

   True   False

10 It is acceptable to code signs and symptoms even when a definitive diagnosis has been confirmed.

   True   False

Chapter Review answers are only available in the TEACH Instructor Resources on Evolve

CHAPTER 3, PART II, PRACTICAL

Identify the first-listed diagnoses and assign the appropriate I-10 codes in the following encounters or visits:

11 Initial office visit for diaper rash

First-listed diagnosis: _____

Code: _____

12 Established patient presents with dyspnea and lower extremity edema. The physician determined that the patient's symptoms were due to an exacerbation of congestive heart failure.

First-listed diagnosis: _____

Code: _____

13 Established patient seen for management of vitamin B12 deficiency and hypertension

First-listed diagnosis: _____

Code: _____

Other diagnoses: _____

Code: _____

14 Patient was admitted as an outpatient for a left arthroscopic knee procedure to repair old anterior cruciate ligament tear.

First-listed diagnosis: _____

Code: _____

15 Patient is admitted to observation for syncope. Patient has diabetes mellitus. After testing, no cardiac or other cause was found.

First-listed diagnosis: _____

Code: _____

Other diagnosis: _____

Code: _____

16 Patient was admitted for pain management following biopsy of the kidney for Stage IV chronic kidney disease.

First-listed diagnosis: _____

Code: _____

Other diagnosis: _____

Code: _____

17 Patient is seen by pulmonologist for surgical clearance for upcoming surgery. Patient has emphysema and is scheduled to have an endarterectomy for severe carotid stenosis on the right.

First-listed diagnosis: _____

Code: _____

Other diagnoses: _____

Codes: _____, _____

18 Patient had an outpatient cystoscopy. The preoperative diagnosis is hematuria. Postoperative diagnosis is hematuria due to bladder cancer.

First-listed diagnosis: _____

Code: _____

Assign the appropriate Z code for the following:

19 Exposure to asbestos _____

20 Personal history of colonic polyps _____

21 Heart transplant status _____

Chapter Review answers are only available in the TEACH Instructor Resources on Evolve

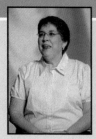

"Don't take for granted that because you know ICD-9-CM that coding ICD-10-CM will come naturally. More codes are required in ICD-10-CM to 'draw the picture' for accurate diagnostic data retrieval. Documentation has to be improved and coders will also need to act as auditors to efficiently retrieve the information needed to complete the billing process."

Sharon J. Oliver, CPC, CPC-I, CPMA
Senior Inpatient Coder
East Tennessee State University Physicians &
Associates
Johnson City, Tennessee

Using ICD-10-CM

Chapter Topics

Organization of the Guidelines

Accurate Coding

Alphabetic Index and Tabular List

Level of Specificity

Integral Conditions

Multiple Coding

Acute and Chronic Combination Codes

Late Effects

Reporting Same Diagnosis Code More Than Once

Laterality

Chapter Review

Learning Objectives

After completing this chapter you should be able to

1 Demonstrate ability to utilize the Alphabetic Index and Tabular List.

2 Understand the steps to accurate coding.

3 Comprehend the organization of the Guidelines.

4 Use both the Alphabetic Index and Tabular List.

5 Outline the need for level of specificity in diagnosis coding.

6 Identify conditions integral to a disease process.

7 Assign multiple codes to a single condition.

8 Report acute and chronic conditions.

9 Demonstrate application of combination codes.

10 Differentiate between residual and late effects.

11 Abstract information that determines if a condition is impending or threatened.

12 Outline the rules when reporting the same diagnosis code more than once.

13 Assign codes based on laterality.

NOTE: *The 2015 ICD-10-CM DRAFT and 2015 ICD-10-PCS DRAFT were used in preparing this text.*

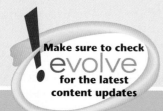

Make sure to check
evolve
for the latest
content updates

ORGANIZATION OF THE GUIDELINES

The *Official Guidelines for Coding and Reporting* have been developed and approved for coding and reporting by the Cooperating Parties for I-10: the American Hospital Association (AHA), American Health Information Management Association (AHIMA), Centers for Medicare and Medicaid Services (CMS), and National Center for Health Statistics (NCHS).

The complete 2015 *ICD-10-CM Official Guidelines for Coding and Reporting* are posted on the Web at www.cdc.gov/nchs/icd/icd10cm.htm. The *Guidelines* are organized into sections. Section I of the Guidelines includes the structure and conventions of the classification and general guidelines that apply to the entire classification, and chapter-specific guidelines that correspond to the chapters as they are arranged in the classification. Section II includes guidelines for selection of principal diagnosis for non-outpatient (hospital) settings. Section III includes guidelines for reporting additional diagnoses in non-outpatient settings. Section IV is for outpatient coding and reporting. Outpatient coders, however, use guidance from throughout the *Official Guidelines for Coding and Reporting* because not all of the coding circumstances are fully explained in Section IV of the Guidelines. Within your learning activities, the number that appears to the left of the guideline is the number of the guideline as listed in the *Official Guidelines for Coding and Reporting.*

ACCURATE CODING

You will be practicing coding using the I-10 throughout this chapter. You need to practice using the steps that are always necessary to assign an I-10 code. If you begin your I-10 coding using these steps, you will develop good coding habits that will last throughout your career.

Steps to Accurate Coding

1. Identify the main term(s) in the diagnostic statement.
2. Locate the main term(s) in the Alphabetic Index (referred to in this material as the Index).
3. Review any subterms under the main term in the Index.
4. Follow any cross-reference instructions, such as *see.*
5. Verify the code(s) selected from the Index in the Tabular List (referred to in this material as the Tabular).
6. Refer to any instructional notations in the Tabular.
7. Assign codes to the highest level of specificity.
8. Code the diagnosis until all elements are completely identified.

ALPHABETIC INDEX AND TABULAR LIST

Guidelines are presented and followed by examples or exercises to illustrate the rule(s). Let's get started with a general coding guideline regarding locating codes in the ICD-10-CM.

ICD-10 OFFICIAL GUIDELINES FOR CODING AND REPORTING

SECTION I.B.

1. Locating a code in the ICD-10-CM

To select a code in the classification that corresponds to a diagnosis or reason for visit documented in a medical record, first locate the term in the Alphabetic Index, and then verify the code in the Tabular List. Read and be guided by instructional notations that appear in both the Alphabetic Index and the Tabular List.

It is essential to use both the Alphabetic Index and Tabular List when locating and assigning a code. The Alphabetic Index does not always provide the full code. Selection of the full code, including laterality and any applicable 7th character can only be done in the Tabular List. A dash (-) at the end of an Alphabetic Index entry indicates that additional characters are required. Even if a dash is not included at the Alphabetic Index entry, it is necessary to refer to the Tabular List to verify that no 7th character is required.

Example of the Use of Both the Alphabetic Index and Tabular List

1. Diagnosis: Hodgkin Disease- see Lymphoma, Hodgkin

   Index: **Lymphoma** (main term)

           Hodgkin (subterm) C81.9

   Tabular: **C81   Hodgkin lymphoma** [category code]

           C81.9   Hodgkin lymphoma, unspecified [subcategory code]

               C81.90   Hodgkin lymphoma, unspecified, unspecified site
   (subclassification code)

   Code: C81.90 Unspecified Hodgkin's disease, unspecified site

Verify C81.90 in the Tabular and read any notes indicated in the Tabular to ensure that the code is complete and correct before assignment.

Example of the Use of Both the Alphabetic Index and Tabular List

2. Diagnosis: Stroke, due to vertebral artery occlusion

   Index: **Stroke** (main term) I63.9

           meaning

              cerebral infarction - code to Infarction, cerebral

   Index: **Infarct, infarction**

           cerebral (*see also* Occlusion, artery cerebral or precerebral, with infarction) I63.9

   Index: **Occlusion, occluded**

           artery (*see also* Embolism, artery) I74.9

              vertebral I65.0-

                 with

                    infarction I63.21-

   Tabular: **I63   Cerebral infarction**

           I63.2   Cerebral infarction due to unspecified occlusion or stenosis of precerebral arteries

               I62.21   Cerebral infarction due to unspecified occlusion or stenosis of vertebral arteries

                   I63.219   Cerebral infarction due to unspecified occlusion or stenosis of unspecified vertebral arteries

LEVEL OF SPECIFICITY

The level of specificity is the level of detail and detail is very important in diagnosis coding. Review the Guideline regarding specificity.

ICD-10 OFFICIAL GUIDELINES FOR CODING AND REPORTING

SECTION I.B.

2. Level of Detail in Coding

Diagnosis codes are to be used and reported at their highest number of characters available.

ICD-10-CM diagnosis codes are composed of codes with 3, 4, 5, 6 or 7 characters. Codes with three characters are included in ICD-10-CM as the heading of a category of codes that may be further subdivided by the use of fourth and/or fifth characters and/or sixth characters, which provide greater detail.

A three-character code is to be used only if it is not further subdivided. A code is invalid if it has not been coded to the full number of characters required for that code, including the 7th character, if applicable.

Examples

Three-Character Code

Diagnosis: Infectious colitis

Index: *Colitis* (acute) (catarrhal) (chronic (noninfective) (hemorrhagic)
    - *see also* Enteritis K52.9

    infectious - *see* Enteritis, infectious

Index: **Enteritis** (acute) (diarrheal) (hemorrhagic) (noninfective) (septic) K52.9

    infectious NOS A09

Tabular: **A09 Infectious gastroenteritis and colitis, unspecified**

Code: A09 Infectious colitis

Four-Character Code

Diagnosis: Subarachnoid hemorrhage, nontraumatic

Index: **Hemorrhage, hemorrhagic** (concealed) R58

    subarachnoid (nontraumatic) - *see* Hemorrhage, intracranial,
        subarachnoid

    intracranial (nontraumatic)

    subarachnoid (nontraumatic) (from) I60.9

Tabular: **I60.9 Nontraumatic subarachnoid hemorrhage, unspecified**

Code: I60.9 Subarachnoid hemorrhage

Five-Character Code

Diagnosis: Aseptic meningitis in leptospirosis

Index: **Leptospirosis** A27.9

Tabular: **A27   Leptospirosis**

    A27.8   Other forms of leptospirosis

    A27.81   Aseptic meningitis in leptospirosis

Code: A27.81 Aseptic meningitis in leptospirosis

Six-Character Code

Diagnosis: Biotinidase deficiency

Index: **Deficiency, deficient**
    biotinidase D81.810

Continued

Tabular: **D81**   **Combined immunodeficiencies**

                D81.8   **Other combined immunodeficiencies**

                      D81.81   **Biotin-dependent carboxylase deficiency**

                              Multiple carboxylase deficiency

                              | EXCLUDES1 | biotin-dependent carboxylase deficiency due to dietary deficiency of biotin (E53.8)

                     D81.810 Biotinidase deficiency

Code: D81.810 Biotinidase deficiency

Seven-Character Code

Diagnosis: Initial encounter for fatigue fracture of vertebra

Index: **Fracture, traumatic**

                   fatigue - *see also* Fracture, stress

                      vertebra M48.40

Tabular: **M48.4 Fatigue fracture of vertebra**

                   The appropriate 7th character is to be added to each code from subcategory M48.4:

                      A initial encounter for fracture

                      D subsequent encounter for fracture with routine healing

                      G subsequent encounter for fracture with delayed healing

                      S sequela of fracture

              M48.40 Fatigue fracture of vertebra, site unspecified

Code: M48.40XA Initial encounter for fatigue fracture of vertebra

---

EXERCISE 4-1   *Level of Specificity in Coding*

Place the code you locate in the Index and Tabular on the line provided:

1 Diagnosis: Recurrent right inguinal hernia, with obstruction

    Index: **Hernia, hernia**l (acquired) (recurrent) _____

                   inguinal (direct) (external) (funicular) (indirect) (internal) (oblique) (scrotal) (sliding) _____

    Tabular: **K40 Inguinal hernia**

                   _____ **Unilateral inguinal hernia, with obstruction without gangrene**

                            _____ **Unilateral inguinal hernia, with obstruction, without gangrene, recurrent**

2 Diagnosis: Primary hypertension

    Index: **Hypertension, hypertensive** (accelerated) (benign) (essential) (idiopathic) (malignant) (systemic) _____

    Tabular: **Essential (primary) hypertension**

                   Includes: high blood pressure hypertension (arterial) (benign) (essential) (malignant) (primary) (systemic)

(Answers are located in Appendix B)

INTEGRAL CONDITIONS

When the signs or symptoms are due to a diagnosed condition, the signs or symptoms are not reported separately. If the signs or symptoms are not due to a diagnosed condition, the signs and symptoms should be reported.

This may require the coder to query the physician regarding the reporting of signs and symptoms that may or may not be routinely associated with a disease process.

ICD-10 OFFICIAL GUIDELINES FOR CODING AND REPORTING

SECTION I.B.

6. Conditions that are not an integral part of a disease process

Additional signs and symptoms that may not be associated routinely with a disease process should be coded when present.

Integral Part of a Disease Process
Example 1

Diagnosis:	Fever and shortness of breath due to pneumonia
Index:	Pneumonia J18.9
Tabular:	**J18.9 Pneumonia, unspecified organism**
Code:	J18.9 Pneumonia

Fever and shortness of breath are common symptoms of pneumonia so additional codes would not be assigned.

Integral Part of a Disease Process
Example 2

Diagnosis:	Abdominal pain that is exacerbated by eating. The patient was diagnosed as having a gastric ulcer.
Index:	**Ulcer, ulcerated, ulcerating, ulceration, ulcerative** stomach (eroded) (peptic) (round) K25.9
Tabular:	**K25 Gastric ulcer** **K25.9 Gastric ulcer, unspecified as acute or chronic, without hemorrhage or perforation**
Code:	K25.9 Gastric ulcer

Abdominal pain that is exacerbated (made worse) by eating is a common symptom of a gastric ulcer.

Not an Integral Part of a Disease Process
Example 1

Diagnosis:	Dehydration and pneumonia
Index:	Pneumonia J18.9
Tabular:	**J18.9 Pneumonia, unspecified organism**
Code:	J18.9 Pneumonia
Index:	**Dehydration** E86.0
Tabular:	**E86 Volume depletion**
	E86.0 Dehydration
Code:	E86.0 Dehydration
Codes:	J18.9 (pneumonia) and E86.0 (dehydration)

Dehydration can result from a wide range of diseases, but not all patients who have pneumonia become dehydrated. Dehydration would be reported with an additional code.

Not an Integral Part of a Disease Process
Example 2

Diagnosis:	Ascites and cirrhosis of the liver
Index:	**Cirrhosis, cirrhotic** (hepatic) (liver) K74.60
	liver K74.60
	alcoholic K70.30
	with ascites K70.31
Tabular:	**K74 Fibrosis and cirrhosis of liver**
	K74.6 Other and unspecified cirrhosis of liver
	K74.60 Unspecified cirrhosis of liver
Code:	K74.60 Cirrhosis of the liver
Index:	**Ascites (abdominal)** R18.8
Tabular:	**R18 Ascites**
	R18.8 Other ascites
	Ascites NOS
	Peritoneal effusion (chronic)
Code:	K74.60 (cirrhosis) and R18.8 (ascites)

Ascites is not present in all patients with cirrhosis of the liver. It would be incorrect to assume that the cirrhosis of the liver was due to alcohol because this was not stated in the diagnosis statement. The ascites should be reported in this case as the patient's treatment may be affected by the ascites.

QUICK CHECK 4-1

1. A patient presents with the chief complaint of headache of three days' duration and frequent urination. Would you report both the headache and urination?

    Yes   No

2. If the patient's medical record stated SOB due to asthma, would you report the SOB?

    Yes   No

(Answers are located in Appendix C)

EXERCISE 4-2 *Integral Conditions*

Without the use of reference material, answer the following:

1 List two common symptoms of appendicitis.

_____

2 List the most common symptom associated with costochondritis.

_____

3 Patient has rheumatoid arthritis and anemia. The anemia is integral to the rheumatoid arthritis.

   True   False

4 Patient has dyspnea due to congestive heart failure. Dyspnea should be assigned as an additional code.

   True   False

Circle the diagnoses that should NOT be coded for the condition in bold typeface:

5 Acute myocardial infarction

   Chest pain

   Shortness of breath

   Congestive heart failure

6 Fractured hip

   Hip pain

   Contusion of hip

(Answers are located in Appendix B)

MULTIPLE CODING

ICD-10 OFFICIAL GUIDELINES FOR CODING AND REPORTING

SECTION I.B.

7. Multiple coding for a single condition

In addition to the etiology/manifestation convention that requires two codes to fully describe a single condition that affects multiple body systems, there are other single conditions that also require more than one code. "Use additional code" notes are found in the Tabular List at codes that are not part of an etiology/manifestation pair where a secondary code is useful to fully describe a condition. The sequencing rule is the same as the etiology/manifestation pair, "use additional code" indicates that a secondary code should be added.

For example, for bacterial infections that are not included in chapter 1, a secondary code from category B95, Streptococcus, Staphylococcus, and Enterococcus, as the cause of diseases classified elsewhere, or B96, Other bacterial agents as the cause of diseases classified elsewhere, may be required to identify the bacterial organism causing the infection. A "use additional code" note will normally be found at the infectious disease code, indicating a need for the organism code to be added as a secondary code.

"Code first" notes are also under certain codes that are not specifically manifestation codes but may be due to an underlying cause. When there is a "code first" note and an underlying condition is present, the underlying condition should be sequenced first.

"Code, if applicable, any causal condition first", notes indicate that this code may be assigned as a principal diagnosis when the causal condition is unknown or not applicable. If a causal condition is known, then the code for that condition should be sequenced as the principal or first-listed diagnosis.

Multiple codes may be needed for sequela, complication codes and obstetric codes to more fully describe a condition. See the specific guidelines for these conditions for further instruction.

Single Code Reporting Manifestation and Etiology

Example 1

Diagnosis: Diabetic retinopathy with type 1 diabetes

In this diagnosis statement, retinopathy is the manifestation (symptom) and diabetes is the etiology (cause) of the retinopathy.

Index: **Diabetes, diabetic** (mellitus) (familial) (sugar) E11.9
                          type 1 E10.9
                                  with
                                        retinopathy E10.319

Tabular: **E10.3   Type 1 diabetes mellitus with ophthalmic complications**

                      E10.31   Type 1 diabetes mellitus with unspecified diabetic retinopathy

                              E10.319   Type 1 diabetes mellitus with unspecified diabetic retinopathy without macular edema

Code: E10.319 Type 1 diabetic retinopathy

Multiple Codes Reporting Manifestation and Etiology (Also Known as Dual Coding)

Example 2

Diagnosis: *Staphylococcal aureus* cellulitis of the face

(Staphylococcal infection is the etiology and cellulitis is the manifestation.)

Index: **Cellulitis** (diffuse) (phlegmonous) (septic) (suppurative) L03.90
                          face NEC L03.211

Tabular: **L03.2   Cellulitis and acute lymphangitis of face and neck**

                      L03.21   Cellulitis and acute lymphangitis of face

                              L03.211   Cellulitis of face

Code: L03.211 Cellulitis of the face

You now must identify the code for the etiology (staphylococcal).

Index: **Infection, infected, infective** (opportunistic) B99.9
                          bacterial NOS A49.9
                                  as cause of disease classified elsewhere B96.89
                                        Staphylococcus B95.8
                                              aureus (methicillin susceptible) (MSSA) B95.61

Tabular: **B95   Streptococcus, Staphylococcus, and Enterococcus as the cause of diseases classified elsewhere**

                      B95.6   Staphylococcus aureus as the cause of diseases classified elsewhere

                              B95.61   Methicillin susceptible Staphylococcus aureus infection as the cause of diseases classified elsewhere (MSSA)

This category of code is to be assigned as an additional or supplementary code to identify the infectious agent in diseases classified elsewhere.

Codes: L03.211 (Cellulitis of face) and B95.61 (Staphylococcus aureus)

EXERCISE 4-3 *Multiple or Combination Coding*

Using multiple codes, fill in the code(s) for the following diagnoses:

1 Chronic prostatitis due to *Streptococcus*

Codes: _____, _____

2 Acute bronchitis due to *Pseudomonas*

Codes: _____, _____

3 Gangrene due to diabetes mellitus, type 1

Code: _____

4 Urinary tract infection due to *Escherichia coli*

Codes: _____, _____

5 Amyloid cardiomyopathy

Codes: _____, _____

(Answers are located in Appendix B)

ACUTE AND CHRONIC

ICD-10 OFFICIAL GUIDELINES FOR CODING AND REPORTING

SECTION I.B.

8. Acute and Chronic Conditions

If the same condition is described as both acute (subacute) and chronic, and separate subentries exist in the Alphabetic Index at the same indentation level, code both and sequence the acute (subacute) code first.

According to the Guideline for acute and chronic conditions, if the condition has separate subentries with the same indentation level for acute and chronic in the Index of I-10, code both the acute and chronic condition, with the acute listed first followed by the chronic condition. For example, Fig. 4-1 illustrates the format of acute pancreatitis and chronic pancreatitis. Acute pancreatitis is K85.9 and chronic pancreatitis is K86.1; in accordance with the Guideline, report K85.9 first followed by K86.1.

```
Pancreatitis (annular) (apoplectic)
      (calcareous) (edematous)
      (hemorrhagic) (malignant)
      (recurrent) (subacute) (suppurative)
      K85.9
   acute K85.9
      alcohol induced K85.2
      biliary K85.1
      drug induced K85.3
      gallstone K85.1
      idiopathic K85.0
      specified NEC K85.8
   chronic (infectious) K86.1
      alcohol-induced K86.0
      recurrent K86.1
      relapsing K86.1
```

FIGURE 4−1 I-10 Index entry for Pancreatitis.

QUICK CHECK 4-2

1. According to Fig. 4-1, what is the code you would reference in the Tabular for the following:
   a. chronic recurrent pancreatitis _____
   b. acute idiopathic pancreatitis _____

(Answers are located in Appendix C)

Acute and Chronic Conditions

Example 1

Diagnosis: Acute and chronic thyroiditis

Index: **Thyroiditis**

        acute E06.0

        chronic E06.5

Note that acute and chronic are at the same indentation level in the Index, and Guideline Section I.B.8. directs the coder to sequence the acute code first, followed by the chronic code when both conditions were being reported.

Tabular: **E06   Thyroiditis**

        E06.0   Acute thyroiditis

        E06.5   Other chronic thyroiditis

Sequence: E06.0, E06.5 Acute and chronic thyroiditis

The acute form of thyroiditis is sequenced before the chronic form.

Acute and Chronic Conditions

Example 2

Diagnosis: Acute and chronic pericarditis

Index: **Pericarditis** (with decompensation) (with effusion)

        acute I30.9

        chronic (nonrheumatic) I31.9

Tabular: **I30   Acute pericarditis**

        I30.9   Acute pericarditis, unspecified

Tabular: **I31   Other diseases of pericardium**

        I31.9   Disease of pericardium, unspecified

            Pericarditis (chronic) NOS

Sequence: I30.9, I31.9 Acute and chronic pericarditis

Both acute and chronic pericarditis are indented at the same level in the Index, requiring that both conditions be reported with the acute condition sequenced first, followed by the chronic condition.

COMBINATION CODES

ICD-10 OFFICIAL GUIDELINES FOR CODING AND REPORTING

SECTION I.B.

9. Combination Code

A combination code is a single code used to classify:

Two diagnoses, or

A diagnosis with an associated secondary process (manifestation)

A diagnosis with an associated complication

Combination codes are identified by referring to subterm entries in the Alphabetic Index and by reading the inclusion and exclusion notes in the Tabular List.

Assign only the combination code when that code fully identifies the diagnostic conditions involved or when the Alphabetic Index so directs. Multiple coding should not be used when the classification provides a combination code that clearly identifies all of the elements documented in the diagnosis. When the combination code lacks necessary specificity in describing the manifestation or complication, an additional code should be used as a secondary code.

Combination Codes

Example 1

Diagnosis: Acute cholecystitis with cholelithiasis

Index: **Cholecystitis** K81.9

> with
>
> > cholelithiasis - *see* Calculus, gallbladder, with cholecystitis

Index: **Calculus**

> gallbladder K80.20
>
> > with
> >
> > > cholecystitis K80.10
> > >
> > > acute K80.00

Tabular: **K80 Cholelithiasis**

> **K80.0   Calculus of gallbladder with acute cholecystitis**
>
> > **K80.00   Calculus of gallbladder with acute cholecystitis without obstruction**

Code: K80.00 Acute cholecystitis with cholelithiasis

The combination code K80.00 fully describes the diagnosis of acute cholecystitis with cholelithiasis.

Example 2

Another example of a diagnosis (streptococcal) and manifestation (pharyngitis or sore throat) reported with a combination code is as follows:

Diagnosis: Streptococcal pharyngitis

Index: **Pharyngitis**

           streptococcal J02.0

Tabular: **J02   Acute pharyngitis**

           Includes: acute sore throat

           J02.0 Streptococcal pharyngitis

              Septic pharyngitis

              Streptococcal sore throat

The single code J02.0 fully describes the diagnosis of streptococcal pharyngitis.

Code: J02.0 Streptococcal pharyngitis

EXERCISE 4-4   *Acute/Chronic and Combination Codes*

Assign combination codes to the following:

1 Pneumonia due to *Hemophilus influenzae*

    Code: _____

2 Candidiasis of the mouth (thrush)

    Code: _____

3 Enteritis due to *Clostridium difficile*

    Code: _____

4 Gastroenteritis due to *Salmonella*

    Code: _____

(Answers are located in Appendix B)

From the Trenches

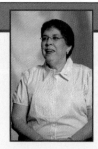

"We have all heard from different authorities that we need to 'brush up' on our anatomy and terminology to appropriately assign ICD-10-CM codes. Guess what!! They're right!!!!"

SHARON

LATE EFFECTS

ICD-10 OFFICIAL GUIDELINES FOR CODING AND REPORTING

SECTION I.B.
10. Sequela (Late Effects)

A sequela is the residual effect (condition produced) after the acute phase of an illness or injury has terminated. There is no time limit on when a sequela code can be used. The residual may be apparent early, such as in cerebral infarction, or it may occur months or years later, such as that due to a previous injury. Examples of sequela include: scar formation resulting from a burn, deviated septum due to a nasal fracture, and infertility due to tubal occlusion from old tuberculosis. Coding of sequela generally requires two codes sequenced in the following order: the condition or nature of the sequela is sequenced first. The sequela code is sequenced second.

An exception to the above guidelines are those instances where the code for the sequela is followed by a manifestation code identified in the Tabular List and title, or the sequela code has been expanded (at the fourth, fifth or sixth character levels) to include the manifestation(s). The code for the acute phase of an illness or injury that led to the sequela is never used with a code for the late effect.

See Section I.C.9. Sequelae of cerebrovascular disease
See Section I.C.15. Sequelae of complication of pregnancy, childbirth and the puerperium
See Section I.C.19. Application of 7ᵗʰ characters for Chapter 19

Late effects codes are not located in a separate chapter in the Tabular. You report late effects when the acute phase of the illness or injury has passed but a residual remains. Sometimes an acute illness or injury leaves a patient with a residual health problem that remains after the illness or injury has resolved. The **residual** is reported **first** and **then** the **late effects** code is assigned to indicate the cause of the residual or late effect of the burn. An example would be scars (residual) that remain after a severe burn (cause).

The term *sequela* means late effect and within the Tabular of the I-10 many codes have a 7th character to identify the sequela (character S), as illustrated in Fig. 4-2. Only one code is necessary to report a sequela (S) of a scalp abrasion because when reporting S00.01XS, you are reporting the residual and late effect with one code.

In other instances, the code(s) only report sequela, as illustrated in Fig. 4-3. In these cases you will need to report the resulting condition with a separate code and the cause (sequela) with a separate code.

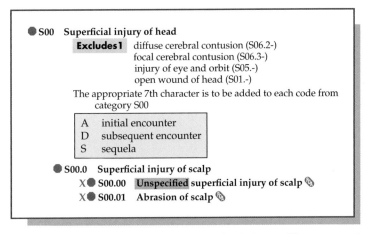

FIGURE 4-2   S00 Superficial injury of head with 7th character "S" to report sequel.

There is no time limit for the development of a residual. It may be evident at the time of the acute illness or it may occur months after an injury. It is also possible that a patient may develop more than one residual. For example, a patient who has had a stroke may develop right-sided hemiparesis (paralysis of one side) and aphasia (loss of ability to communicate).

A person cannot have a current right hip fracture (such as S72.001A) and a late effect of a right hip fracture (such as S72.001S) at the same time. The code is either a current injury or a condition caused by a prior injury. It cannot be both.

SEQUELAE OF INFECTIOUS AND PARASITIC DISEASES (B90-B94)

Note: Categories B90-B94 are to be used to indicate conditions in categories A00-B89 as the cause of sequelae, which are themselves classified elsewhere. The 'sequelae' include conditions specified as such; they also include residuals of diseases classifiable to the above categories if there is evidence that the disease itself is no longer present. Codes from these categories are not to be used for chronic infections. Code chronic current infections to active infectious disease as appropriate.

Code first condition resulting from (sequela) the infectious or parasitic disease

● **B90** **Sequelae of tuberculosis**
Condition resulting from tuberculosis

  B90.0 **Sequelae of central nervous system tuberculosis**

  B90.1 **Sequelae of genitourinary tuberculosis**

  B90.2 **Sequelae of tuberculosis of bones and joints**

  B90.8 **Sequelae of tuberculosis of other organs**
    Excludes2 sequelae of respiratory tuberculosis (B90.9)

  B90.9 **Sequelae of respiratory and unspecified tuberculosis**
    Sequelae of tuberculosis NOS

  B91 **Sequelae of poliomyelitis**
    Excludes1 postpolio syndrome (G14)

  B92 **Sequelae of leprosy**

FIGURE 4-3 B90-B94 Sequelae of Infectious and Parasitic Diseases.

EXERCISE 4-5 Residual and Cause

Write the term(s) that represent the residual and the cause terms on the lines provided:

1 Scars of the face resulting from third-degree burns suffered 1 year ago

Residual: _____

Cause: _____

2 Constrictive pericarditis due to old tuberculosis infection

Residual: _____

Cause: _____

3 Residual foreign body in femur due to gunshot injury years ago

Residual: _____

Cause: _____

4 Mental retardation due to previous poliomyelitis

Residual: _____

Cause: _____

5 Leg pain resulting from old fracture of femur

Residual: _____

Cause: _____

Identify the residual and cause terms and then code the following:

6 Arthritis following pathological fracture of the right femur 3 years ago

Residual: _____

Cause: _____

Codes: _____, _____

7 Sensorineural deafness due to previous meningitis

Residual: _____

Cause: _____

Codes: _____, _____

(Answers are located in Appendix B)

REPORTING SAME DIAGNOSIS CODE MORE THAN ONCE

ICD-10 OFFICIAL GUIDELINES FOR CODING AND REPORTING

SECTION I.B.

12. Reporting Same Diagnosis Code More than Once

Each unique ICD-10-CM diagnosis code may be reported only once for an encounter. This applies to bilateral conditions when there are no distinct codes identifying laterality or two different conditions classified to the same ICD-10-CM diagnosis code.

If the medical documentation indicates that the patient has two different conditions that are both included in one diagnosis code, report the diagnosis code only once.

Although each diagnosis code may be reported only once per encounter, each code can be reported more than once per patient. For example, a patient presents on Tuesday for an office visit and the diagnosis is pneumonia. The physician prescribes antibiotics for 10 days. The patient returns 5 days later, stating that she has not improved. The physician orders a culture and, based on the culture, orders a different antibiotic. The medical necessity for all services to this patient was the pneumonia diagnosis.

LATERALITY

ICD-10 OFFICIAL GUIDELINES FOR CODING AND REPORTING

SECTION I.B.

13. Laterality

Some ICD-10-CM codes indicate laterality, specifying whether the condition occurs on the left, right or is bilateral. If no bilateral code is provided and the condition is bilateral, assign separate codes for both the left and right side. If the side is not identified in the medical record, assign the code for the unspecified side.

Some body parts and organs occur in pairs; for example, kidneys, femurs, and femoral arteries. Other body parts and organs are singular in physiology; for example, bladder, spine, and aorta. Laterality refers to paired organs. Unilateral means one side of a pair, and bilateral means both sides of a pair. Laterality is an important concept in diagnostic coding because it can help define the scope of the disorder.

For some organs, laterality is addressed in only part of the ICD-10-CM classification. Laterality is not a component for code selection in pneumonia, but laterality is a component for code selection for neoplasms of the lung.

Laterality is usually straightforward, but as you become more adept at coding, you will see that there are some complex laterality situations. For example, the spine is a unilateral body part, but for some vertebral procedures, laterality is reported because the procedure can be performed on right, left, or both sides of the individual vertebra.

In the I-10, left and right (laterality) are indicated by the final character. For example, Fig. 4-4 illustrates M70.84, soft tissue disorder related to overuse or pressure to the hand. The right hand is designated with character "1," the left hand is indicated by "2," and unspecified hand is indicated with "9." If the service was provided to both hands, assign a code for the right hand and another code for the left hand.

● **M70.84 Other soft tissue disorders related to use, overuse and pressure of hand**

M70.841 **Other soft tissue disorders related to use, overuse and pressure, right hand**

M70.842 **Other soft tissue disorders related to use, overuse and pressure, left hand**

M70.849 **Other soft tissue disorders related to use, overuse and pressure, unspecified hand**

FIGURE 4–4 Laterality of codes in I-10.

In other instances, bilaterality can be reported with a single code, for example, H52.22 Regular astigmatism (see Fig. 4-5).

● **H52.22 Regular astigmatism**
　　　　H52.221 Regular astigmatism, right eye
　　　　H52.222 Regular astigmatism, left eye
　　　　H52.223 Regular astigmatism, bilateral
　　　　H52.229 Regular astigmatism, unspecified eye

FIGURE 4−5 Bilaterality of codes in ICD-10.

TOOLBOX

Marilyn is a 56-year-old female who is employed as a data entry specialist at the location hospital. Her job requires her to utilize a computer keyboard for extended periods of time frequently throughout the day. During an office visit to her primary care provider, she complains of pain in her hands that wakes her up at night. She is diagnosed with bilateral soft tissue disorder of her hands. Her physician has prescribed a splint to immobilize her hands.

QUESTION
Using Fig. 4-4, which I-10 code or codes would you report for this office visit? _____

▼ **ANSWER**

M70.841 and M70.842

CHAPTER REVIEW

CHAPTER 4, PART I, THEORY

Without the use of reference material, answer the following:

1 List two of the four cooperating parties that agree on coding principles: _____

2 Fill in the missing words in the Steps to Accurate Coding:
   a Identify the main _____ in the diagnostic statement.
   b Locate the main term(s) in the _____ Index.
   c Review any _____ under the main term in the Index.
   d Follow any _____ _____ instructions, such as *see also*.
   e Verify the code(s) selected from the Index (Volume _____) in the Tabular List (Volume _____) (referred to in this text as the Tabular).
   f Refer to any instructional notations in the _____.
   g Assign codes to the highest level of _____. For example, if a fourth digit is available, you cannot assign only a three-digit code, and if a fifth digit is available, you cannot assign only a four-digit code.
   h Code the diagnosis until all _____ are completely identified.

3 A combination code is a single code used to classify _____.
   a two diagnoses
   b a diagnosis with an associated manifestation
   c a diagnosis with an associated complication
   d all of the above

4 Additional signs and symptoms that may not routinely be associated with the disease process being reported should be coded when present.

   True   False

5 In the outpatient setting, an impending condition should be coded as if it actually exists.

   True   False

6 When separate codes exist to identify acute and chronic conditions, the chronic code is sequenced first.

   True   False

7 It is acceptable to use only the Alphabetic Index to assign I-10 codes.

   True   False

8 When sequencing codes for residuals and late effects, the residual is sequenced first followed by a late effect code.

   True   False

9 A code is invalid if it has not been coded to the full number of characters available for that code.

   True   False

10 The *Official Guidelines for Coding and Reporting* are updated annually.

   True   False

Chapter Review answers are only available in the TEACH Instructor Resources on Evolve

CHAPTER 4, PART II, PRACTICAL

List the following:

11 List two common symptoms associated with kidney stones. _____

12 List two common symptoms associated with pneumonia. _____

Assign I-10 codes to the following diagnoses:

13 Acute and chronic prostatitis

  Codes: _____, _____

14 Headache, stiff neck, and fever due to viral meningitis

  Code: _____

15 Acute and chronic pyelonephritis

  Codes: _____, _____

16 Abdominal pain due to acute and chronic cholecystitis

  Code: _____

17 Urinary tract infection due to *Proteus mirabilis*

  Codes: _____, _____

18 Cerebrovascular accident, TIA

  Code: _____

19 Traumatic osteoarthritis of the wrist due to fracture 5 years ago

  Codes: _____, _____

20 Dysphagia due to previous cerebrovascular accident, nontraumatic

  Code: _____

21 Respiratory syncytial virus (RSV) infection

  Code: _____

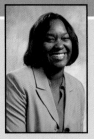

CHAPTER 5

What will be the initial challenges for implementing ICD-10-CM?

"Training, training, and training of physicians and staff. Because the structure of ICD-10 is more specific and the codes look different, the mindset has to change. Documentation must be even more detailed than before."

Letitia Patterson, MPA, CPC, CCS-P
Consultant
A Coder's Resource
Chicago, Illinois

Chapter-Specific Guidelines (ICD-10-CM Chapters 1-10)

Chapter Topics

Certain Infectious and Parasitic Diseases

Neoplasms

Diseases of the Blood and Blood-Forming Organs and Certain Disorders Involving the Immune Mechanism

Endocrine, Nutritional, and Metabolic Diseases

Mental, Behavioral and Neurodevelopmental Disorders

Diseases of the Nervous System

Diseases of the Eye and Adnexa

Diseases of the Ear and Mastoid Process

Diseases of the Circulatory System

Diseases of the Respiratory System

Chapter Review

Learning Objectives

After completing this chapter you should be able to

1 Review certain infectious and parasitic disease codes.

2 Analyze neoplasm codes.

3 Assess the blood and blood-forming organs and certain disorders involving the immune mechanism codes.

4 Examine the endocrine, nutritional, and metabolic diseases codes.

5 Understand the mental, behavioral and neurodevelopmental disorder codes.

6 Examine the diseases of the nervous system codes.

7 Analyze the diseases of the eye and adnexa codes.

8 Comprehend the organization and reporting of the ear and mastoid process codes.

9 Recognize the diseases of the circulatory system codes.

10 Evaluate the diseases of the respiratory system codes.

11 Demonstrate the ability to report diagnoses with I-10 codes for Chapters 1-10.

NOTE: The 2015 ICD-10-CM DRAFT and 2015 ICD-10-PCS DRAFT were used in preparing this text.

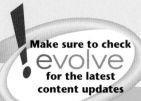

Make sure to check **evolve** for the latest content updates

CERTAIN INFECTIOUS AND PARASITIC DISEASES

Chapter 1 in the I-10 Tabular is Certain Infectious and Parasitic Diseases (A00-B99), which classifies diseases according to the etiology (cause) of the disease. Because infectious and parasitic conditions can affect various parts of the body, the chapter contains a wide variety of codes and complex terminology.

In this chapter there are many instances of combination coding and multiple coding. Remember: **Combination coding** is when one code fully describes the conditions and/ or manifestations. **Multiple coding** is when it takes more than one code to fully describe the condition, circumstance, or manifestation, and then sequencing of multiple codes is considered.

Examples

Combination Coding

Diagnosis:	Candidiasis infection of the mouth
Index:	**Candidiasis,** candidal, mouth B37.0
Tabular:	**B37.0 Candidal stomatitis**
Code:	B37.0 Candidiasis infection of the mouth

B37.0 fully describes the diagnosis.

Multiple Coding

Diagnosis:	Urinary tract infection due to *Escherichia coli (E. coli)*
Index:	**Infection,** infected, infective; urinary (tract) NEC N39.0
Tabular:	**N39.0 Urinary tract infection, site not specified** Use additional code (B95-B97), to identify infectious agent.

Code N39.0 does not fully describe the condition. The instructions in the Tabular for code N39.0 state that you are to also code the organism causing the urinary tract infection. To locate a causative organism, you locate the main term "Infection" in the Index and then the subterm of "bacterial" followed by the subterm "as cause of disease classified elsewhere," and then the specific organism, which in the example is *Escherichia coli.*

Index:	**Infection,** bacterial, as cause of disease classified elsewhere, Escherichia coli B96.2
Tabular:	**B96 Other bacterial agents as the cause of diseases classified elsewhere** **B96.2** Escherichia coli [E. coli] **as the cause of diseases classified elsewhere**

The urinary tract infection is sequenced first, followed by the bacterial organism.

Codes:	N39.0, B96.2 Urinary tract infection due to *Escherichia coli (E. coli)*

Multiple coding is necessary to fully describe the infection of the urinary tract and the causative organism, *E. coli.*

A00-A09	Intestinal infectious diseases
A15-A19	Tuberculosis
A20-A28	Certain zoonotic bacterial diseases
A30-A49	Other bacterial diseases
A50-A64	Infections with a predominantly sexual mode of transmission
A65-A69	Other spirochetal diseases
A70-A74	Other diseases caused by chlamydiae
A75-A79	Rickettsioses
A80-A89	Viral and prion infections of the central nervous system
A90-A99	Arthropod-borne viral fevers and viral hemorrhagic fevers

FIGURE 5-1   Blocks in the A codes of the I-10.

Resistant Infections

ICD-10 OFFICIAL GUIDELINES FOR CODING AND REPORTING

SECTION I.C. Chapter-Specific Coding Guidelines
1.c. Infections resistant to antibiotics

Many bacterial infections are resistant to current antibiotics. It is necessary to identify all infections documented as antibiotic resistant. Assign a code from category Z16, Resistance to antimicrobial drugs, following the infection code only if the infection code does not identify drug resistance.

A Codes (A00-A99)

The A codes include the blocks illustrated in Fig. 5-1.

Antibiotics are used to kill the bacteria that cause disease, but many antibiotics that were historically effective against bacteria are no longer effective. Most bacteria have become resistant to some antibiotics, but other bacteria are resistant to many antibiotics (multiresistant organisms, MROs, or superbugs). Those antibiotics that have been widely prescribed are no longer effective—for example, methicillin-resistant *Staphylococcus aureus* (MRSA), multi-drug-resistant *Mycobacterium* tuberculosis (MDR-TB), and vancomycin-resistant *Enterococcus* (VRE). Penicillin-resistant *Streptococcus pneumonia* has also increased worldwide. When reporting an infection that is antibiotic resistant, report the infection first followed by Z16.- (Infection with drug-resistant microorganism). This is the mechanism by which drug-resistant microorganisms are tracked. *Staphylococcus aureus* is the exception to the Z16.- rule. For *Staphylococcus aureus*, specific codes designate the status of resistance to methicillin:

B95.61	**Methicillin susceptible Staphylococcus aureus infection as the cause of diseases classified elsewhere (MSSA)**
B95.62	**Methicillin resistant Staphylococcus aureus infection as the cause of diseases classified elsewhere (MRSA)**

QUICK CHECK 5-1

1. What category code would you reference when reporting MRSA? _____
2. What is the drug resistance in VRE? _____
3. What does the S stand for in MRSA? _____

(Answers are located in Appendix C)

Sepsis, Severe Sepsis, and Septic Shock

SIRS is an inflammatory condition, also known as systemic inflammatory response syndrome. The inflammation is a response to microorganisms in the tissue, blood, lungs, skin, or urinary system. SIRS is diagnosed when two or more of the following are present:

- hypothermia or fever (<97°F or >100°F or <38°C or >36°C)
- tachycardia (>90-100 bpm)
- increased respiratory rate (>20 breaths per minute or $PaCO_2$ < 32 mm Hg)
- increased or decreased white blood count (<4000 or >12,000)

SIRS is classified as **severe sepsis** when there is organ dysfunction, hypotension, or collection of fluids in the tissues (hypoperfusion). To report severe sepsis, you would report a code from subcategory R65.2 but remember that severe sepsis can only be reported if severe sepsis is documented in the patient health record. The provider will make the diagnosis of SIRS. If the documentation indicates that the patient has SIRS and organ dysfunction and that the organ dysfunction is related to a condition other than SIRS, severe sepsis is not reported. There must be a documented correlation between the SIRS and the organ dysfunction to report severe sepsis. It will require at least three codes to report severe sepsis: a code for the underlying systemic infection, a code from subcategory R65.2, and a code or codes to report organ dysfunction. When the microorganism is not documented, report A41.9, Sepsis, unspecified.

Septic shock is a circulatory failure that represents a type of organ dysfunction. Report the underlying infection first, followed by R65.21, Severe sepsis with septic shock, and codes for any organ dysfunction documented in the health record. Code R65.21 is never assigned as the first-listed diagnosis because it is a result of an underlying infection; therefore, the infection is the first-listed diagnosis followed by the severe sepsis.

ICD-10 OFFICIAL GUIDELINES FOR CODING AND REPORTING

SECTION I.C.
1.d. Sepsis, Severe Sepsis, and Septic Shock

2) Septic shock

(a) Septic shock generally refers to circulatory failure associated with severe sepsis, and therefore, it represents a type of acute organ dysfunction.

For cases of septic shock, the code for the systemic infection should be sequenced first, followed by code R65.21, Severe sepsis with septic shock or code T81.12, Postprocedural septic shock. Any additional codes for the other acute organ dysfunctions should also be assigned. As noted in the sequencing instructions in the Tabular List, the code for septic shock cannot be assigned as a principal diagnosis.

Septic shock indicates the presence of severe sepsis. Code R65.21, Severe sepsis with septic shock, must be assigned if septic shock is documented in the medical record, even if the term severe sepsis is not documented.

3) Sequencing of severe sepsis

If severe sepsis is present on admission, and meets the definition of principal diagnosis, the underlying systemic infection should be assigned as principal diagnosis followed by the appropriate code from subcategory R65.2 as required by the sequencing rules in the Tabular List. A code from subcategory R65.2 can never be assigned as a principal diagnosis.

When severe sepsis develops during an encounter (it was not present on admission) the underlying systemic infection and the appropriate code from subcategory R65.2 should be assigned as secondary diagnoses.

Severe sepsis may be present on admission but the diagnosis may not be confirmed until sometime after admission. If the documentation is not clear whether severe sepsis was present on admission, the provider should be queried.

SIRS may develop as a result of a procedure and becomes a complication of the medical care the patient received. In these instances, report a postprocedural infection first, followed by a code for the specific infection.

Examples

- Subcategory T80.2 Infections following infusion, transfusion, or therapeutic injection, report an additional code to identify the specific infection; such as sepsis [A41.9]
- Subcategory T81.4 Infection following a procedure; report an additional code to identify infection
- Subcategory O86.0 Infection of obstetric surgical wound, report an additional code (B95-B97) to identify infectious agent

ICD-10 OFFICIAL GUIDELINES FOR CODING AND REPORTING

SECTION I.C.
1.d. Sepsis, Severe Sepsis, and Septic Shock
1) Coding of Sepsis and Severe Sepsis

(a) Sepsis

For a diagnosis of sepsis, assign the appropriate code for the underlying systemic infection. If the type of infection or causal organism is not further specified, assign code A41.9, Sepsis, unspecified organism.

A code from subcategory R65.2, Severe sepsis, should not be assigned unless severe sepsis or an associated acute organ dysfunction is documented.

(i) Negative or inconclusive blood cultures and sepsis

Negative or inconclusive blood cultures do not preclude a diagnosis of sepsis in patients with clinical evidence of the condition, however, the provider should be queried.

(ii) Urosepsis

The term urosepsis is a nonspecific term. It is not to be considered synonymous with sepsis. It has no default code in the Alphabetic Index. Should a provider use this term, he/she must be queried for clarification.

(iii) Sepsis with organ dysfunction

If a patient has sepsis and associated acute organ dysfunction or multiple organ dysfunction (MOD), follow the instructions for coding severe sepsis.

(iv) Acute organ dysfunction that is not clearly associated with the sepsis

If a patient has sepsis and an acute organ dysfunction, but the medical record documentation indicates that the acute organ dysfunction is related to a medical condition other than the sepsis, do not assign a code from subcategory R65.2, Severe sepsis. An acute organ dysfunction must be associated with the sepsis in order to assign the severe sepsis code. If the documentation is not clear as to whether an acute organ dysfunction is related to the sepsis or another medical condition, query the provider.

(b) Severe sepsis

The coding of severe sepsis requires a minimum of 2 codes: first a code for the underlying systemic infection, followed by a code from subcategory R65.2, Severe sepsis. If the causal organism is not documented, assign code A41.9, Sepsis, unspecified organism, for the infection. Additional code(s) for the associated acute organ dysfunction are also required.

Due to the complex nature of severe sepsis, some cases may require querying the provider prior to assignment of the codes.

ICD-10 OFFICIAL GUIDELINES FOR CODING AND REPORTING

SECTION I.C.

1.d. Sepsis, Severe Sepsis, and Septic Shock

4) Sepsis and severe sepsis with a localized infection

If the reason for admission is both sepsis or severe sepsis and a localized infection, such as pneumonia or cellulitis, a code(s) for the underlying systemic infection should be assigned first and the code for the localized infection should be assigned as a secondary diagnosis. If the patient has severe sepsis, a code from subcategory R65.2 should also be assigned as a secondary diagnosis. If the patient is admitted with a localized infection, such as pneumonia, and sepsis/severe sepsis doesn't develop until after admission, the localized infection should be assigned first, followed by the appropriate sepsis/severe sepsis codes.

5) Sepsis due to a postprocedural infection

(a) Documentation of causal relationship

As with all postprocedural complications, code assignment is based on the provider's documentation of the relationship between the infection and the procedure.

(b) Sepsis due to a postprocedural infection

For such cases, the postprocedural infection code, such as, T80.2, Infections following infusion, transfusion, and therapeutic injection, T81.4, Infection following a procedure, T88.0, Infection following immunization, or O86.0, Infection of obstetric surgical wound, should be coded first, followed by the code for the specific infection. If the patient has severe sepsis the appropriate code from subcategory R65.2 should also be assigned with the additional code(s) for any acute organ dysfunction.

(c) Postprocedural infection and postprocedural septic shock

In cases where a postprocedural infection has occurred and has resulted in severe sepsis and postprocedural septic shock, the code for the precipitating complication such as code T81.4, Infection following a procedure, or O86.0, Infection of obstetrical surgical wound should be coded first followed by code R65.20, Severe sepsis without septic shock. A code for the systemic infection should also be assigned.

If a postprocedural infection has resulted in postprocedural septic shock, the code for the precipitating complication such as code T81.4, Infection following a procedure, or O86.0, Infection of obstetrical surgical wound should be coded first followed by code T81.12-, Postprocedural septic shock. A code for the systemic infection should also be assigned.

6) Sepsis and severe sepsis associated with a noninfectious process (condition)

In some cases a noninfectious process (condition), such as trauma, may lead to an infection which can result in sepsis or severe sepsis. If sepsis or severe sepsis is documented as associated with a noninfectious condition, such as a burn or serious injury, and this condition meets the definition for principal diagnosis, the code for the noninfectious condition should be sequenced first, followed by the code for the resulting infection. If severe sepsis, is present a code from subcategory R65.2 should also be assigned with any associated organ dysfunction(s) codes. It is not necessary to assign a code from subcategory R65.1, Systemic inflammatory response syndrome (SIRS) of non-infectious origin, for these cases.

If the infection meets the definition of principal diagnosis it should be sequenced before the non-infectious condition. When both the associated non-infectious condition and the infection meet the definition of principal diagnosis either may be assigned as principal diagnosis.

Only one code from category R65, Symptoms and signs specifically associated with systemic inflammation and infection, should be assigned. Therefore, when a non-infectious condition leads to an infection resulting in severe sepsis, assign the appropriate code from subcategory R65.2, Severe sepsis. Do not additionally assign a code from subcategory R65.1, Systemic inflammatory response syndrome (SIRS) of non-infectious origin.

See Section I.C.18. SIRS due to non-infectious process

TOOLBOX

Robert has sepsis resulting from a postprocedural infection that is now complicating his care.

QUESTIONS

1. Sepsis resulting from a postprocedural infection is considered a
   _____.
2. If the documentation stated that Robert's sepsis was severe, you would reference what subcategory for code assignment? _____
3. When reporting severe sepsis, you would also report what dysfunction?
   _____

▼ **ANSWERS**

1. complication, 2. R65.2, 3. organ dysfunction

B Codes (B00-B99)

The B codes include viral infections, mycoses (fungi), protozoal (microscopic animals), helminthiases (parasitic worms), pediculosis (louse), acariasis (mites), sequelae of infectious disease, and other infectious agents. The B codes are illustrated in Fig. 5-2. Common infectious categories within the B codes are herpes (B00), chickenpox (B01), herpes zoster (shingles, B02), measles (B05), and German measles (Rubella, B06).

Viral Hepatitis

Viral hepatitis is reported with codes in the B15-B19 range, which are divided based on with or without hepatic coma and the type of hepatitis. For example, B15 reports acute hepatitis A and B16 reports acute hepatitis B.

- **Hepatitis A** (HAV) was formerly called epidemic, infectious, short-incubation, or acute catarrhal jaundice hepatitis, and the primary transmission mode is the oral–fecal route.
- **Hepatitis B** (HBV) was formerly called long-incubation period, serum, or homologous serum hepatitis. Transmission modes are through blood from infected persons and from body fluids of infected mother to neonate.
- **Hepatitis C** (HCV), caused by the hepatitis C virus and is primarily transfusion associated.

B00-B09	Viral infections characterized by skin and mucous membrane lesions
B10	Other human herpesviruses
B15-B19	Viral hepatitis
B20	Human immunodeficiency virus [HIV] disease
B25-B34	Other viral diseases
B35-B49	Mycoses
B50-B64	Protozoal diseases
B65-B83	Helminthiases
B85-B89	Pediculosis, acariasis and other infestations
B90-B94	Sequelae of infectious and parasitic diseases
B95-B97	Bacterial and viral infectious agents
B99	Other infectious diseases

FIGURE 5–2 Blocks in the B codes of the I-10.

- **Hepatitis D** (HDV), also called delta hepatitis and is caused by the hepatitis D virus in patients formerly or currently infected with hepatitis B.
- **Hepatitis E** (HEV) is also called enterically transmitted non-A, non-B hepatitis. The primary transmission mode is the oral–fecal route, usually through contaminated water.

EXERCISE 5-1   *A Code Infectious and Parasitic Diseases*

Code the following infectious diseases:

1 Viral gastroenteritis

Code: _____

2 Severe sepsis due to *Pseudomonas* with septic shock

Codes: _____, _____

3 Acute poliomyelitis

Code: _____

(Answers are located in Appendix B)

Human Immunodeficiency

B20 reports human immunodeficiency virus diseases and includes AIDS (acquired immune deficiency syndrome), which is caused by HIV (human immunodeficiency virus). HIV affects certain white blood cells (T-4 lymphocytes) and destroys the ability of the cells to fight infections, making patients susceptible to a host of infectious diseases (e.g., *Pneumocystis carinii pneumonia* [PCP], Kaposi's sarcoma, and lymphoma). AIDS-related complex (ARC) is an outdated term for lesser infections associated with HIV. Additional code(s) are reported to identify all the manifestations of AIDS. It is extremely important that only confirmed HIV cases are reported. The assignment of the AIDS code prior to confirmation may cause the patient many unwarranted problems if the patient does not have AIDS. Confirmation does not mean that a serology or culture for HIV is positive, but rather that the physician has documented that the patient is HIV positive or has HIV-related illnesses.

If the encounter is for an HIV-related condition, the first-listed diagnosis is B20 with additional codes to report the HIV-related condition(s). If the encounter is for an HIV-disease patient for other than the HIV or an HIV-related condition, the reason for the encounter is the first-listed diagnosis followed by B20. There are times when a patient is documented to be HIV-positive based on serology or culture but has no symptoms. Report this asymptomatic HIV status with Z21, Asymptomatic HIV status. However, once a patient has AIDS, report B20; never report R75 (inconclusive) or Z21 (asymptomatic). If the patient is known to have been exposed to HIV but has not tested positive for HIV and has no HIV symptoms, report Z20.6. If the serology for HIV is inconclusive, report R75.

If an HIV-positive patient is pregnant and the encounter is for an HIV-related illness, the first-listed diagnosis is O98.7, HIV disease complicating pregnancy, childbirth, and the puerperium, followed by B20 and codes for the HIV-related illness. If the patient's status is asymptomatic HIV, report O98.7 and Z21 (asymptomatic HIV).

If the patient presents for HIV testing, report Z11.4, Encounter for screening for HIV. Additional codes may be assigned for any known high-risk behavior, such as:

- Z72.51   High risk heterosexual behavior
- Z72.52   High risk homosexual behavior
- Z72.53   High risk bisexual behavior

If the patient has signs or symptoms when presenting for HIV screening, report the signs and symptoms and if counseling is provided during the encounter, report Z71.7, HIV counseling. When the patient returns for the results of the HIV screening and the results are negative, report Z71.7.

ICD-10 OFFICIAL GUIDELINES FOR CODING AND REPORTING

SECTION I.C.1.
Chapter 1: Certain Infectious and Parasitic Diseases (A00-B99)

a. Human Immunodeficiency Virus (HIV) Infections

1) Code only confirmed cases

Code only confirmed cases of HIV infection/illness. This is an exception to the hospital inpatient guideline Section II, H.

In this context, "confirmation" does not require documentation of positive serology or culture for HIV; the provider's diagnostic statement that the patient is HIV positive, or has an HIV-related illness is sufficient.

2) Selection and sequencing of HIV codes

(a) Patient admitted for HIV-related condition

If a patient is admitted for an HIV-related condition, the principal diagnosis should be B20, Human immunodeficiency virus [HIV] disease followed by additional diagnosis codes for all reported HIV-related conditions.

(b) Patient with HIV disease admitted for unrelated condition

If a patient with HIV disease is admitted for an unrelated condition (such as a traumatic injury), the code for the unrelated condition (e.g., the nature of injury code) should be the principal diagnosis. Other diagnoses would be B20 followed by additional diagnosis codes for all reported HIV-related conditions.

(c) Whether the patient is newly diagnosed

Whether the patient is newly diagnosed or has had previous admissions/encounters for HIV conditions is irrelevant to the sequencing decision.

(d) Asymptomatic human immunodeficiency virus

Z21, Asymptomatic human immunodeficiency virus [HIV] infection status, is to be applied when the patient without any documentation of symptoms is listed as being "HIV positive," "known HIV," "HIV test positive," or similar terminology. Do not use this code if the term "AIDS" is used or if the patient is treated for any HIV-related illness or is described as having any condition(s) resulting from his/her HIV positive status; use B20 in these cases.

(e) Patients with inconclusive HIV serology

Patients with inconclusive HIV serology, but no definitive diagnosis or manifestations of the illness, may be assigned code R75, Inconclusive laboratory evidence of human immunodeficiency virus [HIV].

(f) Previously diagnosed HIV-related illness

Patients with any known prior diagnosis of an HIV-related illness should be coded to B20. Once a patient has developed an HIV-related illness, the patient should always be assigned code B20 on every subsequent admission/encounter. Patients previously diagnosed with any HIV illness (B20) should never be assigned to R75 or Z21, Asymptomatic human immunodeficiency virus [HIV] infection status.

(Note from author: State laws may have rules for coding and submitting AIDS diagnosis. Example: Under New York State Law, confidential HIV-related information can only be given to people the patient allows to have it by signing a written release or to people who need to know the HIV status in order to provide medical care and services.)

Continued

(g) HIV Infection in Pregnancy, Childbirth and the Puerperium

During pregnancy, childbirth or the puerperium, a patient admitted (or presenting for a health care encounter) because of an HIV-related illness should receive a principal diagnosis code of O98.7-, Human immunodeficiency [HIV] disease complicating pregnancy, childbirth and the puerperium, followed by B20 and the code(s) for the HIV-related illness(es). Codes from Chapter 15 always take sequencing priority.

Patients with asymptomatic HIV infection status admitted (or presenting for a health care encounter) during pregnancy, childbirth, or the puerperium should receive codes of O98.7- and Z21.

(h) Encounters for testing for HIV

If a patient is being seen to determine his/her HIV status, use code Z11.4, Encounter for screening for human immunodeficiency virus [HIV]. Use additional codes for any associated high risk behavior.

If a patient with signs or symptoms is being seen for HIV testing, code the signs and symptoms. An additional counseling code Z71.7, Human immunodeficiency virus [HIV] counseling, may be used if counseling is provided during the encounter for the test.

When a patient returns to be informed of his/her HIV test results and the test result is negative, use code Z71.7, Human immunodeficiency virus [HIV] counseling.

If the results are positive, see previous guidelines and assign codes as appropriate.

EXERCISE 5-2 | *B Code Viral Infections*

Code the following viral diseases:

1 Candidal vaginal infection

Code: _____

2 Post-chickenpox myelitis

Code: _____

3 Unspecified parvovirus infection

Code: _____

4 Oral thrush

Code: _____

5 Body louse (pediculosis) infestation

Code: _____

(Answers are located in Appendix B)

NEOPLASMS

Chapter 2 of the I-10 contains codes C00-D49 to report neoplasms. There are extensive Guidelines that must be understood and followed to correctly code neoplasms.

ICD-10 OFFICIAL GUIDELINES FOR CODING AND REPORTING

SECTION I.C.2.
Chapter 2: Neoplasms (C00-D49)

General guidelines

Chapter 2 of the ICD-10-CM contains the codes for most benign and all malignant neoplasms. Certain benign neoplasms, such as prostatic adenomas, may be found in the specific body system chapters. To properly code a neoplasm it is necessary to determine from the record if the neoplasm is benign, in-situ, malignant, or of uncertain histologic behavior. If malignant, any secondary (metastatic) sites should also be determined.

Primary malignant neoplasms overlapping site boundaries

A primary malignant neoplasm that overlaps two or more contiguous (next to each other) sites should be classified to the subcategory/code .8 ('overlapping lesion'), unless the combination is specifically indexed elsewhere. For multiple neoplasms of the same site that are not contiguous such as tumors in different quadrants of the same breast, codes for each site should be assigned.

Malignant neoplasm of ectopic tissue

Malignant neoplasms of ectopic tissue are to be coded to the site of origin mentioned, e.g., ectopic pancreatic malignant neoplasms involving the stomach are coded to pancreas, unspecified (C25.9).

The neoplasm table in the Alphabetic Index should be referenced first. However, if the histological term is documented, that term should be referenced first, rather than going immediately to the Neoplasm Table, in order to determine which column in the Neoplasm Table is appropriate. For example, if the documentation indicates "adenoma," refer to the term in the Alphabetic Index to review the entries under this term and the instructional note to "see also neoplasm, by site, benign." The table provides the proper code based on the type of neoplasm and the site. It is important to select the proper column in the table that corresponds to the type of neoplasm. The Tabular List should then be referenced to verify that the correct code has been selected from the table and that a more specific site code does not exist.

See Section I.C.21. Factors influencing health status and contact with health services, Status, for information regarding Z15.0, codes for genetic susceptibility to cancer.

a. Treatment directed at the malignancy

If the treatment is directed at the malignancy, designate the malignancy as the principal diagnosis.

The only exception to this guideline is if a patient admission/encounter is solely for the administration of chemotherapy, immunotherapy or radiation therapy, assign the appropriate Z51.-- code as the first-listed or principal diagnosis, and the diagnosis or problem for which the service is being performed as a secondary diagnosis.

b. Treatment of secondary site

When a patient is admitted because of a primary neoplasm with metastasis and treatment is directed toward the secondary site only, the secondary neoplasm is designated as the principal diagnosis even though the primary malignancy is still present.

c. Coding and sequencing of complications

Coding and sequencing of complications associated with the malignancies or with the therapy thereof are subject to the following guidelines:

1) Anemia associated with malignancy

When admission/encounter is for management of an anemia associated with the malignancy, and the treatment is only for anemia, the appropriate code for the malignancy is sequenced as the principal or first-listed diagnosis followed by the appropriate code for anemia (such as code D63.0, Anemia in neoplastic disease).

Continued

appropriate code for the malignancy is sequenced as the principal or first-listed diagnosis followed by code D63.0, Anemia in neoplastic disease.

5) Complication from surgical procedure for treatment of a neoplasm

When an encounter is for treatment of a complication resulting from a surgical procedure performed for the treatment of the neoplasm, designate the complication as the principal/first-listed diagnosis. See guideline regarding the coding of a current malignancy versus personal history to determine if the code for the neoplasm should also be assigned.

6) Pathologic fracture due to a neoplasm

When an encounter is for a pathological fracture due to a neoplasm, and the focus of treatment is the fracture, a code from subcategory M84.5, Pathological fracture in neoplastic disease, should be sequenced first, followed by the code for the neoplasm.

If the focus of treatment is the neoplasm with an associated pathological fracture, the neoplasm code should be sequenced first, followed by a code from M84.5 for the pathological fracture.

m. Current malignancy versus personal history of malignancy

When a primary malignancy has been excised but further treatment, such as an additional surgery for the malignancy, radiation therapy or chemotherapy is directed to that site, the primary malignancy code should be used until treatment is completed.

When a primary malignancy has been previously excised or eradicated from its site, there is no further treatment (of the malignancy) directed to that site, and there is no evidence of any existing primary malignancy, a code from category Z85, Personal history of malignant neoplasm, should be used to indicate the former site of the malignancy.

See Section I.C.21. Factors influencing health status and contact with health services, History (of)

n. Leukemia, Multiple Myeloma, and Malignant Plasma Cell Neoplasms in remission versus personal history

The categories for leukemia, and category C90, Multiple myeloma and malignant plasma cell neoplasms, have codes indicating whether or not the leukemia has achieved remission. There are also codes Z85.6, Personal history of leukemia, and Z85.79, Personal history of other malignant neoplasms of lymphoid, hematopoietic and related tissues. If the documentation is unclear, as to whether the leukemia has achieved remission, the provider should be queried.

See Section I.C.21. Factors influencing health status and contact with health services, History (of)

o. Aftercare following surgery for neoplasm

See Section I.C.21. Factors influencing health status and contact with health services, Aftercare

p. Follow-up care for completed treatment of a malignancy

See Section I.C.21. Factors influencing health status and contact with health services, Follow-up

q. Prophylactic organ removal for prevention of malignancy

See Section I.C. 21, Factors influencing health status and contact with health services, Prophylactic organ removal

r. Malignant neoplasm associated with transplanted organ

A malignant neoplasm of a transplanted organ should be coded as a transplant complication. Assign first the appropriate code from category T86.-, Complications of transplanted organs and tissue, followed by code C80.2, Malignant neoplasm associated with transplanted organ. Use an additional code for the specific malignancy.

QUICK CHECK 5-2

1. According to the Neoplasm Guidelines, you would report a category _____ code for a patient in leukemia remission and code _____ for a personal history of leukemia.
2. When an encounter for a pathological fracture is due to a neoplasm, and if the focus of treatment is the fracture, a code from subcategory_____ should be sequenced first, followed by the code for the _____.

(Answers are located in Appendix C)

Neoplasm Classifications and Staging

In the I-10, neoplasms are classified as:

■ **C00-C96, Malignant:** A cancerous tumor that grows worse over time by invading surrounding tissue, is aggressive in manner, and may metastasize.

    Primary site: Original site of the tumor

    Secondary site: Metastasized from the original site

■ **D00-D09, Ca in situ (CIS):** Latin for "in its place," a cancerous tumor in its original place that has not invaded surrounding tissues

■ **D10-D3A, Benign:** A tumor that does not invade surrounding tissue, is not metastatic, and is not aggressive

■ **D37-D48, Uncertain:** A neoplasm that is not clearly benign or malignant and over time may or may not become more aggressive

■ **D49, Unspecified Behavior:** A neoplasm of unspecified morphology and behavior, such as growth NOS, neoplasm NOS, or tumor NOS. This classification does not include neoplasm of uncertain behavior (D37-D48).

The first step in assigning a code(s) for a neoplasm is to determine if the neoplasm is malignant, in situ, benign, or of uncertain or unspecified behavior and then identify any secondary (metastatic) sites.

Neoplasms are staged, which means that they are evaluated for placement on a common grading scale based on the level of invasion.

Staging

Example
Staging for endometrial, cervical, and ovarian malignancies is staged based on if the malignancy is:
- Stage I, Confined to corpus
- Stage II, Involves corpus and cervix
- Stage III, Extends outside uterus but not outside true pelvis
- Stage IV, Extends outside true pelvis or involves rectum or bladder

Staging

Example
Staging for renal cancer
- Stage I, tumor of kidney capsule only
- Stage II, tumor invading renal capsule/vein but within fascia
- Stage III, tumor extending to regional lymph node/vena cava
- Stage IV, other organ metastasis

	Malignant Primary	Malignant Secondary	Ca in situ	Benign	Uncertain Behavior	Unspecified Behavior
aryepiglottic fold	C13.1	C79.89	D00.08	D10.7	D37.05	D49.0
hypopharyngeal aspect	C13.1	C79.89	D00.08	D10.7	D37.05	D49.0
laryngeal aspect	C32.1	C78.39	D02.0	D14.1	D38.0	D49.1
marginal zone	C13.1	C79.89	D00.08	D10.7	D37.05	D49.0
arytenoid (cartilage)	C32.3	C78.39	D02.0	D14.1	D38.0	D49.1
fold — see Neoplasm, aryepiglottic						
associated with transplanted organ	C80.2	—	—	—	—	—
atlas	C41.2	C79.51	—	D16.6	D48.0	D49.2
atrium, cardiac	C38.0	C79.89	—	D15.1	D48.7	D49.89
auditory						
canal (external) (skin) A81	C44.20-	C79.2	D04.2-	D23.2-	D48.5	D49.2
internal	C30.1	C78.39	D02.3	D14.0	D38.5	D49.1
nerve	C72.4-	C79.49	—	D33.3	D43.3	D49.7
tube	C30.1	C78.39	D02.3	D14.0	D38.5	D49.1
opening	C11.2	C79.89	D00.08	D10.6	D37.05	D49.0
auricle, ear — see also Neoplasm, skin, ear	C44.20-	C79.2	D04.2-	D23.2-	D48.5	D49.2
auricular canal (external) — see also Neoplasm, skin, ear	C44.20-	C79.2	D04.2-	D23.2-	D48.5	D49.2
internal	C30.1	C78.39	D02.3	D14.0	D38.5	D49.2

FIGURE 5-3   I-10 Neoplasm Table.

The pathology report and staging information will be documented in the medical record. To assign a diagnosis code to a neoplasm:

1. Identify the morphology or histologic type of the neoplasm documented. Examples of histology types are carcinoma, adenocarcinoma, sarcoma, melanoma, lymphoma, lipoma, and adenoma.
2. If the histologic type is known, reference the type in the Neoplasm Table.
3. Determine the appropriate column in the Neoplasm Table, as illustrated in Fig. 5-3.
4. Reference the code in the Tabular List.

Sequencing and Complications. When treatment is directed at the primary site of the neoplasm, designate the **primary** site as the first-listed diagnosis. If the treatment is directed at the secondary site of the neoplasm, designate the **secondary** site as the first-listed diagnosis. When the encounter is only for chemotherapy (Z51.11), immunotherapy (Z51.12), or radiation therapy (Z51.0), assign the category Z51 code as the first-listed diagnosis and a code for the malignancy as the secondary diagnosis.

Sequencing

Example

Patient presents for immunotherapy for a malignant, primary neoplasm of the trigone of the bladder. Report:

- Z51.12 (Immunotherapy)
- C67.0 (Malignant neoplasm of trigone of bladder)

If the encounter is for the management and treatment of a complication associated with a neoplasm, the first-listed diagnosis is the complication with additional code(s) to report the neoplasm.

Sequencing

Example

A patient with a malignant, primary neoplasm of the pylorus has been receiving chemotherapy and develops dehydration as a side effect of the chemotherapy. The encounter is only for treatment of the dehydration. Report:

- Complication: E86.0 (Dehydration)
- Adverse effect: T45.1X5A (Adverse effect of antineoplastic)
- Neoplasm: C16.4 (Malignant neoplasm of pylorus)

ICD-10 OFFICIAL GUIDELINES FOR CODING AND REPORTING

SECTION I.C.

2.c. Coding and sequencing of complications

1) Anemia associated with malignancy

When admission/encounter is for management of an anemia associated with the malignancy, and the treatment is only for anemia, the appropriate code for the malignancy is sequenced as the principal or first-listed diagnosis followed by the appropriate code for the anemia (such as code D63.0, Anemia in neoplastic disease).

2) Anemia associated with chemotherapy, immunotherapy and radiation therapy

When the admission/encounter is for management of an anemia associated with an adverse effect of the administration of chemotherapy or immunotherapy and the only treatment is for the anemia, the anemia code is sequenced first followed by the appropriate codes for the neoplasm and the adverse effect (T45.1X5, Adverse effect of antineoplastic and immunosuppressive drugs).

When the admission/encounter is for management of an anemia associated with an adverse effect of radiotherapy, the anemia code should be sequenced first, followed by the appropriate neoplasm code and code Y84.2, Radiological procedure and radiotherapy as the cause of abnormal reaction of the patient, or of later complication, without mention of misadventure at the time of the procedure.

According to the Guidelines, when an encounter is for anemia associated with a malignant neoplasm, and the treatment is only for the anemia, report "anemia in neoplastic disease" with D63.0 secondary to the neoplasm code. This supports the note that follows D63.0, which states to "Code first neoplasm (C00-D49)."

Tabular:
    D63   Anemia in chronic diseases classified elsewhere
    D63.0   Anemia in neoplastic disease
        Code first neoplasm (C00-D49)

Anemia

Example

A patient with a malignant, primary neoplasm of the pylorus has been receiving chemotherapy and develops aplastic anemia from the chemotherapy. The encounter is only for treatment of the anemia. Report:

- Complication: D61.1 Drug-induced aplastic anemia
- Adverse effect: T45.1X5A (Adverse effect of antineoplastic)
- Neoplasm: C16.4 (Malignant neoplasm of pylorus)

If, however, the encounter is only for the management of the neoplasm, report the malignancy first.

   If, during the encounter for the chemotherapy, the patient develops a side effect, such as nausea, report a code from category Z51 as the first-listed followed by a code(s) for the malignancy and a code for the adverse effect of antineoplastic drug, and a code for the nausea.

History of Z Codes. A code from category Z85 reports a personal history of malignant neoplasm. These history codes report a malignant neoplasm that has been excised or eradicated and is no longer present. Be careful in determining whether the physician is indicating a personal past and current history of the malignancy or a true personal past history.

   As long as the neoplasm is being treated with adjunctive therapy (another treatment used in conjunction with the primary treatment, for example, chemotherapy, radiotherapy, medication) following surgical removal of the cancer (primary treatment), report the neoplasm as if it still exists. You would not assign a "history of" Z code because the neoplasm is the reason for the treatment. Instead, the neoplasm is reported as a current or active disease.

EXERCISE 5-3   *Neoplasm Codes*

Assign diagnosis codes to the following:

1 A patient is admitted for chemotherapy for primary ovarian cancer. Two codes are needed for this case: one for the encounter for chemotherapy and the other for the malignant, primary, ovarian neoplasm.

   Codes: _____, _____

2 A patient is admitted for radiation therapy for metastatic bone cancer. The patient had a mastectomy for breast cancer 3 years earlier. There is a code for the admission for management of the radiation therapy, a code to report the secondary neoplasm, and a code for the personal history of a malignant neoplasm of the breast.

   Codes: _____, _____, _____

3 A patient is admitted with chest pain, shortness of breath, and a history of bloody sputum. Diagnostic x-ray film shows a mass in the bronchial tube. A diagnostic bronchoscopy is performed and is positive for cancer. The pathology report states "metastatic carcinoma of bronchus, primary unknown." The patient chooses to undergo chemotherapy.

   a What is the description of the first-listed diagnosis? _____

   b What is the subsequent diagnosis description? _____

Continued

c Is the metastatic carcinoma of the bronchus a primary or secondary malignant neoplasm?

_____

d What are the diagnosis codes for this case?

Codes: _____ , _____

4 A patient is admitted with uncontrolled nausea and vomiting after chemotherapy treatment for lung cancer.

a How many codes would be needed to accurately report this case? _____

b What is the first-listed diagnosis? _____ Code for first-listed DX:_____

c What is the code for the adverse effect? _____ Code for adverse effect:_____

d What is the secondary diagnosis? _____ Code for secondary DX: _____

5 Anemia due to gastric cancer

Codes: _____ , _____

(Answers are located in Appendix B)

Unknown or Unspecified Site. If there is a **known** secondary site, a code must be assigned to the primary site or the history of a primary site. It is possible for the primary site to be unknown and the secondary site to be known.

Example

Diagnosis: Metastatic bone cancer

This statement indicates that the bone cancer is a secondary neoplasm, but there is no indication of the location of the primary site.

Neoplasm
Table: bone C79.51 (Secondary)
              unknown primary site or unspecified C80

Tabular: **C79.5   Secondary malignant neoplasm of bone and bone marrow**

              C79.51   Secondary malignant neoplasm of bone

Tabular: **C80   Malignant neoplasm without specification of site**

              C80.1   Malignant neoplasm, unspecified

Codes: C79.51, C80.1 Metastatic bone cancer (if the treatment is for the secondary site)

              C80.1, C79.51 Metastatic bone cancer (if the treatment or diagnostic workup is for the primary site)

The sequencing of the primary and secondary neoplasms is dependent on the treatment circumstances documented in the health record. If treatment was directed toward the secondary malignancy, the code for the secondary malignancy would be sequenced first. If treatment was focused on determining the site of the unknown primary malignancy, the code for the unknown primary site would be sequenced first.

EXERCISE 5-4   *More Neoplasms*

Assign I-10 codes for the following neoplasms:

1 Multiple myeloma

Code: _____

2 Carcinoma in situ, cervix

Code: _____

3 Cancer of the sigmoid colon with spread to the peritoneum

Codes: _____, _____

4 Adenocarcinoma of the prostate with metastasis to the bone

Codes: _____, _____

5 Metastatic cancer to the brain; primary unknown (treatment directed to metastatic site)

Codes: _____, _____

6 Metastatic carcinoma of the breast to the lungs; the breast carcinoma has been removed by mastectomy

Codes: _____, _____

7 Mr. Jensen is status post colon resection 3 months ago for sigmoid colon cancer and is now admitted for adjunct chemotherapy.

Codes: _____, _____

(Answers are located in Appendix B)

DISEASES OF THE BLOOD AND BLOOD-FORMING ORGANS AND CERTAIN DISORDERS INVOLVING THE IMMUNE MECHANISM

Chapter 3, Diseases of the Blood and Blood-Forming Organs and Certain Disorders Involving the Immune Mechanism, in the I-10 contains codes in the range of D50-D89, as illustrated in Fig. 5-4.

D50-D53	Nutritional anemias
D55-D59	Hemolytic anemias
D60-D64	Aplastic and other anemias and other bone marrow failure syndromes
D65-D69	Coagulation defects, purpura and other hemorrhagic conditions
D70-D77	Other disorders of blood and blood-forming organs
D78	Intraoperative and postprocedural complications of the spleen
D80-D89	Certain disorders involving the immune mechanism

FIGURE 5-4   Blocks in I-10, Chapter 3, Diseases of the Blood and Blood Forming Organs and Certain Disorders Involving the Immune Mechanism (D50-D89).

Anemia

The **anemia** codes (D50-D64) are often reported diagnosis codes because anemia is a common blood disease. Anemia is the main term under which you will find the many subterms that relate to anemia. In addition to there being numerous subterms for anemia, many of those subterms have lengthy additional subterms listed, as illustrated in Fig. 5-5.

There are two anemias that are easy to confuse—anemia of chronic disease and chronic simple anemia. These two diagnostic statements do not have the same meaning. In anemia of chronic disease, the word "chronic" describes the nature of the disease that is the cause of the anemia—for example, anemia due to neoplastic disease. The neoplasm is the chronic disease causing the anemia. If anemia was the reason for the encounter, report anemia in neoplastic disease (D63.0) and then assign the appropriate code to report the neoplasm. In the diagnostic statement chronic, simple anemia, the word "chronic" describes simple anemia. Let's see what difference these diagnostic statements make in code assignment.

```
Anemia (essential) (general) (hemoglobin
      deficiency) (infantile) (primary)
      (profound) D64.9
   with (due to) (in)
      disorder of
         anaerobic glycolysis D55.2
         pentose phosphate pathway D55.1
      koilonychia D50.9
   achlorachydric D50.8
   achrestic D53.1
   Addison (-Biermer) (pernicious) D51.0
   agranulocytic —see Agranulocytosis
   amino-acid-deficiency D53.0
   aplastic D61.9
      congenital D61.09
      drug-induced D61.1
      due to
         drugs D61.1
         external agents NEC D61.2
         infection D61.2
         radiation D61.2
      idiopathic D61.3
      red cell (pure) D60.9
         chronic D60.0
         congenital D61.01
         specified type NEC D60.8
         transient D60.1
      specified type NEC D61.89
      toxic D61.2
   aregenerative
      congenital D61.09
   asiderotic D50.9
   atypical (primary) D64.9
   Baghdad spring D55.0
   Balantidium coli A07.0
   Biermer's (pernicious) D51.0
   blood loss (chronic) D50.0
      acute D62
```

FIGURE 5–5 Anemia subterms in I-10 Index.

Anemia

Example 1

Diagnosis: Anemia of chronic disease

In this diagnosis statement, you do not know what the chronic disease is.

Index: **Anemia**
            due to (in) (with)
            chronic disease classified elsewhere NEC D63.8

Tabular: **D63   Anemia in chronic diseases classified elsewhere**
                D63.8   Anemia in other chronic diseases classified elsewhere

Code: D63.8 Anemia of chronic disease

If there is any question about the classification of the anemia, check with the physician.

Anemia

Example 2

Diagnosis: Chronic simple anemia
Index: **Anemia D64.9**, chronic simple D53.9

In this example, the Index does indicate a subterm that further directs you to chronic simple D53.9.

Tabular: **D53.9   Nutritional anemia, unspecified**
                Simple chronic anemia

Code: D53.9   Chronic simple anemia

Coagulation Defects, Purpura, and Other Hemorrhagic Conditions

Codes in the range D65-D69 report coagulation defects (such as defibrination syndrome and hemophilia). Many of these coagulation defects are congenital conditions, such as Von Willebrand's disease, but there are also acquired coagulation defects, such as those caused by anticoagulant therapies (warfarin, heparin). Some conditions can be either congenital or acquired, such as primary thrombophilia, also known as primary hypercoagulable state. Extensive terms that are included in the code description are common in these code blocks, as illustrated in Fig. 5-6.

D68.2   Hereditary deficiency of other clotting factors
*Blood clotting disorders caused by hereditary
deficiencies of one or more clotting factors*
AC globulin deficiency
Congenital afibrinogenemia
Deficiency of factor I [fibrinogen]
Deficiency of factor II [prothrombin]
Deficiency of factor V [labile]
Deficiency of factor VII [stable]
Deficiency of factor X [Stuart-Prower]
Deficiency of factor XII [Hageman]
Deficiency of factor XIII [fibrin stabilizing]
Dysfibrinogenemia (congenital)
Hypoproconvertinemia
Owren's disease
Proaccelerin deficiency

FIGURE 5-6   Terms following code description in I-10.

Other Disorders of Blood and Blood-Forming Organs (D70-D77)

The conditions in the D70-D77 blocks report blood disorders, such as neutropenia, eosinophilia, elevated white blood count, and diseases of the spleen. Category D72 reports disorders of the white blood cells, such as lymphocytopenia, basophilia, and other abnormal leukocytes. Category D78 reports intraoperative and postprocedural complications of the spleen, such as hemorrhage, hematoma, puncture, laceration, and other complications. Codes in the D80-D89 range reports immune disorders, such as hereditary antibody defects and deficiencies that are associated with other major defects (Wiskott-Aldrich syndrome, Di George's syndrome, etc.).

EXERCISE 5-5   *Diseases of the Blood and Blood-Forming Organs*

Assign codes for the following:

1 Pernicious, congenital, anemia

Code: _____

2 Acquired afibrinogenemia

Code: _____

3 Hemophilia A

Code: _____

4 Acute blood-loss anemia

Code: _____

5 Benign familial polycythemia

Code: _____

(Answers are located in Appendix B)

ENDOCRINE, NUTRITIONAL, AND METABOLIC DISEASES

ICD-10 OFFICIAL GUIDELINES FOR CODING AND REPORTING

SECTION I.C.4.

Chapter 4: Endocrine, Nutritional, and Metabolic Diseases (E00-E89)

a. Diabetes mellitus

The diabetes mellitus codes are combination codes that include the type of diabetes mellitus, the body system affected, and the complications affecting that body system. As many codes within a particular category as are necessary to describe all of the complications of the disease may be used. They should be sequenced based on the reason for a particular encounter. Assign as many codes from categories E08 – E13 as needed to identify all of the associated conditions that the patient has.

1) Type of diabetes

The age of a patient is not the sole determining factor, though most type 1 diabetics develop the condition before reaching puberty. For this reason type 1 diabetes mellitus is also referred to as juvenile diabetes.

2) Type of diabetes mellitus not documented

If the type of diabetes mellitus is not documented in the medical record the default is E11.-, Type 2 diabetes mellitus.

Continued

3) Diabetes mellitus and the use of insulin

If the documentation in a medical record does not indicate the type of diabetes but does indicate that the patient uses insulin, code E11, Type 2 diabetes mellitus, should be assigned. Code Z79.4, Long-term (current) use of insulin, should also be assigned to indicate that the patient uses insulin. Code Z79.4 should not be assigned if insulin is given temporarily to bring a type 2 patient's blood sugar under control during an encounter.

4) Diabetes mellitus in pregnancy and gestational diabetes

See Section I.C.15. Diabetes mellitus in pregnancy.

See Section I.C.15. Gestational (pregnancy induced) diabetes

5) Complications due to insulin pump malfunction

(a) Underdose of insulin due to insulin pump failure

An underdose of insulin due to an insulin pump failure should be assigned to a code from subcategory T85.6, Mechanical complication of other specified internal and external prosthetic devices, implants and grafts, that specifies the type of pump malfunction, as the principal or first-listed code, followed by code T38.3X6-, Underdosing of insulin and oral hypoglycemic [antidiabetic] drugs. Additional codes for the type of diabetes mellitus and any associated complications due to the underdosing should also be assigned.

(b) Overdose of insulin due to insulin pump failure

The principal or first-listed code for an encounter due to an insulin pump malfunction resulting in an overdose of insulin, should also be T85.6-, Mechanical complication of other specified internal and external prosthetic devices, implants and grafts, followed by code T38.3X1-, Poisoning by insulin and oral hypoglycemic [antidiabetic] drugs, accidental (unintentional).

Chapter 4 in the Tabular of the I-10 describes diseases or conditions affecting the endocrine system. The blocks in Chapter 4 are displayed in Fig. 5-7. The endocrine system involves glands that are located throughout the body and are responsible for secreting hormones into the bloodstream.

Frequently used codes in Chapter 4 are E08-E13, Diabetes mellitus. The diabetes mellitus codes are combination codes that include the type of diabetes mellitus as well as any complications due to diabetes. When you locate "Diabetes" in the Index, you will note that

E00-E07	Disorders of thyroid gland
E08-E13	Diabetes mellitus
E15-E16	Other disorders of glucose regulation and pancreatic internal secretion
E20-E35	Disorders of other endocrine glands
E36	Intraoperative complications of endocrine system
E40-E46	Malnutrition
E50-E64	Other nutritional deficiencies
E65-E68	Overweight, obesity and other hyperalimentation
E70-E88	Metabolic disorders
E89	Postprocedural endocrine and metabolic complications and disorders, not elsewhere classified

FIGURE 5-7 Blocks in the I-10, Chapter 4, Endocrine, Nutritional, and Metabolic Diseases (E00-E90).

Example

Diagnosis:	Type 1 diabetes mellitus with retinopathy with macular edema
Index:	**Diabetes**, type 1, with, retinopathy, with macular edema E10.311
Tabular:	**E10 Type 1 diabetes mellitus**

E10.3   Type 1 diabetes mellitus with ophthalmic complications

E10.31   Type 1 diabetes mellitus with unspecified diabetic retinopathy

E10.311   Type 1 diabetes mellitus with unspecified diabetic retinopathy with macular edema

there are many subterms that must be carefully reviewed before referencing the code in the Tabular.

The health care providers usually document the type of diabetes mellitus. You should not assume that because a patient is receiving insulin that he or she is a type 1 diabetic because a type 2 diabetic may also receive insulin. Type 1 diabetes usually develops before the patient reaches puberty and for that reason, type 1 is also referred to as juvenile diabetes as indicated in Fig. 5-8.

If the type of diabetes is not stated in the documentation, query the physician or assign a default code for type 2 diabetes mellitus (E11.-). Note in Fig. 5-9 that the Includes note following E11 indicates that the code includes "diabetes NOS." If the medical documentation does not indicate the type of diabetes but does indicate that the patient is currently using insulin, you also report E11.- . If the documentation indicates that the patient has been routinely using insulin, assign Z79.4 to report the current long-term use of insulin. You would not report Z79.4 if the patient was given insulin on a temporary basis, such as to bring the blood sugar under control during an encounter.

An insulin pump is used to administer insulin to a diabetic, as shown in Fig. 5-10. It may malfunction and provide an underdose or overdose of insulin. The malfunction is a complication and is reported with three codes—one to report the mechanical complication, one to report an underdose or overdose, and one to report the patient's type of diabetes mellitus.

● **E10   Type 1 diabetes mellitus**

Includes	brittle diabetes (mellitus)
	diabetes (mellitus) due to autoimmune process
	diabetes (mellitus) due to immune mediated pancreatic islet beta-cell destruction
	idiopathic diabetes (mellitus)
	juvenile onset diabetes (mellitus)
	ketosis-prone diabetes (mellitus)
Excludes1	diabetes mellitus due to underlying condition (E08.-)
	drug or chemical induced diabetes mellitus (E09.-)
	gestational diabetes (O24.4-)
	hyperglycemia NOS (R73.9)
	neonatal diabetes mellitus (P70.2)
	postpancreatectomy diabetes mellitus (E13.-)
	postprocedural diabetes mellitus (E13.-)
	secondary diabetes mellitus NEC (E13.-)
	type 2 diabetes mellitus (E11.-)

FIGURE 5–8   Type 1 diabetes mellitus is reported with E10 codes.

● **E11   Type 2 diabetes mellitus**

Includes   diabetes (mellitus) due to insulin secretory defect
diabetes NOS
insulin resistant diabetes (mellitus)

Use additional code to identify any insulin use (Z79.4)

Excludes 1   diabetes mellitus due to underlying condition
(E08.-)
drug or chemical induced diabetes mellitus
(E09.-)
gestational diabetes (O24.4-)
neonatal diabetes mellitus (P70.2)
postpancreatectomy diabetes mellitus (E13.-)
postprocedural diabetes mellitus (E13.-)
secondary diabetes mellitus NEC (E13.-)
type 1 diabetes mellitus (E10.-)

FIGURE 5–9   Default code for diabetes not otherwise specified—E11, Type 2 diabetes mellitus.

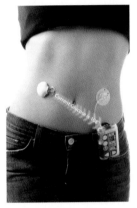

FIGURE 5–10   Insulin pump used to administer insulin.

Example

Underdose

T85.6-	Mechanical complication of the pump (first-listed diagnosis)
T38.3X6-	Underdosing of insulin
E11.- -	Type 2 diabetes mellitus

Example

Overdose

T85.6-	Mechanical complication of the pump (first-listed diagnosis)
T38.3X1-	Unintentional poisoning by insulin
E11.- -	Type 2 diabetes mellitus

If the underdosing or overdosing created additional complications, these complications are also reported.

EXERCISE 5-6 *Endocrine, Nutritional, and Metabolic Diseases*

Fill in the codes for the following:

1 Addison's disease

Code: _____

2 Dehydration

Code: _____

3 Diabetes mellitus with hypoglycemic coma

Code: _____

4 Graves' disease with thyrotoxic crisis

Code: _____

5 Chronic Diabetic foot ulcer (diabetic peripheral angiopathy, no gangrene), in patient with diabetes mellitus, type 1, out of control

Codes: _____, _____, _____, _____

6 Malnutrition

Code: _____

(Answers are located in Appendix B)

MENTAL, BEHAVIORAL AND NEURODEVELOPMENTAL DISORDERS

Chapter 5 in the Tabular of the I-10 is Mental, Behavioral and Neurodevelopmental Disorders. The blocks in this chapter are displayed in Fig. 5-11.

Your understanding of the definitions of these mental disorders is necessary to code accurately. When assigning codes from Chapter 5, you need to take extra care to select the appropriate code(s) and report only those diagnoses that are documented in the medical record. Mental disorders can be difficult to code because physicians are not always as specific in the diagnostic statements as might be required by the codes in the I-10 chapter. When in

F01-F09	Mental disorders due to known physiological conditions
F10-F19	Mental and behavioral disorders due to psychoactive substance use
F20-F29	Schizophrenia, schizotypal, delusional, and other non-mood psychotic disorders
F30-F39	Mood [affective] disorders
F40-F48	Anxiety, dissociative, stress-related, somatoform and other nonpsychotic mental disorders
F50-F59	Behavioral syndromes associated with physiological disturbances and physical factors
F60-F69	Disorders of adult personality and behavior
F70-F79	Intellectual disabilities
F80-F89	Pervasive and specific developmental disorders
F90-F98	Behavioral and emotional disorders with onset usually occurring in childhood and adolescence
F99	Unspecified mental disorder

FIGURE 5–11 Blocks in I-10, Chapter 5, Mental, Behavioral and Neurodevelopmental Disorders (F01-F99).

doubt, always check with the physician. Just one term in the medical record can make a big difference in the code(s) you assign.

Mental disorders in the I-10 are grouped based on the etiology in cerebral disease, brain injury, or other injury leading to the cerebral dysfunction. These dysfunctions may be a result of disease, injury, or secondary, such as in a systemic disease or disorder that affects the brain as one of multiple organs.

Dementia

Dementias are reported based on whether the dementia is documented to be vascular (F01), classified elsewhere (F02), or unspecified type (F03). There is a "Code first the underlying physiological condition . . ." at both F01 and F02, directing the coder to report the condition or sequela that resulted in the dementia first. The underlying condition (etiology) is listed first, followed by the dementia code.

Dementia

Example
The medical record indicates that the patient has Alzheimer's disease with early onset (G30.0) that resulted in dementia without behavioral disturbances (F02.80)—report G30.0, F02.80.

The Excludes1 note following F02, Dementia in other diseases classified elsewhere, gives direction to the coder to NEVER report G31.83, Dementia with Parkinsonism, with F02. This Excludes1 note is used when two conditions cannot occur together, such as a congenital or acquired condition—it can only be one or the other, not both. The same is true for G31.83, which reports dementia **with** Parkinsonism—you cannot report dementia twice. The combination code G31.83 reports the dementia and the Parkinsonism in one code. The Excludes2 note indicates what is not included in the code. The Excludes2 at F02 states that vascular dementia (F01.5) is not a part of the condition and that it is possible for the patient to have both dementia (F02.8-) and vascular dementia (F01.5-), and it is acceptable to assign both codes. There are many Excludes1 and Excludes2 notes throughout Chapter 5 of the I-10.

Substance Use

The category to report alcohol-related disorders or dependence is F10, and the codes are selected based on if the condition is documented to be alcohol abuse, dependence, dependence with withdrawal, or unspecified use. F10 may be assigned with Y90.-, Evidence of alcohol involvement determined by blood alcohol level, based on the documentation level in the medical record. The levels are displayed in Fig. 5-12. Take a moment now to review the codes in the F11-F19 range used to report opioids, cannabis, sedatives, cocaine, stimulants, hallucinogens, nicotine, and others.

Psychological Disorders

Codes F20-F29 report schizophrenia, schizotypal (social isolation and odd behaviors), delusional, and other non-mood psychotic disorders. Codes F30-F39 report mood and

> ● **Y90**   **Evidence of alcohol involvement determined by blood alcohol level**
>
>   *Code first* any associated alcohol related disorders (F10)
>
> **Y90.0**   Blood alcohol level of less than 20 mg/100 ml
>
> **Y90.1**   Blood alcohol level of 20-39 mg/100 ml
>
> **Y90.2**   Blood alcohol level of 40-59 mg/100 ml
>
> **Y90.3**   Blood alcohol level of 60-79 mg/100 ml
>
> **Y90.4**   Blood alcohol level of 80-99 mg/100 ml
>
> **Y90.5**   Blood alcohol level of 100-119 mg/100 ml
>
> **Y90.6**   Blood alcohol level of 120-199 mg/100 ml
>
> **Y90.7**   Blood alcohol level of 200-239 mg/100 ml
>
> **Y90.8**   Blood alcohol level of 240 mg/100 ml or more
>
> **Y90.9**   Presence of alcohol in blood, level not specified

FIGURE 5–12   Supplementary codes to report blood alcohol level.

non-mood disorders. Mood disorders are also known as affective disorders with the main characteristic of disturbance in mood, most commonly anxiety, depression, and bipolar disorders. Codes F40-F99 report phobias, obsessive-compulsive disorders, adjustment disorders, amnesias, hypochondrias (health anxiety), mental retardation, etc. There are many Excludes notes throughout these codes and conditions that are or are not included when reporting the codes.

ICD-10 OFFICIAL GUIDELINES FOR CODING AND REPORTING

SECTION I.C.5.

Chapter 5: Mental, Behavioral and Neurodevelopmental disorders (F01 – F99)

a. Pain disorders related to psychological factors

Assign code F45.41, for pain that is exclusively related to psychological disorders. As indicated by the Excludes 1 note under category G89, a code from category G89 should not be assigned with code F45.41

Code F45.42, Pain disorders with related psychological factors, should be used with a code from category G89, Pain, not elsewhere classified, if there is documentation of a psychological component for a patient with acute or chronic pain.

See Section I.C.6. Pain

Psychological Pain

Pain that is exclusively psychological is reported with F45.41, Pain disorder with related psychological factors. This code may also be assigned in conjunction with a code from the category G89, Pain, NEC, if there is a psychological component to the pain.

EXERCISE 5-7   *Mental, Behavioral and Neurodevelopmental Disorders*

Now you have a chance to show your skill by coding the following:

1 Alzheimer's dementia with aggressive behavior

Codes: _____, _____

2 Depression with anxiety

Code: _____

3 Profound mental retardation

Code: _____

4 Anorexia nervosa

Code: _____

5 Delirium tremens due to withdrawal in alcohol-dependent patient

Code: _____

6 Withdrawal from heroin dependence, daily use

Code: _____

(Answers are located in Appendix B)

DISEASES OF THE NERVOUS SYSTEM

Chapter 6 of the Tabular I-10 is Diseases of the Nervous System and describes diseases or conditions affecting the central nervous system and the peripheral nervous system. Fig. 5-13 displays Chapter 6 blocks.

The chapter contains some combination codes in which one code identifies both the manifestation and the etiology.

G00-G09	Inflammatory diseases of the central nervous system
G10-G14	Systemic atrophies primarily affecting the central nervous system
G20-G26	Extrapyramidal and movement disorders
G30-G32	Other degenerative diseases of the nervous system
G35-G37	Demyelinating diseases of the central nervous system
G40-G47	Episodic and paroxysmal disorders
G50-G59	Nerve, nerve root and plexus disorders
G60-G65	Polyneuropathies and other disorders of the peripheral nervous system
G70-G73	Diseases of myoneural junction and muscle
G80-G83	Cerebral palsy and other paralytic syndromes
G89-G99	Other disorders of the nervous system

FIGURE 5-13   Blocks in I-10, Chapter 6, Diseases of the Nervous System (G00-G99).

Combination Codes

Example

Diagnosis: Pneumococcal meningitis

This diagnostic statement means the meningitis is due to pneumococcal bacteria.

Index: **Meningitis,** pneumococcal G00.1
Tabular: **G00   Bacterial meningitis, not elsewhere classified**
                      G00.1   Pneumococcal meningitis
Code: G00.1 Pneumococcal meningitis

Code G00.1 includes the manifestation of meningitis and also the etiology of pneumococcal organism. No separate code is required to report the organism in this diagnostic statement.

In Chapter 6 of the I-10, you will also locate conditions that are manifestations of other diseases.

Manifestations

Example

Diagnosis: Rheumatoid neuritis with localized amyloidosis
Index: **Neuritis (rheumatoid)** M79.2; amyloid, any site E85.4 [G63]

Entries such as E85.4 [G63] instruct you to report the neuritis [E85.4] first, followed by the polyneuropathy in disease classified elsewhere [G63]. Both codes need to be verified in the Tabular.

Tabular: **G63   Polyneuropathy in diseases classified elsewhere**
Tabular: **E85   Amyloidosis**
                      E85.4   Organ-limited amyloidosis
                            Localized amyloidosis
Codes: E85.4, G63 Rheumatoid neuritis with localized amyloidosis

Pain (Non-Psychological)

ICD-10 OFFICIAL GUIDELINES FOR CODING AND REPORTING

SECTION I.C.6.
Chapter 6: Diseases of Nervous System (G00-G99)

b. Pain - Category G89

1) General coding information

Codes in category G89, Pain, not elsewhere classified, may be used in conjunction with codes from other categories and chapters to provide more detail about acute or chronic pain and neoplasm-related pain, unless otherwise indicated below.

If the pain is not specified as acute or chronic, post-thoracotomy, postprocedural, or neoplasm-related, do not assign codes from category G89.

A code from category G89 should not be assigned if the underlying (definitive) diagnosis is known, unless the reason for the encounter is pain control/management and not management of the underlying condition.

When an admission or encounter is for a procedure aimed at treating the underlying condition (e.g., spinal fusion, kyphoplasty), a code for the underlying condition (e.g., vertebral

Continued

fracture, spinal stenosis) should be assigned as the principal diagnosis. No code from category G89 should be assigned.

(a) **Category G89 Codes as Principal or First-Listed Diagnosis**

Category G89 codes are acceptable as principal diagnosis or the first-listed code:

- When pain control or pain management is the reason for the admission/encounter (e.g., a patient with displaced intervertebral disc, nerve impingement and severe back pain presents for injection of steroid into the spinal canal). The underlying cause of the pain should be reported as an additional diagnosis, if known.

- When a patient is admitted for the insertion of a neurostimulator for pain control, assign the appropriate pain code as the principal or first-listed diagnosis. When an admission or encounter is for a procedure aimed at treating the underlying condition and a neurostimulator is inserted for pain control during the same admission/encounter, a code for the underlying condition should be assigned as the principal diagnosis and the appropriate pain code should be assigned as a secondary diagnosis.

(b) **Use of Category G89 Codes in Conjunction with Site Specific Pain Codes**

(i) **Assigning Category G89 and Site-Specific Pain Codes**

Codes from category G89 may be used in conjunction with codes that identify the site of pain (including codes from chapter 18) if the category G89 code provides additional information. For example, if the code describes the site of the pain, but does not fully describe whether the pain is acute or chronic, then both codes should be assigned.

(ii) **Sequencing of Category G89 Codes with Site-Specific Pain Codes**

The sequencing of category G89 codes with site-specific pain codes (including chapter 18 codes), is dependent on the circumstances of the encounter/admission as follows:

- If the encounter is for pain control or pain management, assign the code from category G89 followed by the code identifying the specific site of pain (e.g., encounter for pain management for acute neck pain from trauma is assigned code G89.11, Acute pain due to trauma, followed by code M54.2, Cervicalgia, to identify the site of pain).

- If the encounter is for any other reason except pain control or pain management, and a related definitive diagnosis has not been established (confirmed) by the provider, assign the code for the specific site of pain first, followed by the appropriate code from category G89.

2) Pain due to devices, implants and grafts

See Section I.C.19. Pain due to medical devices

3) Postoperative Pain

The provider's documentation should be used to guide the coding of postoperative pain, as well as *Section III. Reporting Additional Diagnoses* and *Section IV. Diagnostic Coding and Reporting in the Outpatient Setting.*

The default for post-thoracotomy and other postoperative pain not specified as acute or chronic is the code for the acute form.

Routine or expected postoperative pain immediately after surgery should not be coded.

(a) **Postoperative pain not associated with specific postoperative complication**

Postoperative pain not associated with a specific postoperative complication is assigned to the appropriate postoperative pain code in category G89.

Continued

(b) **Postoperative pain associated with specific postoperative complication**

Postoperative pain associated with a specific postoperative complication (such as painful wire sutures) is assigned to the appropriate code(s) found in Chapter 19, Injury, poisoning, and certain other consequences of external causes. If appropriate, use additional code(s) from category G89 to identify acute or chronic pain (G89.18 or G89.28).

4) **Chronic pain**

Chronic pain is classified to subcategory G89.2. There is no time frame defining when pain becomes chronic pain. The provider's documentation should be used to guide use of these codes.

5) **Neoplasm Related Pain**

Code G89.3 is assigned to pain documented as being related, associated or due to cancer, primary or secondary malignancy, or tumor. This code is assigned regardless of whether the pain is acute or chronic.

This code may be assigned as the principal or first-listed code when the stated reason for the admission/encounter is documented as pain control/pain management. The underlying neoplasm should be reported as an additional diagnosis.

When the reason for the admission/encounter is management of the neoplasm and the pain associated with the neoplasm is also documented, code G89.3 may be assigned as an additional diagnosis. It is not necessary to assign an additional code for the site of the pain.

See Section I.C.2 for instructions on the sequencing of neoplasms for all other stated reasons for the admission/encounter (except for pain control/pain management).

6) **Chronic pain syndrome**

Central pain syndrome (G89.0) and chronic pain syndrome (G89.4) are different than the term "chronic pain," and therefore codes should only be used when the provider has specifically documented this condition.

See Section I.C.5. Pain disorders related to psychological factors

There are many codes to report localized pain throughout the I-10 by coding the pain to the specific site of the pain.

EXAMPLE SITE-SPECIFIC PAIN CODES

- chest pain (R07.1-R07.9)
- ear pain (H92.0-)
- eye pain (H57.1-)
- headache (R51)
- joint pain (M25.5-)
- limb pain (M79.6-)
- lumbar region pain (M54.5)
- pelvic and perineal pain (R10.2)
- shoulder pain (M25.51-)
- spine pain (M54.-)
- throat pain (R07.0)
- tongue pain (K14.6)

Category R52 reports unspecified pain that is acute, chronic, generalized, or not otherwise specified. Acute (G89.0/G89.1) or chronic (G89.2), post-thoracotomy, post-procedural, or neoplasm-related (G89.3) pain that does not have a more specific code is reported with a code from category G89. The default for post-thoracotomy and other post-procedural pain is "acute pain." You do not report routine post-procedural pain because that pain is a usual and expected condition. The G89 category code can be reported with the site-specific pain codes, if the assignment of G89 adds additional information. For example, if a site-specific code was reported but that code did not indicate if the pain was acute or chronic, both the site-specific code and a code from category G89 are reported.

If the underlying reason for the pain is known, the more specific pain code should be assigned, such as tongue pain, K14.6, or spine pain, M54.0-, rather than a general pain code.

If the reason for the encounter is solely for management of **pain** with no treatment or management of the underlying condition, the G89 code is the first-listed. If known, additional codes are assigned for the underlying cause of the pain. If the patient presents only for treatment of the **underlying** condition and no treatment or management was provided for pain, the underlying condition is the first-listed diagnosis and no pain code is assigned.

Some patients have chronic pain, such as chronic back, leg, or arm pain. One treatment option for conditions that result in chronic pain is a neurostimulator, which is an implantable device that delivers electrical energy directly to the nerve fibers and blocks the pain sensation from reaching the brain. When an encounter is for the insertion of a neurostimulator, report the pain as the first-listed diagnosis. When the insertion is for the treatment of the underlying condition, report the underlying condition as the first-listed diagnosis.

Dominant and Nondominant Sides

ICD-10 OFFICIAL GUIDELINES FOR CODING AND REPORTING

SECTION I.C.6.

Chapter 6: Diseases of Nervous System (G00-G99)

a. Dominant/nondominant side

Codes from category G81, Hemiplegia and hemiparesis, and subcategories, G83.1, Monoplegia of lower limb, G83.2, Monoplegia of upper limb, and G83.3, Monoplegia, unspecified, identify whether the dominant or nondominant side is affected. Should the affected side be documented, but not specified as dominant or nondominant, and the classification system does not indicate a default, code selection is as follows:

- For ambidextrous patients, the default should be dominant.
- If the left side is affected, the default is non-dominant.
- If the right side is affected, the default is dominant.

Codes in categories G81, Hemiplegia and hemiparesis, and G83, Other paralytic syndromes, are reported based on if the plegia (paralysis) is of the patient's dominant side. If the medical record does not indicate if the patient is left-hand or right-hand dominant, report the condition as occurring on the dominant side if the paralysis is on the right side. If the patient is ambidextrous (both left- and right-handed), report the default of dominant. These categories of codes are assigned when the paralysis is from an unspecified cause. The codes are also assigned in multiple coding to report paralysis from any cause. These codes are not assigned to report congenital cerebral palsy or hemiplegia/hemiparesis that is due to a sequela of cerebrovascular disease.

EXERCISE 5-8 *Diseases of the Nervous System and Sense Organs*

Assign codes for the following:

1 Meningitis due to *Proteus morganii*

Codes: _____, _____

2 Multiple sclerosis

Code: _____

3 Bell's palsy

Code: _____

4 Seizure complex, febrile with status epilepticus

Code: _____

(Answers are located in Appendix B)

DISEASES OF THE EYE AND ADNEXA

Chapter 7 of the I-10 is Diseases of the Eye and Adnexa (H00-H59). The chapter contains the blocks shown in Fig. 5-14.

Note that at the beginning of Chapter 7 of the I-10, there are significant Excludes2 notes indicating all the conditions that are not included in the H00-H59 codes. For example, diabetes mellitus-related eye conditions are reported with E09.3-, E10.3-, E11.3-, and E13.3-. The terminology within Chapter 7 is complex, so a good medical dictionary is a must when reporting services with these H codes.

Figs. 5-15, 5-16, and 5-17 illustrate the structure of the eye, ocular adnexa, eyelid, and lacrimal apparatus.

Hordeolum and Chalazion

Hordeolum is an inflammatory infection of the sebaceous glands at the base of the eyelashes (stye) and if external (externum) is reported with H00.01-, and if internal (internum) is reported with H00.02-. Chalazion is also an infection of the eyelid that forms a mass on the eyelid. These codes (H00.1) are based on location of right or left eye and upper, lower, or unspecified eyelid.

H00-H05	Disorders of eyelid, lacrimal system and orbit
H10-H11	Disorders of conjunctiva
H15-H22	Disorders of sclera, cornea, iris and ciliary body
H25-H28	Disorders of lens
H30-H36	Disorders of choroid and retina
H40-H42	Glaucoma
H43-H44	Disorders of vitreous body and globe
H46-H47	Disorders of optic nerve and visual pathways
H49-H52	Disorders of ocular muscles, binocular movement, accommodation and refraction
H53-H54	Visual disturbances and blindness
H55-H57	Other disorders of eye and adnexa
H59	Intraoperative and postprocedural complications and disorders of eye and adnexa, not elsewhere classified

FIGURE 5-14 Chapter 7, H codes from the I-10.

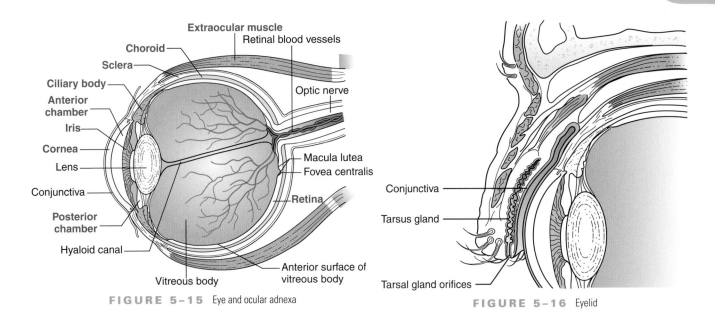

FIGURE 5–15 Eye and ocular adnexa

FIGURE 5–16 Eyelid

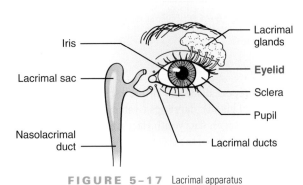

FIGURE 5–17 Lacrimal apparatus

Entropion and Ectropion

Entropion is an inward turning (inversion) of the margin of the eyelid as shown in Fig. 5-18. Entropion can be unspecified (H02.00-), a result of a scar or tightening (cicatricial, H02.01-), mechanical (lack of muscle support, H02.02-), senile (due to aging, H02.03-), or spastic (spasm of muscle, H02.04-). Trichiasis is the ingrowing of hairs of the eyelashes and when present without entropion is reported with H02.05-. **Ectropion** is the pulling away (eversion) of the eyelid as shown in Fig. 5-19, and the codes are divided as the entropion codes are: unspecified (H02.10-), cicatricial (H02.11-), mechanical (H02.12-), senile (H02.13-), or spastic (H02.14-).

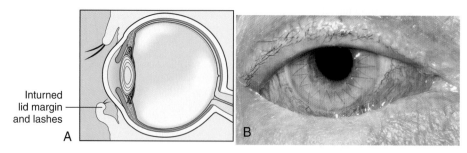

FIGURE 5–18 Entropion is an inward turning of the eyelid. (Note that the patient in B has undergone corneal transplantation.)

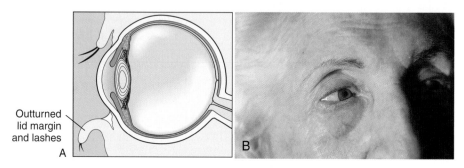

FIGURE 5–19 Ectropion is an outward sagging of the eyelid.

Lacrimal System

Codes to report disorders of the lacrimal system, such as dacryoadenitis (inflammation of the lacrimal gland), dacryops (watery eye), epiphora (overflow of tears due to stricture of the lacrimal passage), dacryolith (lacrimal calculus), are reported with codes from category H04.

The remainder of the codes to report conditions of the eye are divided based on the location, such as orbit, conjunctiva, sclera, cornea, etc.

EXERCISE 5-9 *Eye and Adnexa*

Assign codes for the following:

1 Primary open-angle glaucoma

Code: _____

2 Stenosis of the right lacrimal sac

Code: _____

(Answers are located in Appendix B)

DISEASES OF THE EAR AND MASTOID PROCESS

The blocks in Chapter 8 of the I-10 are displayed in Fig. 5-20.

The codes in the Diseases of the Ear and Mastoid Process are H60-H95 and are divided based on the structure of the ear (external, middle and mastoid, and inner, see Fig. 5-21) and intraoperative/postprocedural complications (H95).

H60-H62	Diseases of external ear
H65-H75	Diseases of middle ear and mastoid
H80-H83	Diseases of inner ear
H90-H94	Other disorders of ear
H95	Intraoperative and postprocedural complications and disorders of ear and mastoid process, not elsewhere classified

FIGURE 5–20   Chapter 8, Ear and Mastoid Process codes from the I-10.

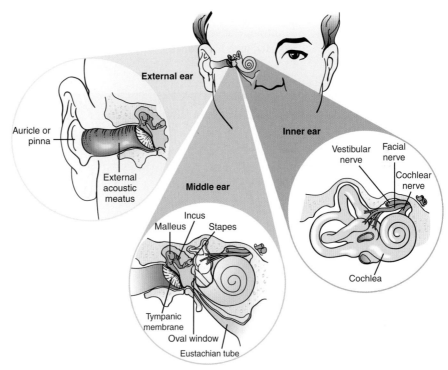

FIGURE 5–21   Auditory System

Ear

External Ear. Conditions of the external ear such as abscess, cellulitis, infection, hematoma, and cholesteatoma (peeling layers of horny epithelium) are reported with categories H60-H62. These codes are based on laterality (right, left, bilateral, unspecified). A common condition reported with these codes is impacted cerumen (ear wax) based on the right, left, bilateral, or unspecified ear (H61.2-).

Middle Ear and Mastoid. Conditions of the middle ear are those such as nonsuppurative otitis media (infection in which clear pale fluid may accumulate), suppurative otitis media (infection with purulent [pus] discharge). If the otitis media is a result of an underlying disease, such as a viral disease, you report the underlying disease first, followed by a code from category H67, Otitis media in diseases classified elsewhere. The Eustachian tubes are part of the middle ear and may become inflamed, infected, or obstructed, and these conditions are reported with H68-H69.

Mastoiditis is an infection of a portion of the temporal bone that is behind the ear (mastoid process) and is caused by an untreated otitis media that results in an infection of the surrounding structures and may even include the brain. Mastoiditis and related conditions are reported with code H70.

Inner Ear. Diseases of the inner ear are reported with codes H80-H83. Otosclerosis is an inherited bone growth that causes hearing loss and is reported with codes H80. Ménière's (H81.-) disease is a vestibular disorder that produces recurring symptoms that include severe and intermittent hearing loss that may include the feeling of ear pressure and pain. The codes are reported based on laterality.

Labyrinthitis is a balance disorder that follows an upper respiratory infection or head injury. The inflammatory process affects the labyrinth that houses the vestibular system of the inner ear. The vestibular system senses changes in head positions.

Intraoperative and postprocedural complications of ear and mastoid process NEC are reported with H95 codes.

EXERCISE 5-10 | *Ear and Mastoid Process*

1 Acute otitis media, right ear

Code: _____

2 Swimmer's ear, left ear

Code: _____

3 Bilateral acute serous otitis media (nonsuppurative)

Code: _____

(Answers are located in Appendix B)

DISEASES OF THE CIRCULATORY SYSTEM

Chapter 9 of the I-10 Tabular, Diseases of the Circulatory System (I00-I99), contains diseases of the heart and blood vessels. The chapter contains the blocks shown in Fig. 5-22.

I00-I02	Acute rheumatic fever
I05-I09	Chronic rheumatic heart diseases
I10-I15	Hypertensive diseases
I20-I25	Ischemic heart diseases
I26-I28	Pulmonary heart disease and diseases of pulmonary circulation
I30-I52	Other forms of heart disease
I60-I69	Cerebrovascular diseases
I70-I79	Diseases of arteries, arterioles and capillaries
I80-I89	Diseases of veins, lymphatic vessels and lymph nodes, not elsewhere classified
I95-I99	Other and unspecified disorders of the circulatory system

FIGURE 5-22 Blocks in I-10, Chapter 9, Diseases of the Circulatory System I00-I99.

ICD-10 OFFICIAL GUIDELINES FOR CODING AND REPORTING

SECTION I.C.9.
Chapter 9: Diseases of the Circulatory System (I00-I99)

a. Hypertension

1) Hypertension with Heart Disease

Heart conditions classified to I50.- or I51.4-I51.9, are assigned to a code from category I11, Hypertensive heart disease, when a causal relationship is stated (due to hypertension) or implied (hypertensive). Use an additional code from category I50, Heart failure, to identify the type of heart failure in those patients with heart failure.

The same heart conditions (I50.-, I51.4-I51.9) with hypertension, but without a stated causal relationship, are coded separately. Sequence according to the circumstances of the admission/encounter.

2) Hypertensive Chronic Kidney Disease

Assign codes from category I12, Hypertensive chronic kidney disease, when both hypertension and a condition classifiable to category N18, Chronic kidney disease (CKD), are present. Unlike hypertension with heart disease, ICD-10-CM presumes a cause-and-effect relationship and classifies chronic kidney disease with hypertension as hypertensive chronic kidney disease.

The appropriate code from category N18 should be used as a secondary code with a code from category I12 to identify the stage of chronic kidney disease.

See Section I.C.14. Chronic kidney disease.

If a patient has hypertensive chronic kidney disease and acute renal failure, an additional code for the acute renal failure is required.

ICD-10 OFFICIAL GUIDELINES FOR CODING AND REPORTING

SECTION I.C.9.
Chapter 9: Diseases of the Circulatory System (I00-I99)

a. Hypertension

4) Hypertensive Cerebrovascular Disease

For hypertensive cerebrovascular disease, first assign the appropriate code from categories I60-I69, followed by the appropriate hypertension code.

5) Hypertensive Retinopathy

Subcategory H35.0, Background retinopathy and retinal vascular changes, should be used with a code from category I10-I15, Hypertensive disease, to include the systemic hypertension. The sequencing is based on the reason for the encounter.

6) Hypertension, Secondary

Secondary hypertension is due to an underlying condition. Two codes are required: one to identify the underlying etiology and one from category I15 to identify the hypertension. Sequencing of codes is determined by the reason for admission/encounter.

7) Hypertension, Transient

Assign code R03.0, Elevated blood pressure reading without diagnosis of hypertension, unless patient has an established diagnosis of hypertension. Assign code O13.-, Gestational [pregnancy-induced] hypertension without significant proteinuria, or O14.-, Pre-eclampsia, for transient hypertension of pregnancy.

Continued

8) Hypertension, Controlled

This diagnostic statement usually refers to an existing state of hypertension under control by therapy. Assign the appropriate code from categories I10-I15, Hypertensive diseases.

9) Hypertension, Uncontrolled

Uncontrolled hypertension may refer to untreated hypertension or hypertension not responding to current therapeutic regimen. In either case, assign the appropriate code from categories I10-I15, Hypertensive diseases.

Hypertension is one of the most common conditions reported with codes from this chapter. The Index contains the Hypertension entry and many levels of subterms. Fig. 5-23 illustrates a portion of the Hypertension entry in the Index.

Hypertension refers to systemic arterial hypertension (high blood pressure) and may be essential (primary) or secondary (due to an underlying condition). **Malignant hypertension** is also known as accelerated hypertension and is a severe form of hypertension, manifested by headaches, blurred vision, dyspnea, and uremia. This type of hypertension usually causes permanent organ damage and has a poor prognosis. **Benign hypertension** is a continuous, mild blood pressure elevation that can usually be controlled by medication. **Unspecified hypertension** has not been specified in the medical record as either benign or malignant.

There is no defined threshold of blood pressure above which an individual is considered hypertensive. Commonly, a sustained diastolic pressure of above 90 mm Hg and a sustained systolic pressure of above 140 mm Hg constitutes hypertension. The physician must document hypertension. A coder cannot report hypertension based solely upon blood pressure readings.

Benign hypertension remains fairly stable over the years and is compatible with a long life, but if untreated it is an important risk factor in coronary heart disease and cerebrovascular disease.

Malignant hypertension is commonly associated with abrupt onset and runs a course measured in months. It causes irreversible organ damage and often ends with renal failure or cerebral hemorrhage. Usually a person with malignant hypertension complains of headaches and vision difficulties, and a blood pressure of 200/140 mm Hg is not uncommon.

Essential hypertension is high blood pressure for which the cause is not known.

Hypertensive heart disease refers to the secondary effects on the heart of prolonged, sustained, systemic hypertension. The heart has to work against increased resistance, and that results in high blood pressure. The primary effect is the thickening of the left ventricle, which eventually may lead to heart failure.

Primary or essential hypertension may be **controlled** (benign) or **uncontrolled** (malignant, untreated, not responding to treatment) and both types are reported with I10. If the hypertension is secondary, report the underlying condition (etiology) with one code and the hypertension with an I15 code. Secondary hypertension is based on if the hypertension is due to renal disorder, endocrine disorder, other secondary hypertension, or unspecified. If the reason for the encounter is due to the hypertension, sequence the hypertension code first followed by the code for the etiology; but, if the encounter is due to etiology, report the etiology first followed by the hypertension code.

Hypertension may last only temporarily (transient), reported with R03.0, Elevated blood pressure reading without diagnosis of hypertension. If the patient has been diagnosed as having high blood pressure, you cannot subsequently assign a transient hypertension code. If the hypertension occurs during and due to pregnancy, assign O13.- or O14.- based on if there is or is not significant proteinuria (large amount of protein in the urine that results from renal disease or other abnormal condition).

Hypertension, hypertensive (accelerated)
        (benign) (essential) (idiopathic)
        (malignant) (systemic) I10
    with
        heart involvement (conditions in
                I51.4-I51.9 due to hypertension) —*see*
                Hypertension, heart
        kidney involvement —*see* Hypertension,
                kidney
    benign, intracranial G93.2
    borderline R03.0
    cardiorenal (disease) I13.10
        with heart failure I13.0
            with stage 1 through stage 4 chronic
                kidney disease I13.0
            with stage 5 or end stage renal disease
                I13.2
        without heart failure I13.10
            with stage 1 through stage 4 chronic
                kidney disease I13.10
            with stage 5 or end stage renal disease
                I13.11
    cardiovascular
        disease (arteriosclerotic) (sclerotic) —*see*
                Hypertension, heart
        renal (disease) —*see* Hypertension,
                cardiorenal
    chronic venous —*see* Hypertension, venous
            (chronic)
    complicating
        childbirth (labor) O10.92
            with
                heart disease O10.12
                    with renal disease O10.32
                renal disease O10.22
                    with heart disease O10.32
                essential O10.02
                secondary O10.42
        pregnancy O16.-
            with edema (*see also* Pre-eclampsia) O14.9-
            gestational (pregnancy induced)
                    (transient) (without proteinuria)
                    O13.-
                with proteinuria O14.9-
                    mild pre-eclampsia O14.0-
                    moderate pre-eclampsia O14.0-
                    severe pre-eclampsia O14.1-
                        with hemolysis, elevated liver
                            enzymes and low platelet
                            count (HELLP) O14.2-
            pre-existing O10.91-
                with
                    heart disease O10.11-
                        with renal disease O10.31-
                        pre-eclampsia O11.-
                    renal disease O10.21-
                        with heart disease O10.31-
                    essential O10.01-
                    secondary O10.41-
        puerperium pre-existing O10.93
            with
                heart disease O10.13
                    with renal disease O10.33
                renal disease O10.23
                    with heart disease O10.33
                essential O10.03
                pregnancy-induced O13.9
                secondary O10.43
    due to
        endocrine disorders I15.2
        pheochromocytoma I15.2
        renal disorders NEC I15.1
            arterial I15.0
        renovascular disorders I15.0
        specified disease NEC I15.8
    encephalopathy I67.4
    gestational (without significant proteinuria)
            (pregnancy-induced) (transient) O13.-
        with significant proteinuria —*see*
                Pre-eclampsia
    Goldblatt's I70.1

FIGURE 5–23 Hypertension entry in the I-10.

Kidney Disease and Hypertension

ICD-10 OFFICIAL GUIDELINES FOR CODING AND REPORTING

SECTION I.C.9.a.

3) Hypertensive Heart and Chronic Kidney Disease

Assign codes from combination category I13, Hypertensive heart and chronic kidney disease, when both hypertensive kidney disease and hypertensive heart disease are stated in the diagnosis. Assume a relationship between the hypertension and the chronic kidney disease, whether or not the condition is so designated. If heart failure is present, assign an additional code from category I50 to identify the type of heart failure.

The appropriate code from category N18, Chronic kidney disease, should be used as a secondary code with a code from category I13 to identify the stage of chronic kidney disease.

See Section I.C.14. Chronic kidney disease.

The codes in category I13, Hypertensive heart and chronic kidney disease, are combination codes that include hypertension, heart disease and chronic kidney disease. The Includes note at I13 specifies that the conditions included at I11 and I12 are included together in I13. If a patient has hypertension, heart disease and chronic kidney disease then a code from I13 should be used, not individual codes for hypertension, heart disease and chronic kidney disease, or codes from I11 or I12.

For patients with both acute renal failure and chronic kidney disease an additional code for acute renal failure is required.

The Guidelines instruct you to assume that there is a cause-and-effect relationship between hypertension and chronic kidney disease reported with N18.-. The physician might not indicate that the hypertension and chronic kidney disease are related, but the coder is to assume this relationship.

Chronic renal failure (CRF), chronic kidney disease (CKD), and chronic renal insufficiency (CRI) when reported with hypertension are reported as follows:

CRF/CKD/CRI + hypertension	I12.9 + N18.9
CKD stage 1 + hypertension	I12.9 + N18.1
CKD stage 2 + hypertension	I12.9 + N18.2
CKD stage 3 + hypertension	I12.0 + N18.3
CKD stage 4 + hypertension	I12.0 + N18.4
CKD stage 5 + hypertension	I12.0 + N18.5
CKD stage 6 or ESRD or on dialysis +	I12.0 + N18.6
Patient with CKD on any type of dialysis	I12.9 + N18.6 + Z99.2

Myocardial Infarction

A myocardial infarction is an acute type of heart attack that occurs when a coronary artery is totally blocked.

- An **STEMI** (ST elevation myocardial infarction) is the most severe type. The "ST" in STEMI refers to a segment in an electrocardiogram (ECG), and when the ST segment is elevated there is heart muscle damage due to occlusion. A STEMI is also known as a Q-wave or transmural myocardial infarction.
- An **NSTEMI** is a non-ST segment acute heart attack and is a less severe type that occurs when the artery is only partially occluded that results in the death of only that portion of the

ICD-10 OFFICIAL GUIDELINES FOR CODING AND REPORTING

SECTION I.C.9.e.
Chapter 9: Diseases of the Circulatory System (I00-I99)

e. Acute myocardial infarction (AMI)

1) ST elevation myocardial infarction (STEMI) and non ST elevation myocardial infarction (NSTEMI)

The ICD-10-CM codes for acute myocardial infarction (AMI) identify the site, such as anterolateral wall or true posterior wall. Subcategories I21.0-I21.2 and code I21.3 are used for ST elevation myocardial infarction (STEMI). Code I21.4, Non-ST elevation (NSTEMI) myocardial infarction, is used for non ST elevation myocardial infarction (NSTEMI) and nontransmural MIs.

If NSTEMI evolves to STEMI, assign the STEMI code. If STEMI converts to NSTEMI due to thrombolytic therapy, it is still coded as STEMI.

For encounters occurring while the myocardial infarction is equal to, or less than, four weeks old, including transfers to another acute setting or a postacute setting, and the patient requires continued care for the myocardial infarction, codes from category I21 may continue to be reported. For encounters after the 4 week time frame and the patient is still receiving care related to the myocardial infarction, the appropriate aftercare code should be assigned, rather than a code from category I21. For old or healed myocardial infarctions not requiring further care, code I25.2, Old myocardial infarction, may be assigned.

2) Acute myocardial infarction, unspecified

Code I21.3, ST elevation (STEMI) myocardial infarction of unspecified site, is the default for unspecified acute myocardial infarction. If only STEMI or transmural MI without the site is documented, assign code I21.3.

3) AMI documented as nontransmural or subendocardial but site provided

If an AMI is documented as nontransmural or subendocardial, but the site is provided, it is still coded as a subendocardial AMI.

See Section I.C.21.3 for information on coding status post administration of tPA in a different facility within the last 24 hours.

4) Subsequent acute myocardial infarction

A code from category I22, Subsequent ST elevation (STEMI) and non ST elevation (NSTEMI) myocardial infarction, is to be used when a patient who has suffered an AMI has a new AMI within the 4 week time frame of the initial AMI. A code from category I22 must be used in conjunction with a code from category I21. The sequencing of the I22 and I21 codes depends on the circumstances of the encounter.

heart muscle that is supplied by the affected artery. The ST segment is not elevated on ECG in the NSTEMI, thus the term non-ST segment myocardial infarction. The NSTEMI is also known as a non-Q wave or non-transmural myocardial infarction.

Category I21, myocardial infarction (MI), requires specific documentation to indicate the infarction site. For example, I21.01 reports the left main coronary artery and I21.11 reports the right coronary artery.

Examples

I21.01 ST elevation (STEMI) myocardial infarction involving left main coronary artery
I21.11 ST elevation (STEMI) myocardial infarction involving right coronary artery

If the documentation does not state the site of the infarction, query the physician as to the location or assign the default code I21.3.

Category I21 STEMI includes the following infarctions:

- cardiac infarction
- coronary artery embolism
- coronary artery occlusion
- coronary artery rupture
- coronary artery thrombosis
- infarction of heart—myocardium or ventricle

Also included in the I21 STEMI is a myocardial infarction specified as acute or with a stated duration of **4 weeks (28 days) or less from acute onset**. Old myocardial infarctions are reported with I25.2 and subsequent myocardial infarctions are reported with I22.-, Subsequent ST elevation (STEMI) and non-ST elevation (NSTEMI) myocardial infarction.

The "Use additional code to identify:" notation at the category I21 directs the coder to also report the following conditions that have a bearing on the AMI with supplementary code(s):

- exposure to environmental tobacco smoke (Z77.22)
- history of tobacco use (Z87.891)
- occupational exposure to environmental tobacco smoke (Z57.31)
- status post administration of tPA (rtPA) in a different facility within the last 24 hours prior to admission to current facility (Z92.82)
- tobacco dependence (F17.-)
- tobacco use (Z72.0)

If a patient has an acute myocardial infarction within four weeks after an initial AMI, report a code from the

- I22 category (Subsequent ST elevation (STEMI) and non-ST elevation (NSTEMI) myocardial infarction)
  and a code from the
- I21 category (ST elevation (STEMI) and non-ST elevation (NSTEMI) myocardial infarction).

The sequencing of the I22 (subsequent MI) and I21 (acute MI) depends on the reason for the encounter. If the patient experiences an AMI and is admitted to the hospital and has a subsequent AMI while in the hospital, report the I21 as the first-listed diagnosis and the I22 as the secondary code. If the same patient is discharged from the hospital and then experiences a subsequent AMI, report the I22 as the first-listed code and the I21 as the secondary code.

EXERCISE 5-11   *Diseases of the Circulatory System*

Assign codes for the following:

1 Congestive heart failure

Code: _____

2 Acute subendocardial infarction, initial episode

Code: _____

3 Treatment for secondary hypertension due to periarteritis nodosa

Codes: _____, _____

4 Cerebral infarction due to arterial thrombosis, brain

Code: _____

5 Subarachnoid hemorrhage

Code: _____

6 Acute renal failure in patient with hypertension

Codes: _____, _____

(Answers are located in Appendix B)

DISEASES OF THE RESPIRATORY SYSTEM

Chapter 10, Diseases of the Respiratory System (J00-J99), in the Tabular includes diseases and disorders of the respiratory tract, beginning with the nasal passages and following a path to the lungs. Note that at the beginning of I-10 Chapter 10 there is an instructional note that covers the entire chapter. The note states, "Use additional code, where applicable, to identify:" followed by a list of conditions and supplementary codes, such as exposure to environmental tobacco smoke (Z77.22).

The blocks in this chapter are as illustrated in Fig. 5-24.

J00-J06	Acute upper respiratory infections
J09-J18	Influenza and pneumonia
J20-J22	Other acute lower respiratory infections
J30-J39	Other diseases of upper respiratory tract
J40-J47	Chronic lower respiratory diseases
J60-J70	Lung diseases due to external agents
J80-J84	Other respiratory diseases principally affecting the interstitium
J85-J86	Suppurative and necrotic conditions of the lower respiratory tract
J90-J94	Other diseases of the pleura
J95	Intraoperative and postprocedural complications and disorders of respiratory system, not elsewhere classified
J96-J99	Other diseases of the respiratory system

FIGURE 5–24   Respiratory system blocks in the I-10.

Assigning ICD-10-CM codes for infectious respiratory diseases, such as pneumonia.

Identifying Infectious Organisms

Example 1

Diagnosis:	Pneumonia due to *Klebsiella pneumoniae*
Index:	**Pneumonia,** broncho-, bronchial, Klebsiella (pneumoniae), J15.0
Tabular:	**J15 Bacterial pneumonia, not elsewhere classified**
	J15.0 Pneumonia due to Klebsiella pneumoniae
Code:	J15.0 Pneumonia due to *Klebsiella pneumoniae*

Code J15.0 is a combination code that includes the disease process (pneumonia) with the causative organism *(Klebsiella pneumoniae)*. In this instance, you would not assign an additional code because the organism is identified in the code J15.0.

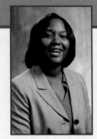

From the Trenches

"Like ICD-9, studying and comprehending the guidelines is imperative in ICD-10. Becoming familiar with chapter-specific guidelines is necessary in knowing when to use the 6th and/or 7th character. These characters are not optional; they are intended for use in recording the information documented in the medical record."

LETITIA

In the following example, two codes are necessary: one to describe the disease process (manifestation) and one to indicate the causative organism (etiology).

Identifying Infectious Organisms

Example 2

Diagnosis:	Acute maxillary sinusitis due to *Hemophilus influenzae*
Index:	Sinusitis (accessory) (chronic) (hyperplastic) (nasal) (nonpurulent) (purulent) J32.9
	acute J01.90 - -
	maxillary J01.00
Tabular:	**J01 Acute sinusitis**
	J01.0 Acute maxillary sinusitis
	J01.00 Acute maxillary sinusitis, unspecified
Index:	**Infection, infected, infective** (opportunistic) B99.9
	Hemophilus
	influenzae
	as cause of disease classified elsewhere B96.3
Tabular:	**B96 Other bacterial agents as the cause of diseases classified elsewhere**
	B96.3 Hemophilus influenzae [H. influenzae] as the cause of diseases classified elsewhere
Codes:	J01.00, B96.3 Acute maxillary sinusitis due to *Hemophilus influenzae*

The manifestation is the first-listed and the etiology is listed second.

EXERCISE 5-12   *Diseases of the Respiratory System*

Assign codes for the following:

1 Croup

Code: _____

2 Treatment for respiratory failure due to congestive heart failure

Codes: _____, _____

3 COPD with chronic bronchitis (without exacerbation)

Code: _____

4 Influenza with acute bronchitis

Code: _____

5 Pneumonia due to *Hemophilus influenzae*

Code: _____

6 COPD with emphysema

Code: _____

7 Aspiration pneumonia

Code: _____

(Answers are located in Appendix B)

CHAPTER REVIEW

CHAPTER 5, PART I, THEORY

Without the use of reference material, answer the following:

1 I-10 assumes a relationship between hypertension and renal failure.

   True   False

2 If a patient is admitted for an HIV-related condition, the first-listed diagnosis is the related condition followed by the diagnosis code B20.

   True   False

3 A Y90 category code would not be assigned to indicate a blood alcohol level.

   True   False

4 Another term to describe malignant hypertension is accelerated hypertension.

   True   False

5 Hypertension that is caused by another condition is called essential hypertension.

   True   False

6 Status asthmaticus can be assigned if the physician documents an acute exacerbation.

   True   False

7 There is no I-10 to report insulin use.

   True   False

8 If a patient receives insulin for diabetes, type 1 diabetes should be reported.

   True   False

9 The site to which a malignant neoplasm has spread is the _____.
   a metastatic site
   b primary site
   c benign site
   d morphology

10 The site in which a malignant neoplasm originated is the _____.
   a metastatic site
   b primary site
   c benign site
   d morphology

CHAPTER 5, PART II, PRACTICAL

Using the I-10 and coding guidelines, assign codes for the following:

11 Combined spinal cord degeneration due to pernicious anemia

   Codes: _____, _____

12 Carcinoma, in situ, of the lip, upper vermilion border

   Code: _____

Chapter Review answers are only available in the TEACH Instructor Resources on Evolve

13 Subacute bacterial endocarditis

Code: _____

14 Acute bronchitis with chronic obstructive bronchitis

Code: _____

15 Group B streptococcal pneumonia

Code: _____

CASE STUDY 1

History of Present Illness

The patient is an 80-year-old female with a known history of advanced metastatic carcinoma of the breast, which was the primary site. (The breast cancer is no longer present but has metastasized to other unspecified areas, which represents a secondary generalized neoplasm.) The patient has been admitted because of increased shortness of breath and severe pain. The pain is worse in her left chest, and this is associated with increased shortness of breath. At the time of admission, the patient is in so much pain that she is unable to remember her history. The patient initially presented for congestive heart failure more than a year earlier. This was subsequently found to be secondary to metastatic breast cancer, after left mastectomy, 3 years ago. The patient had previously been on chemotherapy.

Course in Hospital

The patient is treated initially with intravenous pain medication to control her pain, and subsequently her condition becomes stable on oral medication. By the time of discharge, the patient is stable on oral Vicodin. She is able to eat. Admission blood urea nitrogen (BUN) was 38 mg/dl with creatinine of 1.3 mg/dl secondary to dehydration. By the time of discharge, these levels have improved. Admission glucose of 225 mg/dl is down to 110 mg/dl at discharge.

Discharge Diagnoses

Uncontrolled pain, secondary to widely metastatic breast carcinoma

Dehydration

Type 2 diabetes mellitus, uncontrolled

MATCHING

16 The first-listed diagnosis _____	**a** E11.65
17 Neoplasm _____	**b** Z85.3
18 Volume depletion _____	**c** E86.0
19 Personal history of neoplasm of breast _____	**d** C80.0
20 Uncontrolled type 2 diabetes _____	**e** G89.3

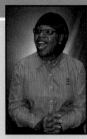

"It is important to study the new guidelines because they will help you to decipher how to select the correct ICD-10 code. . . . Make sure that you keep updated on current changes and the implementation of different phases regarding the ICD-10 transition."

Genieve R. Nottage, MBA, BSHA, CPC-I, CPMA, CMRS, CMBS

CEO/Owner
Chronicles Billing Inc.
Stockbridge, Georgia

Chapter-Specific Guidelines (ICD-10-CM Chapters 11-14)

Chapter Topics

Diseases of the Digestive System

Diseases of the Skin and Subcutaneous Tissue

Diseases of the Musculoskeletal System and Connective Tissue

Diseases of the Genitourinary System

Chapter Review

Learning Objectives

After completing this chapter you should be able to

1 Examine the digestive system coding.

2 Review coding the skin and subcutaneous tissue diseases.

3 Understand diseases of the musculoskeletal system and connective tissue coding.

NOTE: *The 2015 ICD-10-CM DRAFT and 2015 ICD-10-PCS DRAFT were used in preparing this text.*

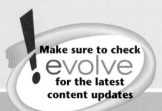

Make sure to check
evolve
for the latest
content updates

DISEASES OF THE DIGESTIVE SYSTEM

Chapter 11, Diseases of the Digestive System, in the Tabular of the I-10 describes diseases or conditions affecting the digestive system. Digestion starts when food is taken into the mouth and follows the gastrointestinal tract until it leaves the body through the anus. The categories in the I-10 are sequenced in a manner that follows that path, starting with disorders of the teeth. The blocks in Chapter 11 are as illustrated in Fig. 6-1.

Hemorrhage

Throughout the chapter, as in other chapters, you must pay close attention to additional characters to be assigned, the use of combination codes, and carefully read the Excludes/Includes notes and any other instructions. Also important in the chapter is the presence of **hemorrhage** (bleeding) and/or perforation associated with the disease. Code K92.2, Gastrointestinal hemorrhage, unspecified, is not assigned when codes for site-specific bleeding exist. Assign this code only when the physician states "gastric hemorrhage," "intestinal hemorrhage," etc., and no further site is specified. Also, because the physician may not always indicate the presence of hemorrhage, the coder must review the record and then clarify the documentation with the physician before code assignment. There are also combination codes to report conditions with hemorrhage.

K00-K14	Diseases of oral cavity and salivary glands
K20-K31	Diseases of esophagus, stomach and duodenum
K35-K38	Diseases of appendix
K40-K46	Hernia
K50-K52	Noninfective enteritis and colitis
K55-K64	Other diseases of intestines
K65-K68	Diseases of peritoneum and retroperitoneum
K70-K77	Diseases of liver
K80-K87	Disorders of gallbladder, biliary tract and pancreas
K90-K95	Other diseases of the digestive system

FIGURE 6-1 Blocks of Chapter 11, Diseases of the Digestive System (K00-K95) of the ICD-10-CM.

Example

Diagnosis:	Diverticulitis of the colon with perforation and abscess with hemorrhage
Index:	**Diverticulitis** (acute), intestine K57.92, large K57.32, with, abscess, perforation, or peritonitis K57.20, with bleeding K57.21
Tabular:	**K57 Diverticular disease of intestine**
	K57.2 Diverticulitis of large intestine with perforation and abscess
	K57.21 Diverticulitis of large intestine with perforation and abscess with bleeding (combination code)
Code:	K57.21 Diverticulitis of colon with perforation and abscess with hemorrhage

If you begin a search for the above diagnosis of "Diverticulitis of the colon with hemorrhage" using the main term "Hemorrhage, gastrointestinal," you are directed to K92.2. When you reference K92.2 in the Tabular, you will find a list of Excludes1 under the code. Note that in the list of Excludes1 is "diverticular disease with hemorrhage (K57.-)." This means that you cannot assign K92.2, gastrointestinal hemorrhage, when there is a mention of diverticulitis of the large intestine (K57.-). If you are reporting a diagnosis of gastrointestinal (GI) hemorrhage with any of the diagnoses listed in the Excludes1 and if the hemorrhage is due to the GI condition, do not report K92.2.

Hemorrhage

Example

Diagnosis:	Gastrointestinal hemorrhage due to acute antral ulcer
Index:	**Ulcer,** antral—*see* Ulcer, stomach
	Ulcer, stomach (eroded) (peptic) (round) K25.9 acute, with, hemorrhage K25.0
Tabular:	**K25 Gastric ulcer**
	K25.0 Acute gastric ulcer with hemorrhage

The combination code K25.0 reports both the acute gastric ulcer and the hemorrhage, so no further code is required to report the GI hemorrhage due to acute antral ulcer.

For a hemorrhage to be reported there does not have to be **active** bleeding; however, there must be documentation in the medical record that supports the fact that active bleeding has occurred and the physician must identify the source of bleeding for a combination code to be assigned.

It is so important to verify code assignment in the Tabular. It is only when you reference the Tabular that you know the Includes and Excludes of a code, which are not listed anywhere else. This is also where you will find additional characters to be assigned. Be certain to always, always check the Tabular before assigning a code.

EXERCISE 6-1   *Diseases of the Digestive System*

Assign I-10 codes for the following:

1 Appendicitis with generalized peritonitis

Code: _____

2 Gastrointestinal bleeding due to acute duodenal ulcer

Code: _____

3 Acute and chronic cholecystitis with cholelithiasis

Code: _____

4 Gastroenteritis

Code: _____

5 Gastroesophageal reflux

Code: _____

(Answers are located in Appendix B)

DISEASES OF THE SKIN AND SUBCUTANEOUS TISSUE

Chapter 12, Diseases of the Skin and Subcutaneous Tissue (L00-L99), in the Tabular of the I-10 describes diseases or conditions of the integumentary system. Conditions affecting the nails, sweat glands, hair, and hair follicles are included in this chapter. Congenital conditions

L00-L08	Infections of the skin and subcutaneous tissue
L10-L14	Bullous disorders
L20-L30	Dermatitis and eczema
L40-L45	Papulosquamous disorders
L49-L54	Urticaria and erythema
L55-L59	Radiation-related disorders of the skin and subcutaneous tissue
L60-L75	Disorders of skin appendages
L76	Intraoperative and postprocedural complications of skin and subcutaneous tissue
L80-L99	Other disorders of the skin and subcutaneous tissue

FIGURE 6-2 Blocks of Chapter 12, Diseases of the Skin and Subcutaneous Tissue (L00-L99) of the ICD-10-CM.

of skin, hair, and nails are classified in category Q80-Q89, Other congenital malformations. Neoplasms of skin are classified in Chapter 2 of I-10. The blocks of Chapter 12 include those displayed in Fig. 6-2.

A "Use additional code" preceding L00 directs the coder to identify the infectious agent (B95-B97) in addition to the code in the categories L00-L08, making multiple coding necessary.

Multiple Coding

Example

Diagnosis:	Cellulitis right small finger due to *Staphylococcus aureus*
Index:	**Cellulitis**, finger (intrathecal) (periosteal) (subcutaneous) (subcuticular) L03.01-
Tabular:	**L03 Cellulitis and acute lymphangitis**
	L03.0 Cellulitis and acute lymphangitis of finger and toe
	L03.01 Cellulitis of finger
	L03.011 Cellulitis of right finger

To locate the code for the causative organism, reference the main term "Infection" in the Index.

Index:	**Infection, infected, infective (opportunistic) B99.9**
	bacterial NOS A49.9
	as cause of disease classified elsewhere B96.89
	Staphylococcus B95.8
	aureus (methicillin susceptible) (MSSA) B95.61
Tabular:	**B95 Streptococcus, Staphylococcus, and Enterococcus as the cause of diseases classified elsewhere**
	B95.6 Staphylococcus aureus as the cause of diseases classified elsewhere
	B96.61 Methicillin susceptible Staphylococcus aureus infection as the cause of diseases classified elsewhere
Codes:	L03.011, B95.61 Cellulitis right small finger due to *Staphylococcus aureus*

The code for the organism is assigned as an additional code and is sequenced after the disease or condition.

Ulcers

Pressure ulcers develop when the circulation to an area is decreased by the application of pressure to the area. Patients restricted to bed or unable to change position often develop pressure ulcers. As the sores ulcerate, the deeper layers of tissue, such as fascia, muscle, and bone, may be affected. Pressure ulcers are graded and reported based on the depth of ulcer and categorized in stages as illustrated in Fig. 6-3. The stages are:

- Stage 1: Erythema (redness) of skin
- Stage 2: Partial loss of skin (epidermis or dermis)
- Stage 3: Full thickness loss of skin (up to but not through fascia)
- Stage 4: Full thickness loss (extensive destruction and necrosis)

Fig. 6-4 illustrates the codes to report pressure ulcer of the left hip that include the stages in the code description.

Non-pressure ulcers typically result from vascular insufficiencies. A note at the beginning of category L97, Non-pressure chronic ulcer of lower limb, not elsewhere classified, directs the coder to report the underlying conditions first, including diabetes, atherosclerosis, chronic venous hypertension, among others. Non-pressure ulcer codes are assigned by the site and depth of the ulcer.

EXERCISE 6-2	*Diseases of the Skin and Subcutaneous Tissue*

Assign I-10 codes for the following:

1 Pruritus vulvae

Code: _____

2 Prickly heat

Code: _____

3 Pustular, generalized psoriasis

Code: _____

4 Decubitus ulcer buttock

Code: _____

5 Dermatitis due to poison ivy

Code: _____

6 Paronychia toe

Code: _____

7 Pilonidal cyst with abscess

Code: _____

(Answers are located in Appendix B)

Stage 1

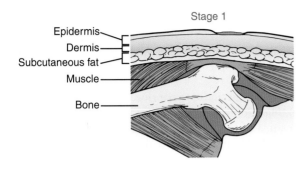

Stage 2

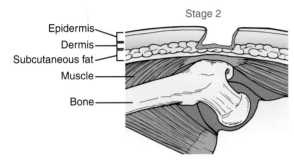

Stage 3

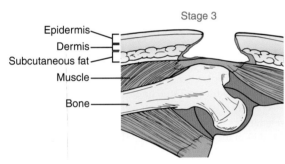

Stage 4

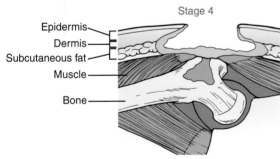

FIGURE 6-3 Stages 1, 2, 3, and 4 of pressure ulcers.

● **L89.22** **Pressure ulcer of left hip**
    L89.220 **Pressure ulcer of left hip, unstageable**
    L89.221 **Pressure ulcer of left hip, stage 1**
        Healing pressure ulcer of left hip back, stage 1
        Pressure pre-ulcer skin changes limited to persistent focal edema, left hip
    L89.222 **Pressure ulcer of left hip, stage 2**
        Healing pressure ulcer of left hip, stage 2
        Pressure ulcer with abrasion, blister, partial thickness skin loss involving epidermis and/or dermis, left hip
    L89.223 **Pressure ulcer of left hip, stage 3**
        Healing pressure ulcer of left hip, stage 3
        Pressure ulcer with full thickness skin loss involving damage or necrosis of subcutaneous tissue, left hip
        MCC when PDx is its own MCC
    L89.224 **Pressure ulcer of left hip, stage 4**
        Healing pressure ulcer of left hip, stage 4
        Pressure ulcer with necrosis of soft tissues through to underlying muscle, tendon, or bone, left hip
        MCC when PDx is its own MCC
    L89.229 **Pressure ulcer of left hip, unspecified stage**
        Healing pressure ulcer of left hip NOS
        Healing pressure ulcer of left hip, unspecified stage

FIGURE 6-4 Left hip pressure ulcer codes by stage.

DISEASES OF THE MUSCULOSKELETAL SYSTEM AND CONNECTIVE TISSUE

Chapter 13, Diseases of the Musculoskeletal System and Connective Tissue, in the I-10 Tabular describes diseases or conditions of the bone, joints, and muscle, and the blocks are displayed in Fig. 6-5.

Most of the codes in Chapter 13 of the I-10 are specific as to site (location on the body) and laterality (right, left, unilateral, bilateral). Fig. 6-6 displays the site and laterality of category M16 that reports bilateral (right and left), unilateral (right or left), and unspecified.

Codes to report previously injured musculoskeletal conditions are located in Chapter 13, and codes to report current injuries are reported with codes from Chapter 19.

M00-M02	Infectious arthropathies
M05-M14	Inflammatory polyarthropathies
M15-M19	Osteoarthritis
M20-M25	Other joint disorders
M26-M27	Dentofacial anomalies [including malocclusion] and other disorders of jaw
M30-M36	Systemic connective tissue disorders
M40-M43	Deforming dorsopathies
M45-M49	Spondylopathies
M50-M54	Other dorsopathies
M60-M63	Disorders of muscles
M65-M67	Disorders of synovium and tendon
M70-M79	Other soft tissue disorders
M80-M85	Disorders of bone density and structure
M86-M90	Other osteopathies
M91-M94	Chondropathies
M95	Other disorders of the musculoskeletal system and connective tissue
M96	Intraoperative and postprocedural complications and disorders of musculoskeletal system, not elsewhere classified
M99	Biomechanical lesions, not elsewhere classified

FIGURE 6–5 Blocks of Chapter 13, Diseases of the Musculoskeletal System and Connective Tissue (M00-M99), of the ICD-10-CM.

● **M16 Osteoarthritis of hip**
   M16.0 Bilateral primary osteoarthritis of hip
● **M16.1 Unilateral primary osteoarthritis of hip**
      Primary osteoarthritis of hip NOS
         M16.10 Unilateral primary osteoarthritis, unspecified hip
         M16.11 Unilateral primary osteoarthritis, right hip
         M16.12 Unilateral primary osteoarthritis, left hip
   M16.2 Bilateral osteoarthritis resulting from hip dysplasia

FIGURE 6–6 Category M16 site and laterality specific.

ICD-10 OFFICIAL GUIDELINES FOR CODING AND REPORTING

SECTION I.C.13.

Chapter 13: Diseases of the Musculoskeletal System and Connective Tissue (M00-M99)

a. Site and laterality

Most of the codes within Chapter 13 have site and laterality designations. The site represents the bone, joint or the muscle involved. For some conditions where more than one bone, joint or muscle is usually involved, such as osteoarthritis, there is a "multiple sites" code available. For categories where no multiple site code is provided and more than one bone, joint or muscle is involved, multiple codes should be used to indicate the different sites involved.

1) Bone versus joint

For certain conditions, the bone may be affected at the upper or lower end, (e.g., avascular necrosis of bone, M87, Osteoporosis, M80, M81). Though the portion of the bone affected may be at the joint, the site designation will be the bone, not the joint.

b. Acute traumatic versus chronic or recurrent musculoskeletal conditions

Many musculoskeletal conditions are a result of previous injury or trauma to a site, or are recurrent conditions. Bone, joint or muscle conditions that are the result of a healed injury are usually found in chapter 13. Recurrent bone, joint or muscle conditions are also usually found in chapter 13. Any current, acute injury should be coded to the appropriate injury code from chapter 19. Chronic or recurrent conditions should generally be coded with a code from chapter 13. If it is difficult to determine from the documentation in the record which code is best to describe a condition, query the provider.

Infectious Arthropathies

Categories M00-M02 report infectious arthropathies due to infections that are either direct or indirect. A **direct** infection is one that invades the synovial tissue as well as the joint and the invasive organism has been identified. There are two types of **indirect** infections:

■ Reactive arthropathy: The microbial infection is identified in the body but the organism and antigen are not identified in the joint

■ Postinfective arthropathy: The microbial antigen (immune response to presence of microbes) is present but the recovery of the organism is not constant and there is no evidence that a microorganism is multiplying

There are three code categories assigned to report infectious arthropathies: M00, M01, and M02.

M00 Reports Direct Infection from a Known Organism. A code from category M00 is reported first followed by a bacterial agent (B95.6-B95.7).

M00

Example

Diagnosis: *Staphylococcal aureus* arthritis of the right wrist joint

Index: **Arthritis, arthritic** (acute) (chronic) (nonpyogenic) (subacute) M19.90
     staphylococcal M00.00 wrist M00.03-

Tabular: **M00   Pyogenic arthritis**
     M00.0   Staphylococcal arthritis and polyarthritis
     Use additional code (B95.6-B95.7) to identify bacterial
     agent
     M00.03   Staphylococcal arthritis, wrist
     M00.031   Staphylococcal arthritis, right wrist

Pyogenic arthritis (M00) is also known as infectious arthritis or septic arthritis and is a serious infection of a joint that can damage both bone and cartilage and has the potential to create septic shock.

M00.031 reports the pyogenic arthritis, but the cause of the infection must still be reported, which in this example is *Staphylococcal aureus*.

Index: **Infection, infected, infective (opportunistic) B99.9**
     bacterial NOS A49.9
     as cause of disease classified elsewhere B96.89
     Staphylococcus B95.8
     aureus (methicillin susceptible) (MSSA) B95.61

Tabular: **B95   Streptococcus, Staphylococcus, and Enterococcus as the cause
     of diseases classified elsewhere**
     **B95.6   Staphylococcus aureus as the cause of diseases
     classified elsewhere**
     **B96.61   Methicillin susceptible Staphylococcus aureus
     infection as the cause of diseases classified
     elsewhere**

Codes: M00.031, B95.61 *Staphylococcal aureus* arthritis of the right wrist joint

There is a "Use additional code" note following M00.0 directing the coder to report a code from B95.61-B95.8. List the disease condition first, followed by the organism causing the infection.

M01 Reports Direct Infection of the Joint Due to Infectious or Parasitic Disease that Is Classified Elsewhere. The infection/parasitic disease is reported first, followed by an M01 code.

M01

Example

The patient presents with paratyphoid fever that has invaded the right shoulder and has resulted in infectious arthritis of the joint due to *Salmonella paratyphi*.

Index: **Arthritis, arthritic** (acute) (chronic) (nonpyogenic) (subacute) M19.90
           due to or associated with
              paratyphoid fever (see also Fever, paratyphoid) A01.4 (see also category M01)

Tabular: **A01** **Typhoid and paratyphoid fevers**
           A01.4 **Paratyphoid fever, unspecified**
               Infection due to Salmonella paratyphi NOS

Tabular: **M01** **Direct infections of joint in infectious and parasitic diseases classified elsewhere**
           M01.X1 **Direct infection of shoulder joint in infectious and parasitic diseases classified elsewhere**
                M01.X11 **Direct infection of right shoulder in infectious and parasitic diseases classified elsewhere**

Code: A01.4, M01.X11 Paratyphoid fever with infectious arthritis of right shoulder

There is a "Code first" following M01 in the Tabular that directs the coder to sequence first the underlying disease followed by the M01 code.

M02 Reports Indirect Infections from an Unknown Organism. The "Code first" note directs coders to report first the underlying disease.

M02

Example

The patient presents with left shoulder swelling, effusion, pain, and instability following immunization. Laboratory results could not confirm the presence of microbial antigens in the joint fluid. Diagnosis is postimmunization infectious arthritis.

Index: **Arthropathy** (see also Arthritis) M12.9
          postimmunization M02.20
            shoulder M02.21-

Tabular: **M02** **Postinfective and reactive arthropathies**
           M02.2 **Postimmunization arthropathy**
               M02.21 **Postimmunization arthropathy, shoulder**
                  M02.212 **Postimmunization arthropathy, left shoulder**

Code: M02.212 Postimmunization arthropathy

Pathological Fractures

ICD-10 OFFICIAL GUIDELINES FOR CODING AND REPORTING

SECTION I.C.13.

Chapter 13: Diseases of the Musculoskeletal System and Connective Tissue (M00-M99)

c. Coding of Pathologic Fractures

7th character A is for use as long as the patient is receiving active treatment for the fracture. Examples of active treatment are: surgical treatment, emergency department encounter, evaluation and continuing treatment by the same or a different physician. While the patient may be seen by a new or different provider over the course of treatment for a pathological fracture, assignment of the 7th character is based on whether the patient is undergoing active treatment and not whether the provider is seeing the patient for the first time.

7th character, D is to be used for encounters after the patient has completed active treatment. The other 7th characters, listed under each subcategory in the Tabular List, are to be used for subsequent encounters for treatment of problems associated with the healing, such as malunions, nonunions, and sequelae.

Care for complications of surgical treatment for fracture repairs during the healing or recovery phase should be coded with the appropriate complication codes.

See Section I.C.19. Coding of traumatic fractures.

A **pathologic** or **spontaneous** fracture is a break in a bone that occurs because of bone disease or a change surrounding the bone tissue that makes the bone weak. A pathologic fracture is serious because healing may be delayed by an underlying bone disease. The fracture is reported in addition to the disease process responsible for the fracture, such as osteoporosis or metastatic cancer of the bone. It is also possible to have a small trauma associated with a pathologic fracture. For example, an elderly woman with severe osteoporosis bumps her hip against the doorway and sustains a hip fracture. This is a pathologic fracture because a person with healthy bones would not have fractured a hip as the result of a slight bump into a doorway. If there is any question about whether a fracture was pathologic or due to trauma, query the physician as to the cause of the fracture. If a pathologic fracture is documented and no other disease process is indicated, review the record or clarify the underlying cause of the fracture with the physician.

Never assign a code for a traumatic fracture and a pathologic fracture of the same bone.

According to the Guidelines for pathological fractures, the 7th character A (initial encounter) is assigned as long as the patient is receiving active treatment for a fracture, such as surgical treatment, emergency treatment, or evaluation/management by a physician other than the original physician. The 7th character D (subsequent encounter) is assigned when all active treatment has been completed. The 7th characters G, K, and P are assigned for subsequent, non-routine encounters (i.e., delayed healing, nonunion, malunion). The 7th character S is reported for a sequela.

ICD-10 OFFICIAL GUIDELINES FOR CODING AND REPORTING

SECTION I.C.13.

Chapter 13: Diseases of the Musculoskeletal System and Connective Tissue (M00-M99)

d. Osteoporosis

Osteoporosis is a systemic condition, meaning that all bones of the musculoskeletal system are affected. Therefore, site is not a component of the codes under category M81, Osteoporosis without current pathological fracture. The site codes under category M80, Osteoporosis with current pathological fracture, identify the site of the fracture, not the osteoporosis.

1) Osteoporosis without pathological fracture

Category M81, Osteoporosis without current pathological fracture, is for use for patients with osteoporosis who do not currently have a pathologic fracture due to the osteoporosis, even if they have had a fracture in the past. For patients with a history of osteoporotic

Continued

fractures, status code Z87.310, Personal history of (healed) osteoporosis fracture, should follow the code from M81.

2) Osteoporosis with current pathological fracture

Category M80, Osteoporosis with current pathological fracture, is for patients who have a current pathologic fracture at the time of an encounter. The codes under M80 identify the site of the fracture. A code from category M80, not a traumatic fracture code, should be used for any patient with known osteoporosis who suffers a fracture, even if the patient had a minor fall or trauma, if that fall or trauma would not usually break a normal, healthy bone.

Pathologic Fracture

Example

Diagnosis:	Pathologic fracture of the first metatarsal, right foot, due to age-related postmenopausal osteoporosis, initial encounter

Index:	**Fracture, pathological** M84.40 -
	   due to
	      osteoporosis M80.80
	         postmenopausal- *see* Osteoporosis postmenopausal, with pathologic fracture

Index:	**Osteoporosis** (female) (male) M81.0
	   postmenopausal,
	      with pathological fracture M80.00
	         metatarsus M80.07-

Tabular:	**M80.0 Age-related osteoporosis with current pathological fracture**
	      Involutional osteoporosis with current pathological fracture
	      Osteoporosis NOS with current pathological fracture
	      Postmenopausal osteoporosis with current pathological fracture
	      Senile osteoporosis with current pathological fracture
	
	      M80.07 Age-related osteoporosis with current pathological fracture, ankle and foot
	         M80.071 Age-related osteoporosis with current pathological fracture, right ankle and foot

Code:	M80.071A Pathologic fracture of the right metatarsal due to age-related postmenopausal osteoporosis, initial encounter

EXERCISE 6-3 *Diseases of the Musculoskeletal System and Connective Tissue*

Assign I-10 codes for the following:

1 Rheumatoid arthritis

Code: _____

2 Pain in the neck

Code: _____

3 Recurrent dislocation, right shoulder

Code: _____

4 Initial encounter for spontaneous fracture left humerus due to metastatic bone cancer; history of cancer of the breast previously excised

Codes: _____ (fracture), _____ (neoplasm), _____ (history of)

(Answers are located in Appendix B)

DISEASES OF THE GENITOURINARY SYSTEM

Chapter 14 in the I-10 Tabular is Diseases of the Genitourinary System (N00-N99). This chapter contains codes to report diagnoses of the male genitalia (N40-N53), female genitalia (N70-N98), breast (N60-N65), and urinary system (N00-N39). One of the most common disorders reported with codes from Chapter 14 are kidney stones located in the Index under the main term, "Calculus."

Kidney Stone

Example

Diagnosis: Flank pain with dysuria and emesis, with 3 renal calculi visible on x-ray.

Index: **Calculus, calculi, calculous**
        kidney N20.0

Tabular: **N20   Calculus of kidney and ureter**

        N20.0   Calculus of kidney

Code: N20.0 Calculus of kidney

Category N18 reports the diagnosis of chronic kidney disease (CKD) according to the stage. When the kidneys are no longer able to adequately filter urine, the patient's CKD is termed end stage renal disease (ESRD). When the patient has ESRD, regular dialysis or a transplanted kidney is required to sustain life. When a patient is receiving dialysis, also report dialysis status (Z99.2). CKD is a common complication of diabetes, and there are combination codes to report CKD due to diabetes. The combination code is listed first, followed by a code that identifies the stage of the CKD.

ICD-10 OFFICIAL GUIDELINES FOR CODING AND REPORTING

SECTION I.C.14.

a. Chronic kidney disease

1) Stages of chronic kidney disease (CKD)

The ICD-10-CM classifies CKD based on severity. The severity of CKD is designated by stages 1-5. Stage 2, code N18.2, equates to mild CKD; stage 3, code N18.3, equates to moderate CKD; and stage 4, code N18.4, equates to severe CKD. Code N18.6, End stage renal disease (ESRD), is assigned when the provider has documented end-stage-renal disease (ESRD).

If both a stage of CKD and ESRD are documented, assign code N18.6 only.

3) Chronic kidney disease with other conditions

Patients with CKD may also suffer from other serious conditions, most commonly diabetes mellitus and hypertension. The sequencing of the CKD code in relationship to codes for other contributing conditions is based on the conventions in the Tabular List.

See I.C.9. Hypertensive chronic kidney disease.

See I.C.19. Chronic kidney disease and kidney transplant complications

CHAPTER REVIEW

CHAPTER 6, PART I, THEORY

Circle the correct answer in each of the following:

1 In order to code a gastrointestinal condition with hemorrhage, active bleeding must be present.

   True   False

2 Which of the following is not included in the blocks of the Digestive System?
   a hernia
   b liver
   c pancreas
   d kidney

3 A pathologic fracture occurs in a bone that is weakened by disease.

   True   False

4 Which of the following is not included in the blocks of the Diseases of the Skin and Subcutaneous Tissue?
   a spondylopathies
   b eczema
   c erythema
   d bullous disorders

Match the following pressure ulcer stages to the correct description of the stage.

5 Stage 1 _____   a full thickness loss of skin (up to but not through fascia)

6 Stage 2 _____   b erythema (redness) of skin

7 Stage 3 _____   c full thickness loss (extensive destruction and necrosis)

8 Stage 4 _____   d partial loss of skin (epidermis or dermis)

9 When a patient with osteoporosis falls and fractures a bone, the Guidelines instruct us to report this as a pathological fracture due to osteoporosis (Category M80), not as a fracture due to an injury.

   True   False

10 Most of the codes in Chapter 13 are specific to site and include laterality.

   True   False

CHAPTER 6, PART II, PRACTICAL

Using an I-10 manual, answer the following questions:

11 Crohn's disease with rectal bleeding

Code: _____

12 Diaphragmatic hernia with gangrene

Code: _____

13 Recurrent dislocation, right shoulder

Code: _____

14 Dermatitis due to poison ivy

Code: _____

15 Paronychia toe

Code: _____

16 Anal fistula

Code: _____

17 Lower gastrointestinal bleeding due to angiodysplasia of colon

Code: _____

18 Diverticulum of appendix

Code: _____

19 Acute and chronic cholecystitis with cholelithiasis

Code: _____

20 Mr. Jones presents to the emergency department with acute abdominal pain. After a thorough examination and diagnostic x-ray film, Mr. Jones is diagnosed with acute small bowel obstruction and taken immediately to surgery.

Code: _____

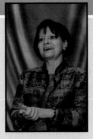

"Education is vital for successful ICD-10 implementation. It is essential to understand the I-10 Official Guidelines and format of the new codes, learn the correct applications which provide specificity, and be able to translate medical record documentation in order to become proficient with this new system."

Patricia Cordy Henricksen, MS, CHCA, CPC-I, CPC, CCP-P, ACS-PM

Auditing and Coding Educator
Soterion Medical Services
Lexington, Kentucky

Chapter-Specific Guidelines (ICD-10-CM Chapters 15-21)

Chapter Topics

Pregnancy, Childbirth, and the Puerperium

Certain Conditions Originating in the Perinatal Period

Congenital Malformations, Deformations, and Chromosomal Abnormalities

Symptoms, Signs and Abnormal Clinical and Laboratory Findings, Not Elsewhere Classified

Injury, Poisoning, and Certain Other Consequences of External Causes

Chapter Review

Learning Objectives

After completing this chapter you should be able to

1   Review the pregnancy, childbirth, and puerperium coding.

2   Report services of certain conditions originating in the perinatal period.

3   Examine the congenital malformations, deformities, and chromosomal abnormalities.

4   Define the rules of symptoms, signs, and abnormal clinical and laboratory findings that are not elsewhere classified.

5   Identify the elements of coding injury, poisonings, and certain other consequences of external causes.

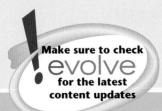
Make sure to check evolve **for the latest content updates**

NOTE: *The 2015 ICD-10-CM DRAFT and 2015 ICD-10-PCS DRAFT were used in preparing this text.*

PREGNANCY, CHILDBIRTH, AND THE PUERPERIUM

Chapter 15, Pregnancy, Childbirth, and the Puerperium (O00-O9A) of the Tabular of the I-10 is a difficult chapter from which to report diagnoses. One reason is that pregnancy and childbirth are natural functions, and physicians often overlook documentation of diagnoses that should be reported. Another reason the coding is complex is that there is extensive use of multiple coding in I-10 Chapter 15. There are instructions throughout this chapter that must be read thoroughly. Obstetric coding can also be difficult because you may not use this chapter as frequently as some of the other chapters, so you won't be as familiar with the notes and coding instructions. Any condition that occurs during pregnancy, childbirth, or the puerperium is considered to be a complication unless the attending physician specifically documents that it neither **affects** the pregnancy nor is **affected by** the pregnancy.

ICD-10 OFFICIAL GUIDELINES FOR CODING AND REPORTING

SECTION I.C.15.
Chapter 15: Pregnancy, Childbirth, and the Puerperium (O00-O9A)

a. General Rules for Obstetric Cases

1) Codes from chapter 15 and sequencing priority

Obstetric cases require codes from chapter 15, codes in the range O00-O9A, Pregnancy, Childbirth, and the Puerperium. Chapter 15 codes have sequencing priority over codes from other chapters. Additional codes from other chapters may be used in conjunction with chapter 15 codes to further specify conditions. Should the provider document that the pregnancy is incidental to the encounter, then code Z33.1, Pregnant state, incidental, should be used in place of any chapter 15 codes. It is the provider's responsibility to state that the condition being treated is not affecting the pregnancy.

c. Pre-existing conditions versus conditions due to the pregnancy

Certain categories in Chapter 15 distinguish between conditions of the mother that existed prior to pregnancy (pre-existing) and those that are a direct result of pregnancy. When assigning codes from Chapter 15, it is important to assess if a condition was pre-existing prior to pregnancy or developed during or due to the pregnancy in order to assign the correct code.

Categories that do not distinguish between pre-existing and pregnancy-related conditions may be used for either. It is acceptable to use codes specifically for the puerperium with codes complicating pregnancy and childbirth if a condition arises postpartum during the delivery encounter.

General Rules of Obstetric Diagnosis Reporting

Chapter 15 codes are never used on the newborn's record because they are only used on the mother's record.

ICD-10 OFFICIAL GUIDELINES FOR CODING AND REPORTING

SECTION I.C.15. a.
Chapter 15: Pregnancy, Childbirth, and the Puerperium (O00-O9A)

2) Chapter 15 codes used only on the maternal record

Chapter 15 codes are to be used only on the maternal record, never on the record of the newborn.

First-Listed Diagnosis in Normal Pregnancy

ICD-10 OFFICIAL GUIDELINES FOR CODING AND REPORTING

SECTION I.C.15.

Chapter 15: Pregnancy, Childbirth, and the Puerperium (O00-O9A)

b. Selection of OB Principal or First-listed Diagnosis

1) Routine outpatient prenatal visits

For routine outpatient prenatal visits when no complications are present, a code from category Z34, Encounter for supervision of normal pregnancy, should be used as the first-listed diagnosis. These codes should not be used in conjunction with chapter 15 codes.

Routine outpatient prenatal visits are reported with codes from category Z34, Encounter for supervision of normal pregnancy, as the first-listed diagnosis. If there is any type of complication, such as those reported with O00-O9A, Z34 codes cannot be reported. For example, if the patient encounter was for the supervision of a normal first pregnancy in the first trimester, assign Z34.01, Encounter for supervision of normal first pregnancy, first trimester.

First-Listed Diagnosis in High-Risk Patients

ICD-10 OFFICIAL GUIDELINES FOR CODING AND REPORTING

SECTION I.C.15.

Chapter 15: Pregnancy, Childbirth, and the Puerperium (O00-O9A)

b. Selection of OB Principal or First-listed Diagnosis

2) Prenatal outpatient visits for high-risk patients

For routine prenatal outpatient visits for patients with high-risk pregnancies, a code from category O09, Supervision of high-risk pregnancy, should be used as the first-listed diagnosis. Secondary chapter 15 codes may be used in conjunction with these codes if appropriate.

Some patients are considered high-risk for complication during pregnancy, such as neonatal death. When encounters are for high-risk patients, report a code from category O09, Supervision of high-risk pregnancy. For example, a patient in her first trimester presents for an office visit with her obstetrician. The patient's first pregnancy ended in neonatal death. Report O09.291, Supervision of pregnancy with other poor reproductive or obstetric history, first trimester.

First-Listed Diagnosis for Delivery

ICD-10 OFFICIAL GUIDELINES FOR CODING AND REPORTING

SECTION I.C.15

Chapter 15: Pregnancy, Childbirth, and the Puerperium (O00-O9A)

b. Selection of OB Principal or First-listed Diagnosis

3) Episodes when no delivery occurs

In episodes when no delivery occurs, the principal diagnosis should correspond to the principal complication of the pregnancy which necessitated the encounter. Should more than one complication exist, all of which are treated or monitored, any of the complications codes may be sequenced first.

Continued

4) When a delivery occurs

When a delivery occurs, the principal diagnosis should correspond to the main circumstances or complication of the delivery. In cases of cesarean delivery, the selection of the principal diagnosis should be the condition established after study that was responsible for the patient's admission. If the patient was admitted with a condition that resulted in the performance of a cesarean procedure, that condition should be selected as the principal diagnosis. If the reason for admission/encounter was unrelated to the condition resulting in the cesarean delivery, the condition related to the reason for the admission/encounter should be selected as the principal diagnosis.

5) Outcome of delivery

A code from category Z37, Outcome of delivery, should be included on every maternal record when a delivery has occurred. These codes are not to be used on subsequent records or on the newborn record.

The outcome of delivery is indicated only on the **mother's** medical record. For example, the mother gives birth to a single live born, reported with Z37.0. The outcome of delivery is only reported once on the mother's record and is not reported on subsequent encounters.

Trimesters

ICD-10 OFFICIAL GUIDELINES FOR CODING AND REPORTING

SECTION I.C.15

Chapter 15: Pregnancy, Childbirth, and the Puerperium (O00-*O9A*)

a. General Rules for Obstetric cases

3) Final character for trimester

The majority of codes in Chapter 15 have a final character indicating the trimester of pregnancy. The timeframes for the trimesters are indicated at the beginning of the chapter. If trimester is not a component of a code it is because the condition always occurs in a specific trimester, or the concept of trimester of pregnancy is not applicable. Certain codes have characters for only certain trimesters because the condition does not occur in all trimesters, but it may occur in more than just one.

Assignment of the final character for trimester should be based on the provider's documentation of the trimester (or number of weeks) for the current admission/encounter. This applies to the assignment of trimester for pre-existing conditions as well as those that develop during or are due to the pregnancy. The provider's documentation of the number of weeks may be used to assign the appropriate code identifying the trimester.

Whenever delivery occurs during the current admission, and there is an "in childbirth" option for the obstetric complication being coded, the "in childbirth" code should be assigned.

4) Selection of trimester for inpatient admissions that encompass more than one trimester

In instances when a patient is admitted to a hospital for complications of pregnancy during one trimester and remains in the hospital into a subsequent trimester, the trimester character for the antepartum complication code should be assigned on the basis of the trimester when the complication developed, not the trimester of the discharge. If the condition developed prior to the current admission/encounter or represents a pre-existing condition, the trimester character for the trimester at the time of the admission/encounter should be assigned.

5) Unspecified trimester

Each category that includes codes for trimester has a code for "unspecified trimester." The "unspecified trimester" code should rarely be used, such as when the documentation in the record is insufficient to determine the trimester and it is not possible to obtain clarification.

Trimesters are indicated on many of the codes in Chapter 15. Trimesters are calculated from the first day of the last menstrual period (LMP) and are as follows:

■ First trimester　　　　　less than 14 weeks 0 days from LMP
■ Second trimester　　　　14 weeks 0 days to less than 28 weeks 0 days from LMP
■ Third trimester　　　　　28 weeks 0 days from LMP until delivery occurs

Specific gestation weeks are assigned category Z3A codes in order to provide additional information about the pregnancy.

Codes from Chapter 15 have priority over codes from other chapters. Although additional codes may be reported for further detail, the Chapter 15 code is first-listed. It is the physician's responsibility to document that the condition or conditions being treated **are not** affecting the pregnancy. In the absence of this documentation, assume the condition **is** affecting the pregnancy.

There are codes for unspecified trimester; however, they should only be used if there is no further information available to determine the correct trimester.

QUICK CHECK 7-1

1. First trimester　　　　less than _____ weeks 0 days from LMP
2. Second trimester　　　_____ weeks 0 days to less than
3. Third trimester　　　　_____ weeks 0 days from LMP
　　　　　　　　　　　　_____ weeks 0 days until delivery occurs

(Answers are located in Appendix C)

There are times when the first-listed diagnosis for a pregnant female will not be a Chapter 15 code:

■ If the physician documents that the pregnancy is **incidental** to the encounter, report Z33.1, Pregnant state, incidental, as a supplemental diagnosis and the reason for the encounter as the first-listed diagnosis.
■ Encounter for a complication at which no delivery occurs, report the complication of pregnancy as the first-listed diagnosis.

There are conditions that are due to pregnancy, and those same conditions that may have been present prior to pregnancy, such as hypertension, are shown in Fig. 7-1. If the category does not state pre-existing or pregnancy-related condition, the category may be assigned to either.

● **O10　Pre-existing hypertension complicating pregnancy, childbirth and the puerperium**

　　Includes　pre-existing hypertension with pre-existing proteinuria complicating pregnancy, childbirth and the puerperium

　　Excludes2　pre-existing hypertension with superimposed pre-eclampsia complicating pregnancy, childbirth and the puerperium (O11.-)

FIGURE 7–1　Pre-existing hypertension.

Peripartum and Postpartum Periods

ICD-10 OFFICIAL GUIDELINES FOR CODING AND REPORTING

SECTION I.C.15.

Chapter 15: Pregnancy, Childbirth, and the Puerperium (O00-O9A)

o. The Peripartum and Postpartum Periods

1) Peripartum and Postpartum periods

The postpartum period begins immediately after delivery and continues for six weeks following delivery. The peripartum period is defined as the last month of pregnancy to five months postpartum.

2) Peripartum and postpartum complication

A postpartum complication is any complication occurring within the six-week period.

3) Pregnancy-related complications after 6 week period

Chapter 15 codes may also be used to describe pregnancy-related complications after the peripartum or postpartum period if the provider documents that a condition is pregnancy related.

4) Admission for routine postpartum care following delivery outside hospital

When the mother delivers outside the hospital prior to admission and is admitted for routine postpartum care and no complications are noted, code Z39.0, Encounter for care and examination of mother immediately after delivery, should be assigned as the principal diagnosis.

5) Pregnancy associated cardiomyopathy

Pregnancy associated cardiomyopathy, code O90.3, is unique in that it may be diagnosed in the third trimester of pregnancy but may continue to progress months after delivery. For this reason, it is referred to as peripartum cardiomyopathy. Code O90.3 is only for use when the cardiomyopathy develops as a result of pregnancy in a woman who did not have pre-existing heart disease.

The time periods of pregnancy are:

- Peripartum   last month of pregnancy to 5 months postpartum
- Postpartum   immediately after delivery to 6 weeks after delivery

If the patient has a pregnancy-related complication after the peripartum and postpartum periods of time, the physician must document that the condition is pregnancy-related in order to assign Chapter 15 codes.

If the mother delivers outside the hospital, report the first-listed diagnosis as Z39.0, Encounter for care and examination of mother immediately after delivery.

Normal Delivery

ICD-10 OFFICIAL GUIDELINES FOR CODING AND REPORTING

SECTION I.C.15.

Chapter 15: Pregnancy, Childbirth, and the Puerperium (O00-O9A)

n. Normal Delivery, Code O80

1) Encounter for full term uncomplicated delivery

Code O80 should be assigned when a woman is admitted for a full-term normal delivery and delivers a single, healthy infant without any complications antepartum, during the delivery, or postpartum during the delivery episode. Code O80 is always a principal diagnosis. It is not

Continued

to be used if any other code from chapter 15 is needed to describe a current complication of the antenatal, delivery, or perinatal period. Additional codes from other chapters may be used with code O80 if they are not related to or are in any way complicating the pregnancy.

2) Uncomplicated delivery with resolved antepartum complication
Code O80 may be used if the patient had a complication at some point during the pregnancy, but the complication is not present at the time of the admission for delivery.

3) Outcome of delivery for O80
Z37.0, Single live birth, is the only outcome of delivery code appropriate for use with O80.

O80 is reported as the first-listed diagnosis for a full-term, uncomplicated delivery of a single, healthy infant without any complications before, during, or after the delivery. If the patient had antepartum complications, but that complication is not present at delivery, you can still report a normal delivery with O80.

The outcome of an **O80** delivery is reported with **Z37.0,** Single live birth. No other outcome of delivery code would be correct to report with O80.

QUICK CHECK 7-2

1. According to the Guidelines, the only birth outcome code that can be reported with O80 is _____.
2. O80 is always listed _____.
3. Additional codes from other chapters may be used with code O80 if they are not related to or are in any way _____ the pregnancy.

(Answers are located in Appendix C)

Ectopic Pregnancy

An ectopic pregnancy is one in which the fertilized ovum implants outside the uterus, usually in the fallopian tube. Ectopic pregnancy includes ruptured ectopic pregnancies and is reported with a code from category O00 based on the location of the pregnancy (abdominal, tubal, ovarian, other, unspecified). If there are any complications with the ectopic pregnancy, report those associated complications with a code from category O08, Complications following ectopic and molar pregnancy.

Hydatidiform Mole

A hydatidiform mole is a tumor of the placenta that secretes hormones (chorionic gonadotropic hormone, CGH) and is shown in Fig. 7-2.

A hydatidiform mole is reported with a category O01 code. Malignant hydatidiform moles are reported with D39.2 (Neoplasm of uncertain behavior of placenta). If there is a complication with the hydatidiform mole, report a code from category O08, Complications following ectopic and molar pregnancy.

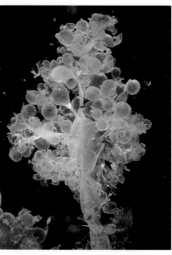

FIGURE 7–2 Hydatidiform mole.

Hypertension in Pregnancy

ICD-10 OFFICIAL GUIDELINES FOR CODING AND REPORTING

SECTION I.C.15.
Chapter 15: Pregnancy, Childbirth, and the Puerperium (O00-O9A)

d. Pre-existing hypertension in pregnancy

Category O10, Pre-existing hypertension complicating pregnancy, childbirth and the puerperium, includes codes for hypertensive heart and hypertensive chronic kidney disease. When assigning one of the O10 codes that includes hypertensive heart disease or hypertensive chronic kidney disease, it is necessary to add a secondary code from the appropriate hypertension category to specify the type of heart failure or chronic kidney disease.

See Section I.C.9. Hypertension.

When hypertension is a pre-existing condition that complicates pregnancy, delivery, or the five-month period after delivery, report the condition with a category O10 code, Pre-existing hypertension complicating pregnancy, childbirth, and the puerperium. The category O10 code is the first-listed diagnosis, and a secondary code is assigned to report any hypertensive heart disease or hypertensive chronic kidney disease.

Pre-Existing Hypertension

Example

A pregnant patient is seen by her obstetrician in her first trimester for a routine prenatal check. The patient has pre-existing stage I hypertensive chronic kidney disease that is complicating her pregnancy.

Report **O10.211**, Pre-existing hypertensive chronic kidney disease complicating pregnancy, first trimester; and **I12.9**, Hypertensive chronic kidney disease with stage 1 through stage 4 chronic kidney disease, or unspecified chronic kidney disease. The notes following code I12.9 state to use an additional code to identify the stage of chronic renal disease; therefore, add **N18.1** (Disease, kidney, chronic, stage 1).

Fetal Conditions

ICD-10 OFFICIAL GUIDELINES FOR CODING AND REPORTING

SECTION I.C.15.

Chapter 15: Pregnancy, Childbirth, and the Puerperium (O00-O9A)

e. Fetal Conditions Affecting the Management of the Mother

1) Codes from categories O35 and O36

Codes from categories O35, Maternal care for known or suspected fetal abnormality and damage, and O36, Maternal care for other fetal problems, are assigned only when the fetal condition is actually responsible for modifying the management of the mother, i.e., by requiring diagnostic studies, additional observation, special care, or termination of pregnancy. The fact that the fetal condition exists does not justify assigning a code from this series to the mother's record.

2) In utero surgery

In cases when surgery is performed on the fetus, a diagnosis code from category O35, Maternal care for known or suspected fetal abnormality and damage, should be assigned identifying the fetal condition. Assign the appropriate procedure code for the procedure performed.

No code from Chapter 16, the perinatal codes, should be used on the mother's record to identify fetal conditions. Surgery performed in utero on a fetus is still to be coded as an obstetric encounter.

Categories O35 and O36 report fetal abnormalities or other fetal problems when these abnormalities or problems affect the care of the mother. If the abnormality or problem is present but does not affect the care of the mother, O35 and O36 are NOT reported. It is only when these conditions exist and do affect the mother's care that O35 or O36 are reported.

TOOLBOX

Carol Jean is a 35-year-old alcoholic in her second trimester with a single fetus. She continues to consume 4-5 drinks daily that contain alcohol. Her OB/GYN is concerned about the slow growth of the fetus and has asked Dr. Zahn, a specialist in fetal alcohol disorders, to provide a consultation regarding suspected fetal alcohol syndrome (FAS).

QUESTIONS

1. When you reference "Pregnancy, complicated by, fetal, damage from, maternal, alcohol addiction," what code are you directed to locate in the Tabular? _____

2. Within the Tabular, the code you reference only has 4 characters, but there are 7th characters to assign to the code. What symbol is placed in the 5th and 6th character position?

   _____

3. What 7th character is assigned to the code to indicate the fetal number?

   _____

4. What would be the code to report the diagnosis for Carol Jean? _____

   ▼ **ANSWERS**

   1. O35.4, 2. XX, 3. 0, 4. O35.4XX0

Diabetes Mellitus in Pregnancy

ICD-10 OFFICIAL GUIDELINES FOR CODING AND REPORTING

SECTION I.C.15.
Chapter 15: Pregnancy, Childbirth, and the Puerperium (O00-O9A)

g. Diabetes mellitus in pregnancy

Diabetes mellitus is a significant complicating factor in pregnancy. Pregnant women who are diabetic should be assigned a code from category O24, Diabetes mellitus in pregnancy, childbirth, and the puerperium, first, followed by the appropriate diabetes code(s) (E08-E13) from Chapter 4.

h. Long term use of insulin

Code Z79.4, Long-term (current) use of insulin, should also be assigned if the diabetes mellitus is being treated with insulin.

i. Gestational (pregnancy induced) diabetes

Gestational (pregnancy induced) diabetes can occur during the second and third trimester of pregnancy in women who were not diabetic prior to pregnancy. Gestational diabetes can cause complications in the pregnancy similar to those of pre-existing diabetes mellitus. It also puts the woman at greater risk of developing diabetes after the pregnancy. Codes for gestational diabetes are in subcategory O24.4, Gestational diabetes mellitus. No other code from category O24, Diabetes mellitus in pregnancy, childbirth, and the puerperium, should be used with a code from O24.4

The codes under subcategory O24.4 include diet controlled and insulin controlled. If a patient with gestational diabetes is treated with both diet and insulin, only the code for insulin-controlled is required.

Code Z79.4, Long-term (current) use of insulin, should not be assigned with codes from subcategory O24.4.

An abnormal glucose tolerance in pregnancy is assigned a code from subcategory O99.81, Abnormal glucose complicating pregnancy, childbirth, and the puerperium.

Poorly controlled diabetes mellitus during pregnancy can lead to serious complications for both the mother and the fetus and may result in miscarriage or stillbirth. **Type 1** diabetes is a condition in which little or no insulin is produced by the body and is controlled with administration of insulin. **Type 2** diabetes is a condition in which too little insulin is produced or the body cannot use the insulin that is produced and is controlled with dietary restrictions and medications and/or insulin.

If the pregnant female has type 2 diabetes mellitus that is well controlled with the use of insulin or oral medication, you would report a code from category **O24**, Diabetes mellitus in pregnancy, childbirth, and the puerperium, as the first-listed diagnosis followed by a code to report the type of diabetes, **E11.9,** Type 2 diabetes mellitus without complications. If the patient's diabetes has been and currently is being controlled with insulin, report **Z79.4,** Long-term (current) use of insulin, as a supplemental code.

Gestational diabetes is a type of diabetes that develops in the second or third trimester of pregnancy in women who did not have either type of diabetes prior to pregnancy. This type of diabetes may be controlled through dietary restrictions or insulin, depending on the severity of the condition and is reported with a code from category O24, Diabetes mellitus in pregnancy, childbirth, and the puerperium. Code Z79.4, Long-term (current) use of insulin, would not be assigned in gestational diabetes.

EXERCISE 7-1 *Pregnancy, Childbirth, and the Puerperium*

Assign I-10 codes for the following:

1 Blighted ovum

Code: _____

2 Incomplete spontaneous abortion, uncomplicated; dilation and curettage (D&C) performed

Code: _____

3 False labor of 38-week pregnancy, undelivered

Code: _____

4 Vaginal delivery of liveborn single infant with fourth-degree perineal laceration; obstetric laceration repaired (include appropriate Z code for outcome of delivery)

Codes: _____ (laceration), _____ (outcome)

5 Obstructed labor due to fetopelvic disproportion; liveborn single infant delivered by lower segment cesarean section

Codes: _____, _____

(Answers are located in Appendix B)

CERTAIN CONDITIONS ORIGINATING IN THE PERINATAL PERIOD

Chapter 16, Newborn (Perinatal) Guidelines (P00-P96), contains codes for the perinatal period, which is before birth through 28 days after birth. The blocks in this chapter are as shown in Fig. 7-3.

P00-P04	Newborn affected by maternal factors and by complications of pregnancy, labor, and delivery
P05-P08	Disorders of newborns related to length of gestation and fetal growth
P09	Abnormal findings on neonatal screening
P10-P15	Birth trauma
P19-P29	Respiratory and cardiovascular disorders specific to the perinatal period
P35-P39	Infections specific to the perinatal period
P50-P61	Hemorrhagic and hematological disorders of newborn
P70-P74	Transitory endocrine and metabolic disorders specific to newborn
P76-P78	Digestive system disorders of newborn
P80-P83	Conditions involving the integument and temperature regulation of newborn
P84	Other problems with newborn
P90-P96	Other disorders originating in the perinatal period

FIGURE 7-3 Blocks in Chapter 16, Certain Conditions Originating in the Perinatal Period (P00-P96).

ICD-10 OFFICIAL GUIDELINES FOR CODING AND REPORTING

CERTAIN CONDITIONS ORIGINATING IN THE PERINATAL PERIOD

SECTION I.C.16.

Chapter 16: Certain Conditions Originating in the Perinatal Period (P00-P96)

For coding and reporting purposes the perinatal period is defined as before birth through the 28th day following birth. The following guidelines are provided for reporting purposes

a. General Perinatal Rules

1) Use of Chapter 16 Codes

Codes in this chapter are <u>never</u> for use on the maternal record. Codes from Chapter 15, the obstetric chapter, are never permitted on the newborn record. Chapter 16 codes may be used throughout the life of the patient if the condition is still present.

Codes from Chapter 16 are only for the **newborn record** and are never reported on the maternal record. These codes do not report congenital malformations, deformities, or chromosomal abnormalities; rather, those conditions are reported with codes in the Q00-Q99 range.

First-Listed Diagnosis

ICD-10 OFFICIAL GUIDELINES FOR CODING AND REPORTING

CERTAIN CONDITIONS ORIGINATING IN THE PERINATAL PERIOD

SECTION I.C.16.a.

Chapter 16: Certain Conditions Originating in the Perinatal Period (P00-P96)

2) Principal Diagnosis for Birth Record

When coding the birth episode in a newborn record, assign a code from category Z38, Liveborn infants according to place of birth and type of delivery, as the principal diagnosis. A code from category Z38 is assigned only once, to a newborn at the time of birth. If a newborn is transferred to another institution, a code from category Z38 should not be used at the receiving hospital.

A code from category Z38 is used only on the newborn record, not on the mother's record.

The first-listed diagnosis on the **newborn** record is a category Z38 code, Liveborn according to place of birth and type of delivery. This category is for use as the first-listed code on the **initial** record of a newborn. It is to be assigned for the initial birth record only, and it is never to be used on the mother's record. For example, Z38.1, Single liveborn infant, born outside hospital, is reported only on the initial newborn record and is never reported on the mother's record.

CONGENITAL MALFORMATIONS, DEFORMATIONS AND CHROMOSOMAL ABNORMALITIES

Chapter 17, Congenital Malformations, Deformations and Chromosomal Abnormalities (Q00-Q99), in the I-10 Tabular describes congenital anomalies and conditions that originate in the perinatal period. The perinatal period extends through the 28 days following birth. The term **perinatal** applies only to the baby and **postpartum** applies to the mother. Codes from Chapter 17 can be assigned beyond the time frame of perinatal period, but as the chapter title indicates, the condition must have **originated** during the perinatal period.

The blocks of Chapter 17 are as illustrated in Fig. 7-4.

Q00-Q07	Congenital malformations of the nervous system
Q10-Q18	Congenital malformations of eye, ear, face and neck
Q20-Q28	Congenital malformations of the circulatory system
Q30-Q34	Congenital malformations of the respiratory system
Q35-Q37	Cleft lip and cleft palate
Q38-Q45	Other congenital malformations of the digestive system
Q50-Q56	Congenital malformations of genital organs
Q60-Q64	Congenital malformations of the urinary system
Q65-Q79	Congenital malformations and deformations of the musculoskeletal system
Q80-Q89	Other congenital malformations
Q90-Q99	Chromosomal abnormalities, not elsewhere classified

FIGURE 7-4   Blocks in Chapter 17, Congenital Malformations, Deformations and Chromosomal Abnormalities (Q00-Q99).

ICD-10 OFFICIAL GUIDELINES FOR CODING AND REPORTING

SECTION I.C.17.
Chapter 17: Congenital malformations, deformations, and chromosomal abnormalities (Q00-Q99)

Assign an appropriate code(s) from categories Q00-Q99, Congenital malformations, deformations, and chromosomal abnormalities when a malformation/deformation or chromosomal abnormality is documented. A malformation/deformation/or chromosomal abnormality may be the principal/first-listed diagnosis on a record or a secondary diagnosis.

When a malformation/deformation/or chromosomal abnormality does not have a unique code assignment, assign additional code(s) for any manifestations that may be present.

When the code assignment specifically identifies the malformation/deformation/or chromosomal abnormality, manifestations that are an inherent component of the anomaly should not be coded separately. Additional codes should be assigned for manifestations that are not an inherent component.

Codes from Chapter 17 may be used throughout the life of the patient. If a congenital malformation or deformity has been corrected, a personal history code should be used to identify the history of the malformation or deformity. Although present at birth, malformation/deformation/or chromosomal abnormality may not be identified until later in life. Whenever the condition is diagnosed by the physician, it is appropriate to assign a code from codes Q00-Q99. For the birth admission, the appropriate code from category Z38, Liveborn infants, according to place of birth and type of delivery, should be sequenced as the principal diagnosis, followed by any congenital anomaly codes, Q00-Q99.

An **anomaly** is an abnormality of a structure or organ. **Congenital** anomaly means that it is an abnormality that one was born with. Some anomalies are noticeable and discovered at birth. In cases of other anomalies, it may be a number of months or even years before the anomaly is diagnosed. If there is a question as to whether a condition was acquired or congenital, you should review the record or query the physician. The physician must document the abnormality, and the abnormality may be either the first-listed diagnosis or an additional diagnosis.

If a patient is admitted for the purpose of birthing, report a code from category Z38, Liveborn infant according to type of birth, and sequence the Z38 code as the first-listed diagnosis. The Z38 code is assigned only once and on the birth record of the newborn because the Z38 code indicates the type of birth. If any other conditions or congenital anomalies are documented, report them as secondary diagnoses.

Newborn Congenital Anomalies

Example

Diagnosis:	Newborn male delivered in the hospital by cesarean section and with Down syndrome (Trisomy 21)
Index:	**Newborn** (infant) (liveborn) (single) Z38.2
	born in hospital Z38.00
	by cesarean Z38.01
Tabular:	**Z38.01 Single liveborn infant, delivered by cesarean**

Next, report the Down syndrome.

Index:	**Down syndrome** Q90.0
Tabular:	**Q90 Down syndrome**

> Use additional code(s) to identify any associated physical conditions and degree of intellectual disabilities (F70-F79).

Q90.9   Down syndrome, unspecified
Trisomy 21 NOS

Codes:	Z38.01, Q90.9, F79 Newborn male delivered by cesarean section in the hospital; Down syndrome

Trisomy 21 is the name for Down syndrome because most Down syndrome is due to a cell having two 21st chromosomes instead of one. When the cells merge, there are three 21st chromosomes, rather than one from each parent. Some cases are due to **mosaicism** in which some cell lines have normal chromosomes and other cell lines have the trisomy 21—resulting in one chromosome from each parent and an additional portion of trisomy 21 from the other parent. There are two types of mosaicism—cellular and tissue. In **cellular mosaicism** there is a mixture of various cells of the same type, and in **tissue mosaicism** one set of cells has normal cells and another has trisomy 21. **Robertsonian translocation** is a condition in which there are irregularities in both the 14th and 21st chromosome in that some of the cells of the 14th chromosome replace some of the cells in the 21st chromosome, and some of the cells in the 21st chromosome replace the cells in the 14th chromosome. Some only have a triplication of the 21st chromosome that is referred to as partial trisomy 21.

All of the codes in Chapter 17 report chromosomal abnormalities, such as Fragile X syndrome (Q99.2), Klinefelter syndrome (Q98.0-Q98.1, Q98.4), and mosaicism (Q91.1,

Q91.5, Q92.1, Q93.1, Q96.3, Q96.4, Q97.2, Q98.7). The physician must document the type of chromosomal abnormalities to enable the coder to correctly assign a diagnosis code. If the documentation is not clear as to the abnormality, query the physician before assigning a code to the abnormality.

EXERCISE 7-2	*Congenital Malformations, Deformations and Chromosomal Abnormalities*

Assign I-10 codes for the following:

1 Congenital absence of the earlobe

Code: _____

2 Newborn male delivered in the hospital via vaginal delivery; undescended bilateral testicles (pediatrician will reevaluate in 6 weeks)

Codes: _____, _____

3 Three-year-old diagnosed with fragile X syndrome

Code: _____

4 Newborn transferred to a facility because of congenital dislocation of right hip (code as the facility transferred to)

Code: _____

(Answers are located in Appendix B)

SYMPTOMS, SIGNS, AND ABNORMAL CLINICAL AND LABORATORY FINDINGS, NOT ELSEWHERE CLASSIFIED

Chapter 18, Symptoms, Signs, and Abnormal Clinical and Laboratory Findings, Not Elsewhere Classified (R00-R99), in the Tabular of the I-10 includes symptoms, signs, abnormal results of investigations, and other ill-defined conditions. Signs and symptoms codes are assigned for encounters until there is a definitive diagnosis. A **sign** is defined as objective evidence of disease that can be observed by the physician. A **symptom** is a subjective observation reported by the patient but not confirmed objectively by the physician.

You assign the codes from Chapter 18 when:

■ no more specific diagnosis can be made after investigation
■ signs and symptoms existing at the time of the initial encounter prove to be transient or a cause cannot be determined
■ a patient fails to return and you have only a provisional diagnosis
■ a case is referred elsewhere before a definitive diagnosis is made
■ a more precise diagnosis is not available for any other reason
■ certain symptoms that represent important problems in the medical care exist and it may be desirable to classify them in addition to the known cause

The blocks for Chapter 18 are displayed in Fig. 7-5.

R00-R09	Symptoms and signs involving the circulatory and respiratory systems
R10-R19	Symptoms and signs involving the digestive system and abdomen
R20-R23	Symptoms and signs involving the skin and subcutaneous tissue
R25-R29	Symptoms and signs involving the nervous and musculoskeletal systems
R30-R39	Symptoms and signs involving the genitourinary system
R40-R46	Symptoms and signs involving cognition, perception, emotional state and behavior
R47-R49	Symptoms and signs involving speech and voice
R50-R69	General symptoms and signs
R70-R79	Abnormal findings on examination of blood, without diagnosis
R80-R82	Abnormal findings on examination of urine, without diagnosis
R83-R89	Abnormal findings on examination of other body fluids, substances and tissues, without diagnosis
R90-R94	Abnormal findings on diagnostic imaging and in function studies, without diagnosis
R97	Abnormal tumor markers
R99	Ill-defined and unknown cause of mortality

FIGURE 7-5　Blocks in Chapter 18, Symptoms, Signs, and Abnormal Clinical and Laboratory Findings, Not Elsewhere Classified (R00-R99).

ICD-10 OFFICIAL GUIDELINES FOR CODING AND REPORTING

SECTION I.C.18.

Chapter 18: Symptoms, signs and abnormal clinical and laboratory findings, not elsewhere classified (R00-R99)

Chapter 18 includes symptoms, signs, abnormal results of clinical or other investigative procedures, and ill-defined conditions regarding which no diagnosis classifiable elsewhere is recorded. Signs and symptoms that point to a specific diagnosis have been assigned to a category in other chapters of the classification.

a. Use of symptom codes

Codes that describe symptoms and signs are acceptable for reporting purposes when a related definitive diagnosis has not been established (confirmed) by the provider.

b. Use of a symptom code with a definitive diagnosis code

Codes for signs and symptoms may be reported in addition to a related definitive diagnosis when the sign or symptom is not routinely associated with that diagnosis, such as the various signs and symptoms associated with complex syndromes. The definitive diagnosis code should be sequenced before the symptom code.

Signs or symptoms that are associated routinely with a disease process should not be assigned as additional codes, unless otherwise instructed by the classification.

c. Combination codes that include symptoms

ICD-10-CM contains a number of combination codes that identify both the definitive diagnosis and common symptoms of that diagnosis. When using one of these combination codes, an additional code should not be assigned for the symptom.

Continued

d. Repeated falls

Code R29.6, Repeated falls, is for use for encounters when a patient has recently fallen and the reason for the fall is being investigated.

Code Z91.81, History of falling, is for use when a patient has fallen in the past and is at risk for future falls. When appropriate, both codes R29.6 and Z91.81 may be assigned together.

e. Coma scale

The coma scale codes (R40.2-) can be used in conjunction with traumatic brain injury codes, acute cerebrovascular disease or sequelae of cerebrovascular disease codes. These codes are primarily for use by trauma registries, but they may be used in any setting where this information is collected. The coma scale codes should be sequenced after the diagnosis code(s).

These codes, one from each subcategory, are needed to complete the scale. The 7th character indicates when the scale was recorded. The 7th character should match for all three codes.

At a minimum, report the initial score documented on presentation at your facility. This may be a score from the emergency medicine technician (EMT) or in the emergency department. If desired, a facility may choose to capture multiple coma scale scores.

Assign code R40.24, Glasgow coma scale, total score, when only the total score is documented in the medical record and not the individual score(s).

f. Functional quadriplegia

Functional quadriplegia (code R53.2) is the lack of ability to use one's limbs or to ambulate due to extreme debility. It is not associated with neurologic deficit or injury, and code R53.2 should not be used for cases of neurologic quadriplegia. It should only be assigned if functional quadriplegia is specifically documented in the medical record.

g. SIRS due to Non-Infectious Process

The systemic inflammatory response syndrome (SIRS) can develop as a result of certain non-infectious disease processes, such as trauma, malignant neoplasm, or pancreatitis. When SIRS is documented with a noninfectious condition, and no subsequent infection is documented, the code for the underlying condition, such as an injury, should be assigned, followed by code R65.10, Systemic inflammatory response syndrome (SIRS) of non-infectious origin without acute organ dysfunction, or code R65.11, Systemic inflammatory response syndrome (SIRS) of non-infectious origin with acute organ dysfunction. If an associated acute organ dysfunction is documented, the appropriate code(s) for the specific type of organ dysfunction(s) should be assigned in addition to code R65.11. If acute organ dysfunction is documented, but it cannot be determined if the acute organ dysfunction is associated with SIRS or due to another condition (e.g., directly due to the trauma), the provider should be queried.

h. Death NOS

Code R99, Ill-defined and unknown cause of mortality, is only for use in the very limited circumstance when a patient who has already died is brought into an emergency department or other healthcare facility and is pronounced dead upon arrival. It does not represent the discharge disposition of death.

You do not report codes from Chapter 18 when a definitive diagnosis is available—for example, this diagnostic statement: "Right lower quadrant abdominal pain due to acute appendicitis." The code for right lower quadrant abdominal pain is R10.31, located in Chapter 18. But because the reason for the pain is the acute appendicitis, you would not include the code for the symptom of abdominal pain; rather you would assign K35.80 for the acute appendicitis—the definitive diagnosis.

You do not report codes from Chapter 18 when the symptom is considered to be routinely associated with a disease process—for example, this diagnostic statement: "Cough and fever with pneumonia." Both cough and fever are symptoms of the pneumonia; therefore, you would not assign codes for either symptom of cough or fever. The only code you would assign would be J18.9 to report pneumonia.

A disease reference book comes in handy until you become more familiar with disease symptoms. If you do not know the symptoms associated with a disease, consult reference material, ask a colleague, or query the physician.

One method to find **abnormal** findings in the Index is to refer the main term "Abnormal" and subterm by specific test.

Abnormal Findings

Example

Diagnosis:	Abnormal liver scan
Index:	**Abnormal, abnormality, abnormalities,** scan, liver R93.2
Tabular:	**R93 Abnormal findings on diagnostic imaging of other body structures**
	R93.2 Abnormal findings on diagnostic imaging of liver and biliary tract
Code:	R93.2 Abnormal liver scan

When reporting complications of surgical or medical care, you must be certain the complications are documented. A surgical complication is one that takes place as a result of the procedure. Just because a complication occurs following a procedure does not mean the complication is a result of the surgery. Do not assume a cause-and-effect relationship. Rather, clarify any questions with the physician.

The term complication as used in I-10 does not imply that improper or inadequate care is responsible for the problem. Also, there is no time limit for the development of a complication. The time the complication presents will dictate the way in which the complication is reported. Be sure to use the Index and follow all instructional notes when locating complication codes. Exclusion notes are extensive in complication codes and often direct the coder to report the complication with a code from another category.

EXERCISE 7-3   *Symptoms, Signs, and Ill-Defined Conditions*

Assign I-10 codes for the following:

1 Fussy infant

Code: _____

2 Pleuritic-type chest pain on breathing

Code: _____

3 Abnormal mammogram

Code: _____

Continued

4 Nonspecific abnormal findings of cervical Papanicolaou smear

Code: _____

5 Elevated blood pressure reading, no diagnosis of HTN

Code: _____

6 Miss Halliday is an 80-year-old woman who presents to the emergency department with a history of abdominal pain, fever, and burning with urination. Urine culture is obtained, and Miss Halliday is admitted for work-up to rule out urosepsis. Urosepsis was ruled out.

Codes: _____, _____, _____

7 Mr. Johnson is admitted to the hospital with chest and epigastric pain. He is evaluated by the emergency department physician with a diagnosis of rule out myocardial infarction. Mr. Johnson is then transferred to a larger facility for further work-up.

Codes: _____ and _____

(Answers are located in Appendix B)

INJURY, POISONING, AND CERTAIN OTHER CONSEQUENCES OF EXTERNAL CAUSES

Injury, poisoning, and certain other consequences of external causes are reported with codes in the S00-T88 range.

The blocks of Chapter 19 are as illustrated in Fig. 7-6.

S00-S09	Injuries to the head
S10-S19	Injuries to the neck
S20-S29	Injuries to the thorax
S30-S39	Injuries to the abdomen, lower back, lumbar spine, pelvis and external genitals
S40-S49	Injuries to the shoulder and upper arm
S50-S59	Injuries to the elbow and forearm
S60-S69	Injuries to the wrist, hand, and fingers
S70-S79	Injuries to the hip and thigh
S80-S89	Injuries to the knee and lower leg
S90-S99	Injuries to the ankle and foot
T07	Injuries involving multiple body regions
T14	Injury of unspecified body region
T15-T19	Effects of foreign body entering through natural orifice
T20-T32	Burns and corrosions
T20-T25	Burns and corrosions of external body surface, specified by site
T26-T28	Burns and corrosions confined to eye and internal organs
T30-T32	Burns and corrosions of multiple and unspecified body regions
T33-T34	Frostbite
T36-T50	Poisoning by, adverse effect of and underdosing of drugs, medicaments and biological substances
T51-T65	Toxic effects of substances chiefly nonmedicinal as to source
T66-T78	Other and unspecified effects of external causes
T79	Certain early complications of trauma
T80-T88	Complications of surgical and medical care, not elsewhere classified

FIGURE 7–6 Blocks in Chapter 19, Injury, Poisoning, and Certain Other Consequences of External Causes (S00-T88).

Code Extensions

ICD-10 OFFICIAL GUIDELINES FOR CODING AND REPORTING

SECTION I.C.19.

Chapter 19: Injury, poisoning, and certain other consequences of external causes (S00-T88)

a. Application of 7th Characters in Chapter 19

Most categories in chapter 19 have a 7th character requirement for each applicable code. Most categories in this chapter have three 7th character values (with the exception of fractures): A, initial encounter, D, subsequent encounter and S, sequela. Categories for traumatic fractures have additional 7th character values. While the patient may be seen by a new or different provider over the course of treatment for an injury, assignment of the 7th character is based on whether the patient is undergoing active treatment and not whether the provider is seeing the patient for the first time.

For complication codes, active treatment refers to treatment for the condition described by the code, even though it may be related to an earlier precipitating problem. For example, code T84.50XA, Infection and inflammatory reaction due to unspecified internal joint prosthesis, initial encounter, is used when active treatment is provided for the infection, even though the condition relates to the prosthetic device, implant, or graft that was placed at a previous encounter.

7th character "A", initial encounter is used while the patient is receiving active treatment for the condition. Examples of active treatment are: surgical treatment, emergency department encounter, and evaluation and continuing treatment by the same or a different physician.

7th character "D" subsequent encounter is used for encounters after the patient has received active treatment of the condition and is receiving routine care for the condition during the healing or recovery phase. Examples of subsequent care are: cast change or removal, an x-ray to check healing status of fracture, removal of external or internal fixation device, medication adjustment, other aftercare and follow up visits following treatment of the injury or condition.

The aftercare Z codes should not be used for aftercare for conditions such as injuries or poisonings, where 7th characters are provided to identify subsequent care. For example, for aftercare of an injury, assign the acute injury code with the 7th character "D" (subsequent encounter).

7th character "S", sequela, is for use for complications or conditions that arise as a direct result of a condition, such as scar formation after a burn. The scars are sequelae of the burn. When using 7th character "S", it is necessary to use both the injury code that precipitated the sequela and the code for the sequela itself. The "S" is added only to the injury code, not the sequela code. The 7th character "S" identifies the injury responsible for the sequela. The specific type of sequela (e.g. scar) is sequenced first, followed by the injury code.

When reporting an S00-T88 code, you would usually also report a secondary code or codes from Chapter 20, External Causes of Morbidity, to indicate the cause of the injury, such as a motor vehicle accident or fall from a ladder. However, there are T codes that include the external cause as part of the code description.

The S00-S99 codes are injuries to specific body areas (head, thorax, hip, etc.) and T07 and T14 are for injuries to unspecified body regions. The remaining T codes report injuries, such as burns, frostbite, poisoning, toxic effects, as well as complications of trauma and surgical/medical care NEC. Most of these codes have 7th character categories to indicate the encounter (initial [A] or subsequent [D] and sequela [S]). The initial encounter is when the patient is receiving active treatment, such as surgical treatment or an office evaluation. The subsequent encounter is for the patient who has received the active treatment and is now receiving routine care during the recovery or healing phase. The sequela is a residual complication or condition that develops as a result of an injury, such as a scar from a burn.

Coding Injuries

> ### ICD-10 OFFICIAL GUIDELINES FOR CODING AND REPORTING
>
> **SECTION I.C.19.**
> **Chapter 19: Injury, poisoning, and certain other consequences of external causes (S00-T88)**
>
> **b. Coding of Injuries**
>
> When coding injuries, assign separate codes for each injury unless a combination code is provided, in which case the combination code is assigned. Code T07, Unspecified multiple injuries should not be assigned in the inpatient setting unless information for a more specific code is not available. Traumatic injury codes (S00-T14.9) are not to be used for normal, healing surgical wounds or to identify complications of surgical wounds.
>
> The code for the most serious injury, as determined by the provider and the focus of treatment, is sequenced first.
>
> **1) Superficial injuries**
>
> Superficial injuries such as abrasions or contusions are not coded when associated with more severe injuries of the same site.
>
> **2) Primary injury with damage to nerves/blood vessels**
>
> When a primary injury results in minor damage to peripheral nerves or blood vessels, the primary injury is sequenced first with additional code(s) for injuries to nerves and spinal cord (such as category S04), and/or injury to blood vessels (such as category S15). When the primary injury is to the blood vessels or nerves, that injury should be sequenced first.

Codes in the S00-T14.9 range are not assigned to report complications of surgical wounds or the normal healing of surgical wounds. For example, if the complication was of burst stitches of an external surgical wound for which there was no specific code, you would report T81.31XA, Disruption of external operation wound, not elsewhere classified; but if the disruption was of an episiotomy wound, you would report the more specific code O90.1, Disruption of perineal obstetric wound.

If the patient has multiple injuries, the physician is to indicate the most serious condition, and it is that condition that is the first-listed diagnosis. Report a code for each injury documented in the medical record. There are rules that indicate when one injury is present, not to report some other types of injuries of the same area. For example, do not report abrasions of an area when there is a more serious injury of the same area, such as abrasions of the knee with fracture of the knee. You would report the fracture but not the abrasions.

When the damage is to the nerve or blood vessel, report the primary injury first and use an additional code if nerve/vessel damage is minor—for example, a puncture wound of the knee in which there was nerve injury. Report the puncture wound as the first-listed diagnosis and additional code(s) for the nerve damage. If, however, the primary injury is to a nerve or blood vessel, report that injury first.

A fracture not indicated as closed or open should be classified as **closed**. If a fracture is not indicated to be displaced or not displaced, report the fracture as displaced. If you have any doubt, query the physician as to the nature of the fracture.

If there is a dislocation and fracture of the same bone, report only the fracture because the fracture is more severe than dislocation.

Coding Fractures

ICD-10 OFFICIAL GUIDELINES FOR CODING AND REPORTING

SECTION I.C.19.
Chapter 19: Injury, poisoning, and certain other consequences of external causes (S00-T88)

c. Coding of Traumatic Fractures

The principles of multiple coding of injuries should be followed in coding fractures. Fractures of specified sites are coded individually by site in accordance with both the provisions within categories S02, S12, S22, S32, S42, S49, S52, S59, S62, S72, S79, S82, S89, S92 and the level of detail furnished by medical record content.

A fracture not indicated as open or closed should be coded to closed. A fracture not indicated whether displaced or not displaced should be coded to displaced.

More specific guidelines are as follows:

1) Initial vs. Subsequent Encounter for Fractures

Traumatic fractures are coded using the appropriate 7th character for initial encounter (A, B, C) while the patient is receiving active treatment for the fracture. Examples of active treatment are: surgical treatment, emergency department encounter, and evaluation and continuing (ongoing) treatment by the same or different physician. The appropriate 7th character for initial encounter should also be assigned for a patient who delayed seeking treatment for the fracture or nonunion.

Fractures are coded using the appropriate 7th character for subsequent care for encounters after the patient has completed active treatment of the fracture and is receiving routine care for the fracture during the healing or recovery phase. Examples of fracture aftercare are: cast change or removal, an x-ray to check healing status of fracture, removal of external or internal fixation device, medication adjustment, and follow-up visits following fracture treatment.

Care for complications of surgical treatment for fracture repairs during the healing or recovery phase should be coded with the appropriate complication codes.

Care of complications of fractures, such as malunion and nonunion, should be reported with the appropriate 7th character for subsequent care with nonunion (K, M, N,) or subsequent care with malunion (P, Q, R).

Malunion/nonunion: The appropriate 7th character for initial encounter should also be assigned for a patient who delayed seeking treatment for the fracture or nonunion.

A code from category M80, not a traumatic fracture code, should be used for any patient with known osteoporosis who suffers a fracture, even if the patient had a minor fall or trauma, if that fall or trauma would not usually break a normal, healthy bone.
See Section I.C.13. Osteoporosis.

The aftercare Z codes should not be used for aftercare for traumatic fractures. For aftercare of a traumatic fracture, assign the acute fracture code with the appropriate 7th character.

2) Multiple fractures sequencing

Multiple fractures are sequenced in accordance with the severity of the fracture.

Dislocation and Fracture

Example

Diagnosis: Traumatic fracture of the right hip with dislocation, initial encounter

Index: **Dislocation,** with fracture—*see* Fracture

The "*see* Fracture" informs the coder that the dislocation is included with the fracture code.

Index: **Fracture,** traumatic, femur, upper end S72.00

Tabular: **S72.00 Fracture of unspecified part of neck of femur**
            Fracture of hip NOS
            Fracture of neck of femur NOS
            S72.001 Fracture of unspecified part of neck of right femur

Code: S72.001A Fractured right hip with dislocation

The S72 category has the 7th characters that are illustrated in Fig. 7-7.

In the Index of the I-10, there is a main entry for "Fracture, pathologic" and "Fracture, traumatic" with subterms by body location (i.e., ankle, clavicle, etc.), due to (i.e., neoplastic disease, specific disease, etc.). If, for example, you reference "Fracture, pathologic, ankle" you are directed to M84.47-, but if you reference "Fracture, traumatic, ankle" you are directed to S82.899. Use caution when locating fracture terms in the Index to ensure you are at the correct subterm. A fracture that is **pathologic** is one that occurs due to disease or weakening of an area, such as osteoporosis, and with pressure that would not ordinarily fracture a bone, such as a bone weakened by osteoporosis fractures. Sometimes, the fractures occur without even a pressure blow of any type; the osteoporotic bone just spontaneously fractures.

Pathological Fracture

Example

Diagnosis: Pathological fracture of the right humerus, due to osteoporosis

Index: Osteoporosis
                with current pathological fracture - M80.00
                    specified type NEC- M81.8
                        with pathological fracture- M80.80
                            humerus - M80.82-

Tabular: **M80   Osteoporosis with current pathological fracture**
                M80.8   Other osteoporosis with current pathological fracture
                    M80.82   Other osteoporosis with current pathological fracture, humerus
                        M80.821 - right humerus

M80.821A Other osteoporosis with current pathological fracture, right humerus

If there are multiple fractures, sequence the fractures in order of severity with the most severe listed first. Query the physician when the severity is not documented.

When there is an aftercare encounter for a fracture (such as cast removal, removal of internal fixation devices), do not assign a Z code (encounters with health care services and health status codes); rather, assign the 7th character of "D" to the fracture code to indicate a subsequent encounter with routine healing.

● **S72   Fracture of femur**

> **Note:** A fracture not indicated as displaced or nondisplaced should be coded to displaced
>
> A fracture not indicated as open or closed should be coded to closed
>
> The open fracture designations are based on the Gustilo open fracture classification
>
> **Excludes1** traumatic amputation of hip and thigh (S78.-)
>
> **Excludes2** fracture of lower leg and ankle (S82.-)
> fracture of foot (S92.-)
> periprosthetic fracture of prosthetic implant of hip (T84.040, T84.041)
>
> The appropriate 7th character is to be added to all codes from category S72

A	initial encounter for closed fracture
B	initial encounter for open fracture type I or II
	initial encounter for open fracture NOS
C	initial encounter for open fracture type IIIA, IIIB, or IIIC
D	subsequent encounter for closed fracture with routine healing
E	subsequent encounter for open fracture type I or II with routine healing
F	subsequent encounter for open fracture type IIIA, IIIB, or IIIC with routine healing
G	subsequent encounter for closed fracture with delayed healing
H	subsequent encounter for open fracture type I or II with delayed healing
J	subsequent encounter for open fracture type IIIA, IIIB, or IIIC with delayed healing
K	subsequent encounter for closed fracture with nonunion
M	subsequent encounter for open fracture type I or II with nonunion
N	subsequent encounter for open fracture type IIIA, IIIB, or IIIC with nonunion
P	subsequent encounter for closed fracture with malunion
Q	subsequent encounter for open fracture type I or II with malunion
R	subsequent encounter for open fracture type IIIA, IIIB, or IIIC with malunion
S	sequela

FIGURE 7-7   The 7th characters of category S72.

Coding Burns and Corrosions

ICD-10 OFFICIAL GUIDELINES FOR CODING AND REPORTING

SECTION I.C.19.
Chapter 19: Injury, poisoning, and certain other consequences of external causes (S00-T88)

d. Coding of Burns and Corrosions

The ICD-10-CM makes a distinction between burns and corrosions. The burn codes are for thermal burns, except sunburns, that come from a heat source, such as a fire or hot appliance. The burn codes are also for burns resulting from electricity and radiation. Corrosions are burns due to chemicals. The guidelines are the same for burns and corrosions.

Current burns (T20-T25) are classified by depth, extent and by agent (X code). Burns are classified by depth as first degree (erythema), second degree (blistering), and third degree (full-thickness

Continued

involvement). Burns of the eye and internal organs (T26-T28) are classified by site, but not by degree.

1) Sequencing of burn and related condition codes

Sequence first the code that reflects the highest degree of burn when more than one burn is present.

a. When the reason for the admission or encounter is for treatment of external multiple burns, sequence first the code that reflects the burn of the highest degree.

b. When a patient has both internal and external burns, the circumstances of admission govern the selection of the principal diagnosis or first-listed diagnosis.

c. When a patient is admitted for burn injuries and other related conditions such as smoke inhalation and/or respiratory failure, the circumstances of admission govern the selection of the principal or first-listed diagnosis.

2) Burns of the same local site

Classify burns of the same local site (three-character category level, T20-T28) but of different degrees to the subcategory identifying the highest degree recorded in the diagnosis.

3) Non-healing burns

Non-healing burns are coded as acute burns.

Necrosis of burned skin should be coded as a non-healed burn.

4) Infected Burn

For any documented infected burn site, use an additional code for the infection.

5) Assign separate codes for each burn site

When coding burns, assign separate codes for each burn site. Category T30, Burn and corrosion, body region unspecified is extremely vague and should rarely be used.

6) Burns and Corrosions Classified According to Extent of Body Surface Involved

Assign codes from category T31, Burns classified according to extent of body surface involved, or T32, Corrosions classified according to extent of body surface involved, when the site of the burn is not specified or when there is a need for additional data. It is advisable to use category T31 as additional coding when needed to provide data for evaluating burn mortality, such as that needed by burn units. It is also advisable to use category T31 as an additional code for reporting purposes when there is mention of a third-degree burn involving 20 percent or more of the body surface.

Categories T31 and T32 are based on the classic "rule of nines" in estimating body surface involved: head and neck are assigned nine percent, each arm nine percent, each leg 18 percent, the anterior trunk 18 percent, posterior trunk 18 percent, and genitalia one percent. Providers may change these percentage assignments where necessary to accommodate infants and children who have proportionately larger heads than adults, and patients who have large buttocks, thighs, or abdomen that involve burns.

7) Encounters for treatment of sequela of burns

Encounters for the treatment of the late effects of burns or corrosions (i.e., scars or joint contractures) should be coded with a burn or corrosion code with the 7th character "S" for sequela.

8) Sequelae with a late effect code and current burn

When appropriate, both a code for a current burn or corrosion with 7th character extension "A" or "D" and a burn or corrosion code with 7th character "S" may be assigned on the same record (when both a current burn and sequelae of an old burn exist). Burns and corrosions do not heal at the same rate and a current healing wound may still exist with sequela of a healed burn or corrosion.

See Section I.B.10 Sequela (Late Effects)

9) Use of an external cause code with burns and corrosions

An external cause code should be used with burns and corrosions to identify the source and intent of the burn, as well as the place where it occurred.

I-10 distinguishes between burns and corrosions. **Burns** are those injuries that result from a heat source, such as a burner on the stove or hot water—thermal burns. Electrical and radiation burns are also considered burns. Burns are reported based on degree of burn—first, second, third; except if the burn is of the eye or internal organ (T26-T28), then the burn is reported by site. **Corrosions** (T20-T25) are a result of chemical contact and are classified by depth, extent, and agent.

Specified sites of burns and corrosions of the external body are reported with T20-T25 codes that are based on degree:

■ First (erythema)
■ Second (blisters, epidermal loss)
■ Third (deep necrosis of underlying tissue or full thickness skin loss)

Sequence the site of the highest degree of burn first. For example, if you are reporting a third-degree burn of the hand and a second-degree burn of the chest wall, sequence the code for the third-degree (the highest degree) chest wall burn first followed by the second-degree hand burn code.

If there are different degrees of burns at the same site, only assign a code to the highest degree. For example, if the documentation indicates there were first- and second-degree burns to the right hand, only report the second-degree burn to the hand because that is the highest of severity. There are also codes used in conjunction with the burn and corrosion codes.

Burns

Example

Diagnosis: First- and second-degree corrosion, due to hydrochloric acid, of the upper back, initial encounter. Location of injury was the patient's private garage attached to his home and the incident was accidental. He was using the acid to remove rust from an iron lawn chair.

Index: **Corrosion** (injury) (acid) (caustic) (chemical) (lime) (external) (internal) T30.4
　　　　　back (lower) T21.44
　　　　　　upper T21.43
　　　　　　　first degree T21.53
　　　　　　　second degree T21.63

Tabular: **T21.6   Corrosion of second degree of trunk**
　　　　　　　Code first (T51-T65) to identify chemical and intent
　　　　　　　Use additional external cause code to identify place (Y92)
　　　　　　T21.63   Corrosion of second degree of upper back

The 6th character "X" is added to allow for the 7th character "A" that indicates an initial encounter.

Code: T21.63XA Second-degree corrosion to the back

Note that the diagnosis includes first- and second-degree corrosion and the code assigned reports only the second-degree corrosion. Report only the highest degree when corrosion or burns are at the same site. The instructional note following T21.6 directs the coder to:

● Code first (T51-T65) to identify chemical and intent.
　　● In this case, T54.2X1A—this is the first-listed diagnosis, followed by the burn code T21.63XA.

- Use additional external cause code to identify place (Y92, Place of occurrence of the external cause).
    - In this case, Y92.015, Private garage of single-family [private] house. The place of occurrence should be recorded only at the initial encounter for treatment.
- The activity code reports the circumstance of the injury.
    - In this case, Y93.H9, Other activity involving property and land maintenance, building, and construction, is assigned to report that the patient was involved in maintenance at the time of the injury.

Codes: T54.2X1A, T21.63XA, Y92.015, Y93.H9

When reporting a burn, report the source of the heat that caused the burn first, followed by a code to report the burn, the place the incident occurred, and the activity being performed at the time of injury.

EXERCISE 7-4   *Burns and Corrosions*

Code the burn, extent of the body surface involved, and percentage of body surface burned using the rule of nines:

1 A 3-year-old receives third-degree burns of the abdomen, 10%, and second-degree burns of the thigh, 5%, after pulling a pot of hot water from stove on herself

Third-degree Code: _____

Second-degree Code: _____

Degree and Percentage Code: _____

X Code: _____

2 Infected third-degree burn, left thigh, 4½%, subsequent early treatment

Third-degree Code: _____

Infected burn Code: _____

Extent Code: _____

3 First- and second-degree burn, right foot, 2¼%, due to bonfire flames

Second-degree Code: _____

Extent Code: _____

X Code: _____

4 Third-degree burn, right hand, 2¼%; excisional debridement performed by physician; patient seen 10 days ago for initial treatment

Third-degree Code: _____

Extent Code: _____

5 Second-degree burn, right forearm, 2%; first-degree burn, right hand, 1%; and third-degree burn, chest wall, 8%, subsequent treatment

Codes: _____, _____, _____, _____

(Answers are located in Appendix B)

Coding Adverse Effects, Poisoning, Underdosing, and Toxic Effects

---

ICD-10 OFFICIAL GUIDELINES FOR CODING AND REPORTING

SECTION I.C.19.
Chapter 19: Injury, poisoning, and certain other consequences of external causes (S00-T88)

e. Adverse Effects, Poisoning, Underdosing and Toxic Effects

Codes in categories T36-T65 are combination codes that include the substance that was taken, as well as the intent. No additional external cause code is required for poisonings, toxic effects, adverse effects and underdosing codes.

1) Do not code directly from the Table of Drugs

Do not code directly from the Table of Drugs and Chemicals. Always refer back to the Tabular List.

2) Use as many codes as necessary to describe

Use as many codes as necessary to describe completely all drugs, medicinal or biological substances.

3) If the same code would describe the causative agent

If the same code would describe the causative agent for more than one adverse reaction, poisoning, toxic effect or underdosing, assign the code only once.

4) If two or more drugs, medicinal or biological substances

If two or more drugs, medicinal or biological substances are reported, code each individually unless a combination code is listed in the Table of Drugs and Chemicals.

5) The occurrence of drug toxicity is classified in ICD-10-CM as follows:
(a) Adverse Effect

When coding an adverse effect of a drug that has been correctly prescribed and properly administered, assign the appropriate code for the nature of the adverse effect followed by the appropriate code for the adverse effect of the drug (T36-T50). The code for the drug should have a 5th or 6th character "5" (for example T36.0X5-) Examples of the nature of an adverse effect are tachycardia, delirium, gastrointestinal hemorrhaging, vomiting, hypokalemia, hepatitis, renal failure, or respiratory failure.

(b) Poisoning

When coding a poisoning or reaction to the improper use of a medication (e.g., overdose, wrong substance given or taken in error, wrong route of administration), first assign the appropriate code from categories T36-T50. The poisoning codes have an associated intent as their 5th or 6th character (accidental, intentional self-harm, assault and undetermined. Use additional code(s) for all manifestations of poisonings.

If there is also a diagnosis of abuse or dependence of the substance, the abuse or dependence is assigned as an additional code.

Examples of poisoning include:

(i) Error was made in drug prescription
Errors made in drug prescription or in the administration of the drug by provider, nurse, patient, or other person.

(ii) Overdose of a drug intentionally taken
If an overdose of a drug was intentionally taken or administered and resulted in drug toxicity, it would be coded as a poisoning.

Continued

(iii) Nonprescribed drug taken with correctly prescribed and properly administered drug
   If a nonprescribed drug or medicinal agent was taken in combination with a correctly prescribed and properly administered drug, any drug toxicity or other reaction resulting from the interaction of the two drugs would be classified as a poisoning.

(iv) Interaction of drug(s) and alcohol
   When a reaction results from the interaction of a drug(s) and alcohol, this would be classified as poisoning.

   See Section I.C.4. if poisoning is the result of insulin pump malfunctions.

(c) Underdosing

Underdosing refers to taking less of a medication than is prescribed by a provider or a manufacturer's instruction. For underdosing, assign the code from categories T36-T50 (fifth or sixth character "6").

Codes for underdosing should never be assigned as principal or first-listed codes. If a patient has a relapse or exacerbation of the medical condition for which the drug is prescribed because of the reduction in dose, then the medical condition itself should be coded.

Noncompliance (Z91.12-, Z91.13-) or complication of care (Y63.6-Y63.9) codes are to be used with an underdosing code to indicate intent, if known.

(d) Toxic Effects

When a harmful substance is ingested or comes in contact with a person, this is classified as a toxic effect. The toxic effect codes are in categories T51-T65.

Toxic effect codes have an associated intent: accidental, intentional self-harm, assault and undetermined.

The codes in the categories T36-T65 report the external causes of adverse effects, poisoning, underdosing, and toxic effects as well as the causative substance; therefore, no additional external cause code is required.

Poisoning

Example

T36.0X1A reports initial encounter for accidental (**unintentional**) poisoning by penicillin

T36.0X2A reports initial encounter for **intentional** self-harm poisoning by penicillin

There are often multiple codes required to completely describe the substances involved. If the causative agent, such as the penicillin, is responsible for multiple reactions, report the agent only once. If multiple substances are involved, report each substance separately, unless there is a combination code to report more than one substance with one code.

The External Causes index and Table of Drugs and Chemicals is used to initially locate the terms, subterms, and codes; but as with all diagnosis coding, you must reference the Tabular before assigning a code. The Table contains classification of drugs and substances to identify adverse effects and poisoning.

Adverse effect occurs when a substance is taken correctly but the patient has a negative reaction to the substance.

Adverse Effect

Example

Amoxicillin is prescribed for a patient with a diagnosis of bronchitis. The patient takes the medicine as prescribed; however, the medication causes a rash (adverse effect).

Poisoning occurs when the medication is incorrectly taken.

Poisoning

Example

Amoxicillin prescribed for a patient with a diagnosis of bronchitis and rather than one tablet, as prescribed, the patient takes 4 tablets and nausea results (poisoning).

The poisoning is due to the improper use of a medication and is assigned a poisoning code from the categories T36-T50.

The Table of Drugs and Chemicals displays the drug name alphabetically on the left under the heading "**Substance**" (Fig. 7-8).

- The code in the first column, "**Poisoning, Accidental (Unintentional),**" is for the substance involved but is not related to an adverse effect.
- The second column is "**Poisoning, Intentional, Self-Harm**" when the external cause is a result of a person intentionally taking the substance.
- The third column is "**Poisoning, Assault**" when there is intentional infliction by another person.
- The fourth column is "**Poisoning, Undetermined**" when the intent is not known.
- The fifth column is "**Adverse Effect**" and was discussed previously.
- The sixth column is "**Underdosing,**" which refers to taking less of the medication than was prescribed.

The codes in the T36-T50 categories report poisoning resulting in adverse effect or underdosing. For example, T49.7, as displayed in Fig. 7-9, illustrates the codes are divided based on accidental, intentional, assault, undetermined, adverse effect, and underdosing. If the underdosing was due to the patient intentionally taking less of the medication than prescribed, report a noncompliance code (Z91.12-, noncompliance, Z91.13-, unintentional).

EXERCISE 7-5   *Poisoning/Table of Drugs and Chemicals*

Using the I-10 manual, assign poisoning T codes to the following:

1 Poisoning by the ingestion of ethanol, subsequent encounter, undetermined cause

    T Code: _____

2 Accidental poisoning by herbicides, subsequent encounter

    T Code: _____

3 Accidental overdose due to therapeutically prescribed valium, initial encounter

    T Code: _____

(Answers are located in Appendix B)

Substance	External Cause (T-Code)					
	① Poisoning, Accidental (Unintentional)	② Poisoning, Intentional Self-Harm	③ Poisoning, Assault	④ Poisoning, Undetermined	⑤ Adverse Effect	⑥ Underdosing
#						
1-propanol	T51.3X1	T51.3X2	T51.3X3	T51.3X4	—	—
2-propanol	T51.2X1	T51.2X2	T51.2X3	T51.2X4	—	—
2,4-D (dichlorophen-oxyacetic acid)	T60.3X1	T60.3X2	T60.3X3	T60.3X4	—	—
2,4-toluene diisocyanate	T65.0X1	T65.0X2	T65.0X3	T65.0X4	—	—
2,4,5-T (trichloro-phenoxyacetic acid)	T60.1X1	T60.1X2	T60.1X3	T60.1X4	—	—
14-hydroxydihydro-morphinone	T40.2X1	T40.2X2	T40.2X3	T40.2X4	T40.2X5	T40.2X6
A						
ABOB	T37.5X1	T37.5X2	T37.5X3	T37.5X4	T37.5X5	T37.5X6
Abrine	T62.2X1	T62.2X2	T62.2X3	T62.2X4	—	—
Abrus (seed)	T62.2X1	T62.2X2	T62.2X3	T62.2X4	—	—
Absinthe	T51.0X1	T51.0X2	T51.0X3	T51.0X4	—	—
beverage	T51.0X1	T51.0X2	T51.0X3	T51.0X4	—	—

FIGURE 7–8 Table of Drugs and Chemicals.

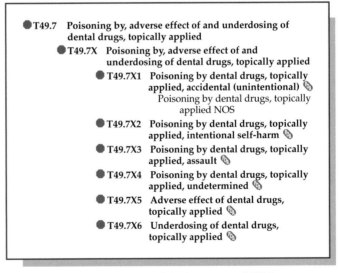

FIGURE 7–9 Poisoning category code T49.7.

Abuse, Neglect, and Other Maltreatment

ICD-10 OFFICIAL GUIDELINES FOR CODING AND REPORTING

SECTION I.C.19.
Chapter 19: Injury, poisoning, and certain other consequences of external causes (S00-T88)

f. Adult and child abuse, neglect and other maltreatment

Sequence first the appropriate code from categories T74.- (Adult and child abuse, neglect and other maltreatment, confirmed) or T76.- (Adult and child abuse, neglect and other maltreatment, suspected) for abuse, neglect and other maltreatment, followed by any accompanying mental health or injury code(s).

If the documentation in the medical record states abuse or neglect it is coded as confirmed (T74.-). It is coded as suspected if it is documented as suspected (T76.-).

For cases of confirmed abuse or neglect an external cause code from the assault section (X92-Y08) should be added to identify the cause of any physical injuries. A perpetrator code (Y07) should be added when the perpetrator of the abuse is known. For suspected cases of abuse or neglect, do not report external cause or perpetrator code.

If a suspected case of abuse, neglect or mistreatment is ruled out during an encounter code Z04.71, Encounter for examination and observation following alleged physical adult abuse, ruled out, or code Z04.72, Encounter for examination and observation following alleged child physical abuse, ruled out, should be used, not a code from T76.

If a suspected case of alleged rape or sexual abuse is ruled out during an encounter code Z04.41, Encounter for examination and observation following alleged physical adult abuse, ruled out, or code Z04.42, Encounter for examination and observation following alleged rape or sexual abuse, ruled out, should be used, not a code from T76.

See Section I.C.15. Abuse in a pregnant patient.

The codes in the categories T74.-, Adult and child abuse, neglect and other maltreatment **confirmed**, or T76.-, Adult and child abuse, neglect and other maltreatment, **suspected**, are to be sequenced first when reporting abuse, neglect, or other maltreatment. You would also report an external cause code from the X92-Y08 categories. If the perpetrator is known, report Y07.-. For example, Y07.01, Husband as perpetrator of maltreatment and neglect.

Only report T74.- when the medical documentation states the abuse, neglect, or other maltreatment is confirmed. If the documentation does not state confirmed, report suspected abuse, neglect, or maltreatment with T76.-.

If the abuse, neglect, or maltreatment is suspected and then is ruled out during an encounter with the physician, report Z04.71 for an adult and Z04.72 for a child:

Z04.71	**Encounter for examination and observation following alleged adult physical abuse**
	Suspected adult physical abuse, ruled out
	  EXCLUDES1 confirmed case of adult physical abuse (T74.-)
	         encounter for examination and observation following alleged adult sexual abuse (Z04.41)
	         suspected case of adult physical abuse, not ruled out (T76.-)

Z04.72   **Encounter for examination and observation following alleged child physical abuse**
Suspected child physical abuse, ruled out
EXCLUDES1   confirmed case of child physical abuse (T74.-)
encounter for examination and observation following alleged child sexual abuse (Z04.42)
suspected case of child physical abuse, not ruled out (T76.-)

Open Wounds, Lacerations, and Punctures

Open wounds, lacerations, and punctures are separate entries within the Index of the I-10. **Open wounds** are located under the main term "Wound."

Open Wound

Example

Diagnosis: Initial encounter for **open wound** of the right knee

Index: **Wound, open**
knee S81.00

Tabular: **S81.00   Unspecified open wound of knee**
                S81.001   Unspecified open wound, right knee

Codes: S81.001A, Initial encounter for open wound of the right knee

Lacerations are located under the main term "Laceration."

Laceration

Example

Diagnosis: Initial encounter for **laceration** of the right knee

Index: **Laceration**
knee S81.019
right, S81.011

Tabular: **S81   Open wound of knee and lower leg**
                S81.0   Open wound of knee
                        S81.01   Laceration without foreign body of knee
                                S81.011   Laceration without foreign body, right knee

Codes: S81.011A, Initial encounter for laceration of the right knee

Puncture

Example

Puncture is located under the main term "Puncture."

Diagnosis: Initial encounter for **puncture** of the right knee

Index: **Puncture**
knee S81.039
right S81.031

Tabular: **S81   Open wound of knee and lower leg**
S81.0   Open wound of knee
S81.03   Puncture wound without foreign body of knee
S81.031   Puncture wound without foreign body, right knee

Codes: S81.031A, Initial encounter for puncture of the right knee

---

EXERCISE 7-6   *Case Study*

History of Present Illness

The patient is a 68-year-old female, status post motor vehicle accident 3 months ago. The patient had an open fracture that was treated initially with traction for 6 to 8 weeks. After initial treatment with traction, the patient was placed in a cast brace. She presents with a complaint of pain in the left femur and inability to bear weight on her leg. The patient was referred from an orthopedic surgeon. The past medical history was significant for no history of myocardial infarction or renal disease and no asthma. The patient had undergone no previous procedures with the exception of debridement of the open fracture. Otherwise the patient's history was unremarkable. The patient was taking no medications and had no known allergies. She underwent a preoperative workup that included a gallium scan.

Physical Examination

The heart, lungs, and abdomen were benign. The left knee had a 30-degree extension lag. There was motion with the knee approximately 30 degrees from horizontal axis to 90 degrees of flexion. The patella was difficult to palpate, and it was very difficult to tell at the time of examination whether motion was occurring at the fracture or whether it was occurring at the knee joint. The vascular examination was unremarkable.

Radiology Data and Course in Hospital

The x-ray film showed nonunion of the left femur. The gallium scan obtained preoperatively was negative, and there was no evidence of infection.

Treatment

On May 14, the patient underwent open reduction and internal fixation of the left femur fracture with a 90-degree dynamic condylar screw and side plate. The patient tolerated the procedure well. She received two units of her own autologous blood at the time of surgery. Postoperatively she was quite anemic due to acute blood loss, with hemoglobin of 6 to 7 mg/dl. The patient was asymptomatic clinically, and her vascular examination was intact. On postoperative day 2, she had motion in the left knee from 0 to 30 degrees of flexion. She was placed in continuous passive motion and was up with physical therapy but non-weight-bearing on the left leg. Physical therapy was tolerated well. The hospital course was benign. The wound was clean and dry, and the neurovascular examination was unchanged. The x-ray films obtained before discharge showed maintenance of alignment of the left femur. The patient's staples were removed on postoperative day 7. She was placed in a cast brace and was discharged home after being independent in physical therapy.

Final Diagnosis

Nonunion of the left femur

Procedure

Open reduction and internal fixation of the left femur with 90-degree screw and site plate

1 Codes: _____, _____

(Answers are located in Appendix B)

Complications

When a patient is admitted for a complication that resulted from medical care or a surgical procedure, the complication is the first-listed.

ICD-10 OFFICIAL GUIDELINES FOR CODING AND REPORTING

SECTION I.C.19.
Chapter 19: Injury, poisoning, and certain other consequences of external causes (S00-T88)

g. Complications of care

1) General guidelines for complications of care

(a) Documentation of complications of care

See Section I.B.16. for information on documentation of complications of care.

2) Pain due to medical devices

Pain associated with devices, implants or grafts left in a surgical site (for example painful hip prosthesis) is assigned to the appropriate code(s) found in Chapter 19, Injury, poisoning, and certain other consequences of external causes. Specific codes for pain due to medical devices are found in the T code section of the ICD-10-CM. Use additional code(s) from category G89 to identify acute or chronic pain due to presence of the device, implant or graft (G89.18 or G89.28).

3) Transplant complications

(a) Transplant complications other than kidney

Codes under category T86, Complications of transplanted organs and tissues, are for use for both complications and rejection of transplanted organs. A transplant complication code is only assigned if the complication affects the function of the transplanted organ. Two codes are required to fully describe a transplant complication: the appropriate code from category T86 and a secondary code that identifies the complication.

Pre-existing conditions or conditions that develop after the transplant are not coded as complications unless they affect the function of the transplanted organs.

See I.C.21. for transplant organ removal status
See I.C.2. for malignant neoplasm associated with transplanted organ.

(b) Kidney transplant complications

Patients who have undergone kidney transplant may still have some form of chronic kidney disease (CKD) because the kidney transplant may not fully restore kidney function. Code T86.1- should be assigned for documented complications of a kidney transplant, such as transplant failure or rejection or other transplant complication. Code T86.1- should not be assigned for post kidney transplant patients who have chronic kidney (CKD) unless a transplant complication such as transplant failure or rejection is documented. If the documentation is unclear as to whether the patient has a complication of the transplant, query the provider.

Conditions that affect the function of the transplanted kidney, other than CKD, should be assigned a code from subcategory T86.1, Complications of transplanted organ, Kidney, and a secondary code that identifies the complication.

For patients with CKD following a kidney transplant, but who do not have a complication such as failure or rejection, *see section I.C.14. Chronic kidney disease and kidney transplant status.*

Continued

4) Complication codes that include the external cause

As with certain other T codes, some of the complications of care codes have the external cause included in the code. The code includes the nature of the complication as well as the type of procedure that caused the complication. No external cause code indicating the type of procedure is necessary for these codes.

5) Complications of care codes within the body system chapters

Intraoperative and postprocedural complication codes are found within the body system chapters with codes specific to the organs and structures of that body system. These codes should be sequenced first, followed by a code(s) for the specific complication, if applicable.

Complications of care must be documented in the medical record by the physician. The medical record must also document the relationship between a procedure and a complication. If the correlation is not documented, the condition is not a complication. You cannot assume there is a correlation as only the provider can indicate that the complication is due to the surgical procedure.

Medical Device, Graft, or Implant. If there is pain due to an implanted medical device, graft, or implant and the physician has documented the correlation in the patient's medical record, report a T code for the external cause. If there is pain due to the presence of the implant, report a G code (G89.18 or G89.28).

Transplant. If a transplanted organ is rejected or there are complications due to the transplanted organ, and the function of the transplanted organ is affected, report a code from category T86. A code must also be reported for the complication that resulted.

EXERCISE 7-7   *Complications*

In the Index, you will find complications of medical and surgical procedures under the main term "Complications."

Code the following complications:

1 Initial encounter for infected breast implants

Code: _____

2 Bone marrow graft, rejection

Code: _____

3 Subsequent encounter for postprocedural stitch abscess

Codes: _____, _____

4 Cardiac pacemaker, (device) mechanical complication, subsequent encounter

Code: _____

(Answers are located in Appendix B)

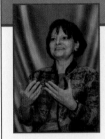

From the Trenches

"Change is the only constant for a medical coder, so it is extremely important to continually pursue education and review payer guidelines and updates."

PATRICIA

⬡ **STOP**   *For 1-10 Chapter 20, see pages 55-59.*

⬡ **STOP**   *For 1-10 Chapter 21, see pages 52-68.*

CHAPTER REVIEW

CHAPTER 7, PART I, THEORY

Circle the correct answer in each of the following:

1 Codes from Chapter _____ report congenital malformation, deformations, and chromosomal abnormalities.
   a 16
   b 17
   c 18
   d 19

2 It is common to use a fifth character of 0 when coding complications related to pregnancy.

   True   False

3 A pathologic fracture occurs in a bone that is weakened by disease.

   True   False

4 The perinatal period extends for 6 weeks following birth.

   True   False

5 Generally you do not assign a code from Chapter 18 if a definitive diagnosis is documented.

   True   False

6 When an accident occurs, an External Cause code should be the first-listed diagnosis.

   True   False

7 If a fracture and dislocation are present at the same site, assign only the fracture code.

   True   False

8 An infected laceration should be coded as a complicated wound.

   True   False

9 A poisoning occurs when a drug has been correctly prescribed and properly administered and the patient develops a reaction.

   True   False

10 When coding a poisoning, the poisoning code is sequenced before any manifestation code.

   True   False

CHAPTER 7, PART II, PRACTICAL

Using an I-10 manual, answer the following questions:

11 Initial encounter for infected breast implants

Code: _____

12 Accidental poisoning by herbicides, subsequent encounter

T Code: _____

13 Uterine fibroids complicating pregnancy, first trimester

Codes: _____, _____

14 Dehiscence cesarean wound. Patient delivered 1 week ago at another facility.

Code: _____

15 Term birth, 2268 grams, delivered by cesarean section, with fetal intrauterine growth retardation; infant's chart

Codes: _____, _____

16 Third-degree burn, right hand, 2¼%; excisional debridement performed by physician; patient seen 10 days ago for initial treatment

Codes: _____ (third degree), _____ (extent)

17 Elevated blood pressure reading, no diagnosis of HTN

Code: _____

18 Three-year-old diagnosed with fragile X syndrome

Code: _____

19 False labor of 38-week pregnancy, undelivered

Code: _____

20 Mrs. Smith is at 32 weeks' gestation and is admitted with severe bleeding with abdominal cramping. An emergency ultrasound is done and fetal monitors are applied. She is diagnosed with total placenta previa with indications of fetal distress. An emergency cesarean section is done, with delivery of a viable male infant.

Codes: _____, _____, _____, _____

CHAPTER 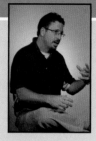 8

"Take some baby steps and figure out where you want to be—then as time progresses, you'll fall into your niche."

John R. Neumann III, RN, CPC
Account Executive
Durham, North Carolina

An Overview of ICD-9-CM

Chapter Topics

The ICD-9-CM

ICD-9-CM Format

Tabular List, Volume 1

Appendices in the Tabular List, Volume 1

Alphabetic Index, Volume 2

Procedures, Volume 3

Chapter Review

Learning Objectives

After completing this chapter you should be able to

1 List the uses of ICD-9-CM.

2 Identify the characteristics of the Tabular List, Volume 1.

3 Identify the characteristics of the Alphabetic Index, Volume 2.

4 Explain the uses of coding conventions when assigning codes.

5 Identify the characteristics of the Procedures Index and Tabular List, Volume 3.

6 Demonstrate use of ICD-9-CM.

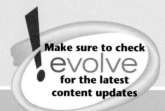
Make sure to check evolve **for the latest content updates**

NOTE: The 2015 ICD-9-CM was used in preparing this chapter.

THE ICD-9-CM

The International Classification of Diseases, 9th Revision, Clinical Modification (ICD-9-CM) is designed for the classification of patient morbidity (sickness) and mortality (death) information for statistical purposes and for the indexing of health records by disease and operations, data storage and retrieval.

The ICD-9-CM is based on the ICD-9, the ninth revision of the official version of the International Classification of Diseases compiled by the World Health Organization (WHO). In February 1977, a committee was convened by the National Center for Health Statistics (NCHS) to provide advice and counsel concerning the development of a clinical modification of the ICD-9. The ICD-9-CM is the resulting clinical modification (CM). The term "clinical" was used to emphasize the intent of the modification to serve as a tool in the area of classification of morbidity data for indexing of diseases, medical care review, ambulatory care, other medical care programs, and basic health statistics.

Through the years, the use of the ICD-9-CM (often called the ICD-9 or I-9) has grown. The Medicare Catastrophic Coverage Act of 1988 (P.L. 100-360) required the submission of the appropriate ICD-9-CM diagnosis codes, with charges submitted to Medicare Part B (outpatient services). The law was later repealed, but the coding requirement still stands.

Although coding was originally designed to provide access to medical records through retrieval for medical research, education, and administration, today codes are used to:
1. Facilitate payment of health services
2. Evaluate patients' use of health care facilities (utilization patterns)
3. Study health care costs
4. Research the quality of health care
5. Predict health care trends
6. Plan for future health care needs

The use and results of coding are widespread and evident in our everyday lives. Many people hear the results of coding on a regular basis and don't even know it. Anytime you listen to the news and hear the newscaster refer to a specific number of AIDS cases in the United States or read a newspaper article about an epidemic of measles, you are seeing the results of ICD-9-CM coding. The ICD-9-CM classification system is totally compatible with its parent system, ICD-9, thus meeting the need for comparability of morbidity and mortality statistics at the international level. This classification system is used to track morbidity and mortality. A classification system means that each condition or disease can be coded to only one code as much as possible to ensure the validity and reliability of data.

Coding must be performed correctly and consistently to produce meaningful statistics. (Refer to Fig. 8-1 for the AAPC Code of Ethics.) To code accurately, it is necessary to have an in-depth knowledge of medical terminology, anatomy and physiology, disease conditions, and pharmacology along with an understanding of the ICD-9-CM coding guidelines, format, and conventions.

Transforming verbal or narrative descriptions of diseases, injuries, conditions, and procedures into numeric designations is a complex activity and should not be undertaken without proper training. Learning to use the ICD-9-CM codes will be a valuable tool to you in any health care career.

AAPC Code of Ethics

Commitment to ethical professional conduct is expected of every AAPC member. The specification of a Code of Ethics enables AAPC to clarify to current and future members, and to those served by members, the nature of the ethical responsibilities held in common by its members. This document establishes principles that define the ethical behavior of AAPC members. All AAPC members are required to adhere to the Code of Ethics and the Code of Ethics will serve as the basis for processing ethical complaints initiated against AAPC members.

AAPC members shall:

- Maintain and enhance the dignity, status, integrity, competence, and standards of our profession.
- Respect the privacy of others and honor confidentiality
- Strive to achieve the highest quality, effectiveness and dignity in both the process and products of professional work.
- Advance the profession through continued professional development and education by acquiring and maintaining professional competence.
- Know and respect existing federal, state and local laws, regulations, certifications and licensing requirements applicable to professional work.
- Use only legal and ethical principles that reflect the profession's core values and report activity that is perceived to violate this Code of Ethics to the AAPC Ethics Committee.
- Accurately represent the credential(s) earned and the status of AAPC membership.
- Avoid actions and circumstances that may appear to compromise good business judgment or create a conflict between personal and professional interests.

Adherence to these standards assures public confidence in the integrity and service of medical coding, auditing, compliance and practice management professionals who are AAPC members.

Failure to adhere to these standards, as determined by AAPC's Ethics Committee, may result in the loss of credentials and membership with AAPC.

FIGURE 8–1   AAPC Code of Ethics. (From American Academy of Professional Coders: AAPC Code of Ethics [website]: www.aapc.com/aboutus/code-of-ethics. aspx. Accessed July 7, 2014.)

EXERCISE 8-1   *What Is ICD-9-CM?*

Using the information presented in this text, complete the following:

1 The ICD-9-CM is designed for the classification of patient _____

   or _____.

2 The ICD-9-CM manual is based on what text developed by the World Health Organization?

   _____

3 The CM in ICD-9-CM stands for _____.

4 List four of the six reasons why the ICD-9-CM codes are used today.

   _____

5 The ICD-9-CM is used to translate what descriptive information into numeric codes?

   _____ or _____

(Answers are located in Appendix B)

ICD-9-CM FORMAT

Volume 1 contains the disease and condition codes and the code descriptions (nomenclature) as well as the Supplementary Classification of Factors Influencing Health Status and Contact with Health Services (V codes) and External Causes of Injury and Poisoning (E codes).

Volume 2 is the Alphabetic Index for Volume 1. Volumes 1 and 2 are used in inpatient and outpatient settings to substantiate the reason for receiving medical services (medical necessity) by assigning diagnosis codes. Volume 3 is used for coding surgical, therapeutic, and diagnostic procedures and is used primarily by hospitals. Today, more than 95 percent of claims are filed electronically using the 5010 claim format required under HIPAA. Examples of the 5010 format can be seen in Figs. D-1 through D-8 (located in Appendix D). ICD-9-CM codes can also be reported on the CMS-1500 insurance claim form (Fig. 8-2). Government and private insurers require diagnostic codes to be submitted to show the medical necessity of services provided.

Depending on the publisher, Volume 2 may be in the front of the ICD-9-CM manual or in the middle of the book. Some publishers have the order as Volume 2, Volume 1, and Volume 3, and other publishers have the order as Volume 1, Volume 2, Volume 3.

To begin the study of ICD-9-CM codes, you will be introduced to the format and content of the volumes. When the review has been completed, you will begin to practice locating codes for various diseases and illnesses using the ICD-9-CM manual. The only way to learn to code is to practice.

Several publishing companies produce versions of the ICD-9-CM manual. All versions are based on the official government version of the ICD-9-CM.

There are four groups whose function it is to deal with in-depth coding principles and practices: Centers for Medicare and Medicaid Services (CMS), which was formerly known as the Health Care Financing Administration (HCFA); National Center for Health Statistics (NCHS); American Health Information Management Association (AHIMA); and American Hospital Association (AHA).

Format

The ICD-9-CM manual is published in three volumes:

Volume 1	Diseases: Tabular List
Volume 2	Diseases: Alphabetic Index
Volume 3	Procedures: Tabular List and Alphabetic Index

TABULAR LIST, VOLUME 1

The Tabular List is Volume 1 of the ICD-9-CM. After referencing the Index (Volume 2), you will locate the code(s) identified in the Tabular. **You can never code directly from the Index.** Rather, you must always reference the Index and then verify the code number in the Tabular. Let's begin by learning about the divisions in the Tabular.

Divisions

Volume 1: Tabular List is the listing of all the codes available for assignment, including their descriptions. When the exact word is not found in the code description in the Tabular List but the descriptive word is found in the Alphabetic Index, you must trust the code provided in the Alphabetic Index to be correct because the Index contains descriptive words that the Tabular **does not.** Not listing all possible descriptive terms in the Tabular saves space.

Anything that can happen, in the way of injury or disease, to a human body has a code in Volume 1. Although there are certainly many things that can happen to us, the people who developed the ICD-9-CM not only included them all but organized them in a systematic way. Volume 1 is separated into two major divisions:

1. Classification of Diseases and Injuries
2. Supplementary Classifications
   ■ Supplementary Classification of Factors Influencing Health Status and Contact with Health Services (V codes) (V01-V91)
   ■ Supplementary Classification of External Causes of Injury and Poisoning (E codes) (E000-E999)

The Supplementary Classifications will be covered in detail in Chapter 9.

HEALTH INSURANCE CLAIM FORM

APPROVED BY NATIONAL UNIFORM CLAIM COMMITTEE (NUCC) 02/12

CARRIER

☐☐☐ PICA   PICA ☐☐☐

1. MEDICARE ☐ (Medicare#)   MEDICAID ☐ (Medicaid#)   TRICARE ☐ (ID#DoD#)   CHAMPVA ☐ (Member ID#)   GROUP HEALTH PLAN ☐ (ID#)   FECA BLK LUNG ☐ (ID#)   OTHER ☐ (ID#)

1a. INSURED'S I.D. NUMBER   (For Program in Item 1)

2. PATIENT'S NAME (Last Name, First Name, Middle Initial)

3. PATIENT'S BIRTH DATE   MM | DD | YY   SEX   M ☐ F ☐

4. INSURED'S NAME (Last Name, First Name, Middle Initial)

5. PATIENT'S ADDRESS (No., Street)

6. PATIENT RELATIONSHIP TO INSURED   Self ☐ Spouse ☐ Child ☐ Other ☐

7. INSURED'S ADDRESS (No., Street)

CITY   STATE

8. RESERVED FOR NUCC USE

CITY   STATE

ZIP CODE   TELEPHONE (Include Area Code) (   )

ZIP CODE   TELEPHONE (Include Area Code) (   )

9. OTHER INSURED'S NAME (Last Name, First Name, Middle Initial)

10. IS PATIENT'S CONDITION RELATED TO:

11. INSURED'S POLICY GROUP OR FECA NUMBER

a. OTHER INSURED'S POLICY OR GROUP NUMBER

a. EMPLOYMENT? (Current or Previous)   YES ☐ NO ☐

a. INSURED'S DATE OF BIRTH MM | DD | YY   SEX   M ☐ F ☐

b. RESERVED FOR NUCC USE

b. AUTO ACCIDENT?   PLACE (State)   YES ☐ NO ☐

b. OTHER CLAIM ID (Designated by NUCC)

c. RESERVED FOR NUCC USE

c. OTHER ACCIDENT?   YES ☐ NO ☐

c. INSURANCE PLAN NAME OR PROGRAM NAME

d. INSURANCE PLAN NAME OR PROGRAM NAME

10d. CLAIM CODES (Designated by NUCC)

d. IS THERE ANOTHER HEALTH BENEFIT PLAN?   YES ☐ NO ☐ If yes, complete items 9, 9a, and 9d.

READ BACK OF FORM BEFORE COMPLETING & SIGNING THIS FORM.

12. PATIENT'S OR AUTHORIZED PERSON'S SIGNATURE I authorize the release of any medical or other information necessary to process this claim. I also request payment of government benefits either to myself or to the party who accepts assignment below.

SIGNED _____   DATE _____

13. INSURED'S OR AUTHORIZED PERSON'S SIGNATURE I authorize payment of medical benefits to the undersigned physician or supplier for services described below.

SIGNED _____

PATIENT AND INSURED INFORMATION

14. DATE OF CURRENT ILLNESS, INJURY, or PREGNANCY(LMP) MM | DD | YY   QUAL.

15. OTHER DATE QUAL.   MM | DD | YY

16. DATES PATIENT UNABLE TO WORK IN CURRENT OCCUPATION FROM MM | DD | YY TO MM | DD | YY

17. NAME OF REFERRING PROVIDER OR OTHER SOURCE
17a.
17b. NPI

18. HOSPITALIZATION DATES RELATED TO CURRENT SERVICES FROM MM | DD | YY TO MM | DD | YY

19. ADDITIONAL CLAIM INFORMATION (Designated by NUCC)

20. OUTSIDE LAB?   YES ☐ NO ☐ $ CHARGES

21. DIAGNOSIS OR NATURE OF ILLNESS OR INJURY Relate A-L to service line below (24E)   ICD Ind.
A. _____ B. _____ C. _____ D. _____
E. _____ F. _____ G. _____ H. _____
I. _____ J. _____ K. _____ L. _____

22. RESUBMISSION CODE   ORIGINAL REF. NO.

23. PRIOR AUTHORIZATION NUMBER

24. A. DATE(S) OF SERVICE From MM DD YY To MM DD YY | B. PLACE OF SERVICE | C. EMG | D. PROCEDURES, SERVICES, OR SUPPLIES (Explain Unusual Circumstances) CPT/HCPCS | MODIFIER | E. DIAGNOSIS POINTER | F. $ CHARGES | G. DAYS OR UNITS | H. EPSDT Family Plan | I. ID. QUAL. | J. RENDERING PROVIDER ID. #

1 | | | | | | | | | | | NPI
2 | | | | | | | | | | | NPI
3 | | | | | | | | | | | NPI
4 | | | | | | | | | | | NPI
5 | | | | | | | | | | | NPI
6 | | | | | | | | | | | NPI

25. FEDERAL TAX I.D. NUMBER   SSN ☐ EIN ☐

26. PATIENT'S ACCOUNT NO.

27. ACCEPT ASSIGNMENT? (For govt. claims, see back)   YES ☐ NO ☐

28. TOTAL CHARGE $

29. AMOUNT PAID $

30. Rsvd for NUCC Use

31. SIGNATURE OF PHYSICIAN OR SUPPLIER INCLUDING DEGREES OR CREDENTIALS (I certify that the statements on the reverse apply to this bill and are made a part thereof.)
SIGNED _____ DATE _____

32. SERVICE FACILITY LOCATION INFORMATION
a. NPI   b.

33. BILLING PROVIDER INFO & PH # (   )
a. NPI   b.

PHYSICIAN OR SUPPLIER INFORMATION

NUCC Instruction Manual available at: www.nucc.org   PLEASE PRINT OR TYPE   APPROVED OMB-0938-1197 FORM 1500 (02-12)

FIGURE 8–2   The CMS-1500 Health Insurance Claim Form.

Classification of Diseases and Injuries. The Classification of Diseases and Injuries is the main part of the ICD-9-CM, Volume 1, Tabular List; it consists of 17 chapters with codes ranging from 001 to 999. Fig. 8-3 illustrates that most chapters are based on body system (e.g., nervous system [Chapter 6], respiratory system [Chapter 8], or digestive system [Chapter 9]). Some chapters are based on the cause or type of disease (e.g., infectious and parasitic diseases [Chapter 1] or neoplasms [Chapter 2]). Fig. 8-4 indicates the format of each chapter.

Chapter. A chapter is the main division in the ICD-9-CM manual.

Section. A section is a group of three-digit categories that represent a group of conditions or related conditions.

CONTENTS

FIGURE 8-3 Volume 1, Diseases: Table of Contents.

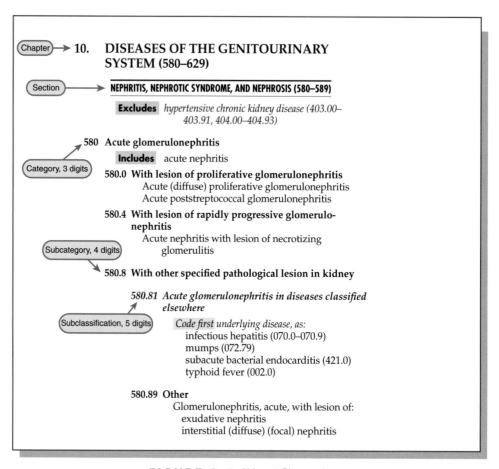

FIGURE 8–4   Volume 1, Diseases: format.

Category. A three-digit category is a code that represents a single condition or disease. There are approximately 100 codes at the category level; most others require a fourth or fifth digit. If you look at the footnote area of your ICD-9-CM manual, you will see there is a symbol that is used to direct the coder to assign further digits.

Subcategory. A four-digit subcategory code provides more information or specificity as compared to the three-digit code in terms of the cause, site, or manifestation of the condition. You must assign the fourth digit if it is available. Always code to the highest level of specificity based on the documentation in the medical record.

Subclassification. A five-digit subclassification code adds even more information and specificity to a condition's description. You must assign the fifth digit if it is available. Instructions on the use of fifth digits may appear at the beginning of a chapter, a section, or third/fourth digit category.

Bold Type

Bold type is used for all codes and titles in the Tabular List in Volume 1.

Example

244.8   Other specified acquired hypothyroidism
Secondary hypothyroidism NEC

Italicized Type

Italicized type is used for all exclusion notes and to identify those codes that are not usually sequenced as the first-listed diagnosis. Italicized type codes cannot be assigned as a first-listed diagnosis because they always follow another code. Italicized codes are to be sequenced in the order specified in the Alphabetic Index, Volume 2, or according to specific coding instructions in the Tabular List, Volume 1, such as "Code first . . ."

Example

420.0   Acute pericarditis in diseases classified elsewhere
Code first underlying disease, as:
actinomycosis (039.8)
amebiasis (006.8)
chronic uremia (585.9)
nocardiosis (039.8)
tuberculosis (017.9)
uremia NOS (586)

EXERCISE 8-2   *ICD-9-CM Chapter Format*

Using ICD-9-CM, Volume 1, Tabular List, locate the first page of Chapter 3 and answer the following questions about the chapter:

1 The name of the chapter: _____

2 The name of the first section: _____

3 The description of the first category: _____

4 The description of the first subcategory: _____

(Answers are located in Appendix B)

The information in this activity was important to your learning because it will enable you to communicate effectively about information in the ICD-9-CM manual using common terminology.

The basic ICD-9-CM code is a three-digit code, as shown in Fig. 8-5. Each code is a rubric (something under which something else is classed). Both the code number and the entry are in bold type. Diagnosis codes always contain at least three digits before the decimal point. If the diagnosis code is "1," it is written 001. Procedure codes from Volume 3 always consist of two

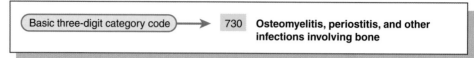

| Basic three-digit category code ⟶ | 730 | Osteomyelitis, periostitis, and other infections involving bone |

FIGURE 8–5 ICD-9-CM three-digit category code.

digits, both placed before the decimal point. You can always tell a procedure code from a diagnosis code by noting the number of digits before the decimal point.

Example

496	Diagnosis code
27.54	Procedure code
461.9	Diagnosis code
21.1	Procedure code

Fourth and Fifth-Digit Specificity. The addition of the fourth and fifth digits to the basic three-digit code provides greater specificity to the numeric designation of the patient's condition and reduces third-party payer (insurance company) returns of claims for further clarification of the diagnosis code(s). When four digits (one digit after the decimal point) are used, they are called **subcategory** codes. If five digits are used (two digits after the decimal point), they are called **subclassification** codes. Fig. 8-6 shows the first three digits of the code used to identify the disease "Osteomyelitis, periostitis, and other infections involving bone"; the fourth digit provides further specificity by distinguishing between acute and chronic osteomyelitis. Pay special attention to the symbols that indicate fourth and fifth digits are to be assigned to the code.

Not all codes have fourth or fifth digits, but when a fourth or fifth digit is available, it must be used. Most ICD-9-CM manuals have a symbol to remind the coder to assign a fourth or fifth digit as shown in Fig. 8-7. As an example of the fifth digit: Code 730.0 appears with a list of fifth digits that are used to identify the location of acute osteomyelitis as:

0 site unspecified
1 shoulder region
2 upper arm
3 forearm
4 hand
5 pelvic region and thigh
6 lower leg
7 ankle and foot
8 other specified sites
9 multiple sites

You indicate that the acute osteomyelitis is located in the patient's shoulder by adding the fifth digit 1 to the 730.0; code 730.01.

CODING SHOT

Remember that the goal is to be as accurate, as complete, and as specific as possible. The code(s) selected must be supported by physician documentation.

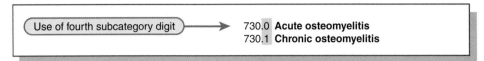

FIGURE 8-6   ICD-9-CM four-digit subcategory code.

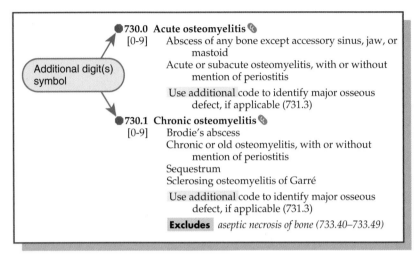

FIGURE 8-7   Use of additional digit(s) symbol.

Fig. 8-8 illustrates how adding the fourth and fifth digits adds specificity to the information about the patient's condition.

The addition of a fourth or fifth digit to a three-digit code provides greater specificity to the diagnosis. Greater specificity decreases the number of third-party-payer returns for further clarification of the diagnosis code(s). Delayed claims result in delayed payment to a physician practice or hospital.

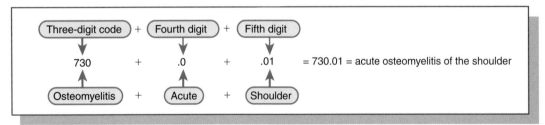

FIGURE 8-8   Specificity in ICD-9-CM codes.

EXERCISE 8-3   *Fifth-Digit Specificity*

Locate the first page of Chapter 13, Diseases of the Musculoskeletal System and Connective Tissue, in the ICD-9-CM manual. Notes immediately following the chapter title indicate the fifth-digit subclassifications and the specific categories with which these fifth digits are used. Read the notes for Chapter 13.

The following is a part of the fifth-digit subclassifications used with categories 711-712, 715-716, 718-719, and 730:

0 site unspecified

1 shoulder region

  Acromioclavicular joint(s)

  Clavicle

  Glenohumeral joint(s)

  Scapula

  Sternoclavicular joint(s)

2 upper arm

  Elbow joint

  Humerus

The various joints of the shoulder region or the elbow joint and humerus of the upper arm are the specific anatomic terms to which the main term refers. The use of the 2 indicates the elbow joint, the humerus, and so forth. These anatomic terms serve to provide further specificity to the code selection.

Locate code 711 in the ICD-9-CM manual, then answer the following:

The patient record states: Pyogenic arthritis in lower leg.

1 What would the correct five-digit code be?

  Code: _____

2 Is the use of the fifth digit optional? _____

3 How is specificity added to ICD-9-CM codes? _____

_____

(Answers are located in Appendix B)

CODING SHOT

Sometimes you will have to go back two or three pages to locate the additional digit that is to be added.

QUICK CHECK 8-1

1. Locate code 719 in the Tabular. Read the notes there. The code for effusion of the knee would be 719.0_. You choose the fifth digit.
   a. 6
   b. 7
   c. 8
   d. 9

2. By reading the notes, how did you identify which of the fifth digits represented "knee"?

   _____

(Answers are located in Appendix C)

APPENDICES IN THE TABULAR LIST, VOLUME 1

Volume 1, Tabular List, contains five appendices:

Appendix A	Morphology of Neoplasms
Appendix B	Glossary of Mental Disorders (Deleted in 2004)
Appendix C	Classification of Drugs by American Hospital Formulary Service List Number and Their ICD-9-CM Equivalents
Appendix D	Classification of Industrial Accidents According to Agency
Appendix E	List of Three-Digit Categories

Appendices are included as a reference for the coder so it is possible to:
1. Provide further information about the patient's clinical picture
2. Further define a diagnostic statement
3. Aid in classifying new drugs
4. Reference three-digit categories

The appendices are titled Appendix A, B, C, D, and E to indicate their positions in the back of Volume 1 of the ICD-9-CM manual.

Appendix A: Morphology of Neoplasms

The World Health Organization has published an adaptation of the International Classification of Diseases for Oncology (ICD-O). The ICD-O contains codes for the **location/site (topography)** and morphology (histology) of tumors. **Morphology** is the study of the form and structure of neoplasms. The morphology codes consist of five digits: the first four identify the histologic type of the neoplasm and the fifth indicates the behavior of the neoplasm.

Examples of **types** of neoplasm are epithelial, papillary, basal cell, and adenoma. Refer to a medical dictionary if you are not familiar with the types of neoplasms presented in Appendix A of the ICD-9-CM.

Examples of the **behaviors** of neoplasms are the terms "benign," "malignant," and "carcinoma in situ." "In situ" means the neoplasm has not spread from another site and is located in its original place without invasion into neighboring tissue. ICD-O codes are used to gather data about the behavior, type, and location of tumors. For example, the coder would assign an ICD-9-CM code from Chapter 2, Neoplasms (140-239); the Certified Tumor Registrar (CTR) would receive a listing of coded data for all neoplasm codes. The CTR would then assign an M code for the morphology (histological type) along with an ICD-O code to indicate the location of the tumor. For example, the coder indicates a breast tumor (basal cell) of the upper-outer quadrant as the diagnosis, using ICD-9-CM code 174.4. The CTR then researches the patient's medical record and assigns an M code (ICD-O) to indicate infiltrating ductal (M8500/3).

The one-digit morphology behavior code is as follows:

/0   Benign

/1   Uncertain whether benign or malignant
      Borderline malignancy

/2   Carcinoma in situ
          Intraepithelial (within the epithelial cells, those cells that cover the internal
              organs and vessels of the body)
      Noninfiltrating (cancer that has not spread to other, adjacent areas)
      Noninvasive (cancer that has not spread outside the original area)

/3   Malignant, primary site

/6   Malignant, metastatic site (secondary site, or site spread to) Secondary site

/9   Malignant, uncertain whether primary or metastatic site (secondary site, or site
          spread to)

A primary site is the originating site of the tumor, and a secondary site is the metastatic site (a spread from the primary to the secondary site).

Appendix B: Glossary of Mental Disorders

The psychiatric terms that appear in ICD-9-CM, Chapter 5, Mental, Behavioral and Neurodevelopmental Disorders, used to be listed in alphabetic order in Appendix B. Appendix B was deleted in 2004. Most psychiatric disorders are classified using the Diagnostic and Statistical Manual of Mental Disorders (DSM-IV).

Appendix C: Drugs

This alphabetized subsection is entitled Classification of Drugs by American Hospital Formulary Services List Number and Their ICD-9-CM Equivalents. (Have you noticed how few short titles there are in the ICD-9-CM!) A division of the American Hospital Formulary Service (AHFS) regularly publishes a coded listing of drugs. These AHFS codes have as many as six digits, with each beginning with a number, then a colon, and then up to four additional digits to provide specificity.

Example

AHFS		ICD-9-CM
8:12.04	Antifungal Antibiotics	**960.1**

Note that the ICD-9-CM code and the AHFS poisoning codes represent the same drug. For example, both AHFS 8:12.04 and ICD-9-CM 960.1 are poisoning by Antifungal Antibiotics. AHFS codes are assigned primarily by pharmacists and are not placed on the insurance forms that you will be responsible to complete.

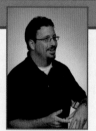

From the Trenches

"Coding is like solving a mystery . . . . I think it is like detective work. There are some easy codes that you'll find very quickly, but there are others that take a great deal of intellect and research to determine whether or not you are actually getting it right."

JOHN

Appendix D: Industrial Accidents

The subsection Classification of Industrial Accidents According to Agency contains three-digit codes to identify occupational hazards. The subsection is divided into the following categories:
1. Machines
2. Means of Transport and Lifting Equipment
3. Other Equipment
4. Materials, Substances, and Radiations
5. Working Environment
6. Other Agencies, Not Elsewhere Classified (NEC)
7. Agencies Not Classified for Lack of Sufficient Data

The identification of occupational hazards is especially important in coding injury or death that is job-related. Statisticians analyze the data and make statements about the risks involved in various occupations based on the data collected from the forms completed by health care workers. Occupational hazard codes are not placed on the insurance or billing forms. Instead, these specialized codes are used by state and federal organizations to summarize data concerning industrial accidents.

Appendix E: Three-Digit Categories

Appendix E is a list of all the three-digit categories in the ICD-9-CM, presented by chapter. The categories are labeled 1 through 17, V01-V91, and E000-E999.

Example

1. INFECTIOUS AND PARASITIC DISEASES
   Intestinal infectious diseases (001-009)

001	Cholera
002	Typhoid and paratyphoid fevers
003	Other salmonella infections
004	Shigellosis
005	Other food poisoning (bacterial)
006	Amebiasis
007	Other protozoal intestinal diseases
008	Intestinal infections due to other organisms
009	Ill-defined intestinal infections

Reviewing Appendix E is a good way to get a quick overview of all of the codes in the ICD-9-CM manual.

EXERCISE 8-4   *The Five Appendices in Volume 1*

Fill in the following:

1 In which appendix of the ICD-9-CM manual would you find the following information?

  a Glossary of Mental Disorders _____

  b Classification of Industrial Accidents According to Agency _____

  c Morphology of Neoplasms _____

  d List of Three-Digit Categories _____

  e Classification of Drugs by American Hospital Formulary Service List _____

2 In which appendix of the ICD-9-CM manual would you find the code to identify an injury resulting from a job-related accident involving a machine? _____

(Answers are located in Appendix B)

ALPHABETIC INDEX, VOLUME 2

The Alphabetic Index is Volume 2 of the ICD-9-CM. As a coder, you will reference the Index first and then locate the code identified in the Index in the Tabular List, Volume 1. Everything in the Index is listed by condition—meaning diagnosis, signs, symptoms, and conditions such as pregnancy, admission, encounter, or complication. Some types of codes

✋ CAUTION *There are terms in the Index that do not appear in the Tabular. For example, "Anton syndrome," 307.9, is listed in the Index but not in the Tabular. Even though the term is not listed in the Tabular description for the code, the code is correct because of the term "Anton syndrome" in the Index.*

may be a little difficult to find, such as those dealing with complications, late effects, and V codes.

The Alphabetic Index consists of three sections:

- Index to Diseases
- Table of Drugs and Chemicals
- Index to External Causes of Injury (E codes)

There are two tables located within the Index to Diseases. These tables are used to better list the subterms under the main term entries of hypertension and neoplasm.

Note: Please refer to the companion Evolve website for the most current guidelines.

ICD-9-CM OFFICIAL GUIDELINES FOR CODING AND REPORTING

SECTION I. **Conventions, general coding guidelines and chapter specific guidelines**

The conventions, general guidelines and chapter-specific guidelines are applicable to all health care settings unless otherwise indicated. The conventions and instructions of the classification take precedence over guidelines.

A. Conventions for the ICD-9-CM

The conventions for the ICD-9-CM are the general rules for use of the classification independent of the guidelines. These conventions are incorporated within the index and tabular of the ICD-9-CM as instructional notes. The conventions are as follows:

1. Format:

The ICD-9-CM uses an indented format for ease in reference

The ICD-9-CM Index utilizes three levels of indentation in the Alphabetic Index. They are the:

- Main terms
- Subterms
- Carryover lines

The main terms are identified by **bold** print and are flush with the left margin of each column. Alphabetization rules apply in locating main terms and subterms in the Alphabetic Index. Numerical entries appear first under the main term or subterm. Each term is followed by the code or codes that apply to the term (Fig. 8-9).

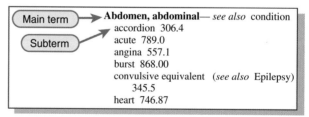

FIGURE 8–9 Main terms are capitalized and in bold print. Subterms are indented two spaces to the right under the term above.

EXERCISE 8-5 *Main Terms*

Underline the main terms to be located in the Alphabetic Index in the following diagnostic statements:

1 Normocytic anemia

2 Acute prostatitis

3 Severe protein calorie malnutrition

4 Granuloma lung

5 Pain in neck

(Answers are located in Appendix B)

The subterms under the main terms are indented to the right. They begin with a lowercase letter and are not bolded. These subterms modify the main term and are called **essential modifiers.** These subterms provide greater specificity for proper code assignment. It is possible for a subterm to be followed by an additional subterm(s). These additional subterms are indented even further to the right.

Example

Incoordination
   esophageal-pharyngeal (newborn) 787.24
   muscular 781.3
   papillary muscle 429.81

The term in parentheses (newborn) is nonessential and merely supplementary. The indented subterms are essential modifiers, such as muscular or papillary muscle.

General adjectives such as "acute," "chronic," "epidemic," or "hereditary" and references to anatomic site, such as "arm," "stomach," and "uterus," will appear as main terms, but they will have a "*see*" or "*see also* condition" reference.

Example

Hereditary—*see* condition
Uterus—*see* condition

Certain subterms are called **connecting words.** These define a relationship between a main term or a subterm and an associated condition or etiology. The connecting words "with" or "without" are located immediately after the main term and before any other subterms. Some additional connecting words are "associated with," "due to," "with mention of" or "in."

Carryover lines are used when there is not enough space on a single line for an entry. They are indented to the right even further than a subterm to avoid confusion, as illustrated in Fig. 8-10.

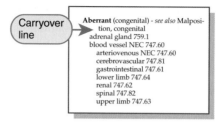

Aberrant (congenital) - *see also* Malposition, congenital
  adrenal gland 759.1
  blood vessel NEC 747.60
     arteriovenous NEC 747.60
     cerebrovascular 747.81
     gastrointestinal 747.61
     lower limb 747.64
     renal 747.62
     spinal 747.82
     upper limb 747.63

Carryover line

FIGURE 8-10 Carryover lines are indented five spaces to the right.

Conventions

The ICD-9-CM manual contains symbols, abbreviations, punctuation, and notations called conventions. Some conventions are used in all three volumes of the ICD-9-CM manual, and others are used in only one or two of the volumes. The ICD-9-CM manual contains a list of the conventions and definitions to be used when assigning codes, usually in the front matter of the manual. It is important that you be familiar with the conventions as you prepare to assign ICD-9-CM codes.

Although the maintenance of the ICD-9-CM is the responsibility of the NCHS (National Center for Health Statistics) and CMS (Centers for Medicare and Medicaid Services), many private companies publish editions of the ICD-9-CM, and each publisher has its own conventions in addition to the standard conventions. For example, some publishers indicate that a fifth digit is required by placing a special symbol next to the code in the index. These additional symbols are helpful to coders but are not a recognized convention.

QUICK CHECK 8-2

What two places could you find information regarding the coding conventions in your publication of ICD-9-CM?
1. _____
2. _____

(Answers are located in Appendix C)

NEC and NOS

ICD-9-CM OFFICIAL GUIDELINES FOR CODING AND REPORTING

SECTION I.A.

2. Abbreviations

  a. Index abbreviations

    NEC "Not elsewhere classifiable"
      This abbreviation in the index represents "other specified" when a specific code is not available for a condition the index directs the coder to the "other specified" code in the tabular.

  b. Tabular abbreviations

    NEC "Not elsewhere classifiable"
      This abbreviation in the tabular represents "other specified". When a specific code is not available for a condition the tabular includes an NEC entry under a code to identify the code as the "other specified" code.
      (See Section I.A.5.a. "Other" codes").

    NOS "Not otherwise specified"
      This abbreviation is the equivalent of unspecified.
      (See Section I.A.5.b., "Unspecified" codes).

The two main abbreviations NEC (not elsewhere classifiable) and NOS (not otherwise specified) are often used and very important.

NEC. NEC is used in both the Alphabetic Index and the Tabular List. In the Alphabetic Index, NEC represents "other specified." When a specific disease or condition is documented and there is not a specific code available, the Index will direct the coder by using the abbreviation NEC to an "other specified" code.

The NEC abbreviation in the Tabular List also means "other specified" and it often is classified to the final digit 8. The code may not fully describe the disease process or medical condition.

Example from Tabular List

244   Acquired hypothyroidism
    Includes: athyroidism (acquired)
                  hypothyroidism (acquired)
                  myxedema (adult) (juvenile)
                  thyroid (gland) insufficiency (acquired)

    244.8   Other specified acquired hypothyroidism
        Secondary hypothyroidism NEC

NOS. NOS (not otherwise specified) is the equivalent of "unspecified." It is used when the information at hand does not permit a more specific code assignment. The coder should query the physician for more specific information so that a more specific code assignment can be made.

Example

159   Malignant neoplasm of other and ill-defined sites within the digestive organs and peritoneum

    159.0   Intestinal tract, part unspecified
        Intestine NOS

From the Trenches

"I try to always keep people aware that we're not just translating an ICD-9 narrative into a code—that's a patient we're dealing with. It's not just a piece of paper, it's not just words we're handling—it's still a patient."

JOHN

Example

NEC

Diagnosis:	Pneumonia due to gram-negative bacteria
Index:	**Pneumonia**
	gram-negative bacteria NEC 482.83
Tabular:	**482.8 Pneumonia due to other specified bacteria**
	482.83 Other gram-negative bacteria
Code:	482.83 Pneumonia due to gram-negative bacteria

Code 482.83 identifies gram-negative bacterial pneumonia that cannot be classified more specifically. The other subclassifications within 482.8 are for anaerobes (482.81), Escherichia coli [E. coli] (482.82), other than gram-negative bacteria (482.83), Legionnaire's disease (482.84), and other specified bacteria (482.89). None of these other subclassifications can be assigned to the diagnostic statement; therefore, 482.83 is the most appropriate code assignment.

NEC can be used in two ways:

1. NEC directs the coder to other classifications, if appropriate. Other subterms or Excludes notes may provide hints as to what the other classifications may be.
2. NEC is used when the ICD-9-CM does not have any codes that provide greater specificity.

Example

NOS

Diagnosis:	Bronchitis
Index:	**Bronchitis** 490
Tabular:	**490 Bronchitis, not specified as acute or chronic**
	Bronchitis NOS
Assign:	490 Bronchitis

The diagnosis was not specified by the physician as acute or chronic; therefore, the "not otherwise specified" code 490 must be assigned. In this situation, it would be appropriate for the coder to query the physician for more specific information.

CODING SHOT

Third-party payers prefer specific codes and do not appreciate a coder's dependence on NOS codes. If the NOS code is the only correct code, you must assign it, but only after a thorough review of all available documentation.

ICD-9-CM OFFICIAL GUIDELINES FOR CODING AND REPORTING

SECTION I.A.

3. Punctuation

[ ] Brackets are used in the tabular list to enclose synonyms, alternative wording or explanatory phrases. Brackets are used in the index to identify manifestation codes.
(See Section I.A.6. "Etiology/manifestations")

( ) Parentheses are used in both the index and tabular to enclose supplementary words that may be present or absent in the statement of a disease or procedure without affecting the code number to which it is assigned. The terms within the parentheses are referred to as nonessential modifiers.

: Colons are used in the Tabular list after an incomplete term which needs one or more of the modifiers following the colon to make it assignable to a given category.

Brackets [ ] Brackets enclose synonyms, alternative wording, or explanatory phrases and are found in the Tabular List.

Example

426.8   **Other specified conduction disorders**
    426.89   **Other**
                    Dissociation:
                        atrioventricular [AV]

Slanted Brackets *[ ]* Slanted brackets used in the Alphabetic Index, Volume 2, are used to enclose the manifestation of the underlying condition. You sequence the code inside the slanted brackets after the underlying condition code.

Example

Diabetic retinal hemorrhage

Hemorrhage, hemorrhagic (nontraumatic) 459.0
    retina, retinal (deep) (superficial) (vessels) 362.81
        diabetic 250.5 *[362.01]*

You sequence the 250.5X (X means the appropriate fifth digit would have to be added) and then 362.01 to indicate that the retinal hemorrhage (the manifestation) was due to diabetes (the underlying disease or etiology).

Parentheses ( ) Parentheses enclose supplementary words (nonessential modifiers) that may be present or absent in the statement of a disease or procedure without affecting code assignment. Parentheses are located in both the Alphabetic Index and the Tabular List.

Example from Tabular List

158   Malignant neoplasm of retroperitoneum and peritoneum
    158.8   Specified parts of peritoneum
        Cul-de-sac (of Douglas)
        Mesentery

The nonessential modifier is "of Douglas." A cul-de-sac is a pouch that is closed at one end. The pouch of Douglas specifically refers to a type of cul-de-sac pouch that is located in the peritoneal cavity between the rectum and the back wall of the uterus (rectouterine pouch).

Example from Alphabetic Index

Ileus (adynamic) (bowel) (colon) (inhibitory) (intestine) (neurogenic) (paralytic) 560.1

The nonessential modifiers are the words "(adynamic) (bowel) (colon) (inhibitory) (intestine) (neurogenic) (paralytic)." Nonessential modifiers are words that may be used to clarify the diagnosis but do not affect code assignment. The code for ileus is 560.1, and the code for adynamic ileus is also 560.1. The addition of the modifier "adynamic" does not affect the code assignment.

EXERCISE 8-6   *Essential/Nonessential Modifier*

Using ICD-9-CM, Volume 2, Alphabetic Index, locate the following main terms and identify if the bolded subterm is an essential or nonessential modifier:

1 Otitis **externa** _____

2 Acute otitis externa _____

3 Streptococcal nasopharyngitis _____

4 Suppurative mastitis _____

5 Congenital spondylolisthesis _____

(Answers are located in Appendix B)

Colon : Colons are located in the Tabular List after an incomplete term that needs one or more of the modifiers that follow in order to make the condition assignable to a given category.

Example

628   **Infertility, female**

     628.4   **Of cervical or vaginal origin**

            Infertility associated with:

               anomaly of cervical mucus

               congenital structural anomaly

               dysmucorrhea

Brace } A brace is used in some publications to enclose a series of terms, each of which is modified by the statement appearing at the right of the brace.

Example

473   **Chronic sinusitis**

     Includes: abscess

               empyema   } (chronic) of sinus (accessory) (nasal)

               infection

               suppuration

ICD-9-CM OFFICIAL GUIDELINES FOR CODING AND REPORTING

SECTION I.A.

4. Includes and Excludes Notes and Inclusion terms

Includes: This note appears immediately under a three-digit code title to further define, or give examples of, the content of the category.

Excludes: An excludes note under a code indicates that the terms excluded from the code are to be coded elsewhere. In some cases the codes for the excluded terms should not be used in conjunction with the code from which it is excluded. An example of this is a congenital condition excluded from an acquired form of the same condition. The congenital and acquired codes should not be used together. In other cases, the excluded terms may be used together with an excluded code. An example of this is when fractures of different bones are coded to different codes. Both codes may be used together if both types of fractures are present.

Inclusion terms: List of terms is included under certain four and five digit codes. These terms are the conditions for which that code number is to be used. The terms may be synonyms of the code title, or, in the case of "other specified" codes, the terms are a list of the various conditions assigned to that code. The inclusion terms are not necessarily exhaustive. Additional terms found only in the index may also be assigned to a code.

Includes. Includes notes appear in the Tabular List, Volume 1, and they further define or provide examples and may apply to the chapter, section, or category. The notes at the beginning of a **chapter** apply to that entire chapter; the notes at the beginning of the **section** apply to that entire section; and the notes at the beginning of the **category** apply to that entire category. You have to refer to the beginning of the chapter or section for any Includes notes that refer to an entire chapter or section because the Includes notes are not repeated within the chapter or section. Includes notes may also be located before or after category codes.

Includes and Excludes notes that apply to codes 001-139 at the beginning of a chapter:

Example

1. INFECTIOUS AND PARASITIC DISEASES (001-139)

Note: Categories for "late effects" of infectious and parasitic diseases are to be found at 137-139.

INCLUDES   diseases generally recognized as communicable or transmissible as well as a few diseases of unknown but possibly infectious origin

EXCLUDES   *acute respiratory infections (460-466)*
carrier or suspected carrier of infectious organism (V02.0-V02.9)
certain localized infections influenza (487.0-487.8, 488.01-488.19)

Includes notes that apply to codes 010-018 at the beginning of a section:

Example

Tuberculosis (010-018)

INCLUDES   infection by Mycobacterium tuberculosis (human) (bovine)

EXCLUDES   *congenital tuberculosis (771.2)*
late effects of tuberculosis (137.0-137.4)

Includes notes that apply to code 006 at the beginning of a category:

Example

006   Amebiasis

INCLUDES   infection due to Entamoeba histolytica

EXCLUDES   *amebiasis due to organisms other than Entamoeba histolytica (007.8)*

Excludes. *Excludes* notes appear in the Tabular List, Volume 1, and indicate terms that are to be coded elsewhere. Excludes notes can be located at the beginning of a chapter or section or below a category or subcategory.

Excludes notes alert the coder to circumstances as in the following three examples:

Example 1

861   Injury to heart and lung

EXCLUDES   *injury to blood vessels of thorax (901.0-901.9)*

This *Excludes* note indicates that injuries to the blood vessels of the thorax are assigned within the codes 901.0-901.9 and are not included within the codes in 861. If a patient had an injury to the thorax along with injury to blood vessels of the thorax, two codes would be assigned.

The code cannot be assigned if an associated condition is present and noted in the Excludes note.

Example 2

463   Acute tonsillitis
    EXCLUDES   *streptococcal tonsillitis (034.0)*

This *Excludes* note indicates that if the tonsillitis is documented as being caused by a streptococcal organism, it would be coded 034.0, not 463.

Example 3

738.4   Acquired spondylolisthesis
        Degenerative spondylolisthesis
        Spondylolysis, acquired
        EXCLUDES   *congenital (756.12)*

This *Excludes* note instructs the coder that congenital spondylolisthesis is not reported with 738.4, but rather with 756.12. As the guidelines state, a code for a congenital condition is excluded from the acquired condition code, and these two codes should not be assigned together.

EXERCISE 8-7   *Excludes*

Using the Tabular List, answer the following questions:

1 Is acute exacerbation of chronic myeloid leukemia assigned code 205.00? _____
   If not, what code is assigned? _____

2 Is rupture of the esophagus assigned code 530.4? _____
   If not, what code is assigned? _____

3 Is congenital clubfoot assigned code 736.71? _____
   If not, what code is assigned? _____

4 Is Shy-Drager syndrome assigned code 333.0? _____
   If not, what code is assigned? _____

5 Is duodenal ulcer included in code category 533? _____
   If not, what code category is assigned? _____

(Answers are located in Appendix B)

> ## ICD-9-CM OFFICIAL GUIDELINES FOR CODING AND REPORTING
>
> **SECTION I.A.**
> **5. Other and Unspecified codes**
>
> **a. "Other" codes**
> Codes titled "other" or "other specified" (usually a code with a 4th digit 8 or fifth-digit 9 for diagnosis codes) are for use when the information in the medical record provides detail for which a specific code does not exist. Index entries with NEC in the line designate "other" codes in the tabular. These index entries represent specific disease entities for which no specific code exists so the term is included within an "other" code.
>
> **b. "Unspecified" codes**
> Codes (usually a code with a 4th digit 9 or 5th digit 0 for diagnosis codes) titled "unspecified" are for use when the information in the medical record is insufficient to assign a more specific code.

Subcategories. Subcategories consist of fourth-digit codes that provide more information or specificity. The specificity may provide insight to the etiology of the disease as well as to the location of the disease or to the manifestation. A manifestation is a symptom or condition that is the result of a disease. A fourth digit of .8 is usually assigned for other specified conditions for that category. A .9 is usually assigned for unspecified conditions of that category, as illustrated in Fig. 8-11.

> **253.8 Other disorders of the pituitary and other syndromes of diencephalohypophyseal origin**
> Abscess of pituitary
> Adiposogenital dystrophy
> Cyst of Rathke's pouch
> Fröhlich's syndrome
> **Excludes** *craniopharyngioma (237.0)*
>
> **253.9 Unspecified**
> Dyspituitarism

FIGURE 8–11   Other specified conditions and unspecified conditions.

Codes in Brackets

ICD-9-CM OFFICIAL GUIDELINES FOR CODING AND REPORTING

SECTION I.A.

6. **Etiology/manifestation convention ("code first", "use additional code" and "in diseases classified elsewhere" notes)**

Certain conditions have both an underlying etiology and multiple body system manifestations due to the underlying etiology. For such conditions, the ICD-9-CM has a coding convention that requires the underlying condition be sequenced first followed by the manifestation. Wherever such a combination exists there is a "use additional code" note at the etiology code, and a "code first" note at the manifestation code. These instructional notes indicate the proper sequencing order of the codes, etiology followed by manifestation.

In most cases the manifestation codes will have in the code title, "in diseases classified elsewhere." Codes with this title are a component of the etiology/manifestation convention. The code title indicates that it is a manifestation code. "In diseases classified elsewhere" codes are never permitted to be used as first listed or principal diagnosis codes. They must be used in conjunction with an underlying condition code and they must be listed following the underlying condition.

There are manifestation codes that do not have "in diseases classified elsewhere" in the title. For such codes a "use additional code" note will still be present and the rules for sequencing apply.

In addition to the notes in the tabular, these conditions also have a specific index entry structure. In the index both conditions are listed together with the etiology code first followed by the manifestation codes in brackets. The code in brackets is always to be sequenced second.

The most commonly used etiology/manifestation combinations are the codes for Diabetes mellitus, category 250. For each code under category 250 there is a use additional code note for the manifestation that is specific for that particular diabetic manifestation. Should a patient have more than one manifestation of diabetes, more than one code from category 250 may be used with as many manifestation codes as are needed to fully describe the patient's complete diabetic condition. The category 250 diabetes codes should be sequenced first, followed by the manifestation codes.

"Code first" and "Use additional code" notes are also used as sequencing rules in the classification for certain codes that are not part of an etiology/manifestation combination.
See – Section I.B.9. "Multiple coding for a single condition".

EXERCISE 8-8   *Etiology/Manifestation*

1 A patient is admitted with a diagnosis of malarial hepatitis.

  a You might not be sure whether the first-listed diagnosis is hepatitis or malaria.

  b Locate the term "Malaria" in the Index. Under the subterm "any type, with," locate "hepatitis 084.9 *[573.2]*." The slanted brackets alert you that *[573.2]* cannot be sequenced as the first-listed diagnosis.

  c Locate the term "Hepatitis" and then the subterm "malarial." Again the entry states 084.9 *[573.2]*.

  d Both Index entries direct you to the first-listed diagnosis of malaria. Hepatitis can be a manifestation of malaria. The slanted brackets in 084.9 *[573.2]* indicate that this hepatitis is a manifestation of the condition malaria. "Hepatitis" is the condition and "malarial" describes the type of hepatitis.

  e In the Tabular locate 084.9. Next locate "malarial" under "Use additional . . ." and then "hepatitis." 084.9 Malaria is the first-listed diagnosis and *[573.2]* hepatitis is the complication, and you would report both (084.9, 573.2) after checking 573.2 in the Tabular, which states *"Hepatitis in other infectious diseases classified elsewhere."*

You do the next one.

2 The patient's record states: endocarditis due to disseminated lupus erythematosus.

  a When you locate the term "Endocarditis, due to, disseminated lupus erythematosus" in the Index, what do you find?

  _____

  b In the Index, locate the main term (condition) "Lupus," the subterm "erythematosus," and the second subterm "systemic." What code are you directed to?

   ICD-9-CM Code: _____

  c What is the title of 710 in the Tabular? _____

  d According to the Includes notes in the Tabular following 710, what does 710 include?

  _____

  e Under the four-digit code 710.0, you are directed to "Use additional code to identify manifestation," which is endocarditis in this case. What code are you directed to?

   ICD-9-CM Code: _____

That "Use additional code . . . " under 710.0 directs you to assign endocarditis (424.91) if the first-listed diagnosis is 710.0 and specified as "with endocarditis."

  Again, the importance of verification in the Tabular is critical. This is where you receive instruction regarding the coding of endocarditis.

  f What four-digit code designates the first-listed diagnosis of "systemic lupus erythematosus"?

   ICD-9-CM Code: _____

  g What are the two codes to be reported for this case?

   ICD-9-CM Codes: _____, _____

(Answers are located in Appendix B)

ICD-9-CM OFFICIAL GUIDELINES FOR CODING AND REPORTING

SECTION I.A.
7. "And"

The word "and" should be interpreted to mean either "and" or "or" when it appears in a title.

SECTION I.A.
8. "With"

The word "with" should be interpreted to mean "associated with" or "due to" when it appears in a code title, the Alphabetic Index, or an instructional note in the Tabular List.

The word "with" in the alphabetic index is sequenced immediately following the main term, not in alphabetical order.

And and With. Although the two words "and" and "with" have similar meanings in everyday language, in ICD-9-CM terminology they have special significance and meanings. "And" means and/or, whereas "with" indicates that two conditions are included in the code and both conditions must be present to report the code.

And

Example

474   Chronic disease of tonsils and adenoids

Code 474 is assigned to identify the disease as one of tonsils and/or adenoids.

With

Example

Diabetes, diabetic (brittle) (congenital) (familial) (mellitus) (severe) (slight) (without complication) 250.0
    with
        coma (with ketoacidosis) 250.3
            due to secondary diabetes 249.3
            hyperosmolar (nonketotic) 250.2
                due to secondary diabetes 249.2
        complication NEC 250.9
            due to secondary diabetes 249.9
            specified NEC 250.8
                due to secondary diabetes 249.8
        gangrene 250.7 *[785.4]*
            due to secondary diabetes 249.7 *[785.4]*
        hyperglycemia - *code to* Diabetes, by type, with 5th digit for not stated as uncontrolled
        hyperosmolarity 250.2
            due to secondary diabetes 249.2
        ketosis, ketoacidosis 250.1
            due to secondary diabetes 249.1
        osteomyelitis 250.8 *[731.8]*

The "Diabetes" entry in the Index of the ICD-9-CM illustrates the use of "with" to direct the coder to the correct codes and the sequence of codes for conditions that may be present with the diabetes.

ICD-9-CM OFFICIAL GUIDELINES FOR CODING AND REPORTING

SECTION I.A.
9. "See" and "See Also"

The "see" instruction following a main term in the index indicates that another term should be referenced. It is necessary to go to the main term referenced with the "see" note to locate the correct code.

A "see also" instruction following a main term in the index instructs that there is another main term that may also be referenced that may provide additional index entries that may be useful. It is not necessary to follow the "see also" note when the original main term provides the necessary code.

Cross References

Cross references provide the coder with possible alternatives or synonyms for a term. There are three types of cross-references:

1. *see*
2. *see* also
3. *see* category

The "*see*" cross-reference is an explicit direction to look elsewhere. It is used for anatomic sites and many modifiers not normally used in the Alphabetic Index. The "*see*" cross-reference is also used to reference the appropriate main term under which all the information concerning a specific disease will be located.

Example

Encephalomeningitis—*see* Meningoencephalitis
Endamebiasis—*see* Amebiasis
Kidney—*see* condition
Leukosis—*see* Leukemia
Lipofibroma (M8851/0)—*see* Lipoma, by site

The "*see also*" cross-reference directs the coder to reference another main term if all the information being searched for cannot be located under the first main term entry.

Example

Laryngoplegia—(*see also* Paralysis, vocal cord) 478.30

The "*see category*" cross-reference directs you to Volume 1, Tabular List, for important information governing the use of the specific code.

Example

Late—*see also* condition
    effect(s) (of)—*see also* condition
        abscess
            intracranial or intraspinal (conditions classifiable to 324)—*see* category 326

EXERCISE 8-9   *See, See Also, See Category*

Using the Alphabetic Index, answer the following questions:

1 Locate the main term "Acquired immunodeficiency syndrome" in the Index. Is there another term for acquired immune deficiency syndrome that may be located in the Index, and if so, what is the term?

_____

2 Locate the main term "Malaria" in the Index. Is there a cross-reference located there?

_____

3 Locate the main term "Itch" in the Index. Is there another term for itch that may be located in the Index, and if so, what is the term?

_____

4 Locate the main term "Polyadenitis" in the Index. Is there another term for polyadenitis that may be located in the Index, and if so, what is the term?

_____

5 Locate the main term "Polypoid" in the Index, and identify cross reference given.

_____

(Answers are located in Appendix B)

Use Additional Code. You add information by assigning an additional code to provide a more complete picture of the diagnosis or procedure. The use of an additional code is mandatory when supporting physician documentation is located in the record.

For example, if you are reporting empyema due to pseudomonas, the codes would be empyema (510.9), due to pseudomonas (041.7). If the organism that is causing the pseudomonas is known, the organism should be reported as indicated in the "Use additional code . . ." located with 510. If no organism has been identified, no additional code is assigned.

Example

510   **Empyema**
Use additional code to identify infectious organism (041.0-041.9)

Code First Underlying Disease. The phrase "Code first underlying disease" is used in the categories in the Tabular List, Volume 1. In some cases, the code, title, and instructions appear in italics to indicate that the underlying disease (etiology) be sequenced first.

Example

366.4   **Cataract associated with other disorders**
366.41   Diabetic cataract
Code first diabetes (249.5, 250.5)

By following this convention, diabetes 249.5X or 250.5X is sequenced first to indicate that the diabetes is the etiology, followed by 366.41 to indicate that the diabetic cataract is the manifestation.

Code, If Applicable, Any Causal Condition. This is an instructional note that appears in the Tabular List. This note instructs the coder to sequence the causal condition (etiology) first. Unlike the instructional note "Code first underlying disease," if no causal condition is present or documented, then the code may be sequenced first.

Example

707   Chronic ulcer of skin
    707.1   Ulcer of lower limbs, except pressure ulcer
        Ulcer, chronic, of lower limb:
           neurogenic of lower limb
           trophic of lower limb
        Code, if applicable, any causal condition first:
           atherosclerosis of the extremities with ulceration (440.23)
           chronic venous hypertension with ulcer (459.31)
           chronic venous hypertension with ulcer and inflammation (459.33)
           diabetes mellitus (249.80-249.81, 250.80-250.83)
           postphlebitic syndrome with ulcer (459.11)
           postphlebitic syndrome with ulcer and inflammation (459.13)

A postphlebitic syndrome with ulcer of the lower limb is the etiology and is reported with 459.11 (postphlebitic syndrome with ulcer) and 707.10 (ulcer of lower limb, unspecified) to report the manifestation.

Notes

Certain main terms are followed by notes that are used to define terms and give coding instructions.

Example

Amputation
    traumatic (complete) (partial)
    Note 06 "Complicated" includes traumatic amputation with delayed healing, delayed treatment, a foreign body, or infection.
    arm 887.4
        at or above elbow 887.2
           complicated 887.3

EXERCISE 8-10 | *Application of Sequencing Rules*

Using the Tabular and instructional notes, assign and sequence the following:

1 In the Tabular, see category 331 and assign code(s) for a patient who has Pick's disease with behavioral disturbances.

⊛ Code(s): _____

2 In the Tabular, see code 484.6 and assign code(s) for a patient with pneumonia due to aspergillosis.

⊛ Code(s): _____

3 In the Tabular, see code 707.1 and assign code(s) for a patient with atherosclerosis of the right lower extremity with an ankle ulcer and necrosis of the muscle.

⊛ Code(s): _____

4 In the Tabular, see code 600.01 and assign code(s) for a patient with benign hypertrophy of the prostate with urinary retention.

⊛ Code(s): _____

5 In the Tabular, see code 713.3 and assign code(s) for a patient with arthropathy of the right shoulder due to erythema multiforme.

⊛ Code(s): _____

(Answers are located in Appendix B)

Notes in the Index list the fifth-digit subclassifications for subcategories—such as the entries "Tuberculosis" or "Diabetes." Only the four-digit code is given for the individual entry, and you must refer to the note following the main term to locate the appropriate fifth-digit subclassification. For example, Fig. 8-12 shows the fifth digits assigned when coding diabetes.

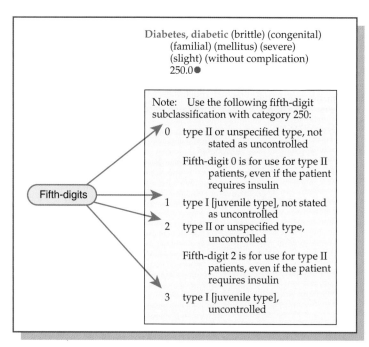

FIGURE 8-12 Index to Diseases, fifth digit, diabetes.

Eponyms

Eponyms (diseases, procedures, or syndromes named for persons) are listed both as main terms in their appropriate alphabetic sequence in the Index and under the main terms "Disease" or "Syndrome." A description of the disease or syndrome is usually included in parentheses following the eponym.

Example

Crigler-Najjar disease or syndrome
  (congenital hyperbilirubinemia) 277.4
Disease
  Crigler-Najjar (congenital hyperbilirubinemia) 277.4
Syndrome
  Crigler-Najjar (congenital hyperbilirubinemia) 277.4

The cross-reference feature will be very helpful to you as you assign ICD-9-CM codes.

EXERCISE 8-11   *Conventions*

Match the convention to the definition:

1 *see* category _____

2 subterms _____

3 *see* _____

4 Notes _____

5 modifiers _____

6 *see also* _____

7 eponym _____

a terms in parentheses or following main terms; they may or may not be essential

b terms indented under main terms, considered essential modifiers

c explicit direction to look elsewhere

d defines and gives instructions

e directs coder to look under another term if all information is not located under the first term

f directs coder to use Volume 1, Tabular List, for additional information

g disease, procedure, or syndrome named for a person

(Answers are located in Appendix B)

EXERCISE 8-12 *More Conventions*

Match the abbreviations, punctuation, symbols, and words to the correct descriptions:

1 [] _____

2 NOS _____

3 : _____

4 italics _____

5 *Excludes* _____

6 Includes _____

7 } _____

8 NEC _____

9 ( ) _____

10 *[ ]* _____

11 bold type _____

a must be modified by an additional term to complete the code description

b used in Volume 2 to enclose the disease manifestation codes that are sequenced after the underlying disease

c typeface used for all codes and titles in Volume 1

d indicates the use of code assignment for "other" when a more specific code does not exist

e encloses a series of terms that modify the statement to the right

f encloses synonyms, alternative words, or explanatory phrases

g equals unspecified

h typeface used for all exclusion notes or diagnosis codes not to be used for first-listed diagnosis

i appears under a code to further define or explain the content

j encloses supplementary words that do not affect the code assignment

k indicates terms that are to be coded elsewhere

Answer the following questions about conventions:

12 Includes and *Excludes* notes have no bearing on the code selection.

    True   False

13 Brackets enclose synonyms, alternative wordings, or explanatory phrases.

    True   False

(Answers are located in Appendix B)

PROCEDURES, VOLUME 3

Procedure codes are located in Volume 3 of the ICD-9-CM. These codes are used only in the hospital setting. You can purchase the ICD-9-CM manual with or without Volume 3.

History

The World Health Organization (WHO) recognized the growing need for a classification of procedures used in medicine and in 1971 sponsored an international working party that was convened by the American Hospital Association to coordinate the recommendations for a classification of procedures, with the primary emphasis on surgery. The International Conference for the 9th Revision of the International Classification of Diseases was convened at WHO Headquarters in Geneva in 1975. From that gathering, a proposal for a classification of procedures was submitted. The recommendations of the working party were to publish the provisional procedures classification as a supplement to the ICD-9. When the I-9 manual was published, a series of separate sections called fascicles (supplements) were also published. Each fascicle provides a classification of a different mode (type) of therapy (e.g., surgery, radiology, and laboratory procedures).

Subsequently, the ICD-9-CM was published in a three-volume set, including Volume 3, Procedures. Volume 3 was drawn primarily from WHO's Fascicle V, Surgical Procedures. At the same time, the codes in Volume 3 were expanded from three to four digits to allow for greater detail.

Volume 3 of the ICD-9-CM manual did not maintain compatibility with the ICD-9 as Volumes 1 and 2 had done. A different approach was taken in the development of Volume 3 that was deemed more appropriate to a classification system that would report surgical and therapeutic procedures.

Format

Volume 3 contains two parts—the Tabular List and the Alphabetic Index. Approximately 90% of the codes in Volume 3 refer to surgical procedures (Fig. 8-13). The remaining 10% of the codes are diagnostic (to diagnose) and therapeutic (to treat) procedures, as shown in Fig. 8-14. For the most part, nonsurgical procedures are segregated from surgical procedures and confined to the codes 87 to 99.

Volume 3 is **not** used in physicians' offices because procedures performed by physicians are reported using the CPT codes. Hospitals use Volume 3 extensively to report procedures provided to inpatients, including surgery, therapy, and diagnostic procedures. Hospitals use the ICD-9-CM codes to bill for inpatient charges (e.g., operating room, room and board, nurses, supplies). For example, a patient is admitted for a total abdominal hysterectomy. The physician would report his or her services and bill for the service of the total abdominal hysterectomy using the CPT code 58150. The hospital would report and bill for facility services for the hysterectomy procedure using the ICD-9-CM procedure code 68.49. The physician and the hospital would report the diagnosis using ICD-9-CM diagnosis codes. If the patient in this example had a diagnosis of chronic endometriosis, both the physician and the hospital would indicate the patient's diagnosis and the reason for their services due to endometriosis of the uterus with 617.0.

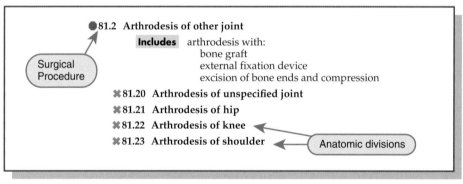

FIGURE 8-13   Volume 3, Surgical procedures.

●88.4 **Arteriography using contrast material**

Includes angiography of arteries
arterial puncture for injection of
contrast material
radiography of arteries (by
fluoroscopy)
retrograde arteriography

Note: The fourth-digit subclassification identifies the
site to be viewed, not the site of injection.

Excludes *arteriography using:*
radioisotopes or radionuclides
(92.01–92.19)
ultrasound (88.71–88.79)
fluorescein angiography of eye (95.12)

Coding Clinic: 1985, Nov-Dec, P14

88.40 **Arteriography using contrast material,
unspecified site**

(Therapeutic procedure)

FIGURE 8–14 Volume 3, Therapeutic procedures.

Example

Physician Codes
    Diagnosis: ICD-9-CM, Vols. 1 and 2
    Procedure: CPT

Inpatient Hospital Codes
    Diagnosis: ICD-9-CM, Vols. 1 and 2
    Procedure: ICD-9-CM, Vol. 3

Outpatient Hospital Codes
    Diagnosis: ICD-9-CM, Vols. 1 and 2
    Procedure: CPT

EXERCISE 8-13 *Table of Contents*

*The Table of Contents, Volume 3 (Fig. 8-15) indicates the 16 chapters in Volume 3. Note that each chapter is
based on a body system, except for Chapters 13 and 16.*

1 What is Chapter 13?
_____

2 What is Chapter 16?
_____

3 What is Chapter 00?
_____

(Answers are located in Appendix B)

Part IV Procedures Volume 3 1205

FIGURE 8–15 Volume 3, Table of Contents.

Tabular List, Volume 3

Volume 3 has abbreviations, punctuation, symbols, and terms similar to those used in Volumes 1 and 2. The following are the conventions, which are the same in all volumes:

1. Abbreviations of NEC and NOS
2. Punctuation symbols: brackets, parentheses, colons, and braces
3. Bold type for all codes and titles
4. Italicized type for all exclusion notes
5. Instructional notations of Includes and Excludes

The term "Code also" has two purposes in Volume 3:

1. To allow the coding of each component of a procedure
2. To allow the coding of the use of special adjunctive (at the same time) procedures or equipment

These instructions are not mandatory, but they serve as a reminder to code these additional procedures if they were performed.

Using the following ICD-9-CM code as an example, let us take a closer look at the code to make sure you understand what the procedure is and how the term "Code also" is used.

Example

42.6   Antesternal anastomosis of esophagus
> Code also any synchronous:
> esophagectomy (42.40-42.42)
> gastrostomy (43.1)

The word "antesternal" will not be located in most medical dictionaries. It is at this time that your skill in medical terminology will help you out. The prefix "ante" means before, and "sternal" refers to sternum. Anastomosis is the joining together of two openings; in this case it is an opening into the esophagus. The location of the opening into the esophagus is above the sternum, which stated in medical terms is antesternal anastomosis of esophagus. The term **"synchronous"** means occurring at the same time; "esophagectomy" is the removal of a part of the esophagus, and "gastrostomy" is the creation of an opening into the stomach. The statement from code 42.6 is translated into "Code also any [esophagectomy or gastrostomy] occurring at the same time." The medical coder needs excellent skills in medical terminology, anatomy, and persistence in the search for accurate definitions of the words used in the medical records. The study of terminology is a lifelong endeavor. There are always new words to be discovered. Just remember to always look up any word you are not certain of and take the time to understand the word in the context in which it is used. If you make a practice of doing this, you will soon find that you have a very dependable medical terminology vocabulary. All coders need excellent medical terminology skills.

The second use of the instruction notation "Code also" is as a reminder to code the use of special adjunctive (accessory) procedures or equipment.

Example

39.21   Caval-pulmonary artery anastomosis
> Code also cardiopulmonary bypass (39.61)

The "Code also" note with code 39.21 directs you to report 39.61 [extracorporeal (outside the body) circulation]. Extracorporeal circulation is an auxiliary procedure performed during heart surgery.

If the procedure or equipment was not used, no additional code would be assigned.

EXERCISE 8-14 *Terminology*

State the definitions of the following terms:

1 cava(l) _____

2 pulmonary _____

3 anastomosis _____

4 cardiopulmonary _____

5 extracorporeal _____

6 What is a caval-pulmonary artery anastomosis? _____

_____

7 What does a heart-lung machine do for a patient who is having a caval-pulmonary artery anastomosis? _____

_____

(Answers are located in Appendix B)

Alphabetic Index, Volume 3

The Index to Procedures is an important complement to the Tabular List of Procedures because the Index contains many procedure terms that do not appear in the Tabular List of Procedures. The list of procedures included in the two-digit category code of the Tabular List of Procedures is not meant to be exhaustive; the terms serve as examples of the content of the category. The Index to Procedures, however, includes most procedure terms currently in use in North America. When the exact word is not located in the Tabular List of Procedures but is located in the Index to Procedures, you must trust that the code listed in the Index to Procedures is correct.

Example

In the Index to Procedures, there is an entry "Gastrostomy," subterm "Janeway," which is a type of gastrostomy. The entry directs you to code 43.19. When you then verify 43.19 in the Tabular List of Procedures, there is no mention of the term Janeway.

Never code directly from the Index to Procedures. After locating a code in the Index, refer to that code in the Tabular List of Procedures for important instructions. Instructions in the form of notes suggesting the use of additional codes and exclusion notes that indicate the circumstances under which a procedure would be coded elsewhere are found only in the Tabular List of Procedures.

The Index to Procedures is arranged primarily by procedure (Fig. 8-16). Procedure codes are numbers only, with no alphabetic characters. The classification is based on a two-digit structure with two additional digits when necessary for greater specificity.

Fig. 8-17 indicates the two-digit category codes, the three-digit subcategory codes, and the four-digit subclassification codes contained in the Tabular List of Procedures. All category codes in Volume 3, Procedures, are **two-digit codes,** whereas all category codes in Volume 1, Tabular List, Disease, are **three-digit codes.**

The sequence of the Index to Procedures is letter-by-letter alphabetic order. Letter-by-letter alphabetizing ignores single spaces and hyphens and produces sequences.

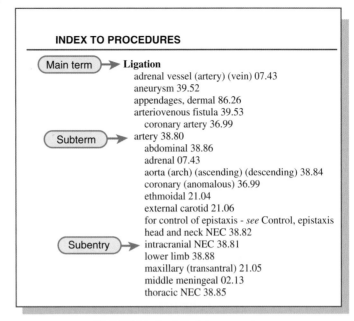

FIGURE 8–16   Index to procedures.

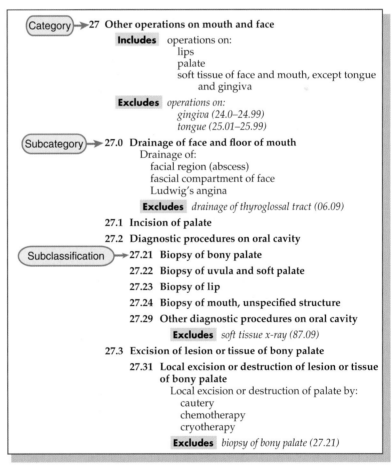

FIGURE 8–17   Volume 3, format.

> **Example**
>
> Opening
>
> open reduction
>
> Upon first consideration, you would think that these two words were not in correct alphabetical order; "open" should come before "opening." The old filer's rule of "nothing comes before something" does not apply here. To alphabetize "opening" and "open reduction," you consider the beginning of the two words as "o-p-e-n"; the fifth letter in "opening" is "i" and the fifth letter in "open reduction" is "r." For alphabetizing purposes, the terms are considered as
>
> opening
>
> openreduction

Numbers, whether Arabic (1, 2, 3), Roman (I, II, III), or ordinal (first, second, third), are all placed in numeric sequence *before* alphabetic characters. Simply stated, numbers come before letters (Fig. 8-18).

The **prepositions** "as", "by", and "with" immediately follow the main term to which they refer. When multiple prepositional references are present, they are listed in alphabetic sequence.

> **Example**
>
> Aneurysmorrhaphy NEC 39.52
>   by or with
>   anastomosis — *see* Aneurysmectomy, with anastomosis, by site
>   clipping 39.51
>   coagulation 39.52
>   electrocoagulation 39.52
>   endovascular graft
>   abdominal aorta 39.71

The Index to Procedures is organized according to main terms, which are printed in bold type. Main terms usually identify the type of procedure performed, rather than the anatomic site involved.

A main term may be followed by a series of terms in parentheses. The presence or absence of these parenthetic terms in the procedure description has no effect on the selection of the code listed for the main term. These parenthetic terms are called **nonessential modifiers**. For example, all of the following words in parentheses are nonessential modifiers.

> **Operation**
>   Beck I (epicardial poudrage) 36.39
>   Beck II (aorta-coronary sinus shunt) 36.39
>   Beck-Jianu (permanent gastrostomy) 43.19

FIGURE 8-18 Numbers alphabetized in the Index.

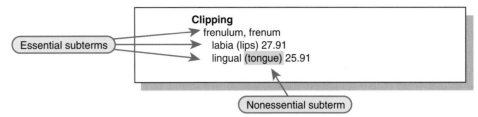

FIGURE 8–19 Essential and nonessential subterms.

Example

Clipping
aneurysm (basilar) (carotid) (cerebellar) (cerebellopontine) (communicating artery)
(vertebral) 39.51

A main term may also be followed by a list of subterms (modifiers) that do have an effect on the selection of the appropriate code for a given procedure. These subterms form individual line entries and describe essential differences in site or surgical technique (Fig. 8-19).

Terms that identify incisions are listed as main terms in the Index to Procedures. If the incision was made only for the purpose of performing further surgery, the instruction "omit code" is given. The incision for the operative approach is bundled into (included in) the surgical code and would not be coded separately. Closure of a surgical wound is not coded separately unless the closure takes place during a separate operative procedure.

Example

Arthrotomy 80.10
as operative approach—*omit* code
with
arthrography—*see* Arthrogram
arthroscopy—*see* Arthroscopy
injection of drug 81.92
removal of prosthesis without replacement—*see* Removal, prosthesis, joint structures
ankle 80.17
elbow 80.12

For some operative procedures it is necessary to record the individual components of the procedure. In these instances the Index to Procedures lists both codes.

Example

Code 57.87 describes the reconstruction of a urinary bladder, and 45.51 indicates the intestinal resection (cutting out of a portion of the intestine) necessary to create an ileal bladder.

Ileal
bladder
closed 57.87 *[45.51]*

It is important to record these codes in the same sequence as that used in the Index to Procedures.

The cross references section provides you with possible modifiers for a term or its synonyms. There are three types of cross references used in the Index to Procedures:

1. The term *"see"* is an explicit direction to look elsewhere. It is used with terms that do not define the type of procedure performed.

Example

Bacterial smear—*see* Examination, microscopic

---

2. The term *"see also"* directs you to look under another main term because all of the information being searched for cannot be located under the first main term entry.

Example

Immunization—*see also* Vaccination

---

3. The term *"see* category" directs you to the Tabular List of Procedures for further information or specific site references.

Example

Osteolysis—*see* category 78.4

Notes are used in the Index to Procedures to list fourth-digit subclassifications for those categories that use the same fourth digit. In these cases, only the three-digit code is given for the individual entry; you must refer to the note following the main term to obtain the appropriate fourth digit. For an example of a note in the Index, see Fig. 8-20.

Examination *(Continued)*
  microscopic (specimen) (of) 91.9 ●

Note: Use the following fourth-digit subclassification with categories 90-91 to identify type of examination:

  1   bacterial smear
  2   culture
  3   culture and sensitivity
  4   parasitology
  5   toxicology
  6   cell block and Papanicolaou smear
  9   other microscopic examination

  adenoid 90.3 ●
  adrenal gland 90.1 ●
  amnion 91.4 ●
  anus 90.9 ●
  appendix 90.9 ●
  bile ducts 91.0 ●

FIGURE 8-20   Note in the Index.

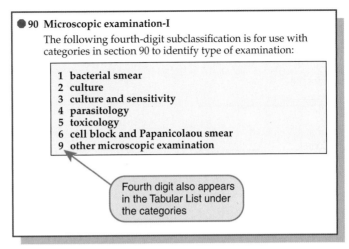

● 90 **Microscopic examination-I**
The following fourth-digit subclassification is for use with
categories in section 90 to identify type of examination:

1 **bacterial smear**
2 **culture**
3 **culture and sensitivity**
4 **parasitology**
5 **toxicology**
6 **cell block and Papanicolaou smear**
9 **other microscopic examination**

Fourth digit also appears
in the Tabular List under
the categories

FIGURE 8-21   Volume 3, Notes, Tabular List.

The fourth-digit subclassification codes also appear in the Tabular List of Procedures with the category codes 90 and 91. See Fig. 8-21 for an example of a note in the Tabular.

Operations named for persons (**eponyms**) are listed both as main terms in their appropriate alphabetic sequence and under the main term "Operation." A description of the procedure or anatomic site affected usually follows the eponym.

Example

Under O:

Operation

Thompson
cleft lip repair 27.54
correction of lymphedema 40.9
quadricepsplasty 83.86
thumb apposition with bone graft 82.69

Under T:

Thompson operation
cleft lip repair 27.54
correction of lymphedema 40.9
quadricepsplasty 83.86
thumb apposition with bone graft 82.69

EXERCISE 8-15   *Procedures, Volume 3*

Code the following using Volume 3 of the ICD-9-CM manual:

1 Flexible sigmoidoscopy

ICD-9-CM Code: _____

2 Vasectomy

ICD-9-CM Code: _____

3 Closed reduction of maxillary fracture

ICD-9-CM Code: _____

4 Transfusion of 2 units packed cells

ICD-9-CM Code: _____

5 Control of epistaxis by cauterization

ICD-9-CM Code: _____

(Answers are located in Appendix B)

CONGRATULATIONS! You have now completed the study of the arrangement of the information in the ICD-9-CM manual. The knowledge you have gained will be used as the foundation that will be built upon in Chapters 9-12. In Chapters 9-12 you will begin further work with the correct assignment and sequencing of ICD-9-CM codes.

CHAPTER REVIEW

CHAPTER 8, PART I, THEORY

Match the appendix to the information contained in the appendix:

1 Appendix A _____   **a** Industrial Accidents

2 Appendix B _____   **b** Classification of Drugs

3 Appendix C _____   **c** Morphology of Neoplasms

4 Appendix D _____   **d** Three-Digit Categories

5 Appendix E _____   **e** Deleted in 2004

Circle the correct answer in each of the following:

6 The ICD-9-CM is designed to classify what two things?
   a sickness and disease
   b symptoms and illness
   c causes of morbidity and mortality
   d diagnosis and disease

7 Which of the following is *not* a stated use for the ICD-9-CM?
   a facilitate payment of health services
   b study health care costs
   c plan for future health care needs
   d evaluate appropriateness of treatment

Match the ICD-9-CM volume number to the correct name of the volume:

8 Volume 1 _____   **a** Tabular List of Procedures and Alphabetic Index to Procedures

9 Volume 2 _____   **b** Diseases: Alphabetic Index
                            c Diseases: Tabular List

10 Volume 3 _____

Identify the format of the chapters in the ICD-9-CM Volume 1, Tabular List, in the proper sequence, from first to last:

11 _____   **a** subcategory

12 _____   **b** chapter

13 _____   **c** subclassification

14 _____   **d** section

15 _____   **e** category

Chapter Review answers are only available in the TEACH Instructor Resources on Evolve

CHAPTER 8, PART II, PRACTICAL

Using the ICD-9-CM manual, answer the following questions:

16 What does the *Excludes* note state under category code 175? _____

_____

17 What does the *Includes* note state under category 444? _____

18 Under category 805, which codes use the subclassification 0-8? _____

19 Would code 362.72 be sequenced as the first-listed diagnosis? _____

Using ICD-9-CM, Volume 1, Tabular List, locate the first pages of Chapter 8 and answer the following questions about the chapter:

20 The name of the chapter: _____

21 The name of the first section: _____

22 The description of the second category: _____

23 The description of the first subcategory: _____

24 The description of the first subclassification: _____

25 What instructional note applies to the entire chapter? _____

26 What *Excludes* note applies to the first section? _____

Underline the main terms to be located in the Alphabetic Index in the following diagnostic statements:

27 Chronic pancreatitis

28 Anal abscess

29 Acute and chronic cholecystitis

30 Abdominal pain

31 Suppurative mastitis

Using ICD-9-CM, Volume 2, Alphabetic Index, locate the following main terms and identify if the bolded subterm is an essential or nonessential modifier:

32 **Chemical** esophagitis _____

33 **Reflux** esophagitis _____

34 **Primary** hyperparathyroidism _____

35 **Uncontrolled** hypertension _____

36 **Congenital** Schatzki's ring _____

Using the Alphabetic Index, answer the following questions:

37 Locate the main term "Roseola infantum" in the Index. The other term for infantum roseola located in the Index is this
   term. _____

38 Locate the main term "Emotional" in the Index. The other term for emotional crisis located in the Index is this term.

_____

Using the Tabular List, answer the following questions.

39 Is acute exacerbation of chronic lymphoid leukemia assigned code 204.00? _____
   If not, what code is assigned? _____

40 Is congenital hydronephrosis assigned code 591? _____

If not, what code is assigned? _____

Using the Tabular and instructional notes, assign and sequence the following code(s):

41 See category 331 and assign code(s) for a patient who has Alzheimer's disease with behavioral disturbances.

_____

42 See code 484.5 and assign code(s) for a patient with pneumonia due to anthrax.

_____

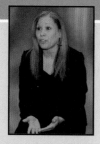

"Professional coding is a job that goes with you. You can work in any state, work in different types of companies, and do many different jobs."

Damaris Ramirez, CPC, CPC-I
National Director for Documentation and Education
EmCare, Inc.—Inpatient Services
Dallas, Texas

ICD-9-CM Outpatient Coding and Reporting Guidelines

Chapter Topics

First-Listed Diagnosis

Additional Diagnoses

V Codes

Specificity

Uncertain Diagnosis

Chronic Diseases

Diagnostic Services

Therapeutic Services

Surgery

Prenatal Visits

Chapter Review

Learning Objectives

After completing this chapter you should be able to

1 Identify the first-listed diagnosis.

2 Demonstrate ability to assign diagnoses codes to unconfirmed conditions.

3 Assign the first-listed diagnosis in the outpatient surgery setting.

4 Report first-listed diagnoses in the observation setting.

5 Validate V code assignment.

6 Apply codes to suspected conditions.

7 Report uncertain diagnoses.

8 Demonstrate ability to report chronic conditions.

9 Examine guidelines for reporting therapeutic services.

10 Evaluate diagnoses reporting for surgical procedures.

11 Identify the Guidelines for reporting prenatal visits.

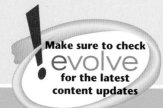

Make sure to check evolve **for the latest content updates**

NOTE: The 2015 ICD-9-CM was used in preparing this chapter.

FIRST-LISTED DIAGNOSIS

The majority of the services that a physician will provide are outpatient services. This chapter introduces you to assigning ICD-9-CM diagnosis codes for outpatient services in accordance with the *ICD-9-CM Official Guidelines for Coding and Reporting*.

Read the following guideline:

ICD-9-CM OFFICIAL GUIDELINES FOR CODING AND REPORTING

SECTION IV. Diagnostic Coding and Reporting Guidelines for Outpatient Services

These coding guidelines for outpatient diagnoses have been approved for use by hospitals/providers in coding and reporting hospital-based outpatient services and provider-based office visits.

Information about the use of certain abbreviations, punctuation, symbols, and other conventions used in the ICD-9-CM Tabular List (code numbers and titles), can be found in Section IA of these guidelines, under "Conventions Used in the Tabular List." Information about the correct sequence to use in finding a code is described in Section I.

The terms encounter and visit are often used interchangeably in describing outpatient service contacts and, therefore, appear together in these guidelines without distinguishing one from the other.

Though the conventions and general guidelines apply to all settings, coding guidelines for outpatient and provider reporting of diagnoses will vary in a number of instances from those for inpatient diagnoses, recognizing that:

> The Uniform Hospital Discharge Data Set (UHDDS) definition of principal diagnosis applies only to inpatients in acute, short-term, long-term care and psychiatric hospitals.

> Coding guidelines for inconclusive diagnoses (probable, suspected, rule out, etc.) were developed for inpatient reporting and do not apply to outpatients.

A. Selection of first-listed condition

> In the outpatient setting, the term first-listed diagnosis is used in lieu of principal diagnosis.

> In determining the first-listed diagnosis the coding conventions of ICD-9-CM, as well as the general and disease specific guidelines take precedence over the outpatient guidelines.

> Diagnoses often are not established at the time of the initial encounter/visit. It may take two or more visits before the diagnosis is confirmed.

> The most critical rule involves beginning the search for the correct code assignment through the Alphabetic Index. Never begin searching initially in the Tabular List as this will lead to coding errors.

Selecting The First-Listed Diagnosis

Examples

1. Established 50-year-old patient was seen in the clinic for acute bronchitis. Patient also received a prescription for refill of medication for hypertension. The first-listed diagnosis is acute bronchitis.
2. Initial office visit for a 36-year-old female complaining of irregular menses. Review of systems identified unexplained weight loss. The first-listed diagnosis is irregular menses.
3. Established patient is a 75-year-old male complaining of substernal chest pain that is relieved with rest. Patient has hypertension, and blood pressure is above baseline on this visit. The first-listed diagnosis is substernal chest pain.

EXERCISE 9-1   *First-Listed Diagnosis*

Identify the term for first-listed diagnosis in the following encounters or visits:

1 Established patient complaining of painful urination and frequency. Patient is a type 2 diabetic. Lab work revealed a urinary tract infection, and blood glucose was within normal limits.

First-listed Diagnosis Term(s): _____

2 Established patient presented to clinic with exacerbation of Crohn's disease. Patient's rheumatoid arthritis is stable. No medication changes were made.

First-listed Diagnosis Term(s): _____

3 Initial office visit for sprained left knee.

First-listed Diagnosis Term(s): _____

4 Initial office visit for patient requiring management of COPD and CHF.

First-listed Diagnosis Term(s): _____

5 Established patient seen for cough, fever, and shortness of breath. Chest x-ray confirmed physician's diagnosis of pneumonia, and patient was sent home on antibiotics.

First-listed Diagnosis Term(s): _____

(Answers are located in Appendix B)

Unconfirmed Diagnosis

Two or More Visits Before a Diagnosis is Confirmed

Examples

1. Initial office visit, 30-year-old woman complains of fatigue, weight gain, and constipation. Lab studies including thyroid function test were ordered. Patient will return in two weeks.

    In this case the only reportable diagnoses are symptom codes as no specific diagnoses have been confirmed during this visit.

    Codes: 780.79 fatigue, 783.1 weight gain, and 564.00 constipation.

2. Follow-up office visit, 30-year-old woman with continued complaints of fatigue, weight gain, and constipation. Lab results confirm that patient has hypothyroidism, and she was started on Synthroid. She will have repeat thyroid function studies on her next visit.

    Code: 244.9 hypothyroidism. The patient was told that she has hypothyroidism and the fatigue, weight gain, and constipation are common symptoms and would likely improve with treatment of her hypothyroidism. No additional treatment was directed at the patient's symptoms.

3. Follow-up office visit, 30-year-old woman is seen following her repeat thyroid function studies, and her hypothyroidism has responded to the Synthroid. She will be maintained on her current dose.

    Code: 244.9 hypothyroidism is the reason for the visit.

EXERCISE 9-2   *Two or More Visits Before a Diagnosis Is Confirmed*

Identify the first-listed diagnosis for the following and assign the correct code(s):

1 Initial office visit for a 28-year-old male with persistent abdominal pain and bloody diarrhea. Patient was scheduled for small-bowel x-rays and colonoscopy. The patient will be seen in the office following the scheduled outpatient procedures.

Codes: _____, _____

2 Follow-up office visit for a 28-year-old male with recent colonoscopy with biopsy and small bowel x-rays. The biopsy and small-bowel x-rays confirmed that the patient had ulcerative colitis. The patient was started on sulfasalazine.

Code: _____

3 Initial office visit for 55-year-old male with fatigue and jaundice. Laboratory tests were ordered. He will return in 1 week for the results.

Codes: _____, _____

4 Follow-up office visit for 55-year-old male with jaundice and fatigue. Diagnostic tests confirm that the patient has hepatitis C. He will be treated with interferon therapy.

Code: _____

(Answers are located in Appendix B)

Outpatient Surgery

ICD-9-CM OFFICIAL GUIDELINES FOR CODING AND REPORTING

SECTION IV.A.

1. Outpatient Surgery

When a patient presents for outpatient surgery, code the reason for the surgery as the first-listed diagnosis (reason for the encounter), even if the surgery is not performed due to a contraindication.

Examples

Outpatient Surgery

Patient presents for an outpatient T&A due to chronic tonsillitis.

First-listed diagnosis: 474.00 Chronic tonsillitis

Outpatient Surgery That has been Canceled

Patient presented for a right inguinal hernia repair. Following assessment of the patient by the nurse, it was discovered that the patient had breakfast and the surgery was canceled and will be rescheduled for next week.

First-listed diagnosis: 550.90 Inguinal hernia (V64.3, surgery not carried out, would also be reported).

EXERCISE 9-3   *First-Listed Diagnosis for Outpatient Surgery*

Identify the term(s) that describe the first-listed diagnosis for the following:

1 A female patient was admitted as an outpatient for elective bilateral tubal ligation. The patient was noted to be wheezing during the nurse's assessment. She was seen by her physician, and her surgery was cancelled because of an exacerbation of her asthma.

    First-listed Diagnosis Term(s): _____

2 A male patient was admitted as an outpatient for transurethral prostatic resection for symptomatic benign prostatic hypertrophy.

    First-listed Diagnosis Term(s): _____

3 A patient was admitted as an outpatient for a cystoscopy for hematuria. The procedure was performed without complications. No abnormality or explanation for the hematuria was found.

    First-listed Diagnosis Term(s): _____

(Answers are located in Appendix B)

Observation Stay

ICD-9-CM OFFICIAL GUIDELINES FOR CODING AND REPORTING

SECTION IV.A.

2. Observation Stay

When a patient is admitted for observation for a medical condition, assign a code for the medical condition as the first-listed diagnosis.

When a patient presents for outpatient surgery and develops complications requiring admission to observation, code the reason for the surgery as the first reported diagnosis (reason for the encounter), followed by codes for the complications as secondary diagnoses.

Observation for a Medical Condition

Example

Patient was admitted for observation due to chest pain. Patient has chronic obstructive pulmonary disease (COPD). After testing, no evidence of cardiac cause was found. Patient was discharged home. Discharge Diagnosis: Noncardiac chest pain.

    First-listed diagnosis: 786.59 Noncardiac chest pain.

Outpatient Surgery with Complication

Example

Patient had a right direct inguinal hernia repair with mesh in the ambulatory surgery center. While in the recovery room, the patient developed atrial fibrillation as a result of the procedure. The patient was admitted for observation and cardiac consult was obtained.

    First-listed diagnosis: 550.90 Right direct inguinal hernia.

EXERCISE 9-4   *Observation Stay*

Identify the term(s) that describe the first-listed diagnosis for the following:

1 A 35-year-old female patient was admitted to observation for severe nausea and vomiting (due to pelvic pain) following diagnostic laparoscopy for pelvic pain.

First-listed Diagnosis Term(s): _____

2 A male patient was admitted to observation following an endoscopic retrograde cholangiopancreatography (ERCP) for acute pancreatitis. Patient has a biliary duct stricture.

First-listed Diagnosis Term(s): _____

3 Patient was admitted for observation because of urinary retention following a dilation and curettage (D&C) for post-menopausal bleeding.

First-listed Diagnosis Term(s): _____

(Answers are located in Appendix B)

ADDITIONAL DIAGNOSES

In the preceding guidelines and exercises, we were concerned primarily with the identification of the first-listed diagnosis. In some cases, additional diagnoses would be reported to describe manifestations, complications, reasons for canceled procedures, and other coexisting conditions.

ICD-9-CM OFFICIAL GUIDELINES FOR CODING AND REPORTING

SECTION IV.
B. Codes from 001.0 through V91.99

The appropriate code or codes from 001.0 through V91.99 must be used to identify diagnoses, symptoms, conditions, problems, complaints, or other reason(s) for the encounter/visit.

The Guidelines state that it is acceptable to use any of the codes throughout the entire Tabular List to identify the reason(s) for an outpatient visit, including the use of V codes. V codes are used more frequently in the outpatient setting. This Guideline is the same as General Coding Guidelines Section I.B.4.

ICD-9-CM OFFICIAL GUIDELINES FOR CODING AND REPORTING

SECTION IV.
C. Accurate reporting of ICD-9-CM diagnosis codes

For accurate reporting of ICD-9-CM diagnosis codes, the documentation should describe the patient's condition, using terminology which includes specific diagnoses as well as symptoms, problems, or reasons for the encounter. There are ICD-9-CM codes to describe all of these.

This Guideline assures data integrity by promoting accurate ICD-9-CM diagnosis codes that are supported by documentation in the health record. It is important to code all the conditions or problems that are being managed during an encounter.

ICD-9-CM OFFICIAL GUIDELINES FOR CODING AND REPORTING

SECTION IV.

D. Selection of codes 001.0 through 999.9

The selection of codes 001.0 through 999.9 will frequently be used to describe the reason for the encounter. These codes are from the section of ICD-9-CM for the classification of diseases and injuries (e.g. infectious and parasitic diseases; neoplasms; symptoms, signs, and ill-defined conditions, etc.).

This Guideline is the same as General Coding Guidelines Section I.B.5 and reaffirms that any code from the ICD-9-CM manual can be used to describe the reason for an encounter or visit.

ICD-9-CM OFFICIAL GUIDELINES FOR CODING AND REPORTING

SECTION IV.

E. Codes that describe symptoms and signs

Codes that describe symptoms and signs, as opposed to diagnoses, are acceptable for reporting purposes when a diagnosis has not been established (confirmed) by the provider. Chapter 16 of ICD-9-CM, Symptoms, Signs, and Ill-defined conditions (codes 780.0-799.9) contain many, but not all codes for symptoms.

This Guideline is the same as General Coding Guidelines Section I.B.6. The examples and exercises used to illustrate the coding of two or more visits before a definite diagnosis can be confirmed shows the use of sign and symptom codes as the reason for the encounter. Remember that you can only code the condition(s) to the highest degree of certainty for a given encounter/visit. This may mean coding symptoms, signs, abnormal test results, or other reasons for the encounter.

ICD-9-CM OFFICIAL GUIDELINES FOR CODING AND REPORTING

SECTION IV.

F. Encounters for circumstances other than a disease or injury

ICD-9-CM provides codes to deal with encounters for circumstances other than a disease or injury. The Supplementary Classification of factors Influencing Health Status and Contact with Health Services (V01.0-V91.99) is provided to deal with occasions when circumstances other than a disease or injury are recorded as diagnosis or problems. *See Section I.C. 18 for information on V codes.*

V CODES

There are 17 chapters in Volume 1, Tabular List, of the ICD-9-CM. Each of the chapters represents a different organ system or type of disease. You will review each of the ICD-9-CM chapters in this text, but first, there are some special codes that you need to know more about—V codes.

ICD-9-CM OFFICIAL GUIDELINES FOR CODING AND REPORTING

SECTION I.C.

18. Classification of Factors Influencing Health Status and Contact with Health Service (Supplemental V01-V91)

Note: The chapter specific guidelines provide additional information about the use of V codes for specified encounters.

a. Introduction

ICD-9-CM provides codes to deal with encounters for circumstances other than a disease or injury. The Supplementary Classification of Factors Influencing Health Status and Contact with Health Services (V01.0 - V91.99) is provided to deal with occasions when circumstances other than a disease or injury (codes 001-999) are recorded as a diagnosis or problem.

There are four primary circumstances for the use of V codes:

1) A person who is not currently sick encounters the health services for some specific reason, such as to act as an organ donor, to receive prophylactic care, such as inoculations or health screenings, or to receive counseling on health related issues.

2) A person with a resolving disease or injury, or a chronic, long-term condition requiring continuous care, encounters the health care system for specific aftercare of that disease or injury (e.g., dialysis for renal disease; chemotherapy for malignancy; cast change). A diagnosis/symptom code should be used whenever a current, acute, diagnosis is being treated or a sign or symptom is being studied.

3) Circumstances or problems influence a person's health status but are not in themselves a current illness or injury.

4) Newborns, to indicate birth status

b. V codes use in any healthcare setting

V codes are for use in any healthcare setting. V codes may be used as either a first listed (principal diagnosis code in the inpatient setting) or secondary code, depending on the circumstances of the encounter. Certain V codes may only be used as first listed, others only as secondary codes.

See Section I.C.18.e, V Codes That May Only be Principal/First-Listed Diagnosis.

Index Locations

In the Tabular, the V codes follow code 999.9. If you have an ICD-9-CM manual available, locate the V codes now. Notice that V codes have only two digits before the decimal point, and a V precedes the number. V codes can be located in the Index like any other code. Often, the most difficult thing about the V code is locating the V code term in the Index. To help you become familiar with how to locate V codes in the Index, review the following most common Index terms for locating V codes:

Admission	Dialysis	Maladjustment	Test
Aftercare	Dissatisfaction	Observation	Transplant
Attention to	with	Problem	Unavailability
Boarder,	Donor	Procedure	of medical
hospital	Examination	(surgical)	facilities
Care (of)	Fitting of	Prophylactic	Vaccination
Carrier	Follow-up	Replacement	
Checking	Health, Healthy	Screening	
Contraception	History	Status	
Counseling	Maintenance	Supervision (of)	

Four Circumstances to Assign

V codes are most often used in outpatient settings, that is, ambulatory care centers, physicians' offices, and outpatient departments of hospitals. There are four circumstances in which V codes are used:

1. When a person who is currently not sick encounters the health services for some specific purpose, such as to act as donor of an organ or tissue, to receive a preventive vaccination, or to discuss a problem that is in itself not a disease or injury. Occurrences such as these are more common among outpatients at health clinics.

Example

The patient is donating a kidney.

Code: V59.4 indicates a donor of a kidney; the donor is not sick but encounters health care
V59   Donors
          V59.4   Kidney

V59 is the category and V59.4 is the subcategory. You would first locate Donor, kidney, in the Index (Volume 2), and then verify code V59.4 in the Tabular List.

Example

A well child receives a polio vaccination.

V04   Need for prophylactic vaccination and inoculation against certain diseases
          V04.0   Poliomyelitis
Code: V04.0 indicates a patient who is not ill but encounters health care for a polio vaccination. V04 is the category and V04.0 is the subcategory.

The Index (Volume 2) entry is "Vaccination, poliomyelitis." If you want to indicate that a child has been in contact with poliomyelitis, assign code V01.2, which has an Index location of "Contact, poliomyelitis."

Example

A student seeks health care to discuss a problem with school.

V62   Other psychosocial circumstances
          V62.3   Educational circumstances
                      Dissatisfaction with school environment
V62 is the category code and V62.3 is the subcategory code.

Code V62.3 indicates a patient who is not ill but encounters health care for a psychosocial circumstance, specifically educational circumstances. The Index location is "Dissatisfaction with, education."

2. A patient with a known disease or injury receives health services for specific treatment of the disease or injury.

Example

A patient with breast cancer reports to the outpatient department of the hospital for a chemotherapy session. The patient is not currently ill but receives health care services for specific treatment of cancer.

Index: **Chemotherapy,** encounter (for) V58.11
Tabular: **V58 Encounter for other and unspecified procedures and aftercare**
            V58.11 Encounter for antineoplastic chemotherapy
Code: V58.11 Chemotherapy treatment

The breast cancer (174.9) would also be coded, but you will learn about the details of that later in Chapter 11; for now, concentrate on the use of the V codes. V codes should not be mistaken for procedure codes. There is an ICD-9-CM procedure code to identify chemotherapy (99.25). Facility policy and the health care setting will determine the assignment of the procedure code.

3. A circumstance or problem is present and influences a patient's health status but is not in itself a current illness or injury. In these situations the V code should be used only as a supplementary or secondary code.

Example

A patient who is allergic to penicillin is admitted to the hospital for treatment of pneumonia using intravenous antibiotic. The patient receives treatment for the pneumonia, but the patient's allergy to penicillin is a special consideration in the treatment received.

Index: **History** (personal) of, allergy to, antibiotic agent NEC V14.1, penicillin V14.0
Tabular: **V14 Personal history of allergy to penicillin**
            V14.0 Penicillin
Code: V14.0 History of allergy to penicillin

Additionally, the pneumonia (486) would be reported as the first-listed diagnosis, but you are focusing only on the use of V codes right now.

4. To indicate the birth status and outcome of the delivery of a newborn.

Example

A live, healthy newborn infant is the result of a vaginal delivery in the hospital.

Index: **Newborn,** single, born in hospital V30.00
Tabular: **V30 Single live born**
Code: V30.00 Vaginal delivery of a single, live-born newborn

The third digit "0" reports born in hospital, and the fourth digit "0" reports delivery without mention of cesarean delivery.

Multiple Gestation Placenta Status (V91)

A new category added to the ICD-9-CM for 2011 was V91 to report multiple gestation placental status. A code from 651.0-651.9 to report multiple gestation is reported first followed by a V91 code to report if the multiples are twins, triplets, quadruplets, or other specified multiples.

EXERCISE 9-5   *V Codes*

Locate the V codes in the ICD-9-CM manual in Volume 2, Alphabetic Index, and then in Volume 1, Tabular List. Code the following:

1 A person who has been in contact with smallpox

Index location: _____

V Code: _____

2 Prophylactic vaccination against smallpox

Index location: _____

V Code: _____

3 Personal history of malignant neoplasm of the tongue

Index location: _____

V Code: _____

Assign the V code for the following:

4 Admission for cardiac pacemaker adjustment

Code: _____

5 Insertion of subdermal implantable contraceptive

Code: _____

6 Personal history of cancer of the prostate

Code: _____

7 Baby in for MMR (measles, mumps, rubella) vaccination

Code: _____

8 Screening mammogram

Code: _____

9 Clinic visit for pre-employment physical examination

Code: _____

(Answers are located in Appendix B)

Observation

> **CAUTION**   *Often, the patient record states that there is a "history of" a disease: for example, "history of diabetes mellitus." This does not mean that the patient no longer has diabetes mellitus but that the patient's medical history includes diabetes mellitus. You would not assign a V code to indicate a previous history of diabetes mellitus but instead would assign the code for the current disease of diabetes mellitus (250.0X). If there is any question regarding the current status of the disease, check with the physician. You may also want to offer some physician education regarding the documentation of past history of diseases.*

Codes from the V71.0-V71.9 series, Observation and evaluation for suspected conditions, are assigned as first-listed diagnoses for encounters or admissions to evaluate the patient's condition when there is some evidence to suggest the existence of an abnormal condition or following an accident or other incident that ordinarily results in a health problem, and where no supporting evidence for the suspected condition is found that requires further treatment. The fact that the patient may be scheduled for continuing observation in the office/clinic setting following discharge does not limit the use of this series of codes.

EXERCISE 9-6   *Observation for Suspected Conditions*

Assign ICD-9-CM codes to the following as directed:

1 The patient fell off his motorcycle when turning too sharply and hit his head on the sidewalk. The patient was wearing a helmet. The examination reveals no outwardly apparent head injury. The only injury noted on examination is abrasion of the elbow. The patient is admitted overnight to the observation unit to rule out head injury.

There will be three codes on this case: one for the **observation** of the head injury (a V code), one for the **abrasion,** and one for the **cause** (falling from motorcycle, reported with an E code).

   a Hospital observation is located in the Index under the main term "Observation." Listed under the main term are the reasons for observation. The subterm is "accident NEC." Check the code in the Tabular. What is the V code?

   Code: _____

   b The second code is for the abrasion to the elbow. When you locate the term "abrasion" in the Index, you are referred to "*see also* Injury, superficial, by site." Locate "Injury, superficial, arm." What is the code for the abrasion?

   Code: _____

   (See the cross reference in the Tabular, and discover whether a fourth digit is needed for specificity.)

   c The E code would be E816.2.

2 A patient is admitted for observation and further evaluation following an alleged rape.

   a There is only one code for this case. What is that V code?

   Code: _____

(Answers are located in Appendix B)

From the Trenches

"In a medical practice, teamwork is the glue that keeps the practice together. With physicians, the back and forth education is priceless. They cannot work without us coders, while we cannot do our job well without their support."

DAMARIS

SPECIFICITY

The addition of fourth and fifth digits to the basic three-digit code category was discussed in Chapter 8. Not all codes have fourth or fifth digits, but when a fourth or fifth digit is available, it must be assigned. Most ICD-9-CM manuals have a symbol to remind the coder to assign the additional digits.

ICD-9-CM OFFICIAL GUIDELINES FOR CODING AND REPORTING

SECTION IV.
G. Level of Detail in Coding

1. ICD-9-CM codes with 3, 4, or 5 digits

ICD-9-CM is composed of codes with either 3, 4, or 5 digits. Codes with three digits are included in ICD-9-CM as the heading of a category of codes that may be further subdivided by the use of fourth and/or fifth digits, which provide greater specificity.

2. Use of full number of digits required for a code

A three-digit code is to be used only if it is not further subdivided. Where fourth-digit subcategories and/or fifth-digit subclassifications are provided, they must be assigned. A code is invalid if it has not been coded to the full number of digits required for that code. *See also discussion under Section I.b.3., General Coding Guidelines, Level of Detail in Coding.*

ICD-9-CM OFFICIAL GUIDELINES FOR CODING AND REPORTING

SECTION IV.
H. ICD-9-CM code for the diagnosis, condition, problem, or other reason for encounter/visit

List first the ICD-9-CM code for the diagnosis, condition, problem, or other reason for encounter/visit shown in the medical record to be chiefly responsible for the services provided. List additional codes that describe any coexisting conditions. In some cases the first-listed diagnosis may be a symptom when a diagnosis has not been established (confirmed) by the physician.

You have already had practice at selecting the first-listed diagnoses, and you know that it is possible for the first-listed diagnosis to be a symptom. The important information in this Guideline is that additional codes should be assigned for any coexisting conditions that are present or treated during that visit or encounter. Sometimes there is more than one symptom that is present.

Examples

1. An established patient was seen for dyspnea on exertion. The patient has hypertension and Graves' disease. No etiology for the dyspnea was determined. Patient's medication prescriptions for hypertension and Graves' disease were refilled.

   Codes: 786.09 dyspnea, 401.9 hypertension, 242.00 Graves' disease.

2. Initial office visit for 55-year-old male with jaundice and fatigue. Laboratory tests were ordered, and patient will return in 1 week for the results.

   Codes: 782.4 jaundice, 780.79 fatigue (either of these diagnoses could be the first-listed diagnosis).

EXERCISE 9-7 *First-Listed Diagnoses and Coexisting Conditions*

Identify the first-listed diagnosis and any coexisting conditions. Assign the ICD-9-CM codes:

1 Patient was seen in the office for a consultation of palpitations. Patient has rheumatoid arthritis. Medications that the patient takes for the arthritis were reviewed to see if they could be the cause of the palpitations.

First-listed Diagnosis Term(s): _____

Code: _____

Other Diagnoses Term(s): _____

Code(s): _____

2 Patient is an established patient with memory loss. Patient also takes medication for diabetes type 2.

First-listed Diagnosis Term(s): _____

Code: _____

Other Diagnoses Term(s): _____

Code(s): _____

3 A new patient was seen for flank pain. He or she was diagnosed with a urinary tract infection and antibiotics were prescribed. Patient has psoriasis, which is stable at this time.

First-listed Diagnosis Term(s): _____

Code: _____

Other Diagnoses Term(s): _____

Code(s): _____

(Answers are located in Appendix B)

UNCERTAIN DIAGNOSIS

ICD-9-CM OFFICIAL GUIDELINES FOR CODING AND REPORTING

SECTION IV.

I. Uncertain diagnosis

Do not code diagnoses documented as "probable", "suspected," "questionable," "rule out," or "working diagnosis" or other similar terms indicating uncertainty. Rather, code the condition(s) to the highest degree of certainty for that encounter/visit, such as symptoms, signs, abnormal test results, or other reason for the visit.

Please note: This differs from the coding practices used by short-term, acute care, long-term care and psychiatric hospitals.

This Guideline states you can only code the condition(s) to the highest degree of certainty for a given encounter/visit in the outpatient setting. This may mean coding symptoms, signs, abnormal test results, or another reason for the encounter.

Examples

1. A chest x-ray is ordered to rule out pneumonia. Patient has cough and fever. The x-ray is normal.

   Codes: 786.2 cough, 780.60 fever. The pneumonia cannot be coded as it is documented as a rule out and has not been confirmed.

2. A 55-year-old male was seen with loss of appetite and jaundice. Further diagnostic studies are needed for suspected cancer of the pancreas.

   Codes: 782.4 jaundice, 783.0 loss of appetite. No code can be assigned for cancer of the pancreas because it is "suspected" and not yet confirmed.

EXERCISE 9-8   *Uncertain Diagnoses*

Identify the diagnoses and ICD-9-CM codes to be assigned.

1 Patient is seen in the office for pain and stiffness of the right knee. X-rays to rule out osteoarthritis were performed.

   Diagnoses Terms and Codes: _____

2 Office visit for established patient with wrist pain and numbness of fingertips. Studies ordered for probable carpal tunnel syndrome.

   Diagnoses Terms and Codes: _____

3 Office consultation for a new patient with amenorrhea and galactorrhea. Studies to rule out pituitary tumor were ordered.

   Diagnoses Terms and Codes: _____

4 Initial visit for a patient with a breast lump. Working diagnosis is breast cancer. Diagnostic workup has been scheduled.

   Diagnosis Term and Code: _____

(Answers are located in Appendix B)

CHRONIC DISEASES

ICD-9-CM OFFICIAL GUIDELINES FOR CODING AND REPORTING

SECTION IV.
J. Chronic diseases

   Chronic diseases treated on an ongoing basis may be coded and reported as many times as the patient receives treatment and care for the condition(s)

Examples

1. Patient is an established patient who is seen for management of asthma and diabetes.
   Codes: 493.90 Asthma, 250.00 Diabetes (either code could be the first listed)

2. Established patient is seen for continued management of systemic lupus erythematosus.
   Code: 710.0 Systemic lupus erythematosus

ICD-9-CM OFFICIAL GUIDELINES FOR CODING AND REPORTING

SECTION IV.
K. Code all documented conditions that coexist

Code all documented conditions that coexist at the time of the encounter/visit, and require or affect patient care treatment or management. Do not code conditions that were previously treated and no longer exist. However, history codes (V10-V19) may be used as secondary codes if the historical condition or family history has an impact on current care or influences treatment.

Examples

1. An established patient is seen in follow-up for coronary artery disease. Patient is also a diabetic on oral medications. The patient had a coronary artery bypass graft 6 months ago. Labs were reviewed and prescriptions for diabetic medications were renewed.

   Codes: 414.00 coronary artery disease, 250.00 diabetes (chronic coexisting conditions that were managed during this visit), V45.81 history of CABG (acceptable to code as this is important in a patient with coronary artery disease).

2. An established patient is seen for management of hypertension and congestive heart failure. Patient has a family history of colonic polyps.

   Codes: 401.9 hypertension, 428.0 congestive heart failure (either could be first-listed diagnosis). No V code is necessary to identify the family history of colonic polyps as it has no bearing on the treatment of hypertension and congestive heart failure.

DIAGNOSTIC SERVICES

ICD-9-CM OFFICIAL GUIDELINES FOR CODING AND REPORTING

SECTION IV.
L. Patients receiving diagnostic services only

For patients receiving diagnostic services only during an encounter/visit, sequence first the diagnosis, condition, problem, or other reason for encounter/visit shown in the medical record to be chiefly responsible for the outpatient services provided during the encounter/visit. Codes for other diagnoses (e.g., chronic conditions) may be sequenced as additional diagnoses.

For encounters for routine laboratory/radiology testing in the absence of any signs, symptoms, or associated diagnosis, assign V72.5 and/or a code from subcategory V72.6. If routine testing is performed during the same encounter as a test to evaluate a sign, symptom, or diagnosis, it is appropriate to assign both the V code and the code describing the reason for the non-routine test.

For outpatient encounters for diagnostic tests that have been interpreted by a physician, and the final report is available at the time of coding, code any confirmed or definitive diagnosis(es) documented in the interpretation. Do not code related signs and symptoms as additional diagnoses.

Please note: This differs from the coding practice in the hospital inpatient setting regarding abnormal findings on test results.

Examples

Diagnostic Services Only

1. Patient encounter for blood typing prior to outpatient surgery tomorrow.

   Code: V72.86 encounter for blood typing

2. Patient is having an MRI of the head to monitor the progression of brain tumor.

   Code: 239.6 brain tumor

3. Patient requested a CBC (complete blood count).

   Code: V72.60 laboratory examination without any sign or symptom documented

4. Patient was seen for shortness of breath and fever with negative x-ray. Patient returned the next day for a CT of chest, which confirmed the presence of pneumonia.

   Code: 486 pneumonia

THERAPEUTIC SERVICES

ICD-9-CM OFFICIAL GUIDELINES FOR CODING AND REPORTING

SECTION IV.

M. Patients receiving therapeutic services only

For patients receiving therapeutic services only during an encounter/visit, sequence first the diagnosis, condition, problem, or other reason for encounter/visit shown in the medical record to be chiefly responsible for the outpatient services provided during the encounter/visit. Codes for other diagnoses (e.g., chronic conditions) may be sequenced as additional diagnoses.

The only exception to this rule is that when the primary reason for the admission/encounter is chemotherapy, radiation therapy, or rehabilitation, the appropriate V code for the service is listed first, and the diagnosis or problem for which the service is being performed listed second.

A therapeutic service is one in which some type of treatment is performed to treat a specific disease. Therapeutic services can range from a medication to a surgical procedure.

Examples

Therapeutic Services Only

1. Patient had an outpatient phlebotomy performed for polycythemia vera.

   Code: 238.4 polycythemia vera

2. Patient received outpatient chemotherapy for breast cancer with metastasis to the axillary lymph nodes.

   Code: V58.11 encounter for chemotherapy, 174.9 breast cancer, and 196.3 metastasis to axillary lymph nodes

3. Patient had monthly B12 shot for pernicious anemia.

   Code: 281.0 pernicious anemia

SURGERY

ICD-9-CM OFFICIAL GUIDELINES FOR CODING AND REPORTING

SECTION IV.

N. Patients receiving preoperative evaluations only

For patients receiving preoperative evaluations only, sequence first a code from category V72.8, Other specified examinations, to describe the pre-op consultations. Assign a code for the condition to describe the reason for the surgery as an additional diagnosis. Code also any findings related to the pre-op evaluation.

Often a surgeon will want a preoperative clearance performed by the patient's primary care provider, often due to a chronic or pre-existing condition. When the primary care provider is reporting the diagnosis for the visit, the first-listed diagnosis must be the appropriate V code to indicate the encounter is for pre-op clearance, followed by the reason for the upcoming surgery, and finally, the condition requiring the clearance. The V code will be one of the following:

V72.81 Preoperative cardiovascular examination

V72.82 Preoperative respiratory examination

V72.83 Other specified preoperative examination

V72.84 Preoperative examination, unspecified

Examples

Preoperative Evaluations Only

1. Patient is seen by cardiologist for surgical clearance for upcoming cataract surgery. The patient has coronary artery disease (CAD) and has a cardiac stent. Patient's medical condition from a cardiac standpoint is stable. Patient can proceed with cataract removal.

   Code: V72.81 preoperative cardiovascular examination, 366.9 cataract, 414.01 coronary artery disease, V45.82 status post cardiac angioplasty

2. Patient is seen by internist for medical clearance for inguinal hernia repair. The patient has a number of chronic medical conditions including hypertension, diabetes type 2, and atrial fibrillation.

   Code: V72.83 other specified preoperative examination, 550.90 inguinal hernia, 401.9 hypertension, 250.00 diabetes type 2, 472.31 atrial fibrillation

---

ICD-9-CM OFFICIAL GUIDELINES FOR CODING AND REPORTING

SECTION IV.

O. Ambulatory surgery

For ambulatory surgery, code the diagnosis for which the surgery was performed. If the postoperative diagnosis is known to be different from the preoperative diagnosis at the time the diagnosis is confirmed, select the postoperative diagnosis for coding, since it is the most definitive.

Examples

1. PRE- AND POSTOPERATIVE DIAGNOSES ARE THE SAME

The patient has an EGD for upper gastrointestinal bleeding. The postoperative diagnosis is upper gastrointestinal bleeding, etiology undetermined.

Code: 578.9

2. PRE- AND POSTOPERATIVE DIAGNOSES ARE DIFFERENT

The patient has an EGD for upper gastrointestinal bleeding. The postoperative diagnosis is gastrointestinal bleeding due to gastric ulcer.

Code: 531.40

PRENATAL VISITS

ICD-9-CM OFFICIAL GUIDELINES FOR CODING AND REPORTING

SECTION IV.

P. Routine outpatient prenatal visits

For routine outpatient prenatal visits when no complications are present, codes V22.0, Supervision of normal first pregnancy, or V22.1, Supervision of other normal pregnancy, should be used as the principal diagnosis. These codes should not be used in conjunction with chapter 11 codes.

Examples

1. FIRST PREGNANCY WITHOUT COMPLICATION

A 25-year-old female presents for initial prenatal visit. This is her first pregnancy. No problems were identified.

Code: V22.0

2. SECOND PREGNANCY WITHOUT COMPLICATION

A 25-year-old female presents for initial prenatal visit. Patient had an uncomplicated vaginal delivery of a term female infant 3 years ago. No problems were identified.

Code: V22.1

3. PRENATAL VISIT WITH COMPLICATION (code from Chapter 11)

A 25-year-old female is seen for a routine prenatal visit. Her laboratory results indicate that she has a urinary tract infection. She is given a prescription for antibiotics and will return in 1 week for repeat urinalysis.

Codes: 646.63, 599.0

EXERCISE 9-9   *Chronic Disease, Diagnostic/Therapeutic Services, Surgery, and Prenatal Visits*

Match each code from the list of codes with the report to which it should be assigned and place the letters for the codes in the correct order:

a 493.90	**c** 710.0	**e** 250.00	**g** V88.01	**i** 692.4	**k** V72.0
b V67.01	**d** V45.81	**f** 414.01	**h** V10.41	**j** V55.3	**l** V58.67

1 A patient with chronic asthma and systemic lupus erythematosus presents to the clinic for an office visit during which the physician assesses the status of the asthma and lupus erythematosus.

   ✇ Code(s): _____

2 A patient with a history of coronary artery bypass graft of the native coronary artery 6 months earlier due to arteriosclerosis. The patient is also evaluated by his internal medicine physician for his longstanding diabetes for which the patient takes insulin. The physician revises the patient's diabetic medications and the Lipitor prescription based on review of laboratory results.

   ✇ Code(s): _____

3 A patient with a colostomy is evaluated by his internist for the patient's complaints of redness and itching at the skin level opening of his colostomy bag. The physician diagnosed dermatitis due to a new brand of skin level plastic seal. He prescribes a topical salve, replaced the seal, and requested the patient to return in 2 weeks if there is not significant improvement.

   ✇ Code(s): _____

4 The patient is examined by the ophthalmologist for an annual eye examination. The patient has no complaints, and the physician indicates the patient's vision is excellent.

   ✇ Code(s): _____

5 A follow-up vaginal pap smear is performed for a patient who is status-post hysterectomy that included the removal of both the cervix and the uterus. The procedure was performed for a primary malignancy. The patient had a previous smear, and both that smear and the current smear were negative for malignancy.

   ✇ Code(s): _____

(Answers are located in Appendix B)

CHAPTER REVIEW

CHAPTER 9, PART I, THEORY

Answer the following questions about the Diagnostic Coding and Reporting Guidelines for Outpatient Services.

1 When a patient is to have outpatient surgery and the surgery is not performed due to contraindication, the reason that the surgery was not performed is the first-listed diagnosis.

    True   False

2 It is appropriate to code the postoperative diagnosis as it is the most definitive diagnosis for ambulatory surgery.

    True   False

3 Chronic diseases that are treated on an ongoing basis should be coded and reported as often as the patient receives treatment and care for the chronic conditions.

    True   False

4 In the physician office it is acceptable to code V codes as a first-listed diagnosis.

    True   False

5 In the outpatient setting it is unacceptable to have a sign or symptom as the first-listed diagnosis.

    True   False

6 When coding an encounter for preoperative evaluation, the reason that the patient is having the surgery or procedure performed is the first-listed diagnosis.

    True   False

7 In the outpatient setting, diagnoses that are documented as "probable," "suspected," "rule out," or "questionable" are coded only to the highest degree of certainty with symptoms, signs, abnormal results, or other reasons for the visit.

    True   False

8 The first-listed diagnosis is defined as the diagnosis that is the most serious.

    True   False

9 It is acceptable to use a code from the ICD-9-CM manual, Chapter 11, in conjunction with V22.0 or V22.1.

    True   False

10 It is acceptable to code signs and symptoms even when a definitive diagnosis has been confirmed.

    True   False

CHAPTER 9, PART II, PRACTICAL

Identify the first-listed diagnoses and assign the appropriate ICD-9-CM codes in the following encounters or visits.

11 Initial office visit for diaper rash

First-listed Diagnosis Term(s): _____   Code: _____

12 Established patient presents with dyspnea and lower extremity edema. The physician determined that the patient's symptoms were due to an exacerbation of congestive heart failure.

First-listed Diagnosis Term(s): _____   Code: _____

13 Established patient seen for management of vitamin B12 deficiency and hypertension

First-listed Diagnosis Term(s): _____   Code: _____

Other Diagnoses Term(s): _____   Code(s): _____

14 Patient was admitted as an outpatient for an arthroscopic knee procedure to repair old anterior cruciate ligament tear.

First-listed Diagnosis Term(s): _____   Code: _____

15 Patient is admitted to observation for syncope. Patient has diabetes mellitus.

After testing, no cardiac or other cause was found.

First-listed Diagnosis Term(s): _____   Code: _____

Other Diagnoses Term(s): _____   Code(s): _____

16 Patient was admitted for pain management following biopsy of the kidney for Stage IV chronic kidney disease.

First-listed Diagnosis Term(s): _____   Code: _____

Other Diagnoses Term(s): _____   Code(s): _____

17 Patient is seen by pulmonologist for surgical clearance for upcoming surgery. Patient has emphysema and is scheduled to have an endarterectomy for severe carotid stenosis on the right.

First-listed Diagnosis Term(s): _____   Code: _____

Other Diagnoses Term(s): _____   Code(s): _____

18 Patient had an outpatient cystoscopy. The preoperative diagnosis is hematuria. Postoperative diagnosis is hematuria due to bladder cancer.

First-listed Diagnosis Term(s): _____   Code: _____

Assign the appropriate V code for the following:

19 Exposure to asbestos _____

20 Personal history of colonic polyps _____

21 Heart transplant status _____

Chapter Review answers are only available in the TEACH Instructor Resources on Evolve

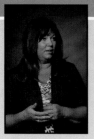

Are there any keys to long-term success in the medical coding field?

"The willingness to keep on learning. Never assume that you know it all . . . after 20+ years in the medical coding field, I still learn new things each day."

Lori Koetje, CCS-P, CPC, CPRC, ACS-GS
Central Billing Office Manager
Lakeshore Health Partners
Holland, Michigan

Using ICD-9-CM

Chapter Topics

Organization of the Guidelines

Level of Specificity

Integral Conditions

Multiple Coding

Acute and Chronic

Combination Codes

Late Effects

Impending or Threatened Condition

Chapter Review

Learning Objectives

After completing this chapter you should be able to

1 Explain the organization of the Guidelines.

2 Determine the level of highest specificity.

3 Identify conditions integral to a disease process.

4 Assign multiple codes to a single condition.

5 Report acute and chronic conditions.

6 Demonstrate application of combination codes.

7 Differentiate between residual and late effects.

8 Abstract information that determines if a condition is impending or threatened.

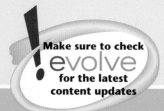
Make sure to check **evolve** for the latest content updates

NOTE: The 2015 ICD-9-CM was used in preparing this chapter.

ORGANIZATION OF THE GUIDELINES

As was discussed in Chapter 9, *Official Guidelines for Coding and Reporting* have been developed and approved for coding and reporting by the Cooperating Parties for ICD-9-CM: the American Hospital Association (AHA), American Health Information Management Association (AHIMA), Centers for Medicare and Medicaid Services (CMS), and National Center for Health Statistics (NCHS).

The complete *ICD-9-CM Official Guidelines for Coding and Reporting* appears on the Evolve website at http://evolve.elsevier.com/Buck/step and is also posted on the Web at www.cdc.gov/nchs/icd/icd9cm_addenda_guidelines.htm#addenda. The Guidelines are organized into sections. Section I of the Guidelines includes the structure and conventions of the classification and general guidelines that apply to the entire classification, and chapter-specific guidelines that correspond to the chapters as they are arranged in the classification. Section II includes guidelines for selection of principal diagnosis for non-outpatient (hospital) settings. Section III includes guidelines for reporting additional diagnoses in non-outpatient settings. Section IV is for outpatient coding and reporting. Outpatient coders, however, use guidance from throughout the *Official Guidelines for Coding and Reporting* because not all of the coding circumstances are fully explained in Section IV of the Guidelines. Appendix I of the Guidelines includes Present on Admission Reporting Guidelines that are guidance for reporting certain conditions in the hospital setting.

QUICK CHECK 10-1

1. Examine your ICD-9-CM manual to determine if the *Official Guidelines for Coding and Reporting* are included in your publication. If so, where are they located? _____

(Answers are located in Appendix C)

The number that appears to the left of the guideline in this text is the number of the guideline as listed in the *Official Guidelines for Coding and Reporting*. For the purposes of this text, the Guidelines will sometimes appear out of order.

In the examples in this text, main terms and subterms are often noted for you after the term enclosed in parentheses to help you locate the terms in the Alphabetic Index. For example, Hodgkin's (main term) disease (subterm) directs you to the location of Hodgkin's disease in the Alphabetic Index like this: "(Hodgkin's, disease)." Remember, the extensive indexing system in the ICD-9-CM allows you many options for locating codes in the Alphabetic Index. The examples and subsequent identification of main terms and subterms represent only one way a term can be located.

You will be practicing coding using the ICD-9-CM throughout this chapter. You need to practice using the steps that are always necessary to assign an ICD-9-CM code. If you begin your ICD-9-CM coding using these steps, you will develop good coding habits that will last throughout your career.

Steps to Accurate Coding

1. Identify the main term(s) in the diagnostic statement.
2. Locate the main term(s) in the Alphabetic Index (Volume 2) (referred to in this text as the Index).
3. Review any subterms under the main term in the Index.
4. Follow any cross-reference instructions, such as *see also*.
5. Verify the code(s) selected from the Index (Volume 2) in the Tabular List (Volume 1) (referred to in this text as the Tabular).
6. Refer to any instructional notations in the Tabular.
7. Assign codes to the highest level of specificity. For example, if a fourth digit is available, you cannot assign only a three-digit code, and if a fifth digit is available, you cannot assign only a four-digit code.
8. Code the diagnosis until all elements are completely identified.

Guidelines are presented and followed by examples or exercises to illustrate the rule(s).

Let's get started with a general coding Guideline:

ICD-9-CM OFFICIAL GUIDELINES FOR CODING AND REPORTING

SECTION I.

B. General Coding Guidelines

1. **Use of Both Alphabetic Index and Tabular List**

   Use both the Alphabetic Index and the Tabular List when locating and assigning a code. Reliance on only the Alphabetic Index or the Tabular List leads to errors in code assignments and less specificity in code selection.

2. **Locate each term in the Alphabetic Index**

   Locate each term in the Alphabetic Index and verify the code selected in the Tabular List. Read and be guided by instructional notations that appear in both the Alphabetic Index and the Tabular List.

Use Both the Alphabetic Index and the Tabular List

Examples

1. Diagnosis: Hodgkin's Disease
   Index: **Hodgkin's** (main term)
                     disease (subterm) 201.9
   Tabular: **201 Hodgkin's disease** [category code]
                     201.9 Hodgkin's disease, unspecified [subcategory code]
   Code: 201.9X Hodgkin's Disease [subclassification code]

Verify 201.9 in the Tabular and note that the code requires a fifth-digit assignment of 0 to 8 to indicate the disease location. You would have missed the required fifth-digit subclassification (indicated by the X in the example) if you had referenced only the Index and not verified the code in the Tabular. You must also always go back to the beginning of the section in the Tabular and read any notes located there. In the case of 201, the section notes (above code 200) indicate the fifth digits to be used with codes 200-202. Code 201.90 is assigned because the type and location of the Hodgkin's disease were both unspecified.

2. Diagnosis: Stroke, due to right vertebral artery occlusion
   Index: **Stroke** (main term) 434.91
   Tabular: **434.9 Cerebral artery occlusion, unspecified**
                     As the occlusion is specified as "due to vertebral artery occlusion," 434.9X, cerebral artery occlusion, unspecified, does not accurately describe the condition. Return to the Index and locate the term "occlusion" to see what other codes might more accurately describe this condition.
   Index: **Occlusion**
                     artery (subterm), vertebral (subterm) 433.2
   Tabular: **433 Occlusion and stenosis of precerebral arteries**
                        0 without mention of cerebral infarction
                        1 with cerebral infarction
                     433.2 Vertebral artery
   Code: 433.21 Stroke, due to right vertebral artery occlusion

The diagnosis statement "fits" or is classifiable to 433.21. You would have incorrectly reported the diagnosis as 434.91 if you had not verified the code in the Tabular. The fifth digit is "1, with cerebral infarction" because a stroke is an infarction. There are no shortcuts in this process: Always check the Tabular.

The level of specificity is the level of detail, and detail is very important in diagnosis coding. Review the Guideline regarding specificity.

LEVEL OF SPECIFICITY

ICD-9-CM OFFICIAL GUIDELINES FOR CODING AND REPORTING

SECTION I.B.

3. Level of Detail in Coding

Diagnosis and procedure codes are to be used at their highest number of digits available.

ICD-9-CM diagnosis codes are composed of codes with 3, 4, or 5 digits. Codes with three digits are included in ICD-9-CM as the heading of a category of codes that may be further subdivided by the use of fourth and/or fifth digits, which provide greater detail.

A three-digit code is to be used only if it is not further subdivided. Where fourth-digit subcategories and/or fifth-digit subclassifications are provided, they must be assigned. A code is invalid if it has not been coded to the full number of digits required for that code. For example, Acute myocardial infarction, code 410, has fourth digits that describe the location of the infarction (e.g., 410.2, Of inferolateral wall), and fifth digits that identify the episode of care. It would be incorrect to report a code in category 410 without a fourth and fifth digit.

ICD-9-CM Volume 3 procedure codes are composed of codes with either 3 or 4 digits. Codes with two digits are included in ICD-9-CM as the heading of a category of codes that may be further subdivided by the use of third and/or fourth digits, which provide greater detail.

Level of Specificity

Examples

1. *Three-Digit Category*

Diagnosis:	Subarachnoid hemorrhage
Index:	**Hemorrhage**, subarachnoid, nontraumatic 430
Tabular:	**430 Subarachnoid hemorrhage** [category code]
Code:	430 Subarachnoid hemorrhage

Diagnosis:	AIDS
Index:	**AIDS** 042
Tabular:	**042 Human immunodeficiency virus (HIV) disease** [category code]
Code:	042 AIDS

   Both of the preceding diagnostic statements are correctly assigned to three-digit category codes because there are no four-digit subcategory codes available within either code.

---

2. *Four-Digit Subcategory*

Diagnosis:	Crohn's disease of large intestine
Index:	**Crohn's disease** (see also Enteritis, regional) 555.9
Tabular:	**555 Regional enteritis (Includes: Crohn's disease)** [category code]
	555.1 Large intestine [subcategory code]
Code:	555.1 Crohn's disease of large intestine

Diagnosis:	Cellulitis of the upper right leg
Index:	**Cellulitis**, leg
Tabular:	**682 Other cellulitis and abscess** [category code]
	682.6 Leg, except foot [subcategory code]
Code:	682.6 Cellulitis of the upper right leg

   Both of the preceding diagnostic statements are correctly assigned to four-digit subcategory codes because no five-digit subclassification codes are available.

Continued

3. *Five-Digit Subclassification*
Diagnosis: RUQ abdominal pain
Index: **Pain,** abdominal
Tabular: **789.0 Abdominal pain** [subcategory code]
              789.01 Right upper quadrant [subclassification code]
Code: 789.01 RUQ abdominal pain

Diagnosis: Bilateral, congenital bowing of femur
Index: **Bowing**
              femur 736.89
              congenital 754.42
Tabular: **754 Certain congenital musculoskeletal deformities** [category code]
              **754.4 Congenital genu recurvatum and bowing of long bones of
              leg** [subcategory code]
              754.42 Congenital bowing of femur [subclassification code]
Code: 754.42 Bilateral, congenital bowing of femur

Both of the preceding diagnostic statements are correctly assigned to five-digit subclassification
codes, having been carried out to the highest level of specificity available.

EXERCISE 10-1   *Level of Specificity in Coding*

Identify the category, subcategory, and subclassifications of the following codes:

1 Diagnosis: Recurrent right inguinal hernia, with obstruction
  Index: **Hernia**
                inguinal 550.9
  Tabular: **550 Inguinal hernia** _____
                    550.1 Inguinal hernia, with obstruction, without mention of gangrene

                    _____

                    550.11 Inguinal hernia, with obstruction, without mention of gangrene, unilateral, recurrent

                    _____

2 Diagnosis: Transient hypertension, 30 weeks' gestation, undelivered
  Index: **Hypertension**
                transient
                of pregnancy (soubrette) 642.3
  Tabular: **642 Hypertension complicating pregnancy, childbirth, and the puerperium**

                    _____

                    642.3 Transient hypertension of pregnancy _____

                    642.33 Antepartum condition or complication _____

(Answers are located in Appendix B)

INTEGRAL CONDITIONS

ICD-9-CM OFFICIAL GUIDELINES FOR CODING AND REPORTING

SECTION I.B.
7. Conditions that are an integral part of a disease process

Signs and symptoms that are associated routinely with a disease process should not be
assigned as additional codes, unless otherwise instructed by the classification.

Integral Part of a Disease Process

Example 1

Diagnosis:	Fever and shortness of breath due to pneumonia
Index:	**Pneumonia** 486
Tabular:	**486 Pneumonia, organism unspecified**
Code:	486 Pneumonia, organism unspecified

Fever and shortness of breath are common symptoms of pneumonia so additional codes would not be assigned.

Integral Part of a Disease Process

Example 2

Diagnosis:	Abdominal pain that is exacerbated by eating. The patient was found to have a gastric ulcer.
Index:	**Ulcer, stomach,** 531.9
Tabular:	**531 Gastric ulcer**
	531.90 Unspecified as acute or chronic, without mention of hemorrhage or perforation
Code:	531.90 Gastric ulcer

Abdominal pain that is exacerbated (made worse) by eating is a common symptom of a gastric ulcer.

ICD-9-CM OFFICIAL GUIDELINES FOR CODING AND REPORTING

SECTION I.B.

8. Conditions that are not an integral part of a disease process

Additional signs and symptoms that may not be associated routinely with a disease process should be coded when present.

Not an Integral Part of a Disease Process

Example 1

Diagnosis:	Dehydration due to pneumonia
Index:	**Pneumonia 486**
Tabular:	**486 Pneumonia, organism unspecified**
Code:	486 Pneumonia, organism unspecified
Index:	**Dehydration 276.51**
Tabular:	**276.5 Volume depletion**
	276.51 Dehydration
Code:	276.51 Dehydration
Codes:	486 (pneumonia) and 276.51 (dehydration)

Dehydration can result from a wide range of diseases, but not all patients who have pneumonia become dehydrated. Dehydration would be assigned as an additional code.

Not an Integral Part of a Disease Process

Example 2

Diagnosis:	Ascites due to cirrhosis of the liver
Index:	**Cirrhosis, cirrhotic**
	liver 571.5
Tabular:	**571.5 Cirrhosis of liver without mention of alcohol**
Code:	571.5 Cirrhosis of liver
Index:	**Ascites 789.59**
Tabular:	**789.59 Other ascites**
Code:	789.59 Ascites
Codes:	571.5 (cirrhosis) and 789.59 (ascites)

Ascites is not present in all patients with cirrhosis of the liver. The ascites should be coded in this case as the patient's treatment may be affected by the ascites.

It is necessary to have strong anatomy, terminology, and pathophysiology skills to know if a condition is an integral part of a disease process.

EXERCISE 10-2 | *Integral and Not Integral Conditions*

Without the use of reference material, answer the following:

1 List two common symptoms of appendicitis.

_____

2 List the most common symptom associated with costochondritis.

_____

3 Patient has rheumatoid arthritis and anemia. The anemia is integral to the rheumatoid arthritis.

   True   False

4 Patient has dyspnea due to congestive heart failure. Dyspnea should be assigned as an additional code.

   True   False

Circle the diagnoses that should NOT be coded for the condition in bold typeface:

5 Acute myocardial infarction
   Chest pain
   Shortness of breath
   Congestive heart failure

6 Fractured hip
   Hip pain
   Contusion of hip

(Answers are located in Appendix B)

MULTIPLE CODING

ICD-9-CM OFFICIAL GUIDELINES FOR CODING AND REPORTING

SECTION I.B.

9. Multiple coding for a single condition

In addition to the etiology/manifestation convention that requires two codes to fully describe a single condition that affects multiple body systems, there are other single conditions that also require more than one code. "Use additional code" notes are found in the tabular at codes that are not part of an etiology/manifestation pair where a secondary code is useful to fully describe a condition. The sequencing rule is the same as the etiology/manifestation pair- "use additional code" indicates that a secondary code should be added.

For example, for infections that are not included in chapter 1, a secondary code from category 041, Bacterial infection in conditions classified elsewhere and of unspecified site, may be required to identify the bacterial organism causing the infection. A "use additional code" note will normally be found at the infectious disease code, indicating a need for the organism code to be added as a secondary code.

"Code first" notes are also under certain codes that are not specifically manifestation codes but may be due to an underlying cause. When a "code first" note is present and an underlying condition is present the underlying condition should be sequenced first.

"Code, if applicable, any causal condition first", notes indicate that this code may be assigned as a principal diagnosis when the causal condition is unknown or not applicable. If a causal condition is known, then the code for that condition should be sequenced as the principal or first-listed diagnosis.

Multiple codes may be needed for late effects, complication codes and obstetric codes to more fully describe a condition. See the specific guidelines for these conditions for further instruction.

Multiple Coding (Also Known as Dual Coding)

Example 1

Diagnosis: Diabetic retinopathy with type 1 diabetes

(Note: Retinopathy is the manifestation and diabetes is the etiology (cause) of the retinopathy or retinal hemorrhage.)

Index: **Retinopathy,** diabetic 250.5 *[362.01]*
                    diabetic 250.5 *[362.01]*

The Index subterm "diabetic" located under "Retinopathy" identifies the code for the etiology as 250.5 and directs you to the code for the manifestation of *[362.01]* retinopathy. The italicized code is never sequenced first as the first-listed diagnosis but is assigned to identify a manifestation.

Tabular: **250 Diabetes mellitus**
                    250.5 Diabetes with ophthalmic manifestations
                            Use additional code to identify manifestation
                        250.51 Type 1, not stated as uncontrolled

Note that the diagnosis of diabetes mellitus will always be reported with a five-digit code because the fifth digit indicates the type of diabetes. See the fifth-digit codes listed after code 250 in the Tabular of your ICD-9-CM.

Code 250.51 is the correct code to describe the diabetes (etiology). The statement "Use additional code to identify manifestation . . ." in the Tabular at 250.5 directs you to assign a code that identifies the manifestation (retinopathy).

Continued

Tabular: **362 Other retinal disorders**
362.0 Diabetic retinopathy
Code first diabetes (249.5, 250.5)
362.01 Background diabetic retinopathy

Note that the "*Code first diabetes (249.5, 250.5)*" directs you to the etiology code (diabetes).

Codes: 250.51, 362.01 Diabetic retinopathy with type 1 diabetes

The multiple codes fully describe the diagnostic statement. The Guideline directs you to place the etiology code first, followed by the manifestation code.

Let's review another example of multiple coding.

Multiple Coding (Also Known as Dual Coding)

Example 2

Diagnosis: Staphylococcal cellulitis of the face
(Staphylococcal infection is the etiology and cellulitis is the manifestation.)

Index: **Cellulitis,** face (any part, except eye) 682.0
Tabular: **682 Other cellulitis and abscess**
682.0 Face
Code: 682.0 Cellulitis of the face

You now must identify the code for the etiology (staphylococcal).

Index: **Infection,** staphylococcal NEC 041.10
Tabular: **041 Bacterial infection in conditions classified elsewhere and of unspecified site**

> **Note:** This category is to be used as an additional code to identify the bacterial agent in diseases classified elsewhere. This category is also used to classify bacterial infections of unspecified nature or site.

041.1 Staphylococcus
041.10 Staphylococcus, unspecified
Codes: 682.0, 041.10 Staphylococcal cellulitis of the face

Note that it is acceptable to sequence the manifestation code first in this example because code 682.0 is not italicized in the Tabular, and the instructional notation listed under category 682 in the Tabular specifically states, "Use additional code to identify organism . . ."

QUICK CHECK 10-2

1. When verifying 682.0 in the Tabular, what note(s) pertaining to infections is stated?

_____

2. In Question 1, is 041.1 a valid code (one that you would report)?
Yes or No?

(Answers are located in Appendix C)

EXERCISE 10-3   *Multiple Coding*

Using multiple codes, fill in the codes for the following diagnoses:

1 Chronic prostatitis due to *Streptococcus*

ICD-9-CM Codes: _____, _____

2 Acute bronchitis due to *Pseudomonas*

ICD-9-CM Codes: _____, _____

3 Gangrene due to diabetes mellitus, type 1, not stated as uncontrolled

ICD-9-CM Codes: _____, _____

4 Urinary tract infection due to *Escherichia coli*

🌐 ICD-9-CM Code(s): _____

5 Amyloid cardiomyopathy

🌐 ICD-9-CM Code(s): _____

(Answers are located in Appendix B)

ACUTE AND CHRONIC

ICD-9-CM OFFICIAL GUIDELINES FOR CODING AND REPORTING

SECTION I.B.

10. Acute and Chronic Conditions

If the same condition is described as both acute (subacute) and chronic, and separate subentries exist in the Alphabetic Index at the same indentation level, code both and sequence the acute (subacute) code first.

See Fig. 10-1 for the format of acute pancreatitis and chronic pancreatitis. Both acute and chronic forms of pancreatitis are subcategorized under code 577. Acute pancreatitis is 577.0 and chronic pancreatitis is 577.1. If the same condition is described as acute and chronic pancreatitis, and occur at the same indentation level in the Alphabetic Index, two codes are required and the acute code is listed first.

577.0 Acute pancreatitis
  Abscess of pancreas
  Necrosis of pancreas:
    acute
    infective
  Pancreatitis:
    NOS
    acute (recurrent)
    apoplectic
    hemorrhagic
    subacute
    suppurative
  Excludes *mumps pancreatitis (072.3)*
577.1 Chronic pancreatitis
  Chronic pancreatitis: Pancreatitis:
    NOS   painless
    infectious   recurrent
    interstitial   relapsing

FIGURE 10–1 Indent level of acute and chronic.

Acute and Chronic Conditions

Example 1

Diagnosis: Acute and chronic thyroiditis
Index: **Thyroiditis**
                 acute 245.0
                 chronic 245.8

Note that acute and chronic are at the same indention level in the Index, and Guideline Section I.B.10. directs the coder to sequence the acute code first, followed by the chronic code if both conditions are being reported.

Tabular: **245 Thyroiditis**
                 245.0 Acute thyroiditis
                 245.8 Other and unspecified chronic thyroiditis
Sequence: 245.0, 245.8 Acute and chronic thyroiditis

Note that the acute form of thyroiditis is sequenced before the chronic form, as directed by Section I.B.10. Guideline.

Acute and Chronic Conditions

Example 2

Diagnosis: Acute and chronic pericarditis
Index: **Pericarditis**
                 acute 420.90
                 chronic 423.8
Tabular: **420 Acute pericarditis**
                 420.9 Other and unspecified acute pericarditis
                     420.90 Acute pericarditis, unspecified
Tabular: **423   Other diseases of pericardium**
                 423.8 Other specified diseases of the pericardium
Sequence: 420.90, 423.8 Acute and chronic pericarditis

Note that while the Index directs you to code 423.8 for chronic pericarditis, when the Tabular is verified, there is no mention of chronic pericarditis. This is an example of a common coding situation in which you must trust the Index to have more descriptive terms than the Tabular. When the condition is both acute and chronic, and both acute and chronic are listed in the Index as separate entries and at the same indentation level, both codes are assigned and the code for acute is sequenced ***first***.

COMBINATION CODES

ICD-9-CM OFFICIAL GUIDELINES FOR CODING AND REPORTING

SECTION I.B.

11. Combination Code

A combination code is a single code used to classify:

Two diagnoses, or

A diagnosis with an associated secondary process (manifestation)

A diagnosis with an associated complication

Combination codes are identified by referring to subterm entries in the Alphabetic Index and by reading the inclusion and exclusion notes in the Tabular List.

Assign only the combination code when that code fully identifies the diagnostic conditions involved or when the Alphabetic Index so directs. Multiple coding should not be used when the classification provides a combination code that clearly identifies all of the elements documented in the diagnosis. When the combination code lacks necessary specificity in describing the manifestation or complication, an additional code should be used as a secondary code.

Combination Codes

Example 1

Diagnosis:	Acute cholecystitis with cholelithiasis
Index:	**Cholecystitis** with calculus (stones in the gallbladder) directs you to *See* Cholelithiasis
Index:	**Cholelithiasis** with, cholecystitis, acute 574.0
Tabular:	**574 Cholelithiasis** **574.0 Calculus of gallbladder with acute cholecystitis**

A fifth-digit subclassification is indicated as 0 for a case without mention of obstruction and as 1 when there is obstruction. There was no mention of obstruction in this case, so assign the fifth digit 0.

Code:	574.00 Acute cholecystitis with cholelithiasis

The single code 574.00 fully describes the diagnosis of acute cholecystitis with cholelithiasis.

Combination Codes

Example 2

Another example of a diagnosis (streptococcal) and manifestation (pharyngitis or sore throat) reported with a combination code is as follows:

Diagnosis:	Streptococcal pharyngitis
Index:	**Pharyngitis,** streptococcal 034.0
Tabular:	**034 Streptococcal sore throat and scarlet fever** **034.0 Streptococcal sore throat**

Septic:	Streptococcal:
angina	angina
sore throat	laryngitis
	pharyngitis
	tonsillitis

The single code 034.0 fully describes the diagnosis of streptococcal pharyngitis.

Code:	034.0 Streptococcal pharyngitis

EXERCISE 10-4 *Combination Codes*

Assign combination codes to the following:

1 Pneumonia due to *Hemophilus influenzae*

ICD-9-CM Code: _____

2 Candidiasis of the mouth (thrush)

ICD-9-CM Code: _____

3 Enteritis due to *Clostridium difficile*

ICD-9-CM Code: _____

4 Gastroenteritis due to *Salmonella*

ICD-9-CM Code: _____

5 Closed fracture of the tibia and fibula

ICD-9-CM Code: _____

(Answers are located in Appendix B)

LATE EFFECTS

Late effects codes are not assigned to a separate chapter in the Tabular. Instead, you must first identify a case as a late effect and then code it as such. You report late effects codes when the acute phase of the illness or injury has passed but a residual remains. Sometimes an acute illness or injury leaves a patient with a residual health problem that remains after the illness or injury has resolved. The **residual** is coded **first** and **then** the **late effects** code is assigned to indicate the cause of the residual. An example would be scars (residual) that remain after a severe burn (cause).

In most instances, two codes will be assigned—one code for the residual that is being treated and one code that indicates the late effect. There is no time limit for the development of a residual. It may be evident at the time of the acute illness or it may occur months after an injury. It is also possible that a patient may develop more than one residual. For example, a patient who has had a stroke may develop right-sided hemiparesis (paralysis of one side) and aphasia (loss of ability to communicate).

A person cannot have a current right hip fracture (820.8) and a late effect of a right hip fracture (905.3) at the same time. The code is either a current injury or a condition caused by a prior injury. It cannot be both. The only exception to this rule is in category 438, Late effects of cerebrovascular disease; this is explained in the following Guideline.

ICD-9-CM OFFICIAL GUIDELINES FOR CODING AND REPORTING

SECTION I.B.

12. Late Effects

A late effect is the residual effect (condition produced) after the acute phase of an illness or injury has terminated. There is no time limit on when a late effect code can be used. The residual may be apparent early, such as in cerebrovascular accident cases, or it may occur months or years later, such as that due to a previous injury. Coding of late effects generally requires two codes sequenced in the following order: The condition or nature of the late effect is sequenced first. The late effect code is sequenced second.

Exceptions to the above guidelines are those instances where the late effect code has been expanded (at the fourth and fifth-digit levels) to include the manifestation(s) **or the classification instructs otherwise**. The code for the acute phase of an illness or injury that led to the late effect is never used with a code for the late effect.

The late effects codes are accessed in the Index under the main term "Late."

ICD-9-CM OFFICIAL GUIDELINES FOR CODING AND REPORTING

SECTION I.C.7.

d. Late Effects of Cerebrovascular Disease

(1) Category 438, Late Effects of Cerebrovascular disease

Category 438 is used to indicate conditions classifiable to categories 430-437 as the causes of late effects (neurologic deficits), themselves classified elsewhere. These "late effects" include neurologic deficits that persist after initial onset of conditions classifiable to 430-437. The neurologic deficits caused by cerebrovascular disease may be present from the onset or may arise at any time after the onset of the condition classifiable to 430-437.

Codes in category 438 are only for use for late effects of cerebrovascular disease, not for neurologic deficits associated with an acute CVA.

(2) Codes from category 438 with codes from 430-437

Codes from category 438 may be assigned on a health care record with codes from 430-437, if the patient has a current cerebrovascular accident (CVA) and deficits from an old CVA.

(3) Code V12.54

Assign code V12.54, Transient ischemic attack (TIA), and cerebral infarction without residual deficits (and not a code from category 438) as an additional code for history of cerebrovascular disease when no neurologic deficits are present.

Residual and Cause

Example

Diagnosis: Aphasia due to a previous cerebrovascular accident

Residual: Aphasia

The aphasia is a condition that remains following the acute illness of the cerebrovascular accident.

Cause: Cerebrovascular accident

This patient had a previous cerebrovascular accident.

Terms to code: Aphasia [residual]

                  Cerebrovascular accident [cause]

The late effect of cerebrovascular accident is reported with a combination code. Locate the terms "Late, effect, cerebrovascular disease, with aphasia" in the Index of the ICD-9-CM and you will be directed to 438.11, which reports both the residual and the cause in one combination code.

EXERCISE 10-5   *Residual and Cause*

Write the term(s) that represent the residual and the cause terms on the lines provided:

1 Scars of the face resulting from third-degree burns suffered 1 year ago

Residual: _____

Cause: _____

2 Constrictive pericarditis due to old tuberculosis infection

Residual: _____

Cause: _____

3 Residual foreign body in femur due to gunshot injury years ago

Residual: _____

Cause: _____

4 Intellectual disabilities due to previous poliomyelitis

Residual: _____

Cause: _____

5 Leg pain resulting from old fracture of femur

Residual: _____

Cause: _____

(Answers are located in Appendix B)

To locate the late effects codes in the Index of the ICD-9-CM, use the entry "Late, effects." There are numerous subterms that describe the various late effects. Review and become familiar with the late effects subterms in the Index.

Assign the code for the acute injury or disease first; then refer to the Index "Late, effects" for that injury or disease. Next, reference the Tabular to ensure the codes are correct and assign any further digits indicated.

EXERCISE 10-6   *Residual and Cause Codes*

Identify the residual and cause terms and then code the following:

1 Traumatic arthritis following fracture of the left ankle 3 years ago

Residual: _____

Code: _____

Cause: _____

Code: _____

2 Dysphasia due to cerebrovascular accident 6 months ago (requires one combination code)

Residual: _____

Cause: _____

Code: _____

3 Sensorineural deafness due to previous meningitis

Residual: _____

Code: _____

Cause: _____

Code: _____

(Answers are located in Appendix B)

IMPENDING OR THREATENED CONDITION

ICD-9-CM OFFICIAL GUIDELINES FOR CODING AND REPORTING

SECTION I.B.

13. Impending or Threatened Condition

Code any condition described at the time of discharge as "impending" or "threatened" as follows:

If it did occur, code as confirmed diagnosis.

If it did not occur, reference the Alphabetic Index to determine if the condition has a subentry term for "impending" or "threatened" and also reference main term entries for "Impending" and for "Threatened."

If the subterms are listed, assign the given code.

If the subterms are not listed, code the existing underlying condition(s) and not the condition described as impending or threatened.

Impending or Threatened Condition

Example 1

Diagnosis:	Threatened abortion
Index:	**Threatened,** abortion 640.0
Tabular:	**640 Hemorrhage in early pregnancy**
	640.0 Threatened abortion
Code:	640.03 Threatened abortion

Fifth-digit 3 indicates an antepartum condition or complication.

Impending or Threatened Condition

Example 2

Diagnosis: Impending myocardial infarction
Index: **Impending,** myocardial infarction 411.1
Tabular: **411 Other acute and subacute forms of ischemic heart disease**
                  411.1 Intermediate coronary syndrome
                          Impending infarction
                          Preinfarction angina
                          Preinfarction syndrome
                          Unstable angina
Code: 411.1 Impending myocardial infarction

If the infarction had occurred, you would have reported it as a confirmed diagnosis by coding myocardial infarction (with the appropriate fifth digit to denote the episode of care).

EXERCISE 10-7   *Uncertain and Impending/Threatened Condition*

Assign codes for the following:

1 Evolving stroke

ICD-9-CM Code: _____

2 Impending delirium tremens

ICD-9-CM Code: _____

3 Threatened miscarriage, unspecified episode of care

ICD-9-CM Code: _____

4 Threatened labor, unspecified episode of care

ICD-9-CM Code: _____

5 Impending coronary syndrome

ICD-9-CM Code: _____

(Answers are located in Appendix B)

CHAPTER REVIEW

CHAPTER 10, PART I, THEORY

Without the use of reference material, answer the following:

1 List two of the four cooperating parties that agree on coding principles:

_____

_____

2 Fill in the missing words in the Steps to Accurate Coding:

   a Identify the main _____ in the diagnostic statement.

   b Locate the main term(s) in the Alphabetic Index (Volume _____).

   c Review any _____ under the main term in the Index.

   d Follow any _____-_____ instructions, such as *see also*.

   e Verify the code(s) selected from the Index (Volume _____) in the Tabular List (Volume _____) (referred to in this text as the Tabular).

   f Refer to any instructional notations in the _____.

   g Assign codes to the highest level of _____. For example, if a fourth digit is available, you cannot assign only a three-digit code, and if a fifth digit is available, you cannot assign only a four-digit code.

   h Code the diagnosis until all _____ are completely identified.

3 A combination code is a single code used to classify:
   a two diagnoses
   b a diagnosis with an associated manifestation
   c a diagnosis with an associated complication
   d all of the above

4 Additional signs and symptoms that may not routinely be associated with the disease process being reported should be coded when present.
   True   False

5 In the outpatient setting, an impending condition should be coded as if it actually exists.
   True   False

6 When separate codes exist to identify acute and chronic conditions, the chronic code is sequenced first.
   True   False

7 It is acceptable to use only the Alphabetic Index to assign ICD-9-CM codes.
   True   False

8 When sequencing codes for residuals and late effects, the residual is sequenced first followed by a late effect code.
   True   False

9 A code is invalid if it has not been coded to the full number of digits available for that code.
   True   False

10 The *Official Guidelines for Coding and Reporting* are updated annually.
   True   False

Chapter Review answers are only available in the TEACH Instructor Resources on Evolve

CHAPTER 10, PART II, PRACTICAL

List the following:

11 List two common symptoms associated with kidney stones. _____

12 List two common symptoms associated with pneumonia. _____

Assign ICD-9-CM codes to the following diagnoses:

13 Acute and chronic prostatitis

ICD-9-CM Codes: _____, _____

14 Headache, stiff neck, and fever due to viral meningitis

ICD-9-CM Code: _____

15 Acute and chronic pyelonephritis

ICD-9-CM Codes: _____, _____

16 Abdominal pain due to acute and chronic cholecystitis

ICD-9-CM Code: _____

17 Urinary tract infection due to *proteus mirabilis*

ICD-9-CM Code(s): _____

18 Impending cerebrovascular accident

ICD-9-CM Code(s): _____

19 Traumatic arthritis wrist due to fracture 5 years ago

ICD-9-CM Code(s): _____

20 Dysphagia due to previous cerebrovascular accident

ICD-9-CM Code(s): _____

21 What is the code for respiratory syncytial virus (RSV)?

ICD-9-CM Code: _____

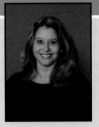

"It is necessary to set yourself apart, to demonstrate a level of professionalism, to ensure your employer that you see coding as a career, rather than just a job. It serves to prove your proficiency and makes you more marketable."

Debbi Miller, RNC, BSN, CPC
Manager, Revenue Integrity
LifePoint Hospitals, Inc.
Brentwood, Tennessee

Chapter-Specific Guidelines (ICD-9-CM Chapters 1-8)

Chapter Topics

Infectious and Parasitic Diseases

Neoplasms

Endocrine, Nutritional, and Metabolic Diseases and Immunity Disorders

Diseases of the Blood and Blood-Forming Organs

Mental, Behavioral and Neurodevelopmental Disorders

Diseases of the Nervous System and Sense Organs

Diseases of the Circulatory System

Diseases of the Respiratory System

Chapter Review

Learning Objectives

After completing this chapter you should be able to

1 Review infectious and parasitic disease codes.

2 Analyze the neoplasms codes.

3 Examine the endocrine, nutritional, metabolic diseases, and immunity disorders codes.

4 Review the blood conditions, mental, behavioral and neurodevelopmental disorders, nervous system, and sense organs codes.

5 Review the circulatory system codes.

6 Review the respiratory system codes.

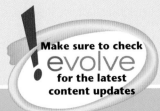

Make sure to check evolve for the latest content updates

NOTE: *The 2015 ICD-9-CM was used in preparing this chapter.*

INFECTIOUS AND PARASITIC DISEASES

Chapter 1 in the ICD-9-CM Tabular is Infectious and Parasitic Diseases, which classifies diseases according to the etiology, or cause, of the disease. Because infectious and parasitic conditions can affect various parts of the body, the chapter contains a wide variety of codes.

In this chapter there are many instances of combination coding and multiple coding. Remember: **Combination coding** applies when one code fully describes the condition. **Multiple coding** applies when it takes more than one code to fully describe the condition, and then sequencing of multiple codes may have to be considered.

From the Trenches

"Always follow the coding guidelines! 'If it's not documented, it wasn't done' is a familiar phrase among coding professionals."

DEBBI

Examples

Combination Coding

Diagnosis:	Candidiasis infection of the mouth
Index:	**Candidiasis,** candidal, mouth 112.0
Tabular:	**112.0 Candidiasis of mouth**
Code:	112.0 Candidiasis infection of the mouth

Code 112.0 fully describes the diagnosis of infection and organism with one code.

Multiple Coding

Diagnosis:	Urinary tract infection due to *Escherichia coli (E. coli)*
Index:	**Infection,** infected, infective; urinary (tract) NEC 599.0
Tabular:	**599.0 Urinary tract infection, site not specified**
	Use additional code to identify organism, such as
	Escherichia coli [E. coli] (041.41–041.49)

Code 599.0 does not fully describe the condition. The instructions in the Tabular for code 599.0 state that you are to also code the organism causing the urinary tract infection. To locate a causative organism, you locate the main term "Infection" in the Index and then the subterm of the specific organism, which in the example is *Escherichia coli*. The urinary tract infection is sequenced first, followed by the bacterial organism.

Index:	**Infection,** infected, infective, Escherichia coli (E. coli) 041.49
Tabular:	**041 Bacterial infection in conditions classified elsewhere and of unspecified site**
	041.4 Escherichia coli [E. coli]
Codes:	599.0, 041.49 Urinary tract infection due to *Escherichia coli (E. coli)*

Multiple coding is necessary to fully describe the infection of the urinary tract and the causative organism, *E. coli.*

Human Immunodeficiency

Another important category in Chapter 1 is 042 Human Immunodeficiency Virus (HIV) Disease. Review the guidelines for HIV codes.

ICD-9-CM OFFICIAL GUIDELINES FOR CODING AND REPORTING

SECTION I.C.1.

a. Human Immunodeficiency Virus (HIV) Infections

1) Code only confirmed cases

Code only confirmed cases of HIV infection/illness. This is an exception to the hospital inpatient guideline Section II, H.

In this context, "confirmation" does not require documentation of positive serology or culture for HIV; the provider's diagnostic statement that the patient is HIV positive, or has an HIV-related illness is sufficient.

2) Selection and sequencing of HIV codes

(a) Patient admitted for HIV-related condition

If a patient is admitted for an HIV-related condition, the principal diagnosis should be 042, followed by additional diagnosis codes for all reported HIV-related conditions.

(b) Patient with HIV disease admitted for unrelated condition

If a patient with HIV disease is admitted for an unrelated condition (such as a traumatic injury), the code for the unrelated condition (e.g., the nature of injury code) should be the principal diagnosis. Other diagnoses would be 042 followed by additional diagnosis codes for all reported HIV-related conditions.

(c) Whether the patient is newly diagnosed

Whether the patient is newly diagnosed or has had previous admissions/encounters for HIV conditions is irrelevant to the sequencing decision.

(d) Asymptomatic human immunodeficiency virus

V08 Asymptomatic human immunodeficiency virus [HIV] infection, is to be applied when the patient without any documentation of symptoms is listed as being "HIV positive," "known HIV," "HIV test positive," or similar terminology. Do not use this code if the term "AIDS" is used or if the patient is treated for any HIV-related illness or is described as having any condition(s) resulting from his/her HIV positive status; use 042 in these cases.

(e) Patients with inconclusive HIV serology

Patients with inconclusive HIV serology, but no definitive diagnosis or manifestations of the illness, may be assigned code 795.71, Inconclusive serologic test for Human Immunodeficiency Virus [HIV].

(f) Previously diagnosed HIV-related illness

Patients with any known prior diagnosis of an HIV-related illness should be coded to 042. Once a patient has developed an HIV-related illness, the patient should always be assigned code 042 on every subsequent admission/encounter. Patients previously diagnosed with any HIV illness (042) should never be assigned to 795.71 or V08.

(g) HIV Infection in Pregnancy, Childbirth and the Puerperium

During pregnancy, childbirth or the puerperium, a patient admitted (or presenting for a health care encounter) because of an HIV-related illness should receive a principal diagnosis code of 647.6X, Other specified infectious and parasitic diseases in the mother classifiable elsewhere, but complicating the pregnancy, childbirth or the puerperium, followed by 042 and the code(s) for the HIV-related illness(es). Codes from Chapter 15 always take sequencing priority.

Patients with asymptomatic HIV infection status admitted (or presenting for a health care encounter) during pregnancy, childbirth, or the puerperium should receive codes of 647.6X and V08.

Continued

(h) Encounters for testing for HIV

If a patient is being seen to determine his/her HIV status, use code V73.89, Screening for other specified viral disease. Use code V69.8, Other problems related to lifestyle, as a secondary code if an asymptomatic patient is in a known high risk group for HIV. Should a patient with signs or symptoms or illness, or a confirmed HIV related diagnosis be tested for HIV, code the signs and symptoms or the diagnosis. An additional counseling code V65.44 may be used if counseling is provided during the encounter for the test.

When a patient returns to be informed of his/her HIV test results use code V65.44, HIV counseling, if the results of the test are negative.

If the results are positive but the patient is asymptomatic use code V08, Asymptomatic HIV infection. If the results are positive and the patient is symptomatic use code 042, HIV infection, with codes for the HIV related symptoms or diagnosis. The HIV counseling code may also be used if counseling is provided for patients with positive test results.

✋ **CAUTION** *This statement is **very** important. You are **never** to code HIV unless you are certain of the diagnosis. This diagnosis stays in the patient's record forever!*

As stated in Guideline Section I.C.1., you do not assign 042 or V08 to a patient's record or insurance claim unless the diagnosis is a **confirmed** diagnosis. The assignment of the code prior to confirmation may cause the patient many unwarranted problems if the patient does not have HIV. Use extreme caution when assigning 042 or V08.

EXERCISE 11-1   *Infectious and Parasitic Diseases*

Code the following infectious diseases:

1 Viral gastroenteritis

    ICD-9-CM Code: _____

2 Septicemia due to *Pseudomonas* with septic shock

    ICD-9-CM Codes: _____, _____, _____

3 Acute poliomyelitis

    ICD-9-CM Code: _____

4 Candidal vaginal infection

    ICD-9-CM Code: _____

(Answers are located in Appendix B)

NEOPLASMS

Chapter 2 in the Tabular of the ICD-9-CM is similar to Chapter 1, Infectious and Parasitic Diseases, in that it classifies diseases according to the etiology, or cause, of the disease. Neoplastic conditions can affect all parts of the body. Before you learn more about what is in Chapter 2, you will review some of the specific terminology by completing the following exercise.

EXERCISE 11-2 *Neoplasms Terminology*

Match the following terms to the correct definitions:

1 neoplasm _____

2 malignant _____

3 primary _____

4 secondary _____

5 benign _____

6 in situ _____

7 uncertain behavior _____

8 unspecified nature _____

9 morphology _____

a Not usually progressive

b Malignancy that is located within the original site of development

c Used to describe a cancerous tumor that grows worse over time

d Study of neoplasms

e Refers to the behavior of a neoplasm as neither malignant nor benign but having characteristics of both malignant and benign neoplasms

f When the behavior or histology of a neoplasm is not known or not specified

g Site to which a malignant tumor has spread

h Site of origin or where the tumor originated

i New tumor growth that can be benign or malignant

(Answers are located in Appendix B)

Neoplasm Codes

Neoplasms are **staged,** which means that they are evaluated for placement on a common grading scale based on the level of invasion. For example, staging for endometrial, cervical, and ovarian malignancies is staged based on if the malignancy (I) is confined to corpus, (II) involves corpus and cervix, (III) extends outside uterus but not outside true pelvis, (IV) extends outside true pelvis or involves rectum or bladder. Staging for renal cancer is staged on Stage I tumor of kidney capsule only, Stage II tumor invading renal capsule/vein but within fascia, Stage III tumor extending to regional lymph/vena cava, or Stage IV other organ metastasis. The pathology report and staging information will be documented in the medical record.

To assign a diagnosis code to a neoplasm is a two-step process:

1. First, locate the morphology or histologic type of the neoplasm in the Index of the ICD-9-CM. Examples of histology types are carcinoma, adenocarcinoma, sarcoma, melanoma, lymphoma, lipoma, adenoma.

2. Once you have located the morphology, review all modifiers and subterms, and then follow the instructions or verify the code listed. Most often you will be instructed to reference the Neoplasm Table in the Index to locate the code, as illustrated in Fig. 11-1.

Although M codes are not assigned in the outpatient setting, M codes are still important because the information will assist you in learning about how neoplasms are classified. In addition, there are coding employees whose job it is to classify neoplasms based on the medical documentation. So a basic knowledge of M codes is important. Mostly, M codes are assigned by the tumor registrar (the person who records morphology information). M codes are not required on insurance forms, but you will see them throughout the Index.

M codes are alphanumeric codes and are listed in Appendix A of the ICD-9-CM manual. The alphanumeric structure of the morphology codes starts with the letter M (for morphology), followed by four digits that indicate the histologic type of neoplasm, and a slash, followed by a fifth digit that indicates the behavior.

SECTION I INDEX TO DISEASES AND INJURIES / Neoplasm, iris

| | Malignant | | | | | |
	Primary	Secondary	Ca in situ	Benign	Uncertain Behavior	Unspecified
Neoplasm *(Continued)*						
iris	190.0	198.4	234.0	224.0	238.8	239.89
ischiorectal (fossa)	195.3	198.89	234.8	229.8	238.8	239.89
ischium	170.6	198.5	—	213.6	238.0	239.2
island of Reil	191.0	198.3	—	225.0	237.5	239.6
islands or islets of Langerhans	157.4	197.8	230.9	211.7	235.5	239.0
isthmus uteri	182.1	198.82	233.2	219.1	236.0	239.5
jaw	195.0	198.89	234.8	229.8	238.8	239.89
bone	170.1	198.5	—	213.1	238.0	239.2
carcinoma	143.9	—	—	—	—	—
lower	143.1	—	—	—	—	—
upper	143.0	—	—	—	—	—
lower	170.1	198.5	—	213.1	238.0	239.2
upper	170.0	198.5	—	213.0	238.0	239.2
carcinoma (any type) (lower) (upper)	195.0	—	—	—	—	—
skin (*see also* Neoplasm, skin, face)	173.30	198.2	232.3	216.3	238.2	239.2
soft tissues	143.9	198.89	230.0	210.4	235.1	239.0
lower	143.1	198.89	230.0	210.4	235.1	239.0
upper	143.0	198.89	230.0	210.4	235.1	239.0
jejunum	152.1	197.4	230.7	211.2	235.2	239.0
joint NEC (*see also* Neoplasm, bone)	170.9	198.5	—	213.9	238.0	239.2

FIGURE 11–1   Neoplasm Table.

Behavior Indicated by Fifth Digit
/0 = Benign
/1 = Uncertain whether benign or malignant
      Borderline malignancy
/2 = Carcinoma in situ
      Intraepithelial
      Noninfiltrating
      Noninvasive
/3 = Malignant, primary site
/6 = Malignant, metastatic site
      Secondary site
/9 = Malignant, uncertain whether primary or metastatic site

The following example shows how the morphology codes are assigned.

ICD-9-CM Codes and Morphology Codes

Example

Diagnosis:	Adenocarcinoma of the upper-outer quadrant right breast with metastasis to the axillary lymph nodes
Index:	**Adenocarcinoma** (M8140/3)—*see also* Neoplasm, by site, malignant
Neoplasm Table:	Breast, upper-outer quadrant, 174.4 (Primary column) Lymph-, lymphatic, gland (Secondary column), axilla, axillary, 196.3

Tabular:	**174 Malignant neoplasm of female breast**
	    174.4 Upper-outer quadrant
	196 Secondary and unspecified malignant neoplasm of lymph nodes
	    196.3 Lymph nodes of axilla and upper limb

Codes:	174.4, 196.3 Adenocarcinoma of the upper-outer quadrant right breast with metastasis to the axillary lymph nodes But wait, you're not finished yet. You have two M codes to assign to this diagnosis before you are finished—one for the primary adenocarcinoma and one for a secondary adenocarcinoma. Both M codes will have the same histologic type of adenocarcinoma, but the fifth digit will be different to indicate the primary and secondary behaviors.
Index:	**Adeno-carcinoma** (M8140/3)—*see also* Neoplasm, by site, malignant
M code:	**Primary** adenocarcinoma of the breast, M8140/**3** (3 indicates primary site)
M code:	**Secondary** adenocarcinoma of the axillary lymph nodes, M8140/**6** (6 indicates secondary site)
ICD-9-CM and M Codes:	174.4, M8140/3, 196.3, M8140/6 Adenocarcinoma of the upper-outer quadrant right breast with metastasis to the axillary lymph nodes

Note that the M codes are sequenced after the ICD-9-CM diagnosis code to which they refer.

The Guidelines provide the following information regarding reporting neoplasms:

ICD-9-CM OFFICIAL GUIDELINES FOR CODING AND REPORTING

SECTION I.C.

2. Chapter 2: Neoplasms (140-239)
General guidelines

Chapter 2 of the ICD-9-CM contains the codes for most benign and all malignant neoplasms. Certain benign neoplasms, such as prostatic adenomas, may be found in the specific body system chapters. To properly code a neoplasm it is necessary to determine from the record if the neoplasm is benign, in situ, malignant, or of uncertain histologic behavior. If malignant, any secondary (metastatic) sites should also be determined.

The neoplasm table in the Alphabetic Index should be referenced first. However, if the histological term is documented, that term should be referenced first, rather than going immediately to the Neoplasm Table, in order to determine which column in the Neoplasm Table is appropriate. For example, if the documentation indicates "adenoma," refer to the term in the Alphabetic Index to review the entries under this term and the instructional note to "see also

Continued

neoplasm, by site, benign." The table provides the proper code based on the type of neoplasm and the site. It is important to select the proper column in the table that corresponds to the type of neoplasm. The tabular should then be referenced to verify that the correct code has been selected from the table and that a more specific site code does not exist.

See Section I. C. 18.d.4. for information regarding V codes for genetic susceptibility to cancer.

a. Treatment directed at the malignancy

If the treatment is directed at the malignancy, designate the malignancy as the principal diagnosis.

The only exception to this guideline is if a patient admission/encounter is solely for the administration of chemotherapy, immunotherapy or radiation therapy, assign the appropriate V58.X code as the first-listed or principal diagnosis, and the diagnosis or problem for which the service is being performed as a secondary diagnosis.

b. Treatment of secondary site

When a patient is admitted because of a primary neoplasm with metastasis and treatment is directed toward the secondary site only, the secondary neoplasm is designated as the principal diagnosis even though the primary malignancy is still present

c. Coding and sequencing of complications

Coding and sequencing of complications associated with the malignancies or with the therapy thereof are subject to the following guidelines:

1) Anemia associated with malignancy

When admission/encounter is for management of an anemia associated with the malignancy, and the treatment is only for anemia, the appropriate anemia code (such as code 285.22, Anemia in neoplastic disease) is designated as the principal diagnosis and is followed by the appropriate code(s) for the malignancy.

Code 285.22 may also be used as a secondary code if the patient suffers from anemia and is being treated for the malignancy.

If anemia in neoplastic disease and anemia due to antineoplastic chemotherapy are both documented, **assign codes for both conditions.**

2) Anemia associated with chemotherapy, immunotherapy and radiation therapy

When the admission/encounter is for management of an anemia associated with chemotherapy, immunotherapy or radiotherapy and the only treatment is for the anemia, the anemia is sequenced first. The appropriate neoplasm code should be assigned as an additional code.

3) Management of dehydration due to the malignancy

When the admission/encounter is for management of dehydration due to the malignancy or the therapy, or a combination of both, and only the dehydration is being treated (intravenous rehydration), the dehydration is sequenced first, followed by the code(s) for the malignancy.

4) Treatment of a complication resulting from a surgical procedure

When the admission/encounter is for treatment of a complication resulting from a surgical procedure, designate the complication as the principal or first-listed diagnosis if treatment is directed at resolving the complication.

d. Primary malignancy previously excised

When a primary malignancy has been previously excised or eradicated from its site and there is no further treatment directed to that site and there is no evidence of any existing primary malignancy, a code from category V10, Personal history of malignant neoplasm, should be used to indicate the former site of the malignancy. Any mention of extension, invasion, or metastasis to another site is coded as a secondary malignant neoplasm to that site. The secondary site may be the principal or first-listed with the V10 code used as a secondary code.

Continued

e. Admission/Encounters involving chemotherapy, immunotherapy and radiation therapy

1) Episode of care involves surgical removal of neoplasm

When an episode of care involves the surgical removal of a neoplasm, primary or secondary site, followed by adjunct chemotherapy or radiation treatment during the same episode of care, the neoplasm code should be assigned as principal or first-listed diagnosis, using codes in the 140-198 series or where appropriate in the 200-203 series.

2) Patient admission/encounter solely for administration of chemotherapy, immunotherapy and radiation therapy

If a patient admission/encounter is solely for the administration of chemotherapy, immunotherapy or radiation therapy assign code V58.0, Encounter for radiation therapy, or V58.11, Encounter for antineoplastic chemotherapy, or V58.12, Encounter for antineoplastic immunotherapy as the first-listed or principal diagnosis. If a patient receives more than one of these therapies during the same admission more than one of these codes may be assigned, in any sequence.

The malignancy for which therapy is being administered should be assigned as a secondary diagnosis.

3) Patient admitted for radiotherapy/chemotherapy and immunotherapy and develops complications

When a patient is admitted for the purpose of radiotherapy, immunotherapy or chemotherapy and develops complications such as uncontrolled nausea and vomiting or dehydration, the principal or first-listed diagnosis is V58.0, Encounter for radiotherapy, or V58.11, Encounter for antineoplastic chemotherapy, or V58.12, Encounter for antineoplastic immunotherapy, followed by any codes for the complications.

f. Admission/encounter to determine extent of malignancy

When the reason for admission/encounter is to determine the extent of the malignancy, or for a procedure such as paracentesis or thoracentesis, the primary malignancy or appropriate metastatic site is designated as the principal or first-listed diagnosis, even though chemotherapy or radiotherapy is administered.

g. Symptoms, signs, and ill-defined conditions listed in Chapter 16 associated with neoplasms

Symptoms, signs, and ill-defined conditions listed in Chapter 16 characteristic of, or associated with, an existing primary or secondary site malignancy cannot be used to replace the malignancy as principal or first-listed diagnosis, regardless of the number of admissions or encounters for treatment and care of the neoplasm.

h. Admission/encounter for pain control/management

See Section I.C.6.a.5 for information on coding admission/encounter for pain control/ management.

V codes are also frequently reported with neoplasms to indicate the history of a malignant neoplasm (V10.00-V10.9). These history codes are used to report a malignant neoplasm that is no longer present. Remember that in the V code section, you were presented with information about documenting a "history of" a disease. Be careful in determining whether the physician is indicating a past and current history of a condition or a true past history. With neoplasms there is often a true "history of" whereby the condition previously existed but is no longer present.

There are also encounter V codes for chemotherapy (V58.11), immunotherapy (V58.12), and radiotherapy (V58.0). When coding an encounter solely for chemotherapy, immunotherapy, or radiotherapy, place the V code first, followed by the active code for the malignant neoplasm, even if that neoplasm has already been removed. As long as the neoplasm is being treated with adjunctive therapy (another treatment used in conjunction with the primary treatment) following a surgical removal of the cancer (primary treatment), you code the neoplasm as if it still exists.

You would **not** assign a "history of" V code because the neoplasm is the reason for the treatment. Instead, the neoplasm is coded as a current or active disease.

EXERCISE 11-3 | *Neoplasm Codes*

Assign diagnosis codes to the following:

1 A patient is admitted for chemotherapy for ovarian cancer.

Two codes are needed for this case: one for the encounter for chemotherapy and the other for the malignant, primary, ovarian neoplasm.

    Locate the code in the Index and verify in the Tabular.

        ICD-9-CM Codes: _____, _____

2 A patient is admitted for radiation therapy for metastatic bone cancer. The patient had a mastectomy for breast cancer 3 years earlier.

There is a code for the admission for radiation management, which will be a V code; a code for the secondary, malignant, bone neoplasm; and a V code for the history of malignant neoplasm of the breast.

        ICD-9-CM Codes: _____, _____, _____

3 A patient is admitted with chest pain, shortness of breath, and a history of bloody sputum. Diagnostic x-ray film shows a mass in the bronchial tube. A diagnostic bronchoscopy is performed and is positive for cancer. The pathology report states "metastatic carcinoma of bronchus, primary unknown." The patient chooses to undergo chemotherapy.

    a What is the description of the first-listed diagnosis? _____

    b What is the subsequent diagnosis description? _____

    c Is the metastatic carcinoma of the bronchus a primary or secondary malignant neoplasm? _____

    d What are the diagnosis codes for this case?

        ICD-9-CM Codes: _____, _____

4 A patient is admitted with uncontrolled nausea and vomiting after chemotherapy treatment for lung cancer.

    a How many codes would be needed to accurately report this case? _____ (plus an E code)

    b What is the first-listed diagnosis? _____

    c What is the secondary diagnosis? _____

    d What is the code for the first-listed diagnosis?

        ICD-9-CM Code: _____

    e What is the code for the secondary diagnosis and the E code?

        ICD-9-CM Codes: _____, _____

(Answers are located in Appendix B)

Unknown Site or Unspecified

There is an entry on the Neoplasm Table that states "unknown site or unspecified." This code, 199.1, is assigned to indicate either an unknown or an unspecified primary or secondary malignancy. If there is a **known** secondary site, a code must be assigned to the primary site or the history of a primary site. It is possible for the primary site to be unknown and the secondary site to be known.

QUICK CHECK 11-1

1. What entry in the Neoplasm Table reports a benign neoplasm of an unspecified site?

_____

(Answers are located in Appendix C)

Unknown Primary Site

Example

Diagnosis: Metastatic bone cancer

This statement indicates that the bone cancer is a secondary neoplasm, but there is no indication of the location of the primary site.

Index:	**Cancer**—*see also* Neoplasm, by site, malignant
Neoplasm Table:	Bone 198.5 (Secondary)
	Unknown site or unspecified 199.1 (Primary)
Tabular:	**198 Secondary malignant neoplasm of other specified site**
	198.5 Bone and bone marrow
Tabular:	**199 Malignant neoplasm without specification of site**
	199.1 Other
Codes:	198.5, 199.1 Metastatic bone cancer (if the treatment is for the secondary site)
	199.1, 198.5 Metastatic bone cancer (if the treatment or diagnostic workup is for the primary site)

The sequencing of the primary and secondary neoplasms is dependent on the treatment circumstances documented in the health record. If treatment was directed toward the secondary malignancy, the code for the secondary would be sequenced first. If treatment was focused on determining the site of the unknown primary malignancy, the code for the unknown site would be sequenced first.

EXERCISE 11-4 *More Neoplasms*

Assign ICD-9-CM codes for the following neoplasms:

1 Multiple myeloma

ICD-9-CM Code: _____

2 Carcinoma in situ, cervix

ICD-9-CM Code: _____

3 Cancer of the sigmoid colon with spread to the peritoneum

ICD-9-CM Codes: _____, _____

4 Adenocarcinoma of the prostate with metastasis to the bone

ICD-9-CM Codes: _____, _____

5 Metastatic cancer to the brain; primary unknown (treatment directed to metastatic site)

ICD-9-CM Codes: _____, _____

6 Metastatic carcinoma of the breast to the lungs; the breast carcinoma has been removed by mastectomy

ICD-9-CM Codes: _____, _____

(Answers are located in Appendix B)

ENDOCRINE, NUTRITIONAL, AND METABOLIC DISEASES AND IMMUNITY DISORDERS

Chapter 3 in the Tabular of the ICD-9-CM describes diseases or conditions affecting the endocrine system. The endocrine system involves glands that are located throughout the body and are responsible for secreting hormones into the bloodstream. Also included in Chapter 3 are diseases or conditions that affect nutritional and metabolic status as well as disorders of the immune system.

One of the frequently used category codes in Chapter 3 is 250, Diabetes Mellitus. When you locate diabetes in the Index, you will note that for many of the subterms, two codes are listed. The 250.XX code is followed by an italicized code in brackets. This is because multiple coding is common for diabetes because both the manifestation (symptom) and the etiology (cause—diabetes) are reported.

Example

Index: **Diabetes,** retinopathy, background, 250.5X *[362.01]*

There are four five-digit subclassifications for use with category 250. It is essential that you read these before assigning codes for diagnosis of diabetes mellitus (DM). The fifth digits identify the type of diabetes: 2 is type 2 or unspecified type, uncontrolled; and 3 is type 1 [juvenile type], uncontrolled. The health care providers usually document the type of diabetes mellitus. You should not assume that because a patient is receiving insulin that he or she is a type 1 diabetic because a type 2 diabetic may be receiving insulin. If there is any question regarding the type of diabetes, query the physician.

In order to appropriately assign the fifth digits 2 or 3, uncontrolled diabetes, the physician must document that the patient's DM is uncontrolled or out of control. If a complication is specified (250.1-250.8), assign the appropriate fourth and fifth digits; do not use the .9 (unspecified).

Example

Diagnosis: Diabetic iritis

Index: **Diabetes, diabetic,** iritis 250.5 *[364.42]*

The first code (250.5) indicates the etiology (diabetes) and the second code *[364.42]* indicates the manifestation (iritis). You need two codes to describe the diagnoses. You will always list the etiology first and then the manifestation.

Tabular: **250.5 Diabetes with ophthalmic manifestations**
            Use additional code to identify manifestation, as:
364.4 Vascular disorders of iris and ciliary body

The Tabular also indicates that a fifth digit should be added for greater specificity.

Tabular: **364.4 Vascular disorders of iris and ciliary body**

364.42 Rubeosis iridis

Even though the 364.42 entry does not specifically indicate iritis, you trust the code that is listed in the Index. You could also reference the main term "Iritis" in the Index and be directed to the same codes.

Index: **Iritis** 364.3, diabetic 250.5 *[364.42]*

You are directed to the same codes.

Codes: 250.50, 364.42 Diabetic iritis

The codes must be sequenced in this order to indicate that the iritis is a manifestation of the diabetes.

To code a disease or condition as a manifestation of DM, it must be stated that the disease or condition is diabetic or due to the diabetes. A cause-and-effect relationship must be stated or evident. If you are unsure of the relationship, you must clarify this relationship with the physician.

If a cause-and-effect relationship is not evident or stated and no further indication of the relationship can be obtained, the following codes would be assigned.

Example

Diagnosis: Diabetes mellitus and iritis

Index: **Diabetes, diabetic** 250.0

Note—Use the following fifth-digit subclassification with category 250:

The Note in the Index directs you to use a fifth digit for greater specificity.

Tabular: **250.0 Diabetes mellitus without mention of complication**

Index: **Iritis 364.3**

Tabular: **364.3 Unspecified iridocyclitis**

Codes: 250.00 Diabetes and 364.3 Iritis

Note that codes (250.00 and 364.3) are individual codes because a cause-and-effect relationship was not established—the iritis is not reported as a manifestation of the diabetes in this case.

EXERCISE 11-5   *Endocrine, Nutritional, and Metabolic Diseases and Immunity Disorders*

Fill in the codes for the following:

1 Addison's disease

ICD-9-CM Code: _____

2 Dehydration

ICD-9-CM Code: _____

3 Diabetes mellitus with hypoglycemic coma

ICD-9-CM Code: _____

4 Graves' disease with thyrotoxic crisis

ICD-9-CM Code: _____

(Answers are located in Appendix B)

DISEASES OF THE BLOOD AND BLOOD-FORMING ORGANS

Chapter 4, Diseases of the Blood and Blood-Forming Organs, in the ICD-9-CM is a short chapter with only 10 categories. The **anemia** category is often used because anemia is the most common blood disease. Anemia is the main term under which you will find the many subterms that relate to anemia. In addition to there being numerous subterms for anemia, many of those subterms have lengthy additional subterms listed under them.

There are two anemias that are easy to confuse—anemia of chronic disease and chronic simple anemia. These two diagnostic statements do not have the same meaning. In anemia of chronic disease, the word "chronic" describes the nature of the disease that is the cause of the anemia, for example, anemia due to neoplastic disease. The neoplasm is the chronic disease causing the anemia. Code anemia (285.22) and then assign the appropriate code to identify the neoplasm. In the diagnostic statement chronic, simple anemia, the word "chronic" describes simple anemia. Let's see what difference these diagnostic statements make in code assignment.

ANEMIA

Example 1

Diagnosis: Anemia of chronic disease

In this diagnosis statement, you do not know what the chronic disease is.

Index: **Anemia**

The Index has a subterm (in, chronic illness, 285.29) that further directs you in the choice of the correct code.

Tabular: **285.2 Anemia of chronic disease**

Code: 285.29 Anemia of other chronic disease

ANEMIA

Example 2

Diagnosis: Chronic simple anemia

Index: **Anemia** 285.9, chronic simple 281.9

In this example, the Index does indicate a subterm that further directs you to chronic simple 281.9.

Tabular: **281.9 Unspecified deficiency anemia**

Code: 281.9 Chronic simple anemia

If there is any question about the classification of the anemia, check with the physician.

EXERCISE 11-6   *Diseases of the Blood and Blood-Forming Organs*

Assign codes for the following:

1 Pernicious anemia

   ICD-9-CM Code: _____

2 Disseminated intravascular coagulation (DIC)

   ICD-9-CM Code: _____

3 Hemophilia

   ICD-9-CM Code: _____

4 Acute blood-loss anemia

   ICD-9-CM Code: _____

5 Familial polycythemia

   ICD-9-CM Code: _____

MENTAL, BEHAVIORAL AND NEURODEVELOPMENTAL DISORDERS

Chapter 5 in the Tabular of the ICD-9-CM is Mental, Behavioral and Neurodevelopmental Disorders. The chapter includes four sections: organic psychotic conditions; other psychoses; neurotic, personality, and other nonpsychotic mental, behavioral and neurodevelopmental disorders; and intellectual disabilities.

Your understanding of the definitions of these mental, behavioral and neurodevelopmental disorders is necessary to enable you to code accurately. When assigning codes from Chapter 5, you need to take extra care to select the appropriate code(s) and report only diagnoses that are documented in the medical record. Mental, behavioral and neurodevelopmental disorders can be difficult to code because physicians are not always as specific in the diagnostic statements as might be required by the codes in the ICD-9-CM chapter. When in doubt, always check with the physician. Just one term in the medical record can make a big difference in the code(s) you use.

Five-Digit Subclassification

A five-digit subclassification is provided for categories 303-305 to indicate the patient's pattern of use of alcohol or drugs:

0	unspecified	
1	continuous:	Alcohol: Refers to daily intake of large amounts of alcohol or regular heavy drinking on weekends or days off from work
		Drugs: Daily or almost daily use of drugs
2	episodic:	Alcohol: Refers to alcoholic binges lasting weeks or months, followed by long periods of sobriety
		Drugs: Indicates short periods between drug use or use on weekends
3	in remission:	Refers either to a complete cessation of alcohol or drug intake or to the period during which decreasing intake leading toward cessation is taking place

CODING SHOT

You should be aware that there is a V code for history of alcoholism (V11.3). Instead of using that code you should use the **alcoholism** code (303.9X) with the fifth digit 3, which specifies in remission. It is rare to assign code V11.3 because the disease of alcoholism cannot be cured, only be in a state of remission.

Another commonly encountered instance is the instruction to "Use additional code to identify the associated neurological condition" or "Use additional code to identify cerebral atherosclerosis." Pay close attention to the instructions given in the Tabular when you see a "Use additional . . ." statement.

Example

Diagnosis:	Arteriosclerotic dementia with delirium
Index:	**Dementia** 294.8, arteriosclerotic (simple type) (uncomplicated) 290.40, with, delirium 290.41
Tabular:	**290 Senile and presenile organic psychotic conditions**
	290.4 Vascular dementia
	Use additional code to identify cerebral atherosclerosis (437.0)
	290.41 Vascular dementia with delirium
Tabular:	**437 Other and ill-defined cerebrovascular disease**
	437.0 Cerebral atherosclerosis
Codes:	290.41, 437.0 Arteriosclerotic dementia with delirium

According to the Guidelines, you are to sequence the etiology before the manifestation; however, if the Tabular directs the manifestation before the etiology, such as in 290, you must adhere to the Tabular direction. The "Use additional code to identify cerebral atherosclerosis (437.0)" is a direction to report the vascular dementia (290.4), which is the manifestation, before the cerebral atherosclerosis, which is the etiology.

EXERCISE 11-7   *Mental, Behavioral and Neurodevelopmental Disorders*

Now you have a chance to show your skill by coding the following:

1 Alzheimer's dementia with aggressive behavior
   ICD-9-CM Codes: _____, _____

2 Depression with anxiety
   ICD-9-CM Code: _____

3 Profound intellectual disabilities
   🔵 ICD-9-CM Code(s): _____

4 Anorexia nervosa
   🔵 ICD-9-CM Code(s): _____

5 Delirium tremens due to chronic alcoholism, continuous
   🔵 ICD-9-CM Code(s): _____

(Answers are located in Appendix B)

DISEASES OF THE NERVOUS SYSTEM AND SENSE ORGANS

Chapter 6 of the Tabular ICD-9-CM is Diseases of the Nervous System and Sense Organs and describes diseases or conditions affecting the central nervous system and the peripheral nervous system. It also includes disorders and diseases of the eyes and ears.

The chapter contains some combination codes in which one code identifies both the manifestation and the etiology.

Combination Codes

Example

Diagnosis: Pneumococcal meningitis

This diagnostic statement means the meningitis is due to pneumococcal bacteria.

Index: **Meningitis,** pneumococcal 320.1

Tabular: **320 Bacterial meningitis**

                320.1 Pneumococcal meningitis

Code: 320.1 Pneumococcal meningitis

Code 320.1 includes the manifestation of meningitis and also the etiology of pneumococcal organism. No separate code is required for the organism in this diagnostic statement.

In Chapter 6 of the ICD-9-CM, you will also locate conditions that are manifestations of other diseases. These categories appear in italics in the Tabular and provide instructions to code the underlying disease process first.

Manifestations

Example

Diagnosis: Chronic iridocyclitis due to sarcoidosis

Index: **Iridocyclitis** NEC 364.3, chronic, in, sarcoidosis 135 *[364.11]*

Entries such as 135 *[364.11]* instruct you to code the sarcoidosis (135) first, followed by the chronic iridocyclitis (364.11). Both codes need to be verified in the Tabular.

Tabular: **135 Sarcoidosis**

Tabular: **364 Disorders of iris and ciliary body**

                364.11 Chronic iridocyclitis in diseases classified elsewhere

                        Code first underlying disease, as:
                            sarcoidosis (135)
                            tuberculosis (017.3)

Codes: 135, 364.11 Chronic iridocyclitis due to sarcoidosis

EXERCISE 11-8   *Diseases of the Nervous System and Sense Organs*

Assign codes for the following:

1 Meningitis due to *Proteus morganii*

ICD-9-CM Code: _____

2 Multiple sclerosis

ICD-9-CM Code: _____

3 Acute otitis media

ICD-9-CM Code: _____

4 Primary open-angle glaucoma, moderate stage

ICD-9-CM Code(s): _____, _____

5 Bell's palsy

ICD-9-CM Code: _____

(Answers are located in Appendix B)

DISEASES OF THE CIRCULATORY SYSTEM

Hypertension

Chapter 7 of the ICD-9-CM Tabular, Diseases of the Circulatory System, contains diseases of heart and blood vessels.

Hypertension is one of the most common conditions coded in this chapter. The Hypertension Table, as shown in Fig. 11-2 (the numbering on Fig. 11-2 will be used as a future reference), is located in the Index. This table provides a complete listing of all conditions due to or associated with hypertension. The first column identifies the hypertensive **condition,** such as accelerated, antepartum, cardiovascular disease, cardiorenal, and cerebrovascular disease. The remaining three columns are Malignant, Benign, and Unspecified and constitute the subcategories of hypertensive disease.

Malignant hypertension is also known as accelerated hypertension and is a severe form of hypertension, manifested by headaches, blurred vision, dyspnea, and uremia. This type

	Malignant	Benign	Unspecified
Hypertension, hypertensive (arterial) (arteriolar) (crisis) (degeneration) (disease) (essential) (fluctuating) (idiopathic) (intermittent) (labile) (low renin) (orthostatic) (paroxysmal) (primary) (systemic) (uncontrolled) (vascular)	401.0	401.1 (#1)	401.9 (#3)
with			
chronic kidney disease	—	—	—
stage I through stage IV, or unspecified	403.00	403.10	403.90
stage V or end stage renal disease	403.01	403.11	403.91
heart involvement (conditions classifiable to 429.0–429.3, 429.8, 429.9 due to hypertension) (*see also* Hypertension, heart)	402.00	402.10	402.90
with kidney involvement - *see* Hypertension, cardiorenal			
renal (kidney) involvement (only conditions classifiable to 585, 587) (excludes conditions classifiable to 584) (*see also* Hypertension, kidney)	403.00	403.10	403.90
with heart involvement - *see* Hypertension, cardiorenal failure (and sclerosis) (*see also* Hypertension, kidney)	403.01	403.11	403.91
sclerosis without failure (*see also* Hypertension, kidney)	403.00	403.10	403.90
accelerated (*see also* Hypertension, by type, malignant)	401.0	—	—
antepartum - *see* Hypertension, complicating pregnancy, childbirth, or the puerperium			
borderline	—	—	796.2
cardiorenal (disease)	404.00	404.10	404.90
with			
chronic kidney disease	—	—	—
stage I through stage IV, or unspecified	404.00	404.10	404.90
and heart failure	404.01	404.11	404.91
stage V or end stage renal disease	404.02	404.12	404.92
and heart failure	404.03	404.13	404.93
heart failure	404.01	404.11	404.91
and chronic kidney disease	404.01	404.11	404.91
stage I through stage IV or unspecified	404.01	404.11	404.91
stage V or end stage renal disease	404.03	404.13	404.93
cardiovascular disease (arteriosclerotic) (sclerotic)	(#2) 402.00	402.10	402.90
with			
heart failure	402.01	402.11	402.91
renal involvement (conditions classifiable to 403) (*see also* Hypertension, cardiorenal)	404.00	404.10	404.90
cardiovascular renal (disease) (sclerosis) (*see also* Hypertension, cardiorenal)	404.00	404.10	404.90

FIGURE 11-2 Hypertension Table, Index to Diseases.

of hypertension usually causes permanent organ damage and has a poor prognosis. **Benign hypertension** is a continuous, mild blood pressure elevation that can usually be controlled by medication. **Unspecified hypertension** has not been specified in the medical record as either benign or malignant.

There is no defined threshold of blood pressure above which an individual is considered hypertensive. Commonly, a sustained diastolic pressure of above 90 mm Hg and a sustained systolic pressure of above 140 mm Hg constitutes hypertension.

Benign hypertension remains fairly stable over the years and is compatible with a long life, but if untreated it is an important risk factor in coronary heart disease and cerebrovascular disease.

Malignant hypertension is commonly associated with abrupt onset and runs a course measured in months. It causes irreversible organ damage and often ends with renal failure or cerebral hemorrhage. Usually a person with malignant hypertension complains of headaches and vision difficulties, and a blood pressure of 200/140 mm Hg is not uncommon.

Essential hypertension is high blood pressure for which the cause is not known.

Hypertensive heart disease refers to the secondary effects on the heart of prolonged, sustained, systemic hypertension. The heart has to work against greatly increased resistance, and, over time, results in heart disease. The primary effect of hypertension is the thickening of the left ventricle, which eventually may lead to heart failure.

There are two sections in this ICD-9-CM chapter that have instructions to "Use additional code to identify presence of hypertension (401-405)." The sections are Ischemic Heart Disease (410-414) and Cerebrovascular Disease (430-438). There are also a number of guidelines that pertain to hypertension or other hypertensive disease processes. Read the hypertension Guidelines that follow.

ICD-9-CM OFFICIAL GUIDELINES FOR CODING AND REPORTING

SECTION I.C.7.

a. Hypertension

Hypertension Table

The Hypertension Table, found under the main term, "Hypertension", in the Alphabetic Index, contains a complete listing of all conditions due to or associated with hypertension and classifies them according to malignant, benign, and unspecified.

1) Hypertension, Essential, or NOS

Assign hypertension (arterial) (essential) (primary) (systemic) (NOS) to category code 401 with the appropriate fourth digit to indicate malignant (.0), benign (.1), or unspecified (.9). Do not use either .0 malignant or .1 benign unless medical record documentation supports such a designation.

2) Hypertension with Heart Disease

Heart conditions (425.8, 429.0-429.3, 429.8, 429.9) are assigned to a code from category 402 when a causal relationship is stated (due to hypertension) or implied (hypertensive). Use an additional code from category 428 to identify the type of heart failure in those patients with heart failure. More than one code from category 428 may be assigned if the patient has systolic or diastolic failure and congestive heart failure.

The same heart conditions (425.8, 429.0-429.3, 429.8, 429.9) with hypertension, but without a stated causal relationship, are coded separately. Sequence according to the circumstances of the admission/encounter.

3) Hypertensive Chronic Kidney Disease

Assign codes from category 403, Hypertensive chronic kidney disease, when conditions classified to category 585 or code 587 are present with hypertension. Unlike hypertension with heart disease, ICD-9-CM presumes a cause-and-effect relationship and classifies chronic kidney disease (CKD) with hypertension as hypertensive chronic kidney disease.

Continued

Fifth digits for category 403 should be assigned as follows:

- 0 with CKD stage I through stage IV, or unspecified.
- 1 with CKD stage V or end stage renal disease.

The appropriate code from category 585, Chronic kidney disease, should be used as a secondary code with a code from category 403 to identify the stage of chronic kidney disease.

See Section I.C.10.a for information on the coding of chronic kidney disease.

4) Hypertensive Heart and Chronic Kidney Disease

Assign codes from combination category 404, Hypertensive heart and chronic kidney disease, when both hypertensive kidney disease and hypertensive heart disease are stated in the diagnosis. Assume a relationship between the hypertension and the chronic kidney disease, whether or not the condition is so designated. Assign an additional code from category 428, to identify the type of heart failure. More than one code from category 428 may be assigned if the patient has systolic or diastolic failure and congestive heart failure.

Fifth digits for category 404 should be assigned as follows:

- 0 without heart failure and with chronic kidney disease (CKD) stage I through stage IV, or unspecified
- 1 with heart failure and with CKD stage I through stage IV, or unspecified
- 2 without heart failure and with CKD stage V or end stage renal disease
- 3 with heart failure and with CKD stage V or end stage renal disease

The appropriate code from category 585, Chronic kidney disease, should be used as a secondary code with a code from category 404 to identify the stage of kidney disease.

See Section I.C.10.a for information on the coding of chronic kidney disease.

5) Hypertensive Cerebrovascular Disease

First assign codes from 430-438, Cerebrovascular disease, then the appropriate hypertension code from categories 401-405.

6) Hypertensive Retinopathy

Two codes are necessary to identify the condition. First assign the code from subcategory 362.11, Hypertensive retinopathy, then the appropriate code from categories 401-405 to indicate the type of hypertension.

7) Hypertension, Secondary

Two codes are required: one to identify the underlying etiology and one from category 405 to identify the hypertension. Sequencing of codes is determined by the reason for admission/encounter.

8) Hypertension, Transient

Assign codes 796.2, Elevated blood pressure reading without diagnosis of hypertension, unless patient has an established diagnosis of hypertension. Assign code 642.3x for transient hypertension of pregnancy.

9) Hypertension, Controlled

Assign appropriate code from categories 401-405. This diagnostic statement usually refers to an existing state of hypertension under control by therapy.

10) Hypertension, Uncontrolled

Uncontrolled hypertension may refer to untreated hypertension or hypertension not responding to current therapeutic regimen. In either case, assign the appropriate code from categories 401-405 to designate the stage and type of hypertension. Code to the type of hypertension.

11) Elevated Blood Pressure

For a statement of elevated blood pressure without further specificity, assign code 796.2, Elevated blood pressure reading without diagnosis of hypertension, rather than a code from category 401.

Kidney Disease and Hypertension

The Guidelines instruct you to assume that there is a cause-and-effect relationship between hypertension and chronic kidney disease reported with category 585 or code 587 with hypertension. The physician might not indicate that the hypertension and chronic kidney disease are related, but the coder is to assume this relationship.

Chronic renal failure (CRF), chronic kidney disease (CKD), and chronic renal insufficiency (CRI) when reported with hypertension are reported as follows:

CRF/CKD/CRI + hypertension	403.90 + 585.9
CKD stage 1 + hypertension	403.90 + 585.1
CKD stage 2 + hypertension	403.90 + 585.2
CKD stage 3 + hypertension	403.90 + 585.3
CKD stage 4 + hypertension	403.90 + 585.4
CKD stage 5 + hypertension	403.91 + 585.5
ESRD or on dialysis + hypertension	403.91 + 585.6
Patient with CKD on any type of dialysis	403.91 + 585.6 + V45.11

Myocardial Infarction

Code 410, acute myocardial infarction (MI), requires a fifth digit assignment and includes specific instructions that must be carefully read.

A fifth digit of 1 indicates an initial episode of care for an MI and can be assigned to the same patient for different encounters by different providers rendering treatment for an initial episode of care for the MI. For example, a patient could be diagnosed with acute MI and be transferred to a larger facility for further investigation and care. The diagnoses reported by both facilities would be the acute MI with the fifth-digit 1.

A fifth digit of 2 indicates subsequent care and is assigned when a patient is readmitted for testing or further care within 8 weeks of the initial episode. For example, a patient had an acute myocardial infarction and was discharged from the hospital. Four weeks later, that same patient was admitted for a cardiovascular procedure. The myocardial infarction would be coded 410.92 to indicate a subsequent episode of care with fifth digit 2. Note that 412 is assigned for a healed (old) myocardial infarction that is not showing any symptoms (asymptomatic). You would not assign a V code history of MI in this situation.

As you review the following examples, refer to Fig. 11-2 for the codes highlighted in each example.

Hypertension

Example 1

Diagnosis: Congestive heart failure **with** benign hypertension

Tabular: **428.0   Congestive heart failure**

401.1   Hypertension, benign (indicated as 1 in Fig. 11-2)

The key word in the above diagnosis statement is "with," which indicates two conditions. Both the congestive heart failure and the benign hypertension are coded because each is a separate condition.

Hypertension

Example 2

Diagnosis: Dilated cardiomyopathy **due to** malignant hypertension

Index: **Hypertension,** cardiovascular disease, 402.00 (indicated as 2 in Fig. 11-2)

Tabular: **402 Hypertensive heart disease**

               402.0 Malignant

               402.00 Without heart failure

In this example, the hypertension caused the cardiomyopathy. The key words here are "due to," which indicates that one condition caused the other condition.

Hypertension

Example 3

Diagnosis: Acute renal failure **with** hypertension

Tabular: **584.9 Acute renal failure,** unspecified

Tabular: **401.9 Hypertension,** unspecified (indicated as 3 in Fig. 11-2)

You would code the hypertension separately because the word "with" is included in the diagnostic statement. Under "Hypertension, renal involvement," in Fig. 11-2, you will see an *Excludes* note. The note indicates that conditions classifiable to 584 (acute renal failure) are excluded from the codes for hypertension with renal involvement. The condition in this example is acute renal failure (584.9); so, you cannot assign a renal involvement hypertension code. Thus, the code for the hypertension in this example is 401.9, Hypertension, unspecified, with code 584.9 for the acute renal failure. The key term included in this diagnosis is "acute" renal failure. See how the coding changes when the term chronic is stated within the diagnosis statement.

Fig. 11-3 shows the portion of the Hypertension Table that includes the secondary hypertension codes. **Secondary hypertension** means that the hypertension is caused by another condition.

	Malignant	Benign	Unspecified
Hypertension, hypertensive *(Continued)*			
renal (disease) (*see also* Hypertension, kidney)	403.00	403.10	403.90
renovascular NEC	405.01	405.11	405.91
secondary NEC	405.09	405.19	405.99
due to			
aldosteronism, primary	405.09	405.19	405.99
brain tumor	405.09	405.19	405.99
bulbar poliomyelitis	405.09	405.19	405.99
calculus			
kidney	405.09	405.19	405.99
ureter	405.09	405.19	405.99
coarctation, aorta	405.09	405.19	405.99
Cushing's disease	405.09	405.19	405.99
glomerulosclerosis (*see also* Hypertension, kidney)	403.00	403.10	403.90
periarteritis nodosa	405.09	405.19	405.99
pheochromocytoma	405.09	405.19	405.99
polycystic kidney(s)	405.09	405.19	405.99
polycythemia	405.09	405.19	405.99
porphyria	405.09	405.19	405.99
pyelonephritis	405.09	405.19	405.99
renal (artery)			
aneurysm	405.01	405.11	405.91
anomaly	405.01	405.11	405.91
embolism	405.01	405.11	405.91
fibromuscular hyperplasia	405.01	405.11	405.91
occlusion	405.01	405.11 #4	405.91
stenosis	405.01	405.11	405.91
thrombosis	405.01	405.11	405.91

Secondary hypertension → (pointing to "secondary NEC")

FIGURE 11-3 Secondary hypertension.

Secondary Hypertension

Example 4

Diagnosis: Secondary, benign hypertension, due to renal artery occlusion

Tabular: **405.11 Hypertension,** secondary, due to renal (artery), occlusion, benign (indicated as 4 in Fig. 11-3)

In this example, the renal artery occlusion caused the hypertension and so is correctly coded to category 405. You would also assign a code to the renal artery occlusion (593.81) because the renal artery occlusion is causing the secondary hypertension.

Code: 593.81, 405.11 Secondary, benign hypertension, due to renal artery occlusion

According to Guideline Section I.C.7.a.7., the sequencing is determined by the reason for admission/encounter.

EXERCISE 11-9	*Diseases of the Circulatory System*

Assign codes for the following:

1 Congestive heart failure

ICD-9-CM Code: _____

2 Acute subendocardial infarction, initial episode

ICD-9-CM Code: _____

3 Secondary hypertension due to periarteritis nodosa

🌐 ICD-9-CM Code(s): _____

4 Cerebral infarction due to thrombosis, brain

🌐 ICD-9-CM Code(s): _____

5 Subarachnoid hemorrhage

🌐 ICD-9-CM Code(s): _____

(Answers are located in Appendix B)

DISEASES OF THE RESPIRATORY SYSTEM

Chapter 8, Diseases of the Respiratory System, in the Tabular includes diseases and disorders of the respiratory tract, beginning with the nasal passages and following a path to the lungs. Note that at the beginning of ICD-9-CM Chapter 8 there is an instructional note that covers the entire chapter. The note states, "Use additional code to identify infectious organism." You should be aware that the organism is already identified in some codes, and in that case, you would not assign an additional code to identify the specific infectious organism.

Identifying Infectious Organisms

Example 1

Diagnosis: Pneumonia due to Klebsiella pneumoniae

Index: **Pneumonia,** Klebsiella pneumoniae, 482.0

Tabular: **482 Other bacterial pneumonia**

          482.0 Pneumonia due to Klebsiella pneumoniae

Code: 482.0 Pneumonia due to *Klebsiella pneumoniae*

Code 482.0 is a combination code that includes the disease process (pneumonia) with the causative organism *(Klebsiella pneumoniae)*. In this instance, you would not assign an additional code because the organism is identified in the code 482.0.

Identifying Infectious Organisms

Example 2

In the following example, two codes are necessary, one to describe the disease process (manifestation) and one to indicate the causative organism (etiology).

Diagnosis: Acute maxillary sinusitis due to *Hemophilus influenzae*

Index: **Sinusitis** (accessory) (nasal) (hyperplastic) (nonpurulent) (purulent) (chronic) 473.9

         acute 461.9

         maxillary 461.0

Tabular: **461 Acute sinusitis**

         461.0 Maxillary

Index: **Infection, infected, infective** (opportunistic), *Hemophilus influenzae* NEC 041.5

Tabular: **041 Bacterial infection in conditions classified elsewhere and of unspecified site**

         041.5 Hemophilus influenzae [H. influenzae]

Codes: 461.0, 041.5 Acute maxillary sinusitis due to *Hemophilus influenzae*

The manifestation is listed first and the etiology is listed second.

Now, let's learn how to code the respiratory condition of chronic obstructive pulmonary disease (COPD), which falls within the category 496 Chronic airway obstruction NEC. The note in the Tabular under code 496 indicates that this code cannot be assigned with any code from categories 491-493 (491 is chronic bronchitis, 492 is emphysema, and 493 is asthma). The *Excludes* note under code 496 indicates that COPD specified "(as) (with) asthma (493.2)" cannot be assigned to code 496; rather, reference 493.2.

Chronic Obstructive Pulmonary Disease

Example

Diagnosis: COPD with asthma

Index: **Asthma, asthmatic** (bronchial) (catarrh) (spasmodic) 493.9, with, chronic obstructive pulmonary disease (COPD) 493.2

Tabular: **493 Asthma**

         493.2 Chronic obstructive asthma

This code is not complete yet because it requires a fifth digit. You have three fifth-digit choices:

0 unspecified

1 with status asthmaticus

2 with (acute) exacerbation

Status asthmaticus is the most severe form of asthma attack and can last for days or weeks. To report the asthma with status asthmaticus, the physician provides specific documentation of the condition. If the clinical condition is severe enough that you suspect that the patient has status asthmaticus, clarification by the physician should be sought.

Code: 493.20 COPD with asthma

EXERCISE 11-10   *Diseases of the Respiratory System*

Assign codes for the following:

1 Croup

ICD-9-CM Code: _____

2 Respiratory failure due to congestive heart failure

ICD-9-CM Codes: _____, _____

3 COPD with chronic bronchitis (without exacerbation)

ICD-9-CM Code: _____

4 Influenza with acute bronchitis

ICD-9-CM Code: _____

5 Pneumonia due to *Hemophilus influenzae*

ICD-9-CM Code: _____

(Answers are located in Appendix B)

CHAPTER REVIEW

CHAPTER 11, PART I, THEORY

Without the use of reference material, answer the following:

1 ICD-9-CM assumes a relationship between hypertension and renal failure.

   True   False

2 If a patient is admitted for an HIV-related condition, the first-listed diagnosis is the related condition followed by the diagnosis code 042.

   True   False

3 A fifth digit of 1 should be assigned to 305.0X for someone who abuses alcohol by binge drinking.

   True   False

4 Another term to describe malignant hypertension is accelerated hypertension.

   True   False

5 Hypertension that is caused by another condition is called essential hypertension.

   True   False

6 A fifth digit of 1 to indicate status asthmaticus can be assigned if the physician documents an acute exacerbation.

   True   False

7 If a patient's diabetes is documented as poorly controlled, a fifth digit for out of control should be assigned.

   True   False

8 If a patient receives insulin for diabetes, type 1 diabetes should be reported.

   True   False

9 The site to which a malignant neoplasm has spread is the:
   a metastatic site
   b primary site
   c benign site
   d morphology

10 The site in which a malignant neoplasm originated is the:
   a metastatic site
   b primary site
   c benign site
   d morphology

CHAPTER 11, PART II, PRACTICAL

Using the ICD-9-CM and coding guidelines, assign codes for the following:

11 Combined spinal cord degeneration due to pernicious anemia

   ICD-9-CM Codes: _____, _____

12 Carcinoma, in situ, of skin of lip, vermilion border

   ICD-9-CM Code: _____

Chapter Review answers are only available in the TEACH Instructor Resources on Evolve

13 Subacute bacterial endocarditis

ICD-9-CM Code: _____

14 Acute bronchitis with chronic obstructive bronchitis

ICD-9-CM Code: _____

15 Group B streptococcal pneumonia

ICD-9-CM Code: _____

16 Alzheimer's disease

ICD-9-CM Code: _____

17 Hypertension with end-stage renal disease

ICD-9-CM Codes: _____, _____

18 Enteritis due to Norwalk virus

ICD-9-CM Code: _____

19 *Pneumocystis* pneumonia in patient with HIV

ICD-9-CM Codes: _____, _____

20 Diabetic foot ulcer in patient with diabetes mellitus, type 1, out of control

ICD-9-CM Codes: _____, _____

21 Inanition

ICD-9-CM Code: _____

22 Neutropenic fever

ICD-9-CM Codes: _____, _____

23 Anemia due to gastric cancer

🌐 ICD-9-CM Code(s): _____

24 Withdrawal from heroin, daily use

🌐 ICD-9-CM Code(s): _____

25 Seizure disorder

🌐 ICD-9-CM Code(s): _____

26 Acute renal failure in patient with hypertension

🌐 ICD-9-CM Code(s): _____

27 COPD with emphysema

🌐 ICD-9-CM Code(s): _____

28 Aspiration pneumonia

🌐 ICD-9-CM Code(s): _____

29 Mr. Jensen is status post colon resection 3 months ago for sigmoid colon cancer and is now admitted for adjunct chemotherapy.

🌐 ICD-9-CM Code(s): _____

Chapter Review answers are only available in the TEACH Instructor Resources on Evolve

CASE STUDY 1

History of Present Illness

This 50-year-old disabled male is a resident of a nursing home who has been admitted because of marked congestion and respiratory distress. He is known to have intellectual disabilities and frequent urinary tract and pulmonary infections. He has a recurrent epileptic disorder that is well controlled on Dilantin.

Physical Examination

On admission, vital signs include a temperature of 101° F, respiratory rate of 32 breaths per minute, heart rate of 82 beats per minute, and blood pressure of 120/70 mm Hg. Examination of the chest reveals bilateral crepitations. There is moderate redness and edema of the scrotal skin.

Laboratory Data and Course in Hospital

His white blood cell count is 8.5; hemoglobin, 12.9 g/dl; polymorphonuclear leukocytes, 64; bands, 19; lymphocytes, 10; monocytes, 6; and eosinophils, 1. Urinalysis shows moderate bacterial and 1+ white blood cell count. Urine culture shows mixed flora. The repeat urine culture shows *Providencia stuartii* sensitive to Fortaz. Sputum culture reveals the presence of methicillin-resistant *Staphylococcus aureus,* sensitive to vancomycin. Chest x-ray film shows bilateral pulmonary infiltrates. Arterial blood gases on room air show a Po_2 of 48, Pco_2 of 30, and pH of 7.50. When repeated with the patient on oxygen, Po_2 is 66, Pco_2 is 36, and pH is 7.45. The patient is treated with intravenous vancomycin and intravenous Fortaz. His pulmonary infiltrate decreases. His oral intake has been somewhat poor, and he has been given intravenous fluids off and on. The nursing staff at the nursing home note that his intake, in terms of eating and taking fluids, is much better. His medications at the nursing home include Dilantin, 200 mg twice a day; Tegretol, 400 mg at 8 AM and 4 PM, and 200 mg at 8 PM; and Cipro, 500 mg twice a day; and his maintenance medications are continued. This patient is being discharged today.

Final Diagnosis

Acute respiratory insufficiency (2)

Bilateral pneumonia due to Staph aureus
(MRSA) (1)

Intellectual disabilities (3)

Epilepsy (6); UTI (4) due to *Providencia stuartii* [gram-negative bacilli (5)]

30 ICD-9-CM Codes: (1)_____, (2)_____, (3)_____, (4)_____,

(5)_____, (6)_____

CASE STUDY 2

History of Present Illness

The patient is an 80-year-old female with a known history of advanced metastatic carcinoma of the breast, which was the primary site. (The breast cancer is no longer present but has metastasized to other unspecified areas, which represents a secondary generalized neoplasm.) The patient has been admitted because of increased shortness of breath and severe pain. The pain is worse in her left chest, and this is associated with increased shortness of breath. At the time of admission, the patient is in so much pain that she is unable to remember her history. The patient initially presented for congestive heart failure more than a year earlier. This was subsequently found to be secondary to metastatic breast cancer, after left mastectomy, 3 years ago. The patient had previously been on chemotherapy.

Course in Hospital

The patient is treated initially with intravenous pain medication to control her pain, and subsequently her condition becomes stable on oral medication. By the time of discharge, the patient is stable on oral Vicodin. She is able to eat. Admission blood urea nitrogen (BUN) was 38 mg/dl with creatinine of 1.3 mg/dl secondary to dehydration. By the time of discharge, these levels have improved. Admission glucose of 225 mg/dl is down to 110 mg/dl at discharge.

Chapter Review answers are only available in the TEACH Instructor Resources on Evolve

Discharge Diagnoses

Uncontrolled pain, secondary to widely metastatic breast carcinoma

Dehydration

Type II diabetes mellitus, uncontrolled

31 What is the first-listed diagnosis and the code for the first-listed diagnosis for this patient?

First-listed Diagnosis Terms and Code: _____

32 What are the other diagnoses for this patient, and what are the codes for these other diagnoses?

Additional Diagnosis Codes:

_____

_____

_____

_____

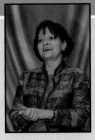
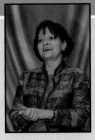

"Qualities that best describe a successful coder would include meticulous attention to detail, a strong sense of honesty and integrity, and perseverance."

Patricia Cordy Henricksen, MS, CHCA, CPC-I, CPC, CCP-P, ACS-PM
Auditing and Coding Educator
Soterion Medical Services
Lexington, Kentucky

Chapter-Specific Guidelines (ICD-9-CM Chapters 9-17)

Chapter Topics

Diseases of the Digestive System

Diseases of the Genitourinary System

Complications of Pregnancy, Childbirth, and the Puerperium

Diseases of the Skin and Subcutaneous Tissue

Diseases of the Musculoskeletal System and Connective Tissue

Congenital Anomalies and Certain Conditions Originating in the Perinatal Period

Symptoms, Signs, and Ill-Defined Conditions

Injury and Poisoning

Chapter Review

Learning Objectives

After completing this chapter you should be able to

1   Examine the digestive system coding.

2   Analyze the genitourinary system coding.

3   Review the pregnancy, childbirth, and puerperium coding.

4   Review the skin and subcutaneous tissue coding.

5   Review musculoskeletal and connective tissue coding.

6   Examine the congenital anomalies and certain conditions originating in the perinatal period coding.

7   Define the rules of symptoms, signs, and ill-defined conditions coding.

8   Identify the elements of coding injuries and poisonings.

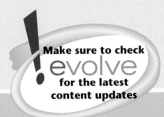
Make sure to check evolve **for the latest content updates**

NOTE: *The 2015 ICD-9-CM was used in preparing this chapter.*

DISEASES OF THE DIGESTIVE SYSTEM

Chapter 9, Diseases of the Digestive System, in the Tabular of the ICD-9-CM describes diseases or conditions affecting the digestive system. Digestion starts when food is taken into the mouth and follows the gastrointestinal tract until it leaves the body through the anus. The categories are sequenced in a manner that follows that path, starting with disorders of the teeth.

Throughout the chapter, as in other chapters, you must pay close attention to fifth-digit assignment, the use of combination codes, and carefully read the *Excludes* notes and any other instructions. Also important in the chapter is the presence of **hemorrhage** (bleeding) associated with the diseases. Codes from category 578, Gastrointestinal hemorrhage, are not assigned when codes for bleeding of any sites mentioned are available. Use this category only when the physician states clearly that the bleeding is due to another condition. The physician may not always indicate the presence of hemorrhage, and the coder must review the record and then clarify the documentation with the physician, then assign the appropriate code(s).

Example

Diagnosis: Diverticulitis of the colon with hemorrhage

Index: **Diverticulitis** (acute), colon (perforated) 562.11, with hemorrhage 562.13

Note that the presence of hemorrhage makes a difference in the code assignment: without hemorrhage, 562.11; with hemorrhage, 562.13.

Tabular: **562 Diverticula of intestine**
                  562.13 Diverticulitis of colon with hemorrhage
                     (a combination code)

Code: 562.13 Diverticulitis of the colon with hemorrhage

If you begin your search for the above diagnosis of "Diverticulitis of the colon with hemorrhage" using the main term "Hemorrhage, gastrointestinal," you will find 578.9. When you reference 578.9 in the Tabular, you will find a long list of *Excludes* under the category code 578. Note that in the list of *Excludes* is "diverticulitis, intestine: large (562.13)" (see arrow below). This means that you cannot assign 578.9, gastrointestinal hemorrhage, when there is mention of diverticulitis of the large intestine (562.13).

578 Gastrointestinal hemorrhage
        EXCLUDES   *that with mention of:*
                        angiodysplasia of stomach and duodenum (537.83)
                        angiodysplasia of intestine (569.85)
                        diverticulitis, intestine:
              →   *large (562.13)*
                               small (562.03)
                        diverticulosis, intestine:
                               large (562.12)
                               small (562.02)
                        gastritis and duodenitis (535.0-535.6)
                        ulcer:
                               duodenal, gastric, gastrojejunal, or peptic (531.00-534.91)

If you are coding a diagnosis of gastrointestinal (GI) hemorrhage with any of the diagnoses listed in the *Excludes* and if the hemorrhage is due to that GI condition, only the combination code would be assigned.

From the Trenches

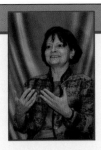

"Education is an ongoing process in the field of coding. . . . Success as a coder involves a thorough understanding of the code set guidelines, as well as knowledge of medical terminology and anatomy."

PATRICIA

Example

Diagnosis: Gastrointestinal hemorrhage due to acute antral ulcer

Index: **Ulcer,** antral—*see* Ulcer, stomach
Ulcer, stomach (eroded) (peptic) (round) 531.9
    acute, with, hemorrhage 531.0

Tabular: **531 Gastric ulcer**
    531.0 Acute with hemorrhage

Code 531.0 is not a complete code. You must assign a fifth digit based on if there was or was not a mention of obstruction. There is no mention of obstruction in the diagnosis, so the fifth digit assigned would be 0, without mention of obstruction, 531.00.

You must now determine if there is any further directive to report the hemorrhage with yet another code. Referencing hemorrhage in the Index, you are directed to 578 again and you note that the *Excludes* notes indicate not to code gastrointestinal hemorrhage with mention of gastric ulcer. So no further code is needed, as the hemorrhage is included in the code for the ulcer (531.00).

Index: **Hemorrhage, hemorrhagic** (nontraumatic) 459.0
    gastrointestinal (tract) 578.9

Tabular: **578 Gastrointestinal hemorrhage**

> EXCLUDES   *that with mention of:*
> *ulcer:*
>   *duodenal, gastric, gastrojejunal, or peptic*
>   *(531.00-534.91)*

Code: 531.00 Gastrointestinal hemorrhage due to acute antral ulcer

CODING SHOT

For a hemorrhage to be reported, there does not have to be **active** bleeding; however, there must be documentation in the medical record that supports the fact that active bleeding has occurred, and the physician must identify the source of bleeding for the combination code to be assigned.

It is so important to verify code assignment in the Tabular. It is only when you check the Tabular that you can know for certain about the Includes and *Excludes*, which are not listed anywhere else. This is also where you will find if a fourth or fifth digit to the code is needed. Be certain to always, always check the Tabular before assigning a code.

EXERCISE 12-1   *Diseases of the Digestive System*

Assign ICD-9-CM codes for the following:

1 Appendicitis with generalized peritonitis

ICD-9-CM Code: _____

2 Gastrointestinal bleeding due to acute duodenal ulcer

ICD-9-CM Code: _____

3 Acute and chronic cholecystitis with cholelithiasis

ICD-9-CM Codes: _____, _____

4 Gastroenteritis

ICD-9-CM Code: _____

5 Gastroesophageal reflux

ICD-9-CM Code: _____

(Answers are located in Appendix B)

DISEASES OF THE GENITOURINARY SYSTEM

Chapter 10, Diseases of the Genitourinary System, in the Tabular of the ICD-9-CM includes conditions and diseases of the male and female genital organs and urinary tract. There are several types of diseases of the kidney (580-589) that are also included in this chapter. For example, nephritis (inflammation of the kidney), nephritic syndrome (proteinuria and water retention), and the stages of kidney disease and failure. Also in this chapter are codes for diseases of the male genital organs (600-608), including codes for disorders and diseases of the prostate. Disorders of the breast (610-612) are also included in this chapter, as well as inflammatory disease and disorders of the female genital tract (614-629).

When you are reporting infections of the urinary tract or the genital organs, you are instructed to use an additional code to identify the organism.

Reporting the Infectious Organism

Example

Diagnosis:	Acute prostatitis due to *Streptococcus*
Index:	**Prostatitis** (congestive) (suppurative) 601.9 acute 601.0
Tabular:	**601 Inflammatory diseases of prostate** **601.0 Acute prostatitis**
Index:	**Infection, infected, infective** (opportunistic) streptococcal NEC 041.00

Tabular:	**041 Bacterial infection in conditions classified elsewhere and of**
	    unspecified site
	    041.0 Streptococcus
	        041.00 Streptococcus, unspecified

Codes:	601.0, 041.00 Acute prostatitis due to *Streptococcus*

EXERCISE 12-2 *Diseases of the Genitourinary System*

Assign ICD-9-CM codes for the following diagnostic statements:

1 Pelvic inflammatory disease (PID)

⊛ ICD-9-CM Code(s): _____

2 Hematuria

⊛ ICD-9-CM Code(s): _____

3 Acute and chronic pyelonephritis

⊛ ICD-9-CM Code(s): _____

4 Benign prostatic hypertrophy (BPH)

⊛ ICD-9-CM Code(s): _____

5 Fibrocystic breast disease

⊛ ICD-9-CM Code(s): _____

(Answers are located in Appendix B)

COMPLICATIONS OF PREGNANCY, CHILDBIRTH, AND THE PUERPERIUM

Chapter 11, Complications of Pregnancy, Childbirth, and the Puerperium, of the Tabular of the ICD-9-CM is probably the most difficult chapter from which to code. One reason is that pregnancy and childbirth are natural functions, and physicians often overlook documentation of diagnoses that should be reported. Another reason the coding is complex is that there is extensive use of multiple coding in the chapter. Also, fifth-digit assignment for pregnancy is often difficult to determine. There are instructions throughout this chapter that must be read thoroughly. Obstetric coding can also be difficult because you may not use this chapter as frequently as some of the other chapters, so you won't be as familiar with the special notes and coding instructions. Any condition that occurs during pregnancy, childbirth, or the puerperium is considered to be a complication unless the attending physician specifically documents that it neither affects the pregnancy nor is affected by the pregnancy.

CODING SHOT

An ectopic pregnancy is one in which the fertilized ovum implants outside the uterus, usually in the fallopian tube. Ectopic and Molar Pregnancy (630-633) contains instructions to use an additional code from category 639 to identify any complication(s).

Category 639, Complications following abortion and ectopic and molar pregnancies, reports genital tract and pelvic infection (639.0), delayed or excessive hemorrhage (639.1), damage to pelvic organs and tissues (639.2), kidney failure (639.3), metabolic disorders (639.4), shock (639.5), embolism (639.6), and other specified complications (639.8), or unspecified complications (639.9). You cannot assign 639, Complications, with any code from categories 634-638 (abortion) because the complications for the abortion are classified according to the fourth-digit subcategory codes. Examples are 635, Legally induced abortion and 635.1, Complicated by delayed or excessive hemorrhage. As stated previously, you assign 639, Complications, to identify any complications related to codes 630-633. You also assign 639, Complications, when the complication is the reason for the medical care, and the abortion, ectopic, or molar pregnancy was treated during a previous episode.

Complications mainly related to pregnancy (640-649) require fifth-digit subclassifications that are of special note:

0 unspecified as to episode of care or not applicable
1 delivered, with or without mention of antepartum condition
2 delivered, with mention of postpartum complication
3 antepartum condition or complication
4 postpartum condition or complication

The fifth digit 0 is assigned when there is no mention of the episode of care or the episode of care is not applicable. To assign the fifth digits 1 and 2, a delivery must have occurred during that inpatient stay. The fifth digit 1 is assigned to cases in which an antepartum condition has or has not been noted. The fifth digits 3 and 4 are reported when no delivery has occurred during that encounter. The fifth digit 3 is reported for antepartum conditions, and the 4 is reported for postpartum conditions. When you review the categories and subcategories throughout the chapter, you will note that many subcategories may indicate that you can use only certain fifth digits with a particular code. For example, with code 641.1, Hemorrhage from placenta previa, the only fifth digits that can be used are 0, 1, or 3. Neither 2 nor 4 can be used because placenta previa occurs **before** a baby is delivered and fifth digits 2 and 4 are assigned **after** delivery.

When reporting multiple diagnoses from one inpatient stay, certain combinations of fifth digits are used to classify that stay or visit. These fifth-digit combinations are:

1 only, or with 2; NOT with 0, 3, or 4
2 only, or with 1; NOT with 0, 3, or 4
3 only, NOT with 0, 1, 2, or 4
4 only, NOT with 0, 1, 2, or 3

Category 650, Normal delivery, cannot be assigned with any other code within the range 630-676 because these codes refer to other than normal delivery. Code 650 is assigned only when all of the following are documented:

- A full-term, single liveborn infant is delivered.
- There are no antepartum or postpartum conditions classifiable to 630-676 (other than normal delivery).
- The presentation is cephalic, requiring minimal assistance and without fetal manipulation or the use of instrumentation.
- An episiotomy may or may not have been performed.

Most deliveries do not meet the requirements for a 650 Normal Delivery code assignment.

Category V27, Outcome of delivery, can be assigned as an additional code to the **mother's record.** Code V27 is indexed under the term "Outcome."

ICD-9-CM OFFICIAL GUIDELINES FOR CODING AND REPORTING

SECTION I.C.11.

b. Selection of OB Principal or First-listed Diagnosis

3) Episodes when no delivery occurs

In episodes when no delivery occurs, the principal diagnosis should correspond to the principal complication of the pregnancy, which necessitated the encounter. Should more than one complication exist, all of which are treated or monitored, any of the complication codes may be sequenced first.

Complicating Pregnancy

Example

Diagnosis: Iron deficiency anemia complicating pregnancy, antepartum

Index: **Pregnancy** (single) (uterine) (without sickness) V22.2
            complicated (by)
               anemia (conditions classifiable to 280-285) 648.2

Tabular: **648.2 Anemia**

This code is not complete because it does not have a fifth-digit assignment and in the Tabular there are instructions to "Use additional code(s) to identify the **condition,**" which means to identify the type of anemia. The Tabular directs you to assign fifth digits 0-4. No delivery has occurred and the condition is stated as being antepartum; therefore, the fifth digit 3 is assigned, 648.23. Next report an additional code to identify the type of anemia.

Index: **Anemia** 285.9, deficiency 281.9, iron (Fe) 280.9

Tabular: **280.9 Iron deficiency anemia, unspecified**

Codes: 648.23, 280.9 Iron deficiency anemia complicating pregnancy, antepartum

The first code, 648.23, indicates that the anemia is a complication of the pregnancy, and the second code, 280.9, identifies the type of anemia (iron deficiency anemia).

Read the following Guidelines that provide direction to the coder regarding sequencing and first-listed diagnosis.

ICD-9-CM OFFICIAL GUIDELINES FOR CODING AND REPORTING

SECTION I.C.

11. Chapter 11: Complications of Pregnancy, Childbirth, and the Puerperium (630-679)

  a. General Rules for Obstetric Cases

    1) Codes from chapter 11 and sequencing priority
    Obstetric cases require codes from chapter 11, codes in the range 630-679, Complications of Pregnancy, Childbirth, and the Puerperium. Chapter 11 codes have sequencing priority over codes from other chapters. Additional codes from other chapters may be used in conjunction with chapter 11 codes to further specify conditions. Should the provider document that the pregnancy is incidental to the encounter, then code V22.2 should be used in place of any chapter 11 codes. It is the provider's responsibility to state that the condition being treated is not affecting the pregnancy.

    2) Chapter 11 codes used only on the maternal record
    Chapter 11 codes are to be used only on the maternal record, never on the record of the newborn.

    3) Chapter 11 fifth-digits
    Categories 640-649, 651-676 have required fifth-digits, which indicate whether the encounter is antepartum, postpartum and whether a delivery has also occurred.

    4) Fifth-digits, appropriate for each code
    The fifth-digits, which are appropriate for each code number, are listed in brackets under each code. The fifth-digits on each code should all be consistent with each other. That is, should a delivery occur all of the fifth-digits should indicate the delivery.

  b. Selection of OB Principal or First-listed Diagnosis

    1) Routine outpatient prenatal visits
    For routine outpatient prenatal visits when no complications are present codes V22.0, Supervision of normal first pregnancy, and V22.1, Supervision of other normal pregnancy, should be used as the first-listed diagnoses. These codes should not be used in conjunction with chapter 11 codes.

Continued

2) Prenatal outpatient visits for high-risk patients

For routine prenatal outpatient visits for patients with high-risk pregnancies, a code from category V23, Supervision of high-risk pregnancy, should be used as the first-listed diagnosis. Secondary chapter 11 codes may be used in conjunction with these codes if appropriate.

3) Episodes when no delivery occurs

In episodes when no delivery occurs, the principal diagnosis should correspond to the principal complication of the pregnancy, which necessitated the encounter. Should more than one complication exist, all of which are treated or monitored, any of the complications codes may be sequenced first.

4) When a delivery occurs

When a delivery occurs, the principal diagnosis should correspond to the main circumstances or complication of the delivery. In cases of cesarean delivery, the selection of the principal diagnosis should be the condition established after study that was responsible for the patient's admission. If the patient was admitted with a condition that resulted in the performance of a cesarean procedure, that condition should be selected as the principal diagnosis. If the reason for the admission/encounter was unrelated to the condition resulting in the cesarean delivery, the condition related to the reason for the admission/encounter should be selected as the principal diagnosis, even if a cesarean was performed.

5) Outcome of delivery

An outcome of delivery code, V27.0-V27.9, should be included on every maternal record when a delivery has occurred. These codes are not to be used on subsequent records or on the newborn record.

c. Fetal Conditions Affecting the Management of the Mother

1) Codes from categories 655 and 656

Codes from categories 655, Known or suspected fetal abnormality affecting management of the mother, and 656, Other known or suspected fetal and placental problems affecting the management of the mother, are assigned only when the fetal condition is actually responsible for modifying the management of the mother, i.e., by requiring diagnostic studies, additional observation, special care, or termination of pregnancy. The fact that the fetal condition exists does not justify assigning a code from this series to the mother's record.

See I.C.18.d. for suspected maternal and fetal conditions not found

2) In utero surgery

In cases when surgery is performed on the fetus, a diagnosis code from category 655, Known or suspected fetal abnormalities affecting management of the mother, should be assigned identifying the fetal condition. Procedure code 75.36, Correction of fetal defect, should be assigned on the hospital inpatient record.

No code from Chapter 15, the perinatal codes, should be used on the mother's record to identify fetal conditions. Surgery performed in utero on a fetus is still to be coded as an obstetric encounter.

d. HIV Infection in Pregnancy, Childbirth and the Puerperium

During pregnancy, childbirth or the puerperium, a patient admitted because of an HIV-related illness should receive a principal diagnosis of 647.6X, Other specified infectious and parasitic diseases in the mother classifiable elsewhere, but complicating the pregnancy, childbirth or the puerperium, followed by 042 and the code(s) for the HIV-related illness(es).

Patients with asymptomatic HIV infection status admitted during pregnancy, childbirth, or the puerperium should receive codes of 647.6X and V08.

e. Current Conditions Complicating Pregnancy

Assign a code from subcategory 648.x for patients that have current conditions when the condition affects the management of the pregnancy, childbirth, or the puerperium. Use additional secondary codes from other chapters to identify the conditions, as appropriate.

f. Diabetes mellitus in pregnancy

Diabetes mellitus is a significant complicating factor in pregnancy. Pregnant women who are diabetic should be assigned code 648.0x, Diabetes mellitus complicating pregnancy, and a secondary code from category 250, Diabetes mellitus, or category 249, Secondary diabetes to identify the type of diabetes.

Code V58.67, Long-term (current) use of insulin, should also be assigned if the diabetes mellitus is being treated with insulin.

Continued

g. Gestational diabetes

Gestational diabetes can occur during the second and third trimester of pregnancy in women who were not diabetic prior to pregnancy. Gestational diabetes can cause complications in the pregnancy similar to those of pre-existing diabetes mellitus. It also puts the woman at greater risk of developing diabetes after the pregnancy. Gestational diabetes is coded to 648.8x, Abnormal glucose tolerance. Codes 648.0x and 648.8x should never be used together on the same record.

Code V58.67, Long-term (current) use of insulin, should also be assigned if the gestational diabetes is being treated with insulin.

h. Normal Delivery, Code 650

1) Normal delivery

Code 650 is for use in cases when a woman is admitted for a full-term normal delivery and delivers a single, healthy infant without any complications antepartum, during the delivery, or postpartum during the delivery episode. Code 650 is always a principal diagnosis. It is not to be used if any other code from chapter 11 is needed to describe a current complication of the antenatal, delivery, or perinatal period. Additional codes from other chapters may be used with code 650 if they are not related to or are in any way complicating the pregnancy.

2) Normal delivery with resolved antepartum complication

Code 650 may be used if the patient had a complication at some point during her pregnancy, but the complication is not present at the time of the admission for delivery.

3) V27.0, Single liveborn, outcome of delivery

V27.0, Single liveborn, is the only outcome of delivery code appropriate for use with 650.

i. The Postpartum and Peripartum Periods

1) Postpartum and peripartum periods

The postpartum period begins immediately after delivery and continues for six weeks following delivery. The peripartum period is defined as the last month of pregnancy to five months postpartum.

2) Postpartum complication

A postpartum complication is any complication occurring within the six-week period.

3) Pregnancy-related complications after 6 week period

Chapter 11 codes may also be used to describe pregnancy-related complications after the six-week period should the provider document that a condition is pregnancy related.

4) Postpartum complications occurring during the same admission as delivery

Postpartum complications that occur during the same admission as the delivery are identified with a fifth digit of "2." Subsequent admissions/encounters for postpartum complications should be identified with a fifth digit of "4."

5) Admission for routine postpartum care following delivery outside hospital

When the mother delivers outside the hospital prior to admission and is admitted for routine postpartum care and no complications are noted, code V24.0, Postpartum care and examination immediately after delivery, should be assigned as the principal diagnosis.

6) Admission following delivery outside hospital with postpartum conditions

A delivery diagnosis code should not be used for a woman who has delivered prior to admission to the hospital. Any postpartum conditions and/or postpartum procedures should be coded.

7) Puerperal sepsis

Code 670.2x, Puerperal sepsis, should be assigned with a secondary code to identify the causal organism (e.g., for a bacterial infection, assign a code from category 041, Bacterial infections in conditions classified elsewhere and of unspecified site). A code from category 038, Septicemia, should not be used for puerperal sepsis. Do not assign code 995.91, Sepsis, as code 670.2x describes the sepsis. If applicable, use additional codes to identify severe sepsis (995.92) and any associated acute organ dysfunction.

j. Code 677, Late effect of complication of pregnancy

1) Code 677

Code 677, Late effect of complication of pregnancy, childbirth, and the puerperium is for use in those cases when an initial complication of a pregnancy develops a sequelae requiring care or treatment at a future date.

Continued

2) After the initial postpartum period

This code may be used at any time after the initial postpartum period.

3) Sequencing of Code 677

This code, like all late effect codes, is to be sequenced following the code describing the sequelae of the complication.

k. Abortions

1) Fifth-digits required for abortion categories

Fifth-digits are required for abortion categories 634-637. Fifth digit assignment is based on the status of the patient at the beginning (or start) of the encounter. Fifth-digit 1, incomplete, indicates that all of the products of conception have not been expelled from the uterus. Fifth-digit 2, complete, indicates that all products of conception have been expelled from the uterus.

2) Code from categories 640-649 and 651-659

A code from categories 640-649 and 651-659 may be used as additional codes with an abortion code to indicate the complication leading to the abortion.

Fifth digit 3 is assigned with codes from these categories when used with an abortion code because the other fifth digits will not apply. Codes from the 660-669 series are not to be used for complications of abortion.

3) Code 639 for complications

Code 639 is to be used for all complications following abortion. Code 639 cannot be assigned with codes from categories 634-638.

4) Abortion with Liveborn Fetus

When an attempted termination of pregnancy results in a liveborn fetus assign code 644.21, Early onset of delivery, with an appropriate code from category V27, Outcome of Delivery. The procedure code for the attempted termination of pregnancy should also be assigned.

5) Retained Products of Conception following an abortion

Subsequent admissions for retained products of conception following a spontaneous or legally induced abortion are assigned the appropriate code from category 634, Spontaneous abortion, or 635 Legally induced abortion, with a fifth digit of "1" (incomplete). This advice is appropriate even when the patient was discharged previously with a discharge diagnosis of complete abortion.

EXERCISE 12-3 *Complications of Pregnancy, Childbirth, and the Puerperium*

Assign ICD-9-CM codes for the following:

1 Blighted ovum

ICD-9-CM Code: _____

2 Incomplete spontaneous abortion; dilation and curettage (D&C) performed

ICD-9-CM Code: _____

3 False labor of 38-week pregnancy, undelivered

ICD-9-CM Code: _____

4 Vaginal delivery of liveborn single infant with fourth-degree perineal laceration; obstetric laceration repaired (include appropriate V code for outcome of delivery)

ICD-9-CM Codes: _____ (laceration), _____ (outcome)

5 Obstructed labor due to cephalopelvic disproportion; liveborn single infant delivered by lower segment cesarean section

ICD-9-CM Codes: _____, _____, _____

(Answers are located in Appendix B)

DISEASES OF THE SKIN AND SUBCUTANEOUS TISSUE

Chapter 12, Diseases of the Skin and Subcutaneous Tissue, in the Tabular of the ICD-9-CM describes diseases or conditions of the integumentary system. This chapter is one of the shorter chapters in the ICD-9-CM manual. Conditions affecting the nails, sweat glands, hair, and hair follicles are included in this chapter. Congenital conditions of skin, hair, and nails are classified in category 757, Congenital anomalies of the integument. Neoplasms of skin are classified in Chapter 2 of ICD-9-CM. When reviewing the first categories, such as 681, 682, and 683, you will note that multiple coding may be necessary for some conditions.

Example

Multiple Coding

Diagnosis: Cellulitis right small finger due to Staphylococcus aureus

Index: **Cellulitis** (diffuse) (with lymphangitis) (*see also* Abscess) 682.9
              finger (intrathecal) (periosteal) (subcutaneous) (subcuticular) 681.00

Tabular: **681 Cellulitis and abscess of finger and toe**
                  681.0 Finger
                      681.00 Cellulitis and abscess, unspecified

There is an instructional note that directs you to identify the organism when assigning code 681.00. To locate the code for the causative organism, reference the main term "Infection" in the Index.

Index: **Infection, infected, infective** (opportunistic) 136.9
              staphylococcal, NEC 041.10
              aureus 041.11

Tabular: **041 Bacterial infection in conditions classified elsewhere and of
                  unspecified site**
                  041.1 Staphylococcus
                      041.11 Methicillin susceptible increase Staphylococcus aureus

The Tabular states at code 681, "Use additional code to identify organism, such as Staphylococcus (041.1)." Code 041.1 must have a fifth-digit assignment before it can be reported, and you would know this only if you verified the code in the Tabular and found that the five-digit code 041.11 specifies Staphylococcus aureus.

Code(s):   681.00, 041.11 Cellulitis right small finger due to Staphylococcus aureus

The code for the organism is assigned as an additional code and is sequenced after the disease or condition.

TOOLBOX

Bryant came to the clinic with a chief complaint of severe itching on his arms after a camping trip 5 days earlier. The physician examined Bryant and diagnosed the condition as dermatitis due to poison sumac.

QUESTIONS
1. What is another name for poison sumac?_____
2. How would you locate the diagnosis in the Index of the ICD-9-CM?

   _____

3. What diagnosis code would you assign to Bryant's service? _____
4. Is sumac included in the terms listed under the code you assigned? _____

   _____

▼ **ANSWERS**

1. *Rhus venenata.* 2. Dermatitis, due to, poison, sumac 3. 692.6 4. Yes

---

EXERCISE 12-4   *Diseases of the Skin and Subcutaneous Tissue*

Assign ICD-9-CM codes for the following:

1 Pruritus

ICD-9-CM Code: _____

2 Heat rash

ICD-9-CM Code: _____

3 Psoriasis

ICD-9-CM Code: _____

4 Decubitus ulcer buttock

ICD-9-CM Codes: _____, _____

5 Dermatitis due to poison ivy

ICD-9-CM Code: _____

(Answers are located in Appendix B)

DISEASES OF THE MUSCULOSKELETAL SYSTEM AND CONNECTIVE TISSUE

Chapter 13, Diseases of the Musculoskeletal System and Connective Tissue, in the ICD-9-CM Tabular describes diseases or conditions of the bone, joints, and muscles. It is important to refer to the note at the beginning of the chapter because that is where you will locate the information on the fifth-digit subclassifications used for categories 711-712, 715-716, 718-719, and 730. If you turn to category 711, you will see the fifth-digit subclassifications again, but not in the same detail as is found at the beginning of the chapter. Most arthropathies (disorders of the joint) are classified in categories 710 through 719 and most dorsopathies (disorders of the back) in categories 720 through 724 in ICD-9-CM.

Example

Fifth Digit

Diagnosis:	Pyogenic arthritis of the wrist
Index:	**Arthritis**, arthritic (acute) (chronic) (subacute), 716.9
	pyogenic organism 711.0
Tabular:	**711 Arthropathy associated with infections**
	711.0 Pyogenic arthritis

Code 711.0 is not valid until you assign a fifth digit to indicate the site of the arthritis. When reviewing the subclassifications, you must know whether the wrist is part of the forearm or part of the hand. Refer to that note at the beginning of the chapter, where you will note that fifth digit "3" reports the forearm includes the radius, ulna, and wrist joint.

Code:	711.03 Pyogenic arthritis of the wrist

Pathologic or spontaneous fracture codes are also located in Chapter 13. A pathologic or spontaneous fracture is a break in a bone that occurs because of bone disease or a change surrounding the bone tissue that makes the bone weak. For a pathologic fracture, you report the fracture and the disease process responsible for the fracture, such as osteoporosis or metastatic cancer of the bone. It is also possible to have a small trauma associated with a pathologic fracture. Suppose, for example, an elderly woman with severe osteoporosis bumps her hip against the doorway and sustains a fractured hip. This may be classifiable as a pathologic fracture because a person with healthy bones would not have fractured a hip as the result of a small trauma such as bumping the hip on a doorway. If there is any question about whether a fracture is pathologic or due to trauma, ask the physician what caused the fracture.

A pathologic fracture is serious because healing may be delayed by the underlying bone disease. Also, if a pathologic fracture is documented and no other disease process is indicated, review the record or clarify with the physician the underlying cause of the fracture. You should never assign a code for a traumatic fracture and a pathologic fracture of the same bone; only code one or the other.

Example

Pathologic Fracture

Diagnosis:	Pathologic fracture of the hip due to severe osteoporosis
Index:	**Fracture** (abduction) (adduction) (avulsion) (compression) (crush) (dislocation)
	(oblique) (separation) (closed) 829.0
	pathologic (cause unknown) 733.10
	hip 733.14
Tabular:	**733.1 Pathologic fracture**
	733.14 Pathologic fracture of neck of femur

A second code will be assigned to identify the underlying disease.

Index:	**Osteoporosis** (generalized) 733.00
Tabular:	**733.0 Osteoporosis**
	733.00 Osteoporosis, unspecified
Codes:	733.14, 733.00 Pathologic fracture of the hip due to severe osteoporosis

The instructions for category 730, Osteomyelitis, periostitis, and other infections involving bone, direct you to identify any organism with an additional code. It is easy to miss the instructions between an *Excludes* note and the list of fifth-digit subclassifications. Highlight these instructions in your ICD-9-CM until you become familiar with their use when coding in this area. If any additional information you add to your code book makes you a better coder—add it.

EXERCISE 12-5   *Diseases of the Musculoskeletal System and Connective Tissue*

Assign ICD-9-CM codes for the following:

1 Rheumatoid arthritis

ICD-9-CM Code: _____

2 Pain in the neck

ICD-9-CM Code: _____

3 Recurrent dislocation, right shoulder

ICD-9-CM Code: _____

4 Spontaneous fracture left humerus due to metastatic bone cancer; history of cancer of the breast previously excised

ICD-9-CM Codes: _____ (fracture), _____ (neoplasm), _____ (history of)

(Answers are located in Appendix B)

CONGENITAL ANOMALIES AND CERTAIN CONDITIONS ORIGINATING IN THE PERINATAL PERIOD

Chapters 14 and 15, Congenital Anomalies and Certain Conditions Originating in the Perinatal Period, in the ICD-9-CM Tabular describe congenital anomalies and conditions that originate in the perinatal period. An **anomaly** is an abnormality of a structure or organ. **Congenital** means that it is an abnormality that one was born with. Some anomalies are noticeable and discovered at birth. In cases of other anomalies, it may be a number of months or even years before they are discovered. If there is any question about whether a condition is acquired or congenital, you can review the record or clarify the case with the physician.

The perinatal period extends through the 28 days following birth. The term **perinatal** applies only to the baby and **postpartum** applies to the mother. Codes from this chapter can still be assigned beyond that time frame, but as the chapter title indicates, the condition must have originated during the perinatal period.

ICD-9-CM OFFICIAL GUIDELINES FOR CODING AND REPORTING

SECTION I.C.

15. Chapter 15: Newborn (Perinatal) Guidelines (760-779)

For coding and reporting purposes the perinatal period is defined as before birth through the 28th day following birth. The following guidelines are provided for reporting purposes. Hospitals may record other diagnoses as needed for internal data use.

a. General Perinatal Rules

1) Chapter 15 Codes

They are <u>never</u> for use on the maternal record. Codes from Chapter 11, the obstetric chapter, are never permitted on the newborn record. Chapter 15 code may be used throughout the life of the patient if the condition is still present.

2) Sequencing of perinatal codes

Generally, codes from Chapter 15 should be sequenced as the principal/first-listed diagnosis on the newborn record, with the exception of the appropriate V30 code for the birth episode, followed by codes from any other chapter that provide additional detail. The "use additional code" note at the beginning of the chapter supports this

Continued

guideline. If the index does not provide a specific code for a perinatal condition, assign code 779.89, Other specified conditions originating in the perinatal period, followed by the code from another chapter that specifies the condition. Codes for signs and symptoms may be assigned when a definitive diagnosis has not been established.

3) Birth process or community acquired conditions

If a newborn has a condition that may be either due to the birth process or community acquired and the documentation does not indicate which it is, the default is due to the birth process and the code from Chapter 15 should be used. If the condition is community-acquired, a code from Chapter 15 should not be assigned.

4) Code all clinically significant conditions

All clinically significant conditions noted on routine newborn examination should be coded. A condition is clinically significant if it requires:

- clinical evaluation; or
- therapeutic treatment; or
- diagnostic procedures; or
- extended length of hospital stay; or
- increased nursing care and/or monitoring; or
- has implications for future health care needs

Note: The perinatal guidelines listed above are the same as the general coding guidelines for "additional diagnoses", except for the final point regarding implications for future health care needs. Codes should be assigned for conditions that have been specified by the provider as having implications for future health care needs. Codes from the perinatal chapter should not be assigned unless the provider has established a definitive diagnosis.

b. Use of Codes V30-V39

When coding the birth of an infant, assign a code from categories V30- V39, according to the type of birth. A code from this series is assigned as a principal diagnosis, and assigned only once to a newborn at the time of birth.

c. Newborn Transfers

If the newborn is transferred to another institution, the V30 series is not used at the receiving hospital.

d. Use of Category V29

1) Assigning a code from category V29

Assign a code from category V29, Observation and evaluation of newborns and infants for suspected conditions not found, to identify those instances when a healthy newborn is evaluated for a suspected condition that is determined after study not to be present. Do not use a code from category V29 when the patient has identified signs and symptoms of a suspected problem; in such cases, code the sign or symptom.

A code from category V29 may also be assigned as a principal code for readmissions or encounters when the V30 code no longer applies. Codes from category V29 are for use only for healthy newborns and infants for which no condition after study is found to be present.

2) V29 code on a birth record

A V29 code is to be used as a secondary code after the V30, Outcome of delivery, code.

e. Use of other V codes on perinatal records

V codes other than V30 and V29 may be assigned on a perinatal or newborn record code. The codes may be used as a principal or first-listed diagnosis for specific types of encounters or for readmissions or encounters when the V30 code no longer applies.

See Section I.C.18 for information regarding the assignment of V codes.

f. Maternal Causes of Perinatal Morbidity

Codes from categories 760-763, Maternal causes of perinatal morbidity and mortality, are assigned only when the maternal condition has actually affected the fetus or newborn.

Continued

The fact that the mother has an associated medical condition or experiences some complication of pregnancy, labor or delivery does not justify the routine assignment of codes from these categories to the newborn record.

g. Congenital Anomalies in Newborns

For the birth admission, the appropriate code from category V30, Liveborn infants according to type of birth, should be used, followed by any congenital anomaly codes, categories 740-759. Use additional secondary codes from other chapters to specify conditions associated with the anomaly, if applicable.

Also, see Section I.C.14 for information on the coding of congenital anomalies.

h. Coding Additional Perinatal Diagnoses

1) Assigning codes for conditions that require treatment

Assign codes for conditions that require treatment or further investigation, prolong the length of stay, or require resource utilization.

2) Codes for conditions specified as having implications for future health care needs

Assign codes for conditions that have been specified by the provider as having implications for future health care needs.

Note: This guideline should not be used for adult patients.

3) Codes for newborn conditions originating in the perinatal period

Assign a code for newborn conditions originating in the perinatal period (categories 760-779), as well as complications arising during the current episode of care classified in other chapters, only if the diagnoses have been documented by the responsible provider at the time of transfer or discharge as having affected the fetus or newborn.

i. Prematurity and Fetal Growth Retardation

Providers utilize different criteria in determining prematurity. A code for prematurity should not be assigned unless it is documented. The 5th digit assignment for codes from category 764 and subcategories 765.0 and 765.1 should be based on the recorded birth weight and estimated gestational age.

A code from subcategory 765.2, Weeks of gestation, should be assigned as an additional code with category 764 and codes from 765.0 and 765.1 to specify weeks of gestation as documented by the provider in the record.

j. Newborn sepsis

Code 771.81, Septicemia [sepsis] of newborn, should be assigned with a secondary code from category 041, Bacterial infections in conditions classified elsewhere and of unspecified site, to identify the organism. A code from category 038, Septicemia, should not be used on a newborn record. Do not assign 995.91, Sepsis, as code 771.81 describes the sepsis. If applicable, use additional codes to identify severe sepsis (995.92) and any associated acute organ dysfunction.

As Guideline Section I.C.15.b. states, code the birth from categories V30-V39, Liveborn infant according to type of birth. The birth code is assigned only once and that is on the birth record of the baby because it indicates the type of birth.

On the baby's birth record the appropriate V code is sequenced first as the first-listed diagnosis. If any other conditions or congenital anomalies are documented, they are reported as secondary diagnoses.

Newborn Congenital Anomalies

Example

Diagnosis:	Newborn male delivered in the hospital by cesarean section and with Down's syndrome
Index:	**Newborn** (infant) (liveborn), single, born in hospital (without mention of cesarean delivery or section) V30.00 with cesarean delivery or section V30.01
Tabular:	**V30 Single liveborn**

The code is not complete until you add a fourth and fifth digit. The fourth digit is "0" for born in the hospital and the fifth digit is "1" for delivered by cesarean delivery. The code would be V30.01. Next, code the Down's syndrome.

Index:	**Syndrome**—*see also* Disease, Down's (mongolism) 758.0
Tabular:	**758 Chromosomal anomalies** **758.0 Down's syndrome**
Codes:	V30.01, 758.0 Newborn male delivered by cesarean section in the hospital; Down's syndrome

In the preceding example, if the baby was transferred to a second facility for treatment of the Down's syndrome, no V code would be assigned by the second facility to identify delivery. The V code can be assigned only once, as the first-listed diagnosis at the birthing facility on the baby's record. The first-listed diagnosis code at the second facility would be Down's syndrome (758.0).

You have to be careful about assigning codes from the 760-763 categories, Maternal Causes of Perinatal Morbidity and Mortality. Many times the mother has a condition, but that condition has no untoward (negative) effect on the baby or fetus. Codes from these categories are to be assigned only when the maternal condition has **affected** the health of the newborn.

EXERCISE 12-6 | *Congenital Anomalies and Certain Conditions Originating in the Perinatal Period*

Assign ICD-9-CM codes for the following:

1 Congenital absence of the earlobe

ICD-9-CM Code: _____

2 Newborn male delivered in the hospital via vaginal delivery; undescended left testicle (will re-evaluate in 6 weeks)

ICD-9-CM Codes: _____, _____

3 Three-year-old diagnosed with fragile X syndrome

ICD-9-CM Code: _____

4 Newborn transferred to a facility because of congenital dislocation of right hip (code as the facility transferred to)

ICD-9-CM Code: _____

(Answers are located in Appendix B)

SYMPTOMS, SIGNS, AND ILL-DEFINED CONDITIONS

Chapter 16, Symptoms, Signs, and Ill-Defined Conditions, in the Tabular of the ICD-9-CM includes symptoms, signs, abnormal results of investigations, and other ill-defined conditions. Signs and symptoms codes are assigned for encounters until there is a definitive diagnosis. A sign is defined as objective evidence of disease that can be observed by the physician. A symptom is a subjective observation reported by the patient but not confirmed objectively by the physician.

You assign the codes from Chapter 16 when:

- No more specific diagnosis can be made after investigation.
- Signs and symptoms existing at the time of the initial encounter prove to be transient or a cause cannot be determined.
- A patient fails to return and you have only a provisional diagnosis.
- A case is referred elsewhere before a definitive diagnosis is made.
- A more precise diagnosis is not available for any other reason.
- Certain symptoms that represent important problems in the medical care exist and it may be desirable to classify them in addition to the known cause.

You do not code from Chapter 16 when a definitive diagnosis is available. Consider, for example, this diagnostic statement: "Right lower quadrant abdominal pain due to acute appendicitis." The code for right lower quadrant abdominal pain is 789.03, located in Chapter 16. But because the reason for the pain is the acute appendicitis, you would not include the code for the symptom of abdominal pain; rather you would assign 540.9 for the acute appendicitis—the definitive diagnosis.

You do not code from Chapter 16 when the symptom is considered to be routinely associated with a disease process. Consider, for example, this diagnostic statement: "Cough and fever with pneumonia." Both cough and fever are symptoms of the pneumonia; therefore, you would not assign codes for either symptom. The only code you would assign would be 486 for the pneumonia.

A disease reference book comes in handy until you become more familiar with disease symptoms. If you do not know the symptoms associated with a disease, consult reference material or ask a colleague.

Finding the codes for **abnormal investigations** in the Index is tricky. The codes are located under the main term "Findings, abnormal, without diagnosis (examination) (laboratory test)." Some entries may also be located under the main term "Elevation," such as blood pressure and body temperature.

Abnormal Findings

Example

Diagnosis:	Abnormal liver scan
Index:	**Findings, abnormal, without diagnosis** (examination) (laboratory test) 796.4
	scan NEC 794.9
	liver 794.8
Tabular:	**794 Nonspecific abnormal results of function studies**
	794.8 Liver
Code:	794.8 Abnormal liver scan

When reporting complications of surgical or medical care, you must be certain the complications are present. A surgical complication is one that takes place as a result of the procedure. Just because a complication occurs following a procedure does not mean the complication is a surgical complication. Do not assume a cause-and-effect relationship. Clarify any doubt or questions with the physician. The term "complication" as used in ICD-9-CM does not imply that improper or inadequate care is responsible for the problem. There is no time limit defined for the development of a complication. At what time it presents will dictate the way in which it is coded. Be sure to use the Index carefully and follow all instructional notes. Exclusion notes are extensive in this section and often direct the coder elsewhere.

EXERCISE 12-7	*Symptoms, Signs, and Ill-Defined Conditions*

Assign ICD-9-CM codes for the following:

1 Fussy infant

ICD-9-CM Code: _____

2 Pleuritic-type chest pain

ICD-9-CM Code: _____

3 Abnormal mammogram

ICD-9-CM Code: _____

4 Seizure

ICD-9-CM Code: _____

5 Elevated blood pressure reading

ICD-9-CM Code: _____

(Answers are located in Appendix B)

INJURY AND POISONING

ICD-9-CM OFFICIAL GUIDELINES FOR CODING AND REPORTING

SECTION I.C.
19. Supplemental Classification of External Causes of Injury and Poisoning (E codes, E800-E999)

Introduction: These guidelines are provided for those who are currently collecting E codes in order that there will be standardization in the process. If your institution plans to begin collecting E codes, these guidelines are to be applied. The use of E codes is supplemental to the application of ICD-9-CM diagnosis codes.

External causes of injury and poisoning codes (categories E000 and E800- E999) are intended to provide data for injury research and evaluation of injury prevention strategies. Activity codes (categories E001-E030) are intended to be used to describe the activity of a person seeking care for injuries as well as other health conditions, when the injury or other health condition resulted from an activity or the activity contributed to a condition. E codes capture how the injury, poisoning, or adverse effect happened (cause), the intent (unintentional or accidental; or intentional, such as suicide or assault), the person's status (e.g. civilian, military), the associated activity and the place where the event occurred.

Some major categories of E codes include:

transport accidents
poisoning and adverse effects of drugs, medicinal substances and biologicals
accidental falls
accidents caused by fire and flames
accidents due to natural and environmental factors

Continued

late effects of accidents, assaults or self injury

assaults or purposely inflicted injury

suicide or self inflicted injury

These guidelines apply for the coding and collection of E codes from records in hospitals, outpatient clinics, emergency departments, other ambulatory care settings and provider offices, and nonacute care settings, except when other specific guidelines apply.

a. General E Code Coding Guidelines

1) Used with any code in the range of 001-V91

An E code from categories E800-E999 may be used with any code in the range of 001-V91, which indicates an injury, poisoning, or adverse effect due to an external cause.

An activity E code (categories E001-E030) may be used with any code in the range of 001-V91 that indicates an injury, or other health condition that resulted from an activity, or the activity contributed to a condition.

2) Assign the appropriate E code for all initial treatments

Assign the appropriate E code for the initial encounter of an injury, poisoning, or adverse effect of drugs, not for subsequent treatment.

External cause of injury codes (E-codes) may be assigned while the acute fracture codes are still applicable.

See Section I.C.17.b.1 for coding of acute fractures.

3) Use the full range of E codes

Use the full range of E codes (E800-E999) to completely describe the cause, the intent and the place of occurrence, if applicable, for all injuries, poisonings, and adverse effects of drugs.

See a.1.), j.), and k.) in this section for information on the use of status and activity E codes.

4) Assign as many E codes as necessary

Assign as many E codes as necessary to fully explain each cause.

5) The selection of the appropriate E code

The selection of the appropriate E code is guided by the Index to External Causes, which is located after the alphabetical index to diseases and by Inclusion and Exclusion notes in the Tabular List.

6) E code can never be a principal diagnosis

An E code can never be a principal (first listed) diagnosis.

7) External cause code(s) with systemic inflammatory response syndrome (SIRS)

An external cause code is not appropriate with a code from subcategory 995.9, unless the patient also has another condition for which an E code would be appropriate (such as an injury, poisoning, or adverse effect of drugs.

8) Multiple Cause E Code Coding Guidelines

More than one E-code is required to fully describe the external cause of an illness, injury or poisoning. The assignment of E-codes should be sequenced in the following priority:

If two or more events cause separate injuries, an E code should be assigned for each cause. The first listed E code will be selected in the following order:

E codes for child and adult abuse take priority over all other E codes. *See Section I.C.19.e., Child and Adult abuse guidelines.*

E codes for terrorism events take priority over all other E codes except child and adult abuse.

Continued

E codes for cataclysmic events take priority over all other E codes except child and adult abuse and terrorism.

E codes for transport accidents take priority over all other E codes except cataclysmic events, and child and adult abuse and terrorism.

Activity and external cause status codes are assigned following all causal (intent) E codes.

The first-listed E code should correspond to the cause of the most serious diagnosis due to an assault, accident, or self-harm, following the order of hierarchy listed above.

9) If the reporting format limits the number of E codes

If the reporting format limits the number of E codes that can be used in reporting clinical data, report the code for the cause/intent most related to the principal diagnosis. If the format permits capture of additional E codes, the cause/intent, including medical mis-adventures, of the additional events should be reported rather than the codes for place, activity or external status.

b. Place of Occurrence Guideline

Use an additional code from category E849 to indicate the Place of Occurrence. The Place of Occurrence describes the place where the event occurred and not the patient's activity at the time of the event.

Do not use E849.9 if the place of occurrence is not stated.

c. Adverse Effects of Drugs, Medicinal and Biological Substances Guidelines

1) Do not code directly from the Table of Drugs

Do not code directly from the Table of Drugs and Chemicals. Always refer back to the Tabular List.

2) Use as many codes as necessary to describe

Use as many codes as necessary to describe completely all drugs, medicinal or biological substances.

If the reporting format limits the number of E codes, and there are different fourth digit codes in the same three digit category, use the code for "Other specified" of that category of drugs, medicinal or biological substances. If there is no "Other specified" code in that category, use the appropriate "Unspecified" code in that category.

If the reporting format limits the number of E codes, and the codes are in different three digit categories, assign the appropriate E code for other multiple drugs and medicinal substances.

3) If the same E code would describe the causative agent

If the same E code would describe the causative agent for more than one adverse reaction, assign the code only once.

4) If two or more drugs, medicinal or biological substances

If two or more drugs, medicinal or biological substances are reported, code each individually unless the combination code is listed in the Table of Drugs and Chemicals. In that case, assign the E code for the combination.

5) When a reaction results from the interaction of a drug(s)

When a reaction results from the interaction of a drug(s) and alcohol, use poisoning codes and E codes for both.

6) Codes from the E930-E949 series

Codes from the E930-E949 series must be used to identify the causative substance for an adverse effect of drug, medicinal and biological substances, correctly prescribed and properly administered. The effect, such as tachycardia, delirium, gastrointestinal hemorrhaging, vomiting, hypokalemia, hepatitis, renal failure, or respiratory failure, is coded and followed by the appropriate code from the E930-E949 series.

Continued

d. Child and Adult Abuse Guideline

1) Intentional injury

When the cause of an injury or neglect is intentional child or adult abuse, the first listed E code should be assigned from categories E960-E968, Homicide and injury purposely inflicted by other persons (except category E967). An E code from category E967, Child and adult battering and other maltreatment, should be added as an additional code to identify the perpetrator, if known.

2) Accidental intent

In cases of neglect when the intent is determined to be accidental E code E904.0, Abandonment or neglect of infant and helpless person, should be the first listed E code.

e. Unknown or Suspected Intent Guideline

1) If the intent (accident, self-harm, assault) of the cause of an injury or poisoning is unknown

If the intent (accident, self-harm, assault) of the cause of an injury or poisoning is unknown or unspecified, code the intent as undetermined E980-E989.

2) If the intent (accident, self-harm, assault) of the cause of an injury or poisoning is questionable

If the intent (accident, self-harm, assault) of the cause of an injury or poisoning is questionable, probable or suspected, code the intent as undetermined E980-E989.

f. Undetermined Cause

When the intent of an injury or poisoning is known, but the cause is unknown, use codes: E928.9, Unspecified accident, E958.9, Suicide and self-inflicted injury by unspecified means, and E968.9, Assault by unspecified means.

These E codes should rarely be used, as the documentation in the medical record, in both the inpatient outpatient and other settings, should normally provide sufficient detail to determine the cause of the injury.

g. Late Effects of External Cause Guidelines

1) Late effect E codes

Late effect E codes exist for injuries and poisonings but not for adverse effects of drugs, misadventures and surgical complications.

2) Late effect E codes (E929, E959, E969, E977, E989, or E999.1)

A late effect E code (E929, E959, E969, E977, E989, or E999.1) should be used with any report of a late effect or sequela resulting from a previous injury or poisoning (905-909).

3) Late effect E code with a related current injury

A late effect E code should never be used with a related current nature of injury code.

4) Use of late effect E codes for subsequent visits

Use a late effect E code for subsequent visits when a late effect of the initial injury or poisoning is being treated. There is no late effect E code for adverse effects of drugs.

Do not use a late effect E code for subsequent visits for follow-up care (e.g., to assess healing, to receive rehabilitative therapy) of the injury or poisoning when no late effect of the injury has been documented.

h. Misadventures and Complications of Care Guidelines

1) Code range E870-E876

Assign a code in the range of E870-E876 if misadventures are stated by the provider. When applying the E code guidelines pertaining to sequencing, these E codes are considered causal codes.

Continued

2) Code range E878-E879

Assign a code in the range of E878-E879 if the provider attributes an abnormal reaction or later complication to a surgical or medical procedure, but does not mention misadventure at the time of the procedure as the cause of the reaction.

i. Terrorism Guidelines

1) Cause of injury identified by the Federal Government (FBI) as terrorism

When the cause of an injury is identified by the Federal Government (FBI) as terrorism, the first-listed E-code should be a code from category E979, Terrorism. The definition of terrorism employed by the FBI is found at the inclusion note at E979. The terrorism E-code is the only E-code that should be assigned. Additional E codes from the assault categories should not be assigned.

2) Cause of an injury is suspected to be the result of terrorism

When the cause of an injury is suspected to be the result of terrorism a code from category E979 should not be assigned. Assign a code in the range of E codes based circumstances on the documentation of intent and mechanism.

3) Code E979.9, Terrorism, secondary effects

Assign code E979.9, Terrorism, secondary effects, for conditions occurring subsequent to the terrorist event. This code should not be assigned for conditions that are due to the initial terrorist act.

4) Statistical tabulation of terrorism codes

For statistical purposes these codes will be tabulated within the category for assault, expanding the current category from E960-E969 to include E979 and E999.1.

Alphabetic Index to External Causes (E Code)

> **🤚 CAUTION** *E codes have their own index. You can locate the E code index in Volume 2, Section III, Index to External Causes of Injury, and then locate the codes you're directed to in the E code Supplementary Classification of Volume 1 (follows the V codes).*

Alphabetic Index to External Causes of Injuries is the **index** for the E codes. The index classifies environmental events (tornadoes, floods), circumstances, and other conditions as the cause of injury and other adverse effects alphabetically. **E codes are never assigned as a first-listed diagnosis.** Rather, E codes are used to clarify injury or adverse effects.

E code terms describe the external circumstances under which an accident, injury, or act of violence occurred. The main terms in the E code index usually represent the type of accident or violence (e.g., assault, collision), with the specific agent or other circumstance listed below the main term. "Collision" in Fig. 12-1 is the type of accident, and listed below Collision are the circumstances of the accident.

You must be sure to read all the information under a term in the E code Index before locating the code in the Tabular. Be sure to check for fourth-digit specificity for railway accidents, motor vehicle traffic and nontraffic accidents, other road vehicle accidents, water transport accidents, and air and space transport accidents shown in the Index of the External Causes.

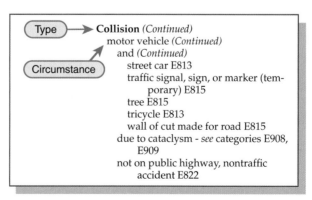

FIGURE 12-1 Section 3, Index to External Causes.

When a code from the E code section is reported, it is **in addition** to an injury code from the Tabular List of the ICD-9-CM. The E code classification is an additional code for greater detail. Most groups of E codes have Includes or *Excludes* notes that provide further detail about assigning the codes. For example, for E845, Accident involving spacecraft, the Includes note states that launching-pad accidents are included, and the *Excludes* note states that the effects of weightlessness in a spacecraft are not included. Be sure to read these notes as you become familiar with what is included or excluded.

The use of the additional digit adds specificity as to who was injured in the accident. For example, if the injured person was the driver of a car involved in a motor vehicle accident, the fifth digit would be 0. If the injured person was a passenger in the vehicle, the fifth digit would be 1.

E codes also permit the classification of environmental events, circumstances, and conditions as the cause of injury, poisoning, and other adverse effects. With E codes, anything that can injure or have an adverse effect on a human body can be coded. The E codes can supply a code if a person is injured while pearl diving (E910.3), injured when a window of a railroad car falls on someone's head (E806.9), or hurt when pecked by a bird (E906.8). They are all in the E codes! These are rather far-fetched examples, granted, but they show how extensive and specific the codes are.

CODING SHOT

Place of occurrence E codes are reported to provide further specificity as to where the accident/external cause occurred. If the place of occurrence is unknown, no code is assigned in accordance with coding guidelines.

Some states have made the assignment of E codes mandatory, and the general use of E codes has increased significantly. At the beginning of Chapter 17, Injury and Poisoning (800-999), the note directs you to "Use E code(s) to identify the cause and intent of the injury or poisoning (E800- E999)." The Occupational Safety and Health Administration (OSHA) and Workers' Compensation are two entities that track the data from E codes to identify the causes of accidents. In states where E code assignment is not mandatory, each facility decides if it will or will not require assignment of E codes.

EXERCISE 12-8   *E Codes*

Using the ICD-9-CM manual, locate the correct E code for each of the following in Volume 2, Alphabetic Index, and then in Volume 1, Tabular List:

1 Railway (E800-E807)

Railway accident involving derailment without antecedent collision, injuring a porter

E code index term(s): _____

ICD-9-CM Code: _____

2 Motor Vehicle Traffic (E810-E819)

Motor vehicle traffic accident due to tire blowout; driver of the car was injured

E code index term(s): _____

ICD-9-CM Code: _____

3 Motor Vehicle Nontraffic (E820-E825)

Driver of an ATV (off-road vehicle) is injured when he collides with a fence

E code index term(s): _____

ICD-9-CM Code: _____

4 Other Road Vehicle (E826-E829)

Horse being ridden, rider injured, and non-motor vehicle collision

E code index term(s): _____

ICD-9-CM Code: _____

5 Water Transport (E830-E838)

Accident to watercraft causing other injury; occupant of small powered boat injured due to collision

E code index term(s): _____

ICD-9-CM Code: _____

(Answers are located in Appendix B)

Table of Drugs and Chemicals

Section II follows the Index in the ICD-9-CM and contains the Table of Drugs and Chemicals, which is an alphabetical listing of poisoning and external causes of adverse effects of drugs and other chemicals. The table headings pertaining to external cause are illustrated in Fig. 12-2.

Accident (E850-E869): Instances of accidental overdose of a drug, wrong substance given or taken, drug taken inadvertently, accidents in the use of drugs and biological agents during medical and surgical procedures, and external causes of poisonings classifiable to 980-989.

Accident

Example

A 35-year-old male is brought to the emergency department with memory disturbance after an accidental exposure to lead paint.

Lead paint	984.0
Memory disturbance	780.93
Accident, intention	E861.5

Substance	Poisoning	External Cause (E Code)				
		Accident	Therapeutic Use	Suicide Attempt	Assault	Undetermined
Acetylcholine (chloride)	971.0	E855.3	E941.0	E950.4	E962.0	E980.4
Acetylcysteine	975.5	E858.6	E945.5	E950.4	E962.0	E980.4
Acetyldigitoxin	972.1	E858.3	E942.1	E950.4	E962.0	E980.4

FIGURE 12-2 Table headings pertaining to external cause.

Therapeutic Use (E930-E949): Instances in which a correct substance properly administered in a therapeutic (treatment) or prophylactic (preventive) dosage has been the external cause of adverse effects.

Therapeutic Use

Example

A 2-year-old male is taken by his mother to the pediatrician for a routine vaccination. That evening the child's temperature is 104ºF, and he is taken by the mother to the emergency department.

Fever	780.60
Unspecified vaccine	E949.9

Suicide Attempt (E950-E959): Instances in which self-inflicted injuries or poisonings have been involved.

Suicide

Example

Rachael broke up with her boyfriend of 6 years. She became so despondent in the days that followed that she wrote a note indicating she was ending her life and took the entire bottle of her mother's prescription of Valium. She was found unconscious later by her mother.

Poisoning, Valium (diazepam)	969.4
Unconscious	780.09
Suicide, intention	E950.3

Assault (E960-E969): Instances in which injury or poisoning has been inflicted by another person with the intent to injure or kill.

Assault

Example

A 42-year-old male presents to his physician with complaints of severe abdominal cramping and pain. After extensive laboratory tests, the physician identifies the source of the problem as high levels of arsenic in the patient's system. The patient's wife was charged with the attempted murder of her husband.

Poisoning, arsenic	985.1
Abdominal pain and cramps	789.00
Assault, intention	E962.1

Undetermined (E980-E989): Instances in which it cannot be determined whether the poisoning or injury was intentional or accidental.

Undetermined

Example

A transient is found comatose under a freeway overpass. Later at the emergency department the patient is found to have high levels of heroin in his system. It is unknown at this time if the overdose was intentional or accidental.

Drug abuse	305.90
Poisoning, heroin	965.01
Coma	780.01
Undetermined, intention	E980.0

A thorough review of the documentation would be done to identify any indication of drug addiction and report if documented in the medical record.

Although certain substances are indexed in the Table of Drugs and Chemicals with one or more subentries, the majority are listed according to one use or state (i.e., solid, liquid, or gas). It is recognized that many substances may be used in various ways, in medicine and in industry, and may cause adverse effects or poisoning. In cases in which the reported data indicate a use or state not in the table, or one that is clearly different from those listed, an attempt should be made to classify the substances in the category that most nearly expresses the reported facts.

Adverse Effects

The coding of adverse effects and poisonings is probably the most difficult part of this chapter. It takes some practice to distinguish between an adverse effect and a poisoning. Because the physician is probably not going to use those specific terms in the diagnostic statement, you must question the physician if you are uncertain whether the diagnosis is an adverse effect or a poisoning.

ICD-9-CM OFFICIAL GUIDELINES FOR CODING AND REPORTING

SECTION I.C.17.

e. Adverse Effects, Poisoning and Toxic Effects

The properties of certain drugs, medicinal and biological substances or combinations of such substances, may cause toxic reactions. The occurrence of drug toxicity is classified in ICD-9-CM as follows:

1) Adverse Effect

When the drug was correctly prescribed and properly administered, code the reaction plus the appropriate code from the E930-E949 series. Codes from the E930-E949 series must be used to identify the causative substance for adverse effect of drug, medicinal and biological substances, correctly prescribed and properly administered. The effect, such as tachycardia, delirium, gastrointestinal hemorrhaging, vomiting, hypokalemia, hepatitis, renal failure, or respiratory failure, is coded and followed by the appropriate code from the E930-E949 series.

Adverse effects of therapeutic substances correctly prescribed and properly administered (toxicity, synergistic reaction, side effect, and idiosyncratic reaction) may be due to (1) differences among patients, such as age, sex, disease, and genetic factors, and (2) drug-related factors, such as type of drug, route of administration, duration of therapy, dosage, and bioavailability.

An **adverse effect** occurs when a drug has been correctly prescribed and properly administered and the patient develops a reaction. Everything has been done correctly by the physician and the patient, but a reaction or adverse effect has occurred because of the drug.

When reporting adverse effects, you code the **effect** first, followed by the E code from the **therapeutic** column in the Table of Drugs and Chemicals. (You use the therapeutic column because the medication was prescribed by the physician as a therapy for a condition.)

Adverse Effect

Example

Diagnosis:	Urticaria due to penicillin (properly taken and prescribed)
Index:	**Urticaria** 708.9, due to, drugs 708.0
Tabular:	**708 Urticaria**
	708.0 Allergic urticaria

You also report the drug using the Table of Drugs and Chemicals.

Table of Drugs:	Penicillin (any type) E930.0
Tabular:	**E930 Antibiotics**
	E930.0 Penicillins
Codes:	708.0, E930.0 Urticaria due to penicillin

The code for the effect (urticaria, 708.0) is listed first and the cause (penicillin, E930.0) next.

The E codes from this section (E930-E949) are considered required E codes. Thus, therapeutic E codes for adverse effects must be assigned. E codes are never assigned as a first-listed diagnosis but are always considered an additional code.

In Fig. 12-3, the Table of Drugs and Chemicals shows that column 1 (Substance) contains the name of the drug or chemical. Column 2 (Poisoning) contains the list of poisoning codes. The remaining five columns are the E codes that are assigned to indicate how the poisoning or adverse effect occurred.

TABLE OF DRUGS AND CHEMICALS

Substance	Poisoning	External Cause (E Code)				
		Accident	Therapeutic Use	Suicide Attempt	Assault	Undetermined
Acetylcholine (chloride)	971.0	E855.3	E941.0	E950.4	E962.0	E980.4
Acetylcysteine	975.5	E858.6	E945.5	E950.4	E962.0	E980.4
Acetyldigitoxin	972.1	E858.3	E942.1	E950.4	E962.0	E980.4
Acetyldihydrocodeine	965.09	E850.2	E935.2	E950.0	E962.0	E980.0
Acetyldihydrocodeinone	965.09	E850.2	E935.2	E950.0	E962.0	E980.0
Acetylene (gas) (industrial)	987.1	E868.1	—	E951.8	E962.2	E981.8
incomplete combustion of - *see* Carbon monoxide, fuel, utility	—	—	—		—	—
tetrachloride (vapor)	982.3	E862.4	—	E950.9	E962.1	E980.9
Acetyliodosalicylic acid	965.1	E850.3	E935.3	E950.0	E962.0	E980.0
Acetylphenylhydrazine	965.8	E850.8	E935.8	E950.0	E962.0	E980.0
Acetylsalicylic acid	965.1	E850.3	E935.3	E950.0	E962.0	E980.0
Achromycin	960.4	E856	E930.4	E950.4	E962.0	E980.4
ophthalmic preparation	976.5	E858.7	E946.5	E950.4	E962.0	E980.4
topical NEC	976.0	E858.7	E946.0	E950.4	E962.0	E980.4
Acidifying agents	963.2	E858.1	E933.2	E950.4	E962.0	E980.4
Acids (corrosive) NEC	983.1	E864.1	—	E950.7	E962.1	E980.6
Aconite (wild)	988.2	E865.4	—	E950.9	E962.1	E980.9
Aconitine (liniment)	976.8	E858.7	E946.8	E950.4	E962.0	E980.4
Aconitum ferox	988.2	E865.4	—	E950.9	E962.1	E980.9
Acridine	983.0	E864.0	—	E950.7	E962.1	E980.6
vapor	987.8	E869.8	—	E952.8	E962.2	E982.8
Acriflavine	961.9	E857	E931.9	E950.4	E962.0	E980.4
Acrisorcin	976.0	E858.7	E946.0	E950.4	E962.0	E980.4
Acrolein (gas)	987.8	E869.8	—	E952.8	E962.2	E982.8
liquid	989.89	E866.8	—	E950.9	E962.1	E980.9
Actaea spicata	988.2	E865.4	—	E950.9	E962.1	E980.9
Acterol	961.5	E857	E931.5	E950.4	E962.0	E980.4
ACTH	962.4	E858.0	E932.4	E950.4	E962.0	E980.4
Acthar	962.4	E858.0	E932.4	E950.4	E962.0	E980.4
Actinomycin (C) (D)	960.7	E856	E930.7	E950.4	E962.0	E980.4
Adalin (acetyl)	967.3	E852.2	E937.3	E950.2	E962.0	E980.2
Adenosine (phosphate)	977.8	E858.8	E947.8	E950.4	E962.0	E980.4
Adhesives	989.89	E866.6	—	E950.9	E962.1	E980.9
ADH	962.5	E858.0	E932.5	E950.4	E962.0	E980.4
Adicillin	960.0	E856	E930.0	E950.4	E962.0	E980.4
Adiphenine	975.1	E855.6	E945.1	E950.4	E962.0	E980.4
Adjunct, pharmaceutical	977.4	E858.8	E947.4	E950.4	E962.0	E980.4

How adverse effect occurred → Therapeutic Use

Drug/chemical name

Poisoning code + How the poisoning occurred

FIGURE 12-3 Section 2, Table of Drugs and Chemicals.

There is a code available for an **unknown adverse effect.** For example, if the physician has documented a reaction due to penicillin and you cannot determine from the record what the exact adverse effect has been, you would report an unknown adverse effect. Adverse effects can be located in the Index under the main term "Effect, adverse," and the subterm "drugs and medicinals, correct substance properly administered 995.20." The correct codes for an unknown adverse effect due to penicillin are 995.20 and E930.0.

A **poisoning** occurs when drugs or other chemical substances are taken not according to a physician's instruction. Poisonings occur in a variety of ways:

- The wrong prescription or dosage is given in error, either during medical treatment or by nonmedical personnel such as the mother or the patient herself or himself.
- The medication is given to the wrong person.
- The medication is taken by the wrong person.
- A medication overdose has occurred.
- Medications (prescription or over-the-counter) have been taken in combination with alcohol or recreational drugs.
- Over-the-counter medications have been taken in combination with prescription medications without physician approval.

ICD-9-CM OFFICIAL GUIDELINES FOR CODING AND REPORTING

SECTION I.C.17.e.

2. Poisoning

(a) Error was made in drug prescription

Error made in drug prescription or in the administration of the drug by provider, nurse, patient, or other person, use the appropriate poisoning code from the 960–979 series.

(b) Overdose of a drug intentionally taken

If an overdose of a drug was intentionally taken or administered and resulted in drug toxicity, it would be coded as a poisoning (960–979 series).

(c) Nonprescribed drug taken with correctly prescribed and properly administered drug

If a nonprescribed drug or medicinal agent was taken in combination with a correctly prescribed and properly administered drug, any drug toxicity or other reaction resulting from the interaction of the two drugs would be classified as a poisoning.

(d) Interaction of drug(s) and alcohol

When a reaction results from the interaction of a drug(s) and alcohol, this would be classified as poisoning.

(e) Sequencing of poisoning

When coding a poisoning or reaction to the improper use of a medication (e.g., wrong dose, wrong substance, wrong route of administration) the poisoning code is sequenced first, followed by a code for the manifestation. If there is also a diagnosis of drug abuse or dependence to the substance, the abuse or dependence is coded as an additional code.

See Section I.C.3.a.6.b. if poisoning is the result of insulin pump malfunctions and Section I.C.19 for general use of E-codes.

✋ CAUTION *You CANNOT use an E code from the therapeutic column (E930–E949) with a poisoning code because they are mutually exclusive (can't be reported together). Something that is therapeutic (intended for treatment) could not be a poisoning (harmful).*

Poisoning codes are found in the Table of Drugs and Chemicals. You must always sequence the poisoning code first, then code any manifestation of the poisoning, such as coma, second. You also assign the corresponding E code from the Table of Drugs and Chemicals. If there is no documentation to indicate the intent so the intent is unknown or if the intent is questionable, code the intent as undetermined E980–E989.

Poisoning

Example

Diagnosis:	Coma due to accidental overdose of Valium (Valium is the brand name for benzodiazepine)

When you reference the main term "Overdose" in the Index, you are directed to the Table of Drugs and Chemicals.

Table of Drugs:	Valium 969.4 (poisoning)
	E853.2 (accidental)
Tabular:	**969 Poisoning by psychotropic agents**
	969.4 Benzodiazepine-based tranquilizers
Tabular:	**E853 Accidental poisoning by tranquilizers**
	E853.2 Benzodiazepine-based tranquilizers
Index:	**Coma** 780.01
Tabular:	**780 General symptoms**
	780.01 Coma
Codes:	969.4, 780.01, E853.2 Coma due to accidental overdose of Valium. Note that the poisoning code (969.4) is sequenced first, followed by the manifestation (780.01) and then the E code (E853.2).

If there has been no manifestation (coma, in the above case) of the poisoning, you would assign only the poisoning code (969.4) with the appropriate E code. When a patient undergoes a poisoning that involves more than one drug or chemical, there could be a different poisoning code and E code for each drug or chemical.

EXERCISE 12-9   *Poisoning/Table of Drugs and Chemicals*

Using the ICD-9-CM manual, assign poisoning codes and E codes to the following:

1 Poisoning by the ingestion of the beverage grain alcohol

ICD-9-CM Codes: _____ (poisoning), _____ (E code)

2 Undetermined poisoning by antifreeze

ICD-9-CM Codes: _____ (poisoning), _____ (E code)

3 Accidental overdose due to therapeutically prescribed valium

⊛ ICD-9-CM Code(s): _____

Manifestations (symptoms or signs) of poisonings and adverse effects of drugs and chemicals are found in Section 1, under the specific symptom or disease. For example, Fig. 12-4 illustrates the location of the symptom Rash in Volume 2, the Alphabetic Index. If the symptom of the drug poisoning or adverse effect is a rash, the subterm "drug (internal use)" directs you to 693.0.

Turn to code 693.0 in Volume 1, Tabular List.

4 What does the description of the ICD-9-CM code state? _____

Note the statement below the code: "Use additional E code to identify drug." In this case the condition is a rash. So when you see this statement, you know you have to identify the drug that caused the rash.

(Answers are located in Appendix B)

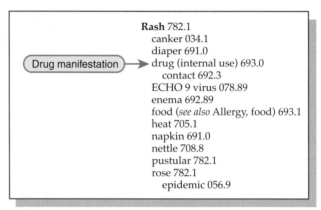

FIGURE 12–4 Index to Diseases, Rash.

Burns

There are numerous guidelines that pertain to injuries and poisonings. It is within this chapter that the codes to report burns are located. First, read the Guidelines on burns:

ICD-9-CM OFFICIAL GUIDELINES FOR CODING AND REPORTING

SECTION I.C.17.

c. Coding of Burns

Current burns (940-948) are classified by depth, extent and by agent (E code). Burns are classified by depth as first degree (erythema), second degree (blistering), and third-degree (full-thickness involvement).

1) Sequencing of burn and related condition codes

Sequence first the code that reflects the highest degree of burn when more than one burn is present.

a. When the reason for the admission or encounter is for treatment of external multiple burns, sequence first the code that reflects the burn of the highest degree.

b. When a patient has both internal and external burns, the circumstances of admission govern the selection of the principal diagnosis or first-listed diagnosis.

c. When a patient is admitted for burn injuries and other related conditions such as smoke inhalation and/or respiratory failure, the circumstances of admission govern the selection of the principal or first-listed diagnosis.

2) Burns of the same local site

Classify burns of the same local site (three-digit category level, 940-947) but of different degrees to the subcategory identifying the highest degree recorded in the diagnosis *[as is illustrated in Fig. 12-5]*.

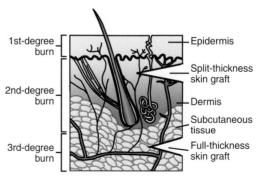

FIGURE 12–5 First-, second-, and third-degree burns

ICD-9-CM OFFICIAL GUIDELINES FOR CODING AND REPORTING

SECTION I.C.17.

c. Coding of Burns

3) Non-healing burns

Non-healing burns are coded as acute burns.

Necrosis of burned skin should be coded as a non-healed burn.

4) Code 958.3, Posttraumatic wound infection

Assign code 958.3, Posttraumatic wound infection, not elsewhere classified, as an additional code for any documented infected burn site.

5) Assign separate codes for each burn site

When coding burns, assign separate codes for each burn site. Category 946 Burns of Multiple specified sites, should only be used if the locations of the burns are not documented.

Category 949, Burn, unspecified, is extremely vague and should rarely be used.

6) Assign codes from category 948, Burns

Burns classified according to extent of body surface involved, when the site of the burn is not specified or when there is a need for additional data. It is advisable to use category 948 as additional coding when needed to provide data for evaluating burn mortality, such as that needed by burn units. It is also advisable to use category 948 as an additional code for reporting purposes when there is mention of a third-degree burn involving 20 percent or more of the body surface.

In assigning a code from category 948:

> Fourth-digit codes are used to identify the percentage of total body surface involved in a burn (all degree).

> Fifth-digits are assigned to identify the percentage of body surface involved in third-degree burn.

> Fifth-digit zero (0) is assigned when less than 10 percent or when no body surface is involved in a third-degree burn.

> Category 948 is based on the classic "rule of nines" [refer to Figs. 12-6 and 12-7] in estimating body surface involved: head and neck are assigned nine percent, each arm nine percent, each leg 18 percent, the anterior trunk 18 percent, posterior trunk 18 percent, and genitalia one percent. Providers may change these percentage assignments when necessary to accommodate infants and children who have proportionately larger heads than adults and patients who have large buttocks, thighs, or abdomen that involve burns.

7) Encounters for treatment of late effects of burns

Encounters for the treatment of the late effects of burns (i.e., scars or joint contractures) should be coded to the residual condition (sequelae) followed by the appropriate late effect code (906.5-906.9). A late effect E code may also be used, if desired.

8) Sequelae with a late effect code and current burn

When appropriate, both a sequelae with a late effect code, and a current burn code may be assigned on the same record (when both a current burn and sequelae of an old burn exist).

d. Coding of Debridement of Wound, Infection, or Burn

Excisional debridement involves surgical removal or cutting away, as opposed to a mechanical (brushing, scrubbing, washing) debridement.

For coding purposes, excisional debridement is assigned to code 86.22.
Nonexcisional debridement is assigned to code 86.28.

The Guidelines for **burns** direct you to sequence the highest degree of burn first. If you are coding a third-degree burn of the hand and a second-degree burn of the chest wall, you would sequence the code for the third-degree burn of the hand first, followed by the second-degree burn of the chest.

If different degrees of burns are documented at the same site, assign a code to the highest degree only. For example, if the patient has first- and second-degree burns to the hand, you would code only the second-degree burn to the hand because that is the highest level of specificity and the most severe.

Facilities may choose to capture data regarding the extent of body area burned. In this case, the Rule of Nines is applied (Figs. 12-6 and 12-7). The Index entry is "Burn . . . 949.0" with a note indicating that the fifth-digit is added with category 948 to indicate the extent of body surface involved (in percentage) with third-degree burns.

Burns are located in the Index by referring to the main term "Burn," subterms according to the site (abdomen or thigh), and finally to the degree of burn (second or third).

Codes from the 948 category can be assigned alone or in combination with other specific burn codes. The inclusion of codes from 948 are important for statistical purposes and may affect reimbursement. The use of the three-digit code 948 indicates a burn condition. The **fourth** digit indicates the **total percentage** of the body that has been burnt—including all first-, second-, and third-degree burns. The **fifth** digit (0-9) indicates the percentage of the body that received **third-degree** burns. It is not the coder's job to calculate the percentages, but you should seek clarification from the physician if documentation is missing or unclear regarding the percentages. Codes 940 through 949 are used for current unhealed burns excluding friction burns and sunburn; these are classified as dermatitis and superficial injury. Necrosis and non-healing burns are coded to acute current burns. Remember it is possible for a patient to have both healed and unhealed burns coded from the same episode of care because burns can heal at a different rate.

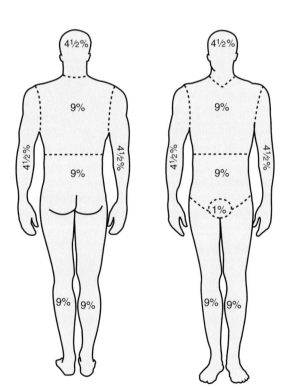

FIGURE 12-6 Rule of nines, adult.

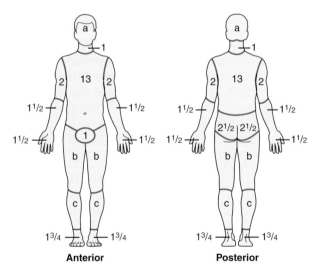

Relative percentage of body surface areas (% BSA) affected by growth

	0 yr	1 yr	5 yr	10 yr	15 yr
a – 1/2 of head	9 1/2	8 1/2	6 1/2	5 1/2	4 1/2
b – 1/2 of 1 thigh	2 3/4	3 1/4	4	4 1/4	4 1/2
c – 1/2 of lower leg	2 1/2	2 1/2	2 3/4	3	3 1/4

FIGURE 12-7 Lund-Browder chart for estimating the extent of burns on children.

Examples:

Diagnosis: First- and second-degree burn to the back

Index: **Burn,** back, second degree 942.24

Tabular: **942 Burn of trunk**
942.2 Blisters, epidermal loss [second degree]

A fifth digit is used to indicate the specific location of the burn to the trunk. In this case, the fifth digit 4 is used to indicate the location, back, 942.24.

Code(s):   942.24 First- and second-degree burn to the back

Note that the diagnosis includes first- and second-degree burns and the code assigned indicates second-degree burns. You code only the highest degree when the burns are at the same site.

Diagnosis: Second-degree burn, 1%, chin, and third-degree burn, 3%, scapular region, for a total of 4% of the body surface

Index: **Burn,** chin, second 941.24

Tabular: **941 Burn of face, head, and neck**
941.2 Blisters, epidermal loss [second degree]

A fifth digit is used to indicate the specific location of the burn to the face, head, or neck. In this case, the fifth digit 4 is used to indicate the location, chin, 941.24. Now, to code the burn to the scapular region:

Index: **Burn,** scapular region, third degree 943.36

Tabular: **943 Burn of upper limb, except wrist and hand**
943.3 Full-thickness skin loss [third degree NOS]

A fifth digit is used to indicate the specific location of the burn. In this case, the fifth digit 6 is used to indicate the location, scapular region, 943.36.

But wait! You need one more code to finish coding this example—one to indicate the total body surface involved.

Index: **Burn**, extent, less than 10%, 948.0

Tabular: **948.0 Burn [any degree] involving less than 10% of body surface**

The fifth digit "0" is required to indicate less than 10% total body surface involved a third-degree burn, 948.00.

Code(s):   943.36, 941.24, 948.00 Third-degree burn, scapular region, and second-degree burn, chin; with the 948.00 indicating that there is less than 10% third-degree burn on less than 10% of the body surface.

E codes for burns are assigned, as per facility policy, for all initial treatments.

EXERCISE 12-10   *Burns*

Code the burn, extent of the body surface involved, and percentage of body surface burned using the rule of nines.

1 A 3-year-old receives third-degree burns of the abdomen, 10%, and second-degree burns of the thigh, 5%, after pulling a pot of hot water on herself

Third-degree Code: _____ Second-degree Code: _____ E Code: _____ Degree

and Percentage (extent) Code: _____

2 Infected third-degree burn, left thigh, 4½%, subsequent treatment

ICD-9-CM Codes: _____ (third degree), _____ (infected burn), _____ (extent)

3 First- and second-degree burn, right foot, 2¼%, due to bonfire

ICD-9-CM Codes: _____ (second degree), _____ (extent), _____ (E code)

4 Non-healing third-degree burn, right hand, 2¼%; excisional debridement performed by physician; patient seen 10 days ago for initial treatment

ICD-9-CM Codes: _____ (third degree), _____ (extent)

5 Second-degree burn, right forearm, 2%; first-degree burn, right hand, 1%; and third-degree burn, chest wall, 8%, subsequent treatment

ICD-9-CM Codes: _____, _____, _____, _____

(Answers are located in Appendix B)

Fractures

Now it is time to learn how to report fractures, so begin by reading the Guidelines on fracture reporting:

ICD-9-CM OFFICIAL GUIDELINES FOR CODING AND REPORTING

SECTION I.C.

17. Chapter 17: Injury and Poisoning (800-999)

a. Coding of Injuries

When coding injuries, assign separate codes for each injury unless a combination code is provided, in which case the combination code is assigned. Multiple injury codes are provided in ICD-9-CM, but should not be assigned unless information for a more specific code is not available. These traumatic injury codes are not to be used for normal, healing surgical wounds or to identify complications of surgical wounds.

The code for the most serious injury, as determined by the provider and the focus of treatment, is sequenced first.

1) Superficial injuries

Superficial injuries such as abrasions or contusions are not coded when associated with more severe injuries of the same site.

2) Primary injury with damage to nerves/blood vessels

When a primary injury results in minor damage to peripheral nerves or blood vessels, the primary injury is sequenced first with additional code(s) from categories 950-957, Injury to nerves and spinal cord, and/or 900-904, Injury to blood vessels. When the primary injury is to the blood vessels or nerves, that injury should be sequenced first.

Continued

b. Coding of Traumatic Fractures

The principles of multiple coding of injuries should be followed in coding fractures. Fractures of specified sites are coded individually by site in accordance with both the provisions within categories 800-829 and the level of detail furnished by medical record content. Combination categories for multiple fractures are provided for use when there is insufficient detail in the medical record (such as trauma cases transferred to another hospital), when the reporting form limits the number of codes that can be used in reporting pertinent clinical data, or when there is insufficient specificity at the fourth-digit or fifth-digit level. More specific guidelines are as follows:

1) Acute Fractures vs. Aftercare

Traumatic fractures are coded using the acute fracture codes (800-829) while the patient is receiving active treatment for the fracture. Examples of active treatment are: surgical treatment, emergency department encounter, and evaluation and treatment by a new physician.

Fractures are coded using the aftercare codes (subcategories V54.0, V54.1, V54.8, or V54.9) for encounters after the patient has completed active treatment of the fracture and is receiving routine care for the fracture during the healing or recovery phase. Examples of fracture aftercare are: cast change or removal, removal of external or internal fixation device, medication adjustment, and follow up visits following fracture treatment.

Care for complications of surgical treatment for fracture repairs during the healing or recovery phase should be coded with the appropriate complication codes.

Care of complications of fractures, such as malunion and nonunion, should be reported with the appropriate codes.

Pathologic fractures are not coded in the 800-829 range, but instead are assigned to subcategory 733.1. *See Section I.C.13.a for additional information.*

2) Multiple fractures of same limb

Multiple fractures of same limb classifiable to the same three-digit or four-digit category are coded to that category.

3) Multiple unilateral or bilateral fractures of same bone

Multiple unilateral or bilateral fractures of same bone(s) but classified to different fourth-digit subdivisions (bone part) within the same three-digit category are coded individually by site.

4) Multiple fracture categories 819 and 828

Multiple fracture categories 819 and 828 classify bilateral fractures of both upper limbs (819) and both lower limbs (828), but without any detail at the fourth-digit level other than open and closed type of fractures.

5) Multiple fractures sequencing

Multiple fractures are sequenced in accordance with the severity of the fracture. The provider should be asked to list the fracture diagnoses in the order of severity.

Fracture is the first section in the chapter, and it contains the codes assigned for fractures caused by trauma. A fracture not indicated as closed or open should be classified as **closed**. If you have any doubt, check with the physician as to the nature of the fracture. A dislocation and fracture of the same bone would be coded to the fracture site because that is the highest level of specificity and fracture is more severe than dislocation. You are also instructed in the Index, under the main term "dislocation" to *see* Fracture, by site. The cross-reference "*see*" is a mandatory instruction that tells you to go to "Fracture" and not to code the dislocation separately. You locate fractures in the Index under "Fracture" and then on the basis of the anatomic location of the fracture.

Examples

Diagnosis:	Fracture, right patella with abrasions of the site
Index:	**Fracture,** patella (closed) 822.0
Tabular:	**822 Fracture of patella** 　**822.0 Closed**
Code(s):	822.0 Fracture, right patella with abrasions of the site

When a fracture is not specified as open or closed, assign a code that indicates a **closed** fracture. You would not assign a code for the dislocation when there is a more severe injury (the fracture) at the same site, as in the following example.

Diagnosis:	Fractured hip with dislocation
Index:	**Dislocation,** with fracture—*see* Fracture by site.

The "*see* Fracture by site" means the dislocation is included with the fracture code.

Index:	**Fracture,** hip (closed) 820.8
Tabular:	**820 Fracture of neck of femur** 　**820.8 Unspecified part of neck of femur, closed**
Code(s):	820.8 Fractured hip with dislocation

Wounds

Wounds (lacerations) are found under the main term "Wound." There are three subcategories in some of the wound codes. These injuries can be classified as:
1. Without mention of complication
2. Complicated
3. With tendon involvement

A **complicated wound** is one that includes documentation of delayed healing, delayed treatment, foreign body, or primary infection.

These codes are for traumatic injuries and should not be reported to identify surgical wounds or ulceration including decubitus and stasis ulcers.

Example

Diagnosis:	Infected wound of the right knee
Index:	**Wound,** knee 891.0 　complicated 891.1
Tabular:	**891 Open wound of knee, leg [except thigh], and ankle** 　**891.1 Complicated**
Code(s):	891.1 Infected wound of the right knee

QUICK CHECK 12-1

In the Index under Wound, what information is included for coding:
a. Penetrating wounds of internal organs
b. Insect bites
c. Crush injuries
d. All of the above

(Answers are located in Appendix C)

Complications

When a patient is admitted for a complication that resulted from medical care or a surgical procedure, the complication is the first-listed. Read the Guideline on complications:

ICD-9-CM OFFICIAL GUIDELINES FOR CODING AND REPORTING

SECTION II.
G. Complications of surgery and other medical care

When the admission is for treatment of a complication resulting from surgery or other medical care, the complication code is sequenced as the principal diagnosis. If the complication is classified to the 996-999 series and the code lacks the necessary specificity in describing the complication, an additional code for the specific complication should be assigned.

EXERCISE 12-11   *Complications*

In the Index, you will find complications of medical and surgical procedures under the main term "Complications."

Code the following complications:

1 Breast implants, infection

ICD-9-CM Code: _____

2 Bone marrow graft, rejection

ICD-9-CM Code: _____

3 Surgical procedures, stitch abscess

ICD-9-CM Code: _____

4 Cardiac pacemaker, (device) mechanical complication

ICD-9-CM Code: _____

(Answers are located in Appendix B)

CHAPTER REVIEW

CHAPTER 12, PART I, THEORY

Circle the correct answer in each of the following:

1 In order to code a gastrointestinal condition with hemorrhage, active bleeding must be present.

   True   False

2 It is common to use a fifth digit of 0 when coding complications related to pregnancy.

   True   False

3 A pathologic fracture occurs in a bone that is weakened by disease.

   True   False

4 The perinatal period extends for 6 weeks following birth.

   True   False

5 Generally you do not assign a code from Chapter 16 if a definitive diagnosis is documented.

   True   False

6 When an accident occurs, an E code should be the first-listed diagnosis.

   True   False

7 If a fracture and dislocation are present at the same site, assign only the fracture code.

   True   False

8 An infected laceration should be coded as a complicated wound.

   True   False

9 A poisoning occurs when a drug has been correctly prescribed and properly administered and the patient develops a reaction.

   True   False

10 When coding a poisoning, the poisoning code is sequenced before any manifestation code.

   True   False

Chapter Review answers are only available in the TEACH Instructor Resources on Evolve

CHAPTER 12, PART II, PRACTICAL

Using an ICD-9-CM manual, answer the following questions:

11 Nephrogenic diabetes insipidus

ICD-9-CM Code: _____

12 Ovarian cyst

ICD-9-CM Code: _____

13 Uterine fibroids complicating pregnancy, 23 weeks' gestation

ICD-9-CM Code: _____

14 Dehiscence cesarean wound. Patient delivered one week ago at another facility.

ICD-9-CM Code: _____

15 Term birth, 2268 grams, delivered by cesarean section, with intrauterine growth retardation

ICD-9-CM Codes: _____, _____

16 Anal fistula

ICD-9-CM Code: _____

17 Lower gastrointestinal bleeding due to angiodysplasia of colon

ICD-9-CM Code: _____

18 Kidney stone

ICD-9-CM Code: _____

19 Paronychia toe

ICD-9-CM Code: _____

20 Pilonidal cyst with abscess

ICD-9-CM Code: _____

21 Osteoarthritis, right knee

ICD-9-CM Code: _____

22 Postlaminectomy syndrome, lumbar

ICD-9-CM Code: _____

23 Bicuspid aortic valve

ICD-9-CM Code: _____

24 Patent ductus arteriosus

ICD-9-CM Code: _____

25 Palpitations

ICD-9-CM Code: _____

26 Lack of appetite

ICD-9-CM Code: _____

27 Infected mosquito bites, both legs

ICD-9-CM Codes: _____, _____

Chapter Review answers are only available in the TEACH Instructor Resources on Evolve

28 Sunburn

ICD-9-CM Codes: _____, _____

29 Hives due to prescription penicillin, which was properly taken

ICD-9-CM Codes: _____, _____

30 Chest pain due to cocaine

ICD-9-CM Codes: _____, _____, _____, _____

Assign the ICD-9-CM codes for the following cases:

31 Mr. Jones presents to the emergency department with acute abdominal pain. After a thorough examination and diagnostic x-ray film, Mr. Jones is diagnosed with acute small bowel obstruction and taken immediately to surgery.

ICD-9-CM Code: _____

32 Mrs. Smith is at 32 weeks' gestation and is admitted with severe bleeding with abdominal cramping. An emergency ultrasound is done and fetal monitors are applied. She is diagnosed with total placenta previa with indications of fetal distress. An emergency cesarean section is done, with delivery of a viable male infant.

ICD-9-CM Codes: _____, _____, _____, _____

33 Miss Halliday is an 80-year-old woman who presents to the emergency department with a history of abdominal pain, fever, and burning with urination. Urine culture is obtained, and Miss Halliday is admitted for workup to rule out urosepsis. Urosepsis was ruled out.

🌐 ICD-9-CM Code(s): _____

34 Mr. Johnson is admitted to the hospital with chest and epigastric pain. He is evaluated by the emergency department physician with a diagnosis of rule out myocardial infarction. Mr. Johnson is then transferred to a larger facility for further workup.

🌐 ICD-9-CM Code(s): _____

CASE STUDY 1

History of Present Illness

The patient is a 68-year-old female, status post motor vehicle accident 3 months ago. The patient had an open fracture that was treated initially with traction for 6 to 8 weeks. After initial treatment with traction, the patient was placed in a cast brace. She presents with a complaint of pain in the left femur and inability to bear weight on her leg. The patient was referred from an orthopedic surgeon. The past medical history was significant for no history of myocardial infarction or renal disease and no asthma. The patient had undergone no previous procedures with the exception of debridement of the open fracture. Otherwise the patient's history was unremarkable. The patient was taking no medications and had no known allergies. She underwent a preoperative workup that included a gallium scan.

Physical Examination

The heart, lungs, and abdomen were benign. The left knee had a 30-degree extension lag. There was motion with the knee approximately 30 degrees from horizontal axis to 90 degrees of flexion. The patella was difficult to palpate, and it was very difficult to tell at the time of examination whether motion was occurring at the fracture or whether it was occurring at the knee joint. The vascular examination was unremarkable.

Laboratory Data and Course in Hospital

The x-ray film showed nonunion of the left femur. The gallium scan obtained preoperatively was negative, and there was no evidence of infection.

Treatment

On May 14, the patient underwent open reduction and internal fixation of the left femur fracture with a 90-degree dynamic condylar screw and side plate. The patient tolerated the procedure well. She received two units of her own autologous blood at the time of surgery. Postoperatively she was quite anemic due to acute blood loss, with hemoglobin of 6 to 7 mg/dl. The patient was asymptomatic clinically, and her vascular examination was intact. On postoperative day 2, she had motion in the left knee from 0 to 30 degrees of flexion. She was placed in continuous passive motion and was up with physical therapy but non-weight-bearing on the left leg. Physical therapy was tolerated well. The hospital course was benign. The wound was clean and dry, and the neurovascular examination was unchanged. The x-ray films obtained before discharge showed maintenance of alignment of the left femur. The patient's staples were removed on postoperative day 7. She was placed in a cast brace and was discharged home after being independent in physical therapy.

Final Diagnosis

Nonunion of the left femur

Procedure

Open reduction and internal fixation of the left femur with 90-degree screw and site plate

35 ICD-9-CM Codes: _____, _____, _____, _____

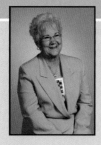

"Teamwork is an essential requirement in our profession. We learn from each other . . . then pass the knowledge on. It is an unbroken cycle."

Nancy Maguire, ACS, CRT, PCS, FCS, HCS-D, APC, AFC
Physician Consultant for Auditing and Education
Winchester, Virginia

Introduction to the CPT and Level II National Codes (HCPCS)

Chapter Topics

The Purpose of the CPT Manual

Updating the CPT Manual

CPT Manual Format

Starting with the Index

History of National Level Codes

Chapter Review

Learning Objectives

After completing this chapter you should be able to

1 Identify the uses of the CPT manual.

2 Name the developers of the CPT manual.

3 Know the importance of using the current-year CPT manual.

4 Identify placement of CPT codes on the CMS-1500 insurance form.

5 Recognize the symbols used in the CPT manual.

6 Identify the content of the CPT appendices.

7 List the major sections found in the CPT manual.

8 Interpret the information contained in the section Guidelines and notes.

9 Describe the CPT code format.

10 Append modifiers.

11 Describe what is meant by unlisted procedures/services.

12 State the purposes of a special report.

13 Review Category II and III CPT codes.

14 Locate the terms in the CPT index.

15 List the major features of Level II National Codes, HCPCS.

16 Demonstrate the ability to assign HCPCS codes.

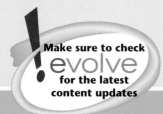

Make sure to check evolve **for the latest content updates**

Some of the CPT code descriptions for physician services include physician extender services. Physician extenders, such as nurse practitioners, physician assistants, and nurse anesthetists, etc., provide medical services typically performed by a physician. Within this educational material the term "physician" may include "and other qualified health care professionals" depending on the code. Refer to the official CPT® code descriptions and guidelines to determine codes that are appropriate to report services provided by non-physician practitioners.

THE PURPOSE OF THE CPT MANUAL

Current Procedural Terminology (CPT), also known as CPT-4, is a coding system developed by the American Medical Association (AMA) to convert widely accepted, uniform descriptions of medical, surgical, and diagnostic services rendered by health care providers into five-digit numeric codes. The use of the CPT codes enables health care providers to communicate both effectively and efficiently with third-party payers (i.e., commercial insurance companies, Medicare, Medicaid) about the procedures and services provided to the patient. For example, on an insurance form you can report a service by entering 21182 rather than "Reconstruction of orbital walls, rims, forehead, nasoethmoid complex following intra- and extracranial excision of benign tumor of the cranial bone (e.g., fibrous dysplasia) with multiple autografts (includes obtaining grafts); total area of bone grafting less than 40 sq cm." By using 21182, you are able to communicate not only quickly but also exactly about a very detailed service.

The majority of CPT codes are referred to as Category I codes and have been approved by the Editorial Panel of the AMA. Category II codes are optional performance measures (e.g., 3014F, screening mammography). Category III codes are temporary codes that identify emerging technologies, services, and procedures (e.g., 0163T, total disc arthroplasty).

Health care providers are reimbursed for the procedures and services rendered based on the codes submitted on a claim form. For an example of placement of the CPT codes on a claim form, refer to the arrow on Fig. 13-1 (24D).

Reporting the correct code is essential because incorrect coding can result in a provider being reimbursed incorrectly or in some cases being penalized by the government for submitting inappropriate claims. The CPT coding system is used by clinics, outpatient hospital departments, ambulatory surgery centers, and third-party payers to describe health care services. Although there are differences in the rules governing coding in various health care settings, CPT codes offer increased compatibility and comparability of data among users and providers, allowing for comparative analysis, research, and reimbursement.

The CPT coding system was first developed and published by the AMA in 1966 as a method of reporting medical and surgical procedures and services using standard terminology. Three editions of *Current Procedural Terminology* were published in the 1970s, and updates and revisions reflected changes in the technology and practices of health care. Use of the CPT manual was increased in 1983 when the Centers for Medicare and Medicaid Services (CMS), formerly the Health Care Financing Administration (HCFA), incorporated CPT codes into the Healthcare Common Procedural Coding System (HCPCS) to provide a uniform system of reporting services, procedures, and supplies. CPT codes are Level I codes and, for the most part, define professional services. Level II National Codes (HCPCS) are alphanumeric codes that are used by providers to report services, supplies, and equipment provided to Medicare and Medicaid patients for which no CPT codes exist.

HCPCS codes may be required even if a CPT Level I is available. Some third-party payers follow Medicare and Medicaid guidelines and may also require HCPCS Level II codes be assigned (e.g., G codes), so HCPCS may be required on non-Medicare and Medicaid patients. Certain HCPCS Level II codes are required by all payers, such as the drug codes, J codes.

UPDATING THE CPT MANUAL

Because the practice of medicine is ever changing, the CPT manual is ever changing. It is updated annually to reflect technologic advances and editorial revisions. It is very important to use the most current CPT manual available so as to provide quality data and ensure appropriate reimbursement. Many revisions to the CPT were necessary to address requirements of the Health Insurance Portability and Accountability Act of 1996 (HIPAA). HIPAA requires the Secretary of Health and Human Services to adopt national uniform standards for the electronic transmission of financial and administrative health information. These standards include a wide variety of health care information. One item that HIPAA requires is a common, concise coding system with clear, expandable definitions. The AMA is meeting this requirement by continuing to make the code definitions more precise.

HEALTH INSURANCE CLAIM FORM

APPROVED BY NATIONAL UNIFORM CLAIM COMMITTEE (NUCC) 02/12

PICA | | | | | | PICA

CARRIER

1. MEDICARE (Medicare#) MEDICAID (Medicaid#) TRICARE (ID#DoD#) CHAMPVA (Member ID#) GROUP HEALTH PLAN (ID#) FECA BLK LUNG (ID#) OTHER (ID#)

1a. INSURED'S I.D. NUMBER (For Program in Item 1)

2. PATIENT'S NAME (Last Name, First Name, Middle Initial)

3. PATIENT'S BIRTH DATE MM DD YY SEX M F

4. INSURED'S NAME (Last Name, First Name, Middle Initial)

5. PATIENT'S ADDRESS (No., Street)

6. PATIENT RELATIONSHIP TO INSURED Self Spouse Child Other

7. INSURED'S ADDRESS (No., Street)

CITY STATE

8. RESERVED FOR NUCC USE

CITY STATE

ZIP CODE TELEPHONE (Include Area Code) ( )

ZIP CODE TELEPHONE (Include Area Code) ( )

9. OTHER INSURED'S NAME (Last Name, First Name, Middle Initial)

10. IS PATIENT'S CONDITION RELATED TO:

11. INSURED'S POLICY GROUP OR FECA NUMBER

a. OTHER INSURED'S POLICY OR GROUP NUMBER

a. EMPLOYMENT? (Current or Previous) YES NO

a. INSURED'S DATE OF BIRTH MM DD YY SEX M F

b. RESERVED FOR NUCC USE

b. AUTO ACCIDENT? YES NO PLACE (State)

b. OTHER CLAIM ID (Designated by NUCC)

c. RESERVED FOR NUCC USE

c. OTHER ACCIDENT? YES NO

c. INSURANCE PLAN NAME OR PROGRAM NAME

d. INSURANCE PLAN NAME OR PROGRAM NAME

10d. CLAIM CODES (Designated by NUCC)

d. IS THERE ANOTHER HEALTH BENEFIT PLAN? YES NO If yes, complete items 9, 9a, and 9d.

READ BACK OF FORM BEFORE COMPLETING & SIGNING THIS FORM.
12. PATIENT'S OR AUTHORIZED PERSON'S SIGNATURE I authorize the release of any medical or other information necessary to process this claim. I also request payment of government benefits either to myself or to the party who accepts assignment below.

SIGNED _____ DATE _____

13. INSURED'S OR AUTHORIZED PERSON'S SIGNATURE I authorize payment of medical benefits to the undersigned physician or supplier for services described below.

SIGNED _____

PATIENT AND INSURED INFORMATION

14. DATE OF CURRENT ILLNESS, INJURY, or PREGNANCY(LMP) MM DD YY QUAL.

15. OTHER DATE QUAL. MM DD YY

16. DATES PATIENT UNABLE TO WORK IN CURRENT OCCUPATION FROM MM DD YY TO MM DD YY

17. NAME OF REFERRING PROVIDER OR OTHER SOURCE

17a. 17b. NPI

18. HOSPITALIZATION DATES RELATED TO CURRENT SERVICES FROM MM DD YY TO MM DD YY

19. ADDITIONAL CLAIM INFORMATION (Designated by NUCC)

20. OUTSIDE LAB? YES NO $ CHARGES

21. DIAGNOSIS OR NATURE OF ILLNESS OR INJURY Relate A-L to service line below (24E) ICD Ind.

A. B. C. D.
E. F. G. H.
I. J. K. L.

22. RESUBMISSION CODE ORIGINAL REF. NO.

23. PRIOR AUTHORIZATION NUMBER

24. A. DATE(S) OF SERVICE From MM DD YY To MM DD YY | B. PLACE OF SERVICE | C. EMG | D. PROCEDURES, SERVICES, OR SUPPLIES (Explain Unusual Circumstances) CPT/HCPCS MODIFIER | E. DIAGNOSIS POINTER | F. $ CHARGES | G. DAYS OR UNITS | H. EPSDT Family Plan | I. ID. QUAL. | J. RENDERING PROVIDER ID. #

1 | | | | | | | | | NPI
2 | | | | | | | | | NPI
3 | | | | | | | | | NPI
4 | | | | | | | | | NPI
5 | | | | | | | | | NPI
6 | | | | | | | | | NPI

PHYSICIAN OR SUPPLIER INFORMATION

25. FEDERAL TAX I.D. NUMBER SSN EIN

26. PATIENT'S ACCOUNT NO.

27. ACCEPT ASSIGNMENT? (For govt. claims, see back) YES NO

28. TOTAL CHARGE $

29. AMOUNT PAID $

30. Rsvd for NUCC Use $

31. SIGNATURE OF PHYSICIAN OR SUPPLIER INCLUDING DEGREES OR CREDENTIALS (I certify that the statements on the reverse apply to this bill and are made a part thereof.)

SIGNED DATE

32. SERVICE FACILITY LOCATION INFORMATION

a. NPI b.

33. BILLING PROVIDER INFO & PH # ( )

a. NPI b.

NUCC Instruction Manual available at: www.nucc.org

PLEASE PRINT OR TYPE

APPROVED OMB-0938-1197 FORM 1500 (02-12)

FIGURE 13-1 The CMS-1500 Health Insurance Claim Form.

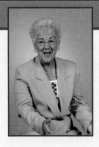

From the Trenches

"Beginners think that if you have the coding books (CPT, ICD-10-CM, ICD-9-CM) you're good to go. I tell them there is a story and history behind each code. . . . They must investigate codes, modifiers, HCPCS codes, and more before a final decision can be made. It is never boring!"

NANCY

Updated editions of the CPT manual are available for purchase in November for use beginning the following January 1.

CHECK THIS OUT ☞ The American Medical Association (AMA) has a website located at www.ama-assn.org.

EXERCISE 13-1 *The Purpose of the CPT Manual*

Complete the following:

1 The CPT manual was developed by the _____.

2 CPT stands for _____.

3 Providers of health care are paid based on the codes submitted for _____ or procedures provided to the patient.

4 The first CPT was published in this year: _____

5 In which year were CPT codes incorporated as Level I codes into the Healthcare Procedure Coding System (HCPCS)?

_____

(Answers are located in Appendix B)

CPT MANUAL FORMAT

The symbols used in the CPT manual are noted on the bottom of each page in the manual along with a short description of the symbol.

In the CPT manual, **new** codes are identified by the bullet (●) symbol that is placed in front of the code. Note the location of this symbol in Fig. 13-2.

New code for service/procedure symbol

●3XXXX Exchange of a previously placed arterial catheter during thrombolytic therapy

FIGURE 13-2 New CPT code symbol.

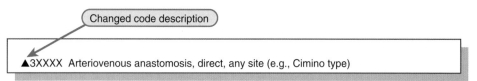

FIGURE 13-3 Changed CPT code symbol.

Pacemaker or ▶Pacing Cardioverter-◀ Defibrillator

A pacemaker system includes a pulse generator containing electronics and a battery, and one or more electrodes (leads). Pulse generators ▶are◀ placed in a subcutaneous "pocket" created in either a subclavicular site ▶or underneath the abdominal muscles just below the ribcage.◀ Electrodes may be inserted through a vein (transvenous) or ▶they may be placed◀ on the surface of the heart (epicardial).▶ The epicardial . . .

FIGURE 13-4 Changed CPT text symbols.

Important Symbols and Appendices

A triangle (▲) placed in front of a code indicates that the description for the code has been **changed** or modified since the previous edition. Changes may be additions, deletions, or revisions in code descriptions (Fig. 13-3).

When the text has changed, a right and a left triangle (▶ ◀) indicate the beginning and end of the text changes, as illustrated in Fig. 13-4.

 QUICK CHECK 13-1

1. Symbols with definitions are located at the bottom of the page in the CPT manual.
   True or False?

(Answers are located in Appendix C)

Appendix A lists all modifiers that are used to alter or modify codes. Modifiers will be discussed in detail later in the chapter and in greater detail in Chapter 14.

Appendix B of the CPT manual contains a complete list of the additions to, deletions from, and revisions of the CPT manual. When a code is listed in Appendix B, the type of change is also listed (Fig. 13-5).

Appendix C of the CPT manual contains clinical examples of many of the Evaluation and Management (E/M) codes (Fig. 13-6).

The examples in Appendix C are meant to offer a broad idea of the type of presenting problem that each code could represent. But a word of caution: Only the patient's record and the services rendered by the physician to a patient determine the level of service provided. Appendix C is not meant to be an exhaustive list of E/M services.

Appendix D in the CPT manual lists all add-on codes. The plus symbol (+) placed in front of a code indicates an **add-on code** (Fig. 13-7).

Add-on codes are never used alone; rather, they are reported with another primary procedure or service code. For example, code 11000 describes a debridement (removal of contaminated tissue) of up to 10% of the body surface. Add-on code 11001 is reported for each additional 10% of the body surface debrided or part thereof. Code 11001 cannot be reported unless code 11000 is reported first. Also notice in Fig. 13-7 that there is a note in parentheses that indicates that code 11001 can be used only in conjunction with code 11000.

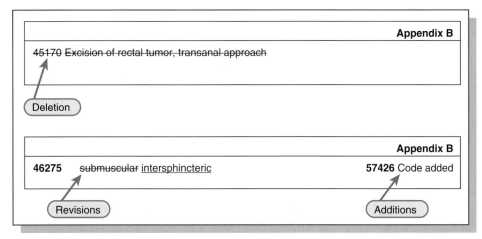

FIGURE 13–5   CPT manual Appendix B, showing types of changes.

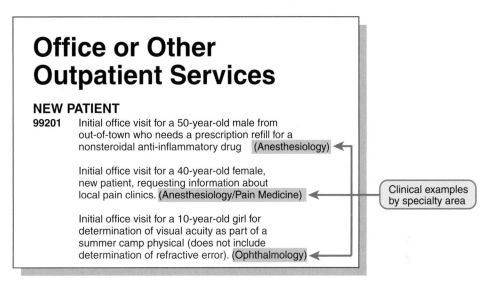

FIGURE 13–6   Appendix C of the CPT manual contains clinical examples in the use of E/M codes.

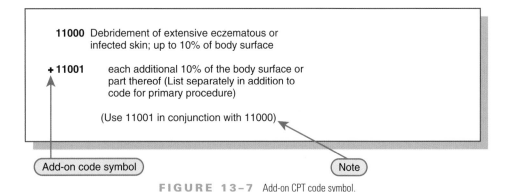

FIGURE 13–7   Add-on CPT code symbol.

Appendix E in the CPT manual contains the complete list of modifier -51 exempt codes. Modifier -51 indicates that more than one (multiple) procedure was performed. The circle with a line through it (⊘) identifies a **modifier -51 exempt** code (Fig. 13-8). Modifier -51 is discussed later in greater detail in Chapter 14.

Appendix F of the CPT manual contains the summary of CPT codes that are Modifier -63 exempt. Modifier -63 identifies procedures that are performed on infants who weigh less than

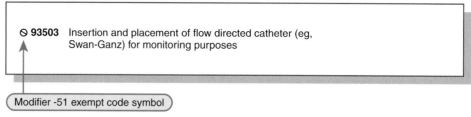

⊘ **93503** Insertion and placement of flow directed catheter (eg, Swan-Ganz) for monitoring purposes

Modifier -51 exempt code symbol

FIGURE 13–8 Modifier -51 exempt CPT code symbol.

4 kg or 8.8 pounds and represents a significant increase in the physician's work and complexity of service/procedure. Services/Procedures submitted with modifier -63 may be reviewed for an increase in reimbursement.

Appendix G is a summary of Moderate (Conscious) Sedation codes identified with a bullseye (⊙) that denotes a procedure that includes moderate (conscious) sedation. For example, 32405, Percutaneous needle biopsy of the lung or mediastinum, has a bullseye before the code indicating that bundled into the code is both the biopsy and any conscious sedation provided. Moderate or conscious sedation is the type that leaves the patient alert enough to follow directions but still sedated enough to alleviate pain.

Appendix H is the Alphabetic Index of Performance Measures by Clinical Condition or Topic and lists the Category II codes. Category II codes are optional tracking codes that are used to identify performance measures of clinical components that may be typically included in evaluation and management services. The codes make it easier to collect data about certain services or test results that contribute to the health and quality of care of the patient. You learn more about Category II codes later in this chapter. As of 2010, the Appendix H was removed from the CPT manual and can be accessed only on the AMA website at www.ama-assn.org.

Appendix I lists the Genetic Testing Code Modifiers but is deleted for 2013.

Appendix J is the Electrodiagnostic Medicine Listing of Sensory, Motor and Mixed Nerves that identify the sensory, motor, and mixed nerves with the corresponding conduction study code. Codes are used to report motor and sensory nerve conduction studies. Appendix J identifies the nerves in each of the nerve groups. Sensory and motor nerves are part of the peripheral nervous system (PNS) and run from the stimulus receptors to the central nervous system (CNS). A table in Appendix J lists the "reasonable maximum number of studies performed per diagnostic category necessary for a physician to arrive at a diagnosis in 90% of the patients with that final diagnosis." The recommended number of studies for each indication (condition) is identified. For example, if the indication was myopathy, it is recommended that the physician perform two needle electromyographies (EMGs), two motor nerve conduction studies (NCS), two sensory NCS, and two neuromuscular junction testings.

Appendix K, Product Pending FDA Approval, contains the lightning bolt symbol (⚡) that identifies codes that are being tracked by the AMA to monitor Food and Drug Administration (FDA) status for approval of a drug. The Internet site www.ama-assn.org provides updates to the list of FDA pending approval codes.

Appendix L, Vascular Families, is a helpful listing of the orders of the vascular families. Listed are the first order, second order, third order branches, and beyond third order branches. The assumption is made that the starting point is the aorta. If the vessel is accessed at some other location, the branches, of course, would not be correct.

Appendix M, Deleted CPT Codes, lists the current-year code to replace a deleted code.

Appendix N, Summary of Resequenced CPT codes. In 2010, the American Medical Association introduced **resequencing**. Historically, the codes within a CPT section have been in numeric order, but that is no longer the case. The pound symbol (#) appears before the resequenced codes (see Fig. 13-9). An example of this resequencing is in the 51725-51798 range where the code and code description for 51797 follow 51729. Code 51797 also appears in correct numeric order, but next to the code a note states "Code is out of numerical sequence. See 51725-51798." See Appendix N of the CPT for a complete list of the resequenced codes.

Appendix O, Multianalyte Assays with Algorithmic Analyses is a listing of codes for advanced diagnostics, such as ovarian oncology code 81500, which assays for two proteins (CA-125 and HE4) for a risk factor.

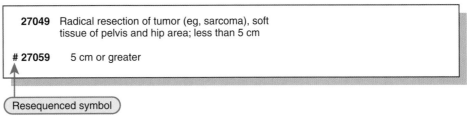

FIGURE 13–9 Resequenced CPT code symbol.

EXERCISE 13-2   *Symbols*

Match the following code symbols with the correct definition:

1 ▲ _____   **a.** beginning and end of text changes

2 ▶◀ _____   **b.** modifier -51 exempt

3 ● _____   **c.** revised procedure description

4 ⊘ _____   **d.** add-on

5 + _____   **e.** moderate (conscious) sedation included

6 ⊙ _____   **f.** pending FDA approval status

7 ⌀ _____   **g.** new

8 Where is a complete list of additions, deletions, and revisions located in the CPT manual? _____

9 Which CPT manual appendix contains a complete list of all modifier -51 exempt codes? _____

10 Which CPT manual appendix contains a complete list of add-on codes? _____

(Answers are located in Appendix B)

CPT Sections

The CPT manual is composed of six chapters into which all codes and descriptions are categorized. These chapters are called **sections.**

THE SECTIONS OF THE CPT MANUAL

- Evaluation and Management   99201-99499
- Anesthesia   00100-01999
- Surgery   10021-69990
- Radiology   70010-79999
- Pathology and Laboratory   80047-89398
- Medicine   90281-99607

The sections are further divided into subsections, subheadings, categories, and subcategories. A **section** is a chapter that covers one of the six topics included in the CPT manual: Evaluation/ Management (E/M), Anesthesia, Surgery, Radiology, Pathology/Laboratory, and Medicine codes. The CPT codes are arranged in numerical order in each section. Let's review these six sections.

Sections are divided into **subsections**. For example, the Surgery section includes subsections of Integumentary, Musculoskeletal, Respiratory, Cardiovascular, and so forth.

Example

Section:	Surgery
Subsection:	Cardiovascular System
Subheading:	Arteries and Veins
Category:	Embolectomy/Thrombectomy
Subcategory:	Arterial, With or Without Catheter

Example

Section:	Surgery
Subsection:	Nervous System
Subheading:	Skull, Meninges, and Brain
Category:	Surgery of Skull Base
Subcategory:	Approach Procedures

EXERCISE 13-3 *Section, Subsection, Subheading, and Category*

To see an example of section, subsection, subheading, and category, locate the code 19000 Puncture aspiration of cyst of breast in the CPT in the Surgery section.

With a CPT beside you, open to the page where CPT code 19000 is located, or referring to Fig. 13-10, find the information on the top of the CPT manual page:

Section. At the top of the page, the word "Surgery" indicates the section. Note that this word is followed by a range of numbers, which is a list of all the code numbers located on that page.

Subsection. Also at the top of the page, the phrase "Integumentary System" indicates the subsection.

Subheading. The word "Breast" indicates the subheading.

Category. The word "Incision" indicates the category.

In summary, the divisions for the previous example are

Section:	Surgery
Subsection:	Integumentary System
Subheading:	Breast
Category:	Incision

Now you try one.

With a CPT manual open to the page that contains code 30100, locate the following information for the 30100 code:

1 Section: _____

2 Subsection: _____

3 Subheading: _____

4 Category: _____

(Answers are located in Appendix B)

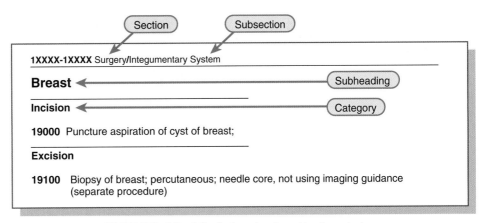

FIGURE 13–10 Section, subsection, subheading, and category.

Subsections, **subheadings, categories,** and **subcategories** are divisions of sections that are based on anatomy, procedure, condition, description, or approach.

Using the section, subsection, subheading, and category information makes it much faster and easier to get around in the CPT manual.

CPT Guidelines

Each section in the CPT manual includes Guidelines. The Guidelines provide specific information about coding in that section and contain valuable information for the coder. Guidelines that are applicable to all codes in the section are found at the beginning of each section (Fig. 13-11).

Notes pertaining to specific codes or groups of codes are listed before or after the codes (Fig. 13-12).

The Guidelines and notes may contain definitions of terms, applicable modifiers, subsection information, unlisted services, special reports information, or clinical examples. Always read the Guidelines and notes before coding to help ensure accurate assignment of the CPT codes.

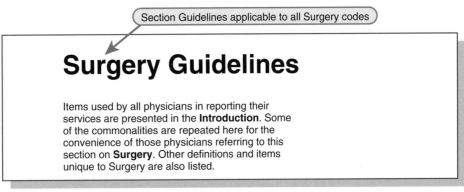

FIGURE 13–11 Section Guidelines.

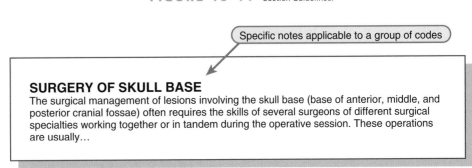

FIGURE 13–12 Specific notes.

EXERCISE 13-4   *Guidelines*

Using the Guidelines for each of the sections, answer the following questions:

1 Write the definition of a chief complaint using the E/M Guidelines.

_____

_____

_____

2 According to the Surgery Guidelines, surgical destruction is a part of a surgical procedure and _____ methods of destruction are not ordinarily listed separately.

3 According to the Radiology Guidelines, who must sign a written report to have the report considered part of the radiologic procedure? _____

4 Under whose supervision are Pathology and Laboratory services provided? _____

5 What is the code listed in the Medicine Guidelines that is to be used to identify materials supplied by the physician that are beyond those ordinarily included in the service provided? _____

(Answers are located in Appendix B)

Code Format

CAUTION *You may not have realized it, but you've just been given a critical clue to coding—the semicolon. The following information will help you understand why the semicolon is so important.*

Procedure and service descriptions are located after the code (Fig. 13-13). These are commonly accepted descriptions of procedures or services that are provided to patients.

There are two types of codes: **stand-alone codes** and **indented codes** (Fig. 13-14).

Only the stand-alone codes have the full description; indented codes are listed under associated stand-alone codes. It is understood that descriptions for indented codes include that portion of the stand-alone code description that precedes the semicolon. The purpose of the semicolon is to save space.

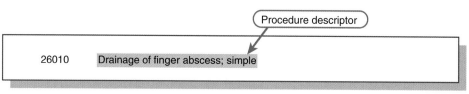

FIGURE 13-13   Code and description format.

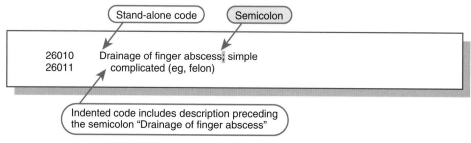

FIGURE 13-14   Stand-alone codes and indented codes.

In Fig. 13-14, the code 26011 is an indented code—the indentation serves to represent the words "Drainage of finger abscess," which appear before the semicolon in CPT code 26010. The semicolon is a powerful tool in the CPT manual; when you see it, be sure to read the words before it carefully.

The words following the semicolon can indicate alternative anatomic sites, alternative procedures, or a description of the extent of the service.

CAUTION *Before assigning an indented code, make sure you refer to the preceding stand-alone code and read the words that precede the semicolon. That is the only way to ensure a full description and select a correct code.*

Example

Alternative Anatomic Site:

27705	Osteotomy; tibia
27707	fibula
27709	tibia and fibula

Alternative Procedure:

31505	Laryngoscopy, indirect; diagnostic (separate procedure)
31510	with biopsy
31511	with removal of foreign body
31512	with removal of lesion
31513	with vocal cord injection

Description of Extent of the Service:

20520	Removal of foreign body in muscle or tendon sheath; simple
20525	deep or complicated

EXERCISE 13-5 | *Code Format*

Complete the following:

1 Describe a stand-alone code.

_____

_____

2 Describe an indented code.

_____

_____

3 Words following the semicolon in stand-alone codes can indicate the following three things:

a _____

b _____

c _____

(Answers are located in Appendix B)

Modifiers

Modifiers provide additional information to the third-party payer about services provided to a patient. At times, the five-digit CPT code may not reflect completely the service or procedure provided. Because numeric codes, not written procedure descriptions, are required by third-party payers, additional numbers or letters may be added to the basic five-digit code to modify the CPT code and provide further specificity. These additional modifiers may be two numbers, two letters, or a letter and a number and are appended, or "tacked on," to the basic five-digit CPT code. In the HCPCS manual, two-place modifiers such as -RC and -F1 are used. Notice the HCPCS modifiers are alpha characters or alphanumeric.

In the CPT system, a modifier is an appended two-digit number, such as:

Example

-62, two surgeons
or
-51, multiple procedures

The two-digit modifier is added to the five-digit CPT code.

Example

Code 43820 is the CPT procedure code for a gastrojejunostomy, without vagotomy (removal of part of the vagus nerve). If two surgeons with different surgical skills participated as primary surgeons, each performing a specific part of the procedure, the procedure code 43820 could be altered by the addition of the modifier -62 to indicate co-surgeons (Fig. 13-15).

The code would be 43820-62 for a gastrojejunostomy, without vagotomy, in which two surgeons participated as primary surgeons. Each physician would submit his or her own bill, indicating code 43820-62.

For a complete listing of all modifiers, see Appendix A in the CPT manual. Refer to Fig. 13-16 for an example of the information found in Appendix A. Further information regarding modifiers is presented throughout the following chapters of this text.

CPT modifiers are listed first in descending numeric order (e.g., -62-50), and CPT modifiers are listed before HCPCS modifiers (e.g., -62-RT) in this book.

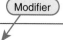

Modifier

62 **Two Surgeons:** When two surgeons work together as primary surgeons performing distinct part(s) of a procedure, each surgeon should report his/her distinct operative work by adding the modifier 62 to the procedure code and any associated add-on code(s) for that procedure as long as both surgeons continue to work together as primary surgeons. Each surgeon should report the co-surgery once using the same procedure code. If additional procedure(s) (including add-on procedure(s)) are performed during the same surgical session, separate codes(s) may also be reported without the modifier 62 added. **Note**: If a co-surgeon acts as an assistant in the performance of additional procedure(s) during the same surgicial session, those services may be reported using separate procedure code(s) with the modifier 80 or modifier 82 added, as appropriate.

FIGURE 13–15 Two-digit modifier.

> Appendix A lists all modifiers with complete directions for use

APPENDIX A
Modifiers

22   **Increased Procedural Services:** When the work required to provide a service is substantially greater than typically required, it may be identified by adding modifier 22 to the usual procedure code. Documentation must support the substantial additional work and the reason for the additional work (ie, increased intensity, time, technical difficulty of procedure, severity of patient's condition, physical and mental effort required). **Note:** This modifier should not be appended to an E/M service.

FIGURE 13-16 Modifiers in Appendix A.

EXERCISE 13-6 *Modifiers*

Using Appendix A of the CPT manual and the information you just learned, answer the following:

1 What is the two-digit modifier that indicates two primary surgeons? _____

2 If the CPT code is 43820 (gastrojejunostomy without vagotomy) and two primary surgeons performed the service, the service could be stated this way: _____, by each surgeon.

Use Appendix A of the CPT manual to list the correct two-digit modifier in the following examples:

3 Bilateral inguinal herniorrhaphy: _____

4 A postoperative ureterotomy patient has to be returned to the operating room (unplanned) for a complication related to the initial procedure during the postoperative period: _____

5 A decision to perform surgery is made during an evaluation and management service on the day before or the day of surgery: _____

6 Multiple procedures performed during the same surgical session: _____

7 A surgical team is required: _____

8 Physician A actively assists physician B during a surgical procedure: _____

(Answers are located in Appendix B)

Unlisted Procedures

When developing the CPT manual, the AMA realized that not every surgical and diagnostic procedure could be listed. There may not be a code for many procedures that are considered experimental, newly approved, or seldom used. In addition, medical advancements often create a variation of procedures currently performed. A procedure or service not found in the CPT manual can be coded as an unlisted procedure if no Category I or III exists to describe the procedure/service provided. For example, when the first heart transplant was performed, there was no code to report the new surgical procedure. Until a code was available, the unlisted code for cardiac surgery was used to report this procedure (Fig. 13-17).

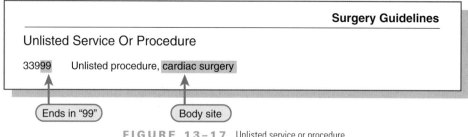

FIGURE 13–17 Unlisted service or procedure.

The Surgery Guidelines have unlisted procedure codes listed by body site or type of procedure. Individually unlisted procedure codes are also at the end of the subsection or subheading to which they refer. For example, at the end of the Cardiovascular System subsection, Heart and Pericardium subheading, is the unlisted cardiac procedure code 33999, and at the end of the Respiratory System subsection, Lungs and Pleura subheading is the unlisted lungs/pleura code 32999.

EXERCISE 13-7   *Unlisted Procedures*

Assuming there is no Category III code available for the procedure you are reporting, using the CPT Guidelines in the front of the sections indicated below, locate the five-digit unlisted procedure code for each of the following:

1 Surgery

Unlisted procedure; middle ear: Code: _____

    arthroscopy: Code: _____

    esophagus: Code: _____

2 Pathology and Laboratory

Unlisted procedure; cytogenetic study: Code: _____

    urinalysis procedure: Code: _____

    chemistry procedure: Code: _____

3 Medicine   Code: _____

Unlisted special service, procedure, or report:

4 Radiology

Unlisted procedure; clinical brachytherapy: Code: _____

Unlisted miscellaneous procedure;   Code: _____
diagnostic nuclear medicine:

(Answers are located in Appendix B)

Category II Codes

Earlier in the chapter you were introduced to Category II codes located on the AMA website, www.ama-assn.org/. Now it is time to take a closer look at the purpose of these codes and how they are reported.

In December of 2006, Congress enacted a law that established a voluntary program within Medicare that paid physicians a bonus for reporting these quality measures. The pay-for-reporting program was the Physician Quality Reporting Initiative (PQRI), later renamed the

Physician Quality Reporting System (PQRS). The measures have been established to determine if the physician is performing certain elements that are considered to be necessary elements of care. For example, patients with diabetes mellitus are at a high risk for heart attack and stroke, and it is very important that these patients control not only their diabetes but also their blood pressure and cholesterol levels. The instruction in the PQRS measure for blood pressure management indicates that at a minimum the diabetic patient's blood pressure is to be reported once in a 12-month period for each patient with diabetes 18-75 years of age. According to the measure, a controlled pressure is less than 140/80 mm Hg.

The **systolic** pressure would be reported with one of the following codes:

3074F	$<$130 mm Hg
3075F	130-139 mm Hg
3077F	$\geq$140 mm Hg ($\geq$ means equal to or greater than)

The **diastolic** pressure would be reported with one of the following codes:

3078F	$<$80 mm Hg
3079F	80-89 mm Hg
3080F	$\geq$90 mm Hg

If the documentation indicated the patient's blood pressure reading was 138/100, you would report 3075F for the systolic pressure and 3080F for the diastolic pressure.

In addition to the code, a modifier may be assigned. There are only 4 modifiers approved for use with Category II codes, and they all report the reason the performance measure was not performed.

1P	medical reasons, such as contraindicated due to adverse drug interaction
2P	patient reason, such as the patient declined for religious reasons
3P	system reasons, such as the equipment to perform the service was not available
8P	not otherwise specified

The measures also state that an E/M code from the CPT or a G code from the HCPCS coding system are the two types of codes permissible with these Category II codes. For example, if 99201 (new patient, office or other patient visit) was reported for a patient with a diagnosis of diabetes and whose blood pressure reading was 128/87 mm Hg. The Category II codes 3074F ($<$130 mm Hg) and 3078F ($<$80 mm Hg) would be reported with 99201 because Category II codes are supplemental codes. HCPCS codes G0270/ G0271 (Medical nutrition therapy) may also be reported with the codes in the range 3074F-3080F.

The diagnoses codes that may be submitted with 3074F-3080F are also listed in the standards for the PQRS measure. For example, E10-E11/250.00-250.09, Diabetes mellitus, and O24/648.00-648.04, Complications of pregnancy, are ranges of diagnosis codes that are acceptable for submitting with 3074F-3080F.

The Category II codes are reported in field 24D on the CMS-1500 paper claim and on the electronic claim (837p) in segment SV1, the professional services segment.

You might wonder why physicians would agree to do all this additional tracking and coding! CMS pays a bonus to physicians who report at least 80% of Medicare encounters with quality measures. The physician's submissions are tracked by the NPI (national provider identification number) because that is the unique physician identification that never changes.

Even if a physician moves from one clinic to another, the NPI for that physician moves right with him or her. The bonus is paid not only on those patients that the physician submits quality measures for but on all Medicare services provided during that 12-month period. For example, if a physician receives $200,000 of Medicare revenue for the year and has reported on at least 80% of his or her encounters for the year with a maximum of three measures per patient (or less if applicable), that physician would receive a $3,000 bonus from CMS. This is a significant amount of money, especially when you consider that this is for reporting measures that the physician would usually perform anyway. The numbers get even more impressive, when applied to a group practice. For example, a clinic has 40 physicians and each generated about $200,000 annually in Medicare revenue. The PQRS bonus could mean an additional $120,000 for the practice. That is a big financial incentive to record, code, and submit the measures. Further, there is nothing a coder likes more than additional codes—it is, after all, great job security!

You can anticipate that these measures will move from voluntary to mandatory, and tracking these measures will be just another element of the ever-changing world of coding.

CHECK THIS OUT 👉 For more information on PQRS, check out www.cms.gov/pqrs/.

Category III Codes

Category III codes report emerging technology and are temporary codes used for up to 5 years. If there is a Category III code for the service or procedure you are reporting, you must use the Category III code, not the Category I unlisted code.

Category I codes (Level 1) are those that are widely used to describe services and procedures that have been approved by the Food and Drug Administration (FDA), if appropriate. Category I codes also relate to services and procedures that have been proven to have clinical effectiveness. Category III codes describe services and procedures that may not have been approved by the FDA, may not be widely offered, and may not have been proven to be clinically effective. The use of the Category III codes allows physicians, other health care professionals, third-party payers, researchers, and health policy experts to identify emerging trends in health care.

Format of Category III Codes. The codes have five digits—four numbers and a letter: for example, 0095T (removal of total disc arthroplasty). Prior to the existence of Category III codes, you would have reported this procedure using an unlisted code, because there was no specific code that described the antiprothrombin antibody. But because there now is a Category III code available that describes it, you must report the antiprothrombin antibody using the Category III code, not an unlisted code from Category I.

Category III codes may or may not eventually receive Category I code status and be placed in the main part of the CPT.

QUICK CHECK 13-2

1. A Category III code would be reported rather than a Category I _____ code.

(Answers are located in Appendix C)

Publication of Category III Codes. New Category III codes are released twice a year (January and July) via the AMA website. The full set of temporary codes is published in the next edition of the CPT in a section following the Medicine section.

Special Reports

Special reports must accompany claims when an unusual, new, seldom used, or Category I unlisted code, or Category III code is submitted. The special report should include an adequate definition or description of the **nature, extent,** and **need** for the procedure or service and the **time, effort,** and **equipment** necessary to provide the service. The special report helps the third-party payer determine the appropriateness of the care and the medical necessity of the service provided.

From the Trenches

What advice do you give to a coder looking to advance or move up?

"Enlarge your circle of influence, investigate other specialties, look to areas of coding compliance, attend workshops, become certified, and continue to learn."

NANCY

QUICK CHECK 13-3

1. Special reports must be submitted with claims for procedures that are unusual, new, seldom used, or use Category I ＿＿＿＿＿＿ codes or Category ＿＿＿＿＿＿ codes.

(Answers are located in Appendix C)

STARTING WITH THE INDEX

The CPT index is located at the back of the CPT manual and is arranged alphabetically. Index headings located at the top right and left corners of the index pages direct the coder to the entries that are included on that page, much like a dictionary. Use of index headings speeds location of the term (Fig. 13-18).

Locating the Terms

Code numbers are displayed in the CPT index in one of the ways shown in the following example.

Example

single code:	38115
multiple codes:	26645, 26650
range of codes:	22305-22325

See Fig. 13-19 for an example of the display in the index using the single, multiple, and range formats.

Single Code

When only one code is stated, you should verify the code in the main (tabular) portion of the CPT manual to ensure its accuracy.

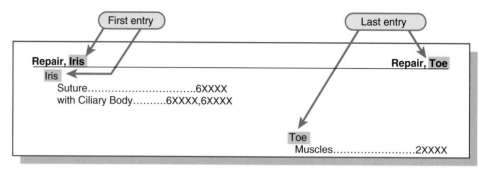

FIGURE 13-18 CPT manual index headings.

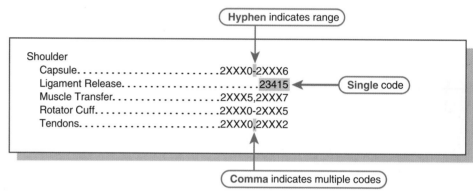

FIGURE 13-19 Code display.

Multiple Codes

The use of a **comma** between code numbers indicates the presence of only those numbers displayed. If more than one code is listed, then all codes must be reviewed in the tabular to make an accurate choice.

Range of Codes

A range is indicated by a **hyphen.** When a range is given in the index, you must look up each code within the range in the tabular of the CPT manual to select the appropriate code from the range. There may even be multiple ranges listed.

The index is in alphabetic order by main terms and is further divided by subterms. Fig. 13-20 illustrates the main term and subterm as used in the index. Having identified the main term of the service or procedure, you can locate the term in the index. When you are just beginning to use the CPT manual, it may be difficult to locate the main term. Not being able to locate a term in the index can be very frustrating, but don't be discouraged if you don't identify the main term on the first try. This is a skill that is learned by practice, and part of the practice is making mistakes. Soon you'll be locating those main terms quickly. Just keep thinking about the service or procedure and looking up the words in the index.

🖐 **CAUTION** *Never code directly from the index. You can't be sure you have the right code until you have located the code in the main portion of the CPT manual and read the information presented there regarding the specifics of the code.*

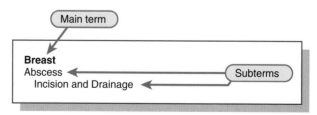

FIGURE 13-20 CPT manual index indicating main terms and subterms.

Some basic location methods will help you to locate these main terms.

LOCATION METHODS

- Service or Procedure
- Anatomic Site
- Condition or Disease
- Synonym
- Eponym
- Abbreviation

Let's take these location methods and apply each one to locating "repair of a fracture of a femur" in the following exercise.

EXERCISE 13-8 *Term Practice*

Service or Procedure

1 When using the service or procedure location method, "repair" would be the main term in "**repair** of a fracture of a femur."

  a Locate "Repair" in the index of the CPT manual. Using this location method, "Repair" is the main term and the subterms are "Fracture" and "Femur."

  b Under the main term "Repair," locate the subterm "Femur." If you were to look under "Repair" and then look for the term "Fracture," you wouldn't find "Fracture," because listed under "Repair" are the anatomic divisions that can be repaired. "Fracture" isn't an anatomic division, so it isn't located under "Repair." It can be just as difficult to locate the correct subterm as it is to find the main term.

Right now, don't be concerned with looking up the codes in the main part of the CPT manual. Concentrate on learning how to locate the main term and subterms in the index of the CPT manual.

Anatomic Site

2 The second method of locating an anatomic site uses the word **"femur"** as the main term, and the subterms are "fracture" and "repair."

  a Locate "Femur" in the index of the CPT manual.

  b Under the main term "Femur," locate the subterm "Fracture."

  c Notice that the entry "Fracture" is further divided based on repair type (e.g., closed treatment) or anatomic location (e.g., distal).

Condition or Disease

3 The third location method focuses on the condition or disease. In this instance you would use the main term **"fracture"** as a condition.

  a Locate the main term "Fracture" in the index.

  b Locate the subterm "Femur."

The use of the first three location methods will usually get you to the applicable codes in the index. If you try each of the first three methods and still can't locate the codes in the index, don't despair; try one of the other location methods: synonym, eponym, or abbreviation.

Synonym

4 The fourth location method involves synonyms. Synonyms are words with similar meanings.

  a Toe joint is a **synonym** for interphalangeal joint or metatarsophalangeal joint. Suppose, then, you couldn't think of the correct medical term, but you could think of the word "toe." In that case, you could look up "Toe" in the CPT manual index, and that entry would direct you to:

  see Interphalangeal Joint, Toe; Metatarsophalangeal Joint; Phalanx

Eponym

5 The fifth location method uses **eponyms.** Eponyms are things that are named after people. For example, the Barr Procedure—a tendon-transfer procedure—was named after the person who developed it.

  a Locate "Barr Procedure" in the CPT manual index. You are directed to:

  See Tendon, Transfer, Leg, Lower

Continued

Abbreviation

6 The sixth location method uses **abbreviations.** Abbreviations are common in medicine for names of drugs, diseases, and procedures.

   a Locate the abbreviation "INH" in the index of the CPT manual. You are directed to:

   See Drug Assay

Medicine uses many synonyms, eponyms, and abbreviations. A good medical dictionary that contains the most common synonyms, eponyms, and abbreviations will be a necessity for you.

Locate each of the following main terms in the CPT manual index, and then locate the subterms and secondary subterms and fill in the code(s) you find there:

MAIN TERM	SUBTERM	SECONDARY SUBTERM	
1 Repair	Abdomen	Suture	Code: _____
2 Femur	Abscess	Incision	Code: _____
3 Fracture	Ankle	Lateral	Codes: _____ - _____

(Answers are located in Appendix B)

You are now ready to put your term location skills to work by doing the next exercise.

EXERCISE 13-9   *Main Term Location*

Identify the main terms in the following examples and write the main term on the line provided. Then locate the main terms and any subterms in the CPT manual index. Write the code listed in the index for that service or procedure on the line provided.

1 Description: Emergency Department Services, Physician Direction of Advanced Life Support

   a Main term: _____

   b Locate the code available in the index of the CPT manual for Emergency Department Services, Physician Direction of Advanced Life Support.

   Code: _____

2 Condition/Disease: Intertrochanteric femoral fracture (closed treatment)

   a Main term: _____

   b Locate the code available in the index of the CPT manual for intertrochanteric femoral fracture (closed treatment).

   Code: _____

3 Procedure: Removal of gallbladder calculi by means of an open procedure

   a Main term: _____

   b Locate the code available in the index of the CPT manual for removal of gallbladder calculi.

   Code: _____

4 Anatomic site: Lung, bullae excision

   a Main term: _____

   b Locate the code available in the index of the CPT manual for excision of bullae of lung.

   Code: _____

(Answers are located in Appendix B)

As you can probably see from this exercise, there are often many ways to locate an item in the index. The same word can serve as a main term or a subterm, depending on the location method you are using. In addition, the annual updating of the CPT results in numerous changes within the index.

You will be locating terms in the CPT manual index throughout your study of this text. For your ready reference, there is also a guideline at the beginning of the index in the CPT manual that contains directions for the use of the CPT manual index. **Appendix B of this text will list not only the correct code answer, but also one index location for that code.** For example, if the correct answer is 99203, the following appears after the code: (Office and/or Other Outpatient Services, New Patient). It is difficult to locate items in the CPT index when you begin coding, so if you get stuck and just cannot locate the index entry, you will be able to find one location following each code in Appendix B of this text.

QUICK CHECK 13-4

1. In the CPT manual there are instructions for using the index. These instructions appear just before the index. The heading on this page is Index, Instructions for the

_____ of the _____ Index.

(Answers are located in Appendix C)

See

"See" is a **cross-reference** term found in the index of the CPT manual. The term directs you to another term or other terms.

"*See*" indicates that the correct code will be found elsewhere.

Example

Anticoagulant   *See* Clotting Inhibitors

EXERCISE 13-10   *See*

Complete the following:

1 Locate the term "Renal Disease Services" in the CPT index. You are directed to

_____.

2 Locate the abbreviation "ANA" in the CPT index. The entry you find is _____.

3 Locate the term "Arm" in the CPT index. You are directed to _____.

(Answers are located in Appendix B)

HISTORY OF NATIONAL LEVEL CODES

CPT coding is only one of a two-part coding system called HCPCS (pronounced hick-picks). The Centers for Medicare and Medicaid Services (CMS), formerly the Health Care Financing Administration, developed the Healthcare Common Procedure Coding System in 1983. The HCPCS is a collection of codes that represents procedures, supplies, products, and services that may be provided to Medicare and Medicaid beneficiaries and to individuals enrolled in private health insurance programs.

Two Levels of Codes

HCPCS is divided into two levels or groups.

Level I codes are CPT codes in the CPT manual, which was developed and is maintained and copyrighted by the AMA. The CPT is the primary coding system used in the outpatient setting to code professional services provided to patients.

Level II codes (National Codes) are approved and maintained jointly by the Alpha-Numeric Workgroup, consisting of the CMS, the Health Insurance Association of America, and the Blue Cross and Blue Shield Association. Level II codes are five-position alphanumeric codes representing physician and nonphysician services and supplies that are not represented in the Level I codes.

There used to be **Level III** codes (Local Codes) that were developed by Medicare carriers or state payers for use at the local (carrier) level. These were five-position alphanumeric codes representing physician and nonphysician services that were not represented in the Level I or Level II codes. Local codes are no longer available since the implementation of HIPAA (Health Insurance Portability and Accountability Act). Some local codes were integrated into the National Codes (HCPCS).

CPT codes do not cover all services that are provided to patients. Allied health care professionals—such as dentists, orthodontists, and various technical support services, such as ambulance services—are not specifically reportable with the CPT coding system. There are also no codes in the CPT system for many of the supplies that are used in patient care (e.g., drugs, durable medical equipment, and orthoses). Reporting of National Codes is mandatory on all Medicare and Medicaid claims submitted for payment for services of the previously listed professionals. Although many of the National Codes were developed for use when reporting for services rendered to Medicare patients, many third-party payers now require that providers use the National Codes when submitting bills for non-Medicare patients too, because the system allows for continuity and specificity. This uniformity also helps the effort to collect uniform health service data.

QUICK CHECK 13-5

1. What is the code range for Drugs? _____

2. In what publication are these codes (from Question 1) published?
   a. HCPCS
   b. CPT
   c. CMT
   d. ICD

(Answers are located in Appendix C)

The first digit in a national code is a letter such as A, B, C, D, E, G, H, J, K, L, M, P, Q, R, S, T, or V that is followed by four numbers. Codes beginning with the letters K, G, Q, and S are for temporary assignment until a definitive decision can be made about appropriate code assignment. The K codes are temporary codes for durable medical equipment, the G codes are temporary codes for procedures and professional services, and the Q codes are temporary codes for procedures, supplies, and Durable Medical Equipment (DME) codes. S codes are temporary Blue Cross/Blue Shield codes that are not valid for Medicare or Medicaid patients. All codes and descriptions are updated annually by the CMS in November for use the following January 1. The alphanumeric listing contains headings of groups of codes, as illustrated in Fig. 13-21.

Note: In Figs. 13-21 through 13-27, and 13-30, the HCPCS codes are samples for the purpose of illustration only. They may not be displayed as such in the current HCPCS manual.

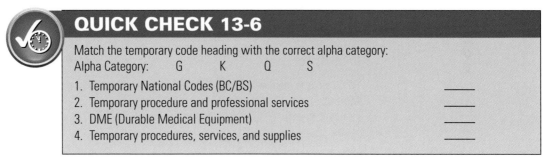

QUICK CHECK 13-6

Match the temporary code heading with the correct alpha category:
Alpha Category: G   K   Q   S

1. Temporary National Codes (BC/BS)   _____
2. Temporary procedure and professional services   _____
3. DME (Durable Medical Equipment)   _____
4. Temporary procedures, services, and supplies   _____

(Answers are located in Appendix C)

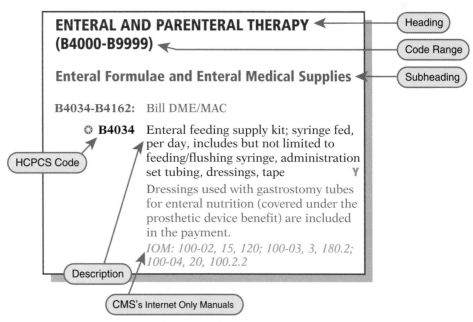

FIGURE 13–21 CMS's Healthcare Common Procedure Coding System (HCPCS), National Codes.

Note that following the heading (in Fig. 13-21) is the range of codes available for assignment in the category. There are also subheadings preceding the codes to identify the type of codes that follow.

National Codes are not used by health care facilities to report services provided to inpatients. Inpatient health care facilities use the diagnosis (from ICD-10-CM/ICD-9-CM) as the basis of payment for their services and assign codes from ICD-10-PCS/ICD-9-CM, Volume 3, for inpatient procedures. The two levels of National Codes are used in outpatient settings (including physicians' offices) where the basis of payment is the service rendered, not the diagnosis.

General Guidelines. The HCPCS manual includes the general guidelines for use of the National Codes, a list of modifiers, the codes, a Table of Drugs, and an index. We begin our study of the HCPCS manual at the index. Publishers of HCPCS manuals have a variety of entries in their individual manuals, so expect to see variations in the number and type of index entries. You have to be able to locate items in the index in order to be able to identify the correct code. The main index terms include tests, services, supplies, orthoses, prostheses, medical equipment, drugs, therapies, and some medical and surgical procedures. The subterms of the index are listed under the main term to which they apply, along with the code.

Example

Blood glucose monitor is found under the entry:

Monitor
   blood glucose, E0607

You then locate the code in the main part of the manual and read any notes that are listed with the code.

General rules for coding using the National Codes are as follows:
1. Never code directly from the index. Always use both the alphanumeric listing and the index.
2. Analyze the statement or description provided that designates the item that requires a code.
3. Identify the main term in the index.
4. Check for relevant subterms under the main term. Verify the meaning of any unfamiliar abbreviations.
5. Note the code(s) found after the selected main term or subterm.
6. After locating the term and the code in the index, verify the code in the tabular to ensure the specificity of the code.
7. In most cases, for each entry a specific code is provided. In some cases, you are referred to a range of codes among which you can locate the required code. You must review the entire range of codes in the tabular to locate the correct entry.

   If you are referred to a single code, locate that code in the tabular. Verify the code and description to be sure that you have selected the correct code to describe the item you are reporting.
8. In all cases, when locating an entry in the index, it is necessary to look at all descriptors under the main term and subterms in order to identify the correct entry and to locate the code in the tabular.

QUICK CHECK 13-7

In the HCPCS index, locate the main term "Aerosol." Identify the subterms that represent:
a. compressor E0571, E0572
b. compressor filter K0178-K0179
c. mask K0180

1. A single code   _____
2. A range of codes   _____
3. Multiple codes   _____

(Answers are located in Appendix C)

CODE GROUPINGS

- A Codes   Transportation Services including Ambulance
  Medical and Surgical Supplies
  Gradient Compression Stockings
  Wound Care
  Respiratory Durable Medical Equipment,
      Inexpensive and Routinely Purchased
  Administrative, Miscellaneous, and Investigational
- B Codes   Enteral and Parenteral Therapy
- C Codes   CMS Hospital Outpatient Prospective Payment System (OPPS)
- D Codes   Dental Procedures (published in Current Dental
  Terminology, CDT)
- E Codes   Durable Medical Equipment
- G Codes   Temporary Procedures/Professional Services
- H Codes   Behavioral Health and/or Substance Abuse Treatment
  Services
- J Codes   Drugs Other Than Chemotherapy
  Chemotherapy Drugs
- K Codes   Temporary Codes Assigned to DME Regional Carriers
- L Codes   Orthotics
  Prosthetics
- M Codes   Other Medical Services
- P Codes   Laboratory Services
- Q Codes   Temporary Codes Assigned by CMS (Procedures, Services,
  and Supplies)
- R Codes   Diagnostic Radiology Services
- S Codes   Temporary National Codes (Established by Private Payers)
- T Codes   Temporary National Codes Established by Medicaid
- V Codes   Vision/Hearing Services

Index. The index is in alphabetical order and includes main terms and subterms (Fig. 13-22). The entries in the index of the National Codes may be listed under more than one main term. For example, surgical kit can be found under the two entries "Kits" and "Surgical," as illustrated in Fig. 13-23.

From the index, you turn to the code in the alphanumeric listing. The entries in the alphanumeric listing further explain what is included in the code.

The venous pressure clamps codes are shown as they appear in the alphanumeric listing in Fig. 13-24. Note that A4918 specifies "each."

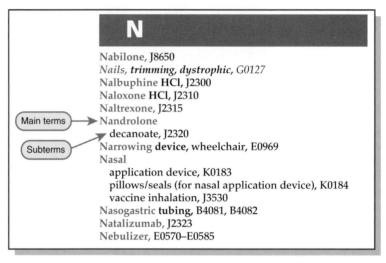

FIGURE 13–22 HCPCS index, National Codes.

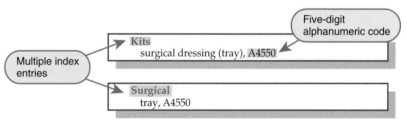

FIGURE 13–23 HCPCS index entries.

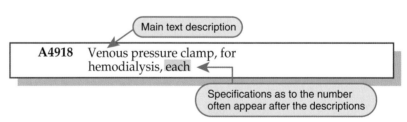

FIGURE 13–24 HCPCS main text display.

There are more than 50 alphabetical modifiers available for assignment to add further specificity to the five-digit national code. For example, modifiers can be used to specify the service provider, specify the anatomic site, or add specificity (Fig. 13-25). Appendix A of the CPT contains some of the Level II, HCPCS/National modifiers.

⚠ **CAUTION** *HCPCS manuals vary considerably depending on publisher.*

Table of Drugs. J codes identify the drugs administered and the amounts or dosages given. The National Codes contain a Table of Drugs (Fig. 13-26) to direct the user to the appropriate drug titles and the corresponding codes. J codes refer to drugs only by generic name. However, if a drug is known only by a brand or trade name, you will be directed to the generic name of the drug and then to the associated J or Q code by a cross-reference system within the table. A *Physicians' Desk Reference* (PDR) is a publication that contains prescribing information on prescription drugs and lists the drugs by generic and brand names. The PDR is a valuable resource for the coder when using the Table of Drugs.

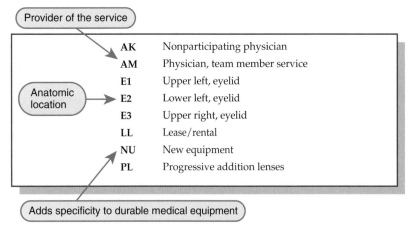

Provider of the service		
AK	Nonparticipating physician	
AM	Physician, team member service	
E1	Upper left, eyelid	
E2	Lower left, eyelid	
E3	Upper right, eyelid	
LL	Lease/rental	
NU	New equipment	
PL	Progressive addition lenses	

Anatomic location

Adds specificity to durable medical equipment

FIGURE 13–25 HCPCS modifiers.

Diazepam	up to 5 mg	IM, IV	**J3360**
Diazoxide	up to 300 mg	IV	**J1730**
Dibent	up to 20 mg	IM	J0500
Dicyclocot	up to 20 mg		J0500
Dicyclomine HCl	up to 20 mg	IM	**J0500**
Didronel	per 300 mg	IV	J1436
Diethylstilbestrol diphosphate	250 mg	IV	**J9165**
Diflucan	200 mg	IV	J1450
Digibind	per vial		J1162
DigiFab	per vial		J1162
Digoxin	up to 0.5 mg	IM, IV	**J1160**
Digoxin immune fab (ovine)	per vial		**J1162**
Dihydrex	up to 50 mg	IV, IM	J1200
	50 mg	ORAL	Q0163
Dihydroergotamine mesylate	per 1 mg	IM, IV	**J1110**
Dilantin	per 50 mg	IM, IV	J1165

Generic drug name → Digoxin

Route → J1160

HCPCS Code

FIGURE 13–26 Example from Table of Drugs.

The Route of Administration column (see Fig. 13-26) lists the most common methods of delivering the referenced generic drug. The official definitions for Level II J codes generally describe administration other than by the oral method. Orally given drugs are not usually provided in a physician's office but are bought at a pharmacy after the visit. Therefore, with a few exceptions, orally delivered drugs are omitted from the Route of Administration column. The following abbreviations and listings are used in the Route of Administration column:

INJ   Injection
IT   Intrathecal
IV   Intravenous
IM   Intramuscular
SC   Subcutaneous
INH   Inhalant solution
VAR   Various routes
OTH   Other routes

QUICK CHECK 13-8

1. Medication Administration Route information is provided with the Table of Drugs and Chemicals.

   True or False?

(Answers are located in Appendix C)

EXERCISE 13-11   *Table of Drugs*

Define the following routes of administration for drugs:

1 Intrathecal _____

_____

2 Intravenous _____

_____

3 Intramuscular _____

_____

4 Subcutaneous _____

_____

5 Inhalant solution _____

_____

(Answers are located in Appendix B)

Routes of Administration of Drugs. Intravenous administration includes all methods, such as gravity infusion, injections, and timed pushes. When several routes of administration are listed, the first listing is the most common method. A "VAR" posting denotes various routes of administration and is used for drugs that are commonly administered into joints, cavities, or tissues, and as topical applications. Listings posted with "OTH" alert the coder to other administration methods, for example, suppositories or catheter injections. Fig. 13-27 illustrates J code information as listed in the tabular.

J1120	Injection, acetazolamide sodium, **up to 500 mg**
	Other: Diamox
	IOM: 100-02, 15, 50
J1160	Injection, digoxin, **up to 0.5 mg**
	NDC: Lanoxin
	IOM: 100-02, 15, 50
J1162	Injection, digoxin immune Fab (ovine), **per vial**
	NDC: Digibind; DigiFab
	IOM: 100-02, 15, 50
J1165	Injection, phenytoin sodium, **per 50 mg**
	Other: Dilantin
	IOM: 100-02, 15, 50

FIGURE 13-27 HCPCS J codes.

Durable Medical Equipment. Durable medical equipment (DME) is equipment used by a patient with a chronic disabling condition, and the term also includes some equipment that is used only temporarily until the patient has healed. Claims for DME and related supplies can be paid only if the items meet the Medicare definition of covered DME and are medically necessary. The determination of medical necessity is made using documentation written by the physician. The documentation can include medical records, a plan of care, discharge plans, and prescriptions or forms explicitly designed to document medical necessity. These forms are referred to as Certificates of Medical Necessity (CMN). An example of a CMN is CMS-848 for a transcutaneous electrical nerve stimulator (Fig. 13-28).

Claims for other items require the use of the CMN, for example, power-operated vehicles, air-fluidized beds, decubitus care pads, seat-lift mechanisms, and paraffin baths.

Physician completion of the required medical documentation ensures that the DME items furnished to a Medicare beneficiary are those specifically needed for the unique medical condition of the patient. The CMS also requires the use of form CMS-484 for the Certification of Medical Necessity—Oxygen (Fig. 13-29).

CHECK THIS OUT 🖝 The forms download website of CMS is www.cms.gov/cmsforms/cmsforms/list.asp#topofpage.

National Physician Fee Schedule. Each fall, the Centers for Medicare and Medicaid Services produces the National Physician Fee Schedule, which lists all HCPCS and CPT codes along with the amount allocated for each service and the covered/noncovered status of each service. A list of fees for drugs is produced on a quarterly basis based on the current Average Sales Price (ASP) of each drug. Fig. 13-30 illustrates a portion of the National Physician Fee Schedule.

CHECK THIS OUT 🖝 The Physician Fee Schedule is on the CMS website at www.cms.gov/PhysicianFeeSched/PFSRVF/list.asp.

DEPARTMENT OF HEALTH AND HUMAN SERVICES
CENTERS FOR MEDICARE & MEDICAID SERVICES

Form Approved
OMB No. 0938-0679

CERTIFICATE OF MEDICAL NECESSITY
CMS-848 — TRANSCUTANEOUS ELECTRICAL NERVE STIMULATOR (TENS)

DME 06.03B

SECTION A Certification Type/Date: INITIAL ___/___/___ REVISED ___/___/___ RECERTIFICATION___/___/___

PATIENT NAME, ADDRESS, TELEPHONE and HIC NUMBER	SUPPLIER NAME, ADDRESS, TELEPHONE and NSC or applicable NPI NUMBER/LEGACY NUMBER
(__ __ __) __ __ __ - __ __ __ __ HICN _____	(__ __ __) __ __ __ - __ __ __ __ NSC or NPI #_____

PLACE OF SERVICE_____	HCPCS CODE	PT DOB ___/___/___ Sex ____ (M/F) Ht. ____(in) Wt ____(lbs.)
NAME and ADDRESS of FACILITY *if applicable (see reverse)*	_____ _____ _____ _____	PHYSICIAN NAME, ADDRESS, TELEPHONE and applicable NPI NUMBER or UPIN (__ __ __) __ __ __ - __ __ __ __ UPIN or NPI #_____

SECTION B   Information in this Section May Not Be Completed by the Supplier of the Items/Supplies.

EST. LENGTH OF NEED (# OF MONTHS): _____ 1-99 *(99=LIFETIME)*   DIAGNOSIS CODES (ICD-9): _____ _____ _____ _____

ANSWERS	ANSWER QUESTIONS 1-6 for purchase of TENS (Circle Y for Yes, N for No,)
Y N	1. Does the patient have chronic, intractable pain?
_____ Months	2. How long has the patient had intractable pain? (Enter number of months, 1 - 99.)
1 2 3 4 5	3. Is the TENS unit being prescribed for any of the following conditions? (Circle appropriate number) 1 - Headache 2 - Visceral abdominal pain 3 - Pelvic pain 4 - Temporomandibular joint (TMJ) pain 5 - None of the above
Y N	4. Is there documentation in the medical record of multiple medications and/or other therapies that have been tried and failed?
Y N	5. Has the patient received a TENS trial of at least 30 days?
____/____/____	6. What is the date that you reevaluated the patient at the end of the trial period?

NAME OF PERSON ANSWERING SECTION B QUESTIONS, IF OTHER THAN PHYSICIAN (Please Print):
NAME: _____TITLE: _____EMPLOYER:_____

SECTION C   **Narrative Description of Equipment and Cost**

(1) Narrative description of all items, accessories and options ordered; (2) Supplier's charge; and (3) Medicare Fee Schedule Allowance for each item, accessory, and option. (see instructions on back)

SECTION D   **PHYSICIAN Attestation and Signature/Date**

I certify that I am the treating physician identified in Section A of this form. I have received Sections A, B and C of the Certificate of Medical Necessity (including charges for items ordered). Any statement on my letterhead attached hereto, has been reviewed and signed by me. I certify that the medical necessity information in Section B is true, accurate and complete, to the best of my knowledge, and I understand that any falsification, omission, or concealment of material fact in that section may subject me to civil or criminal liability.

PHYSICIAN'S SIGNATURE_____ DATE _____/_____/_____

Form CMS-848 (09/05)

FIGURE 13-28 CMS Certificate of Medical Necessity—TENS.

DEPARTMENT OF HEALTH AND HUMAN SERVICES
CENTERS FOR MEDICARE & MEDICAID SERVICES

Form Approved
OMB No. 0938-0534

CERTIFICATE OF MEDICAL NECESSITY
CMS-484 — OXYGEN

DME 484.03

SECTION A	Certification Type/Date: INITIAL ___/___/___ REVISED ___/___/___ RECERTIFICATION___/___/___

PATIENT NAME, ADDRESS, TELEPHONE and HIC NUMBER

(_ _ _) _ _ _ - _ _ _ _ HICN _____

SUPPLIER NAME, ADDRESS, TELEPHONE and NSC or applicable NPI NUMBER/LEGACY NUMBER

(_ _ _) _ _ _ - _ _ _ _ NSC or NPI #_____

PLACE OF SERVICE_____	HCPCS CODE	PT DOB ___/___/___ Sex ____ (M/F)

NAME and ADDRESS of FACILITY
if applicable (see reverse)

_____
_____
_____
_____

PHYSICIAN NAME, ADDRESS, TELEPHONE and applicable NPI NUMBER or UPIN

(_ _ _) _ _ _ - _ _ _ _ UPIN or NPI #_____

SECTION B	**Information in This Section May Not Be Completed by the Supplier of the Items/Supplies.**

EST. LENGTH OF NEED (# OF MONTHS): _____ 1-99 *(99=LIFETIME)*   DIAGNOSIS CODES (ICD-9): _____ _____ _____ _____

ANSWERS	ANSWER QUESTIONS 1-9. (Circle Y for Yes, N for No, or D for Does Not Apply, unless otherwise noted.)
a)_____mm Hg b)_____% c)___/___/___	1. Enter the result of most recent test taken on or before the certification date listed in Section A. Enter (a) arterial blood gas PO2 and/or (b) oxygen saturation test; (c) date of test.
1 2 3	2. Was the test in Question 1 performed (1) with the patient in a chronic stable state as an outpatient, (2) within two days prior to discharge from an inpatient facility to home, or (3) under other circumstances?
1 2 3	3. Circle the one number for the condition of the test in Question 1: (1) At Rest; (2) During Exercise; (3) During Sleep
Y N D	4. If you are ordering portable oxygen, is the patient mobile within the home? If you are not ordering portable oxygen, circle D.
_____LPM	5. Enter the highest oxygen flow rate ordered for this patient in liters per minute. If less than 1 LPM, enter a "X".
a)_____mm Hg b)_____% c)___/___/___	6. If greater than 4 LPM is prescribed, enter results of most recent test taken on 4 LPM. This may be an (a) arterial blood gas PO2 and/or (b) oxygen saturation test with patient in a chronic stable state. Enter date of test (c).
ANSWER QUESTIONS 7-9 **ONLY** IF PO2 = 56–59 OR OXYGEN SATURATION = 89 IN QUESTION 1	
Y N	7. Does the patient have dependent edema due to congestive heart failure?
Y N	8. Does the patient have cor pulmonale or pulmonary hypertension documented by P pulmonale on an EKG or by an echocardiogram, gated blood pool scan or direct pulmonary artery pressure measurement?
Y N	9. Does the patient have a hematocrit greater than 56%?

NAME OF PERSON ANSWERING SECTION B QUESTIONS, IF OTHER THAN PHYSICIAN (Please Print):
NAME: _____TITLE: _____EMPLOYER:_____

SECTION C	**Narrative Description of Equipment and Cost**

(1) Narrative description of all items, accessories and options ordered; (2) Supplier's charge and (3) Medicare Fee Schedule Allowance for each item, accessory and option. (See instructions on back.)

SECTION D	**Physician Attestation and Signature/Date**

I certify that I am the treating physician identified in Section A of this form. I have received Sections A, B and C of the Certificate of Medical Necessity (including charges for items ordered). Any statement on my letterhead attached hereto, has been reviewed and signed by me. I certify that the medical necessity information in Section B is true, accurate and complete, to the best of my knowledge, and I understand that any falsification, omission, or concealment of material fact in that section may subject me to civil or criminal liability.

PHYSICIAN'S SIGNATURE _____ DATE _____/_____/_____

Form CMS-484 (09/05)

FIGURE 13–29 CMS Certificate of Medical Necessity—Oxygen.

HCPCS	Description	Status Code	Conversion Factor
A0021	Outside state ambulance serv	I	$36.0666
A0080	Noninterest escort in non er	I	$36.0666
A0090	Interest escort in non er	I	$36.0666
A0100	Nonemergency transport taxi	I	$36.0666
A0110	Nonemergency transport bus	I	$36.0666
A0120	Noner transport mini-bus	I	$36.0666
A0130	Noner transport wheelch van	I	$36.0666
A0140	Nonemergency transport air	I	$36.0666
A0160	Noner transport case worker	I	$36.0666
A0170	Noner transport parking fees	I	$36.0666
A0180	Noner transport lodgng recip	I	$36.0666
A0190	Noner transport meals recip	I	$36.0666
A0200	Noner transport lodgng escrt	I	$36.0666
A0210	Noner transport meals escort	I	$36.0666
A0380	Basic life support mileage	X	$36.0666
A0382	Basic support routine suppls	X	$36.0666
A0384	Bls defibrillation supplies	X	$36.0666
A0390	Advanced life support mileag	X	$36.0666
A0392	Als defibrillation supplies	X	$36.0666

FIGURE 13–30 Example of CMS's National Physician Fee Schedule Relative Value File indicates HCPCS code and description along with the conversion factor for that code for the following year.

EXERCISE 13-12 *National Codes*

With information provided in this chapter, complete the following:

1 HCPCS is divided into two levels. List the names of the levels, in order, and the level numbers:

a _____

Level _____

b _____

Level _____

2 There are four groups of codes that are used by CMS for temporary assignment until a definitive decision can be made about the correct code assignment. What are the alphabetic letters of these four groups of codes? _____,

_____, _____, and _____

3 Are all HCPCS modifiers numeric? _____

4 What alphabetic group of codes is used to reference drugs in the HCPCS? _____

5 The term "route of administration" generally describes the administration of drugs by methods other than

_____.

6 What group of codes is used to reference durable medical equipment in the National Codes?

_____

Continued

Use Fig. 13-24 through Fig. 13-26 to answer the following questions:

7 What is the modifier for each of the following (Fig. 13-25)?

   a New equipment _____

   b Lower left eyelid _____

   c The services of a physician who was a member of a team that provided service _____

8 What is the route of administration of dicyclomine (HCL) (Fig. 13-26)? _____

9 What is the amount of diazepam for code J3360 (Fig. 13-26)? _____

10 What is the J code for an injection of diazoxide (Fig. 13-26)? _____

11 What is the code available for a venous pressure clamp (Fig. 13-24)? _____

(Answers are located in Appendix B)

CHAPTER REVIEW

CHAPTER 13, PART I, THEORY

Do not use your CPT manual for this part of the review.

1 CPT stands for _____.

2 The CPT manual often reflects the technologic advances made in medicine with these codes:

_____

3 The CPT manual is ever changing and is updated annually to reflect technologic advances and

editorial _____.

4 What type of code ends with 99? _____

5 Coding information that pertains to an entire section is located in the _____.

6 These codes provide supplemental information and do not substitute for a Category I code:

_____

7 What is the name of the two-digit number or a digit and a number that is located after the CPT code number and provides

more detail about the code? _____

8 Where is a list of all the modifiers located? _____

9 When using an unlisted or Category III code, third-party payers usually require the submission of what?

_____

10 Additions, deletions, and revisions are listed in which Appendix? _____

11 A listing of all add-on codes is located in which Appendix? _____

12 The symbol used between two code numbers to indicate that a range is available is a

_____.

Using Fig. 13-31, identify the category, section, subheading, and subsection.

13 _____

14 _____

15 _____

16 _____

17 The symbol that indicates a product is pending FDA approval is the _____.

18 A complete list of the codes designated with the symbol that indicates a product is pending FDA approval is listed in this

appendix of the CPT manual: _____

19 The Genetic Testing Code Modifiers are listed in this appendix of the CPT manual: _____

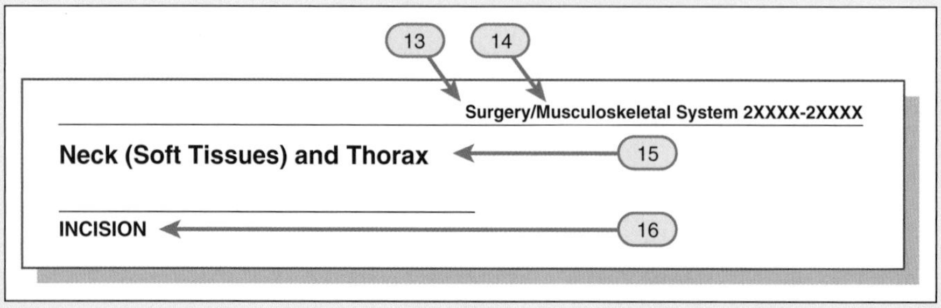

FIGURE 13–31 Identify the section, subsection, subheading, and category.

CHAPTER 13, PART II, PRACTICAL

Use your CPT manual for this part of the review. Using Appendix A of the CPT manual, list the correct two-digit modifiers for the following services:

20 Repeat procedure by the same individual: _____

21 Surgical care only: _____

22 Anesthesia by the surgeon: _____

23 Bilateral procedure: _____

Assuming there is no Category III code for the unlisted procedure you are reporting, locate the following unlisted procedure codes using the Surgery Guidelines:

24 Orbit: Code: _____

25 Rectum: Code: _____

26 Lips: Code: _____

27 General musculoskeletal: Code: _____

Using the index of the CPT manual, locate and write on the line an example of each of the following types of code display:

28 Single code: _____

29 Multiple code: _____

30 Range: _____

Using the index of the CPT manual, locate the following terms and write what the index note directs you to do:

31 T4 Total: _____

32 SHBG: _____

33 Radius: _____

34 Physical Therapy: _____

Using the index of the CPT manual, locate the code(s) for the following (you do not need to check the codes in the tabular for this exercise):

35 Repair, Abdomen: _____

36 Bypass Graft, Excision, Abdomen: _____

37 Catheterization, Arteriovenous Shunt, Initial Access: _____

38 Cystotomy, with Drainage: _____

39 Fracture, Femur, Intertrochanteric, Closed Treatment: _____

40 Alveoloplasty: _____

41 Duodenotomy: _____

Using the index of the HCPCS manual, locate the code(s) following these terms:

42 Enoxaparin sodium: _____

43 Cast, hand restoration: _____

44 Hydraulic patient lift: _____

45 Positioning seat: _____

46 Speech assessment: _____

47 Whirlpool equipment: _____

48 Transportation, corneal tissue: _____

49 Orthotic devices, Legg-Perthes: _____

50 Contraceptive, cervical cap: _____

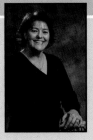

"As you develop your skills, you can move into dozens of different areas of specialization. Pay close attention to the areas of your work where you feel most inclined to excel and explore. You're likely to be very happy there!"

Jane A. Tuttle, CPC-I, CCS-P
Coding Education Endeavors
Westford, Massachusetts

Modifiers

Learning Objectives

After completing this chapter you should be able to

1 Recognize modifiers.

2 Understand the purpose of modifiers.

3 Assign Increased Procedural Services modifier -22.

4 Assign Unusual Anesthesia modifier -23.

5 Assign Unrelated E/M Services by the Same Physician or Other Qualified Health Care Professional During a Postoperative Period modifier -24.

6 Assign Significant Separately Identifiable E/M Service by the Same Physician or Other Qualified Health Care Professional on the Same Day of the Procedure or Other Service modifier -25.

7 Assign Professional Component modifier -26.

8 Assign Mandated Services modifier -32.

9 Assign Preventive Services modifier -33.

10 Assign Anesthesia by Surgeon modifier -47.

11 Assign Bilateral Procedures modifier -50.

12 Assign Multiple Procedures modifier -51.

13 Assign Reduced Services modifier -52.

14 Assign Discontinued Procedure modifier -53.

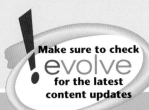

Make sure to check
evolve
for the latest
content updates

CPT MODIFIERS

Modifiers inform third-party payers of circumstances that may affect the way payment is made. Appendix A of the CPT manual lists the full description for all modifiers and the circumstances for their use.

Modifiers indicate the following types of information:

■ Altered service

    Service greater than usually required

    Unusual circumstances

    Part of a service

    Discontinued services

■ Bilateral procedure

■ Multiple procedures

- Professional part of the service/procedure only
- More than one physician/surgeon

Modifiers complete the story for insurance carriers to determine reimbursement. Consider using a modifier when the CPT code does not complete the story.

CODING SHOT

For the purposes of this text, when there are multiple CPT modifiers assigned to one code, list the modifiers from highest to lowest, for example, -78-50.

The CPT modifiers are shown in Fig. 14-1.

-22, Increased Procedural Services

Modifier -22 indicates that the service was greater than usual and required increased physician work above and beyond normal. A special report must accompany the use of modifier -22 to explain how the service was greater. Documentation should indicate the time it usually takes to perform the service and the significant increase in that time due to documented factors. For example, if it normally takes 45 minutes to provide the service, but because of the extent and complications 90 minutes was required. Modifier -22 is reported with surgical codes. Turn to Appendix A in the CPT manual and read the description of this modifier.

The use of modifier -22 indicates that the service provided was significantly greater than the service described in the CPT code. A few additional minutes spent on a procedure does not warrant the use of this modifier. The medical record must contain documentation that substantiates that the service was unusual in some way, such as statements about the increased risk to the patient, the difficulty of the procedure, excessive blood loss, or other statements to indicate the occurrence of an unusually difficult situation. Examples include:

- Excessive blood loss.
- Extensive well-documented adhesions in abdominal surgery.
- Trauma extensive enough to complicate the procedure and the complication is not reported separately.
- Other pathologies, tumors, malformations that directly interfere with the procedure but are not reported separately.
- The service rendered was significantly more complex than described for the code description.

Modifier -22 is overused, so it comes under particularly close scrutiny by third-party payers, especially as there is usually a payment increase of 20% to 30% for services that qualify for the use of modifier -22. When reporting modifier -22, be sure that you have the documentation to support the claim. When the third-party payer receives a claim that includes a service to which modifier -22 has been added, the claim is sent to an individual who reviews the claim. Appropriate documentation must, therefore, accompany the claim—an operative report, a pathology report, office notes, hospital chart notes, and so forth.

CPT Modifiers

-22	-26	-50	-54	-58	-66	-79	-90
-23	-32	-51	-55	-59	-76	-80	-91
-24	-33	-52	-56	-62	-77	-81	-92
-25	-47	-53	-57	-63	-78	-82	-99

FIGURE 14-1 CPT modifiers.

When assigning modifier -22, additional charges are added based on the increase in physician work, and the documentation that supports the higher charge is contained in the medical record.

Avoid routine use of modifier -22, as the modifier should be reported only when a surgeon provides a service that is greater than usually required and a secondary code that would claim the additional work cannot be reported. The use of specialized technology (e.g., laparoscope or laser) does not automatically qualify for use of modifier -22. Abuse of the modifier will attract unwanted scrutiny. Repeated misuse could trigger an audit.

CMS develops rules to promote correct coding methods and to control improper coding leading to inappropriate payment. CMS develops coding policies based on the CPT manual, national and local policies, coding guidelines developed by national societies, analysis of standard medical and surgical practices, and a review of current coding practices. These rules are only for beneficiaries of government programs, such as Medicare, but many third-party payers have adopted many of the guidelines. Within this text, reference will be made to the CMS rules as follows:

CMS RULES

The Medicare Claims Processing Manual 100-04, Chapter 12, 20.4.6 (www.cms.gov/manuals/downloads/clm104c12.pdf) states that the fees for services represent the average work effort and practice expenses required to provide a service. For any given procedure code, there could be a typical range of work effort and practice expense required to provide the service. Thus, carriers may increase or decrease the payment for a service only under very unusual circumstances based upon review of medical records and other supporting documentation.

Modifier -22 is valid for codes with global periods of 0, 10, or 90 days. Modifier -22 is not valid for "XXX" global period indicators, which includes E/M, radiology, laboratory, pathology, and most medicine codes.

QUICK CHECK 14-1

1. According to The Medicare Claims Processing Manual 100-04, Chapter 12, 20.6, Updating Factor for Fee Schedule Services (www.cms.gov/manuals/downloads/clm104c12.pdf), claims processing contractors must maintain at least _____ full calendar years of fee schedules and related pricing data, regardless of the number of updates or pricing periods.

(Answers are located in Appendix C)

-23, Unusual Anesthesia

Modifier -23 is used by an anesthesiologist to indicate a service for which general anesthesia was used when normally the anesthesia would have been local or regional. Turn to Appendix A in the CPT manual and read the description of this modifier.

This modifier can only be assigned with codes in the Anesthesia section (00100-01999) by an anesthesiologist/nurse anesthetist. This modifier is added to the primary procedure that would not usually require general anesthesia services such as 62270 (Spinal puncture, lumbar, diagnostic). The anesthesia code for 62270 is 00635 (Anesthesia for procedures in the lumbar region; diagnostic or therapeutic lumbar puncture). Code 00635-23 indicates that someone other than the anesthesiologist is performing the lumbar puncture and that this procedure usually does not require anesthesia services. Some payers may require documentation to support the need for anesthesia services.

QUICK CHECK 14-2

1. Which of the following may be an example of "unusual anesthesia" circumstances?
   a. Simple open wound repair on the face of a 2-year-old who is unable to sit still for the repair
   b. Pelvic exam on a developmentally challenged woman who is unable to cooperate
   c. Cast application for fracture care of a combative Alzheimer's patient
   d. All of the above

(Answers are located in Appendix C)

-24, Unrelated Evaluation and Management Service by the Same Physician or Other Qualified Health Care Professional During a Postoperative Period

Modifier -24 is used only with E/M codes. Turn to Appendix A in the CPT manual and read the description of this modifier.

Modifier -24 reports services that were performed during a postoperative period but were unrelated to recovery from the surgical procedure. Surgical procedures have a package of services, such as preoperative, procedure (intraoperative), and normal follow-up care. If an E/M service unrelated to the surgical procedure is provided to a patient during the postoperative period, the third-party payer would think that the service was part of the surgical package and deny payment. Modifier -24 is added to indicate that the E/M service was not part of the surgical package (global period) but was an unrelated service. The postoperative period of a major surgical procedure is usually 90 days; a minor surgery, 10 days. Payment for the surgical procedure includes postoperative care of the patient during these periods.

You can also use modifier -24 with the General Ophthalmological Service codes 92002-92014 for eye evaluations, even though these codes are located in the Medicine section. Ophthalmologists report new and established medical examinations using 92002-92014.

CODING SHOT

Modifier -24 requests payment for an unassociated E/M within a global period. The diagnosis code would indicate that the reason for the service was unrelated to the surgical procedure.

For example, a male patient is within the 10-day global period for an incision and drainage of a skin abscess. The patient presents to the physician's office for a wound check and also to ask the physician to evaluate a mole on his chest that has changed color. The postoperative visit is reported with 99024 (no charge code), and the evaluation of the mole is reported with 9921X-24 to indicate a medically necessary E/M service unrelated to the incision and drainage of the skin abscess. The diagnosis code reported with the E/M service for the mole would indicate the medical necessity of the service, such as D23.5 for a benign neoplasm of the skin of the chest wall.

-25, Significant Separately Identifiable E/M Service by the Same Physician or Other Qualified Health Care Professional on the Same Day of the Procedure or Other Service

Modifier -25 is used to report an E/M service on a day when another service was provided to the patient by the same individual. Turn to Appendix A in the CPT manual and read the description of this modifier.

CMS RULES

If reporting services for a Medicare patient, modifier -25 could be added to an E/M code when a decision for surgery was made on the same day as a procedure with a global surgical package of 0-10 days or procedures not covered by global surgery rules (global indicator of XXX) if the E/M service is not associated with the decision to perform a minor surgical procedure whether the patient is a new or established patient. Modifier -57 would be added to an E/M code when the service resulted in a decision for surgery on the day before or the day of a procedure with a global surgical package of 90 days.

To assign modifier -25 correctly, there must be a medical necessity to provide a separate, additional E/M service on the same day a procedure was performed or another service was provided. The medical necessity for this additional E/M service must be documented in the patient's medical record. If you do not add modifier -25 to the additional E/M code for service on the day of a procedure, the third-party payer would disallow the charge because it would be thought to be the evaluation/management portion of the procedure. By adding modifier -25, you are stating that the service was separate from the procedure or original service. Use of modifier -25 increases the potential of receiving payment for the service. For example, a physician provided a dialysis service to a hospital inpatient. In addition, the physician provided a separate discharge service (not related to the dialysis). You would report the dialysis service (procedure) and also report the inpatient service (discharge), adding the modifier -25 to the discharge service.

The modifier can also be assigned when additional E/M services are provided on the same day to the same patient. For example, if a patient came into the office for a visit early in the day and then later in the day returned for a separate unrelated E/M service. You report both services using E/M codes and add modifier -25 to the second E/M code. If the services were for the same related condition as seen in the earlier service, documentation for both services would be considered to assign only one E/M code for that day.

Let's review a couple other examples of the use of modifier -25. A patient presents for repair of a laceration (12042, intermediate laceration repair) and the questions asked by the physician were related only to the laceration repair. In this case, the E/M service is included in the laceration repair service and not reported separately. However, if the physician documented the patient had elevated blood pressure and a history of hypertension and the physician evaluated and treated the hypertensive condition, modifier -25 would be added to the E/M code. Diagnosis code I10/401.X (hypertension) would be reported as the diagnosis for the E/M service. The laceration repair would have a trauma diagnosis for open wound, and as such, the diagnosis code would support the medical necessity for the laceration repair. In this example, both the E/M service (with -25) and the laceration repair are reported with diagnosis codes that indicate the medical necessity of both services.

-26, Professional Component

Modifier -26 is used to designate a physician (professional) component of procedures that have a professional and technical component, such as the interpretation of ultrasounds or x-rays. Turn to Appendix A in the CPT manual and read the description of this modifier.

Modifier -26 is usually used with radiology service because radiology services often have two components—professional component and technical component. An example of the technical component is an independent radiology facility that takes the x-rays (technical component) and sends them to a private radiologist who reads the x-rays and writes a report of the findings (professional component). The physician's services would be reported with modifier -26 added to the code for the x-ray, indicating that only the professional component of the x-ray service was provided, as in the following:

A 35-year-old white female was seen in the emergency department following a fall from a horse. She complained of pain in her right clavicle and shoulder. The emergency physician ordered a complete x-ray of the clavicle. The radiologist provided the report with a diagnosis of a fractured clavicle. The physician component of the x-ray for the radiologist would be reported with 73000-26.

EXERCISE 14-1   *Modifiers -22 through -26*

Using the CPT, ICD-10-CM and/or ICD-9-CM manuals, code the following:

1 The surgeon performed a repair of an enterocele using an abdominal approach (57270) on a morbidly obese patient, and because of the patient's obesity, the procedure took a significant amount of additional time to perform (50 minutes added to the normal time usually required).

   CPT Code and Modifier: _____

2 During a radical orchiectomy with abdominal exploration for an extensive primary, malignant neoplasm (54535) of the left descended testis, the patient began to hemorrhage (a complication). After considerable time and effort, which extended the surgery by 60 minutes, the hemorrhage was controlled.

   CPT Code and Modifier: _____

   ICD-10-CM Codes: _____, _____

   (ICD-9-CM Codes: _____, _____)

3 An extremely anxious and combative elderly man presented to the outpatient same-day surgery unit for a gastroscopy due to hematemesis and suspected peptic ulcer. The patient was unable to cooperate. The physician determined that, because of the patient's advanced Alzheimer's, general anesthesia during this procedure, which usually does not require anesthesia, was the best approach to use with the patient. What modifier would the anesthesiologist report when reporting this service?

   Modifier: _____

   ICD-10-CM Codes: _____, _____, _____, _____

   (ICD-9-CM Codes: _____, _____, _____)

4 Dr. Foster admitted a patient to a skilled nursing facility because of the patient's advanced dementia due to Alzheimer's disease (during the global period for a herniorrhaphy that Dr. Foster performed). What modifier would be added to the admission service?

   Modifier: _____

   ICD-10-CM Codes: _____, _____

   (ICD-9-CM Codes: _____, _____)

5 A patient came to the office twice in one day to see the same physician for unrelated problems. What modifier would be added to the code for the second office visit?

   Modifier: _____

6 A 60-year-old female patient is referred to a radiology laboratory by her general physician. The laboratory takes the x-rays requested and sends them on to a radiologist to interpret and to develop the written report that is sent to the general physician. If you were coding for the radiologist, what modifier would you add to indicate the service provided by the radiologist?

   Modifier: _____

(Answers are located in Appendix B)

-32, Mandated Services

Modifier -32 indicates a service that is required by some third-party entity. Turn to Appendix A in the CPT manual and read the description of this modifier.

This modifier is not used to report a second opinion requested by a patient, a family member, or another physician. Modifier -32 is reported only when a service is mandated. For example, the police require a suspected rape or abuse victim to have certain tests. These are mandated services to which modifier -32 would be added. Another common use of modifier -32 is to indicate that a third-party payer or Workers' Compensation mandated a physical examination of a covered patient. The third-party payer usually waives the deductible and copayment for the patient and usually pays 100% of these mandated services.

-33, Preventive Service

The Patient Protection and Affordable Care Act (PPACA) requires health insurance coverage of preventive services and immunizations without cost. US Preventive Services Task Force (USPSTF) grades preventive services:

Grade A: High certainty that the net benefit is substantial

Grade B: High certainty that the net benefit is moderate or there is a moderate certainty that the net benefit is moderate to substantial

Example of service:
- Grade A
- Topic: Blood pressure screening
- Description: The USPSTF recommends screening for high blood pressure in adults aged 18 and older.

Task Force list located at: www.uspreventiveservicestaskforce.org/uspstf/uspsabrecs.htm

-47, Anesthesia by Surgeon

Modifier -47 is used to report a surgical procedure in which the surgeon administered regional or general anesthesia to the patient. Turn to Appendix A in the CPT manual and read the description of this modifier.

There are times, although they occur infrequently, when a physician acts as both the anesthesiologist and the surgeon. For example, a closed reduction of a mandibular fracture performed in the office under intravenous sedation/general anesthesia would be reported with 21451 for the procedure and 21451-47 as a separate line item for the anesthesia/sedation.

CMS RULES

Medicare does not reimburse the surgeon for anesthesia service when he/she is the performing surgeon.

If the third-party payer allowed payment for modifier -47, payment would be made based on the **time** spent administering the anesthetic. The surgeon acting as an anesthesiologist would report modifier -47 with the surgery code. Modifier -47 is added only to surgery codes and is never added to anesthesia codes.

-50, Bilateral Procedures

If the same procedure is performed on a mirror-image organ of the body (such as right and left kidneys), modifier -50, indicating a bilateral procedure, would be reported. Turn to Appendix A in the CPT manual and read the description of this modifier.

For example, an arthroplasty (total knee replacement, 27447 and 27447-50) for both left and right knees at the same operative session would be reported using the modifier -50.

Another example in which the same services may be performed on two sides would be a bilateral breast procedure (e.g., bilateral, simple complete mastectomy, 19303 and 19303-50).

It is very important to determine how the third-party payer wants bilateral procedures submitted on the claim form, on a single line or multiple lines. One payer may require two codes to be displayed for the bilateral procedure (such as 27447 and 27447-50) for which they would reimburse 100% for the first code and 50% for the second code. Another payer may require that bilateral procedures be reported with only one code (27447-50) and would reimburse 150% based on that one code with modifier -50 representing two services. Still other payers want the service reported as 27447-RT and 27447-LT.

> 🖐 **CAUTION** *Some CPT codes are for bilateral procedures and do not require a bilateral modifier. For example, 27395 is for bilateral lengthening of the hamstring tendon. It would be incorrect to place a bilateral modifier on 27395. Code 92020 (gonioscopy) is also a bilateral procedure and use of modifier -50 would be inappropriate.*

CMS RULES

Medicare does not accept two line items to describe a bilateral procedure. Medicare rules direct the coder to use one line with modifier -50 and 1 unit of service. For example, submit 27447-50 rather than 27447, 27447-50.

Be sure to find out whether your third-party payer wants the surgical code to be used once with the modifier (code plus modifier -50) or used twice (code alone and code plus modifier -50) or whether the procedure should be listed twice.

-51, Multiple Procedures

During any given operative session, more than one procedure may be performed. This is referred to as "multiple procedures" and is indicated by modifier -51. Turn to Appendix A in the CPT manual and read the description of this modifier.

Assign modifier -51 when multiple procedures, other than the E/M services, are performed on the same day or at the same session by the same provider. When reporting multiple surgeries, the primary procedure (the procedure with the highest relative value unit) should be listed first on the claim.

For example, a benign skin lesion is excised from a patient's chest (diameter over 4.0 cm) and closure of the defect using layered closure. The service is reported with **11406** (Excision, benign lesion including margins, except skin tag [unless listed elsewhere], trunk, arms or legs; excised diameter over 4.0 cm) and **12032-51** (Layer closure of wounds of scalp, axillae, trunk and/or extremities [excluding hands and feet]; 2.6 cm to 7.5 cm).

CMS RULES

After the first eligible procedure is reimbursed at 100% of Medicare's allowance, the remaining procedures are reimbursed at 50% up to four additional procedures. No documentation is required. After the fifth procedure, the procedures will be considered 'by report' and documentation is then required.

(Medicare Claims Processing Manual, Chapter 12, 40.6. (www.cms.gov/manuals/downloads/clm104c12.pdf))

You have to be careful when coding multiple procedures because CPT codes include many different procedures bundled together in one code. For example, code 58200 is a total abdominal hysterectomy, but it also includes a partial vaginectomy (removal of the vagina) with para-aortic and pelvic lymph node sampling, with or without removal of tube(s), and with or without removal of ovary(ies). It would be incorrect to report each service separately because they are included (bundled) in the description for code 58200. Listing the subsequent procedures separately (unbundling) is considered fraud by a third-party payer. Unbundling is assigning multiple codes when one code would fully describe the service or procedure. The assigning of multiple codes results in increased reimbursement.

QUICK CHECK 14-3

1. What is the symbol in the CPT manual that indicates modifier -51 should not be used?

_____

(Answers are located in Appendix C)

However, if one code does not describe all of the procedures performed, and the secondary procedure is not considered a minor procedure that is incidental to the major procedure (and therefore bundled into the major procedure), each additional procedure may be reported by using the multiple procedure modifier (-51). For example, a patient has a laminectomy with lumbar disc removal (for a herniated disc), reported with 63030. The patient also has an arthrodesis (stabilization of the area where the disc was removed), reported with 22612. Both services would be reported, and modifier -51 would be added to the lesser of the two services.

There are three significant times when multiple procedures are reported:
1. Same Operation, Different Site
2. Multiple Operation(s), Same Operative Session
3. Procedure Performed Multiple Times

Same Operation, Different Site. Multiple procedures are reported using modifier -51 when the same procedure is performed on different sites. For example, a patient has an excision of a 1.5-cm benign lesion from the forearm and at the same time has an excision of a 3-cm benign lesion from the neck. In this case, the reporting would be 11423 for the 3-cm lesion and 11402-51 for the 1.5-cm lesion. List the most resource-intensive (expensive) procedure first, without a modifier.

Example
The payer reimburses $175.96 for 11423 and $140.54 for 11402. The difference in reimbursement is significant based on the order of the codes.

11423, 11402-51 = $175.96 + $70.27 (50% of $140.54) payment is **$246.23**

11402, 11423-50 = $140.54 + $87.98 (50% of $175.96) payment is **$228.52**

The difference in reimbursement is $17.71 for submission of just these two services in an incorrect order.

Multiple Operation(s), Same Operative Session. Multiple procedures (-51) are also reported when more than one procedure is performed during the same operative session.

The primary procedure during the surgical session would be paid at the full fee, the second procedure during the same session would usually be paid at 50% of the fee, and the third procedure would usually be paid at 25% of the fee. Again, when you are coding procedures for payment, it is important that you put the most resource-intensive procedure first, without a modifier, and then list the subsequent procedures in order of complexity, remembering to use the -51 modifier for all subsequent procedures. This process of assigning the -51 modifier helps to ensure that optimal reimbursement occurs.

Procedure Performed Multiple Times. Multiple procedures are also reported when the same procedure code identifies a service performed more than once during a single operative session. There are two ways to report procedures performed multiple times, depending on the requirements of the third-party payer. One way is to use the code number only once but to list the number of times it is performed (number of units). For example, if a patient had a repair of two flexor tendons of the leg, you would report 27658 × 2 units. Units are used because the code description states "each" tendon, and two tendons were repaired. The other way to code this would be to list 27658 once without a modifier and again with modifier -51 (i.e., 27658-51).

Third-party payers require submission of codes in various formats with various modifiers. HCPCS (Healthcare Common Procedure Coding System) modifiers indicate the right side (-RT) and left side (-LT) and the system also has modifiers that indicate the digits of the foot and hand:

-FA	Left hand, thumb	-TA	Left foot, great toe
-F1	Left hand, second digit	-T1	Left foot, second digit
-F2	Left hand, third digit	-T2	Left foot, third digit
-F3	Left hand, fourth digit	-T3	Left foot, fourth digit
-F4	Left hand, fifth digit	-T4	Left foot, fifth digit
-F5	Right hand, thumb	-T5	Right foot, great toe
-F6	Right hand, second digit	-T6	Right foot, second digit
-F7	Right hand, third digit	-T7	Right foot, third digit
-F8	Right hand, fourth digit	-T8	Right foot, fourth digit
-F9	Right hand, fifth digit	-T9	Right foot, fifth digit

CMS RULES

For all Medicare claims, the modifiers specifying the digit must be reported.

You will find some of the more common HCPCS modifiers on the front inside cover of the Professional Edition of the CPT manual and in Appendix A of the CPT manual. HCPCS modifiers add specificity and, for that reason, are required by many payers.

CODING SHOT

For the purposes of this text, HCPCS modifiers are listed in ascending alphabetic order when added to a code. For example, -AK-GT. If there are also CPT modifiers added to the code, list the CPT modifiers first (highest to lowest) followed by the HCPCS modifiers (ascending alphabetic order).

All of the variations in format can be a bit confusing when you begin coding, so let's stop here for a moment and review a few of the more common configurations that affect -50, -51, and reporting of units (times symbol).

Examples

Modifier -50 (Bilateral)

The physician performs a surgical sinus endoscopy with total ethmoidectomy, 31255, on the left and right ethmoid sinuses (bilateral).

1. Using modifier -50, the service would be usually reported:
   31255 and 31255-50
2. Using the HCPCS modifiers for sides (-LT, left side, and -RT, right side), the service would be reported:
   31255-LT and 31255-RT
3. Using the one-line format, the service would be reported:
   31255-50

The most specific method of reporting is the second format, as it indicates not only the number of procedures, but also the side of the body.

Modifier -51 (multiple)

The physician percutaneously repairs a distal phalangeal fracture of the second and third fingers of the left hand, with skeletal fixation (26756).

1. Using modifier -51, the service would be reported:
   26756 and 26756-51
2. Using the HCPCS modifiers for fingers (-F1, left hand, second digit, and F2, left hand, third digit), the service would be reported:
   26756-F1 and 26756-F2
3. Using the times symbol, the service would be reported:
   26756×2

You can see that the most specific method of reporting is again the second format, as it indicates the procedure, hand, and digit.

The use of the times symbol is another area of confusion when you first begin coding.

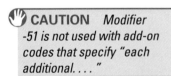

CAUTION *Modifier -51 is not used with add-on codes that specify "each additional. . . ."*

Times Symbol (×)

The physician performs a skin biopsy on five skin lesions.
   11100 (first lesion) and 11101×4 (second through fifth lesions)

Look for the word **"each"** in the code description as a hint to use the times symbol. The code description for 11101 states "**each** separate/additional lesion . . . ," with the "each" being the hint to use the times symbol.

Another example of the use of the times symbol is in pathology codes because some payers want multiple specimens reported in units. For example, the pathologist examines three tissue specimens.
   88302 (first specimen) and 88302×2 (second and third specimens)

The number of units is placed in Block 24G (Units) on the CMS-1500 form.

CODING SHOT

As always, be aware that the payers dictate how providers are to submit for payment of services. For example, some payers may not want providers to submit modifier -51 for the same operation performed on different sites but instead, modifier -59 (Distinct Procedural Service). Usually, however, the standard is to require -51 for the three significant times when multiple procedures are provided.

TOOLBOX

Carter was brought to the pediatrician for DTaP and MMR vaccinations and an annual school physical prior to beginning first grade. During the examination, the physician provided counseling to the mother regarding the vaccinations. The physician also identified a 1-cm mole on Carter's left thigh and after discussion and consent from the mother, excised the lesion. The pathology report later indicated benign tissue.

Reporting would be:
  MMR: 90707 ($35), 90460 ($25)
  DTaP: 90700 ($20), 90461 ($12)
  Preventative examination: 99383 ($72)
  Lesion excision: 11401 ($113)

QUESTIONS

1. In what order would you submit these codes?

   _____

2. Are any modifiers necessary on these codes?

   _____

▼ ANSWERS

1. 11401, 99383, 90707, 90460, 90700, 90461 (most expensive to least expensive)
2. Yes, 99383-25; -51 is not added to any of these codes

-52, Reduced Services

Modifier -52 is used to indicate that a service was provided but was reduced in comparison to the full description of the service. Turn to Appendix A in the CPT manual and read the description of this modifier.

An example of a circumstance in which modifier -52 would be reported is a surgical procedure for the removal of an abdominal carcinoma in which the patient was anesthetized and the excision begun but then was terminated by the physician because the metastasis was too far advanced. When modifier -52 is reported, additional documentation, such as operative reports and/or physician explanation of the reason for the reduced service, will speed the reimbursement process, as the third-party payer usually wants to know the reason for the reduction before making payment.

CODING SHOT

Modifier -52 may or may not affect reimbursement. Some payers decrease the payment if the procedure was not completed, and others pay in full once anesthesia has been administered to the patient.

Example

A physician performed a hammer toe correction (28285) but the tendon was already split (the surgeon usually has to perform this), thereby decreasing the work necessary by the surgeon. In this case, only a portion of the usual procedure was completed. The service would be reported with 28285 with modifier -52.

Example

The operative report indicates: "Excision of ischial pressure ulcer, without ostectomy." Assign 15946 (Excision, ischial pressure ulcer, with ostectomy) with modifier -52. Modifier -52 indicates that all the procedure components were not entirely completed because the code indicated "with ostectomy" and the operative reported stated "without ostectomy."

CMS RULES

Do not assign modifier -52 with E/M services. Medicare does not recognize the modifier for this purpose, according to the Medicare Carriers Manual Section 15501. Instead, use unspecified E/M code 94999 and submit documentation that explains why less than the normal service was completed.

EXERCISE 14-2   *Modifiers -32 through -52*

Using the CPT, ICD-10-CM and/or ICD-9-CM manuals, code the following using the two code format for codes to which you add -50 or -51:

1 Workers' Compensation referred a patient to a physician for a mandatory examination to determine the legitimacy of a claim (insurance certification). What modifier would be added to the code for the examination service?

   Modifier: _____

   ICD-10-CM Code: _____

   (ICD-9-CM Code: _____)

2 Dr. Ramus administers regional anesthesia by intravenous injection (also known as a Bier block) for a surgical procedure on the patient's lower arm. Dr. Ramus then performs the surgical procedure. What modifier would be added to the surgical code?

   Modifier: _____

3 A patient underwent bilateral carpal tunnel surgery. When you assign a code, what modifier would you be certain to use?

   Modifier: _____

   ICD-10-CM Codes: _____, _____

   (ICD-9-CM Code: _____)

4 Destruction of primary, malignant lesion of neck, 4 cm in diameter (17274, $142.43), with destruction of primary, malignant lesion of arm, 4 cm in diameter (17264, $78.40).

   CPT Codes and Modifier: _____, _____

   ICD-10-CM Codes: _____, _____

   (ICD-9-CM Codes: _____, _____)

5 Bilateral supratentorial burr holes (61154) for chronic, subdural hematomas.

   CPT Codes and Modifier: _____, _____

   ICD-10-CM Code: _____

   (ICD-9-CM Code: _____)

6 Treatment of two tarsal bone fractures, without manipulation (each 28450).

   CPT Codes and Modifier: _____, _____

7 What is the code for a bilateral total knee replacement (arthroplasty)?

   CPT Codes and Modifier: _____, _____

8 Which modifier describes a procedure that was reduced at the direction of the physician?

   Modifier: _____

Continued

For Questions 9 and 10, list the three formats that may be required by third-party payers:

9 What are the codes for bilateral arthrotomy of the elbows (24006)?

One code listed twice with CPT modifier: _____, _____

One code listed once with CPT modifier: _____

One code listed twice with HCPCS modifiers: _____, _____

10 The code for a radical mastectomy is 19305. List three ways the bilateral modifier could be used to indicate that a bilateral procedure was performed, depending on the third-party payer's preferences.

One code listed twice with CPT modifier: _____, _____

One code listed once with CPT modifier: _____

One code listed twice with HCPCS modifiers: _____, _____

(Answers are located in Appendix B)

-53, Discontinued Procedure

Modifier -52 describes circumstances in which services were reduced at the direction of the physician, whereas modifier -53 describes circumstances in which a procedure was stopped because of the patient's status. Turn to Appendix A in the CPT manual and read the description of this modifier.

An example of the correct assignment of modifier -53 would be when a patient had received anesthesia and the procedure was underway. The patient then developed arrhythmia that could not be controlled. The physician discontinued the procedure because of the risk continuation presented to the patient. The code for the surgical procedure would be reported along with modifier -53 to indicate that although the procedure was begun, it was discontinued due to the patient's status. The key to proper reporting of modifier -53 is that the patient has been prepared for surgery, anesthetized, and the surgeon discontinued the procedure.

Modifier -53 is **not** used to report services:

■ When the patient cancels the procedure
■ With E/M codes
■ With any code that is based on time (e.g., critical care codes)

Attach a cover note and state the percentage of the procedure that was completed and why the procedure had to be stopped. For example, "Only 50% of procedure was completed. The procedure was stopped because patient developed arrhythmia that could not be controlled."

CMS RULES

Modifier -53 should be used to report a failed or terminated colonoscopy. When a colonoscopy is attempted, but not completed, it should not be reported as a sigmoidoscopy but as discontinued colonoscopy procedure 45378-53.

Modifiers -54, -55, and -56

There may be times when a surgeon performs only the surgery (modifier -54) and requests another physician to perform the preoperative evaluation (modifier -56) and/or the postoperative care (modifier -55). When reporting his or her own individual services, each physician would use the same procedure code for the surgery, letting the modifier indicate to the third-party payer the part of the surgical package that each personally performed.

Example

19303	Mastectomy, simple, complete
19303-54	Mastectomy, simple, complete, **surgery** (intraoperative) only
19303-56	Mastectomy, simple, complete, **preoperative** evaluation only
19303-55	Mastectomy, simple, complete, **postoperative** care only

-54, Surgical Care Only

Modifier -54 indicates the surgical care portion of a surgical procedure (intraoperative). Use modifier -54 only with codes from the Surgery section (10021-69990). Turn to Appendix A in the CPT manual and read the description of this modifier.

Modifier -54 is used correctly only when there has been a **transfer** of responsibility for care from one physician to another. This transfer takes place by means of a transfer order that is signed by both physicians and kept in the patient's medical record. Modifier -54 is not used for minor surgical procedures but for major procedures that involve follow-up care as a part of the service of the surgery (surgery package). Although third-party payers vary, the payment for only the surgical procedure is usually about 70% of the total payment for the procedure, with 10% for the physician who provides the preoperative service, and 20% for the physician who provides the postoperative care.

CODING SHOT

Modifier -54 usually results in reimbursement to the surgeon for the intraoperative percentage of the global package payment. However, some payers also include the preoperative service as a part of the intraoperative care portion. In these cases, you would submit a statement to indicate the preoperative service was provided by another physician.

-55, Postoperative Management Only

Another part of a surgical package is the postoperative care. The amount of postoperative care that is considered part of a surgery varies according to the complexity of the surgery, with 0, 10, or 90 days being the most commonly used number of postoperative days. Turn to Appendix A in the CPT manual and read the description of this modifier.

Modifier -55 is used only for services provided to the patient after discharge from the hospital. To report services by another physician provided while the patient is still in the hospital, use E/M codes (99231-99233, subsequent hospital care) because the payment to the operating physician (70%) assumes that the operating physician provides the care until the patient is discharged from the hospital.

You report the postoperative services by adding modifier -55 to the surgical code. For example, a patient had a nephrolithotomy (calculus removed from kidney), reported with 50060, and then the operating physician transferred to a second physician the postoperative care after the patient's discharge from the hospital. The operating physician would report services using 50060-54, and the physician providing the postoperative care would report 50060-55, with the date of the surgery. The claim is not submitted until after the first postoperative office visit. The physicians use the same surgery code (50060). In this way, the third-party payer knows that the two physicians are splitting the care of the patient into surgical care and postoperative care after discharge.

Modifier -55 should result in reimbursement of the postoperative percentage for the global package. This percentage is based on how many days had passed after the operation before the care was transferred from the first physician to the second physician. Care must be officially transferred from the physician providing the surgical care to the physician providing the postoperative care by way of a transfer order that is kept in the medical record.

When different physicians in a group practice participate in the care of a patient, the group reports the entire global package (no modifier). The physician who performs the surgery is indicated on the claim as the performing physician.

-56, Preoperative Management Only

The third part of a surgical service is the preoperative care. If a physician provides only the preoperative management to a patient in preparation for surgery, the service is reported with modifier -56 added to the surgical code. Turn to Appendix A in the CPT manual and read the description of this modifier.

Before a patient undergoes surgery, a physical examination is performed to determine whether the patient is physically able to withstand the procedure. This examination is the preoperative workup or preop. When one physician performs the preoperative workup and another physician performs the surgery, both physicians report the services using the surgical procedure code with the correct modifier. For example, in preparation for a nephrolithotomy, the patient's local physician performs the preoperative care (50060-56), an itinerate (visiting) surgeon performs the surgery (50060-54), and the local physician performs the postoperative care (50060-55).

CMS RULES

Modifier -56 is never used for services reported to Medicare, as Medicare considers the preoperative service to be part of the surgery and bundles the payment into the surgical payment.

-57, Decision for Surgery

Modifier -57 is reported with an E/M code to indicate the day the decision to perform a major surgery was made. Turn to Appendix A in the CPT manual and read the description of this modifier.

Modifier -57 can be reported not only with E/M codes (99201-99499) to indicate the initial decision to perform a procedure or service but also with the ophthalmologic codes (92002-92014) located in the Medicine section. Modifier -57 requests payment for an E/M service outside of the global package for a major procedure when the decision to perform the surgery was made during the E/M service.

At the present time, not all modifiers are recognized by all third-party payers. Some third-party payers have agreed to pay a physician separately from the surgical package for the initial evaluation of a condition during which the decision to perform surgery was made. Modifier -57 is used to let the payer know that payment for this initial evaluation should be made in addition to payment for surgery.

⚠️ **CAUTION** *Don't make the all too common mistake of adding -57 to codes from the Surgery section. Modifier -57 is never added to surgical codes; rather, it is added only to E/M codes.*

E/M services provided the **day before** or the **day of** a major surgery are included in the global package. There are some exceptions, such as when the service is the patient's initial visit to the physician. To receive payment for these initial visits, modifier -57 is reported to indicate the decision for surgery was made the day before or the day of the **major** procedure and modifier -25 is used to indicate the day of a **minor** procedure.

CODING SHOT

Note that the description of modifier -57 does not indicate whether the decided-upon procedure is diagnostic or therapeutic, minor or major. These guidelines are established by the third-party payers.

CMS RULES

Medicare states that the carrier is to pay for an E/M service on the day of or on the day before a procedure with a 90-day global surgical period if the physician uses CPT modifier -57. Without modifier -57 the service will not be paid.

-58, Staged or Related Procedure or Service by the Same Physician or Other Qualified Health Care Professional During the Postoperative Period

Modifier -58 notifies the payer that a subsequent surgery was planned or staged at the time of the first surgery. Turn to Appendix A in the CPT manual and read the description of this modifier.

The procedure must have been intended to include the original procedure plus one or more subsequent procedures. For example, multiple skin grafts are often done in stages to allow adequate healing time between procedures. The modifier is added to the subsequent submissions of the code when the second or related service is performed during the global period to inform the third-party payer that the service was staged. Modifier -58 can also be used if a therapeutic procedure is performed because of the findings of a diagnostic procedure. For example, a patient may have a surgical breast biopsy, and if the pathology report indicates that the specimen is malignant, the patient may elect to have an immediate radical mastectomy. The mastectomy may be performed during the postoperative period of the biopsy. Modifier -58 indicates to the third-party payer that the second surgery was therapeutic treatment that followed the original diagnostic procedure, and full payment would usually be made for the mastectomy. A new postoperative period would start after the mastectomy, and any postoperative care provided to the patient would be part of the surgical package for the mastectomy.

✋ **CAUTION** *There are some codes that include multiple sessions in the code description. For example, 67141 and 67145 include "1 or more sessions" in the code description. Modifier -58 is not appropriate with these multiple session codes.*

CODING SHOT

Modifier -58 requests full payment for a subsequent procedure that may have been planned in follow-up, at the time of the first surgery, or performed as a more extensive procedure subsequent to the first surgery. A new global period begins with each subsequent procedure modified with -58.

Example
A lesion was excised and determined to be malignant. The patient was returned to the operating room a few days later for a re-excision of the malignancy. Report the re-excision with modifier -58 because the second procedure was performed within the global period of the first procedure and related to the first procedure.

Example
A patient required a toe amputation due to gangrene. On follow-up, the surgeon determined the patient requires further amputation, this time of his entire foot because the original procedure did not completely remove the gangrenous tissue. If the second amputation occurs within the postoperative period of the first amputation, the second amputation would be reported with modifier -58 as it is related to the first procedure.

-59, Distinct Procedural Service

Modifier -59 is reported to indicate that services that are usually bundled into one payment were provided as separate services. Turn to Appendix A in the CPT manual and read the description of this modifier.

As the code description notes, modifier -59 is used to identify the following:

- Different session
- Different procedure or surgery
- Different site or organ system
- Separate incision/excision
- Separate lesion
- Separate injury or area of injury in extensive injuries

Modifier -59 is reported with codes from all sections of the CPT manual except E/M codes.

CMS RULES

Medicare has lists of codes that cannot be reported together called National Correct Coding Initiatives (NCCI edits). These edits have been established to ensure that providers do not report services that are included in a pre-established bundle. For example, the same physician would not report a standard preoperative visit related to a major surgical procedure and then report separately the surgery and follow-up care. All three services—preoperative, intraoperative, postoperative—are bundled together in one major surgical CPT code. The use of modifier -59 indicates that the service was not a part of another service but, indeed, was a distinct service. For example, a colonoscopy utilizing a snare (45385) and a colonoscopy with hot biopsy forceps (45384) would usually not be reported together because both codes would be in the edits, but if -59 was appended to 45384, the surgeon would be indicating that distinct services were provided.

Modifiers -X{EPSU} Effective January 1, 2015, the Centers for Medicare and Medicaid Services (CMS) is establishing four new HCPCS modifiers collectively referred to as modifiers -X{EPSU} to define subsets of modifier -59.

- **-XE Separate Encounter.** A service that is distinct because it occurred during a separate encounter.
- **-XS Separate Structure.** A service that is distinct because it was performed on a separate organ/structure.
- **-XP Separate Practitioner.** A service that is distinct because it was performed by a different practitioner.
- **-XU Unusual Non-Overlapping Service.** Use of a service that is distinct because it does not overlap usual components of the main service.

While CMS will continue to recognize modifier -59, CPT instructions state that modifier -59 should not be used when a more descriptive modifier is available, such as one of the modifiers -X{EPSU}.

CHECK THIS OUT ☞ For more details about modifiers -X{EPSU}, check out http://www.cms.gov/Regulations-and-Guidance/Guidance/Transmittals/Downloads/R1422OTN.pdf

CODING SHOT

Modifier -59 requests payment for a procedure performed on the same day as another procedure that normally would not be reimbursed separately, e.g., a biopsy of one site and an excision of another site.

A note of caution is that modifier -59 has been abused by providers and excessively submitted. The Office of the Inspector General has targeted the submission of this modifier in the past. That means random audits of physician claim submission were conducted.

EXERCISE 14-3   *Modifiers -53 through -59*

Using the CPT, ICD-10-CM and/or ICD-9-CM manuals, code the following:

1 Mrs. Knight has a diagnostic surgical biopsy of deep cervical lymph nodes on May 8, and the pathology report comes back showing secondary malignancy with the primary site unknown. Mrs. Knight elects to have a lymphadenectomy on May 11. What modifier would be used with the lymphadenectomy code?

Modifier: _____

ICD 10-CM Codes: _____, _____

(ICD-9-CM Codes: _____, _____)

2 The intraoperative service for a total esophagectomy without reconstruction (43124)

CPT Code and Modifier: _____

3 The postoperative care only for a radical mastectomy including pectoral muscles, axillary, and internal mammary lymph nodes (19306)

CPT Code and Modifier: _____

4 The procedure in question 3 when only the preoperative service is provided

CPT Code and Modifier: _____

(Answers are located in Appendix B)

-62, Two Surgeons

Modifier -62 indicates two surgeons acted as co-surgeons. Turn to Appendix A in the CPT manual and read the description of this modifier.

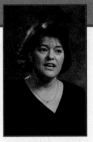

From the Trenches

"Learning to use the CPT manual effectively as a tool is one of the best skills I can teach my students to develop. . . . I always advise them to start with a strong foundation by taking classes in medical terminology, anatomy, and physiology."

JANE

To assign modifier -62 correctly, two physicians of different specialties must have worked together as co-surgeons and each surgeon must have dictated his/her own operative report. If one physician assists another physician, the service cannot be reported using modifier -62. Co-surgeons use different skills during the surgery. Many third-party payers require documentation showing the medical necessity of co-surgeons. The operative reports document each surgeon's participation and clearly show the distinct services each performed. Modifier -62 is correctly reported when two physicians are necessary to complete one surgical procedure, each completing a distinct portion of the procedure. For example, a cardiologist and a general surgeon may install a pacemaker, with the general surgeon preparing the implantation site, the cardiologist inserting and activating the pacemaker, and the general surgeon closing the site. Each physician would report his/her service using the pacemaker insertion code with modifier -62.

CODING SHOT

Modifier -62 will usually cue the payer to reimburse at 125% of the fee schedule, which is then divided, half for each surgeon.

Example

A patient diagnosed with bladder cancer undergoes a radical cystectomy and ureteroileal ileal conduit (passage to divert urine from the kidney to the exterior). A general surgeon opens the surgical area to view, then a urologist removes the bladder. The general surgeon creates an ureteroileal conduit and the general surgeon closes the incisions. Each physician reports 51585 (complete cystectomy) with modifier -62. The surgeons would be paid a combined 125% of the fee schedule amount for the code (62.5% each).

-63, Procedure Performed on Infants Less than 4 kg

Modifier -63 is used to identify procedures provided to a neonate or infant up to 4 kg (8.8 lbs). Turn to Appendix A in the CPT manual and read the description of this modifier.

Do not use modifier -63 with the Integumentary System codes (10030-19499). Parenthetical notes also follow some codes in the 20005-69990 range and direct the coder not to report -63 with certain codes.

Procedures on neonates or infants with a body weight of less than 4 kg (8.8 lbs) are more complex than procedures that are performed on neonates or infants with a body weight of more than 4 kg.

QUICK CHECK 14-4

1. Would modifier -63 be reported with codes 49491-49496? Why or why not?

_____

(Answers are located in Appendix C)

-66, Surgical Team

Modifier -66 is used with very complex surgical procedures that require several physicians, usually of different specialties, to complete the procedure. Turn to Appendix A in the CPT manual and read the description of this modifier.

A surgical team consists of physicians (more than two), technicians, and other trained personnel who function together to complete a complex procedure. For example, teams are usually used in organ transplant surgeries, with each member of the team completing the same function at each surgery. Each physician on the team reports the procedure code with modifier -66. Third-party payers will often increase the total reimbursement for a team. The reimbursement is divided among the physicians on the basis of a prearranged agreement.

CODING SHOT

Modifier -66 will cue the payer that payment for a procedure should be increased by whatever the contract allows to be divided by all surgeons involved.

> **Example**
> A patient is admitted for an artificial heart transplant (33935, heart-lung transplant with recipient cardiectomy-pneumonectomy). A team of cardiologists, general surgeons, and thoracic surgeons performs the surgery and each dictates a description of the procedure. Each surgeon would report 33935 with modifier -66. Each surgeon not only dictates his or her portion of the surgery but also submits his or her own claim.

-76, Repeat Procedure or Service by Same Physician or Other Qualified Health Care Professional

Modifier -76 is assigned to report services or procedures that are being repeated by the same physician. Turn to Appendix A in the CPT manual and read the description of this modifier.

The modifier is reported to indicate to third-party payers that the services are not duplicate services and the bill is not a duplicate bill. Sometimes these repeat services are provided on the same day as the previous service, and without the use of modifier -76, the third-party payer would assume a duplicate bill had been submitted. When modifier -76 has been submitted, documentation to establish medical necessity may be requested by the third-party payer.

CODING SHOT

Modifier -76 requests payment for a service that was repeated. If the modifier was not used, the subsequent service would be denied as a duplicate service.

-77, Repeat Procedure by Another Physician or Other Qualified Health Care Professional

Modifier -77 reports services or procedures that are repeated and are provided by an individual other than the individual who originally provided the service or procedure. Turn to Appendix A in the CPT manual and read the description of this modifier.

Modifier -77 reports to the third-party payer that the services are not duplicate services and, therefore, the bill is not a duplicate bill. Sometimes these repeat services are provided on the same day as the original service or during the postoperative period. Without the use of modifier -77, the third-party payer would assume a duplicate bill had been submitted. When modifier -77 has been assigned, documentation must accompany the claim in order to establish the medical necessity for the procedure.

CODING SHOT

Modifier -77 requests payment for a service that was repeated. If the modifier was not used, the subsequent service would be denied as a duplicate service.

> ✋ **CAUTION** *CMS stated that the increased use of both -76 and -77 indicates possible inappropriate assignment with E/M services, and closer monitoring will be given to the submission of these two modifiers.*

If only a portion of the original service or procedure is repeated, you would also assign modifier -52 to indicate a reduced service.

-78, Unplanned Return to the Operating/Procedure Room by the Same Physician or Other Qualified Health Care Professional Following Initial Procedure for a Related Procedure During the Postoperative Period

Modifier -78 is assigned to indicate a circumstance in which a patient is returned to the operating room for surgical treatment of a complication that resulted from the first procedure. Turn to Appendix A in the CPT manual and read the description of this modifier.

Modifier -78 is appended to the subsequent procedure code to indicate to the third-party payer that the second surgery was necessary because of complications resulting from the first operation. For many third-party payers, only the surgery portion (intraoperative) of the surgical package is paid when the -78 modifier is reported. The patient remains within the postoperative period of the first operation for any further preoperative or postoperative care. For example, if the patient were to develop a second set of complications stemming from the original surgery, you would again report the procedure performed to treat the second complication and add modifier -78 to the code. This way, the third-party payer continues to know that the complication requiring surgery originated from the original surgery during the global period.

✋ **CAUTION** *If there were a complication, you would report -78 (Unplanned Return to the Operating/Procedure Room) and -76 (Repeat Procedure or Service by Same Physician or Other Qualified Health Care Professional). For example, if a patient who has an open heart coronary artery bypass graft procedure (Service 1) returns to the operating room for tamponade (fluid accumulation in the pericardium) twice on the same day (Services 2 and 3), modifier -76 would be appended to the procedure as follows:*

Service 1
33510   Coronary artery bypass graft

Service 2
35820-78   Exploration for postoperative hemorrhage, chest

Service 3
35820-78-76   Repeat exploration for postoperative hemorrhage, chest

Services 2 and 3 procedures should be reimbursed at the intraoperative rate, but the global period would continue from the first session and would not start over again.

CODING SHOT

Modifier -78 will cue the payer to reimburse the procedure at the intraoperative percent of the service. The patient remains in the global period for the initial surgery.

An "operating/procedure" room is defined as a place of service specifically equipped and staffed for the sole purpose of performing procedures. For example, a cardiac catheterization suite, a laser suite, or an endoscopy suite. It does not include a patient's room, a minor treatment room, a recovery room, or intensive care unit (unless the patient's condition was so critical there was insufficient time for transport to an operating room).

-79, Unrelated Procedure or Service by the Same Physician or Other Qualified Health Care Professional During the Postoperative Period

CAUTION *Do not use modifier -79 with staged procedures (use modifier -58) or with procedures that are related to the original procedure. If the service is provided during the post-operative period of a major surgical procedure, billing separately for services included in the surgical package is fraudulent.*

Modifier -79 explains that a patient requires surgery for a condition totally unrelated to the condition for which the first operation was performed. Turn to Appendix A in the CPT manual and read the description of this modifier.

For example, the patient had an appendectomy and 2 weeks later had a gallbladder episode that necessitates removal of the gallbladder. Modifier -79 would be placed on the cholecystectomy code, indicating that the subsequent procedure was unrelated to the first procedure. The diagnosis codes for the two procedures would also be different, further indicating the two procedures were unrelated.

CODING SHOT

Modifier -79 requests payment for the full fee of the subsequent service because it was unassociated with the first procedure. A new global period should start when -79 is submitted.

-80, Assistant Surgeon

A surgical assistant is one who provides service (an extra pair of hands) to the primary surgeon during a surgical procedure. Turn to Appendix A in the CPT manual and read the description of this modifier.

The assistant surgeon's services are reported using the same code as the primary surgeon's, but modifier -80 is added to alert the third-party payer to the assistant surgeon's status. Usually, the assistant surgeon receives 15% to 30% of the usual charge for a surgery when acting in the assistant capacity. Not all payers allow for an assistant surgeon on all procedures. A preauthorization for surgery should be completed before surgery to determine if the payer will reimburse for an assistant surgeon.

CODING SHOT

Preauthorization does not guarantee payment, as the payer can always deny the approval upon review.

CAUTION *A physician assistant providing assist at surgery would use the HCPCS modifier -AS, not modifier -80.*

-81, Minimum Assistant Surgeon

Modifier -81 indicates an assistant surgeon who provides services that are less extensive than those described by modifier -80. Turn to Appendix A in the CPT manual and read the description of this modifier.

Modifier -81 is not commonly used, although there are times when an assistant surgeon is present and assists for only a portion of the procedure. This minimal assistant surgeon service is then reported by adding -81 to the surgical code. Some third-party payers define a minimal assistant surgeon as a nurse practitioner, physician's assistant, or other specialized clinical nursing personnel, but according to the CPT definition, the service is provided by a physician acting in a minimal capacity. You should receive written directives from the third-party payer before reporting -81 for individuals other than a physician.

Many third-party payers do not pay for a minimum assistant surgeon. For example, Medicare will pay for a minimum assistant only on rare occasions in which medical necessity can be proven. Usually, the minimum assistant surgeon receives 10% of the usual charge for a surgery.

-82, Assistant Surgeon (When Qualified Resident Surgeon Not Available)

Modifier -82 is assigned when the hospital in which the procedure was performed has an affiliation with a medical school and has a residency program, but no resident was available to serve as an assistant surgeon. Residents are physicians who are completing a required surgical training period in the hospital during which the residents serve as employees of the hospital who are there to receive training and provide assistance to physicians as part of the hospital's agreement with the medical school. Hospitals that have affiliations with medical schools are considered teaching facilities. Turn to Appendix A in the CPT manual and read the description of this modifier.

Do not confuse modifier -80 (assistant surgeon) with -82 when reporting services.

CODING SHOT

Medicare does not pay for an assistant surgeon if the hospital has a residency program.

Modifier -82 has very limited use and requires supporting documentation that the patient's condition was such that the service required an assistant surgeon and that a qualified resident was not available.

EXERCISE 14-4   *Modifiers -62 through -82*

Using the CPT, ICD-10-CM and/or ICD-9-CM manuals, indicate the correct modifier and diagnosis codes where indicated:

1 Dr. Edwards, a cardiologist, and Dr. Mathews, a general surgeon, worked together as primary surgeons on a complex surgical case. What modifier would be added to the CPT surgery codes for the services of both Dr. Edwards and Dr. Mathews?

Modifier: _____

2 A team of physicians with different specialties, along with a highly skilled team of technical personnel, performed a liver transplant for a patient with chronic viral hepatitis C that has resulted in cirrhosis of the liver. Which modifier would indicate the surgical team concept?

Modifier: _____

ICD-10-CM Codes: _____, _____

(ICD-9-CM Codes: _____, _____)

3 Dr. Stenopolis served as a surgical assistant to Dr. Edwards in a quadruple bypass procedure. Dr. Stenopolis' services were reported by using this modifier:

Modifier: _____

4 In the middle of the bypass procedure in Question 3, the patient experienced severe complications. Dr. Edwards asked Dr. Loren to come into the operating room to temporarily assist with the surgery to stabilize the patient. What modifier would be used when reporting the service Dr. Loren provided?

Modifier: _____

5 A patient had a hernia repair and two days later returned to the operating room for a dehiscence of the incision. When coding the secondary hernia repair, which modifier would you add onto the surgical code?

Modifier: _____

6 If Mr. Smith undergoes an appendectomy on June 8, and then a cholecystectomy is performed on August 16 by the same surgeon, what modifier would be placed on the cholecystectomy code?

Modifier: _____

7 What modifier would you add to a code to indicate that a basic procedure performed by another physician was repeated?

Modifier: _____

(Answers are located in Appendix B)

-90, Reference (Outside) Laboratory

Modifier -90 is used to indicate that services of an outside laboratory were used. Turn to Appendix A in the CPT manual and read the description of this modifier.

This modifier is reported with Pathology and Laboratory codes to report that the procedures were performed by someone other than the treating or reporting physician.

CMS RULES

Medicare does not allow physicians to bill for outside laboratory services and then reimburse the outside laboratory for those services. If the outside laboratory provides the services, the outside laboratory must report the services.

-91, Repeat Clinical Diagnostic Laboratory Test

Modifier -91 reports a laboratory test that was performed on the same day as the original laboratory test. Turn to Appendix A in the CPT manual and read the description of this modifier.

This modifier is correctly assigned when a laboratory test has been repeated so as to produce multiple test results. It cannot be assigned if the lab equipment malfunctioned or if there was a problem with the specimen, because this would result in third-party payers' paying for laboratory errors. Also, do not assign the modifier for services performed because a subsequent test was done to confirm the results of the initial test. The modifier also cannot be assigned when there is a series of test results, such as those performed in allergy testing.

-92, Alternative Laboratory Platform Testing

Modifier -92 reports those incidents when a kit or transportable instrument is used in a laboratory test. For example, a single-use, disposable HIV kit (86701-86703). Turn to Appendix A in the CPT manual and read the description of this modifier.

-99, Multiple Modifiers

Modifier -99 is needed only if the third-party payer does not accept multiple modifiers. This is the case with some computerized insurance submissions. Turn to Appendix A in the CPT manual and read the description of this modifier.

On the CMS-1500 insurance claim form (Fig. 14-2) there is space for multiple modifiers. Third-party payers vary in terms of how they require multiple modifiers to be reported, so be certain to check with the payer before submitting multiple modifiers.

EXERCISE 14-5   *Modifiers -90 through -99*

Using the CPT manual, code the following:

1 What is the modifier that indicates that multiple modifiers apply? _____

2 What modifier would be added to the laboratory procedure code to indicate testing by an outside laboratory? _____

3 The medical record indicated that the physician had an established patient go to the lab for a blood panel in the morning, and in the afternoon had the patient return to the lab for another blood panel so as to produce multiple test results. What modifier

would you add to the code for the panel? _____

(Answers are located in Appendix B)

FIGURE 14-2 Multiple modifiers on the CMS-1500 insurance claim form.

CHAPTER REVIEW

CHAPTER 14, PART I, THEORY

Complete the following:

1 When more than two physicians, with technicians and specialized equipment, work together to complete a complicated procedure and each physician has a specific portion of the surgery to complete, they are termed what?

_____

2 Can modifier -22 be assigned to 99291, 99292 codes?

Yes   No

3 This modifier indicates an increased service and is overused and results in an increase in payment of 20% to 30%. As such, the assignment of this modifier comes under particularly close scrutiny by third-party payers. What is this

modifier? _____

4 When modifier -54 is assigned, payment for the _____ portion of the surgical procedure is being requested.

5 Joan is a new coder at the local clinic. You have been assigned to review her coding before it is submitted to the third-party payer. You note that she assigned modifier -32 to E/M consultation code 99244. The medical record indicates that the request for the second opinion was made by the patient's spouse. Is Joan correct in modifier -32 assignment? Why or

why not? _____

6 Which of these statements is true about modifier -59?
   a It is only appended to E/M codes.
   b It is only appended to other than E/M codes.

7 What is the weight in pounds of a 4-kilogram infant?
   a 7.9
   b 8.8
   c 8.9
   d 9.1

8 Which of the following two statements are NOT true about modifier -53?
   a Describes circumstances based on the patient's preoperative condition
   b May be used to describe those times when the physician elects to terminate a procedure due to the well-being of the patient
   c Describes circumstances in which the patient canceled the procedure
   d May be used to describe ASC reporting of previously scheduled procedure that is partially reduced as a result of extenuating circumstances

9 Modifier -57 can be added to Surgery section codes.

True   False

10 When adding multiple CPT modifiers to a code, you would list the modifiers from:
   a Highest to lowest
   b Lowest to highest
   c Makes no difference which is listed first

Chapter Review answers are only available in the TEACH Instructor Resources on Evolve

CHAPTER 14, PART II, PRACTICAL

Using your CPT manual, identify the modifier for the following descriptions:

11 Repeat procedure or service by same physician _____

12 Two surgeons _____

13 Professional component _____

14 Multiple modifiers _____

15 Distinct procedural service _____

16 Mandated service _____

17 Significant identifiable E/M service provided by the same individual on the same day as another service or procedure

_____

18 Minimum assistant surgeon _____

19 Repeat procedure by another individual _____

20 Unrelated procedure or service by the same individual during the postoperative period _____

21 Unusual anesthesia _____

22 Unplanned return to the operating room for a related procedure during the postoperative period _____

23 Surgical care only _____

24 Reduced service _____

25 Surgical team _____

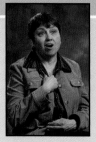

"I think having a goal of being a lifelong learner is important. One also has to have a great degree of integrity. It takes knowledge and character to adhere to the correct way to do things and not be swayed by other factors, such as how to 'get it paid.'"

Joan E. Wolfgang, MEd, RHIT, CPC, COC, CPC-I, CCA
Faculty
Milwaukee Area Technical College
Milwaukee, Wisconsin

Evaluation and Management (E/M) Services

Chapter Topics

Contents of the E/M Section

Three Factors of E/M Codes

Various Levels of E/M Service

An E/M Code Example

Using the E/M Codes

Documentation Guidelines

Chapter Review

Learning Objectives

After completing this chapter you should be able to

1 Identify and explain the three factors of E/M code assignment.

2 Differentiate between a new and an established patient.

3 Differentiate between an inpatient and an outpatient.

4 Explain the levels of E/M service.

5 Review the key components.

6 Analyze the key component history.

7 Analyze the key component examination.

8 Analyze the key component medical decision making.

9 List contributory factors.

10 Analyze code information.

11 Analyze the types of E/M codes.

12 Identify CMS Documentation Guidelines.

13 Demonstrate the ability to code E/M services.

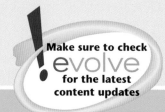

Make sure to check **evolve** for the latest content updates

CONTENTS OF THE E/M SECTION

The information in Chapter 13 described the basic format of the CPT manual. The information and exercises in this chapter will familiarize you with the first section of the CPT manual, Evaluation and Management (E/M). Locate the index in the E/M section of the CPT manual, titled Evaluation and Management (E/M) Services Guidelines. It provides a listing of headings and subheadings for the categories and subcategories of Evaluation and Management services as illustrated in the table below.

Office or Other Outpatient Services		**Prolonged Services**	
New Patient	99201-99205	With Direct Patient Contact	99354-99357
Established Patient	99211-99215	Without Direct Patient Contact	99358-99359
Hospital Observation Services		Standby Services	99360
Observation Care Discharge Services	99217	**Case Management Services**	
Initial Observation Care	99218-99220	Anticoagulation Management	99363-99364
Subsequent Observation Care	99224-99226	Medical Team Conferences	99366-99368
Hospital Inpatient Services		**Care Plan Oversight Services**	99374-99380
Initial Hospital Care	99221-99223	**Preventive Medicine Services**	
Subsequent Hospital Care	99231-99233	New Patient	99381-99387
Observation or Inpatient Care Services	99234-99236	Established Patient	99391-99397
Hospital Discharge Services	99238-99239	Counseling Risk Factor Reduction and Behavior	99401-99420
Consultations		Change Intervention	
Office or Other Outpatients Consultations	99241-99245	**Non-Face-to-Face Services**	
Inpatient Consultations	99251-99255	Telephone Services	99441-99443
Emergency Department Services	99281-99285	On-line Medical Evaluation	99444-99449
Other Emergency Services	99288	**Special E/M Services**	99450-99456
Critical Care Services	99291-99292	**Newborn Care Services**	99460-99463
Nursing Facility Services		Delivery/Birthing Room Attendance and	99464-99465
Initial Nursing Facility Care	99304-99306	Resuscitation Services	
Subsequent Nursing Facility Care	99307-99310	**Inpatient Neonatal Intensive Care Services and Pediatric**	
Nursing Facility Discharge Services	99315-99316	**and Neonatal Critical Care Services**	
Other Nursing Facility Services	99318	Pediatric Critical Care Patient Transport	99466-99486
Domiciliary, Rest Home (e.g., Boarding Home), or		Inpatient Neonatal and Pediatric Critical Care	99468-99476
Custodial Care Services		Initial and Continuing Intensive Care Services	99477-99486
New Patient	99324-99328	**Care Management Services**	99487-99490
Established Patient	99334-99337	Chronic Care Management Services	99490
Domiciliary, Rest Home (e.g., Assisted	99339-99340	Complex Chronic Care Management Services	99487, 99489
Living Facility), or Home Care Plan		**Transitional Care Management Services**	99495-99496
Oversight Services		**Advance Care Planning**	99497-99498
Home Services		**Other E/M Services**	99499
New Patient	99341-99345		
Established Patient	99347-99350		

THREE FACTORS OF E/M CODES

Code assignment in the E/M section varies according to three factors:
1. Place of service
2. Type of service
3. Patient status

Place of Service

The first factor you must consider in code assignment is the place of service (Fig. 15-1).

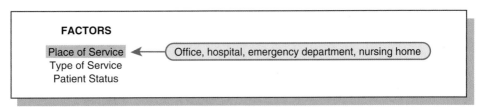

FACTORS

Place of Service ← Office, hospital, emergency department, nursing home
Type of Service
Patient Status

FIGURE 15–1   Place of service.

Place of service explains the setting in which the services were provided to the patient. Codes vary depending on the place of the service. Places of service can be a physician's office, hospital, emergency department, nursing home, and so on.

Type of Service

The second factor in code assignment is the type of service (Fig. 15-2).

Type of service is the reason the service is requested or performed. Examples of types of service are consultation, admission, newborn care, and office visit.

■ **Consultation** is a written or verbal request from one provider/physician to another to obtain an opinion and/or advice about a diagnosis or management options.

■ **Admission** is attention to an acute illness or injury that results in admission to a hospital.

■ **Newborn care** is the evaluation and determination of care management of a newly born infant.

■ **Office visit** is a face-to-face encounter between a physician and a patient to allow for primary management of the patient's health care status.

Patient Status

The third factor in code assignment is patient status (Fig. 15-3).

The four types of patient **status** are new patient, established patient, outpatient, and inpatient. Codes are often grouped in the CPT manual according to the type of patient involved.

■ **New** patient is one who has not received professional services from the physician or another physician of the exact same specialty and subspecialty in the same group within the past 3 years.

■ **Established** patient is one who has received professional services from the physician or another physician of the exact same specialty and subspecialty in the same group within the past 3 years.

■ **Outpatient** is one who has not been formally admitted to a health care facility or a patient admitted for observation.

■ **Inpatient** is one who has been formally admitted to a health care facility.

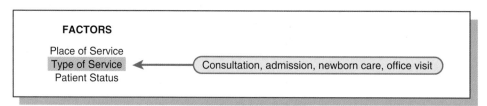

FIGURE 15–2 Type of service.

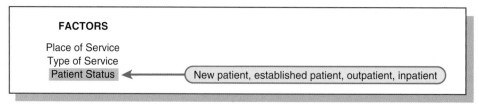

FIGURE 15–3 Patient status.

EXERCISE 15-1   *Three Factors of E/M Codes*

Using a CPT manual, locate the subsection Office and Other Outpatient Services and then the category New Patient in the E/M section to answer the following questions:

1 Where is the place of service? _____

2 What is the type of service? _____

3 What is the patient status? _____

4 What is the first code number listed under the subheading New Patient?

   CPT Code: _____

5 Each code represents a different level of service. How many codes are listed under Office or Other Outpatient Services for a

   new patient? _____

6 How many codes are listed for the established patient in the Office or Other Outpatient Services category? _____

(Answers are located in Appendix B)

Medical Records Documentation

Patient information is located in the medical record. This information is referred to as **documentation**. The documentation in the medical record has many uses, such as evaluation of the patient's treatment, communications regarding the patient's health care, reimbursement claims, review of the use of the health care facility, research/education, and legal documentation. Seven organizations (American Health Information Management Association, American Hospital Association, Managed Care and Review Association, American Medical Association, American Medical Peer Review Association, Blue Cross and Blue Shield Association, and the Health Insurance Association of America) developed minimum documentation guidelines, as follows:

1. The medical record should be complete and legible.
2. Documentation of each encounter should include the date, reason for encounter, appropriate history and physical examination, review of ancillary services, assessment, and plan of care with provider signature and date.
3. Past and present diagnoses should be accessible to the treating and/or consulting physician.
4. The reasons for and results of x-rays, lab tests, and other ancillary services should be clear.
5. Relevant risk factors should be identified.
6. The patient's progress and response to treatment, any change in treatment or change in diagnosis, and any patient noncompliance should be documented.
7. A written plan of treatment should include, when appropriate, treatments and medications, specifying frequency and dosage, any referrals or consultations, patient or family education, and any specific instructions for follow-up care.
8. Documentation should report the intensity of the patient evaluation and/or the treatment, including thought processes and the complexity of the medical decision making.
9. All entries should be dated and authenticated by provider or provider extender.
10. The CPT and ICD-10-CM/ICD-9-CM codes reported on the insurance claim or billing statement should reflect (**support**) the documentation in the medical record.

VARIOUS LEVELS OF E/M SERVICE

The levels of E/M service are based on documentation located in the patient's medical record supporting various amounts of skill, effort, time, responsibility, and medical knowledge used by the physician to provide the service to the patient. The levels of service are based on **key components** (history, examination, and medical decision-making complexity) and **contributory factors** (counseling, coordination of care, nature of presenting problem, and time). The components contain a great deal of information that you need to know before you learn about factors. Let's look at each of these components and factors individually.

Key Components

- History
- Examination
- Medical decision making

The key components of history, examination, and medical decision making reflect the clinical information that is recorded by the physician in the patient's medical record. Key components are present in every patient case except counseling encounters, which are discussed later in the chapter. Key components enable you to choose the appropriate level of service. New patient encounters, consultations, emergency department visits, and admissions require documentation of all three of the key components. Subsequent visits such as daily hospital visits or outpatient visits for an established patient require that only two of the three key components be present for assignment to a given code. For example, to assign code 99214—established patient, office visit—at least two of the three key components must be documented in the patient's medical record.

> **Example**
>
> 99214   Office or other outpatient visit for the evaluation and management of an established patient, which requires **at least two of these three key components:**
>
> - **a detailed history;**
> - **a detailed examination;**
> - **medical decision making of moderate complexity.**

Office, New Patient

According to the E/M Guidelines, the following categories/subcategories must meet or exceed the stated level of the key components:
- Office or Other Outpatient Services, New Patient
- Initial Observation Care, New or Established Patient
- Initial Hospital Care, New or Established Patient
- Office or Other Outpatient Consultations, New or Established Patient
- Observation or Inpatient Care Services, New or Established Patient
- Inpatient Consultations, New or Established Patient
- Emergency Department Services, New or Established Patient
- Initial Nursing Facility Care, New or Established Patient
- Domiciliary, Rest Home (e.g., Boarding Home), or Custodial Care Services, New Patient
- Home Services, New Patient

Of the following categories/subcategories, **two** of the **three** key components must be met or exceeded before the code may be assigned:

- Office or Other Outpatient Services, Established Patient
- Subsequent Observation Care, New or Established Patient
- Subsequent Hospital Care, New or Established Patient
- Subsequent Nursing Facility Care, New or Established Patient
- Domiciliary Care, Rest Home (e.g., Boarding Home), or Custodial Care Services, Established Patient
- Home, Established Patient

History. The history is the subjective information the patient tells the physician based on the four elements of a history—chief complaint (CC); history of present illness (HPI); review of systems (ROS); and past, family, and social history (PFSH). The history contains the information the physician needs to appropriately assess the patient's condition. Not all histories have all elements. The inclusion of each of the elements and the extent to which each of the elements is contained in a history are determined by the physician, based on the need for more or less subjective information, and will determine the extent of the history level. The documentation of the history is found in the patient's medical record and is recorded by the physician.

Ancillary staff (nurses, physician assistants, and so forth) are allowed to document some of the history, such as chief complaint and past, family, and social histories, but the physician must authenticate the entries (physician must evaluate the form and indicate in the medical record that the form has been reviewed). Also, a physician can have the patient complete a form composed of questions concerning the review of systems; however, the physician must authenticate the information.

THE FOUR ELEMENTS OF A HISTORY

- Chief Complaint (CC)
- History of Present Illness (HPI)
- Review of Systems (ROS)
- Past, Family, and/or Social History (PFSH)

History Elements. You need to be able to identify the various elements and levels of a history by reading the notes entered into the medical record by the physician.

1. **Chief Complaint (CC)** is a concise statement describing the symptom, problem, condition, diagnosis, physician-recommended return, or other factor that is the reason for the encounter, usually stated in the patient's words.

2. **History of Present Illness (HPI)** is a chronological description of the development of the patient's present illness from the first sign and/or symptom or from the previous encounter to the present. The HPI may include the elements identified in the following example:

Example

Location: thoracic spine (site on body)

Quality: burning, throbbing (characteristics)

Severity: on a scale of 1 to 10, an 8 (intensity)

Duration: 3 days (how long is an episode or how long has the problem existed)

Timing: throughout the day, continuously, at night, in the morning, etc., the frequency (when does it occur)

Context: when bending over (under what circumstances does it occur)

Modifying factors: better when lying down (what circumstances make it better or worse)

Associated signs and symptoms: weakness (what else is present that relates to chief complaint)

The HPI must be documented in the medical record by the physician.

TOOLBOX

Juanita presents to her family physician today with complaints of sharp stomach pain (5/10, 5 on a severity scale of 10) for 6 days, usually in the afternoon after her afternoon coffee.

HISTORY OF PRESENT ILLNESS (HPI)
1. Location (site on body)
2. Quality (characteristic: throbbing, sharp)
3. Severity (1/10 or how intense)
4. Duration (how long for problem or episode)
5. Timing (when it occurs)
6. Context (under what circumstances does it occur)
7. Modifying factors (what makes it better or worse)
8. Associated signs and symptoms (what else is happening when it occurs)

QUESTION

An E/M audit form would have the HPI elements listed as in the audit form on the left. The coder checks off each element of the HPI as documented in the medical record. Check off the HPI elements on the audit form based on Juanita's record.

How many elements did you count?

▼ ANSWER

4. (Location, Severity, Duration, Modifying factors, Quality, Timing)

3. **Review of Systems (ROS)** is an inventory of body systems obtained through a series of questions seeking to identify signs and/or symptoms that the patient may be experiencing or has experienced. According to Huffman's *Health Information Management,** the "ROS is an inventory of systems to reveal subjective symptoms that the patient either forgot to describe or which at the time seemed relatively unimportant. In general, an analysis of the subjective findings will indicate the nature and extent of examination required." The inventory of systems may be made by means of a questionnaire filled out by the patient or ancillary staff; but the physician *must* evaluate the questionnaire and document in the medical record that the questionnaire has been reviewed in order for it to qualify as an ROS. For the purposes of an ROS, the following systems are recognized*:

- Constitutional symptoms
  Usual weight, recent weight changes, fever, weakness, fatigue
- Eyes (Ophthalmologic)
  Glasses or contact lenses, last eye examination, visual glaucoma, cataracts, eyestrain, pain, diplopia, redness, lacrimation, inflammation, blurring
- Ears, Nose, Mouth, Throat (Otolaryngologic)
  Ears: hearing, discharge, tinnitus, dizziness, pain
  Nose: head colds, epistaxis, discharges, obstruction, postnasal drip, sinus pain
  Mouth and Throat: condition of teeth and gums, last dental examination, soreness, redness, hoarseness, difficulty in swallowing
- Cardiovascular
  Chest pain, rheumatic fever, tachycardia, palpitation, high blood pressure, edema, vertigo, faintness, varicose veins, thrombophlebitis
- Respiratory
  Chest pain, wheezing, cough, dyspnea, sputum (color and quantity), hemoptysis, asthma, bronchitis, emphysema, pneumonia, tuberculosis, pleurisy, last chest radiograph (note: also shortness of breath)
- Gastrointestinal
  Appetite, thirst, nausea, vomiting, hematemesis, rectal bleeding, change in bowel habits, diarrhea, constipation, indigestion, food intolerance, flatus, hemorrhoids, jaundice
- Genitourinary
  Urinary: frequent or painful urination, nocturia, pyuria, hematuria, incontinence, urinary infection
  Genito-reproductive: male—venereal disease, sores, discharge from penis, hernias, testicular pain or masses; female—age at menarche and menstruation (frequency, type, duration, dysmenorrhea, menorrhagia; symptoms of menopause), contraception, pregnancies, deliveries, abortions, last Papanicolaou smear
- Musculoskeletal
  Joint pain or stiffness, arthritis, gout, backache, muscle pain, cramps, swelling, redness, limitation in motor activity

*Definitions from Huffman E: *Health Information Management,* 10th ed. Revised by the American Medical Record Association. Berwyn, IL, Physician's Record Company, 1994, pp 57-62.

■ Integumentary (skin and/or breast)
Skin: rashes, eruptions, dryness, cyanosis, jaundice, changes in skin, hair, or nails**
Breast: lumps, dimpling, nipple discharge**

■ Neurologic (neurological)
Faintness, blackouts, seizures, paralysis, tingling, tremors, memory loss

■ Psychiatric
Personality type, nervousness, mood, insomnia, headache, nightmares, depression

■ Endocrine
Thyroid trouble, heat or cold intolerance, excessive sweating, thirst, hunger, or urination, blood sugar levels

■ Hematologic/Lymphatic
Anemia, easy bruising or bleeding, past transfusions

■ Allergic/Immunologic
Sneezing, itching eyes, rhinorrhea, nasal obstruction, or recurrent infections

4. **Past, Family, and Social History (PFSH)^**

■ Past history is the patient's past experience with illnesses, operations, injuries, and treatments that includes significant information about:
Prior major illnesses and injuries
Prior operations
Prior hospitalizations
Current medications
Allergies (e.g., drug, food)
Age-appropriate immunization status
Age-appropriate feeding/dietary status

■ Social history is an age-appropriate review of past and current activities that includes significant information about:
Marital status and/or living arrangements
Current employment
Occupational history
Military history
Use of drugs, alcohol, and tobacco
Level of education
Sexual history
Other relevant social factors

■ Family history is a review of medical events in the patient's family that includes significant information about:
The health status or cause of death of parents, siblings, and children
Specific diseases related to problems identified in the Chief Complaint or History of the Present Illness, and/or System Review
Diseases of family members that may be hereditary or place the patient at risk

Three of the elements of a history (HPI, ROS, and PFSH) are included to varying degrees in all patient encounters. The degree or level of HPI, ROS, and PFSH is determined by the chief complaint or presenting problem of the patient.

**Modified from Huffman E: *Health Information Management,* 10th ed. Revised by the American Medical Record Association. Berwyn, IL, Physician's Record Company, 1994, pp 57-62.
^Definitions from 2015 CPT, Evaluation and Management Guidelines, pp 6-7. CPT codes, descriptions, and materials only are © 2014 American Medical Association.

History Levels. Now that you have reviewed the elements of a history, you are prepared to choose a history level. There are four history levels; the level is based on the extent of the history during the history-taking portion of the physician-patient encounter.

The history of present illness (HPI) must be documented by the physician or nonphysician practitioner (NPP) billing for the service.

HISTORY LEVELS

■ Problem focused
■ Expanded problem focused
■ Detailed
■ Comprehensive

1. **Problem focused:** The physician focuses on the chief complaint and a brief history of the present problem of a patient.

   A brief history would include a review of the history regarding pertinent information about the present problem or chief complaint. Brief history information would center around the severity, duration, and/or symptoms of the problem or complaint. The brief history does not have to include the past, family, or social history or a review of systems. A brief HPI includes 1-3 of the eight elements.

2. **Expanded problem focused:** The physician focuses on a chief complaint, obtains a brief history of the present problem, and also performs a problem pertinent review of systems. The expanded problem focused history does not have to include the past, family, or social history.

   This history would center around specific questions regarding the system involved in the presenting problem or chief complaint. The review of systems for this history would cover the organ system most closely related to the chief complaint or presenting problem and any related or associated organ system. For example, if the presenting problem or chief complaint is a red, swollen knee, the system reviewed would be the musculoskeletal system.

3. **Detailed:** The physician focuses on a chief complaint, obtains an extended history of the present problem (4 or more of the 8 elements), an extended review of systems, and a pertinent PFSH.

   The system review in this history is extended, which means that positive responses and pertinent negative responses relating to multiple organ systems should be documented.

4. **Comprehensive:** This is the most complex of the history types: the physician documents the chief complaint, obtains an extended history of the present problem, does a complete review of systems, and obtains a complete PFSH.

For a summary of the elements required for each level of history (according to the 1995 Documentation Guidelines), see Fig. 15-4.

Some third-party payers have established standards for the number of elements that must be documented in the medical record to qualify for a given level of service. For example, a third-party payer may state that to qualify as a comprehensive history the medical record must document that an extended HPI was conducted and that it included four of the eight elements (e.g., location, quality, severity, duration), a complete ROS, including a review of at least 10 of the 14 organ systems, and a complete review of all three areas of the PFSH.

History Elements

Chief Complaint (CC)
Reason for the encounter in the patient's words

History of Present Illness (HPI)
Location
Quality
Severity
Duration*
Timing
Context
Modifying factors
Associated signs and symptoms

Review of Systems (ROS)
Constitutional symptoms (fever, weight loss, etc.)
Ophthalmologic (eyes)
Otolaryngologic (ears, nose, mouth, throat)
Cardiovascular
Respiratory
Gastrointestinal
Genitourinary
Musculoskeletal
Integumentary (skin and/or breast)
Neurological
Psychiatric
Endocrine
Hematologic/Lymphatic
Allergic/Immunologic

Past, Family, and/or Social History (PFSH)
Past major illnesses, operations, injuries, and treatments
Family medical history for heredity and risk
Social activities, both past and current

Elements Required for Each Level of History

		Problem Focused	Expanded Problem Focused	Detailed	Comprehensive
History	HPI	Brief 1-3	Brief 1-3	Extended 4+	Extended 4+
	ROS	None	Problem-pertinent 1	Extended 2-9	Complete 10+
	PFSH	None	None	Pertinent 1	Complete 2-3

* Duration is not listed in the CPT E/M Guidelines, but listed in the 1995 Documentation Guidelines.

FIGURE 15-4 History elements required for each level of history.

CODING SHOT

When selecting a history level, the choice goes to the lowest level. For example, if the HPI is a level 2, the ROS is a level 2, but the PFSH is a level 1, the history level is 1. Another example is if the HPI is a level 3, the ROS is a level 2, and the PFSH is a level 2, the history is a level 2.

QUICK CHECK 15-3

1. Which levels of history require the documentation of the Chief Complaint (CC)?
   a. Problem focused
   b. Expanded problem focused
   c. Detailed
   d. Comprehensive
   e. All of the above

(Answers are located in Appendix C)

EXERCISE 15-2 *History Levels*

Using the CPT manual, locate the Office or Other Outpatient Services subsection, New Patient category, to identify the history level on each of the following codes:

CODE	HISTORY LEVEL
1 99201	_____
2 99202	_____
3 99203	_____
4 99204	_____
5 99205	_____

(Answers are located in Appendix B)

Examination. The patient has presented the physician with the **subjective** information regarding the complaint or problem in the history portion of the encounter; now the physician will do an examination of the patient to provide **objective** information, "hands-on" (those findings observed by the physician) about the complaint or problem. The physician then documents the objective findings in the patient record.

Examination Levels. The examination levels have the same titles as the history levels—problem focused, expanded problem focused, detailed, and comprehensive. The four levels are used to indicate the extent and complexity of the patient examination.

EXAMINATION LEVELS

- Problem focused
- Expanded problem focused
- Detailed
- Comprehensive
  1. **Problem focused:** Examination is limited to the affected body area or organ system identified by the chief complaint.
  2. **Expanded problem focused:** A limited examination is made of the affected body area or organ system and other symptomatic or related body area(s)/organ system(s).
  3. **Detailed:** An extended examination is made of the affected body area(s) and other symptomatic or related organ system(s).

4. **Comprehensive:** This is the most extensive examination; it encompasses a general multi-system examination and should include findings about 8 or more of the 12 organ systems.

Some third-party payers, such as Medicare, have guidelines for the comprehensive examination that state that only organ systems qualify when determining the level for the comprehensive examination and that body areas do not qualify.

Fig. 15-5 summarizes the elements required for each level of examination. These elements include various body areas (BAs) and organ systems (OSs). The elements also include an assessment of a patient's general condition, which is indicated by the patient's general appearance, vital signs, and the like.

Examination Elements

Constitutional* (OS)
Blood pressure, sitting
Blood pressure, lying
Pulse
Respirations
Temperature
Height
Weight
General appearance

***Body Areas* (BA)**
Head (including the face)
Neck
Chest (including breasts and axillae)
Abdomen
Genitalia, groin, buttocks
Back
Each extremity

***Organ System* (OS)**
Ophthalmologic (eyes)
Otolaryngologic (ears, nose, mouth, throat)
Cardiovascular
Respiratory
Gastrointestinal
Genitourinary
Musculoskeletal
Integumentary (skin)
Neurologic
Psychiatric
Hematologic/Lymphatic/Immunologic

Elements Required for Each Level of Examination

	Problem Focused	Expanded Problem Focused	Detailed	Comprehensive
Examination	Limited to affected BA or OS	Limited to affected BA or OS and other related OS(s)	Extended of affected BA(s) and other related OS(s)	General multi-system (OSs only)
# of OS/BA	1	2-7 limited	2-7 extended	8+

*Constitutional is NOT in the CPT manual but is in the 1995 Documentation Guidelines (DGs). In the DGs, constitutional is listed as the first organ system for a total of 12 organ systems. Most third-party payers allow for the counting of the constitutional elements to identify the level of the examination. The constitutional examination is placed at the top of the examination elements in this text to provide a list of the various constitutional elements.

FIGURE 15–5   Examination elements required for each level of examination.

EXERCISE 15-3 *Examination Levels*

Using the CPT manual, locate the Office or Other Outpatient Services subsection, New Patient category, to identify the examination levels for each of the following codes:

CODE **EXAMINATION LEVELS**

1 99201 _____

2 99202 _____

3 99203 _____

4 99204 _____

5 99205 _____

(Answers are located in Appendix B)

The patient's medical record will reflect the number of systems examined in a brief statement of the findings. The examination would include the examination elements and the number and extent of elements required for the physician to arrive at the diagnosis. For example, if a patient came to a physician with the complaint of a small foreign object lodged in the eye, the physician would not usually need to do a cardiologic examination. The extent of the examination is based on what needs to be done to treat the patient.

Now you need to pull all the information on history and examination together so that it is usable information. What better way to do that than to use the information in the practical application of an exercise?

EXERCISE 15-4 *Examination Elements*

Label each of the following as body area (BA) or organ system (OS):

1 Skin _____

2 Head _____

3 Eyes _____

4 Ears _____

5 Nose _____

6 Mouth _____

7 Throat _____

8 Neck _____

9 Thorax, anterior and posterior _____

10 Breasts _____

11 Lungs _____

12 Heart _____

13 Abdomen _____

14 Genitourinary _____

15 Vagina _____

16 Arm _____

17 Musculoskeletal _____

18 Lymphatics _____

19 Psychiatric _____

20 Neurologic _____

Continued

Read the following patient record:

21 A new patient, an 8-year-old female, is brought into the office by her mother, who states that the child has an earache in her right ear. Mother reports that the child has been complaining of pain in right ear with a severity of 8 of 10 for the past 2 days. Exam: Child appears to be in only minor distress. Vitals: Temperature, 101° F. Tympanic membrane red, fluid noted in right ear. Health history reviewed. Diagnosis: Acute serous otitis media.

From the patient record, we can identify the history elements as follows:

HISTORY ELEMENTS	PATIENT RECORD
CC:	Earache in the right ear
HPI:	Complaining of pain in the right ear with a severity of 8 of 10 for the past 2 days
	Location: Right ear
	Quality: Aching
	Severity: 8 of 10
	Duration: Two days
PFSH:	Health history reviewed. (The patient information form completed by the mother contains the information that the physician reviewed, along with questions to the patient.)
ROS:	Ears (one organ system)

In this case, the physician focused on the chief complaint and did a brief history centered on gathering information about the present illness. Referring to the description of history levels summarized in Fig. 15-4 or discussed in the E/M Guidelines, answer the following question:

a What is the history level for this case? _____

Now let's establish the level of examination:

EXAMINATION	PATIENT RECORD
General Survey:	Child appears to be in only minor distress
Vital Signs:	Temperature, 101° F
Body Areas/Organ Systems	Ears (one organ system)

In this case, the physician focused on constitutional (temperature and general appearance) and one organ system (ears). Referring to the description of examination levels summarized in Fig. 15-5 or discussed in the E/M Guidelines, answer the following question:

b What is the examination level for this case? _____
That wasn't so difficult, was it? Okay, now you do one.

Read the following patient record:

22 A 68-year-old female established patient presents to the office today with a "cold" of 9 days' duration. Patient reports that she has had a dry, hacking cough and nasal congestion for the past 6 days and a fever for the past 3 days. She states that she is unable to sleep due to the cough, fever, and aching. She appears to be in minor distress. Personal and family history are negative for respiratory problems. Temperature is 100° F; blood pressure 150/90; pulse 93 and regular. Lungs clear to percussion and auscultation. Examination of head and ears, normal; nose, mucous membranes inflamed with postnasal phlegm. Diagnosis: Sinusitis. Plan: Patient was advised to drink fluids, take aspirin as needed for pain, obtain bed rest, and to return if symptoms have not improved in 5 days.

Continued

Locate the information in the patient record that matches the history element and place the information on the lines provided:

HISTORY ELEMENTS   **PATIENT RECORD**

CC: _____

_____

_____

HPI: _____

_____

_____

PFSH: _____

_____

_____

ROS: _____

_____

_____

With the information you placed on the preceding lines, choose the correct history level:

a What is the history level for this case? _____

Locate the information in the patient record that matches the examination, and place the information on the lines provided:

EXAMINATION   **PATIENT RECORD**

General Survey: _____

Vital Signs: _____

_____

_____

_____

Body Areas/Organ Systems: _____

With the information you placed on the preceding lines, choose the correct examination level:

b What is the examination level for this case? _____

(Answers are located in Appendix B)

Medical Decision Making. The key component of medical decision making (MDM) is based on the complexity of the decision the physician must make about the patient's diagnosis and care. Complexity of decision making is based on three elements:

1. Number of diagnoses or management options. The options can be minimal, limited, multiple, or extensive.
2. Amount and/or complexity of data to review. The data can be minimal or none, limited, moderate, or extensive.

3. Risk of complication or death if the condition goes untreated. Risk can be minimal, low, moderate, or high.

Levels. The extent to which each of these elements is considered determines the levels of MDM complexity.

MEDICAL DECISION-MAKING COMPLEXITY LEVELS

■ Straightforward
■ Low
■ Moderate
■ High

1. **Straightforward decision making:** minimal diagnosis and management options, minimal or none for the amount and complexity of data to be reviewed, and minimal risk to the patient of complications or death if untreated.
2. **Low-complexity decision making:** limited number of diagnoses and management options, limited data to be reviewed, and low risk to the patient of complications or death if untreated.
3. **Moderate-complexity decision making:** multiple diagnoses and management options, moderate amount and complexity of data to be reviewed, and moderate risk to the patient of complications or death if untreated.
4. **High-complexity decision making:** extensive diagnoses and management options, extensive amount and complexity of data to be reviewed, and high risk to the patient for complications or death if the problem is untreated.

Management Options. According to the 1995 E/M Documentation Guidelines, documentation of management options in the medical record is as follows:

1. For each encounter, an assessment, clinical impression, or diagnosis should be documented. It may be explicitly stated or implied in documented decisions regarding management plans or further evaluation.
   ■ For a presenting problem with an established diagnosis, the record should reflect whether the problem is (a) improved, well controlled, resolving, or resolved; or (b) inadequately controlled, worsening, or failing to change as expected.
   ■ For a presenting problem without an established diagnosis, the assessment or clinical impression may be stated in the form of differential diagnoses or as a "possible," "probable," or "rule out" (R/O) diagnosis.
   ■ Note: Physician/Provider coders do not code "rule out," "possible," or "probable" diagnosis; rather they code the presenting symptoms and/or complaints unless there is a definitive diagnosis rendered.
2. The initiation of, or changes in, treatment should be documented. Treatment includes a wide range of management options, including patient instructions, nursing instructions, therapies, and medications.
3. If referrals are made, consultations requested, or advice sought, the record should indicate to whom or where the referral or consultation has been made or from whom the advice is requested.

Data to Be Reviewed. The following are some basic documentation guidelines for the amount and complexity of data to be reviewed:

1. If a diagnostic service (test or procedure) is ordered, planned, scheduled, or performed at the time of the E/M encounter, the type of service (e.g., laboratory or radiology) should be documented.
2. The review of laboratory, radiology, or other diagnostic tests should be documented. An entry in a progress note such as "WBC elevated" or "chest x-ray negative" is acceptable. Alternatively, the review may be documented by initialing and dating the report containing the test results.
3. A decision to obtain old records or to obtain additional history from the family, caregiver, or other source to supplement that obtained from the patient should be documented.

4. Relevant findings from the review of old records or the receipt of additional history from the family, caregiver, or other source should be documented. If there is no relevant information beyond that already obtained, that fact should be documented. A notation of "old records reviewed" or "additional history obtained from family" without elaboration is insufficient.

5. The results of discussion of laboratory, radiology, or other diagnostic tests with the physician who performed or interpreted the study should be documented.

6. The direct visualization and independent interpretation of an image, tracing, or specimen previously interpreted by another physician should be documented.

Risk. Some basic documentation guidelines for risk of significant complications, morbidity, or mortality include the following:

1. Comorbidities (secondary conditions), underlying diseases, or other factors that increase the complexity of medical decision making by increasing the risk of complications, morbidity, or mortality should be documented.

2. If a surgical or invasive diagnostic procedure is ordered, planned, or scheduled at the time of the E/M encounter, the type of procedure (e.g., laparoscopy) should be documented.

3. If a surgical or invasive diagnostic procedure is performed at the time of the E/M encounter, the specific procedure should be documented.

4. The referral for or decision to perform a surgical or invasive diagnostic procedure on an urgent basis should be documented or implied.

Examples of the levels of risk may be found in Table 15-1.

When you select one of the four types of complexity of medical decision making—straightforward, low, moderate, or high—the documentation in the medical record must support the selection in terms of the number of diagnoses or management options, amount and/or complexity of data to be reviewed, and risks. Two of the three elements in Fig. 15-6 must be met or exceeded to qualify for a level of medical decision making.

Refer to Fig. 15-6 for an overview of medical decision making. Given the information in the medical record, you would consider the information in the context of the complexity of the diagnosis and management options, data to be reviewed, and risks to the patient in order to choose the complexity of MDM. Let's look at an example of choosing the MDM level.

TABLE 15–1

LEVELS OF RISK

Level of Risk	Presenting Problem or Problems
Minimal (Level 1)	One self-limited or minor problem (e.g., insect bite, tinea corporis)
Low (Level 2)	Two or more self-limited or minor problems
	One stable chronic illness (e.g., well-controlled hypertension or non-insulin dependent diabetes, cataract, benign prostatic hypertrophy)
	Acute, uncomplicated illness or injury (e.g., cystitis, allergic rhinitis, simple sprain)
Moderate (Level 3)	One or more chronic illnesses with mild exacerbation, progression, or side effects of treatment
	Two or more stable chronic illnesses
	Undiagnosed new problem with uncertain prognosis (e.g., lump in breast)
	Acute illness with systemic symptoms (e.g., pyelonephritis, pneumonitis, colitis)
High (Level 4)	One or more chronic illnesses with severe exacerbation, progression, or side effects of treatment
	Acute or chronic illnesses or injuries that pose a threat to life or body function (e.g., multiple trauma, acute myocardial infarction, pulmonary embolus, severe respiratory distress, progressive severe rheumatoid arthritis, psychiatric illness with potential threat to self or others, peritonitis, acute renal failure)
	An abrupt change in neurologic status (e.g., seizure, transient ischemic attack, weakness, or sensory loss)

Medical Decision-Making Elements

Number of Diagnoses or Management Options
Minimal
Limited
Multiple
Extensive

Amount or Complexity of Data to Review
Minimal/None
Limited
Moderate
Extensive

Risk of Complications or Death IF Condition Goes Untreated
Minimal
Low
Moderate
High

Elements Required for Each Level of Medical Decision Making

	Straightforward	Low	Moderate	High
Number of DX or management options	Minimal	Limited	Multiple	Extensive
Amount or complexity of data	Minimal/None	Limited	Moderate	Extensive
Risks	Minimal	Low	Moderate	High

FIGURE 15-6 Decision making elements required for each level of medical decision making complexity. Two of the three elements must be met or exceeded to qualify for a level of medical decision making.

CODING SHOT

When selecting an MDM level, the choice is the majority. For example, if the number of diagnosis management options is a level 2, the amount of data is a level 2, but the risk is a level 1, the MDM level is 2. Another example is if the number of management options is a level 1, the amount of data is a level 3, and the risk is a level 2, the MDM is a level 2. This is different than the history in which the lowest level directed the level choice; in the MDM the level is the highest two.

Example 1

An established patient's outpatient medical record indicates the following: Female patient fell and scraped arm; problem focused history and examination were done. The patient states that she slipped on the ice on the walk outside her home approximately 3 hours earlier. The area of abrasion appears to be relatively clean, with no foreign materials imbedded. There appears to be only minimal cutaneous damage. The area was washed and a dressing applied.

1. **Diagnosis and management options** for an abrasion (clean and dress). (Options are minimal, limited, multiple, or extensive.)

    As a coder, you think about how many various options are open to the physician to diagnose the problem and decide how to manage this patient's care—minimal, limited, multiple, extensive? The management of an abrasion is fairly clear—clean and dress the wound; therefore, the diagnosis and management options are minimal.

2. **Data to review** to provide service. (Data can be minimal/none, limited, moderate, or extensive.)

    Think about how much and how complex the information (data) would be that the physician must obtain, review, and analyze to care for this patient—minimal/none, limited, moderate, or extensive? The amount of data to review would be minimal/none for an abrasion.

3. **Risk** if not treated. (Risk can be minimal, low, moderate, or high.)

    As a coder, you think about how great a risk there is that the patient would die or encounter severe complications (e.g., infection), morbidity (additional diseases such as gangrene), or mortality (death) if the abrasion was not treated—minimal, low, moderate, or high? The risk of death or of complications is minimal.

The diagnosis and management options are minimal, data are minimal/none, and risk is minimal. Consideration of these three elements has placed this patient's care into a straightforward MDM complexity level.

The history level is stated to be problem focused and the examination level is problem focused. The patient was an established patient seen as an outpatient. Carefully look at each of the items set in boldface type in code 99212 below. The place of service, type of service, type of history, type of examination, and complexity level of the MDM are identified in the description of the code.

99212	**Office or other outpatient** visit for the evaluation and management of an **established patient** that requires at least two of these three key components:
	● **a problem focused history**
	● **a problem focused examination**
	● **straightforward medical decision making**

CPT code 99212 is the correct code for this service.

Example 2

The patient's record states the following: Unknown (new) patient presenting to the office with chest pain (R07.9/788.50). A comprehensive history was taken and a comprehensive examination performed. The physician ordered an electrocardiogram (ECG), laboratory reports, and x-rays.

The MDM complexity level must be chosen:

1. **Diagnosis and management options** for a cardiac origin could be myocardial infarction, angina, or heart block. Gastrointestinal origin could be reflux or an ulcer. Respiratory origin could be a pulmonary embolism or pleuritis. (Diagnosis and management options can be minimal, limited, multiple, or extensive.)

   What do you think it would take for the physician to decide on the diagnosis or management options for this patient? There are many possibilities of origin for the chest pain; therefore, the diagnosis and management options are extensive.

2. **Data to review** in order for the physician to provide service. (Data can be minimal/none, limited, moderate, or extensive.) How much data would the physician have to obtain through current tests and how much review and analysis of previous records would be necessary to provide services to the patient—minimal/none, limited, moderate, extensive? In this case, the patient's care requires moderate data review, including laboratory reports, radiology reports, and ECG. You very well may have chosen the data review level of extensive rather than moderate and that is acceptable. Once you are in the medical office and have the patient's full medical record available to review, the choice of the amount of data that was reviewed becomes easier to identify.

3. **Risk** if left untreated. (Risk can be minimal, low, moderate, or high.) If the patient's condition was not treated, what do you think the risk of death or serious complication would be—minimal, low, moderate, or high? This patient would have a high risk of death or severe complications if this condition was left untreated.

   The extensive diagnosis and management options and high risk to the patient mean that two of the three elements have been met. So this patient's care is considered to have a high level of MDM complexity. A new patient with a comprehensive history and examination together with a high MDM complexity assigns this case to code 99205.

EXERCISE 15-5   *Medical Decision-Making Complexity*

A new patient's record states that an initial office visit was made for the evaluation and management of a 48-year-old male with recurrent low back pain from a herniated disc, with pain radiating to the leg (myelopathy). A detailed history and a detailed examination were performed.

Using the information above, identify the following factors in the case:

1 Diagnosis and management options for recurrent low back pain radiating to the leg. (Options can be minimal, limited, multiple, or extensive.)

_____

2 Data to review in order to provide service. (Data can be minimal/none, limited, moderate, or extensive.) Only the current record is available.

_____

3 Risk if left untreated. (Risk can be minimal, low, moderate, or high.)

_____

4 Two of the three elements have been met to qualify this patient for what level of MDM complexity? (Complexity can be straightforward, low, moderate, or high.)

_____

5 The patient record indicates that a detailed history was taken and a detailed examination was performed. When this is combined with the level of MDM complexity you arrived at for this patient, what is the correct CPT code for the case?

CPT Code: _____

ICD-10-CM Code: _____ (ICD-9-CM Code: _____)

Now, let's look again at two cases for which you previously established the history and examination levels:

6 A new patient, an 8-year-old female, is brought into the office by her mother, who states that the child has an earache in the right ear. Mother reports that the child has been complaining of pain in right ear with a severity of 8 of 10 for the past 2 days. Child appears to be in only minor distress. Temperature, 101° F. Tympanic membranes red, fluid noted in right ear. Health history reviewed. Diagnosis: Acute serous otitis media.

What is the MDM level for this patient? _____

What diagnosis code would be reported for this patient? _____

ICD-10-CM Code: _____

(ICD-9-CM Code: _____)

7 A 68-year-old female established patient presents to the office today with a "cold" of 9 days' duration. Patient reports that she has had a dry, hacking cough and nasal congestion for the past 6 days and a fever for the past 3 days. She states that she is unable to sleep due to the cough, fever, and aching. She appears to be in minor distress. Personal and family history are negative for respiratory problems. Temperature is 100° F; blood pressure 150/90; pulse 93 and regular. Lungs clear to percussion and auscultation. Examination of head and ears, normal; nose, mucous membranes inflamed with postnasal phlegm. Diagnosis: Acute sinusitis. Plan: Patient was advised to drink fluids, take aspirin as needed for pain, obtain bed rest, and return if symptoms have not improved in 5 days.

What is the MDM level for this patient? _____

What diagnosis code would be reported for this patient? _____

ICD-10-CM Code: _____

(ICD-9-CM Code: _____)

(Answers are located in Appendix B)

There is certainly a great amount of information that must be considered in order to choose the correct E/M code! Only with practice can you expect to remember all of the various elements and levels within each component. Each medical facility has its own procedure for identifying the level of E/M service; some facilities require the physician to identify all the components of service, whereas other facilities require the component information to be abstracted from the medical record by support personnel. Either way, you need to be knowledgeable about all components of E/M codes, and it really does get easier with practice!

From the Trenches

"I tell people that while the study and practice of medicine is considered a science, the coding is an art. There are often varying ways to do things, dependent on different circumstances. Attention to detail is important, but flexibility is also necessary."

JOAN

STOP *You have examined each of the three key components and seen how they apply to the assignment of an E/M code. You will be referring to the information as you are presented with additional cases. Make note of the important points and remember that the information about the key components is in the E/M Guidelines in the CPT manual.*

Now that you are familiar with the key components of history, examination, and medical decision making, let's review the contributory factors.

Contributory Factors

There are three contributory factors: counseling, coordination of care, and the nature of the presenting problem. Contributory factors are those conditions that help the physician determine the extent of the history, examination, and decision making (key components) necessary to treat the patient. Contributory factors may or may not be considered in every patient case.

CONTRIBUTORY FACTORS

- Counseling
- Coordination of care
- Nature of presenting problem

Counseling. Counseling is a service that physicians provide to patients and their families. It involves discussion of diagnostic results, impressions, and recommended diagnostic studies; prognosis; risks and benefits of treatment; instructions for treatment; importance of compliance with treatment; risk factor reduction; and patient and family education. Some form of counseling usually takes place in all physician-patient encounters, and this was factored into the codes when they were developed by the AMA. Only when counseling is the reason for the encounter or consumes most of the visit time (more than 50% of the total time) is counseling considered a component of code assignment. The following statement is made often within the codes in the E/M section:

Counseling and/or coordination of care with other physicians, other qualified health care professionals or agencies are provided consistent with the nature of the problem(s) and the patient's and/or family's needs.

Coordination of Care. Coordination of care with other health care providers or agencies may be necessary for the care of a patient. In coordination of care, a physician might arrange for other services to be provided to the patient, such as arrangements for admittance to a long-term nursing facility.

Nature of the Presenting Problem. This is the foundation of the level assigned. The presenting problem is the patient's chief complaint or the situation that leads the physician to determining the level of care necessary to diagnose and treat the patient. The CPT describes the **presenting problem** as a disease, condition, illness, injury, symptom, sign, finding, complaint, or other reason for the encounter, with or without a diagnosis being established at the time of the encounter. There are five types of presenting problems:

- Minimal
- Self-limited
- Low severity
- Moderate severity
- High severity

1. **Minimal:** A problem may not require the presence of the physician, but a service is provided under the physician's supervision. A minimal problem is a blood pressure reading, a dressing change, or another service that can be performed without the physician being immediately present.

2. **Self-limited:** Also called a minor presenting problem, a self-limited problem runs a definite and prescribed course, is transient (it comes and goes), and is not likely to permanently alter health status, or the presenting problem has a good prognosis with management and compliance.

3. **Low severity:** The risk of complete sickness (morbidity) without treatment is low, there is little or no risk of death without treatment, and full recovery without impairment is expected.

4. **Moderate severity:** The risk of complete sickness (morbidity) without treatment is moderate, there is moderate risk of death without treatment, and an uncertain prognosis or increased probability of impairment exists.

5. **High severity:** The risk of complete sickness (morbidity) without treatment is high to extreme, there is a moderate to high risk of death without treatment, or there is a strong probability of severe, prolonged functional impairment.

The patient's medical record should contain the physician's observation concerning the complexity of the presenting problem(s). Your responsibility is to identify the words that correctly indicate the type of presenting problem.

Direct face-to-face and **unit/floor time** are two measures of time. Outpatient visits are measured as direct face-to-face time. Direct face-to-face time is the time a physician spends directly with a patient during an office visit obtaining the history, performing an examination, and discussing the results. Inpatient time is measured as unit/floor time and is used to describe the time a physician spends in the hospital setting dealing with the patient's care. Unit/floor time includes care given to the patient at the bedside as well as at other settings on the unit or floor (e.g., the nursing station). It is an often-heard comment that physicians get paid a great deal of money just for stopping in to see a hospitalized patient. However, what is not realized is that the physician spends additional time reviewing the patient's records, test results, and writing orders for the patient's care.

Time in the E/M section is referred to in statements such as this one that is located with code 99203:

Usually, the presenting problem(s) are of moderate severity. Typically, 25 minutes are spent face to face with the patient and/or family.

These statements concerning time are used when counseling and/or coordination of care represent more than **50% of the time spent with a patient.** The times referred to in these statements are the basis of the selection of the E/M code. For example: An established patient returns for an office visit to get the results of tests. The physician spends 25 minutes going over the unfavorable results of the tests. The physician discusses various treatment options, the prognosis, and the risks of treatment and of treatment refusal. The correct code would be 99214, in which the time statement is, "Typically, 25 minutes are spent face to face with the patient and/or family." The physician must either document the beginning and ending time in the patient's medical record or document the total time spent and how much was spent in counseling in order to be able to consider time in the code assignments.

✋ CAUTION *Time was not included in the CPT manual before 1992 but was incorporated to assist with the selection of the most appropriate level of E/M services. The times indicated with the codes are only **averages** and represent a simple estimate of the possible duration of a service.*

EXERCISE 15-6   *Presenting Problem*

Match the presenting problem to the severity level in the patient:

a minimal   **b** self-limited   **c** low   **d** moderate   **e** high

1 Four-year-old female established patient presents with slight pain in right ear, of 2 days' duration. Physician diagnosed a minor infection and prescribed antibiotic for acute exudative otitis media.

  Level of Presenting Problem: _____

  ICD-10-CM Code: _____ (ICD-9-CM Code: _____)

2 Eighty-six-year-old woman who has a history of chronic obstructive pulmonary disease (COPD) and is oxygen-dependent comes in because of dizziness and weakness. Diagnosis is acute exacerbation of COPD.

  Level of Presenting Problem: _____

  ICD-10-CM Codes: _____, _____

  (ICD-9-CM Codes: _____, _____)

3 Established patient, 71 years old, with shortness of breath on exertion and a history of congestive cardiomyopathy.

  Level of Presenting Problem: _____

  ICD-10-CM Codes: _____ (shortness of breath), _____ (cardiomyopathy, congestive)

  (ICD-9-CM Codes: _____ (shortness of breath), _____ (cardiomyopathy, congestive))

4 Fourteen-year-old presents with moderate pain in left thumb after a fall from his skateboard. Diagnosis is sprain of left thumb.

  Level of Presenting Problem: _____

  ICD-10-CM Codes: _____ (sprain), _____ (external cause), _____ (activity)

  (ICD-9-CM Codes: _____ (sprain), _____ (external cause), _____ (activity))

5 Established patient, 34 years old, presents for a blood pressure check due to her malignant hypertension.

  Level of Presenting Problem: _____

  ICD-10-CM Code: _____ (ICD-9-CM Code: _____)

6 Physician recommends an over-the-counter medication for patient with seasonal grass allergic reaction.

  Level of Presenting Problem: _____

  ICD-10-CM Code: _____ (ICD-9-CM Code: _____)

(Answers are located in Appendix B)

AN E/M CODE EXAMPLE

With the CPT manual open to the first page of the E/M section, locate the notes above the 99201 code. These notes highlight the incidents in which codes in that particular category are appropriate for assignment. The notes above 99201 indicate that the codes that follow the notes are appropriate for use in coding services provided in a "physician's office or in an outpatient or other ambulatory facility."

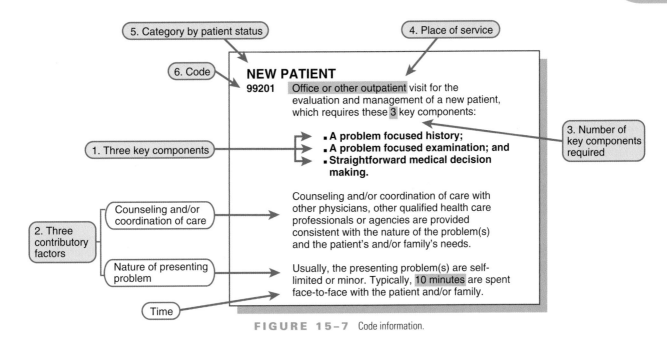

FIGURE 15-7 Code information.

The information also directs you to other code subsections if the patient classification is not correct. As an example of this directional feature, the notes above 99201 state, "For services provided in the emergency department, see 99281-99285."

Fig. 15-7 shows the first code for a new patient under the category New Patient under subsection Office or Other Outpatient Services. Review Fig. 15-7 carefully before continuing. Note the location of each important piece of information.

Locate the following items in Fig. 15-7:

1. Three key components
2. Three contributory factors
3. Number of key components required
4. Place of service
5. Category by patient status
6. Code

USING THE E/M CODES

Now you are going to use the information you have learned about codes in the E/M services section as you continue to identify the differences among the codes.

Office and Other Outpatient Services

New Patient. The first subsection in the E/M section is Office and Other Outpatient Services, New Patient Category (99201-99205).

You will recall from information presented earlier that a new patient is defined as one who has not received professional services from the physician or another physician of the exact same specialty and subspecialty in the same group within the past 3 years. A physician must spend more time with a new patient—obtaining the history, conducting the examination, and considering the data—than with an established patient. Consider that the established patient is probably known to the physician, and the person's medical records are available, but with a new patient none of this is available to the physician. For these reasons, the cost of a new patient office visit is higher, so third-party payers reimburse the physician at a higher rate for new patient services than for the same type of service when it is provided to an established patient.

EXERCISE 15-7 *New Patient Services*

Using the CPT manual and the ICD-10-CM and/or ICD-9-CM manuals, fill in the blanks with the correct words:

1 For code 99203, the history level is _____, the examination is _____, and the MDM is of _____ complexity.

2 For code 99204, the history level is _____, the examination is _____, and the MDM complexity is _____.

3 For code 99205, the history level is _____, the examination is _____, and the MDM complexity is _____.

Code the following cases for new patients:

4 A 53-year-old new patient presents for an initial office visit to discuss a surgical vasectomy for sterilization. The history and examination are detailed and the MDM is of low complexity.

  CPT Code: _____

  ICD-10-CM Code: _____ (ICD-9-CM Code: _____)

5 A 4-year-old new patient presents for the removal of sutures from an appendectomy incision made 10 days earlier in another city. The physician conducts a brief history and examination prior to removing the stitches.

  CPT Code: _____

  ICD-10-CM Code: _____ (ICD-9-CM Code: _____)

6 A 23-year-old man who is a new patient has an initial office visit for severe depression *(report as first-listed diagnosis)* that has led to frequent thoughts of suicide in the past several weeks and is acute today. More than an hour is spent discussing the patient's problems and options. Past medical history is negative. The social history reveals that the patient suffers from sleeplessness *(report as an additional diagnosis);* smokes between two and two and a half packs of unfiltered cigarettes a day and has for 5 years *(report as tobacco abuse);* drinks 10 to 12 cups of coffee; and denies current use of drugs. (The actual patient record continues and indicates that a comprehensive history and examination was conducted; high MDM complexity.)

  CPT Code: _____

  ICD-10-CM Codes: _____, _____, _____, _____

  (ICD-9-CM Codes: _____, _____, _____, _____)

7 A new patient, a 10-year-old boy, is brought in by his father for a knee injury sustained in a hockey game. The knee is swollen and the patient is in apparent pain. A detailed history and examination are obtained. A diagnosis of medial collateral sprain of the right knee is made. Low MDM complexity.

  CPT Code: _____

  ICD-10-CM Codes: _____, _____

  (ICD-9-CM Codes: _____, _____)

8 A 41-year-old woman, new to the office, complains of headache and rhinitis of 4 days' duration. The patient states that she has had a problem with her allergies during this season for years. An expanded problem-focused history and examination are done. Straightforward MDM complexity. The diagnosis was grass pollen allergy.

  CPT Code: _____

  ICD-10-CM Code: _____ (ICD-9-CM Code: _____)

(Answers are located in Appendix B)

Established Patient. The second category of codes in subsection Office and Other Outpatient Services is for the established patient in an outpatient setting (99211-99215). You will recall that the definition of an established patient is one who has received professional services from the physician or another physician of the exact same specialty and subspecialty in the same group within the past 3 years.

Code 99211 reports services provided in the office and for which the physician may not be present during the service but is in the office suite and is immediately available. Further, the employee providing the service must have the credentials necessary to provide the service, and the service must be part of a documented treatment plan. The physician should sign the documentation of the service.

QUICK CHECK 15-4

1. Could a physician assign 99211 to report a patient encounter?

   Yes or No?

(Answers are located in Appendix C)

EXERCISE 15-8   *Established Patient Services*

Fill in the blanks with information from codes in the Established Patient category:

1 99211: This minimal service level does not exist in the New Patient category because a new patient is seen by the physician. The established patient may or may not be seen by the physician. Read the description and information for code 99211 in the CPT manual. Would an established patient returning for a simple blood pressure check be appropriately reported as 99211?

_____

2 A 42-year-old established patient presents for an office visit with complaints of severe vaginal itching and moderate pain. During the expanded problem focused history, the patient states that several weeks earlier she had noted a slight itching, which has increased in severity. Yesterday, she noted a lesion on her genitalia. Burning and painful urination have increased over the past 5 days accompanied by rectal itching. She has tried a variety of over-the-counter ointments and creams, which induced no improvement. The patient states that she has had several yeast infections in the past that had been successfully treated by her previous physician. Personal history indicates several prior urinary infections. No discharge noted. A problem focused examination of the external genitalia reveals a lesion, which had previously ruptured, located on the vulva. Bacterial and viral smears are done. The MDM complexity is straightforward. The patient is advised that the smears would be back in 24 hours and that a treatment plan would be developed based on the reports. (The smear was positive for a bacterial infection, for which antibiotics were prescribed.)

CPT Code: _____

3 A 17-year-old football player comes to the clinic for a 50 mg gold injection for a left anterior cruciate knee sprain that occurred last week. The injection was given by the nurse. Only the nurse sees this established patient. (Code only the E/M service and diagnosis.)

CPT Code: _____

ICD-10-CM Code: _____ (ICD-9-CM Code: _____)

4 A 53-year-old established patient complains of frequent fainting. The history and examination are comprehensive, and the MDM is of high complexity.

CPT Code: _____

ICD-10-CM Code: _____ (ICD-9-CM Code: _____)

5 A 61-year-old established patient is seen for medication management of malaise and fatigue produced by hypertensive medication. An expanded problem focused history and examination are done, and the MDM is of moderate complexity.

CPT Code: _____

ICD-10-CM Codes: _____, _____, _____, _____

(ICD-9-CM Codes: _____, _____, _____, _____)

6 An established 31-year-old patient presents with an irritated infected skin tag. A problem focused history and examination are done. MDM complexity is low.

CPT Code: _____

ICD-10-CM Code: _____ (ICD-9-CM Code: _____)

7 An established 48-year-old woman has had diarrhea for the past 5 days. Her temperature is 101° F. An expanded problem focused history and examination are done. MDM complexity is low.

CPT Code: _____

ICD-10-CM Code: _____ (ICD-9-CM Code: _____)

(Answers are located in Appendix B)

Remember, it takes a lot of practice to learn to code. It is not a skill that is quickly acquired. You need to have patience and know that practice, practice, practice is the only thing that will make this skill yours.

Hospital Observation Services

The codes in the Hospital Observation subsection (99217-99226) identify initial observation care, subsequent observation care, or observation discharge services. The services in the observation subsection are for patients who are in a hospital on observation status.

Observation is a status used for the classification of a patient who does not have an illness severe enough to meet acute inpatient criteria and does not require resources as intensive as an inpatient but does require hospitalization for a short period of time. Patients are also admitted to observation so further information can be obtained about the severity of the condition and to determine whether the patient can be treated on an outpatient basis. In some hospitals in some parts of the country, observation status is conducted in the temporary care unit (TCU). Generally observation status can be designated anywhere in the hospital; however, the patient is considered an outpatient.

The observation codes are for new or established patients. Each code from the range 99218-99220 requires all three of the key components to establish a level of service.

If a patient is admitted to the hospital as an inpatient after having been admitted earlier the same day as an observation patient, you do not report the observation status separately. The services provided during observation become part of (are bundled into) the initial inpatient hospital admission code.

QUICK CHECK 15-5

1. Are observation codes 99218-99220 and 99224-99226 reported for inpatient or outpatient

   services? _____

(Answers are located in Appendix C)

Observation Care Discharge Services. The Observation Care Discharge Services code (99217) includes the final examination of the patient upon discharge from observation status. Discussion of the hospital stay, instructions for continued care, and preparation of discharge records are also bundled into the Observation Care Discharge Services code. The code is used only with patients who are discharged on a day that follows the first day of observation.

Initial Observation Care. Initial Observation Care codes (99218-99220) designate the beginning of observation status in a hospital. Again, the hospital does not need to have a formal observation area, since the designation of observation status is dependent on the severity of illness of the patient. These codes also include development of a care plan for the patient and periodic reassessment while on observation status. Observation admission can be reported only for the first day of the service. If the patient is admitted and discharged on the same day, a code from the range 99234-99236, Observation or Inpatient Care Services, is assigned to report the service. If the patient is in the hospital overnight but remains there for a period that is **less than 48 hours,** the first day's service is reported with a code from the range 99218-99220, Initial Observation Care, and the second day's service is coded

99217, Observation Care Discharge Services. If the patient is on observation status for **longer than 48 hours**, the first day is reported with a code from the range 99218-99220, Initial Observation Care; the second day is reported with a code from the range 99224-99226, Subsequent Observation Care; and the third day is coded 99217, Observation Care Discharge Services.

Services performed in sites other than the observation area (e.g., clinic, nursing home, emergency department) and that precede admission to observation status are included in (bundled into) the Initial Observation Care codes and are not to be reported separately.

For example, an established patient was seen in the physician's office for frequent fainting of unknown origin. The history and examination were comprehensive and the MDM complexity was moderate. The code for the office visit would be 99215. But the physician decided to admit the patient immediately to observation status until a further determination could be made as to the origin of the fainting. You would assign a code from the Hospital Observation Services subsection, Initial Observation Care subheading, to report the physician's service of admission to observation status (99219) and would not separately report the office visit (99215).

If a patient is admitted to observation status and then becomes ill enough to be admitted to the hospital, an Initial Hospital Care code (99221-99223), not an observation code, is assigned to report services.

Subsequent Observation Care. Subsequent observation services are reported with codes in the 99224-99226 range. The codes report the physician's services for day 2 to the date of discharge. The code assignment is based on the documented level of at least two of the three key components (history, examination, and complexity of medical decision making). These codes indicate the time the physician typically spends providing the service. (Note that these are resequenced codes.)

> ✋ **CAUTION**   *Observation or Inpatient Care Services (including admission and discharge service), codes 99234-99236, have a very specific purpose: to report services for a patient who is admitted to and discharged from observation or inpatient status on the **same day**. All the services provided to the patient—same-day office services, observation care, and discharge—are bundled into one code from the 99234-99236 range.*

CMS RULES

When reporting physician services (99234-99236), Medicare requires a patient to be admitted to observation status for **more than 8 hours** and discharged on the same date of service. A period of 8 hours or less is reimbursed as initial observation status (99218-99220), even if the patient is discharged on the same date.

EXERCISE 15-9   *Hospital Observation Services*

Using the CPT manual and the ICD-10-CM and/or ICD-9-CM manuals, code the following:

1 A patient was in an automobile accident and is complaining of a minor headache and no other apparent injuries. History gathered from bystanders states that patient was not wearing a seat belt and hit his head on the windshield. A 15-minute loss of consciousness was noted. The patient was diagnosed with a concussion. The patient was then admitted for 24-hour observation to rule out head injury. A comprehensive history and examination were performed. The MDM was of moderate complexity.

      CPT Code: _____

      ICD-10-CM Codes: _____, _____

      (ICD-9-CM Codes: _____, _____)

(Answers are located in Appendix B)

Hospital Inpatient Services

Hospital Inpatient Services codes (99221-99239) report a patient's status as an inpatient in a hospital or partial hospital setting and, therefore, identify the hospital setting as the place where the physician renders service to the patient. An **inpatient** is one who has been formally admitted to an acute health care facility.

Note that within the subsection Hospital Inpatient Services, all the subheadings **except** Hospital Discharge Services are divided on the basis of the three key components of history, examination, and MDM complexity. Further, within this subsection only Subsequent Hospital Care codes do not require all three key components to be at the level described in the code. For example, the key components for code 99222 are a comprehensive history, a comprehensive examination, and a moderate level of MDM complexity. If the case you are coding has a comprehensive history and a comprehensive examination but a low complexity of MDM, you cannot assign code 99222 to the case; instead, you would have to assign the lower level code of 99221, which has a low complexity of MDM because the codes require three of the three key components to assign the code to a service.

The subsection of Hospital Inpatient Services is divided into two subheadings.
1. Initial Hospital Care
2. Subsequent Hospital Care

Initial Hospital Care. Initial Hospital Care codes are used to report the initial service of admission to the hospital by the **admitting physician.** Only the admitting physician can report the Initial Hospital Care codes. These codes reflect services in any setting (office, emergency department, nursing home) that are provided in conjunction with the admission to the hospital. For example, if the patient is seen in the office and subsequently is admitted to the hospital the same day, the office visit is bundled into the initial hospital care service. All services provided in the office may be taken into account when selecting the appropriate level of hospital admission. This means that if the physician performed a comprehensive examination in the office, that level of examination is considered when determining the level of the hospital admission service.

EXERCISE 15-10 *Initial Hospital Care*

Fill in the missing words or codes for the following:

1 Which Initial Hospital Care code has a comprehensive history with a straightforward or low complexity of MDM?

CPT Code: _____

2 Which code has a time component of 70 minutes?

CPT Code: _____

3 Code 99222 has a _____ history and examination level and a _____ MDM complexity.

4 An 80-year-old woman has inflammation of the kidneys and renal pelvic area. She is complaining of hematuria, dysuria, and pyuria. She is in good general health other than this condition. She has had some previous workup for this condition as an outpatient but is now being admitted for a cystoscopy. In the patient's history, the physician noted the patient's chief complaints and described the bright red nature of the hematuria, the severe discomfort associated with the dysuria, including burning and itching, and her other symptoms of frequency and urgency. The patient had stated that her symptoms had begun gradually over the past 2 weeks but had become more intense in the past 48 hours. The physician documented the patient's positive responses and pertinent negative responses in his review of her cardiovascular, respiratory, genitourinary, musculoskeletal, neurologic, and endocrine systems. Her past history relating to urinary and renal problems was reviewed. The physical examination noted the complete findings relative to her reproductive system as well as to her urinary system. An examination of her back and related musculoskeletal structures was included because she complained of mild back pain as well. After completing the detailed history and examination, the physician concluded with a diagnosis of acute cystitis and acute pyelitis, possibly associated with endometritis. The MDM complexity was low. The patient was reassured and told to expect a short stay once the exact problem was pinpointed.

CPT Code: _____

ICD-10-CM Codes: _____, _____

(ICD-9-CM Codes: _____, _____)

(Answers are located in Appendix B)

Subsequent Hospital Care. Subsequent Hospital Care (99231-99239) is the second subheading of codes in the Hospital Inpatient Services subsection. The Subsequent Hospital Care codes are used by physicians to report daily hospital visits while the patient is hospitalized.

The first Subsequent Hospital Care code is 99231. Typically, the 99231 level implies that the patient is in stable condition and is responding well to treatment. Subsequent codes in the subsection indicate (in the "Usually, the patient…" area) the status of the patient, such as stable/unstable or recovering/unresponding. Be certain to read the contributory factors area for each code in this subheading.

A general rule of thumb for subsequent hospital services is as follows:

■ Level 1 The patient is recovering and improving.
■ Level 2 The patient has a minor complication or inadequate response to the current therapy.
■ Level 3 The patient is unstable, has a significant complication, or has developed a new problem.

The patient's medical record should indicate the patient's progress from the status indicated in the previous note.

Several physicians, of different specialties, can report the subsequent care codes on the same day. This is called concurrent care. **Concurrent care** is being provided when more than one physician provides service to a patient on the same day for different conditions. An example of concurrent care is a circumstance in which physician A, a cardiologist, treats the patient for a heart condition and at the same time physician B, an oncologist, treats the patient for a cancer condition. The patient's attending (admitting) physician maintains the primary responsibility for the overall care of the patient, no matter how many other physicians are providing services to the patient, unless a formal transfer of care has occurred.

An **attending physician** is a doctor who, on the basis of education, training, and experience, is granted medical staff membership and clinical privileges by a health care organization to perform diagnostic and therapeutic procedures in the facility. An attending physician is legally responsible for the care and treatment provided to a patient. The attending physician may be a patient's personal physician or may be a physician assigned to a patient who has been admitted to a hospital through the emergency department. The attending physician is usually a provider of primary care, such as a family practitioner, internist, or pediatrician, but the attending physician may also be a surgeon or another type of specialist. In an academic medical center, the attending physician is a member of the academic or medical school staff who is responsible for the supervision of medical residents, interns, and medical school students and oversees the care the residents, interns, or students provide to the patients.

CODING SHOT

Note that there is no comprehensive history or comprehensive examination level in the codes in the Subsequent Hospital Care subheading because the comprehensive level of service would have been provided at the time of admission. Also note that only two of the three key components must be met or exceeded to assign a subsequent hospital code.

Observation or Inpatient Care Services (Including Admission and Discharge Services). Codes in the 99234-99236 range report services provided when the patient is admitted and discharged on the **same day**. For example, when the patient is admitted to inpatient status from observation status on the same date of service. Codes in this range require that all three of the key components must be at or exceed the level stated in the code description. These codes include both the admission service and the discharge service. Bundled into the admission are services that were provided in another location, such as the physician's office, nursing facility, or emergency department. This means that the services provided in these other locations are considered when assigning a code from the 99234-99236 range.

Hospital Discharge Services. Inpatient Hospital Discharge Services (99238, 99239) are reported on the final day of services for a **multiple-day** stay in a hospital setting. The service reflects the final examination of the patient as appropriate, follow-up instructions to the patient, and arrangements for discharge, including completion of discharge records. The codes are based on the time spent by the physician in handling the final discharge of the patient, and the time spent must be documented in the medical record.

The Hospital Discharge Services codes are not assigned if the physician is a consultant, unless the primary physician transfers complete care to the consultant. If a consulting physician is following the patient for a separate condition, those services would require a subsequent hospital care code. Only the attending physician, not the consultant, is responsible for completion of the final examination, follow-up instructions, and arrangements for discharge and discharge records. Because these additional services are included in the Hospital Discharge codes, only the attending physician's services can be reported using the codes.

Code 99239, discharge management greater than 30 minutes, requires documentation of time spent performing the discharge instructions. If no indication of time is noted in the documentation, the lowest level of discharge service is reported.

QUICK CHECK 15-6

1. What is the one criterion for selecting a hospital discharge day management code?

_____

(Answers are located in Appendix C)

EXERCISE 15-11   *Hospital Discharge Services*

Fill in the blanks:

1 What are the times indicated for each of the Hospital Discharge Services codes?

_____

2 According to the category notes in Hospital Discharge Services, does the time spent by the physician arranging for the final hospital

discharge of the patient have to be continuous? _____

(Answers are located in Appendix B)

Consultation Services

We all need advice once in a while—maybe for a problem or situation that we cannot find a solution to. Perhaps we think we are doing the right thing but want another person's advice or view to make certain we are following the best course of action. Physicians need opinions and advice, too, and when they do, they ask another physician for an opinion or advice on the treatment, diagnosis, or management of a patient. The physician asking for the advice or opinion is making a **request for consultation** and is the **requesting** physician. The physician giving the advice is providing a consultation and is the **consultant.** Consultations can be provided to both outpatients and inpatients. The CPT manual has different codes for each of the two types of patient consultation—outpatient and inpatient.

"Request for consultation" used to be termed "referral"; making a referral means that the referring physician is asking for the advice or opinion of another physician (a consultation). However, some third-party payers have chosen to define **referral** to mean a total transfer of the care of a patient. In other words, if a patient is referred by physician A to physician B, physician A is expecting physician B to evaluate and treat (assume care for) the patient for the condition for which the patient is being referred. The services of physician B would then **not** be reported using consultation codes. On the other hand, if physician A makes a **request for a consultation** to physician B, it is expected that physician B will provide physician A with his or her advice or opinion and that the patient will return to physician A for any necessary treatment. Physician B would then report his or her services using consultation codes. Although these semantics (use of words) may seem unimportant, they make a difference in the codes you assigned to report the services.

In the Consultation subsection (99241-99255), there are two subheadings of consultations:
1. Office or Other Outpatient Consultations
2. Inpatient Consultations
These subheadings define the location in which the service is rendered; the patient is an outpatient or an inpatient.

Only one initial consultation is reported by a consultant for the patient on each admission, and any subsequent service is reported using codes from the Subsequent Hospital Care codes (99231-99233) or Office or Other Outpatient Services, Established Patient (99211-99215). If more than one consultation is ordered on an inpatient, each consultant may report the initial consultation using the Inpatient Consultation codes (99251-99255).

A **consultation** is a service provided by a physician whose opinion or advice regarding the management or diagnosis of a specific problem has been requested. The consultant provides a written report of the opinion or advice to the attending physician and documents the opinion and services provided in the medical record; the care of the patient is thus complete. Sometimes the attending physician will request the consultant to assume responsibility for a specific area of the patient's care. For example, a consultant may be asked by the attending physician to see an inpatient regarding the care of the patient's diabetes while the patient is hospitalized for gallbladder surgery. After the initial consultation, the attending physician may ask the consultant to continue to monitor the patient's diabetic condition. The consultant assumes responsibility for management of the patient in the specific area of diabetes. Subsequent visits made by the consultant would then be reported using the codes from the subheading Subsequent Hospital Care or Subsequent Nursing Facility Care.

Documentation in the medical record for a consultation must show a request from a physician for an opinion or the advice of a consultant for a specific condition. Findings and treatments rendered during the consultation must be documented in the medical record by the consulting physician and communicated to the requesting physician. The consulting physician can order tests and services for a patient, but the medical necessity of all tests and services must be indicated in the medical record.

Office or Other Outpatient Consultations. The Office or Other Outpatient Consultations codes (99241-99245) report consultative services provided to a patient in an office setting, including hospital observation services, home services, custodial care, and services that are provided in a domiciliary, rest home, or emergency department. Outpatient consultations include consultations provided in the emergency department because the patient is considered an outpatient in the emergency department setting. The codes are for both new and established patients. The codes in this subsection are of increasing complexity, based on the three key components and any contributory factors.

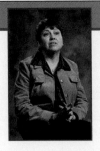

From the Trenches

"Keep the lines of communication open with fellow students, former instructors, co-workers, and the medical staff for whom you code. If you can establish yourself as someone who is dedicated to doing your work with integrity, interacts with respect, and is always willing to help out, you will be successful."

JOAN

Inpatient Consultations. The codes in the Inpatient Consultations subheading (99251-99255) report services by physicians in inpatient settings. This subheading is used for both new and established patients and can be reported only one time per patient admission, per consulting physician, per specialty.

After the initial consultation report, the subsequent hospital or nursing facility codes would be assigned to report services.

The office and inpatient consultation codes (99241-99255) require documentation in the medical record to support all three of the key components listed in the code description. For example, 99243, office consultation, requires a detailed history and examination as well as a low level of medical decision making complexity. Let's say the documentation indicated a detailed history and examination but only a straightforward level of medical decision making. Code 99243 could not be reported because only two of the three key components were at the correct level. The lower level code, 99242, would be assigned.

Various people request consultations on a recommended treatment or diagnosis. Insurance companies or other third-party payers may request a consultation regarding a diagnosis, prognosis, or treatment plan for a patient. These types of consultations are also reported based on the location of the service—office or inpatient. If the consultation is mandated, such as those required by an insurance company, add modifier -32 (Mandated Service) to the code. This modifier is only added if the consultation is mandated by an official body.

For office consultations, a written or verbal request stating results is sent to the requesting physician. This is not necessary with an inpatient because the physicians share the patient's medical record and the inpatient consultant would dictate a consultation report to be included in the medical record.

QUICK CHECK 15-8

1. Can time be utilized to determine a consultation level of service rather than the key components?

   Yes or No?

(Answers are located in Appendix C)

CMS RULES

CMS no longer recognizes CPT consultation codes (ranges 99241-99245 and 99251-99255) for Part B payment for office/outpatient and inpatient facility settings.

EXERCISE 15-12 *Consultation Services*

Using the CPT manual and the ICD-10-CM and/or ICD-9-CM manuals, code the visit in the following scenarios:

1 A 56-year-old female was sent at the request of her primary care physician (PCP) to the oncologist for his opinion regarding the treatment options. The patient had had a right breast carcinoma 6 years earlier but over the past 4 months had developed progressively more painful back pain. In the physician's HPI it was noted that the pain was in the mid-back, with the patient rating it an 8 in intensity on a scale of 1 to 10. However, when the pain started, she thought it was about a 4 on the same scale. The pain has caused her to have neck and leg pains as well, as she has adjusted her walking stance in order to alleviate the pain. She responded to the physician's questions in the review of 10 of her organ systems. Her past medical and surgical history was noted, including the fact that her mother and one sister had also had breast cancer. A comprehensive history was taken. She had worked as a legal secretary up until 2 weeks earlier but is now on sick leave. The comprehensive physical examination performed by the physician was a complete multi-system review of 12 organ systems. The physician ordered a series of radiographic and laboratory tests and reviewed her recent spine x-ray series, which revealed multiple pathologic vertebral compression fractures. The MDM complexity was moderate.

    CPT Code: _____

    ICD-10-CM Codes: _____, _____

    (ICD-9-CM Codes: _____, _____)

2 A 45-year-old man was sent by his PCP to an orthopedic surgeon's office to render an opinion for acute pain and stiffness in his right elbow. In his problem focused history, the physician noted that the man was a farmer and used his right hand and arm repeatedly, lifting heavy objects. The patient had no other complaints and reported to be in otherwise excellent health. The patient described the pain as severe and unrelenting, and it prevented him from using his arm. The problem focused physical examination noted the man's slightly swollen right elbow, with marked pain on movement. No other problems were noted with his right upper extremity. The physician diagnosed the problem as elbow tendinitis and bursitis, recommended warm compresses, and gave the patient a prescription for an anti-inflammatory medication. The MDM complexity was straightforward.

    CPT Code: _____

    ICD-10-CM Codes: _____, _____

    (ICD-9-CM Codes: _____, _____)

3 A 72-year-old man was seen in the internal medicine clinic as an outpatient for medical clearance prior to the replacement of his right knee due to localized primary osteoarthritis. The patient had a history of essential hypertension and mild coronary artery disease. The internist noted, during the expanded problem focused history, that the patient had no complaints relative to his hypertension or heart disease. His blood pressure appeared to be controlled by his medication and low-salt diet. The patient denied any chest pain or discomfort either while working or at rest. In the physician's review, his cardiovascular and respiratory systems appeared to be negative. The physician performed an expanded problem focused physical examination of his head, neck, chest, and abdomen but found no major problems related to his cardiovascular or respiratory system. The internist confirmed the diagnoses previously established and made no changes in the management of either condition. The MDM complexity was straightforward.

    CPT Code: _____

    ICD-10-CM Codes: _____, _____, _____, _____

    (ICD-9-CM Codes: _____, _____, _____, _____)

4 A 52-year-old patient was sent to a surgeon for an office consultation concerning bleeding internal hemorrhoids. A problem focused history and examination were performed. The consultant recommended treating with medication after a straightforward MDM.

    CPT Code: _____

    ICD-10-CM Code: _____ (ICD-9-CM Code: _____)

Continued

5 A 60-year-old man was seen in consultation by a cardiologist in the clinic for complaints of dyspnea, fatigue, and lightheadedness. His history included the insertion of a pacemaker 6 years earlier. He also had a history of mitral regurgitation. The cardiologist performed a comprehensive cardiology physical examination, including cardiac monitoring, pacemaker evaluation, and review of his associated respiratory status. Noted in the comprehensive history were a variety of complaints the patient had in addition to the past pacemaker insertion and current mitral valve regurgitation diagnosed by cardiac catheterization. The physician reviewed the patient's medical history, from the first signs of problems 6 years earlier until the present. His review of systems elicited positive findings in the cardiovascular, respiratory, gastrointestinal, genitourinary, musculoskeletal, and neurologic systems. The other systems had negative responses. The physician had multiple management options concerning the pacemaker function but also had to consider new valvular problems that might have been present as well as related gastrointestinal symptoms. Extensive tests that had been performed recently were reviewed, and additional testing was ordered. The MDM complexity was moderate.

CPT Code: _____

ICD-10-CM Codes: _____ (dyspnea), _____ (fatigue), _____ (dizziness),

_____ (mitral insufficiency), _____ (Z code for status, cardiac device, pacemaker)

(ICD-9-CM Codes: _____ (dyspnea), _____ (fatigue), _____ (dizziness),

_____ (mitral insufficiency), _____ (V code for status, cardiac device, pacemaker))

6 A 65-year-old man had recently undergone a prostatectomy for prostate cancer. Since the surgery, his previously controlled atrial fibrillation had become a problem again. A cardiologist was called in for an inpatient consultation; he reviewed the patient's present status, including the duration and severity of his symptoms. The cardiologist's review of systems related strictly to the cardiovascular system during an expanded problem focused history. The expanded problem focused physical examination concentrated on the man's neck, chest, and abdomen and attempted to elicit all cardiovascular pathology. The consultant suggested that the atrial fibrillation could be controlled better with a different medication. The MDM complexity was straightforward.

CPT Code: _____

ICD-10-CM Code: _____ (ICD-9-CM Code: _____)

7 An internist requested an inpatient consultation from an orthopedic surgeon to evaluate a 35-year-old female who had been in a motor vehicle accident. After reviewing the multiple x-ray reports and the documentation generated by the emergency department physicians, the paramedics' progress notes from the scene of the accident, and the history and physical examination produced by the internist, the orthopedist performed a complete review of systems; complete past, family, and social history; and extended details of the history of the present illness in a comprehensive history review. The comprehensive physical examination was a complete musculoskeletal and neurologic examination with a review of all other organ systems. Based on the patient's multiple fractures and internal injuries, the orthopedist concluded that the patient needed immediate surgery to repair and control the life-threatening conditions that existed. The MDM complexity was high. A neurosurgeon and a general surgeon were also asked to see the patient immediately and possibly to assist in surgery. (Code only the orthopedic consultation.)

CPT Code: _____

8 A 55-year-old patient was injured at work when he fell from a house roof and struck his head. He was admitted for a right frontal parietal craniotomy with removal of a subdural hematoma. After 5 days of rapid recovery from this surgery, a consultation was requested regarding a drug reaction that produced a rash on his upper torso. The physician conducted a brief HPI during the expanded problem focused history, in addition to an ROS focused on the patient's condition. The expanded problem focused examination included three body areas and one organ system. The MDM complexity was straightforward.

CPT Code: _____

9 A 10-year-old was admitted 4 days ago for tympanotomy. Postsurgically, the child developed febrile seizures of unknown origin. A pediatric consultation was requested. The HPI was extended with a complete ROS. A complete PFSH was elicited from the mother as part of a comprehensive history. A comprehensive examination was conducted on all body areas and organ systems. The MDM complexity was high.

CPT Code: _____

ICD-10-CM Code: _____ (ICD-9-CM Code: _____)

Continued

10 A cardiologist was asked by a family practitioner to see an 80-year-old male inpatient a second time. One week prior, the patient, who had multiple other medical problems, had suffered an anterior wall myocardial infarction. Despite following the medical management suggested by the cardiologist, the patient continued to have angina and ventricular tachycardia. The cardiologist closely examined all of the documentation and test results that had been generated in the past week and performed a complete ROS and an extended HPI during the detailed interval history. The detailed physical examination performed was a complete cardiovascular system examination. Based on the subjective and objective findings, the cardiologist concluded that more aggressive medical management was in order. Given the patient's multiple problems coupled with the new threat of cardiorespiratory failure, the patient was immediately transferred to the intensive care unit. The MDM was of high complexity.

    CPT Code: _____

    ICD-10-CM Code: _____ (ICD-9-CM Code: _____)

11 The attending physician had requested an inpatient consultation on a 10-year-old admitted 7 days earlier for tympanotomy. Postsurgically, the patient developed fever and seizures. An initial consultation diagnosis was febrile seizure. Now, on day 7, the child's temperature had returned to normal but the child had had a recurrence of seizures of increased severity. A follow-up consultation was requested. The consultant performed a detailed history and physical examination. The MDM was of high complexity.

    CPT Code: _____

    ICD-10-CM Code: _____ (ICD-9-CM Code: _____)

12 Dr. Jones asked Dr. Williams to confirm the diagnosis of tetralogy of Fallot in a 6-day-old male infant prior to cardiovascular surgery. The patient was seen in the office, where Dr. Williams performed an initial comprehensive history and physical examination on the infant and reviewed the results of the extensive tests already performed. The consultant confirmed the diagnosis and concluded that the child's problem was of high severity and recommended immediate surgery. The MDM complexity was moderate.

    CPT Code: _____

    ICD-10-CM Code: _____ (ICD-9-CM Code: _____)

13 The 45-year-old female's insurance company required a second opinion regarding the degenerative disc disease of her lumbar spine. One orthopedic surgeon had recommended a laminectomy. A second orthopedic surgeon was consulted in the office and performed an expanded problem focused history and physical examination, particularly of her musculoskeletal and neurologic systems. Based on his findings and the conclusive findings of a recent myelogram, the second orthopedic surgeon was quick to conclude that the laminectomy was a reasonable course to follow. The MDM complexity was straightforward.

    CPT Code: _____

14 A third-party payer sought consultation for confirmation about a patient's ability to return to work after the removal of a subdural hematoma 2 months previously. The patient's primary physician had stated that the patient was not yet able to return to his employment, and the third-party payer wanted a second opinion. The patient stated that he continued to have severe and incapacitating headaches and was unable to return to work. A comprehensive history and physical examination were performed in the office. The MDM was of moderate complexity, based on physician findings.

    CPT Code: _____

(Answers are located in Appendix B)

Emergency Department Services

Emergency Department Services codes (99281-99288) are assigned for new or established patients when services are provided in an emergency department (ED) that is a part of a hospital and the ED is available 24 hours a day. These patients are presenting for immediate attention. The codes are assigned for patients without appointments. Emergency Department Services codes are not assigned for patients at the hospital on observation status, even if the observation unit is located in or near the emergency department.

Codes 99281-99285 are based on the type of service the physician performs in terms of the history, the examination, and the complexity of the MDM. These codes require all three of the key components to be assigned. In addition to this information within each code, note that the paragraph at the end of each code that begins with "Usually, the presenting problem(s) are of . . . " identifies the immediacy of the care. For example, 99283 indicates that the presenting problem is of "moderate severity," whereas 99285 indicates that the presenting problem is of "high severity and poses an immediate significant threat to life . . . " Sometimes the patient's clinical condition poses an immediate threat to life, making it possible for the physician to use the higher level code even if it may not be possible to perform the required history and physical examination.

QUICK CHECK 15-9

1. What are the times associated with codes 99281-99285? _____

2. If a patient presents to the emergency department in a clinically life-threatening state that prevents the physician from performing a complete history or physical examination, could the code 99285 still be reported?

   Yes or No?

(Answers are located in Appendix C)

Critical care provided to a patient in the emergency department is reported using additional codes from the Critical Care Service code section, which we will discuss later in this chapter.

If a patient initially treated in the emergency department requires admittance to the hospital, the patient's attending physician would serve as the admitting physician.

Emergency department codes can be assigned to report the services not only of the ED physician, but also of any physician who cares for a patient in the ED. For example, if the patient's primary care physician (PCP) meets the patient in the ED or is called into the ED, and the PCP cares for the patient in the ED, not admitting the patient to the hospital, then the PCP reports the services using either ED codes or outpatient established patient codes. Note that in this instance, the PCP is NOT a consultant but is serving as the patient's physician in the emergency room location.

Also, ED physicians do not admit patients to a hospital. If a patient is seen in the ED and has to be admitted to the hospital, the patient's PCP or other designated physician will admit the patient. An example of a designated physician would be a hospitalist. A **hospitalist** is a hospital-based physician who only sees patients in the hospital and assumes the responsibility of the primary care physician for hospitalized patients. This is a relatively new approach to hospital coverage but is fast gaining popularity.

Other Emergency Department Services. The Other Emergency Department Services subheading is at the end of the Emergency Department Services subsection, and the code located there (99288) reports the services of a physician based at the hospital who provides two-way communication with the ambulance or rescue team. This physician provides direction and advice to the team as they attend the patient en route to the emergency department.

The subheading notes contain examples of the types of medical services the physician might direct. Be certain to read these notes so you understand the types of services the code refers to.

EXERCISE 15-13 *Emergency Department Services*

Use the information contained in the code descriptions in the Emergency Department Services subsection to answer the questions in this exercise.

1 The severity of the presenting problem for Code 99281 would usually be _____.

2 The severity of the presenting problem for Code 99284 would usually be _____.

3 The severity of the presenting problem for Code 99283 would usually be _____.

4 The severity of the presenting problem for Code 99282 would usually be _____.

Code the following:

5 A patient in the emergency department has extreme acute chest pains and goes into cardiac arrest. The emergency department physician is unable to obtain a history or perform a physical examination because the patient's condition is critical. The MDM is of high complexity.

    CPT Code: _____

    ICD-10-CM Code: _____ (ICD-9-CM Code: _____)

6 An elderly patient in the emergency department has a temperature of 105° F and is in acute respiratory distress. Symptoms include shortness of breath, chest pain, cyanosis, and gasping. The physician is unable to obtain a history or perform a comprehensive physical examination because the patient's condition is critical. The MDM complexity is high.

    CPT Code: _____

    ICD-10-CM Code: _____ (ICD-9-CM Code: _____)

7 A child presents to the emergency department with his parents after being bitten by a dog. The child is in extreme pain and bleeding from a wound on the forearm. The animal has not been located to quarantine for rabies. An expanded problem focused history is obtained and an expanded problem focused physical examination is performed. The MDM complexity is moderate because of the possibility of rabies.

    CPT Code: _____

8 The physician directs the emergency medical technicians via two-way communications with an ambulance en route to the emergency department with a patient in apparent cardiac arrest.

    CPT Code: _____

(Answers are located in Appendix B)

Critical Care Services

Critical Care Services codes (99291, 99292) identify services that are provided during medical emergencies to patients over 71 months of age who are either critically ill or injured. These codes require the physician to be constantly available to the patient and providing services exclusively to that patient. For example, a patient who is in shock or cardiac arrest would require the physician to provide bedside critical care services. Critical care is often, but not required to be, provided in an acute care setting of a hospital. Acute care settings are intensive care units, coronary care units, emergency departments, and similar critical care units of a hospital. Codes in this subsection are listed according to the time the physician spends providing critical care to the patient. The time calculation is not just the face-to-face time the physician spends with the patient. The review of records and diagnostic results at the time of the encounter should also be counted in determining the time spent in providing critical care to the patient.

The time the physician spends in providing other procedures must be deducted from the total critical care time. For example, if an adult patient is intubated during critical care, the time spent on the intubation (31500) is deducted from the total critical care time because the physician will report the intubation service separately.

The total critical care time, per day, the physician spends in care of the patient is stated in one amount of time, even if the time was not continuous. Code 99291 is reported only once a day for the first 30 to 74 minutes of critical care, and 99292 is reported for each additional 30 minutes beyond 74 minutes. If the critical care is less than 30 minutes, an E/M code would be assigned to report the service.

Total Duration of Critical Care Time	CPT Codes Reported
Less than 30 minutes	appropriate E/M code
30-74 minutes	99291 × 1
75-104 minutes	99291 × 1 and 99292 × 1
105-134 minutes	99291 × 1 and 99292 × 2
135-164 minutes	99291 × 1 and 99292 × 3
165-194 minutes	99291 × 1 and 99292 × 4
195 minutes or longer	99291 and 99292 as appropriate

As an example, if a physician sees a critical care patient for 74 minutes and then leaves and returns for 30 minutes of critical care at a later time in the same day, the coding would be for 104 minutes of care. The coding for 104 minutes would be:

99291 for the 74 minutes

99292 for the additional 30 minutes

CODING SHOT

Most third-party payers will not pay for more than one physician at a time for critical care services.

There are service codes that are bundled into the Critical Care Services codes. These services are normally provided to stabilize the patient. An example of this bundling is as follows: A physician starts ventilation management (94002) while providing critical care services to a patient in the intensive care unit of a hospital. The ventilator management is not reported separately but, instead, is considered to be bundled into the Critical Care Services code. The notes preceding the critical care codes in the CPT manual list the services and procedures bundled into the codes. If the physician provided a service at the same time as critical care and that service is not bundled into the code, the service could be reported separately. Some third-party payers may require the use of modifier -25 with the critical care codes when reporting a service that is not bundled into the Critical Care Services. You will know what is bundled into the codes because this information is listed either in the extensive description of the code or in the notes preceding the code. Be certain to read these notes, as they contain many exclusions and inclusions for these codes.

If the patient is in a critical care unit but is stable, you report the services using codes from the Hospital Inpatient Services subsection, Subsequent Hospital Care subheading or from the Consultations subsection, Inpatient subheading.

QUICK CHECK 15-10

1. List two types of service and the CPT codes for the services that are bundled into critical care services.

Such as: Chest x-rays (71010, 71015, 71020)

_____

_____

(Answers are located in Appendix C)

EXERCISE 15-14   *Critical Care Services*

Fill in the information for the following:

1 Critical care is provided to the patient for 70 minutes.

🌐 CPT Code(s): _____

2 Can code 99292 be reported without code 99291? _____

3 A physician is called to the intensive care unit to provide care for a patient who has received second-degree burns over 50% of his body. The physician provides support for 2 hours. After leaving the unit, the physician returns later that day to provide an additional hour of critical care support to the patient.

🌐 CPT Code(s): _____

🌐 ICD-10-CM Code(s): _____   (🌐 ICD-9-CM Code(s): _____)

(Answers are located in Appendix B)

Nursing Facility Services

A **nursing facility** is not a hospital but does have inpatient beds and a professional health care staff that provides health care to persons who do not require the level of service provided in an acute care facility.

A **skilled nursing facility** (SNF) is one that has a professional staff that often includes physicians and nurses. The patients of a skilled nursing facility require less care than that given in an acute care hospital, but more care than that provided in a nursing home. Skilled nursing facilities are also called skilled nursing units, skilled nursing care, or extended care facilities. Professional and practical nursing services are available 24 hours a day. Rehabilitation services, such as occupational therapy, physical therapy, and speech therapy, are available on a daily basis. A skilled nursing facility was previously called an extended care facility. Patients may stay for several weeks in a skilled nursing facility before returning home or being transferred to an intermediate care facility for long-term care. Skilled nursing facilities provide care for individuals of all ages, even though the majority of services are provided to geriatric patients.

An **intermediate care facility** provides regular, basic health services to individuals who do not need the degree of care or treatment provided in a hospital or a skilled nursing facility. Residents, because of their mental or physical conditions, require assistance with their activities of daily living, such as bathing, dressing, eating, and ambulating. Intermediate care facilities generally provide long-term care, usually over several years. Professional and practical nursing services are available on a 24-hour basis. Activities, social services, and dietary and other therapies are available on a daily basis. The majority of residents of intermediate care facilities are geriatric individuals or individuals of any age with developmental disabilities.

The **long-term care facility** describes health and personal services provided to ill, aged, disabled, or mentally handicapped individuals for an extended period of time. Other types of facilities are better described as skilled or intermediate care facilities.

Four subheadings of nursing facility services are available: Initial Nursing Facility Care, Subsequent Nursing Facility Care, Nursing Facility Discharge Services, and Other Nursing Facility Services.

Initial Nursing Facility Care. Initial Nursing Facility Care codes (99304-99306) do not distinguish between new and established patients. These codes report services provided by the physician at the time of admission or re-admission. Assessments by physicians play a central role in the development of the resident's individualized care plan. The care plan is developed by an interdisciplinary care team using the Resident Assessment Instrument (RAI) and the Minimum Data Set (MDS).

CHECK THIS OUT ☞ The MDS forms are located on the CMS website at www.cms. gov/NursingHomeQualityInits/Downloads/MDS20MDSAllForms.pdf.

Subsequent Nursing Facility Care. Subsequent Nursing Facility Care codes (99307-99310) do not distinguish between a new and an established patient. These codes reflect services provided by a physician on a periodic basis when a resident does not need a comprehensive assessment. Typically, such a resident has not had a major change in his or her condition since the previous physician visit but requires ongoing management of a chronic condition or treatment of an acute short-term problem. The higher level codes are assigned to patients with new problems or significant changes in existing problems.

Nursing Facility Discharge Services. The Nursing Facility Discharge Services codes (99315, 99316) report the services the physician renders to the patient on the day of discharge. The codes are assigned based on the amount of time documented for discharge management. Code 99315 is assigned if 30 minutes or less or when no time is documented. Code 99316 is reported for documented time of greater than 30 minutes. The time spent need not be continuous or spent entirely with the patient but must be documented. The physician may conduct a final physical examination, give instructions to the patient's caregivers, and prepare all necessary discharge documentation, referral forms, and medication orders.

Other Nursing Facility Services. Other Nursing Facility Services contains only one code, 99318, and reports the annual nursing facility assessment provided by the physician. By law, the nursing facility must conduct a comprehensive assessment of each resident at least once a year and determine if there is any significant change in the resident's physical or mental condition. As with many subheadings throughout the E/M section, if a patient is admitted to a nursing facility but the service was started elsewhere, such as a physician's office or emergency department, all the evaluation and management services provided to the patient in these other locations are considered part of the nursing facility code. For example, a patient was seen in the hospital emergency department, where a comprehensive history and examination were performed for a condition that required high MDM complexity (99285, Emergency Department Services). The physician made the decision to admit the patient to a nursing facility on the same day. Rather than reporting 99285 (Emergency Department Services), you would report the same level service from the subheading Initial Nursing Facility Care, 99306.

Nursing Facility Services codes are also assigned for services in a type of place you would not think would apply—psychiatric residential treatment centers. The center must be a stand-alone facility or a separate part of a facility that provides group living facilities and must have 24-hour staffing. Nursing Facility Services codes identify evaluation and management services. If a physician also provides medical psychotherapy, you would report those services separately.

When a patient has been in the hospital and is discharged from the hospital to a nursing facility, all on the same day, you can report the hospital discharge (99238-99239) and the nursing facility admission (99304-99306) separately. This is also true for same-day services for patients who are discharged from observation status (99217) and admitted to a nursing facility (99304-99306).

EXERCISE 15-15 *Nursing Facility Services*

Answer the following:

1 According to the code description for 99305, the usual level of severity of the problem(s) that required admission to the nursing

facility is: _____

2 A 72-year-old male patient is transferred to a nursing facility from a hospital after suffering a cerebrovascular accident (stroke) with cerebral infarction. The patient needs a comprehensive assessment before his active rehabilitation plan can be started. A comprehensive history is gathered by the internist, including the patient's chief complaint of left-sided weakness on his dominant side, an extended HPI, and a complete ROS. Details of the patient's past, family, and social history add information to the care-planning process. The internist performs a comprehensive multisystem physical examination. After much deliberation with the multidisciplinary rehabilitation team, the physician determines that the patient is ready for active rehabilitation. The physician also writes orders to continue treatment of the patient's other medical conditions, including hypertension and diabetes. The MDM complexity is high.

CPT Code: _____

ICD-10-CM Codes: _____, _____, _____

(ICD-9-CM Codes: _____, _____, _____)

Using the following information within the code descriptions in the Subsequent Nursing Facility Care subheading, match the medical decision making complexity in the description of the code with the code:

3 99307 _____   **a** moderate
4 99308 _____   **b** low
5 99309 _____   **c** straightforward

Code the following:

6 Subsequent follow-up care is provided for a comatose patient transferred to a long-term care center from the hospital. The resident had a brain injury and shows no signs of consciousness on examination but appears to have developed a minor upper respiratory tract infection with a fever and cough. The physician performs an expanded problem focused interval history (by way of nursing staff notes) and physical examination, including neurologic status, respiratory status, and status of related organ systems. Because the physician is concerned that the existing respiratory infection could progress to pneumonia, appropriate treatment is ordered. The MDM complexity is moderate.

CPT Code: _____

ICD-10-CM Codes: _____, _____, _____

(ICD-9-CM Codes: _____, _____, _____)

(Answers are located in Appendix B)

Domiciliary, Rest Home (e.g., Boarding Home), or Custodial Care Services

These codes (99324-99337) are divided into subheadings based on the patients' status as new or established service provided. The codes are arranged in levels based on the documentation in the patient's medical record. Time estimates are established for codes in this category.

These codes are reported for the evaluation and management of residents who reside in a domiciliary, rest home, or custodial care center. Generally, health services are not available on site, nor are any medical services included in the codes. These facilities provide residential care, including lodging, meals, supervision, personal care, and leisure activities, to persons who, because of their physical, mental, or emotional condition, are not able to live independently. Such facilities might include alternative living residences, assisted living facilities, retirement centers, community-based living units, group homes, or residential treatment centers. These facilities provide custodial care for residents of all ages.

Domiciliary, Rest Home (e.g., Assisted Living Facility), or Home Care Plan Oversight Services

Codes 99339, 99340 apply to services provided to a patient who is being cared for at home and not enrolled with a home health care agency. These patients are being cared for by family members, health care professionals, and other types of caregivers. These codes are not reported if the patient is receiving his or her care from a home health agency, hospice program, or nursing facility. When reporting these codes the patient is not present, rather the physician is developing a care plan or overseeing the care of the patient. The physician's time may be reported if the time was over 15 minutes within a calendar month. Code 99339 reports 15-29 minutes, and 99340 reports 30 minutes or more. Again, these codes are only reported once for each calendar month.

Home Services

Health care services can also be provided to patients in their homes. Times have been established for this category of services. Note that there is a statement about typical time located under the code description in the paragraph that begins, "Usually, the presenting problem(s) is . . . " Never report a code based on time unless at least 50% of the time was spent on counseling or coordinating care. The codes (99341-99350) for these services are also divided into categories for new and for established patients.

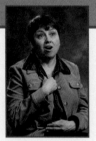

From the Trenches

"I have found that there is definitely a sense of family among coders. Like all families, we don't always agree on everything, but we care about each other's thoughts and challenges . . . and know that there is always someone out there that can be there for you, whether it is a coding dilemma or a bigger, career-type decision."

JOAN

EXERCISE 15-16 | *Home Services*

Code the following scenario:

1 A 64-year-old established female patient has diabetes mellitus and has been having problems adjusting her insulin doses. She has had an onset of dizziness and sensitivity to light. The physician makes a home visit during which he gathers a brief HPI and a problem-pertinent ROS during the problem focused history. The problem focused physical examination focuses on the body systems currently affected by the diabetes. The physician finds the patient's condition to be moderately severe and the MDM complexity is straightforward.

CPT Code: _____

(Answers are located in Appendix B)

Prolonged Services

In the Prolonged Services subsection there are three subheadings:

■ Prolonged Physician Service *With* Direct Patient Contact
■ Prolonged Physician Service *Without* Direct Patient Contact
■ Standby Services

Prolonged Physician Services With or Without Direct Patient Contact.
Prolonged Physician Services codes (99354-99357, 99359) are all add-on codes. Note the plus symbol (1) beside all codes in the 99354-99359 range. Because add-on codes can be reported only with another code, all Prolonged Physician Services codes are intended to be used only in addition to other codes to show an extension of some other service. The time is to be documented in the medical record to support the submission of the Prolonged Care code(s). The following example illustrates the use of these codes.

Example

An established patient with a history of COPD presents, in an office visit, with acute bronchospasm and moderate respiratory distress. The physician conducts a problem focused history followed by a problem focused examination, which shows a respiratory rate of 30, and labored breathing and wheezing are heard in all lung fields. Office treatment is initiated; it includes intermittent bronchial dilation and subcutaneous epinephrine. The service requires the physician to have intermittent direct contact with the patient over a 2-hour period. The MDM complexity is low.

✋ **CAUTION**   *If you hadn't carefully read the notes preceding the Prolonged Services codes, you would not know that there are many rules that govern the calculation of time when determining the codes.*

The office visit service would be reported using the office visit code 99212 (which has 10 minutes as the usual time); but the additional time the physician spent providing service to the patient over and above that which is indicated in code 99212 would have to be reported using a prolonged service code.

As the notes indicate, the first 30 minutes of prolonged services are not even counted but are considered part of the initial service. So you cannot use a prolonged services code until after the first 30 minutes of the prolonged services have been provided. The physician, therefore, has to spend 30 minutes with the patient in prolonged services before it is possible to report any prolonged service time.

The reporting on this service is as follows:

  120 minutes spent with patient

<u>−10</u> minutes for the usual time in 99212

  110 minutes remaining

According to the grid before 99354, for 105 minutes or more you are to report 99354 × 1 and 99355 × 2.

The time the physician spends providing the prolonged services does not have to be continuous, as is the situation in this example; the physician monitored the patient on an intermittent basis, coming into the room to check on the patient and then leaving the room.

But let's change this case a bit and see how the coding changes. If the physician spent 70 minutes with the patient, you could code only the first hour at 99354. The additional 10 minutes beyond the first 60 are not coded separately. Remember that you would need at least 15 minutes beyond the first hour to code for the time beyond the first hour. For help in applying these codes, refer to the table preceding the codes; there you can locate the total time your physician spent with the patient and see an example of the correct coding.

The direct Prolonged Physician Services codes describe services that require the physician to have **direct contact** with the patient; but the Prolonged Physician Services Without Direct Patient Contact codes describe services during which the physician is not in direct contact with the patient. For example, a physician evaluates an established patient, a 70-year-old female with dementia, in an office visit. The physician then spends an extensive amount of time discussing the patient's condition, her treatment plan, and other recommendations with the daughter of the patient. The services would be reported by using an office visit code for the patient evaluation and the appropriate prolonged service without direct contact code for the time spent with the daughter.

Prolonged Physician Services codes are most often reported with the higher level E/M codes, which themselves carry longer time frames. According to the CPT notes for Prolonged Physician Services, these codes are add-on codes and are reported in addition to another E/M code.

Prolonged Physician Services With Direct Patient Contact codes are divided on the basis of whether the services were provided to an outpatient or an inpatient.

Standby Services. The code (99360) for Standby Services is reported when a physician, at the request of another physician, is standing by in case his or her services are needed. The standby physician cannot be rendering services to another patient during this time. The standby code is reported in increments of 30 minutes. The 30-minute increments referred to here really mean from the first minute to the 30th minute and do not have any of the complicated rules for reporting time that exist for reporting prolonged services.

An important note concerning the standby code is that this code is reported only when there is a documented request in the patient's medical record and **no service** is performed and there is **no direct contact** with the patient. This code is not reported when a standby status ends, and the standby physician provides a service to a patient. The service the physician provides is reported as any other service would be, even though it began as a standby service.

CODING SHOT

To report standby services, there must be a written request for standby services in the medical record.

Read the notes before Code 99360 before completing Exercise 15-17.

EXERCISE 15-17   *Prolonged and Standby Services*

Using the notes in the subsections, answer the following:

1 Does the time the physician spends with the patient in prolonged, direct contact have to be continuous? _____

2 Can a code from the Prolonged Services subsection be reported alone? _____

3 If the prolonged contact with the patient lasts less than 30 minutes, is the time reported separately? _____

4 The codes in the Prolonged Services With Direct Patient Contact subheading are based not only on the time the physician spends with the patient, but also on another factor. What is that other factor? _____

5 Are the codes in the subheading Prolonged Services Without Direct Patient Contact categorized according to the place of service?

_____

6 According to the notes in the Standby Services subsection, can a physician report the time spent in proctoring (monitoring) another physician? _____

(Answers are located in Appendix B)

Case Management Services

The Case Management Services subsection (99363-99368) consists of codes used by physicians to report anticoagulant therapy and coordination of care services with other health care professionals.

Anticoagulant Management. The codes report anticoagulant services using Warfarin/Coumadin. Anticoagulants inhibit coagulation of the blood and are prescribed to patients with various thromboembolic disorders. Patients on this medication are monitored by means of blood tests and adjustments are then made in the blood thinner dosage if the physician determines the clotting levels are not ideal. Codes 99363 and 99364 report the monitoring services provided on an outpatient basis for the initial 90 days of therapy (with a minimum of eight assessments) and each subsequent 90 days of therapy (with at least three assessments). Any period less than 60 continuous outpatient days is not reported.

Medical Team Conferences. The medical team must include at least three qualified health care professionals from different specialties. The team members must have all performed a face-to-face evaluation or treatment of the patient within the previous 60 days. Codes 99366-99368 are divided based on if the patient and/or family is/are present in the conference with the participation of the physician and non-physician health care professionals.

EXERCISE 15-18 *Case Management Services*

Complete the following:

1 What is the time component specified in the Medical Team Conference codes from the Case Management Services subsection?

_____

2 What are the three Medical Team Conference codes? _____

(Answers are located in Appendix B)

Care Plan Oversight Services

At times, health care professionals are asked to manage a complex case that involves an individual such as a hospice patient or a patient who is homebound and receives the majority of his or her health care from visiting nurses. When regular communication is necessary between the nurses and the physician to discuss revising the care plan, coordinating the treatment plan with other professionals, or adjusting the therapies, codes from the Care Plan Oversight Services subsection (99374-99380) report these additional services. The codes are divided according to whether the supervision is of a patient being cared for by home health workers or a patient in a hospice or nursing facility. The codes are also divided based on the length of time of the service—either 15 to 29 minutes or 30 minutes or more. Reporting is by time over a month-long period.

Preventive Medicine Services

Preventive Medicine Services codes (99381-99429) report the routine evaluation and management of a patient who is healthy and has no complaint. The codes in this subsection report a routine physical examination provided at the patient's request, such as a well-baby check-up. Preventive Medicine codes are intended to identify comprehensive services, not a single system review. The codes are reported for infants, children, adolescents, and adults; they differ according to the age of the patient and whether the patient is a new or an established patient.

CODING SHOT

If the physician should encounter a problem or abnormality during the course of a preventive service, and the problem or abnormality requires significant additional service, you can also code an office visit code with a modifier -25 added. The modifier -25 is added to indicate that a significant, separately identifiable E/M service was performed by the physician on the same day as the preventive medicine service. If you did not add the modifier -25, the third-party payer would think that you had made an error and were reporting both a preventive medicine service code and an office visit code for the same service. Only with the use of the modifier -25 can you convey that the services were indeed separate.

Note that in the code descriptions for both the New Patient and the Established Patient categories, the terms "comprehensive history" and "comprehensive examination" are used. These terms are not the same as the ones used with other E/M codes (99201-99350). Here, "comprehensive" means a complete history and a complete examination, as is conducted during an annual physical. The comprehensive examination performed as part of the preventive medicine E/M service is a multisystem examination, but the extent of the examination is determined by the age of the patient and the risk factors identified for that individual.

EXERCISE 15-19 *Preventive Medicine Services*

Complete the following:

1 According to the notes in the Preventive Medicine Services subsection, the extent and focus of the services provided, whether to a new or established patient, will depend largely upon what factor? _____

2 If, during the preventive medicine evaluation, a problem is encountered that requires the physician to perform a problem focused E/M service, what modifier would be appended to the code? _____

(Answers are located in Appendix B)

Counseling Risk Factor Reduction and Behavior Change Intervention. These codes (99401-99429) are for both new and established healthy patients. The services are based on whether individual or group counseling is provided to the patient and on the amount of time the service requires. Codes in this category report a physician's services to a patient for risk factor interventional counseling, such as a diet and exercise program, smoking cessation, or contraceptive management.

Non-Face-to-Face Services

These codes are divided into Telephone Services (99441-99443) and On-Line Medical Evaluation (99444–99449) assigned to report services provided by a physician or other qualified professional. To report these same services provided by a non-physician, assign Medicine codes 98966-98969. The notes and the code descriptions for these codes indicate that the telephone or online service cannot originate from a related assessment that was provided within the previous seven days or result in an appointment within the next 24 hours or the soonest available appointment. The telephone services are reported based on the documented time, and the online service is reported only once for the same episode of care during a seven-day period. Interprofessional Telephone/Internet Consultations (99446-99449) are codes a consultant reports for an assessment and management services requested by the patient's attending or primary. During this service, there is no face-to-face contact between the patient and consultant. Usually, these services are provided in an urgent or emergency situation. The patient may be new or established with the consultant, with a new or worsening problem, and has not been seen in a face-to-face encounter within the last 14 days. The consultant reviews the medical documentation and any available assessments, such as imaging studies, and the review is bundled into the codes and not reported separately.

Although most payers and CMS do not currently reimburse for telephone services, some payers do, such as Workers' Compensation. Even if a payer does not reimburse, you should still submit all the codes necessary to completely explain the service. This type of historical data is used to analyze services provided and may, in the future, result in changes to reimbursement.

Special Evaluation and Management Services

The codes in this subsection (99450-99456) are used to report evaluations for life or disability insurance baseline information. The services can be performed in any setting for either a new or an established patient. The codes vary, based on whether the service is for an examination for life or disability insurance and whether the examination is done by the physician treating the patient's disability or by someone other than the treating physician.

EXERCISE 15-20 *Special Evaluation and Management Services*

Answer the following:

1 An insurance examination was conducted by the physician for a new patient for a term life insurance policy. From what subheading would you select a code to report this service? _____

2 A 50-year-old man was referred for a disability examination. The patient had been injured at work when he slipped off a ladder and fell from a height of 10 feet, landing on his back. He has not returned to work since that time 6 months ago. The patient had been under the care of a physician from another state and was referred by the insurance company for the assessment of the patient's ability to return to work. His primary physician had stated that this patient will be unable to return to his previous work as a bricklayer. From what subheading would you select a code to report this service? _____

3 What is the difference between the two codes in the Work Related or Medical Disability Evaluation Services codes?

_____

_____

_____

4 A 58-year-old man was seen by his private physician for an examination as part of his claim for long-term medical disability. The patient has chronic obstructive lung disease with severe emphysema and has been unable to work during the past year. The physician completed all the necessary documentation required by the insurance company, including his opinion that the patient would be unable to work in the future, as his pulmonary function is markedly impaired, in spite of continual respiratory and pharmacologic therapy.

CPT Code: _____

ICD-10-CM Codes: _____ (medical exam for insurance certification), _____ (COPD with emphysema)

(ICD-9-CM Codes: _____ (medical exam for insurance certification), _____ (COPD with emphysema))

(Answers are located in Appendix B)

Newborn Care Services

Newborn Care Services codes (99460-99465) report services to normal newborns. Note that there are three history and examination codes; one is specifically for a newborn assessment and discharge from a hospital or birthing room on the same date (99463), one is for hospital or birthing room deliveries (99460), and one is for other than a hospital or birthing center (99461). The initial services are reported on a per day basis. Subsequent services are reported with 99462. If the physician provides a discharge service to a newborn discharged subsequent to the admission date, you would choose a code from the Hospital Inpatient Services subsection, Hospital Discharge Services subheading (99238, 99239).

Delivery/Birthing Room Attendance (99464, 99465) codes report the attendance of a physician, at the request of the delivering physician, to provide the initial stabilization of a newborn or for the resuscitation/ventilation of the newborn. The request for physician attendance must be documented in the patient's medical record.

Inpatient Neonatal Intensive Care and Pediatric and Neonatal Critical Care Services (99466-99486)

Pediatric Critical Care Patient Transport. These codes (99466, 99467) report face-to-face services provided to a pediatric patient (24 months of age or younger). During the provision of these services, the patient is being transported from one facility to another. The codes are time-based. Codes 99485 and 99486 report supervision by a control physician with the first 30 minutes reported with 99485 and each additional 30 minutes reported with 99486. If the physician is in physical attendance for less than 30 minutes, the service is not reported with these transportation codes.

> ✋ **CAUTION** *Bundled into the codes are routine monitoring evaluations, such as heart rate and blood pressure. Other services provided before transport and nonroutine services provided during transport may be reported separately.*

Inpatient Neonatal and Pediatric Critical Care. Codes 99468-99476 report initial and subsequent critical care services to neonatal and pediatric patients. The codes are based on the age of the patient:

- Neonate, 28 days or younger
- Pediatric, 29 days through 24 months of age or 2 years through 5 years

The name of the intensive care unit does not matter in the assignment of these codes. The services can be provided in a pediatric intensive care unit, neonatal critical care unit, or any of the many other names that these types of intensive care units have. **Bundled** into the codes are many services you would anticipate would be used in the support of a critically ill neonate or pediatric patient (for example, arterial catheters, nasogastric tube placement, endotracheal intubation, and invasive electronic monitoring of vital signs). The notes preceding the codes list bundled services, descriptions, and codes for services (for example, blood transfusion, 36440). To ensure that you do not unbundle, you will need to refer back to these lists of bundled services. If the physician performed a service not listed in the bundle, you would report the service separately. Other notes indicating bundled services appear in the code descriptions. For example, cardiac and/or respiratory support is bundled into some of the codes.

Initial and Continuing Intensive Care Services. When a neonate or infant is **not** considered critically ill but still needs intensive observation and other intensive care services, the Initial and Continuing Intensive Care Services codes (99477-99486) are reported. These codes are not based on the age of the patient, but are based on weight.

- Very low birth weight (VLBW) is less than 1500 grams (less than 3.3 pounds)
- Low birth weight (LBW) is 1500-2500 grams (3.3-5.5 pounds)
- Normal birth weight is 2501-5000 grams (5.51-11.01 pounds)

The assignment of these codes changes when the neonate/infant weight changes. The codes from the subsection are reported only once in every 24-hour period (same day). There are no hourly service codes as there are in other critical care codes.

EXERCISE 15-21   *Newborn Care and Neonatal/Pediatric Critical Care Services*

Answer the following:

1 What does the abbreviation VLBW mean? _____

2 What code would you assign to report the face-to-face service provided by a physician during an interfacility transport of a critically ill patient who is 16 months of age? The service was for 60 minutes.

    CPT Code: _____

3 A normal newborn was admitted to the hospital on Saturday morning and was discharged Saturday evening. The physician provided evaluation and management services including the admission and the discharge. What code would you assign to report the physician service?

    CPT Code: _____

4 The physician provided a subsequent inpatient service to a 3-year-old critically ill patient.

    CPT Code: _____

5 The physician provided an intensive care service to an infant of 1450 grams on the patient's second day of the hospital stay.

    CPT Code: _____

(Answers are located in Appendix B)

Care Management Services (99487-99490)

Chronic Care Management Services (99490) Reporting of 99490 requires the patient to have two or more chronic conditions that are expected to last at least 12 months or result in death. There is a risk of death or functional decline. A comprehensive care plan is established, implemented, revised, or monitored. At least 20 minutes of physician directed staff time is provided during the month.

Complex Chronic Care Management Services (99487, 99489) Codes 99487 and 99489 report complex chronic care management services provided during a month. In addition to compliance with chronic care criteria, there is development of or substantial revision of a comprehensive care plan. The MDM is of moderate to high complexity and includes at least 60 minutes of physician directed clinical staff time. The CPT notes identify extensive criteria for assignment of these codes. The codes are time-based of at least 60 minutes per calendar month and each additional 30 minutes.

Transitional Care Management Services (99495-99496)

Codes 99495 and 99496 are transitional care management codes that are based on the number of days after discharge from a medical facility and if the medical decision making complexity is moderate or high. The service involves the management of the various available care options for the patient. These codes can be assigned for a new or established patient and require an initial face-to-face visit, patient contact, and reconciliation of the patient's medications during a specified time frame.

Advance Care Planning (99497-99498)

Advance Care Planning codes report face-to-face services with a patient or the patient's surrogate and a physician or other qualified health care professional to counsel and discuss advance directives regarding medical treatment; for example, Medical Orders for Life-Sustaining Treatment (MOLST). When reporting these codes, there is no active management of the problem(s) during the reported time. Services are reported based on the first 30 minutes and each additional 30-minute increment. These codes may be reported with select E/M codes, such as 99201-99215.

Other Evaluation and Management Services

Other Evaluation and Management Services (99499) is the last subsection in the E/M section. Code 99499 is an unlisted code that is used to indicate that there is no other code that accurately represents the services provided to the patient. A special report would accompany the unlisted E/M service code. 99499 should be reported if the key components of an E/M service do not meet the lowest level of a category (e.g., 99221).

Coding Practice

CONGRATULATIONS! Good job! You have been through all of the E/M codes and are now familiar with the basics of CPT code arrangement. Can you imagine how well you would know your favorite novel if you read it several times a month? Well, coders use their CPT manuals every day and become very familiar with the information in the guidelines, notes, and descriptions of the codes. Please be sure to locate the code in the CPT manual and read all notes, guidelines, and descriptions about each code you work with. In this way, you will build a solid knowledge foundation.

Now let's begin to do some coding that will require you to combine all the information you have learned as you begin to code patient cases.

EXERCISE 15-22 *Coding Practice*

Code the following:

1 A new patient is seen in the office for an earache (otalgia). The history and examination are problem focused and the MDM complexity is straightforward. The diagnosis was acute mastoiditis.

CPT Code: _____

ICD-10-CM Code: _____ (ICD-9-CM Code: _____)

2 An established patient is seen in the office of an ENT (ear-nose-throat) specialist with the chief complaint of otalgia. The physician completes a problem focused history and physical examination of the head, eyes, ears, nose, and throat. To the physician, this is a straightforward case of acute otitis media, and prescription medications are ordered. The MDM complexity is straightforward.

CPT Code: _____

ICD-10-CM Code: _____ (ICD-9-CM Code: _____)

3 An established patient is seen in the office for a blood pressure check, which is done by the physician's nurse.

CPT Code: _____

4 Lilly Wilson, a new patient, is seen by the physician in the skilled nursing facility for an initial nursing facility assessment. Mrs. Wilson recently suffered a cerebral thrombosis with residual dysphagia and paresis of the left extremities. She was transferred from the acute care hospital to the skilled nursing facility for concentrated rehabilitation. Mrs. Wilson also has arteriosclerotic heart disease with a permanent pacemaker in place, rheumatoid arthritis, urinary incontinence, and macular degeneration in her right eye. The physician, who did not know Mrs. Wilson prior to her transfer, performs a comprehensive history and physical examination. Given the patient's multiple diagnoses and the moderate amount of data the physician has to review, the MDM is of a high level of complexity.

CPT Code: _____

5 John Taylor is a 16-year-old outpatient who is a new patient to the office. John complains of severe pustule facial acne. The history and physical examination are expanded problem focused. The physician must consider related organ systems in addition to the integumentary system in order to treat the condition properly. With the minimal number of diagnoses to consider and the minimal amount of data to review, the physician's decision making is straightforward with regard to the plan of care.

CPT Code: _____

ICD-10-CM Code: _____ (ICD-9-CM Code: _____)

6 Jan Sharp, an established patient, has an office appointment because she needs a new dressing on the laceration on her arm. The physician's nurse changes the dressing.

CPT Code: _____

7 Anna Rall is seen in the emergency department, complaining of pressure in her chest and the feeling that her heart is racing. After her vital signs are taken, an immediate electrocardiogram is performed, and her heart rate is found to be in excess of 160 beats per minute, with increased activity at the atrioventricular junction. After performing a comprehensive history and physical examination, the physician continues to evaluate the patient, who has been placed on continuous electrocardiographic monitoring. The emergency department physician documents the diagnosis of paroxysmal nodal tachycardia and calls a cardiologist for a consultation and possible admission of the patient to the hospital. Given the uncertainty of the diagnosis and the various other possible options, the physician's decision making is at a highly complex level. (Code only the emergency department physician's services.)

CPT Code: _____

ICD-10-CM Code: _____ (ICD-9-CM Code: _____)

8 A physician is called to the intensive care unit at the local hospital to care for Joe West, a patient in coronary crisis. The physician spends an hour at the patient's bedside, stabilizing him.

CPT Code: _____

9 The physician is preparing to leave the hospital after seeing Joe West but is called back to the intensive care unit to see and stabilize another patient, Ted Keel. The service to the patient takes 1½ hours.

CPT Codes: _____ , _____

Continued

10 An established patient, Harriet Turner, comes into the office for a follow-up visit. She had been prescribed medication for her recent onset of depression, but since her last visit, when the dosage was increased, she has felt that the medication is making her sleepy and lethargic. Considering the other factors such as other medical problems and drug interactions, the physician spends 25 minutes with the patient performing a detailed history and physical examination. After reviewing the details as well as recent laboratory work, the physician concludes that a different medication should be prescribed. The physician's decision making is moderately complex, given the possible medical complications that could arise.

CPT Code: _____

11 Dr. Welton calls Dr. Stouffer to perform a consultation on Carol Jones for advice on the management of her diabetes. Mrs. Jones is hospitalized for a hysterectomy, which had been an uncomplicated procedure, but is experiencing a slow recovery 4 days postop. Her abdominal wound does not appear to be healing well and her blood sugar has been fluctuating each day. Dr. Stouffer, who has never met Mrs. Jones before, performs a comprehensive, multisystem physical examination and completes a comprehensive history with a complete review of systems and extensive past medical history review. Dr. Stouffer recommends a new insulin regimen in addition to other medications to manage what might be a postoperative wound infection. Dr. Stouffer's medical decision making is of moderate complexity because he has to consider multiple diagnoses, a moderate amount of data, and the moderate risk of complications that Mrs. Jones could develop.

CPT Code: _____

(Answers are located in Appendix B)

CONGRATULATIONS! Now you're coding! Be sure to check your answers as you complete each activity. If you identify a code incorrectly, go back and read the CPT manual information again.

DOCUMENTATION GUIDELINES

Medicare recipients account for the majority of patients receiving services in the American health care system. Thus, any change by the third-party payer, Medicare, has dramatic effects on the health care system. One such change that currently is in development is the documentation necessary when submitting a claim for Evaluation and Management services provided to a Medicare patient. The Medicare program is the responsibility of the Centers for Medicare and Medicaid Services (CMS), formerly the Health Care Financing Administration (HCFA). Several years ago, CMS determined that there should be a nationally uniform requirement for documentation contained in the patient record when submitting charges for E/M services. The CMS developed a set of standards for documentation of E/M services. The standards are informational items that must be in the patient record to substantiate a given level of service. The standards are called the **Documentation Guidelines**. These guidelines apply only to E/M services and only to patients covered by Medicare and Medicaid. E/M services represent 50% of all services provided to these patients. The importance of the guidelines cannot be underestimated. Whatever guidelines the CMS institutes for patients have a dramatic effect on the systems in health care and will soon spread to other third-party payers, who will then begin to require the same or similar documentation.

History of the Development of Guidelines

The CMS published the first set of documentation guidelines in 1995, but did not require compliance for payment of claims. The 1995 Documentation Guidelines are posted on the Evolve website for this text (see Appendix A for free access information). The 1995 guidelines are easier to understand because they are not lengthy or complex. The documentation guidelines (DG) present information about what must be contained in the medical record for that information to "qualify" as documentation. For example, one DG states, "The CC, ROS and PFSH may be listed as separate elements of history, or they may be included in the description of the history of the present illness." This means that the

GENERAL MULTI-SYSTEM EXAMINATION

To qualify for a given level of multi-system examination, the following content and documentation requirements should be met:

- **Problem Focused Examination**—should include performance and documentation of one to five elements identified by a bullet (•) in one or more organ system(s) or body area(s).

- **Expanded Problem Focused Examination**—should include performance and documentation of at least six elements identified by a bullet (•) in one or more organ system(s) or body area(s).

- **Detailed Examination**—should include at least six organ systems or body areas. For each system/area selected, performance and documentation of at least two elements identified by a bullet (•) is expected. Alternatively, a detailed examination may include performance and documentation of at least twelve elements identified by a bullet (•) in two or more organ systems or body areas.

- **Comprehensive Examination**—should include at least nine organ systems or body areas. For each system/area selected, all elements of the examination identified by a bullet (•) should be performed, unless specific directions limit the content of the examination. For each area/system, documentation of at least two elements identified by a bullet is expected.

FIGURE 15-8   1997 Documentation Guidelines for general multisystem examination requirements.

location in the documentation of the chief complaint; review of systems; and past, family, or social history is not important, but what is important is that each of these items is documented in the record. Another example of the content of the 1995 guidelines is a DG for a general multisystem examination as: "The medical record for a general multisystem examination should include findings about 8 or more of the 12 organ systems." The documentation guidelines provide further clarification as to the documentation required to assign a level to the history, examination, and medical decision making as stated in the medical record.

A new set of guidelines was published in July 1997 for implementation January 1, 1998. The 1997 set of guidelines was intended to be the standard used when reviewing claims for payment and is also posted on the Evolve website for this text (see Appendix A for free access information). If the physician did not have the documentation required in the guidelines, payment would be adjusted based on what was actually in the medical record. The guidelines were so complex and required such extensive revision of medical record-keeping practices that the AMA (American Medical Association), on behalf of its physician members, requested an extension of the implementation date to allow time for education about the guidelines and for the CMS to meet with representatives of the AMA to reconsider the guidelines. Although the CMS rescinded the requirement for strict compliance with the guidelines, they continue random review of claims, based on whichever set of guidelines (1995 or 1997) the provider has elected to use.

The 1997 Documentation Guidelines specify the information that must be documented in the medical record for an E/M service to qualify for a given level of service. Fig. 15-8 illustrates the examination requirements for a general multisystem examination under the 1997 Documentation Guidelines. Note that for an examination to qualify as an expanded problem focused examination, the medical record must document that the physician performed at least six of the elements identified by a bullet (•) in Fig. 15-9. If the medical record documents that only five of the elements identified by a bullet were performed, the examination would have to be reported at the lower problem focused examination level.

A revised set of guidelines, published in 2000, took into consideration some of the suggestions put forth by the AMA. At the time of the publication of this text, the CMS and the

AMA were still in discussions regarding which set of documentation guidelines would become the standard for documenting E/M services.

CHECK THIS OUT 👉 The CMS has its own website: www.cms.gov/Outreach-and-Education/Medicare-Learning-Network-MLN/MLNEdWebGuide/EMDOC.html. You will find many articles regarding documentation guidelines for E/M services if you do a search of the CMS website.

Although the guidelines will continue to be revised, documentation guidelines will be a part of the standard for the medical record now and in the future for Medicare and Medicaid patients. You can anticipate that, as a coder, you will be required to learn about and follow these documentation guidelines.

General Multi-System Examination

System/Body Area	Elements of Examination
Constitutional	• Measurement of **any three of the following seven** vital signs: (1) sitting or standing blood pressure, (2) supine blood pressure, (3) pulse rate and regularity, (4) respiration, (5) temperature, (6) height, (7) weight (may be measured and recorded by ancillary staff) • General appearance of the patient (e.g., development, nutrition, body habitus, deformities, attention to grooming)
Eyes	• Inspection of conjunctivae and lids • Examination of pupils and irises (e.g., reaction to light and accommodation, size and symmetry) • Ophthalmoscopic examination of optic disks (e.g., size, C/D ratio, appearance) and posterior segments (e.g., vessel changes, exudates, hemorrhages)
Ears, Nose, Mouth, and Throat	• External inspection of ears and nose (e.g., overall appearance, scars, lesions, masses) • Otoscopic examination of external auditory canals and tympanic membranes • Assessment of hearing (e.g., whispered voice, finger rub, tuning fork) • Inspection of nasal mucosa, septum, and turbinates • Inspection of lips, teeth, and gums • Examination of oropharynx: oral mucosa, salivary glands, hard and soft palates, tongue, tonsils, and posterior pharynx
Neck	• Examination of neck (e.g., masses, overall appearance, symmetry, tracheal position, crepitus) • Examination of thyroid (e.g., enlargement, tenderness, mass)

FIGURE 15–9 1997 Documentation Guidelines of the general multisystem elements.

CHAPTER REVIEW

CHAPTER 15, PART I, THEORY

Without using the CPT manual, complete the following:

1 Is examination of the back an organ system or body area examination? _____

2 The four types of patient status are_____, _____, _____,

   and _____.

3 The first outpatient visit is called the _____ visit, and the second visit is called the

   _____ visit.

4 The first three factors a coder must consider when coding are patient _____, _____,

   and _____.

5 How many types of histories are there? _____

6 Which history is more complex: the problem focused history or the expanded problem focused history?

   _____

7 The four types of examinations, in order of difficulty (from least difficult to most difficult), are as follows:

   a _____

   b _____

   c _____

   d _____

8 The examination that is limited to the affected body area is the _____.

9 What does VLBW stand for? _____

10 What medical decision making involves a situation in which the diagnosis and management options are minimal,
    data amount and complexity that must be reviewed are minimal/none, and there is a minimal risk to the patient of

    complications or death? _____

11 What term is used to describe a patient who has been formally admitted to a hospital?

    _____

CHAPTER 15, PART II, PRACTICAL

Using the CPT manual and the ICD-10-CM and/or ICD-9-CM manuals, identify the codes for the following cases:

12 The physician provides initial intensive care service for the evaluation and management of a critically ill newborn (5 days old) inpatient for one day.

CPT Code: _____

13 A 55-year-old man is seen by the dermatologist for the first time and complains of two cystic lesions on his back. Considering that the patient is otherwise healthy and has a primary care physician caring for him, the dermatologist focuses the history of the present illness on the skin lesions (problem focused history) and focuses the problem focused physical examination on the patient's trunk. The physician concludes with straightforward decision making that the lesions are sebaceous cysts. The physician advises the patient that the lesions should be monitored for any changes but that no surgical intervention is warranted at this time.

CPT Code: _____

ICD-10-CM Code: _____

(ICD-9-CM Code: _____)

14 A 68-year-old woman visits her internist again complaining of angina that seems to have worsened over the past 3 days. The patient had had an acute anterior wall myocardial infarction (MI) 2 months earlier. One month after the acute MI, she began to have angina pectoris. The patient also states that she thinks the medications are causing her to have gastrointestinal problems while not relieving her symptoms. She had refused a cardiac catheterization after her MI to evaluate the extent of her coronary artery disease. The physician performs a detailed history and a detailed physical examination of her cardiovascular, respiratory, and gastrointestinal systems. The physician indicates that the decision-making process is moderately complex, given the number of conditions it is necessary to consider.

CPT Code: _____

15 A 22-year-old woman visits the gynecologist for the first time since relocating from another state last year. The patient wants a gynecologic examination and wants to discuss contraceptive options with the physician (think Preventive Medicine Services!). The physician collects pertinent past and social history related to the patient's reproductive system and performs a pertinent systems review extended to a limited number of additional systems. The physician completes the history with an extended history of her present physical state. A physical examination includes her cardiovascular and respiratory systems with an extended review of her genitourinary system. Given the patient's history of not tolerating certain types of oral contraceptives in the past, the physician's decision making involves a limited number of management options, all with low risk of morbidity to the patient.

CPT Code: _____

ICD-10-CM Codes: _____ (exam), _____ (counseling, for contraceptive maintenance)

(ICD-9-CM Codes: _____ (exam), _____ (counseling, for contraceptive maintenance))

16 An established patient is admitted on observation status for influenza symptoms and extreme nausea and vomiting. The patient is dehydrated and has been experiencing dizziness and mental confusion for the past 2 days. Prior to this episode the patient was well but became acutely ill overnight with these symptoms. Given the abrupt onset of these symptoms, the physician has to consider multiple possible causes and orders a variety of laboratory tests to be performed. The patient is at risk for a moderate number of complications. The MDM complexity is moderate. A comprehensive history is collected, and a comprehensive head-to-toe physical examination is performed.

CPT Code: _____

ICD-10-CM Codes: _____, _____, _____, _____

(ICD-9-CM Codes: _____, _____, _____, _____)

17 A physician visits another patient on observation status who has severe influenza. The decision is made to admit the patient, whose condition has worsened and who is not responding to the therapy initiated on the observation unit. The physician performs a detailed history and a detailed physical examination to reflect the patient's current status. The patient's problem is of low severity but requires ongoing active management, with possible surgical consultation. The MDM complexity is low.

CPT Code: _____

18 An 8-month-old infant, who is a new patient, is brought in by her mother for diaper rash. The physician focuses on the problem of the diaper rash for the problem focused history and examination. The MDM complexity is straightforward.

CPT Code: _____

ICD-10-CM Code: _____

(ICD-9-CM Code: _____)

19 A 33-year-old man is brought to his private physician's office by his wife. The man, who is an established patient, has been experiencing severe leg pain of 2 weeks' duration. In the past 2 days, the patient has experienced fainting spells, nausea, and vomiting. The patient has had multiple other vague complaints over the past month that he dismissed as unimportant, but his wife is not so sure, and she describes his general health as deteriorating. The physician performs a comprehensive multisystem physical examination after performing a complete review of systems and a complete past medical, family, and social history, with an extended history of the present illness (comprehensive history). The physician has to consider an extensive number of diagnoses, orders a variety of tests to be performed immediately, and indicates the MDM complexity to be high.

CPT Code: _____

ICD-10-CM Codes: _____ (leg pain), _____ (fainting), _____ (nausea with vomiting)

(ICD-9-CM Codes: _____, _____, _____)

20 A 42-year-old woman, who is an established patient, visits her family practitioner with the chief complaint of a self-discovered breast lump. She describes a feeling of fullness and tenderness over the mass that has become more pronounced in the past 2 weeks. Because the patient is otherwise healthy and has had a physical within the past 6 months, the physician focuses his attention on the breast lump during the taking of a problem focused history and the performance of a problem focused physical examination. The physician orders an immediate mammography to be performed and a follow-up appointment in 5 days. The physician has given the patient no other options and indicates that the MDM complexity is straightforward.

CPT Code: _____

ICD-10-CM Code: _____

(ICD-9-CM Code: _____)

21 Contusion of left knee and right elbow due to fall from roof. (Do not assign External Cause codes.)

ICD-10-CM Codes: _____, _____

(ICD-9-CM Codes: _____, _____)

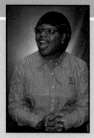

Why did you choose coding as a profession?

"I enjoy surgery and reading about the different approaches that it entails. Your profession should be something that you are passionate about."

Genieve R. Nottage, MBA, BSHA, CPC-I, CPC

Educator/Consultant
Chronicles Billing Inc.
Locust Grove, Georgia

Anesthesia

Chapter Topics

Types of Anesthesia

Anesthesia Section Format

Formula for Anesthesia Payment

Concurrent Modifiers

Unlisted Anesthesia Code

Other Reporting

Chapter Review

Learning Objectives

After completing this chapter you should be able to

1 Define types of anesthesia.

2 Explain the format of the Anesthesia section and subsections.

3 Understand the anesthesia formula.

4 Identify other reporting issues.

5 Demonstrate ability to report anesthesia services.

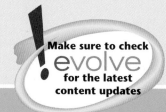

Make sure to check
evolve
for the latest
content updates

TYPES OF ANESTHESIA

The Anesthesia section is a specialized section that is used by an anesthesiologist, anesthetist, or other physician to report the provision of anesthesia services, usually during surgery. **Anesthesia** means induction or administration of a drug to obtain partial or complete loss of sensation. **Analgesia** (absence of pain) is achieved so that a patient may have surgery or a procedure performed without pain. Types of anesthesia may be general, regional, local, or monitored anesthesia care (MAC). Moderate (conscious) sedation is not reported with anesthesia codes but rather is reported with Medicine codes. Local anesthesia is usually administered by the surgeon.

The practice of anesthesiology is not limited to administration of anesthesia for the surgical patient. The American Society of Anesthesiologists (ASA) defines the practice of anesthesiology as dealing with but not limited to the following:

- The management of procedures for rendering a patient insensible to pain and emotional stress during surgical, obstetrical, and other diagnostic and therapeutic procedures.
- The evaluation and management of essential physiologic functions under the stress of anesthetic and surgical manipulations.
- The clinical management of the patient unconscious from whatever cause.
- The evaluation and management of acute or chronic pain.
- The management of problems in cardiac and respiratory resuscitation.
- The application of specific methods of respiratory therapy.
- The clinical management of various fluid, electrolyte, and metabolic disturbances.*

Take a moment and consult a good medical dictionary under the entry "anesthesia." You will find that in addition to the definition of the term anesthesia, a wide variety of types of anesthesia are defined. Some types of anesthesia are named for the site of the anesthesia administration, such as sacral, lumbar, and caudal. Other types of anesthesia are named for the category of anesthesia, such as freezing (frost) for cryoanesthesia. Some of the more commonly used anesthesia terms are endotracheal, epidural, regional, and patient-controlled analgesia.

- **Endotracheal** anesthesia is accomplished by insertion of a tube into the nose or mouth, and passing the tube into the trachea for ventilation, as illustrated in Fig. 16-1.
- **Epidural** anesthesia is the injection of an anesthetic agent into the epidural spaces between the vertebrae, also known as peridural, or epidural block.
- **Spinal** or intraspinal anesthesia refers to anesthesia produced by an injection of local anesthetic into the subarachnoid space around the spinal cord.
- **General** anesthesia is a state of unconsciousness that is accomplished by the use of a drug or combination of drugs administered intramuscularly, rectally, intravenously, or by inhalation.
- **Regional** anesthesia interrupts the sensory nerve conductivity in a region of the body and is produced by a field block (forming a wall of anesthesia around the site by means of local injections) or nerve block (injection of the area close to the site). Nerve block is also known as block, block anesthesia, or conduction anesthesia. Although not a type of anesthesia, a procedure used by anesthesiologists for treatment of a postdural puncture headache is a blood patch, also known as an epidural blood patch (EBP). A **blood patch** procedure is when a cerebrospinal fluid leak is closed by means of an injection of the patient's blood into the epidural space at or near the area of the dural puncture that was accessed during spinal anesthesia.
- **Local** anesthesia can be accomplished by means of application of an anesthetic agent (such as lidocaine) placed directly on the area involved (**topical** anesthesia) or local infiltration through subcutaneous injection of an anesthetic agent. Lidocaine can be subcutaneously injected, as illustrated in Fig. 16-2.

---

*Definitions excerpted from the *2014 Relative Value Guide*, © 2013 of the American Society of Anesthesiologists. All Rights Reserved. *Relative Value Guide is a registered trademark of the American Society of Anesthesiologists.* A copy of the full text can be obtained from ASA, 520 N. Northwest Highway, Park Ridge, IL, 60068-2573.

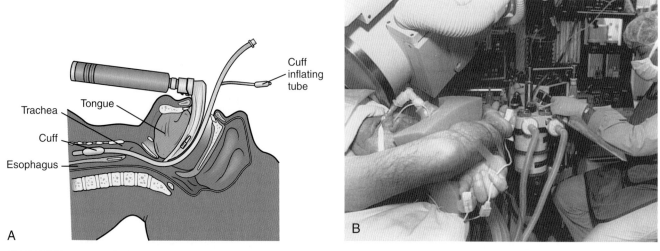

A

B

FIGURE 16–1 **A,** Placement of endotracheal tube for administration of anesthesia. **B,** General endotracheal anesthesia is a support system of major importance.

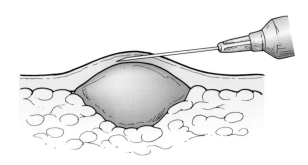

FIGURE 16–2 Administration of local anesthesia.

■ **Patient-controlled analgesia** (PCA) is a system that allows the patient to administer an analgesic drug such as morphine to control pain.

A device is attached to a pump holding the drug and the patient can depress a handheld button to administer a dose of the drug (Fig. 16-3). In this way, the patient can control the amount of the drug and the frequency of administration. PCA is considered a hospital service and not generally reported by a physician. Refer to individual payer guidelines for instructions to report PCA management.

QUICK CHECK 16-1

1. In the index of the CPT, you would reference this main term and these two subterms to locate a

   blood patch code. _____

(Answers located in Appendix C)

Each type of anesthesia will be covered in depth, but generally speaking, the types of anesthesia are:

■ **Monitored Anesthesia Care** (MAC)

MAC is provided by an anesthesiologist or CRNA. The patient is monitored, and if necessary, sedation is provided; even general anesthesia.

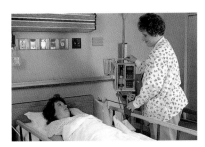

FIGURE 16-3 Patient-controlled sedation machine.

■ **General anesthesia**
Used for cases that requires deep sedation, such as open heart surgery or complicated abdominal surgery. The patient is usually intubated. The patient is in a deep state of sedation and is not arousable or able to communicate or follow commands. Several different types of medication may be used during general anesthesia, including drugs for analgesia (pain relief), sedation, amnesiacs (to lessen awareness), and paralytics for muscle relaxation to prevent movement or reflexive action by the patient during procedures.

■ **Regional anesthesia**
Regional anesthesia uses injection to target the nerves of the area being treated.

■ **Spinal and epidural anesthesia**
Spinal anesthesia is administered into the cerebral spinal fluid or epidural area of the spine that corresponds with the area being treated. Spinals are generally used for procedures below the waist. Epidural catheters are often placed to facilitate administration of medication into the spinal region.

Moderate (Conscious) Sedation

Moderate or conscious sedation is a type of sedation that can be provided by a surgeon or the surgeon's staff while the surgeon is performing a procedure; it provides a decreased level of consciousness that does not put the patient completely to sleep. This level of consciousness allows the patient to breathe without assistance and to respond to stimulation and verbal commands. A trained observer must be present when moderate sedation services are provided by the same physician performing the therapeutic or diagnostic service in order to assist the physician in monitoring the patient. The codes to report conscious sedation are located in the Medicine section (99143-99150), not in the Anesthesia section. Codes 99143-99145 report the moderate sedation services when the service is provided by the same physician performing the diagnostic or therapeutic service and requires the presence of an independent trained observer. The codes are divided based on the patient's age of under or over 5 years of age and the duration of the service. Codes 99148-99150 report moderate sedation services when the anesthesia service is provided by a physician other than the health care professional performing the service. These codes are divided based on the patient's age of under or over 5 years of age and the duration of the service. Bundled into these codes is the assessment of the patient, establishment of intravenous access, administration of the sedation agent, sedation maintenance, monitoring of patient vital signs, and recovery from anesthesia.

The code descriptions for the Moderate (Conscious) Sedation codes include the term "intraservice time." **Intraservice** time begins with the administration of the sedation agent, requires continuous face-to-face attendance by the physician, and ends when the personal contact by the physician ends. The time the physician spends with the patient in assessment of the patient prior to administration of the sedation and the time in recovery is not included in the intraservice time.

CODING SHOT

Moderate (conscious) sedation codes are only reported when the physician performing the procedure administers the sedation and an independent trained observer assists.

CAUTION *Do not confuse conscious sedation with monitored anesthesia care. Conscious sedation is administered by the surgeon or another physician; MAC is provided by an anesthesiologist or CRNA.*

Moderate or conscious sedation methods are much less invasive than anesthesia services that provide the complete loss of consciousness. For example, for a colonoscopy, a physician could administer an intravenous sedation, such as meperidine (Demerol), morphine, or diazepam (Valium). The patient would be monitored closely as the medication is administered so that the appropriate level of sedation is reached. After the procedure, the physician may administer a drug intravenously to reverse the effects of the sedation. The patient would have this procedure in an outpatient setting and be able to go home after the procedure. Moderate sedation is included in many CPT codes and, as such, is not reported separately. The bullseye (⊙) is displayed to the left of the codes in the CPT manual that include the moderate/conscious sedation bundled into the code. For example, the codes in the 33206-33208 range report insertion of a new or replacement of a permanent pacemaker and include moderate sedation. Appendix G in the CPT manual lists the codes that include moderate sedation.

ANESTHESIA SECTION FORMAT

Most anesthesia codes are divided first by anatomic site and then by specific type of procedure, as shown in Fig. 16-4.

The last four subsections in Anesthesia—Radiologic Procedures (01916-01936), Burn Excisions or Debridement (01951-01953), Obstetric (01958-01969), and Other Procedures (01990-01999)—are not organized by anatomic division. The CPT codes in the Radiologic Procedures subsection report anesthesia service when radiologic services are provided to the patient for diagnostic or therapeutic reasons.

Example

Therapeutic reason: 01925 Anesthesia for therapeutic interventional radiological procedures involving the arterial system; carotid and coronary

Diagnostic reason: 01922 Anesthesia for non-invasive imaging or radiation therapy

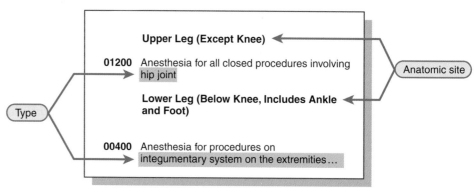

FIGURE 16-4 Anatomic divisions in Anesthesia section.

Anesthesia providers may be a(n):

- Anesthesiologist
- Certified registered nurse anesthetist (CRNA)
- Anesthesiologist's assistant (who may not work without oversight of anesthesiologist)
- Resident (cannot bill if the case is performed without the participation of another anesthesia provider)
- Student registered nurse anesthetist (billing is based on specific rules for each payer depending on the payer's definition of medical direction)

EXERCISE 16-1 *Anesthesia Format*

Complete the following exercise:

1 Which subsections are *not* divided by anatomic site? _____

_____

2 What is analgesia? _____

3 What is anesthesia? _____

4 Name three types of anesthesia: _____, _____, and _____.

5 What is the type of sedation that enables the patient to maintain breathing for himself/herself?

_____

6 In what section of the CPT are the sedation codes identified in Question 5 located?

_____

(Answers are located in Appendix B)

FORMULA FOR ANESTHESIA PAYMENT

When an anesthesiologist provides an anesthesia service to a patient, the preoperative, intraoperative/intraservice (care during surgery), and postoperative care are all included in the CPT code. These services include the usual preoperative and postoperative visits (on day of surgery) to the patient by the anesthesiologist; the routine intraoperative care, such as administration of fluids and/or blood; and the usual monitoring services. The care also includes the patient's history taken by the anesthesiologist, ventilation establishment, and administration of preoperative and postoperative medications. Monitoring services include blood pressure, temperature, arterial oxygen levels (oximetry), exhalation of carbon dioxide (capnography), and spectrometry (blood analysis). The intraoperative care includes intubation to administer anesthesia. Postoperative care usually includes pain management. Some pain management is reported separately, e.g., spinal injection for significant postoperative pain. If the anesthesiologist provides care that is unusual or beyond that which would usually be provided, these services can be reported in addition to the basic anesthesia service. For example, if the patient requires intraoperative cardiac monitoring, the anesthesiologist may insert a Swan-Ganz catheter, as illustrated in Fig. 16-5.

A Swan-Ganz catheter is not a normal service provided during a surgery, so it could be reported using a code from the Medicine section for placement of a flow-directed catheter (93503). Some payers will require modifier -59 (distinct procedural service) be appended to the catheter code if another central line is also placed. The time necessary to insert the catheter is not counted in the anesthesia time because the service of the insertion is reported separately and is considered a surgical procedure. Reporting the insertion separately and also adding the insertion time to the anesthesia service would result in double payment for the insertion service.

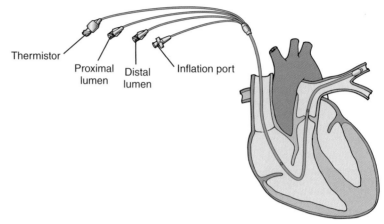

Thermistor

Proximal lumen

Distal lumen

Inflation port

FIGURE 16–5 Swan-Ganz catheter.

QUICK CHECK 16-2

1. Where is the information regarding inclusive anesthesia service located within the CPT manual?

_____

(Answers are located in Appendix C)

What makes anesthesia coding different from any other coding is the way in which anesthesia services are billed. There is a standard formula for payment of anesthesia services that is, for the most part, nationally accepted. The formula is base units + time units + modifying units (B + T + M) × conversion factor. Let's look at each of these elements in more detail.

Another tool is the ASA CROSSWALK book from the American Society of Anesthesiologists and it provides anesthesia coders with a comprehensive list of CPT codes that link to the corresponding anesthesia code(s). This book also lists the base value of each anesthesia service. CPT codes are located in the crosswalk book enabling the anesthesia coder to select the service with the highest base value for submission. The book also lists alternative codes, allowing the anesthesia coder to make the most specific selection. The anesthesia crosswalk book is updated by the ASA annually.

B Is for Base Unit

The ASA publishes a *Relative Value Guide*®(RVG), which contains codes for anesthesia services and the base unit value for each anesthesia code. The CPT manual also contains these anesthesia service codes in the Anesthesia section. Italicized comments appear in the American Society of Anesthesiologists' *Relative Value Guide*® to clarify code assignment, as illustrated in Fig. 16-6. These italicized comments are not part of the CPT manual.

CODING SHOT

Anesthesia is paid based on:
- Base units +
- Time units +
- Modifying units (if allowed) × conversion factor

INTRATHORACIC

CPT Code	CPT Descriptor	Base Unit Value
00500	Anesthesia for all procedures on esophagus......................................	15 + TM
	(*RVG Comment: Code 00500 describes anesthesia for open procedures on the esophagus.*)	
00520	Anesthesia for closed chest procedures; (including bronchoscopy) not otherwise specified..	6 + TM
	(*RVG Comment: For transvenous pacemaker insertion, report code 00530.*)	

FIGURE 16-6 The *Relative Value Guide*® contains italicized comments that do not appear in the code description in the CPT. (Excerpted from *2014 Relative Value Guide*®, © 2013 of the American Society of Anesthesiologists. All Rights Reserved. *Relative Value Guide is a registered trademark of the American Society of Anesthesiologists*. A copy of the full text can be obtained from ASA, 1061 American Lane, Schaumburg, Illinois, 60173-4973.)

CMS's Base Units. The RVG is not a fee schedule (a list of charges for services) but instead compares anesthesia services with each other. For example, anesthesia services provided for a biopsy of a sinus are less complicated than services provided for a radical sinus surgery. A team of physicians with expertise in anesthesiology developed the comparisons and assigned numerical values to each service, termed the **base unit value** (Fig. 16-7). Annually, CMS also publishes a list of the base unit values for the codes, as illustrated in Fig. 16-8.

The CMS's base unit value is accepted as the standard in the United States for most third-party payers.

Base unit value

LOWER LEG (BELOW KNEE, INCLUDES ANKLE AND FOOT)

CPT Code	CPT Descriptor	Base Unit Value
01462	Anesthesia for all closed procedures on lower leg, ankle, and foot...........	3 + TM
01464	Anesthesia for arthroscopic procedures of ankle and/or foot	3 + TM
01470	Anesthesia for procedures on nerves, muscles, tendons, and fascia of lower leg, ankle, and foot; not otherwise specified	3 + TM
01472	repair of ruptured Achilles tendon, with or without graft........................	5 + TM
01474	gastrocnemius recession (eg, Strayer procedure)	5 + TM

FIGURE 16-7 The ASA's *Relative Value Guide*® lists the Base Unit value for the codes. (Excerpted from *2014 Relative Value Guide*®, © 2013 of the American Society of Anesthesiologists. All Rights Reserved. *Relative Value Guide is a registered trademark of the American Society of Anesthesiologists*. A copy of the full text can be obtained from ASA, 1061 American Lane, Schaumburg, Illinois, 60173-4973.)

Code	Base Unit Value
00100	5
00102	6
00103	5
00104	4
00120	5
00124	4
00126	4
00140	5
00142	4
00144	6
00145	6
00147	4
00148	4
00160	5
00162	7
00164	4
00170	5
00172	6
00174	6
00176	7
00190	5
00192	7
00210	11

FIGURE 16–8 CMS's annual list of base units.

One coding circumstance unique to anesthesia coding occurs when multiple surgical procedures are performed during the same session. In this case, only the procedure with the highest base unit value is assigned. For example, if during the same surgical procedure session a clavicle biopsy (base unit value of 3) and a radical mastectomy (base unit value of 5) are performed, the base unit value for both procedures becomes 5. The anesthesia service is then reported with only the code for the higher base unit value.

CMS RULES

For Medicare, anesthesia service involving multiple procedures is reported with the CPT anesthesia code for the procedure with the highest base unit value. The actual total time for all procedures is reported. Only one anesthesia code can be reported. There is an exception for the add-on codes for burn excision or debridement (01953) and obstetrics (01968, 01969).

The pricing for add-on anesthesia codes is different than other payers because only the base unit value of the add-on code is allowed and all anesthesia time is reported with the primary anesthesia code. There is an exception to this rule when reporting obstetrical anesthesia, as both the base unit value and time units for the primary and add-on, obstetrical codes are reported.

T Is for Time

Anesthesia services are provided based on the time during which the anesthesia was administered and calculated, in total minutes. The timing is started when the anesthesiologist begins preparing the patient to receive anesthesia and is in constant attendance with the patient, continues through the procedure, and ends when the patient is turned over to the post-anesthesia caregivers. The minutes during which anesthesia was administered are recorded in the patient record. Carriers independently determine the amount of time that is considered a unit. Often, 15 minutes equal a unit, but for some carriers, 1, 10, or 30 minutes equals a unit.

CMS RULES

For Medicare, time units are computed by dividing the reported actual anesthesia service time by 15 minutes and then rounding to one decimal place. No time units are reported for anesthesia CPT codes 01953 and 01996. Medicare reimburses for anesthesia services based on a combination of time and base units multiplied by a geographic-area-specific conversion factor.

The start time on the anesthesia record should match the time reported on the claim form. The recorded time on all records must be the same:

- Anesthesia record
- CRNA, anesthesiologist, or resident billing slip
- Time on all documents submitted to insurance company

When completing the Medicare claim, always record the actual time—that is, the time the anesthesia provider spent personally attending the patient. Many private payers also require actual time, so it is necessary to verify time submission requirements with each payer.

Private payers may or may not reimburse CRNA services, or they may require these services be reported under the supervising anesthesiologist's name and NPI (National Provider Identification) number. You must verify the method for submission for each payer.

When preparing the claim, always record the actual time that indicates the ending time of personal attendance. The time is illustrated in Fig. 16-9, *A*. The stop time is when the patient can be safely turned over to a non-anesthesia provider. This generally does not occur in the operating room.

The start time on the anesthesia record should match the time reported on the claim form and indicate the beginning time of the service. Note that Fig. 16-9, *B* illustrates the medical document that contains the pre-anesthesia evaluation that the provider completes prior to the start of surgery.

From the Trenches

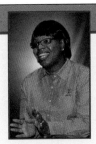

"Continue to educate yourself. Don't second guess your initial thoughts, only code what is documented."

GENIEVE

M Is for Modifying Unit

As the name implies, modifying units reflect circumstances or conditions that change or modify the environment in which the anesthesia service is provided. There are two base-modifying factors: qualifying circumstances codes and physical status modifiers.

Qualifying Circumstances. At times, anesthesia is provided in situations that make the administration of the anesthesia more difficult. These types of cases include those that are performed in emergency situations and those dealing with patients of extreme age. They also include services performed during the use of controlled hypotension or the use of total body hypothermia (refer to Fig. 16-10). The Qualifying Circumstances codes begin with 99 and

AUTHORIZED FOR LOCAL REPRODUCTION

MEDICAL RECORD–ANESTHESIA

PROCEDURE

ITEM	START	STOP
Anesthesia		
Procedure		

DATE   OR NO.   PAGE OF   SURGEON(S)

PRE-PROCEDURE
☐ Identified ☐ ID Band ☐ Questioning
☐ Chart Review ☐ Permit Signed
☐ NPO Since
Pre-anesthetic State: ☐ Calm
☐ Awake ☐ Asleep
☐ Apprehensive ☐ Confused
☐ Uncooperative ☐ Unresponsive

PATIENT SAFETY
☐ Anes. Machine # _____ Checked
☐ Safety Belt On ☐ Axillary Roll
☐ Arm Restraints ☐ Arms Tucked
☐ Pressure points checked and padded
☐ Eye Care: ☐ Ointment ☐ Saline
☐ Taped ☐ Pads ☐ Goggles

MONITORS AND EQUIPMENT
☐ Steth ☐ Esoph ☐ Precord ☐ Other
☐ Non-Invasive B/P ☐ Nerve Stimulator
☐ Continuous EKG ☐ V Lead EKG
☐ Pulse Oximeter ☐ Oxygen Analyzer
☐ End Tidal CO₂ ☐ Resp Gas Anlyzr
☐ Temp _____ ☐ EEG
☐ Warming Blanket ☐ Fluid Warmer
☐ Airway Humidifier ☐ _____
☐ NG/OG Tube ☐ Foley Catheter
☐ Art Line _____
☐ CVP _____
☐ PA Line _____
☐ IV(s) _____
☐ _____

ANESTHETIC TECHNIQUES
Method: ☐ General ☐ Spinal
☐ Epidural ☐ Caudal ☐ Brachial
☐ Bier Block ☐ Ankle Blk ☐ M.A.C.
General: ☐ Pre-O₂ ☐ L.T.A.
☐ Rapid Sequence ☐ Cricoid Pressure
☐ Intravenous ☐ Inhalation
☐ Intramuscular ☐ Rectal
Regional: ☐ Position _____
☐ Prep _____ ☐ Local _____
☐ Needle _____
☐ Drug(s) _____
☐ Dose _____ ☐ Attempts x _____
☐ Site _____ ☐ Level _____
☐ Catheter _____ ☐ See Remarks

AIRWAY MANAGEMENT
☐ Intubation ☐ Oral ☐ Nasal
☐ Direct Vision ☐ Magill's ☐ Blind
☐ Diff. see Rmks ☐ Fiber Op ☐ Stylet
☐ Attempts x ___ ☐ Blade _____
☐ Tube size ___ ☐ Endobronchial
☐ Regular ☐ RAE ☐ Armored ☐ Laser
☐ Cuffed ☐ Min. occ. pres. ☐ Air ☐NS
☐ Uncuffed, leaks at ___ cm H₂O
☐ Secured at _____ ☐ ET CO₂ Present
☐ Breath Sounds _____
☐ Circuit: ☐ Circle ☐ Non-rebreathing
☐ Airway: ☐ Oral ☐ Nasal ☐ Natural
☐ Mask Case ☐ Via Tracheostomy
☐ Nasal Cannula ☐ Simple O₂ Mask

RECOVERY ROOM
Time	B/P	O₂ Sat.
☐ PACU	P	R T
☐ ICU ☐ L&D		

☐ Awake ☐ Spont Resp ☐ Oral Airway
☐ Asleep ☐ Ventilator ☐ Nasal Airway
☐ Stable ☐ Extubated ☐ Face Shield O₂
☐ Unstable ☐ Intubated ☐ T-Piece O₂

CONTROLLED DRUGS
Drug	Used	Destroyed	Returned

Provider   Witness

TIME:

AGENTS ☐ Hal ☐ Enf ☐ Iso (%)															TOTALS	
☐ N₂O ☐ Air (L/min)																
Oxygen (L/min)																
( )																
( )																
( )																
( )																
( )																

FLUIDS

| Urine (ml) | | | | |
| EBL (ml) | | | | |

MONITORS
EKG
% O₂ Inspired (FIO₂)
O₂ Saturation (SaO₂)
End Tidal CO₂
Temp: ☐ °C ☐ °F

VITAL SIGNS

Baseline Values

B/P   P   R

200
180
160
140
120
100
80
60
40
20

SYMBOLS

✕ ANESTHESIA

⊙ OPERATION

∨∧ B/PCUFF PRESSURE

⊥⊤ ARTERIAL LINE PRESSURE

Δ MEAN ARTERIAL PRESSURE

● PULSE

O SPONTANEOUS RESP

∅ ASSISTED RESP

⊗ CONTROLLED RESP

T TOURNIQUET

VENT
Tidal Vol. (ml)
Resp. Rate
Peak Pres. (cm H₂O)
PEEP (cm H₂O)

Symbols for Remarks
Position

ANESTHESIA PROVIDER(S)

REMARKS

PATIENT'S IDENTIFICATION (For typed or written entries give: Name–last, first, middle: ID No. (SSN or other); hospital or medical facility.)

ANESTHESIA
Medical Record
OPTIONAL FORM 517 (7–95)
Prescribed by GSA/ICMR
FPMR (41 CFR) 101–11.203(b)(10)

A

FIGURE 16–9A Anesthesia medical record.

PRE-ANESTHESIA EVALUATION

AGE	SEX	HEIGHT	WEIGHT	PRE-PROCEDURE VITAL SIGNS			
	☐ M ☐ F	in./cm.	lb./kg.	B/P	P	R	T

PROPOSED PROCEDURE

PREVIOUS ANESTHESIA/OPERATIONS *(If none, check here ☐)*　　　　　CURRENT MEDICATIONS *(If none, check here ☐)*

FAMILY HISTORY OF ANESTHESIA COMPLICATIONS *(If none, check here ☐)*　　ALLERGIES *(If NKDA, check here ☐)*

AIRWAY/TEETH/HEAD AND NECK

HISTORY FROM
☐ PARENT/GUARDIAN　☐ POOR HISTORIAN　☐ CHART
☐ SIGNIFICANT OTHER　☐ PATIENT

SYSTEM	WNL	COMMENTS	PERTINENT STUDY RESULTS
RESPIRATORY Asthma　Pneumonia Bronchitis　Productive cough COPD　Recent cold Dyspnea　SOB Orthopnea　Tuberculosis	☐	Tobacco Use: ☐ No ☐ Yes ____ Pack/Day for ____ Years	Chest X-ray　　Pulmonary Studies
CARDIOVASCULAR Angina　MI Arrhythmia　Murmur CHF　MVP Exercise Tolerance　Pacemaker Hypertension　Rheumatic fever	☐		EKG
HEPATO/GASTROINTESTINAL Bowel obstruction　Jaundice Cirrhosis　N&V Hepatitis　Reflux/heartburn Histal hernia　Ulcers	☐	Ethanol Use: ☐ No ☐ Yes Frequency_____	
NEURO/MUSCULOSKELETAL Arthritis　Paresthesia Back problems　Syncope CVA/stroke　Seizures DJD　TIAs Headaches　Weakness Loss of consciousness Neuromuscular disease Paralysis	☐		
RENAL/ENDOCRINE Diabetes Renal failure/Dialysis Thyroid disease Urinary retention Urinary tract infection Weight loss/gain	☐		
OTHER Anemia Bleeding tendencies Hemophilia Pregnancy Sickle cell trait Transfusion history			

PROBLEM LIST/DIAGNOSES	ASA PS	LAB STUDIES	Hgb/HcT/CBC	Electrolytes	Urinalysis
	1				
	2				
PLANNED ANESTHESIA/SPECIAL MONITORS	3	Other			
	4				
	5				
	E	**POST-ANESTHESIA NOTE**			

PRE-ANESTHESIA MEDICATIONS ORDERED

SIGNATURE OF EVALUATOR(S)

Signed　　　　　　　　　　　　　Date　　　Time

OPTIONAL FORM 517 BACK

B

FIGURE 16-9B Anesthesia medical record, pre-anesthesia evaluation and post-anesthesia notes.

V. Qualifying Circumstances: (More than one may be reported)

CPT Code	CPT Descriptor	Base Unit Value
+99100	Anesthesia for patient of extreme age, younger than 1 year and older than 70... (List separately in addition to code for primary anesthesia procedure)	1
+99116	Anesthesia complicated by utilization of total body hypothermia.. (List separately in addition to code for primary anesthesia procedure)	5
+99135	Anesthesia complicated by utilization of controlled hypotension.. (List separately in addition to code for primary anesthesia procedure)	5
+99140	Anesthesia complicated by emergency conditions (specify).. (List separately in addition to code for primary anesthesia procedure)	2
	(An emergency is defined as existing when delay in treatment of the patient would lead to a significant increase in the threat to life or body part.)	

FIGURE 16–10 Qualifying Circumstances with relative value. (Excerpted from *2014 Relative Value Guide®*, © 2013 of the American Society of Anesthesiologists. All Rights Reserved. *Relative Value Guide is a registered trademark of the American Society of Anesthesiologists.* A copy of the full text can be obtained from ASA, 1061 American Lane, Schaumburg, Illinois, 60173-4973.)

are considered **adjunct codes,** which means that the codes can never be reported alone but must be used in addition to another code to provide additional information. A Qualifying Circumstances code is reported in addition to the anesthesia procedure code. Qualifying Circumstances codes are located in two places in the CPT manual: the Medicine section and the Anesthesia section Guidelines. In both locations the plus symbol is located next to the codes (99100-99140), indicating their status as add-on codes.

STOP   *You were just presented with some very important information about the use of certain codes in the CPT manual. The plus (+) symbol next to any CPT code—not just next to Qualifying Circumstances codes—indicates that that code cannot be used alone. Throughout the remaining sections of the CPT manual, the plus symbol will appear to caution you to use the code only as an adjunct code (with other codes).*

When used, the Qualifying Circumstances code is reported in addition to the primary anesthesia procedure code. For example, if anesthesia was provided for an 80-year-old patient during a corrective lens procedure, the reporting would be:

00142	Anesthesia for procedures on eye; lens surgery
99100	Anesthesia for 80-year-old patient

The RVG lists the Qualifying Circumstances codes along with the relative value for each code (see Fig. 16-10).

The CPT index lists the Qualifying Circumstances codes under Anesthesia, Special Circumstances.

Physical Status Modifiers. The second type of modifying unit used in the Anesthesia section is the physical status modifier (refer to Fig. 16-11). These modifiers indicate

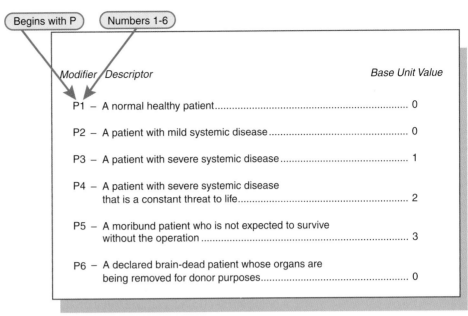

FIGURE 16–11 Physical status modifiers. (Excerpted from *2014 Relative Value Guide*®, © 2013 of the American Society of Anesthesiologists. All Rights Reserved. *Relative Value Guide is a registered trademark of the American Society of Anesthesiologists.* A copy of the full text can be obtained from ASA, 1061 American Lane, Schaumburg, Illinois, 60173-4973.)

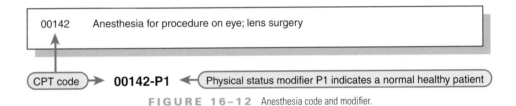

FIGURE 16–12 Anesthesia code and modifier.

the patient's condition at the time anesthesia was administered and identify the level of complexity of the services provided to the patient. For instance, anesthesia service to a gravely ill patient is much more complex than the same type of service to a normal, healthy patient. The physical status modifier is not assigned by the coder but is determined by the anesthesiologist and documented in the anesthesia record. The physical status modifier begins with the letter "P" and contains a number from 1 to 6 (see Fig. 16-11).

Note that the relative value for P1, P2, and P6 is zero because these conditions are considered not to affect the service provided. A physical status modifier is used after the five-digit CPT code and is illustrated in Fig. 16-12.

Summing It Up!

Most health care facilities have software that automatically performs the conversion calculations based on the various conversion factors and unit designations. However, you still need to understand the process used to convert the anesthesia formula into the anesthesia payment. Let's put the elements of the equation to practical use by applying the equation (B + T + M) to a case.

An 84-year-old female (qualifying circumstance for extreme age, value 1) with severe hypertension (value of 1) has a 4-cm malignant lesion removed from her right knee (base value of 3). The total time of anesthesia service was 60 minutes, and the carrier indicates a unit is 15 minutes (4 units). The anesthesiologist recorded that the patient's physical status at the time of the procedure was P3 for a severe systemic disease (relative value of 1), for the severe hypertension.

3	base procedure value
4	time units
2	modifiers: physical status = 1; extreme age = 1
9	total units

The coding that identifies all elements of this case would be:

00400-P3	Anesthesia for procedure of integumentary system of knee for a patient with severe systemic disease (severe hypertension)
99100	Anesthesia for an 84-year-old patient
9	Units at the third-party payer established rate per unit

Conversion Factor. A conversion factor is the dollar value of each unit. Each third-party payer issues a list of conversion factors. The lists vary with geographic location because the cost of practicing medicine varies from one region to another. Fig. 16-13 shows an example of a third-party payer's (CMS) anesthesia conversion factors. Note that North Dakota is $21.80 per unit and Manhattan, NY, is $25.21 per unit, as it is less expensive to provide anesthesia services in Grand Forks, ND, than it is to provide the same services in Manhattan, NY.

The conversion factor for the locale is multiplied by the number of units for the procedure. For example, the previous case had 9 units. If the anesthesiologist was located in Manhattan, NY, and the conversion factor is $25.21, the total for the procedure would be 226.89 (9 × $25.21). If the same services were provided in North Dakota, with the conversion factor of $21.80, the total for the procedure would be $196.20 (9 × $21.80).

CHECK THIS OUT ☞ The CMS website posts the anesthesia base unit values and conversion factors at www.cms.gov/center/anesth.asp

Multiple Procedures

- When multiple surgical procedures are performed during a single anesthetic administration, the anesthesia code that represents the highest base value unit procedure is reported. The time reported is the combined total for all procedures.
- Assign the code for procedure of highest base value unit.
- Indicate cumulative start/stop time for all surgical procedures performed.

Anesthesia time for a medically necessary surgical procedure performed during the same intra-operative session as a cosmetic procedure should be split and reported separately.

CODING SHOT

According to Medicare rules, modifier -50 would not be used on anesthesia CPT codes. It would be used on anesthesia surgical procedures, performed by anesthesiologists, such as femoral continuous blocks for pain management for bilateral knee replacement (64448-59-50), in addition to the ASA code or anesthesia CPT code.

Locality Name	Anesthesia Conversion Factor
Manhattan, NY	25.21
NYC suburbs/Long I., NY	25.80
Queens, NY	25.92
Rest of New York	21.84
North Carolina	21.93
North Dakota	21.80

FIGURE 16–13 2014 CMS Anesthesia Conversion Factors.

EXERCISE 16-2   *Modifiers and Time in Anesthesia*

Complete the following:

1 If the anesthesia service was provided to a patient who had mild systemic disease, what would the physical status modifier

likely be? _____

2 If the same service was provided to a patient who had severe systemic disease, what would the physical status modifier likely

be? _____

3 Anesthesia complicated by utilization of total body hypothermia

Code: _____

4 When filling out the claim, always record the _____ time, which indicates the ending time of the time spent personally attending to the patient for anesthesia services.

5 _____ time is that time when the anesthesia care of the patient can be safely turned over to a non-anesthesia provider. This generally never happens in the operating room.

6 The _____ time on the anesthesia record should match the time reported on the claim form and indicates the beginning time of the anesthesia service.

(Answers are located in Appendix B)

CONCURRENT MODIFIERS

Some third-party payers require additional modifiers to indicate how many cases an anesthesiologist was performing or directing at one time. Certified registered nurse anesthetists (CRNAs) may administer anesthesia to patients under the direction of a licensed physician, or they may work independently. An anesthesiologist may medically direct up to four cases at the same time (concurrently). If a physician directs more than four cases, it is referred to as medical supervision. Medical direction means the directing anesthesiologist is present at the induction and emergence from anesthesia, for all key portions of the procedure, and is immediately available in case of an emergency. The CRNA would be with the patient the entire time.

CMS RULES

When medical direction occurs, certain documentation must be submitted for services for Medicare patients. The documentation must support that certain services were personally performed by the physician. These include:
1. Pre-anesthesia examination and evaluation
2. Prescription of an anesthesia plan
3. Personally participates in the most demanding procedures in the anesthesia plan, including induction and emergence
4. Ensures that any procedures in the anesthesia plan that he or she does not perform are performed by a qualified anesthetist
5. Monitors the course of anesthesia administration at frequent intervals
6. Remains physically present and available for immediate diagnosis and treatment of emergencies
7. Provides indicated post-anesthesia care (42 C.F.R. 415.110 Conditions for Payment: Medically directed anesthesia services)

Additional modifiers that define the types of providers involved in anesthesia are:

-**AA**   Anesthesia services performed personally by an anesthesiologist

-**AD**   Medical supervision by a physician; more than 4 concurrent anesthesia procedures

-**G8**   Monitored anesthesia care (MAC) for deep, complex, complicated, or markedly invasive surgical procedure

-**G9**   Monitored anesthesia care for patient who has a history of severe cardiopulmonary condition

-**QK**   Medical direction of two, three, or four concurrent anesthesia procedures involving qualified individuals

-**QS**   Monitored anesthesia care service

-**QX**   Certified registered nurse anesthetist (CRNA) service, with medical direction by a physician

-**QY**   Medical direction of one certified registered nurse anesthetist (CRNA) by an anesthesiologist

-**QZ**   CRNA service, without medical direction by a physician

These modifiers are not CPT modifiers but HCPCS modifiers and further define the anesthesia services provided. Anesthesia modifiers are always placed first after the CPT anesthesia code. These anesthesia modifiers are pricing modifiers and are listed first to assure correct reimbursement.

QUICK CHECK 16-3

1. What is the difference between modifiers QX and QY? _____

_____

_____

_____

(Answers are located in Appendix C)

EXERCISE 16-3   *Modifiers*

Using Appendix A of the CPT manual, identify the following CPT modifiers:

1 Increased Procedural Services _____

2 Unusual Anesthesia _____

Using the descriptions for the preceding HCPCS modifiers, answer the following questions. Which modifier would be used to identify:

3 Medical supervision by a physician of more than 4 concurrent anesthesia procedures? _____

4 Monitored anesthesia care service? _____

5 CRNA medical direction by a physician? _____

(Answers are located in Appendix B)

UNLISTED ANESTHESIA CODE

In the Anesthesia section, an unlisted procedure code is available and is located under the Other Procedures subsection in the Anesthesia section. When there is no CPT code to indicate the anesthesia services, the unlisted Anesthesia code (01999) may be reported.

EXERCISE 16-4 *Anesthesia Codes*

Complete the following:

1 What is the unlisted anesthesia procedure code?

Code: _____

Locate anesthesia procedures in the CPT manual index under the entry "Anesthesia" and then subtermed by the anatomic site. Write the CPT index location on the line provided (e.g., Anesthesia, Thyroid). Then locate the code(s) identified in the Anesthesia section of the CPT manual. Choose the correct code(s) and write the code(s) on the line provided.

2 Needle biopsy of the thyroid (neck)

Index location: _____

Code: _____

3 Cesarean section, delivery only

Index location: _____

Code: _____

4 Transurethral resection of the prostate

Index location: _____

Code: _____

5 Repair of cleft palate

Index location: _____

Code: _____

6 Repair of ruptured Achilles tendon without graft

Index location: _____

Code: _____

Using the following information and the B + T + M formula, calculate the payment for the anesthesia services.

For the following questions a time unit will be 15 minutes. Base unit value for each case is provided within the questions. Refer to Fig. 16-13 for the conversion factors used in these questions; to Fig. 16-10 for the value of the Qualifying Circumstances; and to Fig. 16-11 for the value of the Physical Status Modifiers.

7 A needle biopsy lasting 15 minutes was conducted in North Dakota on a normal, healthy 75-year-old patient. The base unit value for the service is 3.

Anesthesia payment: _____

8 A patient with diabetes mellitus, controlled by diet and exercise, undergoes a 60-minute anesthesia period for a transurethral resection of the prostate (base unit value of 5). Calculate the anesthesia rate if the procedure were performed in the following locales:

a Manhattan _____

b North Carolina _____

9 A cesarean section was conducted in Alfred, NY, on a patient with preeclampsia (1 modifying unit). The base unit value for the service is 7. Calculate the anesthesia rates for procedures lasting two different lengths of time (refer to Fig. 16-13 for conversion rates):

a 30-minute procedure _____

b 45-minute procedure _____

(Answers are located in Appendix B)

OTHER REPORTING

Return to Operating Room

If a patient is returned to the operating room on the same day for the same or a related procedure, and the same individual is performing the second procedure, report the service with modifier -76. For example, the anesthesiologist provides the service for an upper gastrointestinal endoscopic procedure and reports the service 00740-AA. Later that day, the patient is returned for a lower intestinal endoscopic procedure. The second service would be reported 00810-AA-76. If that second procedure was performed by another anesthesiologist, the second service would be reported 00810-AA-77.

Pre-Anesthetic Examination

If the pre-anesthetic examination was provided by an anesthesiologist for a patient who did not undergo surgery, the E/M service would be reported for consideration for reimbursement.

TOOLBOX

The patient presents for transabdominal repair of a diaphragmatic hernia. The patient has severe diabetes, but the surgeon indicates the patient is stable and able to undergo the procedure. The anesthesiologist provides medical direction for one CRNA.

QUESTIONS

1. What modifier identifies the medical direction for the anesthesiologist? _____

2. What code reports anesthesia services for a transabdominal repair of a diaphragmatic hernia? _____

3. What would be the physical status modifier documented in the medical record? _____

▼ ANSWERS

1. -QY, 2. 00756, 3. P3

CHAPTER REVIEW

CHAPTER 16, PART I, THEORY

Complete the following:

1 Anesthesia services are based on _____ time the patient is under the anesthesiologist's care. Calculation of units of time is determined by the third-party payer.

2 Anesthesia time begins when the anesthesiologist _____, _____ continues _____ the procedure, and ends when _____.

3 According to the Anesthesia Guidelines, what is the one modifier that is not used with anesthesia procedures? _____ _____

4 "P1" is an example of what type of modifier? _____

5 What word means "in a dying state"? _____

6 What word means "affecting the body as a whole"? _____

7 The letter "P" in combination with what number indicates a brain-dead patient? _____

8 What type of circumstance identifies a component of anesthesia service that affects the character of the service? _____

9 Anesthesia procedures are divided by what type of site? _____

10 According to the Anesthesia Guidelines, the Separate or Multiple Procedures section, when multiple surgical procedures are performed during a single anesthetic administration, the anesthesia code representing the most _____ procedure is reported and the time reported is the _____ for all procedures.

11 Is it true that a physician who personally administers the anesthesia to the patient upon whom he or she is operating cannot bill the third-party payer? _____

12 What is the name of the guide that is published by the American Society of Anesthesiologists and provides the weights of various anesthesia services? _____

CHAPTER 16, PART II, PRACTICAL

Using your CPT manual, identify the modifier for the following descriptions:

13 Anesthesia for tendon repair of the shoulder, normal, healthy patient

Anesthesia Code: _____

14 Anesthesia for a cesarean hysterectomy following neuraxial labor anesthesia, normal, healthy patient

Anesthesia Codes: _____, _____

15 Anesthesia for a missed abortion procedure in which the mother is in grave danger of death

Anesthesia Code: _____

16 Cranioplasty for a depressed skull fracture, simple, extradural, for a patient with mild diabetes, well-controlled

Anesthesia Code: _____

17 Total hip replacement in a 75-year-old patient with hypertension that is well controlled with medication

Anesthesia Codes: _____, _____

18 Burn excision of 5% of the total body surface with skin grafting of the abdomen. Patient is 9 months old and in stable condition.

Anesthesia Codes: _____, _____

19 Hospital management of a continuous epidural drug delivery system for 5 days

Anesthesia Code: _____

20 Arthroscopic total wrist replacement in a normal, healthy patient

Anesthesia Code: _____

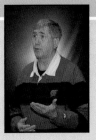

"Learn conflict resolution skills that use a 'win-win' approach and create the proper atmosphere for resolving differences and working together as a team. Maintain a positive sense of self-esteem."

Robert H. Ekvall, PhD, CCS, COC, CPC
Coder/Biller
Scripps Green Hospital
La Jolla, California

Surgery Guidelines and General Surgery

Chapter Topics

Introduction to the Surgery Section

Notes and Guidelines

Unlisted Procedures

Special Reports

Separate Procedure

Surgical Package

General Subsection

Chapter Review

Learning Objectives

After completing this chapter you should be able to

1   Understand the Surgery section format.

2   Locate notes and Guidelines in the Surgery section.

3   State the use of the unlisted procedure codes.

4   Interpret elements of a special report.

5   Examine the separate procedure designation.

6   Analyze the contents of a surgical package.

7   Determine the contents of the General Subsection.

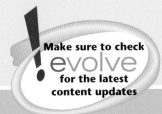

Make sure to check
evolve
for the latest
content updates

INTRODUCTION TO THE SURGERY SECTION

The Surgery section is the largest in the CPT manual. The codes range from 10021 to 69990. Surgery is divided into subsections. Most Surgery subsections are defined according to medical specialty or body system (e.g., integumentary or respiratory). Take a moment to review the Surgery subsections of the CPT manual so you have an understanding of the content of this important section.

Within the Surgery section, some of the more complex subsections are the Integumentary, Musculoskeletal, Respiratory, Cardiovascular, Digestive, and Female Genital subsections. Before we get into the details of the subsections, let's look at the general information that is pertinent to the entire Surgery section.

NOTES AND GUIDELINES

Guidelines are found at the beginning of each of the CPT sections. The section Guidelines define terms that are necessary to know for appropriately interpreting and reporting the procedures and services contained in the section. The following is an example of the type of information located in the Surgery Guidelines:

- Services: A reference explaining how to assign E/M codes
- CPT Surgical Package Definition: Defines what is included in the surgical procedure
- Follow-up Care for Diagnostic Procedures: Defines follow-up care for diagnostic services
- Follow-up Care for Therapeutic Surgical Procedures: Defines follow-up care for therapeutic surgical services
- Supplied Materials: Describes how and when to report supplies
- Reporting More Than One Procedure/Service: Identifies situations in which it may be appropriate to use modifiers for multiple services provided on the same day
- Separate Procedure: How to assign codes with this designation
- Unlisted Service or Procedure: Unlisted service codes from the Surgery section
- Special Report: What to include and when to submit a special report
- Surgical Destruction: Clarifies that destruction can be accomplished by any method, and that there are limited exceptions when the method is coded separately

An index at the beginning of each subsection within the Surgery section, lists subheadings, categories, and subcategories with instructional notes.

QUICK CHECK 17-1

1. A listing of subsections that have instructional notes is not included in the Surgical section Guidelines.

   True or False?

(Answers are located in Appendix C)

The **Guidelines** contain information that you will need to know in order to correctly code in the section, and most of the information is not repeated elsewhere in the section. So always review the Guidelines before coding in the section. Remember that with each new edition of the CPT manual, you will need to review the Guidelines for any changes. The changes are indicated by the "New or Revised Text" symbols used throughout the CPT manual (Fig. 17-1).

Reporting More Than One Procedure/Service

▶ When a physician performs more than one procedure/service on the same date, during the same session, or during a postoperative period (subject to the "surgical package" concept), several CPT modifiers may apply. (See Appendix A for definition.) ◀

New or revised text symbol

FIGURE 17–1 New or revised text symbol.

Note that the content of the figures is only for illustration, and the current year CPT may not display the information as stated in these text figures.

Common throughout the CPT manual are notes. Notes may appear before subsections (Fig. 17-2), subheadings (Fig. 17-3), categories (Fig. 17-4), and subcategories (Fig. 17-5).

The information in the notes indicates the special instructions unique to particular codes or groups of codes. The notes are extremely important because the information contained in

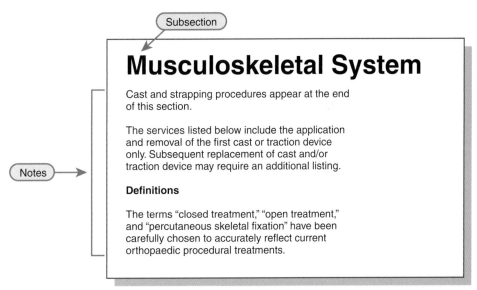

Subsection

Musculoskeletal System

Cast and strapping procedures appear at the end of this section.

The services listed below include the application and removal of the first cast or traction device only. Subsequent replacement of cast and/or traction device may require an additional listing.

Definitions

The terms "closed treatment," "open treatment," and "percutaneous skeletal fixation" have been carefully chosen to accurately reflect current orthopaedic procedural treatments.

Notes

FIGURE 17–2 Subsection notes.

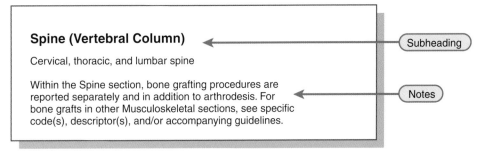

Spine (Vertebral Column)

Cervical, thoracic, and lumbar spine

Within the Spine section, bone grafting procedures are reported separately and in addition to arthrodesis. For bone grafts in other Musculoskeletal sections, see specific code(s), descriptor(s), and/or accompanying guidelines.

Subheading

Notes

FIGURE 17–3 Subheading notes.

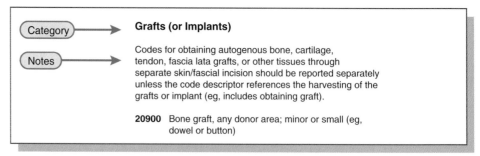

FIGURE 17-4   Category notes.

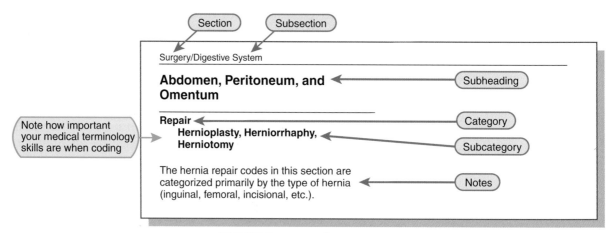

FIGURE 17-5   Subcategory notes.

them is not usually available in the section Guidelines. Always make it a practice to read any notes available before coding. If notes are present, they must be followed if the coding is to be accurate. Make it a practice to write in your coding manuals. Highlight important points, make notes in the margins, and personalize your coding manual. You will find these personal annotations are very helpful as you code.

Additional information is enclosed in parentheses, called parenthetical phrases or expressions. They sometimes follow the code or group of codes and provide further information about codes that may be applicable. For example, 42120, Resection of the palate or extensive resection of a lesion, is followed by information about codes you would assign if reconstruction of the palate followed the resection (Fig. 17-6).

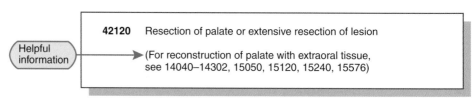

FIGURE 17-6   Additional helpful information in parentheses.

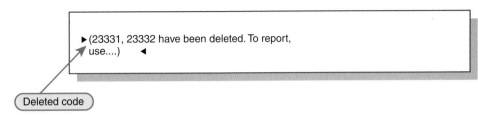

▶(23331, 23332 have been deleted. To report, use....) ◀

Deleted code

FIGURE 17-7 Deleted codes in parentheses.

Deleted codes are also indicated in the CPT manual, enclosed in parentheses. Often the code that is to be used in place of the deleted code will be listed (Fig. 17-7). Appendix B of the CPT manual has a summary of code additions, deletions, and revisions for the current year.

Also note in Fig. 17-7 that the arrows at the beginning and end of the information indicate that the information is new or has been revised for the current edition.

UNLISTED PROCEDURES

The Surgery Guidelines contain many unlisted procedure codes, presented by anatomic site. These unlisted codes are presented in numeric order by their location in the Surgery section Guidelines and in the subsections by body system. For example, the unlisted procedure code for procedures of the forearm or wrist, 25999, is located in the Surgery Guidelines and also at the end of the subheading Forearm and Wrist. The unlisted codes identify procedures or services throughout the Surgery section for which there is no CPT code. If a Category III code is available for the unlisted service you are reporting, you must use the Category III code, not the unlisted Category I code. Reimbursement for Category III codes will vary by payer.

QUICK CHECK 17-2

1. Before you can assign an unlisted code, you must first be certain there is no more specific code and that there is not a Category _____ code available.

(Answers are located in Appendix C)

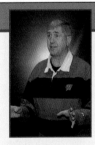

From the Trenches

"Understand all the different types of devices/tools and what they are generally used for so you can learn which CPT codes were involved in the surgery."

ROBERT

EXERCISE 17-1   *Unlisted Procedures*

Using the CPT manual, locate the unlisted procedure codes in the Surgical Guidelines and identify the unlisted procedure codes for the following anatomic areas:

1 Musculoskeletal system, general

Code: _____

2 Inner ear

Code: _____

3 Skin, mucous membrane, and subcutaneous tissue

Code: _____

4 Leg or ankle

Code: _____

5 Nervous system

Code: _____

6 Eyelids

Code: _____

(Answers are located in Appendix B)

SPECIAL REPORTS

✋ **CAUTION**   *Unlisted codes are assigned only after thorough research fails to reveal a more specific code.*

When using an unlisted procedure code to report a surgical service, a special report describing the procedure must accompany the claim. According to the CPT manual, "Pertinent information *[in the special report]* should include an adequate definition or description of the **nature, extent,** and **need** for the procedure, and the **time, effort,** and **equipment** necessary to provide the service."

Example

When the first total disc arthroplasty (artificial disc) was performed there was no code to report the service, so a special report would have been submitted. The report contained a detailed description of the procedure, why it was being performed, the extent of the procedure, the length of time the procedure required, and the equipment necessary. Later, there was a Category III code to describe this procedure (0090T). When the procedure gained approval, 0090T was deleted and a Category I code was created.

Medical supplier representatives may be of assistance to you in obtaining the information necessary to support the use of the new technique used during the procedure.

SEPARATE PROCEDURE

Some procedure codes will have the words "separate procedure" after the descriptor. The term "separate procedure" does not mean that the procedure was the only procedure that was performed; rather, it is an indication of how the code can be assigned. Locate code 19100 in the CPT manual. The breast biopsy code 19100 has the words "(separate procedure)" after the description. Procedures followed by the words "separate procedure" (in parentheses) are considered **minor** procedures that are reported only when they are the only services performed or when they are performed with another major procedure but at a different site or unrelated to the major procedure. When the minor procedure is performed in conjunction with a related major procedure, the minor procedure is considered incidental and is bundled into the code for the major procedure.

Example

Separate procedure bundled into the major procedure: Breast biopsy (19100) has "separate procedure" after it. If a breast biopsy was performed in conjunction with a modified radical mastectomy (19307), only the mastectomy would be reported. Because the breast biopsy and the mastectomy were conducted on the same body area during the same surgery, the breast biopsy would be considered a minor procedure that was incidental and would be bundled into the major procedure of the mastectomy. Exception: A scenario when the "separate procedure" would not be bundled can be illustrated in the following example. A patient has a percutaneous breast biopsy (19100) performed and then is brought back to the operating room for extensive tissue removal by subcutaneous mastectomy (19304) on the same day. The second procedure would have modifier -58 (Staged or related procedure or service by the same individual during the postoperative period) appended to the code (19304-58).

Example

Two separate procedures: If a breast biopsy (19100 a separate procedure) was performed in conjunction with an esophagoscopy (43200), both the breast biopsy and the esophagoscopy would be reported. The breast biopsy and the esophagoscopy were performed on different body areas and, as such, the breast biopsy would not be bundled into the esophagoscopy procedure.

Example

Separate procedure bundled into the major procedure. Salpingo-oophorectomy (58720—removal of tubes and ovaries) has "separate procedure" after it. If a salpingo-oophorectomy was performed in conjunction with an abdominal hysterectomy (removal of the uterus, 58150), only the hysterectomy would be reported. Because the salpingo-oophorectomy and the abdominal hysterectomy were conducted on the same body area, the salpingo-oophorectomy would be bundled into the more major procedure of the hysterectomy.

Example

Two separate procedures: If a salpingo-oophorectomy (58720—separate procedure) was performed in conjunction with an esophagoscopy (43200), both the salpingo-oophorectomy and the esophagoscopy would be reported. Because the salpingo-oophorectomy and the esophagoscopy were conducted on different body areas, the salpingo-oophorectomy is considered a separate procedure, not a minor procedure incidental to a major procedure.

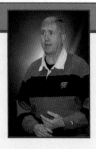

From the Trenches

"Learn how to read and abstract a medical report to know which CPT codes apply to what occurred in the operation, surgery, or medical procedure. Doctors don't often use the words that the CPT code describes."

ROBERT

QUICK CHECK 17-3

1. When a minor procedure is performed with a more major procedure of the same area, you would report both the minor and major procedure.

   True or False?

(Answers are located in Appendix C)

SURGICAL PACKAGE

Often, the time, effort, and services rendered when accomplishing a procedure are bundled together to form a surgical package. Payment is made for a package of services and not for each individual service provided within the package. The CPT manual describes the surgical package as including the operation itself, local anesthesia, and "typical postoperative follow-up care," one related E/M encounter prior to the procedure, and immediate follow-up care, including written orders. Read the information regarding the surgical package in the Surgery Guidelines and highlight the "included" elements because you will be referring back to this information as you report surgical services.

The surgical package contains the components of:

- Preoperative visits
- Intraoperative services
- Complications following surgery
- Post-operative visits
- Supplies
- Miscellaneous service—dressing changes, catheter removal, etc.

Local anesthesia is defined as local infiltration, metacarpal/digital block, or topical anesthesia. Follow-up care for complications, exacerbations (a worsening), recurrence, and the presence of other diseases that require additional services is not included in the surgical package. General anesthesia for surgical procedures is not part of the surgical package; general anesthesia services are reported separately by the anesthesiologist.

Third-party payers have varying definitions of what constitutes a surgical package and varying policies about what is included in the surgical package. Surgical packages also define the services for which you can or cannot submit additional charges because the rules of the surgical package define what is and is not included with the surgical procedure. Included in the definition of the surgical package are routine preoperative and postoperative care—including minor complications—and up to a predefined number of days before and after the surgery. Reimbursement policies vary from payer to payer because of the way each payer defines each surgical package. For instance, Medicare states that they averaged the costs associated with additional services for complications and added payments for those services into the initial surgical payment. Other commercial payers determine the reimbursement based on services associated only with performing the surgery and choose to let costs for services for complications be reported separately. The period of time following each surgery that is included in the surgery package is established by the third-party payer and is referred to as the **global (post-operative) surgery** period. The global period is usually **90** days for major surgery and **10** days for minor surgery.

Fig. 17-8 shows CPT codes 10080 and 10081 for incision and drainage of a pilonidal cyst. The third-party payer may indicate that code 10080 has zero days for the global surgical package, so you would charge for any additional services that were provided in addition to the 10080 incision and drainage itself. The payer may indicate that 10081 has 10 days for the global surgical package that would include routine follow-up care and services (such as removal of sutures) at no charge. You must know the number of days in the global service for a code to correctly bill for the services that are not included in the bundle and to be certain not to bill for services that were included in the surgical package.

CHECK THIS OUT ☞ The Physician's Fee Schedule Relative Value Files are located on the CMS website at www.cms.gov/PhysicianFeeSched/PFSRVF/list.asp. It is within these files that the global days for each surgical procedure is located.

One last coding guideline that you have to know before you begin to code surgical procedures pertains to materials and supply codes. When **materials** or **supplies** over and above those usually used in an office visit have been used, you code and charge for these materials and supplies in addition to charging for the office visit or procedure. For example, when a physician does a wound repair during an office visit and uses a surgical tray, the surgical tray may be identified by CPT code 99070. Code 99070 is listed in the Medicine section, Special Services, Procedures, and Reports subsection, Miscellaneous Services.

CMS RULES

HCPCS code A4550 also reports the use of a surgical tray. Third-party payers who pay separately for a surgical tray usually want the HCPCS "A" code to report the tray. Some third-party payers pay separately for a surgical tray. Medicare does not pay separately for specific kit trays.(Medicare Claims Processing Manual, Chapter 12, Section 20.4.4-Supplies, B3-15900.2 (www.cms.gov/manuals/downloads/clm104c12.pdf))

The following examples recap two major guidelines concerning surgical packages:
1. Surgical packages for procedures usually include the preoperative service, the procedure (intraoperative), related services, and routine postoperative services. Payers vary in their interpretation of the global surgical package. Although most follow the CPT guidelines, some payers, such as Medicare, expand the services that are included in the surgical package to include treatment of complications by the same physician.

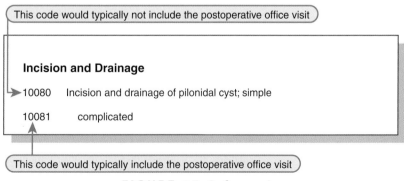

This code would typically not include the postoperative office visit

Incision and Drainage

10080   Incision and drainage of pilonidal cyst; simple

10081   complicated

This code would typically include the postoperative office visit

FIGURE 17–8 Surgery package.

Example

An established patient, Mary Smith is referred to a surgeon for excessive menstrual bleeding. The surgeon decides a hysterectomy is necessary and schedules the surgical procedure for 2 weeks later. The surgeon plans to recheck Mary in the office the day before surgery. The initial visit, at which the decision is made to perform surgery, is billable, but the preoperative visit on the day before surgery is bundled into the surgical package, as is the procedure itself and any routine follow-up.

2. Complications are usually added on a service-by-service basis.

CMS RULES

Medicare includes care for complications related to the primary surgical procedure in the global reimbursement and does not reimburse separately for the complications. If the complication requires a return to the operating room, the procedure is separately reported with modifier -78 (Unplanned return to the operating/procedure room by the same physician following initial procedure for a related procedure during the postoperative period) and the initial surgery global period continues. Most private payers follow the Medicare rules.

Even though the routine follow-up care is at no charge, the service is still coded to indicate that the service was provided. CPT code 99024 (Postoperative follow-up visit, included in global service) alerts the third-party payer that the services were rendered but the services were included in a surgical package and not charged for.

From the Trenches

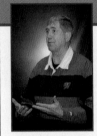

"We see the importance of networking and assisting each other as we seek answers/solutions to complex coding scenarios. . . . There are so many complexities to coding where there are no easy answers as we seek to code correctly and ethically."

ROBERT

Example

A patient undergoes a wound repair that is coded 12014 (the third-party payer indicated that there was a 10-day surgical package for this code) and 5 days afterwards sees the physician for routine follow-up care of the wound. The fee statement for the office visit at which the routine follow-up care is provided would be:

99024	Postoperative follow-up visit	No charge

However, if the patient returned during the global period because of a breakdown in the skin around the surgical wound (dehiscence) but with no signs of infection, and the patient was returned to the operating room at which time the physician trimmed the skin margins around the wound and resutured the wound, you would report and charge for this complication during the global period with:

12020-78	Dehiscence, simple closure	$xx.xx

If a patient undergoes the repair of a 7.9-cm wound that is coded 12004 (the third-party payer indicated that there was no surgical package for this code) and sees the physician a few days later for routine follow-up care, the service is coded and charged for.

12004	Wound repair, 7.9 cm	$xx.xx
99070	Surgical tray	$xx.xx
99212	Office visit	$xx.xx

CMS RULES

Medicare assigns 12004 a 0-day global period. Medicare does not reimburse separately for supplies.

Inclusion or exclusion of a procedure in the CPT manual does not imply any health insurance coverage or reimbursement policy. Although the CPT manual includes guidelines on usage, third-party payers may interpret and accept the use of CPT codes and the guidelines in any manner they choose.

EXERCISE 17-2 *Surgical Package*

Answer the following:

1 What are the three parts of a surgery bundled into a surgical package?

a _____

b _____

c _____

2 Is general anesthesia included in the surgical package? _____

3 Do all third-party payers follow the same reimbursement guidelines for the global packages? _____

(Answers are located in Appendix B)

GENERAL SUBSECTION

The General subsection contains codes for fine needle aspirations (10021, 10022), excluding bone marrow aspirations (see code 38220). The codes are divided based on whether **imaging guidance** was used during the aspiration. A **fine needle aspiration** is used to withdraw fluid that contains individual cells, as illustrated in Fig. 17-9. The needle is inserted into the area being biopsied and moved several times to take multiple samples without withdrawing the needle. The aspirated fluid/cells are then examined by a pathologist using a microscope (88172, 88173, or 88177). This type of biopsy is not to be confused with a needle core biopsy, such as that identified by 19100, percutaneous breast biopsy using a **needle core,** in which a core of suspicious tissue is removed for examination, or the biopsy represented in 19101, breast biopsy using an open incision, which reports a procedure in which the biopsy site is exposed to the surgeon's view and a sample of the lesion is removed. Notes following codes 10021-10022 indicate several other codes that are used to report percutaneous needle biopsies based on what was biopsied.

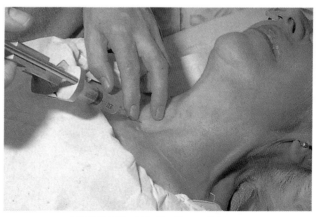

FIGURE 17–9 Fine needle biopsy.

EXERCISE 17-3   *General Subsection*

Using the CPT manual, report the services for the following:

1 The physician palpates a cyst on the right breast and performs a fine needle aspiration in the office.

Code: _____

2 A patient presents to the outpatient surgical center at the clinic for a fine needle aspiration of the thyroid. Ultrasound guidance is utilized during the aspiration.

Code aspiration: _____

Code ultrasound guidance: _____

(Answers are located in Appendix B)

CHAPTER REVIEW

CHAPTER 17, PART I, THEORY

Now is an excellent time to put all your newly learned coding skills to work by completing a Chapter Review.

1 What is the largest section of the six CPT manual sections? _____

2 Does Medicare reimburse for every surgical tray?

   Yes   No

3 The subsections in the Surgery section are usually divided according to _____.

4 These are found at the beginning of each section and contain information specific to the section: _____
   _____

5 This symbol indicates new or revised text within the current edition of the CPT manual: _____

6 Information within parentheses is referred to as _____ expression or phrase.

7 Before assigning this type of code, you must be certain that a more specific Category I or a Category III code is not available: _____

8 This report contains the nature, extent, need, time, effort, and at times equipment necessary to provide a service:
   _____

9 This designation within the CPT manual indicates a procedure that is only reported when it is performed as the only procedure or when another procedure performed at the same time is unrelated to this procedure. This is a _____ procedure.

10 When time, effort, and services are bundled together, they form a _____ package.

11 _____ anesthesia is defined as local infiltration, metacarpal/digital block, or topical anesthesia.

12 According to Medicare guidelines, _____ complications of a surgical procedure are usually included in the reimbursement for a major surgical procedure.

13 Code _____ is a CPT code that can be assigned to report a surgical tray.

14 Code _____ is a HCPCS code that can be assigned to report a surgical tray.

15 This code reports a postoperative follow-up visit that is included in the global service: _____

Chapter Review answers are only available in the TEACH Instructor Resources on Evolve

CHAPTER 17, PART II, PRACTICAL

With the use of the CPT manual Surgery Guidelines, answer the following:

16 _____ destruction is a part of a surgical procedure, and different methods of destruction are not ordinarily listed separately.

17 Care of the condition for which a diagnostic procedure was performed or of other _____ conditions is not included and may be listed separately.

18 There are "Notes" in the Burns, _____ Treatment category.

19 The only code in the Operating Microscope subsection is _____.

20 Follow-up care for therapeutic surgical procedures includes only that care which is usually part of the _____ _____.

According to the parenthetical information that follows code 10022:

21 The four codes for radiological supervision and interpretation are _____, _____, _____, and _____.

22 For evaluation of fine needle aspirate, see _____, _____, _____.

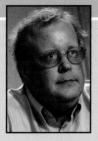

"Get to know what your doctors are doing—how they do procedures and how they document. . . . You can get all the codes correct up front. It sets the stage for anything you have to do with the insurance companies later."

Christopher P. Galeziewski, CPC
Coding Compliance Specialist
Coding Compliance Department
Kelsey-Seybold Clinic
Houston, Texas

Integumentary System

Chapter Topics

Integumentary System

Format

Skin, Subcutaneous, and Accessory Structures

Nails, Pilonidal Cyst and Introduction

Repair (Closure)

Burns

Destruction

Breast Procedures

Chapter Review

Learning Objectives

After completing this chapter you should be able to

1 Describe the format of the Integumentary System in the CPT manual.

2 Identify the elements of coding Skin, Subcutaneous, and Accessory Structures services.

3 Review the main services in Nails, Pilonidal Cyst and Introduction.

4 Identify the major factors in Repair.

5 State the important coding considerations in destruction and breast procedures.

6 Demonstrate the ability to code integumentary services and procedures.

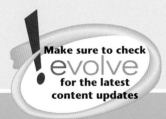

Make sure to check **evolve** for the latest content updates

INTEGUMENTARY SYSTEM

The Integumentary System subsection includes codes assigned by many different physician specialties. There is no restriction on who reports the codes from this or any other subsection. You may find a family practitioner using the incision and drainage, debridement, or repair codes; a dermatologist using excision and destruction codes; a plastic surgeon using skin graft codes; or a surgeon using breast procedure codes.

You will learn about the Integumentary System subsection by first reviewing the subsection format and then learning about coding the services and procedures in the subsection.

QUICK CHECK 18-1

1. Dermatologists are the only providers who utilize the codes in the Integumentary System subsection of the CPT manual.
   True or False?

(Answers are located in Appendix C)

FORMAT

The subsection is formatted on the basis of anatomic site and category of procedure. For example, an anatomic site is "Neck" and a category of procedure is "Repair."

The subsection Integumentary contains the subheadings:

- Skin, Subcutaneous, and Accessory Structures
- Nails
- Pilonidal Cyst
- Introduction
- Repair (Closure)
- Destruction
- Breast

Each subheading is further divided by category. For example, the subheading Skin, Subcutaneous, and Accessory Structures is divided into the following categories:

- Introduction and Removal
- Incision and Drainage
- Debridement
- Paring or Cutting
- Biopsy
- Removal of Skin Tags
- Shaving of Epidermal or Dermal Lesions
- Excision—Benign Lesions
- Excision—Malignant Lesions

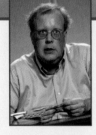

From the Trenches

"[Documentation] comes down to semantics. Certain words mean certain things. . . . That's what insurance companies look for to describe what type of test or work effort was done to determine the patient's illness."

CHRIS

SKIN, SUBCUTANEOUS, AND ACCESSORY STRUCTURES

Introduction and Removal (10030)

Code 10030 is assigned to report percutaneous image-guided fluid drainage of a collection, such as an abscess, seroma, cyst, hematoma, or lymphocele, from soft tissue. The collection is by means of a catheter and reported once for each individual collection drained. Image guidance is included and not reported separately.

Incision and Drainage

Incision and Drainage (I&D) codes (10040-10180) are divided according to the condition for which the I&D is being performed. Acne surgery, abscess, carbuncle, boil, cyst, hematoma, and wound infection are just some of the conditions for which a physician uses I&D (Fig. 18-1). The physician opens the lesion to allow drainage. Also included under this heading is a **puncture aspiration** code (10160), which describes inserting a needle into a lesion and withdrawing the fluid (aspiration). Whichever method is used—incision or aspiration—the contents of the lesion are drained. Packing material may be inserted into the opening or the wound may be left to drain freely. A tube or strip of gauze, which acts as a wick, may be inserted into the wound to facilitate drainage.

The I&D codes are first divided according to the condition and then according to whether the procedure was simple/single or complicated/multiple. The medical record would indicate the condition and complexity of the I&D. Verify the body area where the incision and drainage was performed for any specific CPT code that could be assigned outside of the range 10040-10180. For example, a simple and complicated finger abscess would be reported with an incision and drainage code (26010, 26011) from the Musculoskeletal System subsection, Hand and Finger, Incision codes. When you reference the index of the CPT manual, under the main term "Abscess" and subterm "Finger," you are directed to the Musculoskeletal System codes. Those codes are the most specific codes to report the incision and drainage of a finger abscess and you are to always assign the most specific code you can locate. Note that in the index of the CPT manual again under the main term "Abscess" and subterm "Skin," you are directed to the Integumentary codes. You should always reference the specific location of the abscess to receive direction to the most correct code(s) and only reference the skin subterm when there is no more specific location provided.

Debridement

Debridement is the removal of infected, contaminated, damaged, devitalized, necrotic, or foreign tissue from a wound. Debridement promotes wound healing by reducing sources of infection and other mechanical impediments to healing. The goal of debridement is to cleanse the wound, reduce bacterial contamination, and provide an optimal environment for wound healing or possible surgical intervention. The usual end point of debridement is removal of pathological tissue and/or foreign material until healthy tissue is exposed. Debridement techniques include, among others, sharp and blunt dissection, curettement, scrubbing, and forceful irrigation. Surgical instruments may include a scrub brush, irrigation device,

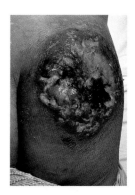

FIGURE 18–1 Massive staphylococcal carbuncle.

electrocautery, laser, sharp curette, forceps, scissors, burr, or scalpel. Prior to debridement, determination of the extent of an ulcer/wound may be aided by the use of probes to determine the depth and to disclose abscess and sinus tracts.

These debridement codes do not apply to debridement of burned surfaces. For debridement of burned surfaces, CPT codes 16000-16036 are reported.

Excision—Debridement

Codes in this category (11000-11047) describe services of debridement based on depth, body surface, condition, and for 11004-11006 by location. The first debridement codes (11000 and 11001) are reported for eczematous debridement. **Eczema** is a skin condition that blisters and weeps, as illustrated in Fig. 18-2.

The dead tissue may have to be cut away with a scalpel or scissors or, in less severe cases, washed with a saline solution. Code 11000 reports debridement of 10% of the body surface or less, and add-on code 11001 reports each additional 10% or part thereof.

Codes 11042-11047 are based on the depth of tissue removed and surface area of the wound. When reporting one wound, report the depth of the deepest level of tissue removed. When reporting multiple wounds, sum the surface area of the wound at the same depth. Do not combine sums of different depths.

Some codes in this category are based on the extent of the debridement of the skin, subcutaneous tissue, muscle fascia, muscle, or bone.

CODING SHOT

Some surgical procedure codes include debridement as a part of the service. You may report a debridement as a separate service when the medical record indicates that a greater than usual debridement was provided. For example, if an extensive debridement of an open fracture was performed when usually a simple debridement would be performed, you report the additional service using a debridement code from the 11010-11012 range.

Introduction to Lesions

Before you learn about coding the various methods of lesion destruction and excision, you need to review a few rules that apply broadly to this commonly performed procedure. After you have learned the general lesion information, you will review each of the destruction and excision methods.

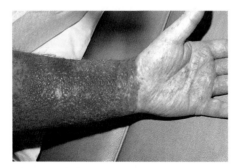

FIGURE 18-2 Eczematous dermatitis.

CMS RULES

According to Medicare LCD for Debridement Services L27373, 03/25/2013, the following is considered when reporting debridement:

1. CPT codes 11000 and 11001 describe removal of extensive eczematous or infected skin. A key word is extensive. Conditions that may require debridement of large amounts of skin include: rapidly spreading necrotizing process (sometimes seen with aggressive streptococcal infections), severe eczema, bullous skin diseases, extensive skin trauma (including large abraded areas with ground-in dirt), or autoimmune skin diseases (such as pemphigus).

2. If there is no necrotic, devitalized, fibrotic, or other tissue or foreign matter present that would interfere with wound healing, the debridement service is not medically necessary. The presence or absence of such tissue or foreign matter must be documented in the medical record.

3. The following procedures are considered part of active wound care management, and are not considered as debridement and are not included in this LCD: Removal of devitalized tissue from wound(s), non-selective debridement, without anesthesia (e.g., wet-to-moist dressings, enzymatic, abrasion), including topical application(s), wound assessment, and instruction(s) for ongoing care.

4. CPT code 11001 is limited to those practitioners who are licensed to perform surgery above the ankle, since the amount of skin required by the code is more than that contained on both feet.

5. Removing a collar of callus (hyperkeratotic tissue) around an ulcer is not debridement of skin or necrotic tissue and should not be billed as such. The service should be billed under CPT code 11055 or 11056. Please refer to NGS LCD Routine Foot Care and Debridement of Nails (L26426) for information regarding these CPT codes. This LCD does not apply to debridement services performed by physical or occupational therapists. For debridement services performed by physical or occupational therapists, please use CPT codes 97597, 97598 and 97602. Providers should refer to NGS LCD for Outpatient Physical and Occupational Services (L26884).

6. Local infiltration, metacarpal/digital block or topical anesthesia are included in the reimbursement for debridement services and are not separately payable. Anesthesia administered by or incident to the provider performing the debridement procedure is not separately payable.

7. Photographic documentation of wounds either immediately before or immediately after debridement is recommended for prolonged or repetitive debridement services (especially those that exceed five extensive debridements per wound (CPT code 11043 and/or 11044)). If the provider is unable to use photographs for documentation purposes, the medical record should contain sufficient detail to determine the extent of the wound and the result of the treatment.

8. Debridement services are now defined by body surface area of the debrided tissue and not by individual ulcers or wounds. For example, debridement of two ulcers on the foot to the level of subcutaneous tissue, total area of 6 sq cm should be billed as CPT code 11042 with unit of service of "1".

Lesion Excision and Destruction. There are many types of lesions of the skin (Fig. 18-3) and many types of treatment for lesions. Types of treatment include **paring** (peeling or scraping), **shaving** (slicing), **excision** (cutting removal), and **destruction** (ablation). To code these procedures properly, you must know the **site, number,** and **size** of the excised lesion(s), as well as whether the lesion is malignant or benign.

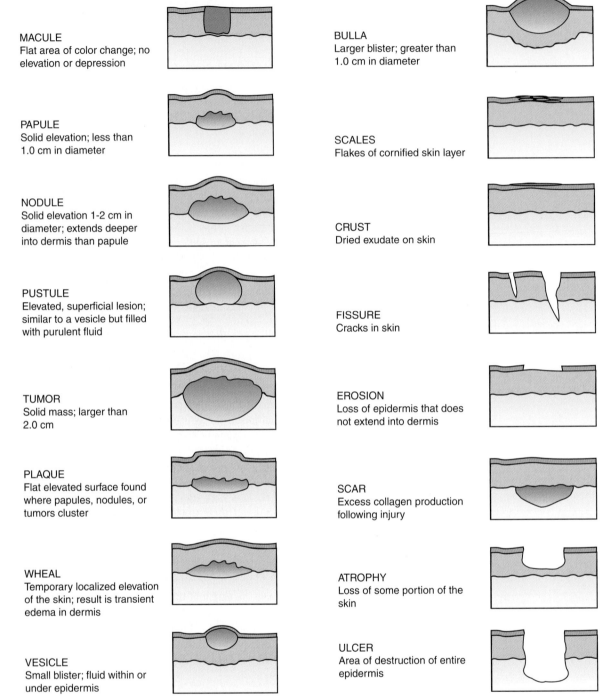

MACULE
Flat area of color change; no elevation or depression

PAPULE
Solid elevation; less than 1.0 cm in diameter

NODULE
Solid elevation 1-2 cm in diameter; extends deeper into dermis than papule

PUSTULE
Elevated, superficial lesion; similar to a vesicle but filled with purulent fluid

TUMOR
Solid mass; larger than 2.0 cm

PLAQUE
Flat elevated surface found where papules, nodules, or tumors cluster

WHEAL
Temporary localized elevation of the skin; result is transient edema in dermis

VESICLE
Small blister; fluid within or under epidermis

BULLA
Larger blister; greater than 1.0 cm in diameter

SCALES
Flakes of cornified skin layer

CRUST
Dried exudate on skin

FISSURE
Cracks in skin

EROSION
Loss of epidermis that does not extend into dermis

SCAR
Excess collagen production following injury

ATROPHY
Loss of some portion of the skin

ULCER
Area of destruction of entire epidermis

FIGURE 18–3 Lesions of the skin.

Prior to excision, the greatest diameter of the lesion is measured. The measurement includes the margin (extra tissue taken from around the lesion) at its narrowest part. Fig. 18-4 illustrates calculations of a 2.0 cm lesion. The size of the margin necessary to completely remove the lesion is based on the physician's judgment. The pathology report is used to identify the size of the lesion only if no other record of the size can be documented because the solution the lesion is stored in shrinks the lesion.

All lesions excised will have a pathology report for diagnosing the removed tissue as malignant or benign; since the codes are divided based on whether the excised lesion is malignant or benign, the billing for the excision is not submitted to the third-party payer until the pathology report has been completed.

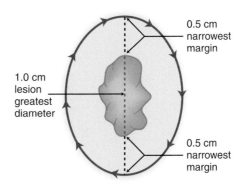

FIGURE 18–4 Calculations of a 2.0 cm lesion.

Codes in the Integumentary System subsection differ greatly in their descriptions. Some codes indicate only one lesion per code, others are for the second and third lesions only, and still others indicate a certain number of lesions (e.g., up to 15 lesions). When reporting multiple lesions, you must read the description carefully to prevent incorrect coding.

If multiple lesions are treated, code the **most complex lesion procedure first followed by the others using modifier -51** to indicate that multiple procedures were performed. Remember that the third-party payer will usually reduce the payment for the services identified with modifier -51; so you want to be certain that you place the service with the highest dollar amount first, without the modifier. If the code description includes multiple lesions (a stated number of lesions), modifier -51 is not necessary. For example, if the code states "2 to 4 lesions" or "more than 4 lesions," modifier -51 is not required.

Closure of Excision Sites. Included in the codes for lesion excision is the direct, primary, or simple closure of the operative site. **Excision** is defined as a full thickness (through the dermis) excision of a lesion and a **simple closure** is nonlayered closure (Fig. 18-5).

Closures can also be **intermediate** (layered; Fig. 18-6) or **complex** (greater than layered). The local anesthesia is included in the excision codes. Any closure other than a simple closure can be reported separately with lesion excision.

Three final notes on treatment of lesions:
1. The shaving of lesions requires no closure because no incision has been made.
2. Excision includes simple closure but may require more complex closure. If more complex closure is required, follow the notes in the CPT manual to appropriately code for these services.
3. Destruction may be by any method, including freezing, burning, chemicals, etc.

Paring or Cutting

Paring or Cutting codes (11055-11057) report the services when a physician removes a benign hyperkeratotic skin lesion such as a callus or corn (Fig. 18-7). Paring codes include removal by peeling or scraping. A small ring-shaped instrument (curette), blade, or similar sharp instrument is used for paring. Bleeding is usually controlled by a chemical that is applied to the surface after removal of the lesion. The codes are divided based on the number of lesions removed.

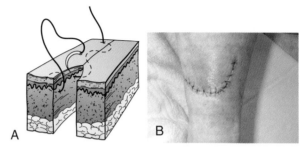

FIGURE 18-5 A and B, Simple closure. (B courtesy Mary Garden.)

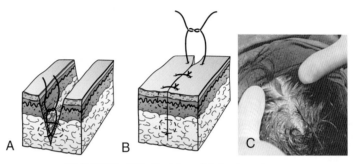

FIGURE 18-6 Intermediate two-layer closure.

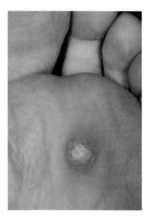

FIGURE 18-7 Corns (clavi) on the plantar surface.

Biopsy

"Biopsy" is a term applied to the procedure of removing tissue for histopathology (study of microscopic tissue changes). Removing a tissue sample of a lesion may be by needle aspiration, incisional biopsy (open, sharp, and partial removal), or by excisional biopsy (complete removal). You would not report **both** a biopsy and an excision performed at the same time as the biopsy

CODING SHOT

Included in the Biopsy codes are codes for biopsies of mucous membranes. A mucous membrane is tissue that covers a variety of body parts, such as the tongue and the nasal cavities.

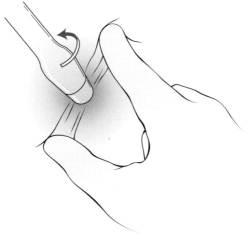

FIGURE 18-8 Punch biopsy.

F.	G.	H.	I.	
$ CHARGES	DAYS OR UNITS	EPSDT Family Plan	ID. QUAL.	
			NPI	
			NPI	
			NPI	
			NPI	
			NPI	
			NPI	
28. TOTAL CHARGE		29. AMOUNT PAID		
$		$		

FIGURE 18-9 Units column (G) of the CMS-1500.

is bundled into the excision service. For CPT lesion biopsy codes, only a portion of the lesion and some of the surrounding tissue is removed. The section of surrounding tissue (margin) is included so the pathologist can compare the normal tissue to the lesion tissue and note the differences.

Many methods are used to obtain biopsies; the method chosen is determined by the size and type of the lesion and the physician's preference. Common biopsy methods are scraping, cutting, and the punch. A punch biopsy is illustrated in Fig. 18-8 and is used to excise a disc of tissue. A punch can also be used in the excision of the entire lesion, so just because the medical record refers to the use of a punch, it does not mean that a biopsy was performed.

Biopsy sites do not necessarily have to be closed; some are so small that they will close readily. Other sites are large enough that closure is required, and simple closure is bundled into the biopsy codes. If closure of the biopsy site is more than a simple closure, you would report the more extensive closure separately. You will learn more about closure later in this chapter.

On the paper CMS-1500 claim form, you would report the number of lesions treated in column 24G., Days or Units, as illustrated in Fig. 18-9.

> **CAUTION** Do not assign modifier -51 with these biopsy codes, as 11100 reports a single lesion, and 11101 is an add-on code for each additional lesion. The correct coding for three lesions would be 11100 for lesion one and 11101 × 2 for lesions two and three.

Skin Tags

Skin tags are flaps of skin (benign lesions) that can appear anywhere, but most often appear on the neck or trunk, especially in older people (Fig. 18-10, *A*). Skin tags are removed in a variety of ways—scissors, blades, ligatures, electrosurgery, or chemicals. **Scissors removal** of a skin tag is illustrated in Fig. 18-10, *B*. Scissoring is often used for tissue column lesions. The forceps grasps the column, and the physician snips the lesion off at its base. Closure is achieved by using sutures or an aluminum chloride solution. In **ligature strangulation,** a thread is tied at the base of the lesion and left there until the tissue dies. The lesion then drops off. Whatever method of removal is used, simple closure is included in the skin tag codes, as is any local anesthesia that is used. Also, note that the codes (11200, 11201) are based on the first 15 lesions and then on each additional 10 lesions (or part thereof) after the first 15. On the CMS-1500 claim form, report the number of lesions treated in 24G., Days or Units (see Fig. 18-9).

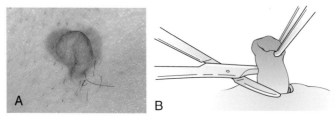

FIGURE 18–10 **A,** Skin tag. **B,** Scissors removal.

CODING SHOT

Do not use modifier -51 (multiple procedure) with skin tag codes, as the codes are based on the number of lesions removed.

Shaving of Epidermal or Dermal Lesions

The **shaving** of a lesion (11300-11313) can be performed by using a scalpel blade or other sharp instrument. The shaving of a lesion is illustrated in Fig. 18-11.

The blade is held horizontal to the skin and an epidermal or dermal lesion is sliced off. Anesthesia and cauterization (electrocautery or chemical cautery) to control bleeding are included in the lesion-shaving codes.

Electrocautery is sometimes used to finish the edges of the shaving, but if electrocautery is the main method by which the lesion was removed, you would assign codes from the Destruction, Benign or Premalignant Lesions category (17000-17250), not from the Shaving category. Electrosurgery used in shaving a superficial lesion burns (destroys) the lesion, so the destruction code would be reported.

The Shaving codes are further defined according to the **location** of the lesion—trunk, neck, nose—and the **size** of the lesion. If more than one lesion was removed, you would add modifier -51 (multiple procedures) to any codes after the first code. For example, if one 2.0-cm lesion was removed from the trunk, and a 1.0-cm lesion was removed from the hand, you would list the 2.0-cm lesion first with no modifier and the 1.0-cm lesion second, with modifier -51 added. Many third-party payers reimburse 100% for the first lesion and 50% for the second lesion, so by placing the more intensive procedure first, you optimize reimbursement.

Excision—Benign Lesions

The CPT manual divides the category of excision of lesions on the basis of whether a lesion is benign or malignant. Although at the time of excision it is not known for certain whether the lesion is benign or malignant, the physician makes an assessment of the lesion's status and usually plans the extent of the excision based on that assessment. The codes in the Excision—Benign Lesions category (11400-11471) are assigned for all benign lesions except skin tags, which you learned about earlier.

The codes include local anesthesia, so do not report local anesthesia separately, as that would be unbundling. The Excision codes also include simple closure (see Fig. 18-5) of the excision site. If the closure is noted in the medical record as being more than simple (intermediate or complex), you would code the more complicated closure using a separate code from Repair subheading (12031-13160).

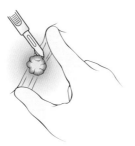

FIGURE 18–11 Shaving of a lesion.

CODING SHOT

You are not to assign the shaving codes if the shaving penetrated through the dermis (full thickness). Full-thickness shavings are to be reported with the excision codes found in the Excision—Benign Lesions or Excision—Malignant Lesions categories.

The codes in the Excision—Benign Lesions category are based on the **location** of the excision (e.g., trunk, scalp, ears, etc.) and the **size** of the lesion (e.g., 0.6-1.0 cm, 1.1-2.0 cm).

CODING SHOT

In excision of either benign or malignant tissue, focus on the dimension of the normal tissue margin excised with the lesion. This normal tissue margin is the determining factor in selecting the correct CPT code.

There are several codes at the end of the category (11450-11471) for excision of the skin and subcutaneous tissue in cases of **hidradenitis** (Fig. 18-12), which is the chronic abscessing and subsequent infection of a sweat gland. The abscess is excised and the wound left open to heal. The hidradenitis codes are based on the abscess location (axillary, inguinal, perianal, perineal, or umbilical) and the complexity of the repair (simple, intermediate, or complex).

Excision—Malignant Lesions

Codes in the Excision—Malignant Lesions subheading (11600-11646) are assigned for malignant lesions and include local anesthesia and simple closure (Fig. 18-13). As with the benign lesion codes, these codes refer to each lesion removed and are divided according to the **location** and **size** of the lesion. If you are coding a lesion removal that has been performed by a method other than excision (e.g., electrosurgery), the notes preceding the Excision codes direct you to the Destruction codes (17260-17286). If the closure is more than simple you would also use a repair code.

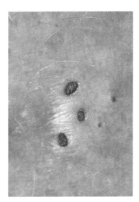

FIGURE 18–12 A hallmark of hidradenitis is the double and triple comedone, a blackhead with two or sometimes several surface openings that communicate under the skin.

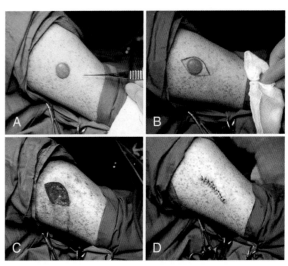

FIGURE 18–13 Excision biopsy technique.

CODING SHOT

If the excision is of a malignant lesion on the eyelid, and if the excision involves more than the skin of the eyelid (lid margin, tarsus, or conjunctiva), do **not** use codes from the Integumentary System chapter of CPT. Instead, you would use a surgery code from the subsection Eye and Ocular Adnexa, Excision category (67800-67850).

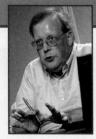

From the Trenches

Would you recommend coding as a profession?

"I would for people who are meticulous and have a mind for detail. . . . People who take pride in their work. Someone who will say, 'I can find things out. I can learn things, and I can make it worthwhile for the physician to employ me.'"

CHRIS

NAILS

Within the Nails category (11719-11765) are codes for the trimming of fingernails and toenails, debridement of nails, removal of nails, drainage of hematomas, biopsies of nails, repair of nails, reconstruction of the nail bed. **Podiatrists** are physicians who specialize in the care of the foot; as such, these physicians use this category of codes extensively. However, all physicians can and do use these codes when providing nail care services to the feet and the hands.

The first code in the Nails category is 11719, which reports the trimming of nails that are not defective. This is a minimal service, and the code reports trimming one fingernail/toenail or many fingernails/toenails. **Debridement** (11720) is a more complex service—the manual cleaning of up to five nails—and it includes the use of various tools, cleaning materials/solutions, and files. You would not report the supplies used for a nail debridement service separately, as these supplies are included in the codes. The two debridement codes are divided according to the number of nails attended to during the service. If the payer requires HCPCS codes, report G0127.

TOOLBOX

Mary presents to the physician for cleaning and trimming of 10 toenails. Mary is handicapped and lives alone and has not had anyone to help her with care of her toenails.

QUESTIONS
1. Which of the following correctly reports the service provided to Mary?
   a. 11720 × 10
   b. 11719 × 10
   c. 11732
   d. 11719
2. Why are you certain this is the correct answer? _____

▼ ANSWERS

1. d, 2. Because the code reports one or many toenail(s)

Avulsion is the separation and removal of the nail plate (11730, 11732), preserving the root so the nail will grow back. An anesthetic is administered, the nail is lifted away from the nail bed, and a portion or all of the nail plate is removed.

Place the number of nails treated in the units column (G) of the CMS-1500 form.

CODING SHOT

Do not use modifier -51 (multiple procedures) with nail removal codes, as there are two codes available: one for a single nail and one for each additional nail. For example, if three nails were removed, you would report: 11730 (for the first nail) and 11732 × 2 (for the second and third nails). Often, third-party payers require the use of HCPCS modifiers (F1-FA to indicate the finger and T1-TA to indicate the toe; Fig. 18-14) and the separate reporting of each digit treated.

A subungual hematoma (blood trapped under the nail) is evacuated by puncturing the nail with an electrocautery needle (11740). The trapped blood and fluid are drained by applying pressure to the top of the nail.

Onychocryptosis (ingrown toenail) is the most common condition of the great toe, as illustrated in Fig. 18-15. The nail grows down and into the soft tissue of the nail fold, causing extreme pain and often infection. Treatment for severe cases is a partial onychectomy (removal of the nail plate and root). The toe is anesthetized and a portion of the nail plate and root is removed (11750-11752). The nail will not grow back where the base has been removed.

CODING SHOT

Use of HCPCS modifiers is very important. For example, nail biopsies (11755) were performed on the left third finger (F2) and the left fourth finger (F3), in addition to the right fourth digit (F8). The reporting would be 11755-F2, 11755-F3, 11755-F8.

F1	Left hand, second digit	T1	Left foot, second digit
F2	Left hand, third digit	T2	Left foot, third digit
F3	Left hand, fourth digit	T3	Left foot, fourth digit
F4	Left hand, fifth digit	T4	Left foot, fifth digit
F5	Right hand, thumb	T5	Right foot, great toe
F6	Right hand, second digit	T6	Right foot, second digit
F7	Right hand, third digit	T7	Right foot, third digit
F8	Right hand, fourth digit	T8	Right foot, fourth digit
F9	Right hand, fifth digit	T9	Right foot, fifth digit
FA	Left hand, thumb	TA	Left foot, great toe

FIGURE 18-14 HCPCS modifiers used to indicate digits of hands and feet.

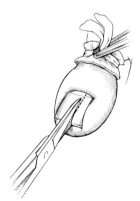

FIGURE 18-15 Removal of ingrown toenail.

Pilonidal Cyst

The codes for the excision of a pilonidal cyst or sinus are 11770-11772. A pilonidal cyst is located in the sacral area and is most often caused by an ingrown hair. The codes are divided according to the complexity of the excision—simple, extensive, or complicated. For a simple cyst, the physician would excise the cyst and suture the skin together. A cyst larger than 2 cm is considered complicated and requires more extensive excision and closure. A complicated excision is very extensive and usually requires reconstructive surgical repair.

Introduction

Within the Introduction category of codes (11900-11983) are lesion injection, tattooing, tissue expansion, contraceptive capsule insertion/removal, and hormone implantation services. Lesions are injected with medication to treat conditions such as acne, keloids (scar tissue), and psoriasis (autoimmune disorder that results in scaly patches). Lesion injection codes are divided according to the number of lesions injected (1-7 or 8+).

CODING SHOT

Lesion injection code 11901 is not an add-on code! You report 11900 for lesion injections numbering one through seven, and 11901 to report injections eight and more. For example, if seven lesions are injected, the service is reported with 11900. If eight lesions are injected, the service is reported with 11901.

Tattooing codes (11920-11922) are also located in the Introduction category. Tattooing is reported on the basis of square centimeters covered. Sometimes physicians use tattooing to disguise birthmarks or scars.

Codes for subcutaneous injection of filling material (11950-11954) are located in the Introduction category and are reported for services such as collagen or silicone injections (injectable dermal implants) used as a wrinkle treatment. The codes are based on the amount of material injected. The procedure is usually repeated at 2 to 3 week intervals until the results are those desired.

Tissue-expander codes (11960-11971) are also located in the Introduction category and report tissue expanders. A tissue expander is an elastic material formed into a sac that is then filled with fluid or air so it expands like a balloon. The expander is placed under the skin and is filled, stretching the skin. Expanders are most often used to prepare a site for a permanent implant. Expanders are also used to assist in the repair of scars and the removal of tattoos by stretching the skin, removing the expander, removing the scar or tattoo, and suturing the skin edges together. The codes are divided according to whether the service is an insertion, a removal, or an expander removal with replacement of a prosthesis.

CODING SHOT

Do not report an expander code from the Introduction category after a mastectomy in which a temporary expander has been inserted. Code 19357 from the reconstruction section of the Integumentary subsection is a combination of the mastectomy and insertion of an expander. If at a later date the expander was replaced with a permanent prosthesis, you would report replacement of tissue expander with permanent prosthesis with 19342.

You will also find insertion of **implantable contraceptive capsules** in the Introduction category. Implantable contraceptive capsules are inserted under the skin by means of a small incision on the upper arm. A capsule is effective for a number of years; at the end of that time, it must be removed. Read the descriptions in the implantable contraceptive capsule codes (11976-11981) carefully, as there are codes for insertion and removal.

In addition to reporting the service of the introduction of the implantable contraceptive capsule, you report the supply of the contraceptive system with HCPCS code J7306 or J7307.

Subcutaneous hormone pellet implantation is commonly used for the insertion of a hormone in a time-release capsule into the buttocks of women requiring hormone replacement therapy after menopause. The code for this implantation is in the Introduction category (11980). The implantation area is anesthetized and the pellet is inserted through a tube. The pellet is completely absorbed into the system and does not need to be removed, as does a contraceptive capsule. However, a new pellet must be inserted every 6 to 9 months, and each reinsertion is reported separately.

EXERCISE 18-1 | *Skin, Subcutaneous, and Accessory Structures*

Apply the information about lesion procedures by coding the following:

1 Paring of three common warts

CPT Code: _____

ICD-10-CM Code: _____ (ICD-9-CM Code: _____)

2 Removal of 15 skin tags

CPT Code: _____

ICD-10-CM Code: _____ (ICD-9-CM Code: _____)

3 Shaving of 1-cm dermal lesion of face

CPT Code: _____

ICD-10-CM Code: _____ (ICD-9-CM Code: _____)

(Answers are located in Appendix B)

REPAIR (CLOSURE)

Repair Factors

When reporting integumentary wound repair, the following three factors must be considered:
1. Length of the wound in centimeters
2. Complexity of the repair
3. Site of the wound repair

Remember **length, complexity,** and **site.** Fig. 18-16 illustrates an example from the CPT manual of these three factors in the wound repair codes.

There are many different types of wounds (Fig. 18-17). Wound repair is classified by the type of repair necessary to repair the wound. There are three types of repair:
1. **Simple:** Superficial wound repair (12001-12021) that involves epidermis, dermis, and subcutaneous tissue (Fig. 18-18) and requires only simple, one-layer suturing. If the simple wound repair is accomplished with tape or adhesive strips, the charge for the closure is included in the E/M service code and would not be reported separately with a repair code. The repair codes are for suture closure.

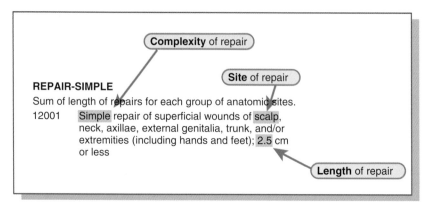

FIGURE 18−16 Wound repair. Note that metric measure is used throughout the CPT manual.

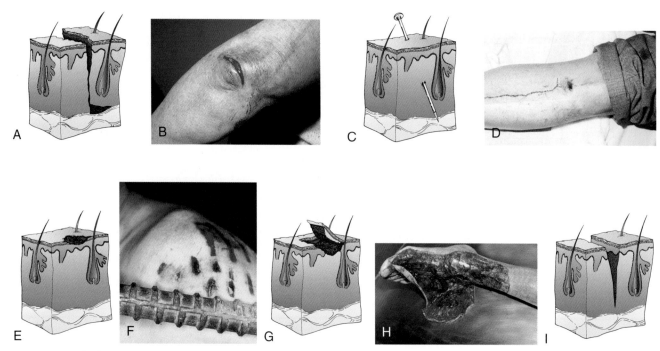

FIGURE 18−17 Types of wounds. **A** and **B**, Laceration. **C** and **D**, Puncture. **E** and **F**, Abrasion. **G** and **H**, Avulsion. **I**, Incision.

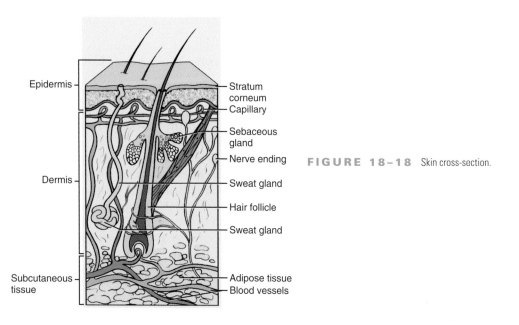

FIGURE 18−18 Skin cross-section.

2. **Intermediate:** Requires closure of one or more layers of subcutaneous tissue and superficial (non-muscle) fascia, in addition to the skin closure. You can report intermediate closure (12031-12057) when the wound has to be extensively cleaned, even if the closure was a single-layer (simple) closure.

3. **Complex:** Involves complicated wound closure including revision, debridement, extensive undermining, stents or retention sutures, and more than layered closure (13100-13160).

From the Trenches

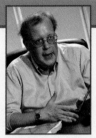

"[It's my job] to make sure physicians are saying [everything] into their microrecorder, or writing it down. You would be surprised how many physicians [diagnose a patient] mentally, as an automatic thing as part of their evaluation of the patient's condition—then they do the medical decision making on how to treat the patient. Sometimes a third of it doesn't even get put down, and the coder can only count that third of information, until it's in the record . . . . I've told doctors 'You dictated this, and this is all you're going to get' so they can see the consequences."

CHRIS

CODING SHOT

HCPCS code **G0168** reports skin closures using adhesives (such as Dermabond, a special glue that is put into the wound, the edges are closed together; a bandage is placed over the wound). Most other third-party payers use the simple repair code to report skin closures using adhesives. Medicare requires G0168.

For each anatomic site, the lengths of wounds are totaled together by complexity (simple, intermediate, complex). All the simple wounds of the same site grouping are reported together; all the intermediate wounds of the same site grouping are reported together; and all the complex wounds of the same site grouping are reported together. The codes group together sites that require similar techniques to repair. For example, 12001 groups superficial scalp, neck, axillae, external genitalia, trunk, and extremities (including hands and feet). When there is more than one repair type, the **most complex** type is listed as the first (primary) procedure. The secondary procedure is then reported using modifier -59 (distinct procedural service).

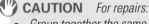

CAUTION *For repairs:*
- Group together the same anatomic **sites,** *such as* face and hand.
- Group together the same **classification,** *such as* simple or intermediate.

The CPT manual notes located under the subheading Repair (Closure) include extensive definitions of each level of repair. These notes must be read carefully before you code repairs.

Repair Component

Three things are considered components (parts) of integumentary wound repair:

1. Simple **ligation** (tying) of small vessels is considered part of the wound repair and is not reported separately. Simple ligation of medium or major arteries in a wound is, however, reported separately.
2. Simple **exploration** of surrounding tissue, nerves, vessels, and tendons is considered part of the wound repair process and is not listed separately.
3. Normal **debridement** (cleaning and removing skin or tissue from the wound until normal, healthy tissue is exposed) is not listed separately.

If the wound is grossly contaminated and requires extensive debridement, a separate debridement procedure may be assigned (11000-11047 for extensive debridement). Fig. 18-19 illustrates a surgical type of debridement.

Tissue Transfers, Grafts, and Flaps

There are many types of grafting procedures that can be performed to correct a defect (e.g., adjacent tissue transfers or rearrangements, skin replacement surgery and skin substitutes, flaps). To understand skin grafting, you must know that the **recipient site** is the area of defect that receives the graft, and the **donor site** is the area from which the healthy skin has been taken for grafting. (If a skin graft is required to close the donor site, the closure is reported as an additional procedure.) A brief description follows of some different types of skin grafting and coding guidelines specific to their assignment.

Adjacent Tissue Transfer or Rearrangement. There are many types of adjacent tissue transfers (14000-14350). Some of them are Z-plasty (Fig. 18-20), W-plasty, V-Y plasty, rotation flaps (Fig. 18-21), and advancement flaps. These procedures are various methods of moving a segment of skin from one area to an adjacent area, while leaving at least one side of the flap (moved skin) intact to retain some measure of blood supply to the graft. Incisions are made, and the skin is undermined and moved over to cover the defective area, leaving the base (connected portion) intact. The flap is then sutured into place.

Adjacent tissue transfers are reported according to the size of the **recipient site.** The size is measured in square centimeters (1 inch equals 2.54 cm). Simple repair of the donor site is included in the tissue transfer code and is not reported separately. If there is a complex closure, or grafting of the donor site, this could be reported separately. Adjacent Tissue Transfer or Rearrangement (14000-14350) in the CPT manual is divided based on the **location** of the defect (trunk or arm) and the **size** of the defect. In addition, there are codes at the end of the category for coding defects that are extremely complicated. When skin grafting is required to cover both the primary defect (results from the excision) and the secondary defect (results from the flap design), the measurements of each defect are added together to determine the code selection for the graft.

Any excision of a lesion that is repaired by adjacent tissue transfer is included in the tissue transfer code. If you reported the excision in addition to the transfer, it would be considered unbundling.

Adjacent tissue transfer codes can be located in the CPT manual index under the main term "Skin" and subterm "Adjacent Tissue Transfer."

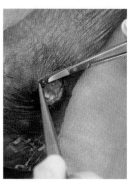

FIGURE 18–19 Surgical debridement for the removal of periwound nonmigratory tissue using a pair of scissors and forceps.

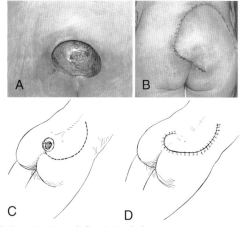

FIGURE 18–21 **A,** Sacral ulcer. **B,** Closure by a large rotation flap based superiorly. **C** and **D,** Outline of flap and rotation downward and medially.

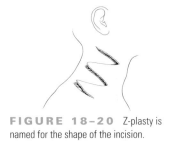

FIGURE 18–20 Z-plasty is named for the shape of the incision.

Skin Replacement Surgery (15002-15278). These codes report surgical site preparation (15002-15261) using a variety of grafting materials and repair methods using skin or skin substitutes. The site of the defect (recipient site) may require surgical preparation before repair, and is reported with 15002-15005 based on the size of repair and site. Free skin grafts (such as 15100/15101 and 15120/15121) are pieces of skin that are either **split thickness** (epidermis and part of the dermis) or **full thickness** (epidermis and all of the dermis) as illustrated in Fig. 18-22. The grafts are completely freed from the donor site and placed over the recipient site. There is no connection left between the graft and the donor site (Fig. 18-23). Free skin grafts are reported by recipient **site, size** of defect, and **type** of repair. The size is measured in square centimeters.

Many of the code definitions in the Skin Replacement Surgery and Skin Substitutes category refer to a measurement in square centimeters and a percentage of body area. The square centimeters measurement is applied to adults and children over 10 years of age, and the percentage of body area is applied to infants and children under the age of 10.

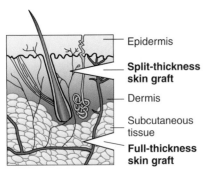

FIGURE 18-22   Split-thickness skin graft and full-thickness skin graft.

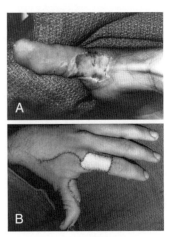

FIGURE 18-23   **A,** Small, localized, full-thickness burn of the first web space. **B,** Immediate postoperative results, after a dorsal metacarpal artery flap was transposed into the defect.

A **pinch graft** (15050) is a small, split-thickness repair. Often a split-thickness graft is referred to in the patient record as STSG, and a full-thickness skin graft as FTSG.

Autografts are grafts that are taken from the patient's body (Fig. 18-24), whereas **allografts** (homografts) are grafts that are taken from a human donor. Epidermal autografts (15110-15116) and dermal **autografts** (15130-15136) are reported based on graft depth, location, and size. Tissue cultured skin autografts (15150-15157) are grafts that are cultured (grown) from the patient's own skin cells, thereby reducing the chances of rejection. **Acellular** dermal replacement (15271-15278) is the use of skin replacement products based on the location and size of repair. **Temporary** allografts are also reported with 15271-15278 based on the location and size of repair. Temporary grafts are used to protect defect sites while healing is taking place (Figs. 18-25 and 18-26). A **permanent** graft may be placed over the site at a later date to complete the repair process.

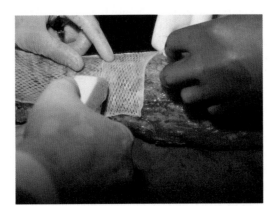

FIGURE 18-24   Appearance during application of meshed autograft.

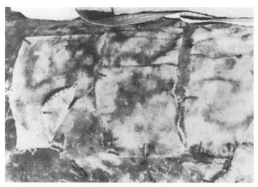

FIGURE 18-25 Three sheets of cultured epithelial autograft are in place on the left anterior thigh, which 3 weeks before was excised to muscle fascia and covered with cadaver allograft.

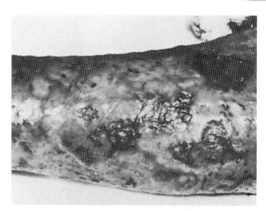

FIGURE 18-26 The same area of left anterior thigh in Fig. 18-25, 1 month after grafting.

Allograft/Tissue Cultured Allogeneic Skin Substitutes (15040-15261) are grafts obtained from a donor genetically different, but of the same species, which include healthy cadaveric donors. Xenografts are grafts taken from a different species (cross species, such as pigskin grafts). Xenografts are also known as heterografts.

Skin Substitute Grafts are reported based on the wound surface area. For areas up to 100 square centimeters (sq cm) of the trunk, arms, or legs, report 15271 for the first 25 sq cm and 15272 for each additional 25 sq cm or part thereof. For areas on the face, scalp, eyelids, mouth, neck, ears, orbits, genitalia, hands, feet, or multiple digits, report 15275 for the first 25 sq cm and 15276 for each additional sq cm. For wound surface areas greater than or equal to 100 sq cm, report 15273/15274 or 15277/15278 based on the location of the area. The supply of the skin substitute graft(s) are reported separately.

Flaps. A physician may develop a donor site at a location far away from the recipient site. The graft may have to be accomplished in stages. The graft code can be assigned more than once when the surgery is performed in stages. Notes specific to this group of codes state that when reporting transfer flaps (in several stages), report the **donor site** when a tube graft (Fig. 18-27) is formed for later use or when a delayed flap is formed before it is transferred (Fig. 18-28). The **recipient site** is reported when the graft is attached to its final site.

In a **delayed graft,** a portion of the skin is lifted and separated from the tissue below, but it stays connected to blood vessels at one end. This keeps the skin viable while it is being moved from one area to another, and at the same time, it allows the graft to get used to living on a small supply of blood. It is hoped that living on a small blood supply will give the graft a better chance of survival when inserted into the recipient site.

There are two categories of codes for flaps. The first category, Flaps (Skin and/or Deep Tissues) (15570-15738), is subdivided based on the type of flap (i.e., pedicle, cross finger, delayed, or muscle flaps) and then by the location of the flap (scalp, trunk, or lips). The codes do not include any extensive immobilization that may be necessary, such as a large plaster cast. Extensive immobilization would be reported in addition to the flap procedure. Also not included in the flap procedure codes is the closure of a donor site, which would be reported in addition to the flap procedure.

The second category, Other Flaps and Grafts (15740-15777), is subdivided based on the type of flap (free muscle, free skin, fascial, or hair transplant).

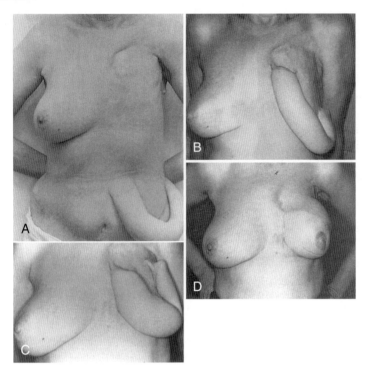

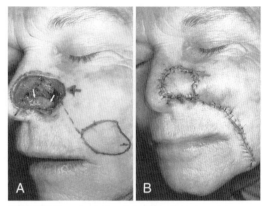

FIGURE 18–28 **A,** A skin and soft tissue defect extends from alar lobule into medial cheek. The cheek advancement flap is designed to repair cheek defect. Separate subcutaneous pedicle transposition flap is designed to resurface the alar lobule after placement of auricular cartilage graft (arrows) along the missing alar margin. **B,** Two flaps are in position.

FIGURE 18–27 **A,** Correction of a radical mastectomy defect with a tube flap, created from the abdominal pannus. **B,** Intermediate inset of the tube flap following separation from its abdominal blood supply. This process of "waltzing" or "walking" a tube-flap from the abdomen to the chest was used by Halsted and Billroth. **C,** Final inset into the sternum before shaping. **D,** The lateral half of the tube flap was then detached laterally and inset into the upper sternum to create the breast shape. This type of reconstruction usually took more than a year to complete, with more than a dozen procedures.

Within the flap codes (15740-15750) the flap (donor site and recipient site remain connected for a period of time) can be an island pedicle or a neurovascular pedicle. The pedicle is the end of the flap that remains connected to the donor area. An **island pedicle flap** contains an artery and vein, and a **neurovascular pedicle flap** contains an artery, vein, and nerve. The term "island" refers to the removal of the fat and subcutaneous tissue prior to implantation into the recipient site. The neurovascular pedicle flap is used when the area of defect requires restoration of sensation in the area; for example, the end of a finger that has sustained damage that destroyed the sensation on the tip of the finger. A neurovascular graft from an adjacent finger could restore sensation to the defective area. A flap from the donor area is freed up and grafted into the recipient area. The connection between the donor and the recipient sites remains in place until the graft has satisfactorily healed, at which time the connection is severed. The donor area may require a separate skin graft, and that graft would be reported separately.

QUICK CHECK 18-2

There are three types of measurements utilized in the Integumentary System subsection of the CPT manual. Match the procedure with the type of measurement.

a. length in cm
b. area in square cm
c. diameter in cm

1. Skin Grafts/Flaps _____
2. Lesion Removal _____
3. Wound Repair   _____

(Answers are located in Appendix C)

Other Procedures

The Other Procedures codes (15780-15879) report a wide variety of repair services, such as abrasion, chemical peel, and blepharoplasty (surgical reconstruction of the eyelid). The codes are often divided based on the site or extent of repair.

Dermabrasion is used to treat acne, wrinkles, or general keratoses (horny growth) (Fig. 18-29). The skin area is anesthetized by a chemical that freezes the area (a cryogen), and the area is sanded down using a motorized brush. The facial dermabrasion codes (15780-15781) are divided according to the surface area of the face treated (total, segmental). Areas other than the face are reported with 15782.

A tattoo can be removed by dermabrasion. The process involves the use of a high-speed mechanical wheel to remove the epidermis and part of the papillary dermis. The service is reported with code 15783.

The **abrasion** codes (15786, 15787) report the use of abrasion to remove a lesion, such as scar tissue, a wart, or a callus. This technique is often used to remove areas of sun-damaged skin. The first abraded lesion is reported with 15786, and each additional four or fewer lesions are reported with 15787.

Chemical peels, also known as chemexfoliation, are treatments in which a chemical is applied to the skin and then removed (Fig. 18-30). The skin surface will then shed its outer layer, much as it does after a sunburn. The treatment is used for cosmetic purposes, such as smoothing the wrinkles around the mouth or removing liver spots (lentigines) (Fig. 18-31). The chemical peel codes (15788-15793) are divided according to whether the peel is on the face or not on the face, in addition to the depth of the peel (epidermal or dermal).

Cervicoplasty, 15819, is a surgical procedure in which the physician removes excess skin from the neck, usually for cosmetic reasons. **Blepharoplasty** (15820-15823), also performed predominantly for cosmetic purposes, is the removal of excess skin and to support the muscles of the upper eyelid. Rhytidectomy is the removal of wrinkles by pulling the skin tight and removing the excess. **Rhytidectomy** codes (15824-15829) report

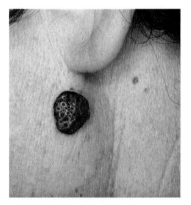

FIGURE 18–29 Large and disfiguring seborrheic keratosis reveals evidence of horn pearls.

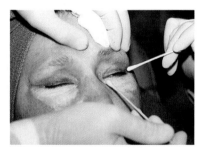

FIGURE 18–30 Chemical peel.

these cosmetic services. Excision of excess skin and subcutaneous tissue of other parts of the body (e.g., abdomen, thigh, buttock, and arm) most commonly due to bariatric surgery is reported with codes in the 15830-15839 range. To report abdominoplasty with panniculectomy (excision of the hanging tissue in the abdominal region [Fig. 18-32]), report 15830 with add-on code 15847.

Grafts for facial nerve paralysis (15840-15845) are procedures in which the physician harvests a graft from some location on the body and places the graft over the area damaged by facial paralysis.

There are also codes in the Other Procedures category for the removal of sutures and for dressing changes (15850-15852) performed under anesthesia.

Lipectomy (liposuction) codes (15876-15879) are divided according to the body area being treated—head, trunk, upper extremities, and lower extremity. If the procedure is performed bilaterally, add modifier -50 to the procedure code.

Pressure Ulcers

Pressure ulcers are also known as decubitus ulcers or bedsores (Fig. 18-33, *A*). Pressure ulcers are located on areas of the body that have bony projections, such as the hips and the area above the tailbone. Pressure on these areas causes decreased blood flow, and sores form. With continued pressure, the sores ulcerate, and deeper layers of tissue, such as fascia, muscle, and bone, may be affected. As illustrated in Fig. 18-33, *B,* the depth of the ulcer is referred to in stages—1, 2, 3, 4. Pressure ulcers commonly occur in patients who are unable to change position or have devices that prevent mobility (splints, casts).

Although a pressure ulcer can be seen, the depth to which the ulceration has penetrated cannot be seen. The ulcer may involve only superficial skin or may affect deeper layers. The treatment for a pressure ulcer (15920-15999) is excision of the ulcerated area to the depth of unaffected tissue, fascia, or muscle.

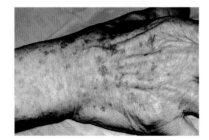

FIGURE 18–31 Lentigines of the hand.

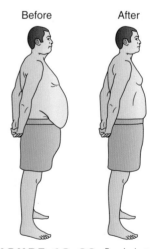

Before   After

FIGURE 18–32 Panniculectomy.

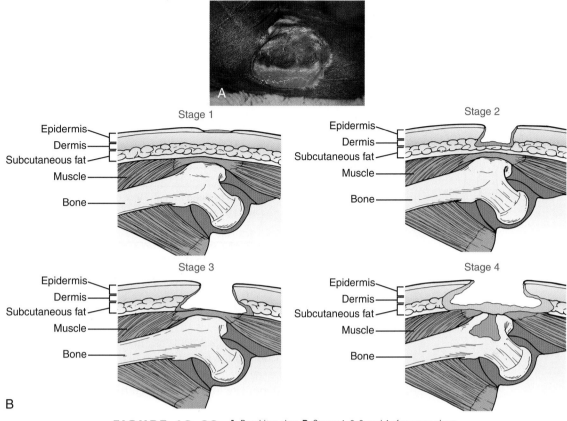

FIGURE 18–33   A, Decubitus ulcer. **B,** Stages 1, 2, 3, and 4 of pressure ulcers.

CODING SHOT

Only an adjacent tissue transfer is bundled into the pressure ulcer codes. If the medical record indicates a myocutaneous flap closure, or a muscle flap, report codes from both the Pressure Ulcer category (15920-15999) and from the Flaps (Skin and/or Deep Tissue) category (15570-15738). Also, if a free skin graft is used to close the ulcer, that closure would be reported separately with a code from the Other Flaps and Grafts category.

You will note that many of the Pressure Ulcer codes have "with ostectomy" as the indented code. An **ostectomy** is the removal of the bone that underlies the ulcer area. The bony prominences are chiseled or filed down to alleviate future pressure. The operative report will indicate if the bone was removed.

Read the code descriptions carefully when coding from the ulcer repair category, as the codes are divided based on the location, type, and extent of closure required.

BURNS

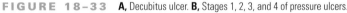

Fig. 18-34 illustrates the Rule of Nines, which is used to calculate the percentage of body area in adults. Fig. 18-35 illustrates the Lund-Browder classification of burns, which is often used to calculate the percentage of body area in infants. Although the Lund-Browder approach

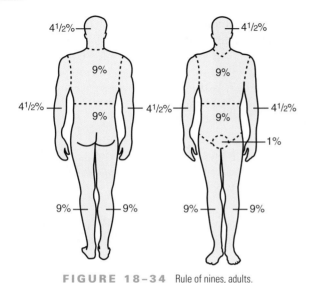

FIGURE 18-34 Rule of nines, adults.

Relative percentage of body surface areas (% BSA) affected by growth

	0 yr	1 yr	5 yr	10 yr	15 yr
a – 1/2 of head	9¹/₂	8¹/₂	6¹/₂	5¹/₂	4¹/₂
b – 1/2 of 1 thigh	2³/₄	3¹/₄	4	4¹/₄	4¹/₂
c – 1/2 of lower leg	2¹/₂	2¹/₂	2³/₄	3	3¹/₄

FIGURE 18-35 Lund-Browder chart for estimating the extent of burns on children.

is similar to the Rule of Nines, adjustments are made in the percentages because an infant's head is larger in proportion to the rest of his or her body. On the job, the medical coder is not required to calculate the percentage, as the physician is to indicate the percentages in the medical record. If the donor site for the graft requires repair by grafting, an additional graft code is used. Simple repair (closure) of the donor site is included in the graft code.

Burns are classified as first, second, or third degree based on the depth of the burn. If the medical documentation indicated a burn of the epidermis, that is a first degree burn, a dermal burn is a second degree, and a subcutaneous level burn is third degree (Fig. 18-36). The documentation should indicate the degree of burn at each location, and the physician should be queried if the degree is not stated.

Burn treatment is unique in that it is common for a patient to undergo multiple dressing changes or debridements (Fig. 18-37) during the healing period. Dressing and debridement codes report either initial or subsequent treatments. Burn dressing and/or debridement codes (16020-16030) are divided based on whether the dressing or debridement is of a small, medium, or large area. The definition of small is less than 5% of the total body surface area, medium is the whole face or whole extremity, or 5% to 10% of the total body surface area, and large is more than one extremity or greater than 10% of the total body area.

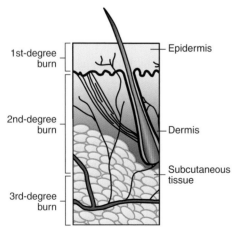

FIGURE 18-36 First-, second-, and third-degree burns.

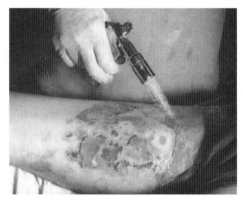

FIGURE 18-37 Burn debridement.

Bundled into codes 16000-16036 is the application of dressing, such as temporary skin replacement. The notes in the Burn, Local Treatment category state 16020-16030 include application of materials (e.g., dressings) not described in codes 15100-15278. Some third-party providers bundle materials, such as Biobrane, into the Burn, Local Treatment codes. Biobrane® is a biosynthetic skin substitute that is constructed of a silicone film with a nylon fabric embedded into the film. Collagen is then embedded into the film and fabric. There are small pores on the skin substitute to make the covering permeable to allow for the application of topical antibiotics during healing.

The Burn category contains codes for **escharotomy** (16035, 16036), a procedure in which the physician cuts through the dead skin that covers the surface when there is a full-thickness burn. The crust covers the surface and diminishes blood flow and healing.

CODING SHOT

Some third-party payers allow you to submit charges for burn care using the first date of service to the last date of service. This allows you to indicate multiples of the same service (e.g., ×5 or ×3). Other payers require you to list each date of service and to report each service separately. For example, if the patient received five burn debridements on five separate days, you would report the CPT code five separate times, once for each day of service.

EXERCISE 18-2   *Repair (Closure) and Burns*

The patient record states: **"simple wound repair 12-cm wound, left hand."**

To locate the code for the repair in the CPT manual Index using the condition method, you first locate the main term **Wound,** and then the subterm **Repair.** Wound is the condition and Repair is the procedure. You then identify the type of repair (i.e., complex, simple).

To locate the code using the service or procedure method, you would first locate the main term, **Repair.** Repair is the service or procedure. The subterm **Wound** is located next, and finally the type (i.e., complex, simple). These are just two of the ways to locate this service in the Index.

From the main term Wound, subterms Repair, Simple, you are directed to a range of codes, 12001-12021. Locate this range in the CPT manual. The notes under the subheading, Repair (Closure), are "must" reading. Also, read the description of the first code in the category (12001). The description specifies that the code includes the term hands, which is what you are looking for. Now locate the correct length (12 cm), and you will have the correct code—12004.

Now you code the following:

The patient record states: complex wound repair on right hand, 3.1 cm.

1 What are the correct codes?

CPT Code: _____

ICD-10-CM Code: _____ (ICD-9-CM Code: _____)

2 After an assault with a knife, a patient requires simple repair of a 3-cm laceration of the neck, simple repair of a 4-cm laceration of the back, simple repair of a 5-cm laceration of the forearm, and complex repair of a 3-cm laceration of the abdomen. (Note: Remember to use modifier -59 with the least intensive repair.)

CPT Codes: _____, _____

3 Harry Torgerson, a 42-year-old construction worker, is injured at work when a box containing wood scraps and shingles falls from a second story scaffolding and strikes him on the left forearm, causing multiple lacerations. Forearm repairs: a 5.1-cm repair of the subcutaneous tissues (intermediate closure) and a 5.6-cm laceration, with particles of shingles and wood materials deeply embedded, (complex closure). There is also a superficial wound of the scalp of 3.1 cm that requires simple closure.

CPT Codes: _____, _____, _____

Continued

4 A patient with multiple healed scars requests they be removed and repaired for cosmetic reasons. The defects include a 100-cm² scar of the right cheek and a 200-cm² defect of the left upper chest. Several split-thickness skin grafts totaling 300 cm² are harvested from the left and right thighs. The scar tissue is cut away, and the sites are prepared for grafting.

Cheek graft: _____

Upper chest graft: _____, _____

Site prep, cheek, 100 cm²: _____

Site prep, chest, 200 cm²: _____, _____

5 The patient had a 20-cm² defect of the right cheek that was repaired with a rotation flap (adjacent tissue transfer).

CPT Code: _____

6 The patient had a 10-cm² malignant neoplasm removed from the forehead. Z-plasty was used to repair this site. How would the excision and repair be coded?

CPT Code: _____

7 A patient has had a portion of his mandible removed due to excision of a malignant tumor. Repair of the site is now performed by use of a myocutaneous flap graft.

CPT Code: _____

8 A patient incurs second- and third-degree burns of the abdomen and thigh (10%) when she pulls a pan of boiling water off the stove. She requires daily debridements or dressing changes for the first week (Monday through Friday, ×5). She is in severe pain and requires anesthesia during these treatments. During the following 2 weeks she will be receiving dressing changes every other day (Monday, Wednesday, Friday, ×6), and it is expected that enough healing will have taken place that anesthesia will not be necessary. What codes would be reported for services during the 3-week treatment period?

Week 1 CPT Code: _____

Weeks 2 and 3 CPT Code: _____

(Answers are located in Appendix B)

DESTRUCTION

The next subheading in the subsection of the Integumentary System is Destruction. The codes report destruction of lesions by means **other than excision.** Codes 17000-17286 are for benign, premalignant, or malignant lesions destroyed by means of electrosurgery (use of various forms of electrical current to destroy the lesion), cryosurgery (use of extreme cold), laser (Light Amplification by Stimulated Emission of Radiation), or chemicals (acids). Read the notes under the Destruction subsection heading because they contain a list of types of lesions. Destruction codes state "any method" and are divided according to type of lesion (benign or malignant). Further divisions are based on the number of lesions destroyed or the size of the area destroyed. The malignant lesions are divided based on location (nose, ear, and so forth) and size (0.6-1.0 cm, and so forth), regardless of the method used.

Codes 17000-17004 report destruction of lesions by the number treated. For example, a patient goes to his or her physician to have 20 lesions removed using cryosurgery reported with 17004. If the patient had six lesions removed, the first one would be reported with 17000 and lesions two through six are reported with 17003 × 5. Careful reading of the coding guidelines is a must for proper reporting of destruction codes.

Mohs Micrographic Surgery

One sophisticated procedure is Mohs micrographic surgery (17311-17315). The method is named after the physician who pioneered the basic microscopic technique, Frederic Mohs, MD. The microscope is used during the surgical procedure to view the lesion and assess its invasion by a single physician acting in two separate and distinct capacities—surgeon and pathologist. If another physician is delegated the role of pathologist, these codes should not be reported. If the lesion is malignant, it is immediately removed. Mohs micrographic surgery is especially useful in cases of large tumors. The procedure involves mapping the exact contour

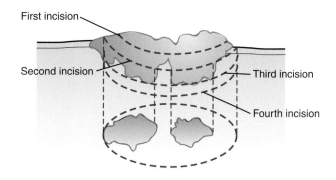

FIGURE 18–38 Mohs micrographic surgical technique.

of the tumor and removing tissue down to the level at which cancerous cells are no longer found. The process involves stages in which the surgeon removes a layer of skin and examines it under a microscope for cancerous cells, then returns to the lesion to remove another layer of skin, again examining it under a microscope (Fig. 18-38). This process is continued until cancerous cells are no longer identified in the layers being removed. The surgeon acts as both the pathologist and the surgeon.

From the Trenches

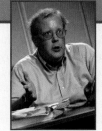

"Find a subspecialty you like . . . [and] if it's a surgical subspecialty, get as many operative reports as you can. Read them. Compare the codes in the book to what's on the operative report. See if you can get into the operating room with the doctors . . . [and] know your sterile field techniques so you know what NOT to touch!"

CHRIS

The codes in the category include the removal of the lesion(s) and pathologic evaluation of the lesion(s). These codes are also divided based on the stage (e.g., first, second) of the surgery and the number of tissue blocks the surgeon takes during the surgery for pathologic examination.

A new patient presents to the dermatologist with a lesion, and the dermatologist performs a biopsy that he then examines in the office using a microscope. His determination is that the lesion is basal cell carcinoma, and he advises the patient to have the lesion removed the same day using Mohs microscopic technique. The patient consents to this and the dermatologist makes arrangements to remove the lesion later that day. According to the notes before 17311, if a biopsy of a suspected skin cancer is "performed on the same day as Mohs surgery because there was no prior pathology confirmation of a diagnosis, then report diagnostic skin biopsy (11100, 11101) and frozen section pathology (88331) with modifier 59 to distinguish from the subsequent definitive surgical procedure of Mohs surgery." This means that you would report 11100-59 and add-on code 11101-59 (biopsy service), if more than one biopsy was performed and 88331-59 (pathology service) because the primary procedure is the Mohs surgery (17311).

QUICK CHECK 18-3

1. The Mohs notes before 17311-17315 indicate repairs are:
   a. bundled
   b. reported separately

(Answers are located in Appendix C)

EXERCISE 18-3 *Destruction*

1 Electrosurgical destruction of a herpetic lesion

CPT Code: _____

2 Cryosurgical destruction of 14 actinic keratoses

CPT Codes: _____, _____ × _____

ICD-10-CM Code: _____ (ICD-9-CM Code: _____)

3 Mohs micrographic surgery by a single physician removing and examining three specimens, first stage of the neck

⊛ CPT Code(s): _____

(Answers are located in Appendix B)

BREAST PROCEDURES

Breast procedures (19000-19499) are divided according to category of procedure (e.g., incision, excision, introduction, repair and/or reconstruction). You must read the documentation to identify the procedure used, such as incisional versus excisional biopsies. In an **incisional biopsy**, an incision is made into the lesion and a small portion of the lesion is taken out. In an **excisional biopsy**, the entire lesion is removed for biopsy. In some cases it may be necessary to mark the lesion preoperatively by placing a marker to identify its exact location (Fig. 18-39). The marker or location device is placed to allow the physician to precisely identify the depth and position of the needle placement to obtain a breast tissue biopsy. After the biopsy, the location device may be left in place to identify the biopsied area on subsequent mammography. Percutaneous breast biopsies are reported with 19081-19086 based on the guidance method. A location device (clip, metallic pellet, wire, needle, radioactive seed) placed without a biopsy is reported with 19281-19288 based on the guidance method.

There are many mastectomy codes, and you need to carefully review the operative report to confirm whether pectoral muscles, axillary lymph nodes, or internal mammary lymph nodes were also removed. This information will be necessary to determine the correct mastectomy code.

A **partial** mastectomy (19301) is one in which only a portion of the breast tissue is removed. If an axillary lymphadenectomy is performed with a partial mastectomy, report the service with 19302. A partial mastectomy is also known as a lumpectomy, segmentectomy, or tylectomy. Fig. 18-40 illustrates the quadrants and axillary tail of the breast. Fig. 18-41 illustrates the simple, modified radical, radical, and partial mastectomies.

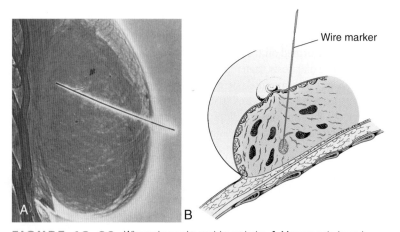

FIGURE 18–39 Wire marker used to mark breast lesion. **A,** Mammography is used to place a preoperative needle used to mark a lesion. **B,** The wire marker serves as a guide for the surgeon to perform the biopsy.

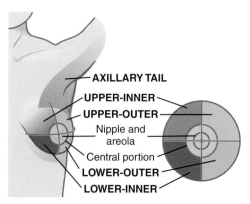

FIGURE 18–40 Female breast quadrants and axillary tail.

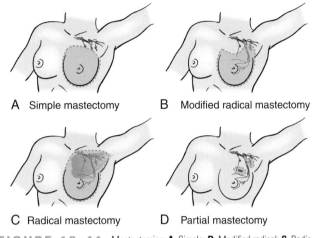

A Simple mastectomy   **B** Modified radical mastectomy

C Radical mastectomy   **D** Partial mastectomy

FIGURE 18–41 Mastectomies: **A,** Simple; **B,** Modified radical; **C,** Radical; **D,** Partial.

A **simple** or **complete** mastectomy (19303) is one in which all of the subcutaneous tissue and breast tissue are removed and the nipple and skin may or may not be removed. A **subcutaneous** mastectomy (19304) is one in which the skin and muscle is left but all the breast tissue is removed.

A **modified radical** mastectomy (19307) is one in which the breast is removed in addition to the axillary lymph nodes, and the pectoralis minor muscle may or may not be removed. The pectoralis major muscle is not removed in the modified radical mastectomy.

A **radical** mastectomy (19305) is one in which the entire breast is removed in addition to the pectoral muscles and axillary lymph nodes (Fig. 18-42). Code 19306 reports another type of radical mastectomy that includes the internal mammary lymph nodes and is also known as an Urban type operation.

A breast lesion is often identified as a result of a screening mammogram, and a breast biopsy is then scheduled. During the biopsy, a specimen is obtained and sent to the pathologist for analysis. This biopsy is reported separately and is not bundled into the screening mammogram or any subsequent procedure. However, if a biopsy is obtained in the operating room and based on the results of the biopsy, a mastectomy is performed, the biopsy is bundled into the mastectomy.

The Repair and/or Reconstruction codes 19316-19396 include codes to report breast reduction (19318), augmentation (breast enlargement, 19324, 19325), and breast reconstruction (19357-19369). The reconstruction for 19357 includes the insertion of a tissue expander and the subsequent expansion. The tissue expander is placed to stretch the skin overlying the breast to allow for insertion of a permanent prosthesis.

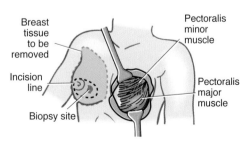

FIGURE 18–42 Mastectomy procedure.

CODING SHOT

Any breast procedure performed on **both** breasts must be reported as a bilateral procedure (modifier -50).

EXERCISE 18-4   *Breast Procedures*

Locate the correct code for the following procedures. Be sure to read all notes in the CPT manual and the description of the code before applying the code.

1 Aspiration of one cyst, breast

   CPT Code: _____

2 Simple, complete bilateral mastectomies

    CPT Code(s): _____

3 Right modified radical mastectomy, including axillary lymph nodes without any muscles

   CPT Code: _____

4 Preoperative placement of one breast wire by magnetic resonance guidance, left breast

   CPT Code: _____

5 Reconstruction of nipple/areola, right breast

   CPT Code: _____

(Answers are located in Appendix B)

CONGRATULATIONS! You made it through the entire Integumentary System subsection! The subsection is quite complicated, and you have done a great job if you understand the basics of these codes. As you use these codes here and on the job, your knowledge will continue to grow.

CHAPTER REVIEW

What are the three things that are considered components of wound repair?

1 _____

2 _____

3 _____

Wound repair codes are determined by what three criteria?

4 _____

5 _____

6 _____

What are the three classifications of wound repair?

7 _____

8 _____

9 _____

10 Modifier -51 indicates what? _____

11 What is the title for the information that precedes each section? _____

12 _____ is the cleansing of an area or wound.

13 A(n) _____ biopsy may be performed to excise a disc of tissue.

14 What is the term for the elastic material formed into a sac that is then filled with fluid or air? _____

_____

15 What is the name of the graft that is taken from the patient's body? _____

16 The major distinction in coding destruction of lesions is whether the lesion is

_____ or _____.

17 The division of malignant lesion excision is based on _____ and _____.

18 What is the procedure used to treat acne or wrinkles by means of sanding? _____

19 In order to report Mohs surgery, the physician would act as the surgeon and the _____.

20 In a(n) _____ biopsy, the entire lesion is removed for biopsy.

CHAPTER 18, PART II, PRACTICAL

Code the following cases for the surgical procedures and office visits only. Do not code the radiology services or laboratory work that may be included.

21 Margaret Wilson, a 26-year-old mother of three (new patient), has routine screening mammography of both breasts. (You do not need to code the mammography.) A shadow is visualized in the right breast. The physician performs a biopsy (needle core). The biopsy indicates malignancy. The patient agrees to and has a mastectomy (simple, complete) 1 week later.

There is no global period on this procedure. Pathology report indicated a primary malignant neoplasm.

CPT Codes: _____, _____

ICD-10-CM Code: _____

(ICD-9-CM Code: _____)

22 Shirley Peters, age 80, an established patient, presents to the office for removal of 12 skin tags.

CPT Code: _____

ICD-10-CM Code: _____

(ICD-9-CM Code: _____)

23 Removal of 180-cm² strawberry nevus of left cheek, autograft with split-thickness skin graft of 180 cm²

CPT Codes: _____, _____, _____, _____

ICD-10-CM Code: _____

(ICD-9-CM Code: _____)

24 Nipple reconstruction

CPT Code: _____

25 Destruction of 0.4-cm malignant lesion of the neck

CPT Code: _____

26 Simple repair of a superficial wound of the genitalia; 2.4 cm

CPT Code: _____

27 Adjacent tissue transfer of chin defect; 9 cm²

CPT Code: _____

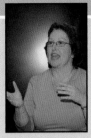

"Be the individual always willing to step in and help. Be the one to recognize issues and have solutions to those issues."

Martha Tracy, CPC, CPC-I
Coding & Compliance Manager
Mid-America Cardiology
Kansas City, Kansas

Musculoskeletal System

Chapter Topics

Format

Fractures and Dislocations

General

Application of Casts and Strapping

Endoscopy/Arthroscopy

Chapter Review

Learning Objectives

After completing this chapter you should be able to

1   Differentiate between fracture and dislocation treatment types.

2   Understand types of traction.

3   Identify services/procedures included in the General subheading.

4   Analyze cast application and strapping procedures.

5   Understand elements of arthroscopic procedures.

6   Demonstrate the ability to code musculoskeletal services and procedures.

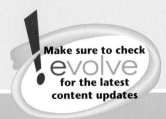

Make sure to check
evolve
for the latest
content updates

FORMAT

The Musculoskeletal System subsection is formatted by anatomic site, such as General, Head, and Neck.

The first subheading in this subsection is General, and it contains procedures that are applicable to many different anatomic sites. The other subheadings are further divided by anatomic site, procedure type, condition, and description. They usually include:

- Incision
- Excision
- Introduction or Removal
- Repair, Revision, and/or Reconstruction
- Fracture and/or Dislocation
- Arthrodesis
- Amputation

Any or all of these categories of procedures may be located under each subheading.

The codes in the Musculoskeletal System subsection are reported extensively by orthopedic surgeons to describe the services provided to restore and preserve the function of the skeletal system. There are many codes, however, that are used frequently by a wide variety of primary care and family practice physicians, such as the splinting, casting, and fracture codes. Your study of the Musculoskeletal subsection of the CPT will focus on the format of the subsection, fracture types and repair, application of casts and strapping, the General subheading, and endoscopic procedures.

Thorough review of the medical record will help you to identify key information necessary for coding. The following tips will help you to choose the most correct code from this subsection:

1. Identify whether the procedure is being performed on soft tissue or bone.
   Many Musculoskeletal System Excision codes to report tumor excision are based on if the tumor is of the:
   - Subcutaneous soft tissue tumors (below the skin but above the deep fascia)
   - Fascial or subfascial soft tissue tumors (within or below deep fascia, but not involving bone)
   - Radical resection of soft tissue tumors (subcutaneous or subfascial but with wide margins, appreciable vessel exploration, and/or repair/reconstruction of nerves)
   - Radical resection of bone tumors (wide margins, appreciable vessel exploration, and/or repair/reconstruction of nerves and complex bone repair/reconstruction)

   Careful reading of Musculoskeletal section guidelines is a must before reporting excision of tumors.

2. Determine whether treatment is for a traumatic injury (acute) or a medical condition (chronic). The diagnosis codes indicating acute or chronic must match the treatment codes. External cause/E codes from ICD-10-CM/ICD-9-CM should also be assigned to describe accidents and injuries.

3. Identify the most specific anatomic site. For example, when coding vertebral procedures, it is necessary to know whether the procedure was for cervical, thoracic, or lumbar vertebrae.

4. Determine whether the code description includes grafting or fixation. If grafting or fixation is not listed within the major procedure code description, each may be reported as an additional procedure.

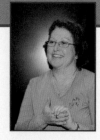

From the Trenches

"Be willing to constantly learn and research questions. Network with other coders, have fun and passion for your job!"

MARTHA

5. Read the code carefully to determine whether it describes a procedure that was on a single site (e.g., each finger). If the same procedure is performed on multiple sites (e.g., multiple fingers), you must indicate the number of units (such as 26060 × 2) or list the code multiple times. HCPCS modifiers are used to identify the digit treated, such as F6 for right hand, second digit.

6. Check any medical terms you do not understand in a medical dictionary or in the Glossary at the back of the book.

FRACTURES AND DISLOCATIONS

Fractures

Fractures are coded by treatment—open, closed, or percutaneous. **Open treatment** of a fracture is made when a surgery is performed in which the fracture is exposed by an incision made over the fracture and the fractured bone is visualized. **Closed treatment** is performed when the physician repairs the fracture without directly visualizing the fracture. The treatment method used—open or closed—depends on the type and severity of the fracture. A closed fracture (Fig. 19-1) may receive either closed, open, or percutaneous fixation, whereas a more complicated compound fracture usually requires an open treatment to provide internal fixation (e.g., wires, pins, screws). Fractures are coded to the specific anatomic site and then according to whether manipulation was performed. All fractures and dislocations are reported based on the reason for the treatment. For instance, if a hip replacement (arthroplasty) is performed for medical reasons, such as **osteoarthritis,** it is reported with 27130, located under the subheading Pelvis and Hip Joint, category Repair, Revision, and/or Reconstruction. The

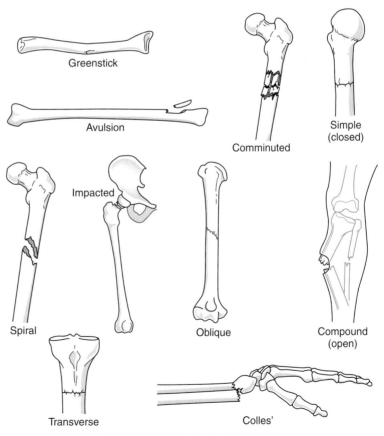

Greenstick

Avulsion

Comminuted

Simple (closed)

Impacted

Spiral

Oblique

Compound (open)

Transverse

Colles'

FIGURE 19-1 Types of fractures.

osteoarthritis that caused the breakdown of the bone of the hip requiring repair was the reason for the treatment. If the hip replacement was performed for a **fracture,** it is reported with 27236, located under the subheading Pelvis and Hip Joint, category Fracture and/or Dislocation. The fracture, which is not a progressive, degenerative disease, was the reason for the treatment.

The CPT manual defines closed, open, and percutaneous treatments as follows:

Closed Treatment: This terminology is used to describe procedures that treat fractures by one of three methods: (1) without manipulation, (2) with manipulation, or (3) with or without traction.

Manipulation is attempted reduction, which is an attempt to maneuver the bone back into proper alignment. The physician may bend, rotate, pull, or guide the bone back into position.

Closed treatment without manipulation is a procedure in which the physician immobilizes the bone with a splint, cast, or other device but without having to manipulate the fracture into alignment. Code 25500 describes a closed treatment of a radial shaft fracture without manipulation. This code is correctly reported when a patient has a broken but stable radial shaft that is not displaced and the physician only applies a cast. Initial casting or splinting services are included in the fracture care, but the supplies used are not. Initial splinting or casting of fractures performed by another physician as the only service can be reported by that physician (i.e., an emergency department physician). If the cast needs to be removed and reapplied during the global period, the surgeon that charged the global fee may report the cast/splint application with 29000-29799 and append modifier -58 (staged or related procedure/service). Only charge for cast removal without reapplication if the physician or physician group is not assuming care for the fracture.

Closed treatment with manipulation is a procedure in which the physician has to reduce (put back in place) a fracture. Code 21320 describes a closed treatment of a nasal bone fracture with stabilization, as illustrated in Fig. 19-2. This code is correctly reported when a patient has a displaced nose that requires manipulation to return it to the normal position. The physician would then apply external and/or internal splints to immobilize the nose.

Open treatment is used when the fracture is opened (exposed to the external environment). In this instance, the fracture (bone) is open to view and internal fixation (pins, screws, etc.) may be used. For example, 23630, open treatment of greater humeral tuberosity fracture, includes internal fixation when performed. The physician opens the site, reduces the fracture, and applies internal fixation, as needed to maintain anatomic position of the fracture.

ICD-10-CM: Fractures are divided based on whether the fracture is pathological (occurred in an area of weakness) or traumatic (due to injury). Fracture codes are reported with a 7th character to indicate whether the fracture care was:

■ Initial or a subsequent encounter
■ Open or closed

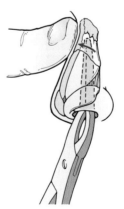

FIGURE 19–2   Realignment and support of nasal fracture.

Open means the fracture has broken through the bone cortex and the bone has been exposed to air (elements).

Closed means the fracture is not exposed to air.

■ Healing was routine or delayed
■ Nonunion

ICD-9-CM: Open treatment can also mean that a remote site (not directly over the fracture) is opened to place a nail (intramedullary) across the fracture site. Fracture is defined as open or closed fracture within the ICD-9-CM, the same as within the ICD-10-CM.

■ **Open** means the fracture has broken through the bone cortex and the bone has been exposed to air (elements).
■ **Closed** means the fracture is not exposed to air.

QUICK CHECK 19-1

1. Which code would be reported for a repair of a femoral shaft fracture using an intramedullary rod?
   a. 27506
   b. 27507

(Answers are located in Appendix C)

Percutaneous skeletal fixation describes fracture treatment that is neither open nor closed. In this procedure, the fracture is not open to view, but fixation (e.g., pin, screw) is placed across the fracture site, usually under x-ray imaging. For example, percutaneous skeletal fixation of a fracture of the great toe, phalanx, or phalanges with manipulation (28496). This procedure is performed entirely percutaneously.

Areas of bones, as Fig. 19-3 illustrates, are important to know when identifying the location of a fracture. For example, there may be an open treatment of a proximal fibula fracture (27784), proximal being closer to the body, or of a distal fibula fracture (27792), distal being further from the body.

CODING SHOT

If the physician attempts a reduction of a fracture but is unable to align the fracture successfully, you still report a reduction service. List the attempted reduction service code and then list the more involved fracture care (i.e., open, endoscopic) the physician successfully performed to reduce the fracture with modifier -58 (staged or related procedure/service) appended.

Traction definitions are as follows:

Traction is the application of pulling force to hold a bone in alignment (Fig. 19-4).

Skeletal traction is the use of internal devices, such as pins, screws, or wires. The devices are inserted into the bone through the skin, with ends of the pins, screws, or wires sticking out through the skin, so traction devices can be attached (Fig. 19-5).

Skin traction involves strapping, elastic wrap, or tape that is fastened to the skin or wrapped around the limb. Weights are then attached to apply force to the fracture (Fig. 19-6).

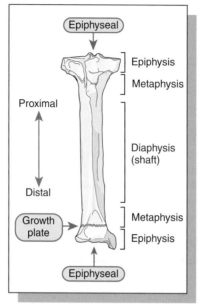

FIGURE 19–3   Areas of the tibia.

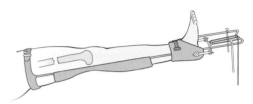

FIGURE 19–4   Traction is the application of a pulling force to hold a bone in alignment.

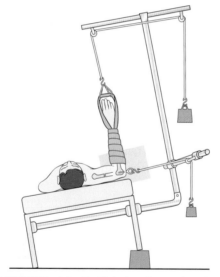

FIGURE 19–5   Skeletal traction uses the patient's bones to secure internal devices to which traction is attached.

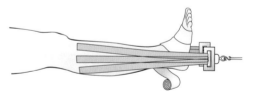

FIGURE 19–6   Skin traction utilizes strapping, wraps, or tape to which traction is attached.

TOOLBOX

Jerry broke his arm when he fell from a tree that he was trimming in his backyard.

QUESTIONS

What three External Cause codes do you assign?_____ (fall = cause), _____ (accident = place), and _____ (activity code)

▼ ANSWERS

ICD-10-CM: W14.XXXA (Fall, from tree, initial encounter), Y92.017 (Accident, house), Y93.H2 (Injury while landscaping); ICD-9-CM: E884.9 (Fall, from, tree); E849.0 (Accident, occurring [at][in] yard, private), E016.1 (Injury while landscaping)

Dislocations

Dislocation is the displacement of a bone from its normal location in a joint (Fig. 19-7), and the treatment of the dislocation injury is to return the bone to its normal location (anatomic alignment) by a variety of methods. For example, if a finger was dislocated and the bone did not protrude through the skin, the physician may administer a digital block (Fig. 19-8) and apply gentle traction until the finger realigns. A splint would then be applied to keep the finger immobile for about 3 weeks. If the shoulder was dislocated, the physician might elevate the arm and rotate the humerus while applying pressure to the head of the humerus. Or the patient might lie face down on a table with the arm hanging off the edge while a weight is attached to the hand; the weight is sufficient to pull the arm back into place (Fig. 19-9). If external measures such as those just described do not relocate the joint, surgical reduction might be indicated.

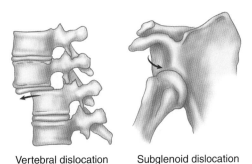

Vertebral dislocation   Subglenoid dislocation

FIGURE 19-7 Vertebral and subglenoid dislocations.

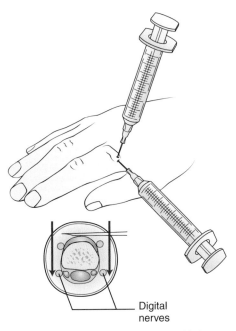

Digital nerves

FIGURE 19-8 Digital nerve block.

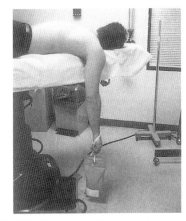

FIGURE 19-9 External technique for relocation of a shoulder (Stimson technique).

QUICK CHECK 19-2

1. According to the Musculoskeletal System notes before 20005, does the type of fracture/ dislocation (i.e., open, closed) determine the type of treatment (e.g., open, closed)?
   Yes or No?

(Answers are located in Appendix C)

EXERCISE 19-1 | *Fractures and Dislocations*

Using the CPT, ICD-10-CM and/or ICD-9-CM manuals, provide the codes for the following:

1 Nasal bone fracture, closed treatment
   CPT Code: _____

2 Uncomplicated, closed treatment of sternum fracture
   CPT Code: _____

3 Interphalangeal joint dislocation of toe, open treatment with internal fixation
   CPT Code: _____

4 Open distal fibula fracture repair with internal fixation
   CPT Code: _____

5 Femoral shaft fracture repair using closed treatment
   CPT Code: _____

6 Percutaneous skeletal fixation of impact fracture of proximal end, femoral neck
   CPT Code: _____

7 Open treatment of shoulder dislocation with closed fracture of the greater humeral tuberosity, non-displaced
   CPT Code: _____
   ICD-10-CM Code: _____ (ICD-9-CM Code: _____)

8 Closed treatment of closed mandibular fracture, including interdental fixation
   CPT Code: _____
   ICD-10-CM Code: _____ (ICD-9-CM Code: _____)

9 Percutaneous skeletal fixation of a closed distal radius fracture
   CPT Code: _____
   ICD-10-CM Code: _____ (ICD-9-CM Code: _____)

10 Closed ankle dislocation, closed treatment
   CPT Code: _____
   ICD-10-CM Code: _____ (ICD-9-CM Code: _____)

(Answers are located in Appendix B)

GENERAL

The first subheading in the Musculoskeletal subsection is General. As the name implies, this subheading includes miscellaneous procedures that are not specific to an anatomic site.

Incision

The first code is 20005, used to report the incision and drainage of a **soft tissue abscess** that is below the deep fascia (subfascial). There are codes in the Integumentary System for incisions that are for skin only. What makes 20005 different from those in the Integumentary System is that 20005 is reported when the abscess is associated with the deep tissue and possibly even down to the bone that underlies the area of abscess. The physician would make an incision into the abscess, explore and clean the abscess, and debride it (remove dead tissue). This procedure is very different from the procedures you report with Integumentary System codes for incision of an abscess.

Wound Exploration

The Wound Exploration codes (20100-20103) report traumatic wounds that result from a penetrating trauma (e.g., gunshot, knife wound). Wound Exploration codes include basic exploration and repair of the area of trauma. These codes are used specifically when the repair requires enlargement of the existing wound for exploration, cleaning, and repair. Included in the Wound Exploration codes are not only the exploration and enlargement of the wound but also debridement, removal of any foreign body(ies), ligation of minor blood vessel(s), and repair of subcutaneous tissues, muscle fascia, and muscle, as would be necessary to repair the wound (Fig. 19-10).

If the wound does not require enlargement, you would report a code from the Integumentary System, Skin Repair codes. If, however, the wound is more severe than a Wound Exploration code would indicate, the repair code would come from the specific repair by anatomic site codes. For example, for a bullet wound to the chest with suspicion of cardiac injury, the treatment will be thoracotomy of any approach, as illustrated in Fig. 19-11, with control of the hemorrhage and repair of any injured intrathoracic organ. The thoracotomy code is located in the subsection Respiratory System under the subheading Lungs. As you can see from this example, you have to assess the extent of the procedure carefully, reading the medical record to ensure you are in the correct area so you can choose the correct code. In the case of the bullet wound to the chest, the wound exploration is included in the thoracotomy and would not be reported separately.

QUICK CHECK 19-3

1. Penetrating wound exploration may be coded from the Musculoskeletal System, Integumentary System, or the appropriate _____ site.

(Answers are located in Appendix C)

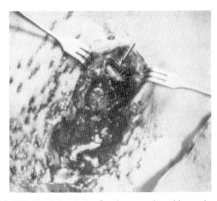

FIGURE 19–10 Gunshot wound requiring exploration.

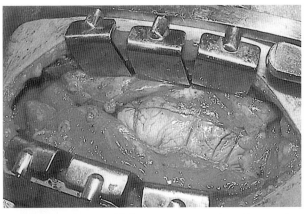

FIGURE 19–11 Median sternotomy was performed because of the position of the entrance wound and the suspicion of cardiac injury. Palpation of the left hemidiaphragm revealed a defect and indicated laparotomy.

Excision

The Excision category (20150-20251) codes are for the biopsies of muscle and bone. The codes are divided based on the type of biopsy (muscle, bone), the depth of the biopsy (superficial, deep), and, in some codes, the method of obtaining the biopsy (e.g., percutaneous needle).

The procedure for a muscle or bone biopsy typically includes the administration of local anesthetic into the biopsy area, an incision into the area allowing exposure of the muscle or bone, removal of tissue for biopsy, and suturing of the area. A **percutaneous biopsy**, as represented in 20206, differs in that the area is not opened to the physician's view. A trocar (hollow needle) or needle is placed into the muscle or bone by passing the needle through the skin and into the muscle or bone and withdrawing a sample. When the percutaneous method is used to obtain a biopsy, the area does not require suturing. If the biopsy is extremely complicated, the surgeon may request the assistance of ultrasound to be able to view the biopsy area during the procedure and receive guidance as to the placement of the needle. Notice the guideline in the CPT following 20206 directs you to the radiology codes if imaging guidance is utilized during the procedure.

Biopsy codes in the Excision category of the General subheading are not to be reported for the excision of tumors of muscle. If the medical record indicates excision of a muscle tumor, you would have to choose a code from the correct Musculoskeletal subsection. For example, 24071 reports excision of a tumor, 3 cm or greater, from the soft tissue of the upper arm or elbow.

Biopsy codes do not include the pathology workup that is performed on the sample.

General Introduction or Removal

Within the Introduction or Removal category there is a wide variety of injection, aspiration, insertion, application, removal, and adjustment codes. Because the category is within the General subheading of the Musculoskeletal subsection, the codes also have a wide application in coding services.

Therapeutic **sinus tract injection** procedure codes are within this category. You may initially think of the nasal sinuses, but these are not the sinuses that are being injected here. The term "sinus" refers to a cyst or abscess inside the body with a tract (known as a fistula) connecting to another surface—internal (to the gut) or external (to the skin). The infection is treated by injecting an antibiotic or other substance into the sinus by way of the sinus tract. With certain sinus injections, a radiologist provides guidance to ensure the correct placement of the needle and the guidance is reported separately. For example, an interstitial abscess located perirectally develops a sinus tract opening perianally may be treated by instilling a caustic substance to stimulate healing. Other methods that may be used in treatment of the sinus tract are the incision or opening of the tract (fistulotomy) to promote healing or excision (fistulectomy) of the tract.

Removal codes located in the Introduction or Removal category (20520-20525) report the removal of a foreign body lodged in muscle or tendon. Recall that the Integumentary System removal codes describe foreign bodies lodged in the skin. **Injection** codes in this category report injections made into a tendon, ligament, or ganglion cyst (cystic tumor). An example of the use of these injection codes would be a corticosteroid injection as a ganglion cyst treatment.

CODING SHOT

You must read the codes carefully. For most injection codes (i.e., 20550, 20551, 20553) the code description states "Injection(s)." This means that one or more injections can be reported with the same code with no modifier.

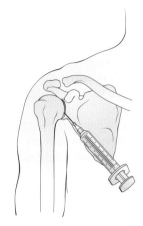

FIGURE 19–12 Arthrocentesis of a joint.

Arthrocentesis is aspiration of a joint (Fig. 19-12), and the codes to report such a service are in the range of 20600-20611. Arthrocentesis is a procedure commonly used in the treatment of joint conditions. The area over the involved joint is injected with anesthetic, a needle is inserted into the joint, and fluid is withdrawn.

Code 20612 reports an aspiration and/or injection of a ganglion cyst, which is a rubbery swelling that may occur anywhere on the body but usually occurs over a joint or tendon of the wrist or foot. The treatment of a ganglion cyst is surgical removal, aspiration, or aspiration with injection of a corticosteroid. Often, ganglion cysts will appear in a cluster and if multiple cysts are treated, report the service with 20612 with modifier -59 appended.

CODING SHOT

The code descriptions for arthrocentesis indicate that the codes can be used for an aspiration, an injection, or both an aspiration and an injection. You would not report the performance of both an aspiration and an injection at the same session by using multiple codes, as that would be unbundling. You would instead report both services using a single code.

The arthrocentesis codes are divided according to whether the joint is small (finger, toe), intermediate (ankle, elbow), or major (shoulder, hip). Note that while the shoulder is a major joint, the acromioclavicular joint, which is a part of the shoulder, is only an intermediate joint. This often leads to incorrectly coding the acromioclavicular joint as a major joint rather than as an intermediate joint. Codes are also divided by with or without guidance.

Lidocaine, Marcaine, and so forth, when used as anesthetics, are not reported separately. Any injected therapeutic drug such as a steroid is reported separately using a HCPCS J code (drug code).

Insertion of wires or pins to repair a bone (20650) is a procedure often used by orthopedic physicians. The procedure is performed using a local or general anesthetic. The bone is drilled through with a power drill and pins and/or wires are placed through the holes in the bone and allowed to emerge through the skin on each side of the bone. A traction device is then attached to the pins or wires to hold the bone immobile while healing takes place (refer to Fig. 19-5). This may sound painful, but actually, the procedure is used to allow well-aligned healing, as well as alleviate pain.

CODING SHOT

The removal of the external skeletal wires or pins is included in the reimbursement for fixation; but for internal fixation removal, report separately using 20670, 20680.

The codes to report the **application** of many of the devices used for fixation of the bones of the body during the healing process—cranial tong, cranial halo, pelvic halo, femoral halo, caliper, stereotactic frame—are located in this category. Each of the applications includes the removal of the device, unless the device is removed by another physician (20665). When the application of these devices is performed through an open surgical procedure, the procedure is referred to as an open reduction with internal fixation (**ORIF**) and uses pins, wires, and screws to stabilize a fracture.

Implant removal codes (20670, 20680) are available for reporting the services of removal of buried wires, pins, rods, etc., previously implanted. If, for example, there is a complication, such as pain, the hardware may be removed. Diagnosis coding must support the necessity of removal of the deep hardware as a complication. If removed during the global period, report the service with modifier -58 (staged) appended to the procedure code. The implant removal codes are divided according to whether the implants are superficial or deep.

External fixation is the application of a device that holds a bone in place, but unlike internal fixation, the device is placed on the outside of the body and pins or wires are placed into the bone from the outside (Fig. 19-13). These wires and pins, when fastened to the bone, hold the device or system immobile. This type of fixation is commonly used with comminuted fractures (fragmented) that are difficult to hold in place. External fixation is used primarily in cases of limb fracture, major pelvic disruption, osteotomy, arthrodesis, bone infection, and bone lengthening.

Codes 20690 and 20692 report whether the device or system is placed on one surface (uniplane) or several surfaces (multiplane). With the uniplane device, two or more pins are inserted above the fracture site and two or more pins are inserted below the fracture site. Multiplane devices are more complicated and are usually reserved for highly complex fractures (see Fig. 19-13).

CODING SHOT

The fixation devices codes are reported in addition to the code for the treatment of the fracture, unless the application code specifically states that fracture repair is included. For example, see code 25545: "Open treatment of ulnar shaft fracture includes internal fixation, when performed." This code specifies both the treatment of the fracture and the fixation. External fixation, if performed, would be reported separately.

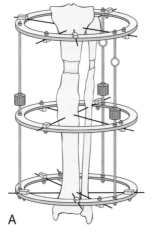
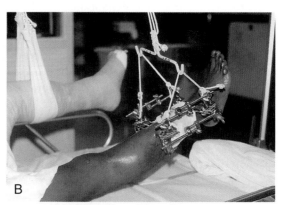

FIGURE 19–13 **A,** External fixation (Ilizarov multiplane). **B,** Example of an external fixation device on the right leg. The left leg is in a splint.

Note also that most of the codes in the Introduction or Removal categories are for **unilateral** services, so if a procedure is bilateral you would assign modifier -50.

If the device is **adjusted,** the service is reported separately (20693). **Removal** of external fixation devices or systems is usually accomplished under anesthesia and is reported separately from the application (20694). However, if the removal does not require return to the operating room, you would not report the service separately but would consider the removal as being bundled into the application code. If the removal was performed outside the global period, some payers may reimburse the removal as an E/M service.

EXERCISE 19-2   *General*

Using the CPT, ICD-10-CM and/or ICD-9-CM manuals, provide the codes for the following:

1 Exploration of a penetrating wound of the left leg

    CPT Code: _____

2 Replantation of right foot after a complete, traumatic amputation

    CPT Code: _____

3 Radical resection of sarcoma of cheek, less than 2 cm

    CPT Code: _____

4 Nonoperative, electrical stimulation of nonhealing femur fracture

    CPT Code: _____

5 Percutaneous needle biopsy of muscle of upper arm in a patient with congenital myotonic muscular dystrophy

    CPT Code: _____

    ICD-10-CM Code: _____ (ICD-9-CM Code: _____)

6 Intra-articular aspiration and injection without guidance of finger joint for primary osteoarthritis

    CPT Code: _____

    ICD-10-CM Code: _____ (ICD-9-CM Code: _____)

(Answers are located in Appendix B)

Grafts (or Implants)

Codes 20900-20938 report the harvesting of bone, cartilage, fascia lata, tendon, or tissue through an incision separate from that used to implant the graft. Graft material is used in a wide variety of repair procedures. For example, if a tibial fracture has failed to heal in 20 weeks, the surgeon may decide that the fracture requires bone grafting to achieve healing. Bone grafting is also used in cases of large defects (>6 cm). Some types of fractures commonly heal with difficulty, so after debridement the surgeon may decide to allow a 5- to 7-day healing period before the bone grafting procedure is performed. The grafts are obtained from the patient or a donor. Donors can be either living or deceased (cadaver). The pieces of bone are shaped into bars or pegs and then used to repair the defect.

Fascia lata grafts are taken from the mid-upper lateral thigh area because the fascia is thickest in this area. Fascia is the fibrous tissue that serves as connective tissue; it may be shaved off with an instrument called a stripper or it may be incised (cut) away. The fascia lata is then used in the repair procedure. Codes for obtaining the fascia lata graft are based on whether a stripper (20920) was used to remove the fascia or whether a more complex removal procedure (20922) was required to obtain the graft material.

Tissue grafts include obtaining of the fat, dermis, paratenon (loose connective tissue from the tendon compartment), and other tissue types. **Spine surgery** codes 20930-20938 report the obtaining and shaping of the tissue, whether from the patient (autograft) or from a donor (allograft). The obtaining and shaping of the spine graft material is reported in addition to reporting the implantation procedure, which is the primary procedure (definitive procedure), unless the description of the major procedure includes a graft.

Other Procedures

Other Procedure codes (20950-20999) report monitoring muscles, bone grafting with microvascular technique, free osteocutaneous flaps with microvascular technique, electronic/ultrasound stimulation, and computer-assisted surgical navigation procedures. **Monitoring of interstitial fluid pressure** (20950) is a procedure in which the physician inserts a device into the muscle compartment to measure the pressure changes within the muscle. Increased pressure in the muscle due to accumulation of fluid causes the blood supply to be compromised.

Bone grafts (20955-20962) are identified by the site from which the graft is obtained. When the bone grafts are removed, the small blood vessels remain attached to the graft. The graft is then inserted and the blood vessels are attached to vessels in the area of implant, using an operating microscope. The use of the operating microscope (69990) is included in the code descriptions for 20955-20962. As a reminder, there is a parenthetical statement following 20962 that states, "(Do not report 69990 in addition to codes 20955-20962)."

Free osteocutaneous flaps (20969-20973) are bone grafts that include the skin and tissue that overlie the bone. The flap has an arterial pedicle that is attached (anastomosed) to an artery on the recipient site. The surgeon then utilizes the skin, tissue, and bone to reconstruct the defect, using an operating microscope. The codes are divided based on which part of the body the flap is taken from.

Codes 20955-20962 are vascularized bone grafts that are used where there are large defects, usually in long bones, where a standard iliac bone graft or other types of nonvascularized bone grafts are not likely to heal.

Electrical or ultrasound stimulation (20974-20979) is used to promote healing. Low-voltage electricity or ultrasound is applied to the skin, and both are often used in the treatment of fractures.

Computer-assisted surgical navigation (20985) is the use of navigational assistance in musculoskeletal procedures. The code is listed in addition to the code for the primary procedure.

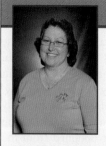

From the Trenches

"The most rewarding part of my job is helping others understand a coding or billing issue, whether they are a patient, employee, physician, or student. I enjoy teaching and mentoring others."

MARTHA

Spinal Instrumentation and Fixation

Within the subheading Spine (Vertebral Column) (22010-22899), services are often based on the cervical (C1-C7), lumbar (L1-L5), and thoracic (T1-T12) spinal areas. For example, codes in the range 22210-22216 identify osteotomy of the cervical, lumbar, or thoracic spinal area. Codes are often further divided based on the exact spinal location. For example, codes in the range 22590-22600 identify arthrodesis of three different cervical areas: occiput-C2, C1-C2, or cervical below the C2 segment. Of special note in the CPT manual is that the C1 is often referred to as the **atlas** and C2 is referred to as the **axis.**

Arthrodesis can be performed with another surgical procedure, such as fracture care or a laminectomy. If arthrodesis is performed with a more major procedure, use modifier -51 on the arthrodesis code to indicate multiple procedures were performed. An exception to this rule is when the code is an add-on code, which is exempt from use with modifier -51. For example, 22614 is used to report an arthrodesis of multiple vertebral segments. A code from the 22600-22612 range reports the first segment, and 22614 is reported for each additional vertebral segment. Modifier -51 is, therefore, not required.

CODING SHOT

When choosing codes for spine procedures, verify whether the code is describing a vertebral segment, the actual bony segment, versus an interspace (the space between two vertebral segments). If reporting a procedure performed at L4-L5, you would choose the primary code to represent L4 and the add-on code to represent L5. If the procedure code description was by interspace, only one code would be assigned.

Spinal instrumentation is used to stabilize the spinal column in some repair procedures. **Segmental instrumentation** is the attachment of a fixative device at each end of the area being repaired and at least one other attachment in the spinal area being repaired (Fig. 19-14). For example, if the repair was at T10 and T11 (thoracic vertebral bodies 10 and 11) and a rod was attached to T7 and L1, the repair rod may also be attached at T8, T9, T10, T11, and T12. **Nonsegmental instrumentation** is the application of the fixative device at each end of the area being repaired, as illustrated in Fig. 19-15. For example, if the repair was of T10, the rod may be attached at T7 and T12.

Many of the instrumentation codes are add-on codes (22840-22848 and 22851) and are reported in addition to the major procedure.

Foot and Toe Repairs

A common procedure performed on the toe is a hallux valgus correction (bunion surgery). Hallux is the great toe and valgus is the angulation of the toe away from the midline, as illustrated in Fig. 19-16.

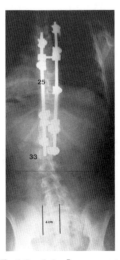

FIGURE 19-14 Decompensated lumbar curve after fusion of thoracic curve only.

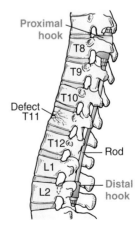

FIGURE 19-15 Fixation at each end of the area to be repaired (nonsegmental spinal instrumentation).

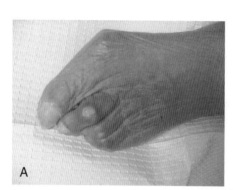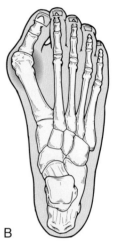

FIGURE 19–16   **A** and **B,** Hallux valgus, or bunion, is a bursa usually found along the medial aspect of the big toe. Most commonly, it is attributed to heredity or to poorly fitting shoes.

A variety of procedures are performed to correct the defect, as represented by codes in the range 28290-28299. For example, the Keller type of procedure is reported with 28292 and describes a procedure in which a wire is inserted through the bones of a toe to hold the bones in correct alignment. Each code description indicates the procedure type that is included, many of which include specific eponyms (names of individuals for whom the procedures are named), so careful reading is necessary to choose the correct bunion repair code.

APPLICATION OF CASTS AND STRAPPING

Application of Casts and Strapping codes (29000-29799) are used for the initial or subsequent treatment of fractures, ligament sprains/tears, and overuse injuries. They may also be reported for the initial stabilization of an injury until definitive restorative treatment can be provided. Because each injury is unique, each cast is unique in terms of size and position. The cast immobilizes the fracture with materials such as plaster, fiberglass, or thermoplastics. Each physician has a preference for the types of cast materials used.

Strapping is the taping of a body part, as illustrated in Fig. 19-17. Strapping is used to exert pressure on a body part to give it more stability, and is used in the treatment of sprains, strains, and dislocations. **Splints** are made of wood, cloth, metal, or plastic, as illustrated in Fig. 19-18, and are used to immobilize, support, or protect a body part, thereby allowing rest and healing. The **removal** of the cast, strapping, or splint is included in each of the Application of Casts and Strapping codes.

CODING SHOT

If a cast, strapping, or splint is applied as a part of a surgical procedure, you do not report codes from the Application of Casts and Strapping subheading because the musculoskeletal surgical procedure codes include the first cast, strapping, or splint as well as its later removal. The surgery, application, and removal are all bundled into the surgical code.

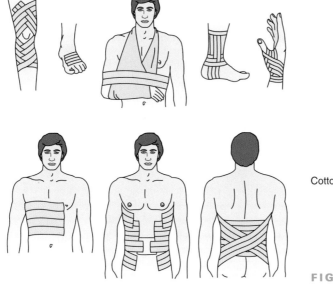

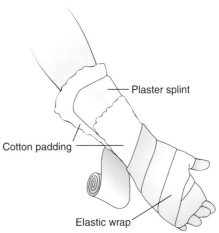

Plaster splint

Cotton padding

Elastic wrap

FIGURE 19–17 Types of strapping.

FIGURE 19–18 Splint used to immobilize a joint or bone.

If the cast, strapping, or splint is applied as a part of a **fracture repair,** the application service is not reported separately. The application service is bundled into all fracture repair codes, as is the removal. If a subsequent cast, strapping, or splint is applied within the follow-up period for either the surgical procedure or the fracture repair, you can bill the application with modifier -58 and also bill for the materials (A4580-A4590). You can bill for a separate office visit during which a second cast, strapping, or splint is applied only if the patient is provided some additional, separate, and significant service. Modifier -25 would be appended to the E/M code.

QUICK CHECK 19-4

1. A replacement cast during the global period of fracture care may require which modifier?

_____

(Answers are located in Appendix C)

You can report the Application of Casts and Strapping codes only when the physician:
- Applies an initial cast, strapping, or splint for stabilization prior to definitive treatment by another provider.
- Applies a subsequent cast, strapping, or splint.
- Treats a sprain or fracture and does not expect to provide any other type of restorative treatment.

The subheading Application of Casts and Strapping is divided into three major categories:
- Body and Upper Extremity
- Lower Extremity
- Removal or Repair (provided by a physician other than the one who initially applied it)

The subcategories of Body/Upper Extremity and Lower Extremity are:
- Casts
- Splints
- Strapping—Any Age

The codes in all subcategories are divided primarily according to the **location** of the cast, splint, or strapping on the body—head, hand, extremity—and often on the **type**—Minerva, Velpeau, static (nonmovable), dynamic (movable).

EXERCISE 19-3 *Application of Casts and Strapping*

Using the CPT and/or HCPCS manuals, provide the codes for the following:

1 Replacement during global period by treating physician of fiberglass shoulder-to-hand (long-arm) cast for a 54-year-old patient

CPT Codes: _____, _____

2 Initial application of a walking-type short leg cast for a sprain

CPT Code: _____

3 Removal of a full leg cast by a physician who did not apply the cast

CPT Code: _____

4 Strapping of a 46-year-old patient's knee

CPT Code: _____

5 Replacement of a thigh-to-toes cast on the right leg of a 35-year-old female patient (Initial visit)

CPT Codes: _____, _____

(Answers are located in Appendix B)

ENDOSCOPY/ARTHROSCOPY

Arthroscopy is often the treatment of choice for many orthopedic surgical procedures. The incisions are smaller, which decreases the risk of infection and speeds recovery time. Several small incisions are made through which lights, mirrors, and instruments are inserted, as illustrated in Fig. 19-19.

The arthroscopy codes are located at the end of the Musculoskeletal subsection. If multiple procedures are performed through a scope, they are reported with modifier -51. Bundled into all surgical arthroscopic procedure codes is the diagnostic arthroscopy. You must not unbundle and report a diagnostic arthroscopy and a surgical arthroscopy if both were performed during the same encounter. Do not report separately services performed during a procedure that are considered part of the procedure, such as shaving, removing, evacuating, casting, splinting, or strapping.

A note preceding the Endoscopy/Arthroscopy codes (29800-29999) states, "When arthroscopy is performed in conjunction with arthrotomy, add modifier -51." This note

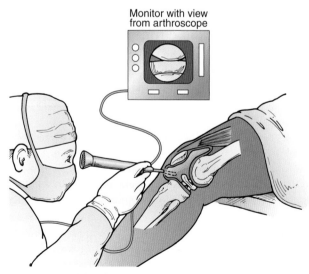

Monitor with view from arthroscope

FIGURE 19–19 Arthroscopy of knee.

indicates that if a surgeon performs an arthroscopy and during the procedure extends the procedure to an arthrotomy, both services are reported. For example, a physician performs an arthroscopic shaving of the articular cartilage and also performs an open capsulotomy (posterior capsular release) of the knee. Both the arthroscopic shaving (29877) and the capsulotomy (27435) would be reported, and to the least expensive procedure add modifier -51 (multiple procedures).

In arthroscopic procedures, it is also correct to report multiple procedures in different compartments in the joint area with one code. For example, in the knee, there are three compartments, the medial, lateral, and patellofemoral. If a meniscectomy (29881) is performed in the medial compartment, and a shaving (29877) is performed in the patellofemoral compartment, only the 29881 is reported as it includes the shaving.

CODING SHOT

When coding arthroscopic procedures of the knee, note the use of **basket forceps,** which indicates a meniscectomy (meniscus removal) rather than a shaving and debridement.

The codes in the Arthroscopy subheading are divided according to body area—elbow, shoulder, knee—and then according to the type and extent of procedure performed. An example of type of service is as follows: 29805 reports an arthroscopy of the shoulder for **diagnostic** purposes, whereas code 29806 is an arthroscopy of the shoulder for a **surgical** repair procedure. Not only are there two different codes for surgical and diagnostic arthroscopic procedures, but also the reimbursement for the surgical procedures is higher than the diagnostic procedure. So great care must be taken to select the code that correctly describes the services supported in the medical record and in code placement. If the procedure began as a diagnostic procedure, which is often the case, and converts to a surgical procedure, only the surgical procedure is reported. The reimbursement for the surgical procedure is higher than the reimbursement for the diagnostic procedure. For example, one payer's reimbursement was $424.86 for the diagnostic procedure (29805) and $979.21 for the surgical procedure (29806).

CODING SHOT

A diagnostic arthroscopy is always included in a surgical arthroscopy.

Note the description for code 29805: "Arthroscopy, shoulder, diagnostic, with or without synovial biopsy (separate procedure)." You will find the statement "separate procedure" several times in the Endoscopy/Arthroscopy subheading because often a minor arthroscopic procedure is part of a more major procedure. You cannot report the service of the minor procedure unless it has been performed as an independent service, addressing a distinctly separate problem. Also note that the parenthetical information indicates the codes "(23065-23066, 23100-23101)" are to be reported if the procedure was done as an open (incisional) procedure rather than as an endoscopic procedure.

EXERCISE 19-4   *Endoscopy/Arthroscopy*

Using the CPT manual, provide the codes for the following:

1 Surgical arthroscopy of ankle, which included extensive debridement

CPT Code: _____

2 Diagnostic knee arthroscopy with a synovial biopsy

CPT Code: _____

3 Diagnostic shoulder arthroscopy

CPT Code: _____

4 Arthroscopic repair of tuberosity fracture of knee with manipulation

CPT Code: _____

5 Surgical arthroscopy of ankle, including drilling and excision of tibial defect

CPT Code: _____

(Answers are located in Appendix B)

CHAPTER REVIEW

CHAPTER 19, PART I, THEORY

Without the use of reference material, complete the following:

1 The Musculoskeletal System subsection is formatted according to what type of sites? _____

2 Which physician subspecialty can report the codes from the Musculoskeletal System subsection? _____

3 List the three types of fracture treatments and briefly describe each: _____

4 It is the _____ of the fracture that determines the method of treatment.

5 _____ is the application of pulling force to hold a bone in place.

6 What is the term that describes the physician's actions of bending, rotating, pulling, or guiding the bone back into place? _____

7 What term is used to mean "put the bone back in place"? _____

8 What term describes a bone that is not in its normal location? _____

9 What term describes the cleaning of a wound? _____

10 This is a hollow needle that is often used to withdraw samples of fluid from a joint: _____

11 Would a biopsy code usually include the administration of any necessary local anesthesia? _____

CHAPTER 19, PART II, PRACTICAL

With the use of the CPT, ICD-10-CM and/or ICD-9-CM manuals, complete the following:

12 Incision of a subfascial soft tissue abscess

CPT Code: _____

13 Radical resection of a 2.7 cm sarcoma of the soft tissue of the upper back

CPT Code: _____

14 Closed treatment of three vertebral process fractures

CPT Code: _____

15 Under general anesthesia, manipulation of a right shoulder joint with external fixation

CPT Code: _____

16 Lengthening of four tendons of elbow

CPT Code(s): _____

17 Incision and drainage of bursa of elbow

CPT Code(s): _____

18 Open treatment of a carpal scaphoid fracture with internal fixation applied

CPT Code(s): _____

19 Arthroplasty of two metacarpophalangeal joints

CPT Code(s): _____

20 Tenotomy of two flexor tendons of a finger using an open procedure

CPT Code(s): _____

21 Amputation, lower arm, using Krukenberg procedure

CPT Code(s): _____

22 Open treatment of radial and ulnar shaft fractures with internal fixation of both radius and ulna

CPT Code(s): _____

23 Osteoplasty for shortening of both radius and ulna for adult Kienböck's disease

CPT Code(s): _____

ICD-10-CM Code: _____

(ICD-9-CM Code: _____)

24 Percutaneous lateral tenotomy for tennis elbow (lateral epicondylitis)

CPT Code(s): _____

ICD-10-CM Code: _____

(ICD-9-CM Code: _____)

25 Replantation of right arm, including the neck of the humerus through the elbow joint, following a complete traumatic amputation

CPT Code(s): _____

ICD-10-CM Code: _____

(ICD-9-CM Code: _____)

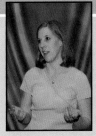

"I really like how my work contributes to higher reimbursement rates and less denials for the physicians. That in turn always improves quality of patient care because we have the resources to provide that based on reimbursement and fewer denials."

Lynda Kross, CPC
Certified Reimbursement Assistant
University Physicians—University of Missouri
Health Care
Columbia, Missouri

Respiratory System

Chapter Topics

Format

Endoscopy

Nose

Accessory Sinuses

Larynx

Trachea/Bronchi

Lungs and Pleura

Chapter Review

Learning Objectives

After completing this chapter you should be able to

1   Differentiate between services reported with codes from the Respiratory System subsection and those reported with codes from other subsections.

2   Explain the effects of extent and approach when reporting endoscopy respiratory procedures.

3   Identify highlights of nasal procedure coding.

4   Analyze the codes to report services to the accessory sinuses.

5   Categorize the codes in the Larynx subheading.

6   Explain the structure of the trachea/bronchi codes.

7   Distinguish the difference amongst the codes assigned to report lungs and pleura services, and procedures.

8   Demonstrate the ability to code respiratory services and procedures.

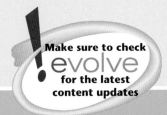

Make sure to check
evolve
for the latest
content updates

FORMAT

The Respiratory System subsection is arranged by anatomic site (e.g., nose, accessory sinus, larynx) and then by procedure (e.g., incision, excision, introduction). Your knowledge of respiratory terminology is important (Fig. 20-1), as you assign codes from the Respiratory System subsection.

In the Musculoskeletal System subsection, arthroscopy codes are placed at the end of the subsection, but in the Respiratory System subsection, the **endoscopy** codes are listed throughout, according to anatomic site. **Fracture repair**, such as that of the nose or sternum, is listed in the Musculoskeletal System subsection, not in the Respiratory System subsection. Procedures that are performed on the **throat** or **mouth** are not located in the Respiratory System subsection but instead are located in the Digestive System subsection.

The Respiratory System subsection contains some codes that may be considered **cosmetic**. It is important to note each of the components performed during the procedure because there are many services bundled into some of these codes. For example, under the subheading Nose and the category Repair, there is code 30400 for rhinoplasty. The rhinoplasty may be performed either through external skin incisions (open) or through intranasal incisions (closed), and both approaches can be reported with 30400. The extent of the procedure varies based on the desired outcome, but a rhinoplasty can include fracturing a deformed septum, repositioning the septum, reshaping and/or augmenting the nasal cartilage, removing fat from the area, performing a layered closure, and applying a splint or cast. If all of these components of a rhinoplasty were performed, they would be bundled into 30420. You have to read all of the notes and the code information carefully to ensure that you do not code components of the procedure separately if there is one code that includes all the components.

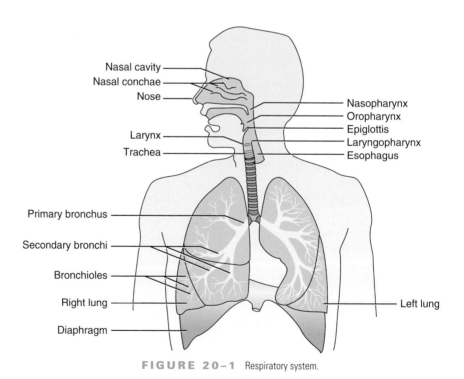

FIGURE 20−1   Respiratory system.

QUICK CHECK 20-1

1. Rhinoplasty can be performed either _____, through external skin incisions, or closed, through _____ incisions.

(Answers are located in Appendix C)

ENDOSCOPY

During endoscopic procedures, a scope is placed through an existing body orifice (opening), or a small incision is made into a cavity for scope placement.

When sinus endoscopies are performed, a scope is placed through the nose into the nasal cavity. Codes for sinus endoscopy (31231-31294) report unilateral (on one side) procedures except in the case of a diagnostic nasal endoscopy, which is unilateral or bilateral. Multiple procedures may be performed within different sinuses (frontal, maxillary, and ethmoid sinuses) during the same operative session. The CPT manual has combined into a single code some multiple sinus procedures commonly performed at the same operative session.

Example

31276   Nasal/sinus endoscopy, surgical with frontal sinus exploration, with or without removal of tissue from frontal sinus

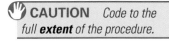

CAUTION *Code to the full **extent** of the procedure.*

Endoscopic procedures may start at one site (such as the nose) and follow through to another site (such as the larynx or bronchial tubes). It is important to choose the code that most appropriately reflects the furthest extent of the procedure. For example, if a direct laryngoscopy is performed, and the scope is progressed past the larynx and includes examination of the trachea, the service is reported with 31515 because the code description states either with or without tracheoscopy. However, if it is necessary to continue the procedure to the bronchial tubes, the service would be reported with 31622 (bronchoscopy). The larynx and trachea must be passed to get to the farthest point (bronchial tubes). In these instances, it is the full extent of the procedure that determines the code assignment.

CAUTION *Code the correct **approach** for the procedure.*

The same surgical procedure may be performed using different approaches. For example, code 32141 describes a **thoracotomy** with "resection-plication (removal/shortening) of bullae (blisters); includes any pleural procedure, when performed." Code 32655 describes a surgical **thoracoscopy** with resection-plication of bullae, includes any pleural procedures when performed. Code 32655 describes the same procedure as 32141, except that 32655 is a procedure performed through very minute incisions utilizing a thoracoscope, whereas code 32141 describes an open incision through the thorax, opening the full operative site to the surgeon. In these instances, it is the approach utilized to perform the procedure that determines the code assignment.

CAUTION *Do not confuse nasal/sinus endoscopic procedures with intranasal procedures. Intranasal procedures may require that surgical instruments be placed into the nose but do not require the use of an endoscope. When an endoscope is used in a nasal/sinus procedure, assign a nasal/sinus endoscopy code.*

Multiple endoscopic procedures may be performed through the same scope during the operative session. When this occurs, each procedure should be reported with modifier -51 (multiple procedures) placed on subsequent procedure(s). For example, a bronchoscopy with biopsy is performed as well as a bronchoscopy with removal of a foreign body. Not only would you report a bronchoscopy with biopsy, but you would also report the removal of a foreign body. The multiple procedure modifier -51 would be placed after the lower priced (least resource-intensive) procedure. The exception to this occurs when the CPT manual offers a code for which the description includes all the separate elements of the procedure bundled into one code.

Remember that a diagnostic endoscopy is always bundled into a surgical endoscopy. For example, if a physician began a diagnostic endoscopic nasal procedure and continued on to complete a surgical procedure, you report only for the surgical procedure. To report both a diagnostic and a surgical nasal endoscopy is unbundling if the diagnostic and surgical procedures are performed on the same nasal space. However, if a diagnostic sinus endoscopy is performed on the right maxillary sinus and a surgical endoscopic maxillectomy on the left, both procedures are reported with appropriate -LT and -RT modifiers because two different procedures were performed.

When reporting laryngoscopic procedures, note that the terms "indirect" and "direct" are often stated in the code description. For example, locate codes 31505, indirect, and 31515, direct in the CPT manual. **Indirect** in 31505 means that the physician used a tongue depressor to hold the tongue down and view the epiglottis (the lid that covers the larynx) with a mirror. The patient vocalizes (says "ah") and the physician can then view the vocal cords. **Direct** in 31515 means that the endoscope is passed into the larynx and the physician looks directly at the larynx through the endoscope. The operative report will indicate whether the procedure was indirect or direct.

Locating Endoscopy Codes. Endoscopy codes can be located in the CPT manual index under "Endoscopy" and then under the anatomic subterm of the site. You can also locate an endoscopic procedure by the anatomic endoscopy title. For example, a bronchial biopsy using endoscopy is listed under "Bronchoscopy" and then under the subterm "Biopsy."

EXERCISE 20-1   *Endoscopy Terminology*

Using the CPT and manual, complete the following:

1 Endoscopic maxillary antrostomy

CPT Code: _____

2 Direct laryngoscopy for removal of fish bone

CPT Code: _____

3 After the airway is sufficiently anesthetized, a flexible bronchoscope is inserted through the mouth and advanced to the bronchus, where a transbronchial biopsy of one lobe is obtained.

CPT Code: _____

4 Diagnostic thoracoscopy of the mediastinal space is accomplished with the use of a flexible endoscope that is inserted through a small incision on the chest (no biopsy was performed).

CPT Code: _____

5 Segmental resection of the right single lung lobe using a flexible endoscope (surgical thoracoscopy)

CPT Code: _____

(Answers are located in Appendix B)

NOSE

Many of the codes in the Nose subheading are reported by physicians who specialize in treating conditions of the nose (otorhinolaryngologist; ear, nose, and throat specialists), but there are also many codes in the subheading that are more widely used. For example, it is in the Nose subheading that you will locate codes for commonly performed office procedures, such as control of nosebleeds, incision of abscesses, removal of foreign objects from the nose (think children!), and removal of nasal cysts and lesions.

Incision

Codes for incision of a nasal abscess (30000, 30020) are divided on whether the abscess is on the nasal mucosa or the septal mucosa. If a nasal abscess is approached from the outside of the nose **(external approach),** you would assign a code from the Integumentary System

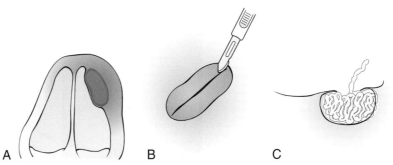

FIGURE 20–2 **A,** Nasal mucosal abscess. **B,** Incision of abscess. **C,** Gauze packed into abscess with end extended outside the abscess, acting as a wick.

subsection; but if the approach is from the inside of the nose **(internal approach),** you would assign a code from the Respiratory System subsection. The medical record will describe the approach to the procedure.

After an abscess has been penetrated, the physician may close the area immediately or place a tube in the incision to ensure that the pus continues to drain from the abscess area. After the drain is removed, the abscess may be packed with gauze, with one end of the packing material left outside the surface to act as a wick, as illustrated in Fig. 20-2, *A-C.*

The insertion and removal of the tube and/or gauze and any required sutures and/or anesthesia are bundled into the code, so you should not report these services separately. You should report any additional supplies over and above those usually used for the procedure by using the Medicine section code for supplies, 99070, or a HCPCS code, as directed by the third-party payer.

Excision

Within the Nose subheading, the Excision category (30100-30160) contains a wide range of procedures that describe removal of tissue from the nose—for example, biopsy, polyp excision, and cyst excision—as well as resection of the turbinate bone.

CODING SHOT

When two procedures are completed during the same surgical session, the most complex procedure is sequenced first.

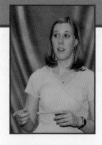

From the Trenches

"When someone expresses an interest in coding, I explain not only what I do day to day but also why coding is so important. Many people don't realize that selecting proper codes is in the patient's best interest as they can give a detailed picture of the patient's medical condition and history."

LYNDA

The **biopsy** code (30100) reports a biopsy that is performed intranasally; but if the procedure was for a biopsy of the skin outside of the nose, you assign the biopsy code 11100 from the Integumentary System.

Nasal polyps develop and mature, causing nasal obstruction (Fig. 20-3, *A*). The physician removes the polyps, usually with a snare, as illustrated in Fig. 20-3, *B.*

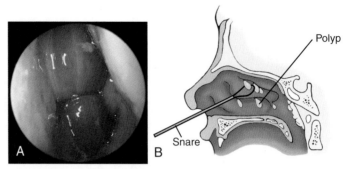

FIGURE 20-3 **A,** Nasal polyp. **B,** A nasal snare is used to remove nasal polyps. The nose is anesthetized, a snare is slipped around the polyp, which is transected, and a forceps is used to remove the polyp.

The excision of **nasal polyps** is reported with one of two codes (30110 and 30115). The difference between the codes is the extent of the excision. Code 30110 reports a simple polyp excision that would usually be performed in the office, whereas 30115 reports a more extensive polyp excision that would usually be performed in a hospital setting.

CODING SHOT

Modifier -50 (bilateral) is assigned when the polyps are removed from both the left and right sides of the nose.

The codes for excision or destruction of **lesions** inside the nose are divided based on the approach—internal or external. Usually, if the approach to the procedure is external, you are referred to the Integumentary System subsection to locate the correct code; but the nasal lesion excision/destruction codes can be assigned for either an external or an internal approach to a lesion.

You have to read the code descriptions carefully to ensure that you understand all of the circumstances that surround assignment of the code, and you have to identify codes such as the lesion excision/destruction that are exceptions to the usual rules.

All methods of lesion destruction, including laser, are included in the Excision codes. Usually, if laser was used in the destruction of a lesion, you would be referred to a separate set of codes just for laser destruction; but with the lesion destruction codes in the Nose category, laser is included as one of the destruction methods.

Turbinates are the bones on the inside of the nose. These bones are shaped like a spiral shell and humidify, warm, and filter the air. These bones are referred to as the nasal conchae. The turbinates are divided into three sections—inferior, middle, and superior (Fig. 20-4). Portions of or all of a turbinate bone may be removed because of chronic congestion or neoplastic growth. Because third-party payers usually do not pay for cosmetic surgical procedures, you must document the medical necessity for noncosmetic procedures carefully to ensure appropriate reimbursement. Watch for and read the extensive notes inside the parentheses throughout this category.

Introduction

Introduction codes (30200-30220) include injection, displacement therapy, and insertion. **Injections** into the turbinates (30200) are therapeutic injections usually performed to shrink the nasal tissue to improve breathing. For example, if a patient has inflamed nasal passages due to an allergic reaction or a deviated septum, the patient may benefit from a steroid injection into the turbinates. **Displacement therapy** (30210) is a procedure in which the physician flushes saline solution into the sinuses to remove mucus or pus. The insertion of a **nasal button** (30220) (as illustrated in Fig. 20-5) is a technique used for a

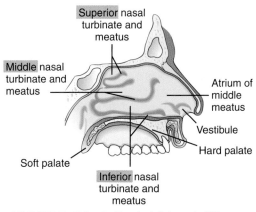

FIGURE 20–4 Superior, inferior, and middle nasal turbinates.

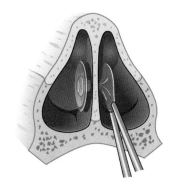

FIGURE 20–5 Insertion of nasal button.

patient who has a perforated septum. The physician places the button into the opening and fastens the button in place with sutures. The button is usually made of silicone or rubber. This technique is used as a method of repairing the septum without surgical grafting.

Removal of a Foreign Body

A variety of objects are inserted into the various orifices (openings) of the body, and the nose is a common place into which these foreign objects are placed. The code to report an office procedure for the removal of a foreign body from the nose is 30300. Codes for more extensive procedures are also available for removal of foreign objects from the nose, such as those requiring general anesthesia (30310) and a more invasive surgical procedure.

Repair

Within the Repair category (30400-30630) are the plastic procedures—rhinoplasty, septoplasty, and septal dermatoplasty. **Rhinoplasty** is a procedure to reshape the nose internally, externally, or both. The codes are divided based on the extent (minor, intermediate, major), on whether the septum was also repaired (septoplasty), and on whether the procedure was an initial or secondary procedure. **Secondary** procedures are those that are performed after an initial procedure. For example, if a rhinoplasty was performed and the results were not as successful as the patient desired, the surgeon could perform a second procedure (secondary) to improve the result.

Septoplasty is rearrangement of the nasal septum. This procedure is commonly performed due to a deviated septum.

CAUTION   *Do not use a septoplasty code if the operative report indicates that only a resection of the inferior turbinate(s) was performed. The resection of the inferior turbinate(s) is reported with 30140 and is not a procedure performed on the septum. The septoplasty code, 30520, is reported when the nasal septum is resected. There is a note enclosed in parentheses following both codes—30140 and 30520—that cautions you to use the correct code, depending on whether the turbinate or the septum was resected.*

Destruction

Destruction can be accomplished by use of ablation. **Ablation** is removal, usually by cutting, or cauterization is performed to remove excess nasal mucosa or to reduce inflammation. The destruction codes (30801, 30802) are divided according to the extent of the procedure—superficial or intramural. **Intramural** is ablation of the deeper mucosa, as compared to **superficial** ablation, which involves only the outer layer of mucosa.

Other Procedures

Codes (30901-30920) for the control of nasal hemorrhage are located in the Other Procedures category and are often reported. The physician may use anterior or posterior pressure to control the hemorrhage. Anterior nasal packing (Fig. 20-6) is the application of pressure using packing to the anterior aspect of the nasal cavity, and posterior nasal packing is the application of pressure to the posterior aspect of the nasal cavity. The nasal pack is inserted via the nasal opening. A balloon may be inserted and inflated to further control bleeding (Fig. 20-7). The codes are divided according to the type and extent of control required.

CODING SHOT

The key to correctly coding nasal hemorrhage is to know the type of control (anterior/posterior) and the level of complexity (simple/complex) utilized by the physician to control the hemorrhage.

There are times when neither cauterization nor packing will control a nasal hemorrhage, and ligation of the bleeding artery is required. Ligation of ethmoidal arteries involves opening the upper side of the nose and locating and tying the ethmoid artery (Fig. 20-8). Ligation of the internal maxillary artery is performed to gain control of nasal hemorrhage by locating and ligating the maxillary artery (Fig. 20-9).

A **therapeutic fracture** of the nasal turbinate is a procedure in which the physician fractures the turbinate bone and then repositions it, under local anesthetic. Repositioning the turbinate(s) often alleviates obstructed airflow caused by enlarged inferior turbinates or a previous fracture that has healed out of alignment and resulted in a deviation of the nose.

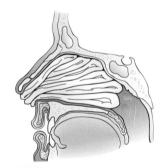

FIGURE 20–6   Anterior nasal packing.

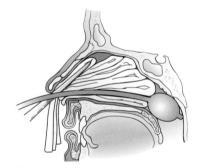

FIGURE 20–7   Posterior nasal packing.

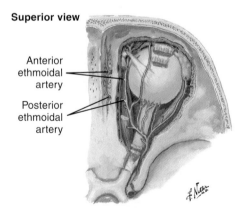

FIGURE 20–8   Ethmoid artery. (Modified from Netter FH: *Atlas of Human Anatomy,* ed 4, Philadelphia, 2006, Saunders.)

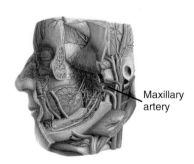

FIGURE 20–9   Maxillary artery.

EXERCISE 20-2 *Nose*

Using the CPT, ICD-10-CM and/or ICD-9-CM manuals, complete the following:

1 Biopsy of an intranasal lesion

CPT Code: _____

ICD-10-CM Code: _____   (ICD-9-CM Code: _____)

2 Primary rhinoplasty including major septal repair due to deviated nasal septum, acquired

CPT Code: _____

ICD-10-CM Code: _____   (ICD-9-CM Code: _____)

3 Anterior control of nasal hemorrhage by means of limited chemical cauterization and simple packing

CPT Code: _____

ICD-10-CM Code: _____   (ICD-9-CM Code: _____)

4 Septoplasty with contouring and grafting

CPT Code: _____

5 Removal of crayon from nose of 5-year-old boy, conducted as an office procedure

CPT Code: _____

(Answers are located in Appendix B)

ACCESSORY SINUSES

Incision

Within the Incision category are codes for services that you would not think of as being incisional. For example, the nasal sinuses can be washed (lavage) with a saline solution introduced through a canula (hollow tube) to remove infection. The Incision category code 31000 describes lavage of the maxillary sinus. Lavage can be performed on both the maxillary and the sphenoid sinuses (Fig. 20-10). If the lavage is of the sphenoid sinus, you report 31002.

CODING SHOT

Use modifier -50 (bilateral) when the lavage is performed on both the left and right maxillary sinuses.

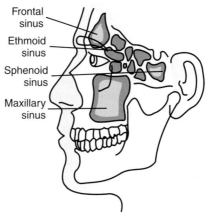

FIGURE 20–10 Paranasal sinuses.

Many of the codes in the Incision category are for sinusotomies. A **sinusotomy** is a procedure in which the physician enlarges the passage or creates a new passage from the nasal cavity into a sinus. This procedure is usually performed due to chronic sinus infection; the procedure improves sinus drainage. The codes are divided according to the extent of the procedure.

EXERCISE 20-3 *Accessory Sinuses*

Using the CPT, ICD-10-CM and/or ICD-9-CM manuals, complete the following:

1 Lavage of the maxillary sinus, bilateral

  CPT Codes: _____ and _____

2 Simple left frontal sinusotomy using an external approach

  CPT Code: _____

3 Unilateral sinusotomy of frontal, ethmoid, and sphenoid

  CPT Code: _____

4 Right radical maxillary sinusotomy

  CPT Code: _____

5 Pterygomaxillary fossa surgery, transfacial approach, due to chronic antritis of maxillary sinus

  CPT Code: _____

  ICD-10-CM Code: _____   (ICD-9-CM Code: _____)

(Answers are located in Appendix B)

LARYNX

The procedures reported with codes in the Larynx subheading (31300-31599) include a wide range of surgical procedures, such as laryngectomy, plastic repair, and nerve destruction.

Excision

Laryngotomy is an incision that is made over the larynx (thyrotomy) to expose the larynx to view. With the larynx exposed, the surgeon can remove a tumor, a laryngocele (air-filled space), or a vocal cord (cordectomy). A laryngotomy can also be performed for diagnostic purposes, without a surgical procedure being performed.

Be careful not to get the codes from the Laryngotomy category confused with the tracheostomy codes located in the Trachea and Bronchi subheading, Incision category, which you will learn more about later in this chapter. The codes from the two categories differ, depending on the **purpose** of the procedure. The Laryngotomy category codes describe procedures in which the surgeon performs a thyrotomy (incision of the larynx through the thyroid cartilage) for the purpose of exposing the larynx. The codes in the Trachea and Bronchi subheading, Incision category, describe a procedure in which the surgeon performs only the tracheostomy, usually to establish airflow, and no procedure or exposure of the larynx is planned or is involved.

Radical neck dissection, as referred to in the codes for laryngectomy, is the removal not only of the larynx but also of lymph glands and/or other surrounding tissue. Many of the codes in the Larynx subheading, Excision category are divided according to whether radical neck dissection was or was not performed. The operative report would indicate the extent of the dissection by referring to excision of lymph nodes in a radical procedure.

Introduction

Intubation is the establishment of an airway. The intubation represented in 31500 is provided on an emergency basis at such time as the patient experiences respiratory failure or the

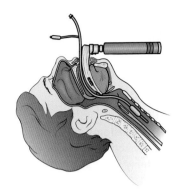

FIGURE 20–11 Endotracheal intubation.

occurrence of an inadequate airway. Fig. 20-11 illustrates endotracheal intubation. The other Introduction code (31502) is for the replacement of a previously inserted tracheotomy tube.

Repair

Within the Repair category are several plastic procedures. A laryngoplasty for a **laryngeal web** is a surgical procedure, usually performed in two stages, for the repair of congenital webbing between the vocal cords. The surgeon removes the webbing and places a spacer between the vocal cords. At a later time, the surgeon will again expose the vocal cords, using the same tracheostomy incision made on the initial procedure, and remove the spacer.

EXERCISE 20-4 *Larynx*

Using the CPT, ICD-10-CM and/or ICD-9-CM manuals, complete the following:

1 Diagnostic laryngotomy

    CPT Code: _____

2 Laryngoplasty, two stages, for repair of congenital laryngeal web, removal of spacer

    CPT Code: _____

3 Emergency establishment of positive airway by means of endotracheal intubation

    CPT Code: _____

4 Subtotal supraglottic laryngectomy with removal of adjacent lymph nodes and tissue due to a primary malignant neoplasm of glossoepiglottic folds

    CPT Code: _____

    ICD-10-CM Code: _____ (ICD-9-CM Code: _____)

5 Pharyngolaryngectomy with radical neck dissection for a primary malignant neoplasm of pharyngeal region

    CPT Code: _____

    ICD-10-CM Code: _____ (ICD-9-CM Code: _____)

(Answers are located in Appendix B)

TRACHEA/BRONCHI

Procedures in the Trachea and Bronchi subheading (31600-31899) include incisions, introductions, and repairs, in addition to the endoscopic procedures.

Incision

Tracheostomy is the most common procedure reported with codes from the Incision category. A tracheostomy can be planned or performed as an emergency procedure. A planned tracheostomy is usually performed when there is a need for prolonged ventilation support, beyond the level of support that can be provided by endotracheal intubation, or when a patient cannot tolerate an endotracheal tube.

Code 31603 is assigned for an emergency **transtracheal** tracheostomy, and 31605 is assigned for an emergency **cricothyroid** membrane tracheostomy. These codes represent two different approaches to establishing an airway. Fig. 20-12 illustrates the transverse (across) incision used in a transtracheal approach; it is made between the cricoid cartilage and the sternal notch. Fig. 20-13 illustrates entry into the trachea using the transtracheal approach. Fig. 20-14 illustrates the vertical incision made for a cricothyroid tracheostomy. Fig. 20-15 shows the entry into the trachea using the cricothyroid approach.

TOOLBOX

Thomas is scheduled to have a tracheostomy because he continues to need ventilator support and is unable to tolerate the endotracheal tube that was inserted yesterday and removed earlier this morning.

QUESTIONS
1. Is this a planned or unplanned tracheostomy? _____
2. If the surgeon performs a cricothyroid tracheostomy, a _____ incision would be made.

▼ **ANSWERS**

1. planned, 2. vertical

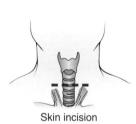

FIGURE 20–12 Transverse incision used in a transtracheal approach.

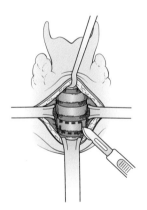

FIGURE 20–13 Transtracheal entry into the trachea using the transtracheal approach.

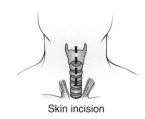

FIGURE 20–14 Vertical incision made for a cricothyroid tracheostomy.

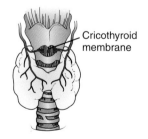

FIGURE 20–15 Cricothyroid entry into the trachea.

Introduction

Codes in the Introduction category (31717-31730) report services of catheterization, naso-tracheal and tracheobronchial aspirations, and transtracheal introduction of dilators, stents, or tubes for oxygen therapy. For an endotracheal intubation, assign 31500 (emergency endotracheal intubation) rather than a code from the Introduction category 31717-31730. For tracheal aspiration under direct vision, assign 31515 from the Endoscopy category.

Code 31720 reports nasotracheal aspiration with a suction catheter for airway clearance. The procedure involves inserting a catheter into the nostril and through the trachea. A saline solution may be introduced to help remove blockage. Report 31725 if a fiberscope is used and the procedure is performed at the patient's bedside. Code 31725 includes moderate sedation.

Excision/Repair

Excision/Repair procedures (31750-31830) in the Trachea and Bronchi subheading include plastic repairs, such as tracheoplasty and bronchoplasty, in addition to the excision of stenosis or of tumors, the suturing of tracheal wounds, scar revision and closure of a tracheostomy.

Tracheoplasty involves the surgical repair of a damaged trachea. The repair may involve reconstruction of the trachea by the use of grafts or splints formed from cartilage taken from other areas of the body or by the use of prostheses. The codes are divided according to the approach used (cervical or thoracic) and the extent and type of repair.

Bronchoplasty is repair of the bronchus and often involves the use of grafting repair or stents. A chest tube may be left in the area as a drain after the procedure and is not reported separately because it is bundled into the code to report the procedure. A grafting procedure is not bundled into the bronchoplasty code 31770 and is reported separately.

EXERCISE 20-5 *Trachea and Bronchi*

Using the CPT, ICD-10-CM and/or ICD-9-CM manuals, complete the following:

1 Emergency tracheostomy, cricothyroid approach

CPT Code: _____

2 Excision of a tumor of the trachea, cervical

CPT Code: _____

3 Catheterization with bronchial brush biopsy (code only the biopsy)

CPT Code: _____

4 Planned tracheostomy in 47-year-old patient with acute respiratory failure

CPT Code: _____

ICD-10-CM Code: _____   (ICD-9-CM Code: _____)

5 Catheterization with bronchial brush biopsy for bronchiolitis, acute

CPT Code: _____

ICD-10-CM Code: _____   (ICD-9-CM Code: _____)

(Answers are located in Appendix B)

LUNGS AND PLEURA

The Lungs and Pleura subheading (32035-32999) includes a wide range of codes to report procedures such as thoracentesis, thoracotomy, and pneumonostomy, in addition to lung transplants and plastic procedures.

Incision

Thoracotomy involves making a surgical incision into the chest wall and opening the area to the view of the surgeon. This is a major surgical procedure during which the patient is under general anesthesia. The codes are divided according to the reason for the procedure, such as biopsy, control of bleeding, cyst removal, foreign body removal, or cardiac massage. The insertion of a chest tube is bundled into the thoracotomy codes.

Excision

The Excision category contains codes for pleurectomy, biopsy, pneumonocentesis, removal, and reconstructive lung procedures.

Pleurectomy is a procedure in which the physician opens the chest cavity to full view. With the chest open and the ribs spread apart by a rib spreader, the parietal pleura is removed. The parietal pleura lines the mediastinum and body walls as illustrated in Fig. 20-16. If a pleurectomy is performed as part of another, more major procedure such as the removal of a lung (pneumonectomy), you would not report the pleurectomy separately. Note that after code 32310, pleurectomy, parietal "separate procedure" warns you not to report a pleurectomy if the pleurectomy was performed as a part of a more major procedure.

Percutaneous needle lung or mediastinum **biopsy** is often performed under radiologic guidance so that correct placement of the needle can be ensured. As with the bronchography procedure described earlier, in the discussion of the Trachea and Bronchi subheading, if radiologic guidance was used, you report the service with a code from the Radiology section. There is a note following code 32405 (biopsy) that directs you to the Surgery section, General subsection, code 10022, when a fine-needle aspiration is performed, which differs from a tissue biopsy. A fine-needle aspiration is a procedure in which fluid is withdrawn for examination.

Removal

Pneumonocentesis is the withdrawal of fluid from the lung by means of an aspirating needle. Air or gas in the pleural cavity is known as pneumothorax and occurs when the lung is traumatically ruptured or an emphysematous bulla ruptures. When the thoracic cavity (intrathoracic) air pressure increases, the pressure on the lung can result in collapse of the lung. The surgeon withdraws the air to allow the lung to reinflate.

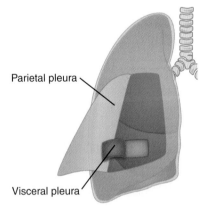

Parietal pleura

Visceral pleura

FIGURE 20-16   Parietal and visceral pleura.

The codes for the removal of the lung are based on how much of the lung is removed—segmentectomy for one segment, lobectomy for one lobe, bilobectomy for two lobes, total pneumonectomy for an entire lung—as well as on the extent of the procedure and the approach.

CODING SHOT

If a part of the bronchus was removed or repaired at the same time as the lobectomy or segmentectomy, report the service with add-on code 32501.

The preferred method of accomplishing a **thoracentesis** is by having the patient sit with arms supported, as illustrated in Fig. 20-17; local anesthesia is administered, a needle is inserted (Fig. 20-18) between the ribs, and fluid is withdrawn. Thoracentesis is performed to withdraw fluid from the pleural space that has accumulated as a result of a variety of conditions, such as congestive heart failure, pneumonia, tuberculosis, or carcinoma.

Thoracentesis may also be performed to insert a **chest tube** as an indwelling method of draining the accumulated fluid in the pleural space (pleural effusion), as illustrated in Fig. 20-19. Local anesthesia is administered, and a small incision is made through the skin, fat, and muscle. The hole is then enlarged by using an instrument, and the tube is inserted into the pleural space. A suture is placed through the skin and tied to the tube. The tube is then secured with tape. The fluid is withdrawn by means of a suction device called a multichamber water-seal suction tube. This therapeutic procedure may be performed when the patient's pleural space contains air or gas (pneumothorax), blood (hemothorax), or a large amount of fluid (pleural effusion). These conditions can be due to trauma, secondary to another disease process, or occur spontaneously.

From the Trenches

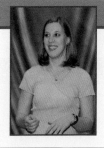

"Certification has made a huge difference in my career. It has allowed me to move up from the follow-up world of payments and denials to the front-end world of reviewing documentation and coding."

LYNDA

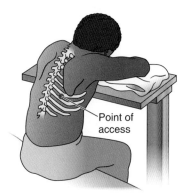

Point of access

FIGURE 20–17 Patient position for a thoracentesis.

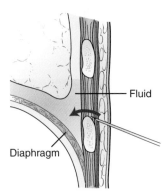

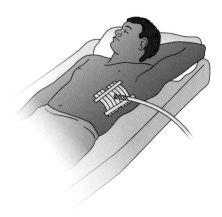

FIGURE 20–18 After administration of local anesthesia, a needle is inserted between the ribs, and fluid is withdrawn (thoracentesis).

FIGURE 20–19 A chest tube may be inserted after thoracentesis to allow for further fluid draining.

Surgical Collapse Therapy; Thoracoplasty

Thoracoplasty is a procedure in which a portion of the internal skeletal support is removed to treat a condition in which pus chronically collects in the chest cavity (chronic thoracic empyema). The procedure is major and requires extensive resecting of the membrane that lines the chest cavity. Gauze is left in the cavity and after several days is removed. Note that code 32905, thoracoplasty, refers to "all stages." The subsequent stages are for the removal of the packing and are bundled into the surgical code.

Pneumonolysis is a procedure that is performed to separate the inside of the chest cavity from the lung to permit the lung to collapse. This procedure was originally used as a treatment for tuberculosis but is now used in the evaluation of pleural diseases, debridement of chronic emphysema, and as a treatment for emphysematous blebs, in addition to other therapeutic treatments.

Pneumothorax injection (32960) is a therapeutic procedure in which the surgeon inserts a needle into the pleural cavity and injects air into the pleural cavity. The pressure in the thoracic cavity is increased and the lung partially collapses. This procedure is sometimes performed to treat tuberculosis. A chest tube may be inserted into the space for further injections of air. You would not report the insertion of the chest tube separately, as the insertion is bundled into the procedure code.

EXERCISE 20-6   *Lungs and Pleura Terminology*

Using the CPT, ICD-10-CM and/or ICD-9-CM manuals, complete the following:

1 Thoracotomy for exploration

   CPT Code: _____

2 Percutaneous needle lung biopsy

   CPT Code: _____

3 Lobectomy and bronchoplasty performed at same surgical session

   CPT Codes: _____, _____

4 Resection of an apical malignant lung neoplasm

   CPT Code: _____

   ICD-10-CM Code: _____   (ICD-9-CM Code: _____)

5 Pneumonostomy with open drainage of abscess (pulmonary necrosis)

   CPT Code: _____

   ICD-10-CM Code: _____   (ICD-9-CM Code: _____)

(Answers are located in Appendix B)

CHAPTER REVIEW

CHAPTER 20, PART I, THEORY

Without the use of reference material, complete the following:

1 The Respiratory System subsection is arranged by _____ site.

2 The procedure in which a scope is placed through a small incision and into a body cavity is called a(n) _____

_____.

3 When coding endoscopic procedures, you must be certain to code to the fullest _____ of the procedure and to code the correct approach for the procedure.

4 If more than one distinct procedure was performed during an endoscopic procedure, what modifier would you add to the lesser-priced service? _____

5 What type of endoscopy is always bundled into a surgical endoscopy? _____

6 A(n) _____ laryngoscopy is performed when a physician uses a tongue depressor to hold the tongue down and views the epiglottis with a mirror.

7 A(n) _____ laryngoscopy is performed when the endoscope is passed into the larynx and the physician can look at the larynx through a scope.

8 An otorhinolaryngologist is a physician who specializes in treating conditions of the _____, _____, and

_____.

9 When coding a nasal abscess or a nasal biopsy of the skin using the external approach, you use codes from the

_____ System subsection.

10 When coding a nasal abscess or a nasal biopsy using the internal approach, you use codes from the _____

_____ System subsection.

11 What are the three sections of turbinates? _____, _____

_____, and _____

12 What is the name of the therapy in which the physician flushes saline solution into the sinuses to remove mucus or pus?

_____

CHAPTER 20, PART II, PRACTICAL

With the use of the CPT, ICD-10-CM and/or ICD-9-CM manuals, code the following procedures. Code only the physician services in this exercise; do not code the laboratory or radiology services.

13 A unilateral, total lung lavage following smoke inhalation

CPT Code: _____

ICD-10-CM Code: _____

(ICD-9-CM Code: _____)

14 Performed as a separate procedure, a parietal pleurectomy for pleurisy with bacterial, nontuberculous effusion

CPT Code: _____

ICD-10-CM Code: _____

(ICD-9-CM Code: _____)

Chapter Review answers are only available in the TEACH Instructor Resources on Evolve

15 Resection of apical lung tumor, secondary site malignant neoplasm, with chest wall resection and reconstruction, unknown primary site

CPT Code: _____

ICD-10-CM Codes: _____, _____

(ICD-9-CM Codes: _____, _____)

16 Removal of a crayon lodged inside nasal passage, office procedure

CPT Code: _____

ICD-10-CM Code: _____

(ICD-9-CM Code: _____)

17 Surgical right nasal cavity endoscopy with polypectomy for nasal polyps

CPT Code: _____

ICD-10-CM Code: _____

(ICD-9-CM Code: _____)

18 Direct, operative laryngoscopy for removal of button lodged in 2-year-old child's larynx

CPT Code: _____

ICD-10-CM Code: _____

(ICD-9-CM Code: _____)

19 Indirect laryngoscopy with biopsy of nodule

❀ CPT Code(s): _____

❀ ICD-10-CM Code(s): _____

(❀ ICD-9-CM Code(s): _____)

20 Internal approach used to drain nasal septum hematoma

❀ CPT Code(s): _____

❀ ICD-10-CM Code(s): _____

(❀ ICD-9-CM Code(s): _____)

21 External, simple, left frontal sinusotomy for chronic frontal sinusitis

❀ CPT Code(s): _____

❀ ICD-10-CM Code(s): _____

(❀ ICD-9-CM Code(s): _____)

22 Surgical sinus endoscopy with sphenoidotomy for acute sphenoidal sinusitis

❀ CPT Code(s): _____

❀ ICD-10-CM Code(s): _____

(❀ ICD-9-CM Code(s): _____)

23 Submucous resection of nose with scoring of cartilage and contouring for an overdevelopment of nasal bones, acquired

❀ CPT Code(s): _____

❀ ICD-10-CM Code(s): _____

(❀ ICD-9-CM Code(s): _____)

24 Jack Rogers developed chest pain and difficulty breathing. He has also been coughing up thick, blood-tinged sputum. A chest radiograph shows an ill-defined mass. A diagnostic bronchoscopy of one lung is performed and a specimen of the endobronchial mass is taken. While the patient remains hospitalized, the pathology report comes back 2 days later positive for primary cancer of upper lobe and a lobectomy is performed.

CPT Code(s): _____

ICD-10-CM Code(s): _____

(ICD-9-CM Code(s): _____)

25 James Wilson has been having difficulty breathing and has had continual chronic ethmoidal sinusitis. Dr. Adams takes James to the operating room to perform a sinus endoscopy with right anterior and posterior ethmoidectomy and removal of polyps.

CPT Code(s): _____

ICD-10-CM Code(s): _____

(ICD-9-CM Code(s): _____)

26 Mary Bronson has a nosebleed that won't stop. She goes to the emergency department, where anterior packing is done to control the anterior nasal hemorrhage. She also has documented benign hypertension.

CPT Code(s): _____

ICD-10-CM Code(s): _____

(ICD-9-CM Code(s): _____)

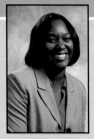

"The world of coding is wide open; coders should explore all available opportunities and find what most interests them."

Letitia Patterson, MPA, CPC, CCS-P
Consultant
A Coder's Resource
Chicago, Illinois

Cardiovascular System

Chapter Topics

Coding Highlights

Cardiovascular Coding in the Surgery Section

Cardiovascular Coding in the Medicine Section

Cardiovascular Coding in the Radiology Section

Chapter Review

Learning Objectives

After completing this chapter you should be able to

1 Understand cardiovascular services reported with codes from the Surgery, Medicine, and Radiology sections.

2 Review cardiovascular coding terminology.

3 Recognize the major differences in the subheadings of the Cardiovascular subsection.

4 Define rules of coding cardiovascular services when using codes from the Medicine section.

5 Identify the major rules of coding cardiovascular services using the Radiology section codes.

6 Demonstrate ability to code Cardiovascular services.

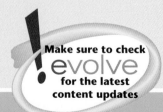
Make sure to check
evolve
for the latest
content updates

CODING HIGHLIGHTS

Cardiology is one of the largest subspecialties in medicine, and numerous modern techniques are used to diagnose and treat cardiac conditions. A **cardiologist** is an internal medicine physician who is specialized in the diagnosis and treatment of conditions of the heart. A cardiologist can further specialize in cardiovascular surgical procedures or other treatment and diagnostic specialties. In a smaller practice a cardiologist may do many of these procedures himself/herself, whereas in a larger practice a cardiologist may be more specialized and provide a more limited number of services.

Coding from Three Sections

When you are reporting cardiology services you will often be using codes from three sections: Surgery, Medicine, and Radiology.

■ The Surgery section contains codes for cardiovascular surgical procedures.
■ The Medicine section contains codes for nonsurgical cardiovascular services.
■ The Radiology section contains diagnostic studies or radiologic visualization codes.

Fig. 21-1 is a list of the section information that is most often used when reporting cardiovascular services. The confusion in coding cardiology usually comes from not understanding the components (parts) of coding cardiovascular services, the various locations of these codes in the CPT manual, and the terminology associated with cardiovascular services. To clarify cardiology coding, let's begin by reviewing the definitions of invasive, noninvasive, electrophysiology, and angiography as they relate to cardiovascular coding.

Invasive

Invasive is entering the body—breaking the skin—to make a correction or for examination. An example of an invasive cardiac procedure is the removal of a tumor from the heart. The chest is opened, the ribs spread apart, the heart fully exposed to the view of the surgeon, and the tumor removed. Another example is the removal of a clot from a vessel. The surgeon usually enters the body percutaneously (through the skin) by means of a catheter that is threaded through the vessel to the location of the clot. The clot can then be pulled out of the vessel through the catheter or can be injected with a substance that dissolves it. Although an open surgical procedure was not used, the body was entered—an invasive procedure. Invasive cardiology procedures are also called **interventional** procedures; some codes are located in the Surgery section for the surgical technique, and others are located in the Medicine section and the Radiology section for the radiologic supervision and guidance, and both codes are reported for the one procedure. Sometimes, one physician provides both components of the procedure and in other instances, two physicians will provide the components.

SURGERY SECTION	MEDICINE SECTION	RADIOLOGY SECTION

Cardiovascular System (33010-37799)
   Heart and Pericardium
   Endoscopy
   Arteries and Veins
   Adjuvant Techniques
	Cardiovascular System (92920-93799)
	   Coronary Therapeutic Services and
	     Procedures
	   Cardiography
	   Cardiovascular Monitoring Services
	   Implantable and Wearable Cardiac Device
	     Evaluations
	   Echocardiography
	   Cardiac Catheterization
	   Intracardiac Electrophysiological Procedures
	   Peripheral Arterial Disease Rehabilitation
	   Noninvasive Physiologic Studies and
	     Procedures
	   Other Procedures
		Diagnostic Radiology (75557-75791)
		   Heart
		   Vascular Procedures
		     Aorta and Arteries
		Diagnostic Ultrasound (various)
		   Ultrasonic Guidance Procedures
		Radiologic Guidance (77001-77022)
		Nuclear Medicine (78414-78499)
		   Cardiovascular System

FIGURE 21-1   A list of the section information that is most often used when reporting cardiovascular services.

Noninvasive

Noninvasive services and procedures—not breaking the skin—are usually performed for diagnostic purposes. Usually, performing these procedures does not require entering the body; rather, they are diagnostic tests that can be performed from outside the body, for example, echocardiography (93303-93355) or cardiography (93000-93278) from the Medicine section.

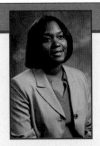

From the Trenches

What qualities best describe a medical coder?

"Detail oriented, investigative and research oriented, patient, and excellent analytical skills."

LETITIA

CODING SHOT

To choose the correct cardiology code, first determine whether the procedure or service was invasive (interventional [percutaneous] or open) or noninvasive.

Electrophysiology

Electrophysiology (EP) is the study of the electrical system of the heart and includes the study of arrhythmias. Diagnostic procedures include procedures such as recordings from inside the heart by placing wire electrodes into the heart percutaneously and by means of an electrogram, recording the electrical activity within the heart. The codes for these invasive diagnostic and therapeutic procedures are located in the Medicine section (93600-93662).

As a treatment for abnormal electrical activity in the heart, more invasive treatments can be performed, such as the placement of a pacemaker, implantable defibrillator, or other devices to regulate the rhythm of the heart. These invasive treatments are surgical procedures, and the codes are located in the Surgery section, Cardiology subsection, Pacemaker or Implantable Defibrillator (33202-33273). There are also Surgery codes for operative procedures to correct electrophysiologic problems of the heart (33250-33266), when the electrical problems are corrected surgically by incision, excision, or ablation. For example, code 33250 reports an operative ablation performed for patients with conduction disorders such as Wolff-Parkinson-White syndrome, in which there is a short circuit between the atria and ventricles. This is a congenital defect that results in rapid heartbeats due to a muscle fiber that remains after the heart developed. This fiber would usually not be present in the normally developed heart and when it is present it interrupts normal conduction. The surgeon ablates the fibers by means of a small wire that destroys the fibers and restores normal heart rhythm. You will be learning more about the electrical conduction system of the heart later in this chapter.

Nuclear

Nuclear cardiology is a diagnostic specialty that plays a very important role in modern cardiology. A physician who specializes in nuclear cardiology uses radioactive radiologic procedures to aid in the diagnosis of cardiologic conditions. When reporting nuclear cardiology services, HCPCS Level II codes will often also be reported. For example, "A" codes report radiopharmaceuticals; "G" codes report the procedures and procedures combined with the supplies, radiopharmaceuticals, and drugs; "J" codes report the drugs; and "Q" codes report contrast agents. For example, if the cardiologist provided a myocardial perfusion imaging, tomography (SPECT) (78452) during a stress test (93015) with two units A9500 (99mTc sestambi, per study dose) and 60 mg of adenosine (J0152), you would report: 78452, 93015, A9500 × 2, and J0152 × 2.

EXERCISE 21-1 *Coding Highlights*

Complete the following:

1 This term means entering the body: _____

2 A cardiologist is a(n) _____ medicine physician who has chosen to specialize in the diagnosis and treatment of conditions of the heart.

3 What three sections of the CPT will you often use to code cardiology services? _____, _____, and _____

4 What type of cardiology enters the body—breaks the skin—to make a correction or for examination? _____

5 What is the term that describes the study of the electrical system of the heart and includes the study of arrhythmias?

_____

6 Physician who specializes in _____ cardiology uses radioactive radiologic procedures to aid in the diagnosis of cardiologic conditions.

(Answers are located in Appendix B)

Now that you are familiar with some of the basic terms and coding of the cardiovascular services and procedures, let's look at the three sections where you will locate the components (parts) of cardiovascular coding: Surgery, Medicine, and Radiology.

CARDIOVASCULAR CODING IN THE SURGERY SECTION

The Cardiovascular System subsection (33010-37799) of the Surgery section contains diagnostic and therapeutic procedure codes that are divided on the basis of whether the procedure was performed on the heart/pericardium or on arteries/veins. The Heart and Pericardium subheading (33010-33999) contains codes for procedures that involve the repair of the heart and coronary vessels, such as placement of pacemakers, repair of valve disorders, and graft/bypass procedures. In the Arteries and Veins subheading (34001-37799) are the same types of procedures but for noncoronary (nonheart) vessels. For example, a thromboendarterectomy is the removal of a thrombus (stationary obstruction) and a portion of the lining of an artery. When a thromboendarterectomy is performed on a coronary artery, you would assign a code from the Heart and Pericardium subheading; but if the procedure was performed on a noncoronary artery, you would assign a code from the Arteries and Veins subheading.

CODING SHOT

The location of the procedure—coronary or noncoronary—is the first step in selecting the correct cardiovascular surgical code, because the CPT codes are divided on the basis of whether a procedure involved coronary or noncoronary vessels.

Heart and Pericardium

The Surgery section, Cardiovascular System subsection, Heart and Pericardium subheading (33010-33999) contains procedures that are performed both percutaneously and through open surgical sites. There are always many revisions and additions in this subheading each year to reflect the many advances in this important specialty. Numerous notes are located throughout the subheading, and they must be read prior to coding. Codes in the Heart and Pericardium subheading are for services provided to repair the heart (Fig. 21-2), pericardium or coronary vessels (Fig. 21-3). Pericardiocentesis codes 33010 and 33011 are divided based on initial or subsequent service.

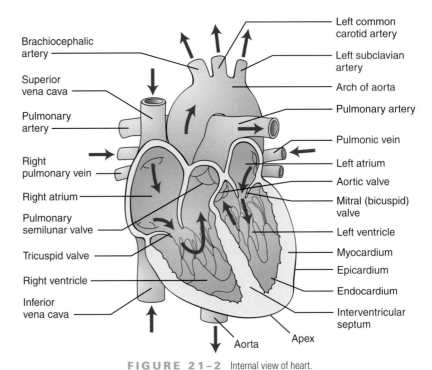

FIGURE 21-2   Internal view of heart.

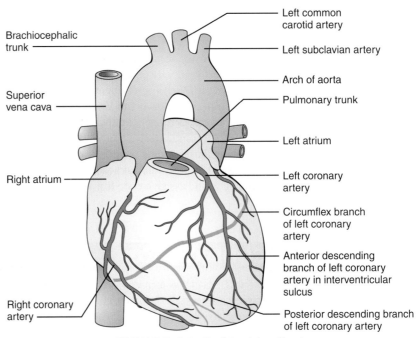

FIGURE 21-3   External view of heart.

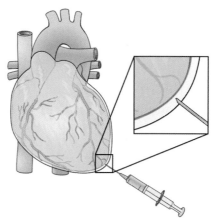

FIGURE 21-4   Pericardiocentesis is the withdrawal of fluid from the pericardium by means of aspiration.

QUICK CHECK 21-1

1. Using Fig. 21-3, name the three main coronary arteries: _____

_____

(Answers are located in Appendix C)

Pericardium

Pericardiocentesis (33010, 33011) is a procedure in which the surgeon withdraws fluid from the pericardial space by means of a needle inserted percutaneously into the space as illustrated in Fig. 21-4. The insertion can be performed using radiologic (ultrasound) guidance—the use of which would be reported with a separate code from the Radiology section. There is a note following the pericardiocentesis codes that states: "(For radiological supervision and interpretation, use 76930)"; that is, ultrasonic guidance for pericardiocentesis, imaging supervision, and interpretation. Watch for these directional features throughout the Cardiovascular System subsection.

The fluid withdrawn during a pericardiocentesis is then examined for microbial agents (such as tuberculosis), neoplasia, or autoimmune diseases (such as lupus or rheumatoid arthritis). The pericardiocentesis codes are divided on the basis of whether the service was initial or subsequent.

A tube pericardiostomy (33015) uses the same procedure described above, but a catheter is left in the pericardial sac/space leading to the outside of the body to allow for continued drainage.

The remaining procedures in the Pericardium category (33020-33050) are open surgical procedures for the removal of clots, foreign bodies, tumors, cysts, or a portion of the pericardium to create a window to allow pericardial fluid to drain into the pleural space.

Cardiac Tumor

A procedure performed to remove a tumor of the pericardium is reported using a code from the Pericardium category (33010-33050), but if a tumor is removed from the heart, you would select a code from the category Cardiac Tumor (33120, 33130). There are only two tumor-removal codes in the Cardiac Tumor category, one for a tumor that is removed from inside the heart (intracardiac) and one for a tumor that is removed from outside the heart (external). Both procedures are open surgical procedures that involve opening the chest, spreading the ribs, and excising the tumor.

Transmyocardial Revascularization

Laser transmyocardial revascularization describes a procedure in which areas of cardiac ischemia (reversible muscle damage) are exposed to a laser beam to create holes in the surface of the heart. This procedure encourages new capillary growth, thereby revitalizing the damaged area by increasing the blood flow in the area. This procedure can be performed alone, as the only surgical procedure performed (33140), or at the time of another open cardiac procedure (add-on code 33141).

Pacemaker or Implantable Defibrillator

A pacemaker and implantable defibrillator (33202-33273) are devices that are inserted into the body to electrically shock the heart into regular rhythm (as illustrated in Figs. 21-5 and 21-6). When a pacemaker is inserted, a pocket is made and a generator and lead(s) are placed inside the chest (Fig. 21-7). Sometimes, only components of the pacemaker are reinserted, repaired, or replaced. You need to know three things about the service provided to correctly code the pacemaker:

1. Where the electrode (lead) is placed: atrium, ventricle, or both ventricle and atrium
2. Whether the procedure involves initial placement, replacement, upgrade or repair of all components or separate components of the pacemaker
3. The approach used to place the pacemaker (epicardial or transvenous)

CODING SHOT

A single pacemaker has one lead (atrium or ventricle), a dual pacemaker has two leads (one lead in the right atrium and one in the right ventricle), and a biventricular pacemaker has three leads (one in the right atrium, one in the right ventricle, and one on the left ventricle via the coronary sinus vein).

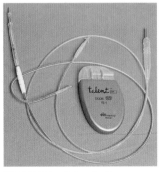

FIGURE 21-5 Permanent cardiac pacemaker unit.

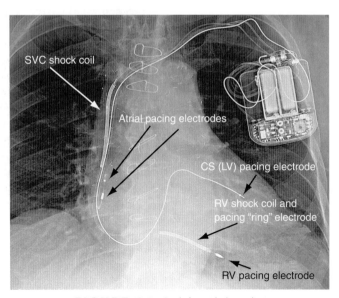

FIGURE 21-6 Left ventricular pacing.

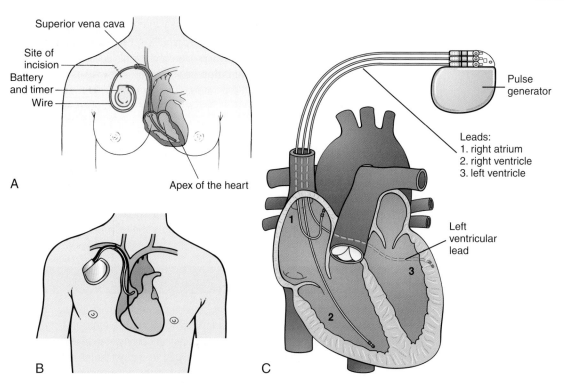

Superior vena cava

Site of incision
Battery and timer
Wire

Apex of the heart

A

B

C

Pulse generator

Leads:
1. right atrium
2. right ventricle
3. left ventricle

Left ventricular lead

FIGURE 21–7 A, Single pacemaker insertion. **B,** Dual chamber pacemaker. **C,** Biventricular pacemaker.

Approaches. The two approaches that are used when inserting a pacemaker are epicardial (on the heart) and transvenous (through a vein), and the codes are divided according to the surgical approach.

1. The **epicardial** approach involves opening the chest cavity and placing a lead on the epicardial sac of the heart. A pocket is formed in either the upper abdomen or under the clavicle, and the pacemaker generator is placed into the pocket. The wires are then connected to the pacemaker generator and the chest area is closed. Codes for the epicardial process are further divided based on the approach to the heart—thoracotomy, upper abdominal (xiphoid region), or endoscopic.

2. The **transvenous** approach involves accessing a vein (subclavian or jugular) and inserting an electrode (lead) into the vein. The pacemaker is affixed by creating a pocket into which the pacemaker generator is placed. The fluoroscopy views the internal structure by means of x-rays. Fluoroscopic guidance is included in 33206-33249. Diagnostic fluoroscopic guidance for diagnostic lead evaluation with lead insertion, replacement, or revision is reported with 76000. Transvenous codes are further divided based on the area of the heart into which the pacemaker is inserted. For example, 33207 (single-lead pacemaker) is reported for transvenous placement of a pacemaker into the ventricle of the heart. If the pacemaker electrodes were placed in both the atrium and ventricle, 33208 (dual-lead pacemaker) is reported.

The documentation in the medical record will indicate whether a pacemaker or implantable defibrillator was inserted or replaced.

The same set of criteria applies to choosing the correct implantable defibrillator codes:

1. Revision or replacement of lead(s)
2. Replacement, repair, removal of components
3. Approach used for insertion or repair

CODING SHOT

A change of batteries in a pacemaker or an implantable defibrillator is a **removal** of the implanted generator and the **reimplantation** (insertion) of a new generator. Both the removal and the reimplantation are reported separately.

If electrophysiology (EP) is used to diagnose a condition that resulted in the insertion of a pacemaker or an implantable defibrillator, the EP is not included in the surgery code reported for the insertion. Rather, the EP is reported separately using the Medicine section codes 93600-93662.

Remember to use modifier -26 on a radiology service when only the professional portion of the service was provided and -TC when only the technical portion was provided.

CODING SHOT

If a patient with a pacemaker or other implantable device is seen by the physician within the 90-day follow-up (global) period for implantation for a problem not related to the implantation, the service for the new problem can be billed. Documentation in the medical record must support the statement that the service is unrelated to the implantation. Append the E/M service code with modifier -24 (unrelated E/M service). If the patient is returned to the operating room for repositioning or replacement of the pacemaker or an implantable defibrillator during the global period by the same physician, modifier -78 would be appended to the code.

EXERCISE 21-2 *Pericardium, Cardiac Tumors, and Pacemakers*

Using the CPT, ICD-10-CM and/or ICD-9-CM manuals, code the following:

1 Allen Jackson gets very tired walking up and down stairs. He has a hard time catching his breath and experiences instances when his heart feels as if it is beating fast. His physician has told him that he will require a pacemaker implantation. Allen goes to surgery and has a single-lead pacemaker implanted with a ventricular lead.

CPT Code: _____

2 Five days after the pacemaker is implanted, Allen (from Question 1) feels very dizzy and his electrocardiogram is showing some abnormalities. His physician returns him to the operating room and discovers that the pacemaker lead is malfunctioning. The pacemaker lead is replaced, and Allen recovers nicely.

CPT Code: _____

3 Five years later, the battery in Allen's pacemaker is found to have become depleted. He is also having some other symptoms that his physician believes necessitate not only a replacement pacemaker, but also an upgrade to a dual-lead device.

CPT Code: _____

4 A new patient with a chief complaint of sharp, intermittent retrosternal pain that is reduced by sitting up or leaning forward is evaluated by a cardiologist. Chest films reveal acute pulmonary edema with acute pericardial effusion. The physician performs a pericardiocentesis. (Code the procedure and diagnoses.)

CPT Code: _____

ICD-10-CM Codes: _____, _____

(ICD-9-CM Codes: _____, _____)

5 Resection of an endocardium primary malignant tumor in which cardiopulmonary bypass is required

CPT Code: _____

ICD-10-CM Code: _____ (ICD-9-CM Code: _____)

(Answers are located in Appendix B)

Electrophysiologic Operative Procedures

Electrophysiology, as you learned earlier in this chapter, is the study of the electrical system of the heart, and most of the codes for the EP tests are in the Medicine section. The codes in the Surgery section (33250-33266) apply to the surgical repair of a defect that causes an abnormal rhythm. Cardiopulmonary bypass is usually required during these major operative procedures in which the chest is opened to expose the heart to the full view of the surgeon. Codes 33265 and 33266 are used to report endoscopic approach for EP procedures. The surgeon maps the locations of the electrodes of the heart and notes the source of the arrhythmia. The source of the arrhythmia is then ablated (separated). The codes are divided on the basis of the need for cardiopulmonary bypass, the reason for the procedure (atrial fibrillation, atrial flutter, etc.), and the approach. Percutaneous electrophysiology is discussed later in this chapter under the heading Intracardiac Electrophysiologic Procedures/Studies.

From the Trenches

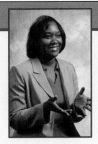

"It is important to be a multi-tasker in the work environment. Also, be as flexible as possible. Learn the basics of the entire practice if the opportunity presents itself."

LETITIA

Patient-Activated Event Recorder

A patient-activated event recorder is also known as a cardiac event recorder or a loop recorder. Codes 33282 and 33284 involve surgical implantation into the subcutaneous tissue of the upper left quadrant. The recorder senses the heart's rhythms, and when the patient presses a button, the device records the electrical activity of the heart. The recording can assist the physician in making a diagnosis of a hard-to-detect rhythm problem. Codes are divided on the basis of whether the device was implanted or removed.

Heart (Including Valves) and Great Vessels

The Heart (Including Valves) and Great Vessels category (33300-33335) contains codes to report the services of repair of cardiac wounds, exploratory (including foreign body removal), and insertion of graft of the aorta or great vessels. The codes are reported with or without cardiopulmonary bypass. Suture repair of the aorta or great vessels (33320-33322) is reported with or without shunt or cardiopulmonary bypass.

Cardiac Valves

The category Cardiac Valves (33361-33478) has subcategory codes of aortic, mitral, tricuspid, and pulmonary valves. The procedures listed are similar for each valve; some are a little more extensive than others. Code descriptions vary depending on whether a cardiopulmonary bypass (heart-lung) machine was used during the procedure. The cardiopulmonary bypass is a resource-intensive procedure that requires a heart-lung machine to assume the patient's heart and lung functions during surgery.

The cardiac valve procedures are located in the CPT manual index under the valve type or under what was done, such as a repair or a replacement. For example, the replacement of an aortic valve is located in the CPT index under "Aorta," subterm "Valve," subterm "Replacement."

The aortic valve controls the flow of blood from the left ventricle to the aorta. When a patient has aortic valve stenosis the flow of blood is restricted. Medications or balloon valve angioplasty are the less invasive treatments; however, valve replacement may be required. Codes 33361-33369 report transcatheter aortic valve replacement (TAVR) and transcatheter aortic valve implant (TAVI). The delivery catheter is inserted into an artery using a percutaneous, open, or transaortic approach. Codes 33361-33365 are divided based on the approach. Codes 33367-33369 are add-on codes that are reported when the TAVR/TAVI are performed in addition to a more primary procedure.

EXERCISE 21-3   *EP, Event Recorder, and Valves*

Using the CPT, ICD-10-CM and/or ICD-9-CM manuals, code the following:

1 Mary Black's echocardiogram and cardiac catheterization show severe mitral stenosis with regurgitation. Her physician believes that because she is symptomatic, she should have her mitral valve replaced. The mitral valve replacement includes cardiopulmonary bypass.

CPT Code: _____

2 Andrew Nelson has a loud heart murmur and, after study, is found to have severe aortic stenosis. He elects to have an aortic valve replacement. He is taken to the operating room and placed on a heart-lung machine. He then has his aortic valve replaced with a prosthetic valve.

CPT Code: _____

3 With the heart exposed through the sternum and the patient's functions supported by a cardiopulmonary bypass, the right atrium is opened and the bigeminal arrhythmia foci are ablated by using electrical current. Bypass is discontinued and the atrium and sternum are closed in the usual fashion.

CPT Code: _____

ICD-10-CM Code: _____ (ICD-9-CM Code: _____)

4 Implantation of a patient-activated cardiac loop device with programming for a diagnosis of palpitations and dizziness.

CPT Code: _____

ICD-10-CM Codes: _____, _____

(ICD-9-CM Codes: _____, _____)

(Answers are located in Appendix B)

Coronary Artery Anomalies

The Coronary Artery Anomalies category (33500-33507) contains codes to report the services of repair of the coronary artery by various methods, such as graft, ligation (tying off), and reconstruction. The codes include endarterectomy (removal of the inner lining of an artery) and angioplasty (blood vessel repair). Do not unbundle the codes and report the endarterectomy or angioplasty separately. Also, the procedures often require the use of cardiopulmonary bypass to allow the surgeon to repair the defect while the heart is without blood flow, which makes a difference in the choice of codes.

Coronary Artery Bypass

Arteries deliver oxygenated blood to all areas of the body, and veins return the blood that is full of waste products. The heart muscle is fed by coronary arteries that encircle the heart. When these arteries clog with plaque (atherosclerosis) (Fig. 21-8), the flow of blood lessens. Sometimes the arteries clog to the point that the heart muscle begins to perform at low levels due to lack of blood (**reversible ischemia**) or actually die (**irreversible ischemia**).

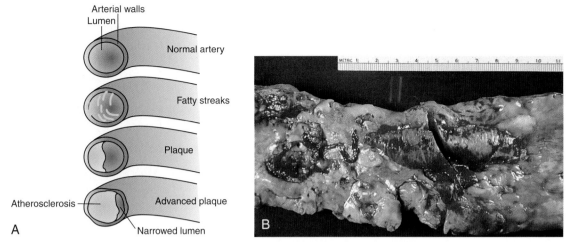

FIGURE 21–8   A, Atherosclerosis. **B,** Atherosclerotic vessel.

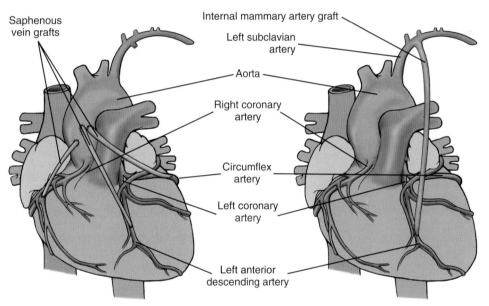

FIGURE 21–9   Coronary artery bypass graft (CABG).

Reversible ischemia means that if the bloodflow is increased to the heart muscle, the heart muscle may again begin to function at normal or near-normal levels. **Coronary artery bypass grafting (CABG)** is one way to increase the flow of blood (as illustrated in Fig. 21-9). The diseased portion of the artery is bypassed by attaching a healthy vessel above and below the diseased area and allowing the healthy vessel to then become the conduit of the blood, thus bypassing the blockage (Fig. 21-10). Blockage can also be pushed to the sides of the coronary arterial walls by a procedure in which a balloon is expanded inside the artery. This procedure is known as a **percutaneous transluminal coronary angioplasty (PTCA)** (Fig. 21-11).

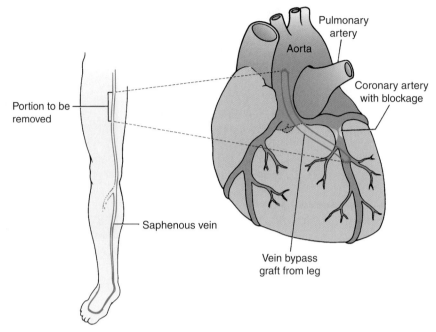

FIGURE 21-10 Coronary artery bypass.

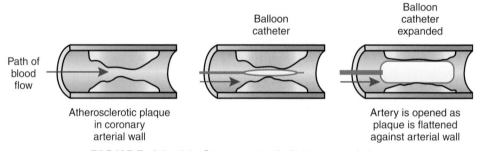

FIGURE 21-11 Percutaneous transluminal coronary angioplasty.

QUICK CHECK 21-2

1. What is the acronym commonly used for coronary artery bypass graft?

_____

(Answers are located in Appendix C)

To correctly report coronary bypass grafts, you must know whether an artery (33533-33548), a vein (33510-33516), or both (33517-33523, plus 33533-33548) are being used as the bypass graft. You must also know how many bypass grafts are being performed. There may be more than one blockage to be bypassed and, therefore, more than one graft. If only a vein is used for the graft (most often the saphenous vein from the leg is harvested and used for this purpose; see Fig. 21-10), the code reflecting the number of grafts would be assigned from the category Venous Grafting Only for Coronary Artery Bypass (33510-33516).

The following exercise will help you understand the differences in coding for bypass grafts using arteries, veins, or both, and for coding anomalies.

EXERCISE 21-4   *Coronary Artery Bypass and Anomalies*

Using the CPT, ICD-10-CM and/or ICD-9-CM manuals, code the following:

1 Two coronary bypass grafts using veins only

   CPT Code: _____

The code for Question 1 came from the category Venous Grafting Only for Coronary Artery Bypass because the bypass was accomplished using a venous graft. If the bypass had been accomplished using an arterial graft, the codes in the category Arterial Grafting for Coronary Artery Bypass would be used to report the service. If both veins and arteries were used to accomplish the bypass, you would report the service by reporting an artery bypass code and a code from the category Combined Arterial-Venous Grafting for Coronary Bypass. Because the title of the category contains the words "arterial-venous," you might think that the codes in the category report both the artery and the vein, but this is not the case. The category codes under "arterial-venous" are used only when a venous graft has been used in addition to an arterial graft, and these arterial-venous codes are used only in combination with the arterial graft codes (33533-33536).

For example, a patient has had a **five-vessel** coronary artery bypass graft, for which two bypasses were accomplished using internal mammary arteries and three bypasses were accomplished using veins (reported with 2A and 2B):

2A Coronary artery bypass using two arterial grafts

   CPT Code: _____

2B Coronary artery bypass using three venous grafts in addition to the arterial grafts for coronary artery disease, native arteries, due to arteriosclerotic coronary heart disease

   CPT Code: _____

   ICD-10-CM Code: _____ (ICD-9-CM Code: _____)

3 Coronary artery bypass of native arteries using one internal mammary artery graft and three venous grafts. Patient has documented arteriosclerotic coronary heart disease and hypertensive heart disease, benign.

   CPT Codes: _____, _____

   ICD-10-CM Codes: _____, _____

   (ICD-9-CM Codes: _____, _____)

(Answers are located in Appendix B)

CODING SHOT

Modifier -51 would not be assigned with the code for the venous grafts because codes 33517-33523 are add-on codes. Parenthetical notations with each code indicate the code is to be used in conjunction with 33533-33548. This means that the venous code is never reported alone but always follows an arterial code.

Arteries and Veins

Code groupings for arteries and veins vary according to procedures such as thrombectomies, aneurysm repairs, bypass grafting, repairs, angioplasties, and all other procedures. Codes in the subheading Arteries and Veins (34001-37799) refer to all arteries and veins except the coronary arteries and veins (Figs. 21-12 and 21-13).

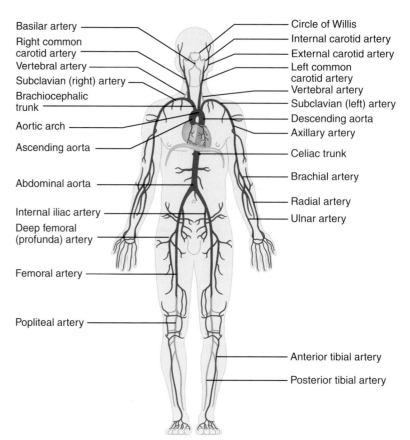

Basilar artery

Right common
carotid artery

Vertebral artery

Subclavian (right) artery

Brachiocephalic
trunk

Aortic arch

Ascending aorta

Abdominal aorta

Internal iliac artery

Deep femoral
(profunda) artery

Femoral artery

Popliteal artery

Circle of Willis

Internal carotid artery

External carotid artery

Left common
carotid artery

Vertebral artery

Subclavian (left) artery

Descending aorta

Axillary artery

Celiac trunk

Brachial artery

Radial artery

Ulnar artery

Anterior tibial artery

Posterior tibial artery

FIGURE 21–12   Arteries of the body.

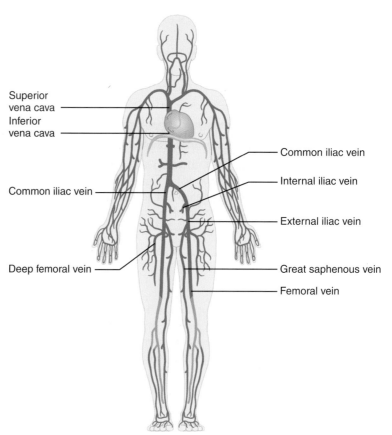

Superior
vena cava

Inferior
vena cava

Common iliac vein

Deep femoral vein

Common iliac vein

Internal iliac vein

External iliac vein

Great saphenous vein

Femoral vein

FIGURE 21–13   Veins of the body.

Vascular Families—Selective or Nonselective Placement

A vascular family can be compared to a tree with branches. The tree has a main trunk from which large branches and then smaller branches grow. The same is true with vascular families. A main vessel is the main trunk, and other vessels branch off from the main vessel. Vessels connected in this manner are considered families.

Catheters, as shown in Fig. 21-14, may have to be placed in vessels for monitoring, removal of blood, injection of contrast materials, or infusion. When coding the placement of a catheter it is necessary to know where the catheter starts and where it ends.

Catheter placement is nonselective or selective. **Nonselective catheter placement** means the catheter or needle is placed directly into an artery or vein (and not manipulated farther along) or is placed only into the aorta from any approach. **Selective catheter placement** means the catheter must be moved, manipulated, or guided into a part of the venous or arterial system other than the aorta or the vessel punctured (that is, into the branches), generally under fluoroscopic guidance. The following codes illustrate nonselective and selective placement:

Example

Nonselective: 36000 Introduction of needle or intracatheter, vein

Selective: 36012 Selective catheter placement, venous system; second order, or more selective, branch

Code 36000 describes the placement of a needle or catheter into a vein with no further manipulation or movement. Code 36012 describes the placement of a catheter into a vein and its manipulation or moving to a second-order vein or farther.

The first note in the Cardiovascular System subsection in the CPT manual (before code 33010) refers to selective placement. The note appears at the beginning of the section because it is very important and applies to the entire Cardiovascular System subsection. When coding selective placement for any procedure, you report the fullest extension into one vascular family, just as you would when coding a gastrointestinal endoscopic procedure, when you report to the farthest extent of the procedure. The same is true of selective placement into a vascular family: Code to the farthest extent of the placement within the vascular family.

The **first order** is the main artery in a vascular family, the **second order** is the branch off the main artery, the **third order** is the next branch off the second order, and so on. A vascular family can have more than one second-order, third-order, and so on, vessel, as illustrated in Fig. 21-15. Note that the first order in Fig. 21-15 is the brachiocephalic artery, the second order is the common carotid artery, and that there are two third-order arteries. If the farthest

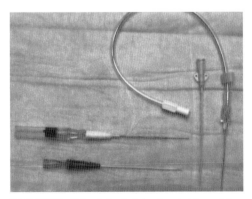

FIGURE 21-14 Catheters for arterial cannulation.

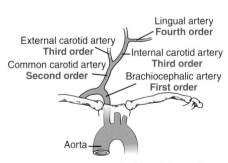

FIGURE 21-15 Brachiocephalic vascular family with first-, second-, third-, and fourth-order vessels.

extent of the placement was to the third order, only the third-order code would be reported. For example, if a catheter was placed into the first-order brachiocephalic artery and from there manipulated through the second-order artery (right common carotid), and finally into the third-order artery (right internal or external carotid), you would report only the third-order artery, with code 36217, which describes an initial third-order placement within the brachiocephalic family.

CODING SHOT

Appendix L of the CPT manual is a listing of the vascular families based on the starting point of the aorta.

If the catheter placement continued from one branch of the brachiocephalic family into another branch of the family, you would report the additional second order, third order, and beyond using an add-on code—36218. Oftentimes, a physician will investigate not only one branch of an artery but several others. Report all subsequent catheter placement to the farthest extent of each placement.

CODING SHOT

Code to the farthest extent of the vascular family using an initial code; then code any additional services of the second order, third order, or beyond by using an add-on code.

Catheter placement codes may vary according to the vascular family into which the catheter is placed. Look at the example of the two codes below and note the difference in vascular families.

Example

36215	Selective catheter placement, arterial system; each first order **thoracic or brachiocephalic** branch, within a vascular family
36245	Selective catheter placement, arterial system; each first order **abdominal, pelvic, or lower extremity artery** branch, within a vascular family

QUICK CHECK 21-3

1. Which CPT Appendix would be a helpful resource for selective vascular coding?

_____

(Answers are located in Appendix C)

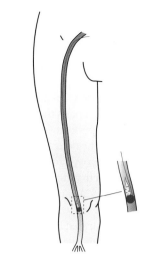

FIGURE 21–16 Embolectomy.

Embolectomy/Thrombectomy

An **embolus** is a mass of undissolved matter that is present in blood and is transported by the blood. A **thrombus** is a blood clot that occludes, or shuts off, a vessel. When a thrombus is dislodged, it becomes an embolus. Thrombectomies or embolectomies are performed to remove the unwanted debris, or clot, from the vessel and allow unrestricted bloodflow. A thrombus or embolus may be removed by opening the vessel and scraping out the debris or by percutaneously placing a balloon within the vessel to push the material aside and out of the vessel (see Fig. 21-11). A catheter may also be used to draw a thrombus or embolus out of the vessel, as illustrated in Fig. 21-16. Embolectomy/Thrombectomy codes (34001-34490) are divided based on the artery or vein in which the clot or thrombus is located (e.g., radial artery, femoropopliteal vein), with the site of incision specified in the code description (e.g., arm, leg, abdominal incision). You can locate these codes in the CPT manual index under "Embolectomy" or "Thrombectomy," subdivided by arteries and veins (e.g., carotid artery, axillary vein).

When more involved procedures such as grafts are performed, inflow and outflow establishment is included in the major procedure codes. This means that if a thrombus is present and a bypass graft is performed, the removal of the thrombus is bundled into the grafting procedure if performed on the same vessel. Also bundled into the aortic procedures is any sympathectomy (interruption of the sympathetic nervous system) or angiogram (radiographic view of the blood vessels).

EXERCISE 21-5   *Embolectomy/Thrombectomy*

Using the CPT, ICD-10-CM and/or ICD-9-CM manuals, code the following:

1 Thrombectomy of the aortoiliac artery, by leg incision

CPT Code: _____

2 Embolectomy, carotid artery, by neck incision

CPT Code: _____

3 Thrombectomy of venous bypass graft, postop complication

CPT Code: _____

ICD-10-CM Code: _____ (ICD-9-CM Code: _____)

(Answers are located in Appendix B)

Vascular Repairs

The category Venous Reconstruction (34501-34530) contains codes for the various repairs made to the vena cava, saphenous vein, and valves of the femoral vein. The repair to valves is made by opening the site and clamping off the vessels. The surgeon then opens the vein and tacks down excess material of the valve with sutures (plication). If there is a defect in the vein, the surgeon repairs the defect with a graft, usually harvested from elsewhere in the body. **Vein repairs** are performed by locating the defective vessel, clamping the vessel off, and bypassing or grafting the defect.

The category Direct Repair of Aneurysm or Excision (Partial or Total) and Graft Insertion for Aneurysm, Pseudoaneurysm, Ruptured Aneurysm, and Associated Occlusive Disease (35001-35152) contains **aneurysm repair** codes that are divided according to the type of aneurysm and the vessel the aneurysm is located in (subclavian artery, popliteal artery). The aneurysm is formed by the dilation of the wall of an artery; it is filled with fluid or clotted blood. During repair, the aneurysm is located, and clamps are placed above and below it. The section containing the aneurysm is then removed or bypassed. The aneurysm codes often refer to a **pseudoaneurysm** (false aneurysm), which is an aneurysm in which the vessel is injured and the aneurysm is being contained by the tissue that surrounds the vessel.

Endovascular aneurysm repair (EVAR) is a technology that involves placing a stent graft, a fabric tube, inside the affected area of the blood vessel accessed through an artery. For example, abdominal aortic aneurysm repair by endovascular technique is reported with codes 34800-34834, and iliac aneurysm endovascular repair is reported with 34900.

Repair, Arteriovenous Fistula category codes (35180-35190) are reported for **fistula repair** and are divided on the basis of whether the fistula (abnormal passage) is congenital, acquired, or traumatic. An arteriovenous fistula occurs when blood flows between an artery and a vein. An example of an acquired arteriovenous fistula is the creation of an arteriovenous connection that is used for a hemodialysis site (Fig. 21-17). In repairing a fistula, the surgeon separates the artery and vein and then patches the area of separation with sutures or a graft.

If an **angioscopy** of the vessel or graft area is performed during a therapeutic procedure, code 35400, Angioscopy (noncoronary vessels or grafts) during therapeutic intervention, is listed in addition to the procedure code. For example, the surgeon performed the repair of an acquired arteriovenous fistula of the neck (35188) and then placed a scope into the artery to determine visually whether the repair was complete. Code 35188 describes the primary therapeutic procedure of repair of the acquired arteriovenous fistula, and 35400 describes the use of the angioscope to accomplish the repair. Note that 35400 is an add-on code and cannot be reported alone, but only in conjunction with another procedure code.

A **transluminal angioplasty** is a procedure in which a vessel is punctured and a catheter is passed into the vessel for the purposes of widening a narrow or obstructed vessel by inflating a balloon. The category codes 35450-35476 are divided on the basis of whether the catheter was passed into the vessel by incising the skin to expose the vessel (open) or by passing the catheter through the skin (percutaneous) into the vessel. Further divisions of the codes are based on the vessel into which the catheter is placed (e.g., iliac, aortic).

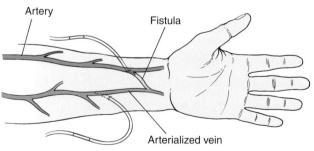

FIGURE 21-17 Hemodialysis.

Bypass Grafts

As with coronary artery bypass grafting (CABG), you must know the type of grafting material used for vascular bypass grafts (Bypass Grafts 35500-35671). Grafts can be vessels harvested from other areas of the body or they may be made of artificial materials. Codes are chosen on the basis of the type of graft and the specific vessel(s) that the graft is being bypassed from and to. For example, 35506 describes a graft that is placed to bypass a portion of the subclavian artery. During this procedure the surgeon sews a harvested vein to the side of the carotid artery and attaches the other end of the vein to the subclavian artery below the damaged area, creating a bypass around the defect.

QUICK CHECK 21-4

1. According to the CPT manual notes for bypass grafts, which of the following procurements is bundled in the bypass?
   a. upper extremity graft
   b. composite graft(s)
   c. saphenous vein graft
   d. femoropopliteal vein graft

(Answers are located in Appendix C)

One way to locate the graft codes in the CPT manual index is to reference "Bypass Graft" and then the subterm type (e.g., carotid, subclavian, vertebral).

Vascular Access

Some treatments are administered through the blood by means of vascular access. For instance, in patients receiving hemodialysis, arteriovenous fistulas may be created for dialysis treatments (see Fig. 21-17). This means that an artificial connection is made between a vein and an artery, allowing blood to flow from the vein through the graft for dialysis (cleansing of waste products) and then be returned to the artery.

Vascular Injection Procedures

 CAUTION *Just for a moment, think about what a difference a seemingly small fact—such as what is included in the vascular injection procedures— makes in the amount received for the procedure over the course of a year! It is your responsibility as the coder to know the rules of coding to ensure appropriate reimbursement for services provided by physicians. Details are important in the business of coding!*

Bundled into the vascular injections (36000-36522) are the following items:
- Local anesthesia
- Introduction of needle or catheter
- Injection of contrast media
- Pre-injection care related to procedure
- Post-injection care related to procedure

Vascular injections bundles do not include the following items:
- Catheter
- Drugs
- Contrast media

For items not bundled into the injection procedure, report each item separately.

Code 99070 (supplies and materials) from the Medicine section or HCPCS supply codes report items such as catheters, drugs, and contrast media if the procedure is performed in the clinic facility. If the procedure is performed in the hospital catheterization laboratory, the hospital-based coder would report the supply.

As previously discussed, knowledge of the vascular families is critical in coding vascular injection procedures because the initial placement and the extent of placement are usually the characteristics that determine the codes. You now know that the initial placement of the catheter is reported first and that add-on codes report any additional services. For example, review the following initial and additional third-order placement code descriptions in this example:

Example

36217	Selective catheter placement, arterial system; **initial** third order or more selective thoracic or brachiocephalic branch, within a vascular family
36218	Selective catheter placement, arterial system; **additional** second order, third order, and beyond, thoracic or brachiocephalic branch, within a vascular family

In the service described in 36217, the physician inserts a needle through the skin and into an artery. The needle has a guidewire attached to it, as illustrated in Fig. 21-18, and when the needle is withdrawn, the guidewire is left inside the artery. The guidewire can then be manipulated into the particular artery. Once the guidewire is in the correct artery, a catheter is threaded into place over the guidewire and into the first-order brachiocephalic artery. The catheter is manipulated through the second-order artery and arrives at the third-order artery, where contrast material is injected into the artery through the catheter and an arteriography is completed.

After the completion of the service described in 36217, the physician pulls the catheter back into the artery and then manipulates the catheter into another third-order artery (36218), where contrast material is again injected into the artery through the catheter and another arteriography is completed.

Figs. 21-19 and 21-20 illustrate vascular coding with a common femoral artery approach.

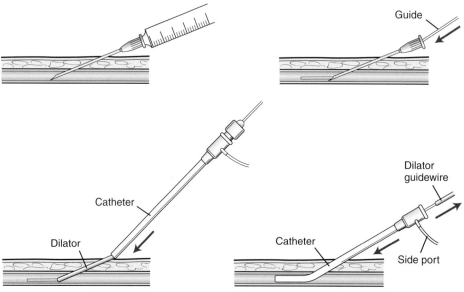

FIGURE 21–18 Catheter insertion.

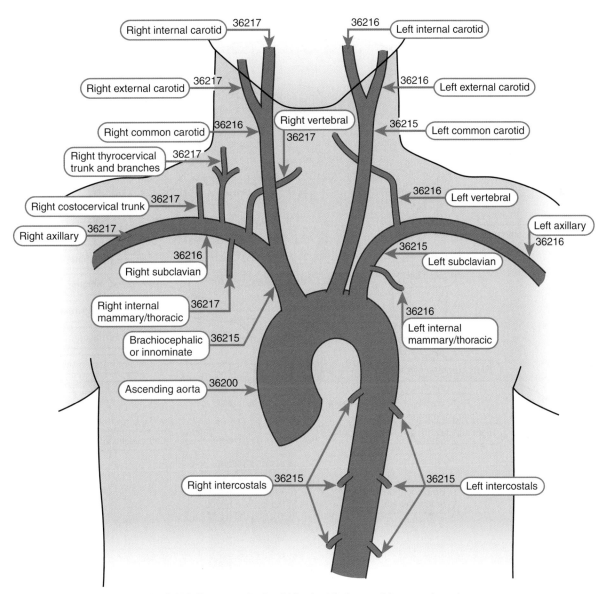

FIGURE 21-19 Arterial Head and Neck approach is common femoral.

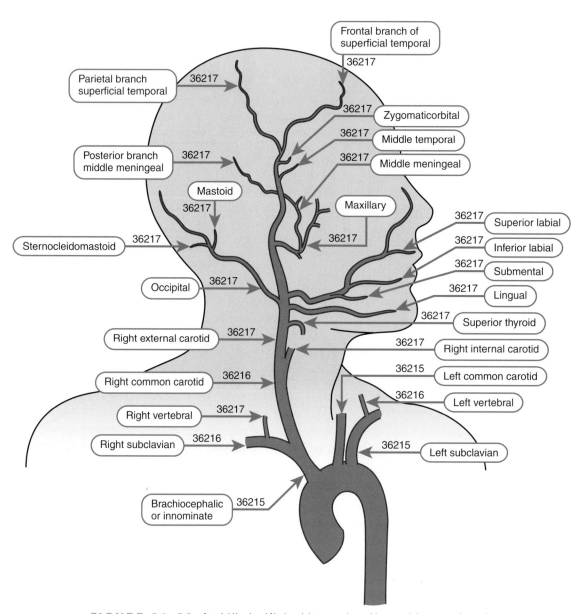

FIGURE 21-20 Arterial Head and Neck—right external carotid approach is common femoral.

EXERCISE 21-6 *Repairs, Grafts, and Vascular Access*

Using the CPT, ICD-10-CM and/or ICD-9-CM manuals, code the following:

1 Bypass graft, with vein; carotid-subclavian

CPT Code: _____

2 Bypass graft, with vein; femoral-popliteal

CPT Code: _____

3 Bypass graft, using Gore-Tex; axillary-axillary

CPT Code: _____

4 Excision, with application of a patch graft, for an aneurysm, common femoral artery

CPT Code: _____

ICD-10-CM Code: _____ (ICD-9-CM Code: _____)

5 From a right femoral artery approach, the catheter is placed in the abdominal aorta and is then threaded into the left external iliac artery where contrast material is injected and angiography is done. The surgeon then pulls back the catheter into the right external iliac where contrast is injected and angiography is completed. The catheter is withdrawn. The patient was diagnosed as having peripheral vascular disease. *(Note: Report the catheterization and radiographic guidance services separately.)*

CPT Codes: _____ LT, _____ (angiography)

ICD-10-CM Code: _____ (ICD-9-CM Code: _____)

(Answers are located in Appendix B)

CARDIOVASCULAR CODING IN THE MEDICINE SECTION

Services in the Cardiovascular subsection of the Medicine section (92920-93799) can be either invasive/noninvasive or diagnostic/therapeutic. The invasive treatments are not a matter of cutting open the body so the surgeon can view it, as was the case in the Cardiovascular subsection of the Surgery section, but are invasive in that there is an incision into or a puncture of the skin. Review the subheadings in the Cardiovascular subsection in the Medicine section of the CPT manual.

Therapeutic Services and Procedures

It is within the Therapeutic Services and Procedures subheading (92920-92998) that you locate many commonly assigned cardiovascular codes, such as cardioversion, infusions, thrombolysis, placement of catheters and stents, atherectomy, and angioplasty. Many of these services used to be performed as open operative procedures, but with the advent of modern techniques, many are now performed by means of percutaneous access. Division of the codes is based on **method** (balloon, blade), **location** (aorta or mitral valve), and **number** (single or multiple vessels).

Thrombolysis, as described in 92975, is a percutaneous procedure in which the physician inserts a catheter into a coronary vessel and injects contrast material into the vessel to further enhance the visualization of a blood clot. The clot is then destroyed by a drug that the physician injects through the catheter. The Medicine section code 92975 represents the total procedure when the thrombolysis is performed in a coronary vessel. If vessels other than the coronary vessels are treated, a code from the Surgery section, Cardiovascular subsection, would be assigned to report a transcatheter infusion for thrombolysis (see 37211-37214).

Intravascular ultrasound of the coronary vessels can be reported using the two codes 92978 and 92979, depending on the number of vessels being diagnosed. A needle is inserted percutaneously into the vessel and a guidewire introduced, followed by an ultrasound probe. The probe allows a two-dimensional image of the inside of the vessel to be viewed on the

---

Angioplasty/Stent

Patient: Marlene Castello   **Number:** 45900   **Room:** Cardiac Cath Lab 5F

DOB: 02/13/43   **Attending Physician:** Dr. Helen Palmer

DATE OF STUDY: 04/06/XX

PROCEDURE: Angioplasty/stent of 80 to 90 percent proximal/mid-right coronary artery stenosis.

INDICATIONS: Chest pain and abnormal Cardiolite stress test.

COMPLICATIONS: None

RESULTS: Successful angioplasty/stent of 80 to 90 percent proximal/mid-right coronary artery stenosis with no residual stenosis at the end of the procedure.

David H. Robinson, MD

David H. Robinson, MD

Cardiology Department

DHR/jkl

FIGURE 21–21 Angioplasty/stent report.

ultrasound monitor. The physician can assess the vessel before and after treatment. The physician may reposition the probe to assess additional vessels, and 92979 is reported to indicate this subsequent placement. Note that both 92978 and 92979 are add-on codes intended to be reported only in conjunction with the primary procedure. For example, intravascular ultrasound with coronary stent placement would be reported as 92928 (placement of stent) and 92978 (intravascular ultrasound).

Intracoronary stent placement (92928, 92929) is performed using a catheter to reinforce a coronary vessel that has collapsed or is blocked. The placement of the stent is usually accomplished with radiographic guidance which is included. The codes are divided on the basis of whether more than one coronary vessel was cleared of obstruction and had a stent placed within it.

Fig. 21-21 illustrates an angioplasty/stent report in which the coronary artery is repaired by placement of a stent. Percutaneous transluminal coronary angioplasty (PTCA) is described in codes 92920 and 92921. The codes are divided on the basis of whether a single vessel or additional vessels are treated during the procedure. Add-on code 92921 (PTCA for each additional vessel) is of interest because it can be assigned not only with 92920, but also with other codes in the category. For example, 92921 can be assigned with 92928, placement of a stent, when a stent is placed in one vessel and the PTCA is performed in a different vessel. If a patient had an intracoronary stent placed in one coronary vessel, report 92928, and if the physician also performed a PTCA on another coronary vessel, report 92921. This is the first time that you have used an add-on code with a code other than the one(s) that appears directly above it in the same group of codes, so be certain to read the code descriptions for each of the codes used in the example and pay special attention to the notes that follow 92921.

CODING SHOT

There are HCPCS modifiers to identify the specific coronary arteries that are treated, such as **-RC,** right coronary; **-LC,** left circumflex; and **-LD,** left anterior descending.

Valvuloplasty can also be performed by inserting a catheter percutaneously. The procedure opens a blocked valve by using a balloon, which is inflated to clear the blockage. Codes 92986-92990 are divided based on the valve being repaired.

The balloon technique is also used to treat congenital heart defects such as vessels that are too narrow. A blade can also be deployed inside the coronary vessels. A special catheter that has a retractable blade is guided into the vessel and the surgeon manipulates the blade to enlarge the area, using ultrasound or fluoroscopic guidance.

Cardiography and Cardiovascular Monitoring Services

This category (93000-93278) of the Cardiovascular System subsection contains frequently assigned codes, such as those for electrocardiograms and heart monitoring, which are certain to be used in most office practices, even if the practice does not include a cardiologist.

The Cardiography subheading codes report electrocardiographic procedures such as stress tests. **Stress tests** are performed to assess the adequacy of the amount of oxygen getting to the heart muscle (at rest and during exercise) and thus indicate the presence or absence of heart disease (Fig. 21-22). The top number on a blood pressure reading is systole (heart muscle is contracting); the bottom number is diastole (heart muscle is relaxing). The heart muscle is fed by three coronary arteries and their branches. If these arteries are clear, the amount of blood going to the muscle is adequate during rest and exercise. The heart muscle is fed only during diastole. Normal blood pressure is about 120/80 mm Hg, and the normal heart rate is about 60-100 beats per minute. During low blood pressure, little blood and oxygen get to the heart.

As the heart beats faster, such as during exercise, the heart rate increases and diastolic pressure time decreases, meaning that there is less time to supply blood to the heart muscle. As the heart beats faster, more oxygen is required. With narrowing of coronary arteries and branches, too little blood may circulate to the heart muscle, supplying even less oxygen than during rest. Chest pain may result as an indication that heart muscle tissue is dying. Indications of heart disease during a stress test are chest pain and a depressed or elevated ST wave segment on the ECG, as illustrated in Fig. 21-23.

The **Holter** monitor, as illustrated in Fig. 21-24, is similar to an electrocardiogram (ECG), as illustrated in Fig. 21-25, in that leads are attached to the patient. There are portable Holter monitors that record the patient's ECG readings for 24 hours. Leads are attached to the chest and to a cassette machine. The monitor converts the ECG readings to sound, and the sound is converted back to an ECG reading when completed. The reading is then sped up to hundreds of times faster than normal by computers. Any reading that varies from a normal reading will be identified. The Q, R, and S waves are related to the contraction of the ventricles of the heart. The QRS waves and heartbeats can be monitored by Holter monitors. Cardiac arrhythmias can be identified using the Holter monitor process. An example of a Holter report is presented in Fig. 21-26.

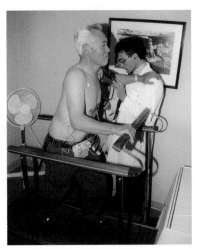

FIGURE 21-22 Stress test.

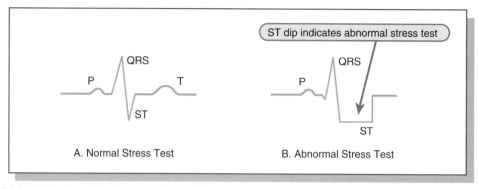

FIGURE 21–23   Normal and abnormal ECG test results. **A,** Normal ECG reading. **B,** Abnormal ECG reading. The ST segment dips. QRS complex and T waves are related to the contraction of the ventricles. Indications of heart disease during a stress test are chest pain and lengthened ST segments.

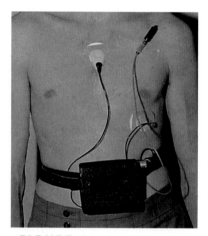

FIGURE 21–24   Holter monitor.

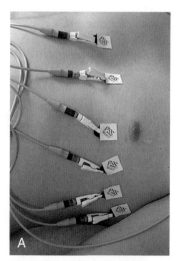
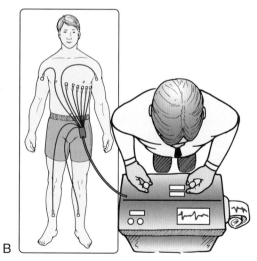

FIGURE 21–25   **A** and **B,** Placement of the electrodes for a standard ECG. The ECG is a visual record of the electrical activity of the heart.

Holter Report

INDICATIONS: Patient with atrial fibrillation on Lanoxin. Patient with known cardiomyopathy.

BASELINE DATA: 84-year-old gentleman with congestive heart failure on Elavil, Vasotec, Lanoxin, and Lasix.

The patient was monitored for 24 hours.

INTERPRETATION: 1. The predominant rhythm is atrial fibrillation. The average ventricular rate is 74 beats per minute, minimal 49 beats per minute, and maximum 114 beats per minute.
2. A total of 4948 ventricular ectopic beats were detected. There were 4 forms. There were 146 couplets with 1 triplet and 5 runs of bigeminy. There were 2 runs of ventricular tachycardia, the longest for 5 beats at a rate of 150 beats per minute. There was no ventricular fibrillation.
3. There were no prolonged pauses.

CONCLUSION: 1. Predominant rhythm is atrial fibrillation with well-controlled ventricular rate.
2. There are no prolonged pauses.
3. Asymptomatic, nonsustained ventricular tachycardia.

Raymond P. Price, MD

Raymond P. Price, MD

Cardiology Department

RPP/lpm

FIGURE 21–26 Holter report.

CODING SHOT

Many CPT monitoring codes cannot be billed with modifiers -TC or -26, as there are individual codes for the professional and technical components.

An ECG is typically conducted by attaching 10 electrodes (leads) to the patient's chest to monitor 12 areas. The ECG provides a reading of the electrical currents of the heart and is a standard test conducted to detect suspected cardiac abnormalities, such as arrhythmias and conduction abnormalities. Codes report the tracing only (the technical component), the interpretation and report only (the professional component), or the entire procedure of tracing and interpretation (the technical and professional components). The medical record will indicate the components provided. Codes 93000-93010 are for the standard 12-lead ECG; the codes are divided on the basis of the component(s) provided.

Codes 93040-93278 report other various ECGs and are divided according to the type of recording and the component(s) provided. Only careful reading will reveal the often slight differences between codes.

Of special note is **signal-averaged electrocardiography (SAECG)** reported with 93278. SAECG is a type of electrocardiography that can help physicians predict certain tendencies to abnormalities such as ventricular tachycardia. The signal is recorded during nine periods, each lasting 10 to 20 minutes, and the computer manipulates the data produced and predicts certain tendencies. The SAECG is a more sophisticated ECG than the standard ECG and is used when a standard ECG is unable to demonstrate the suspected conductive abnormalities.

CODING SHOT

If only the interpretation and report are done with an SAECG, report 93278-26 to indicate that only the professional component was provided.

Telephonic transmission of an external patient-activated electrocardiogram records irregular rhythms. The readings can then be sent to the physician by means of a telephone to transmit the information, which is subsequently printed for the physician's review. Third-party payers usually restrict the payment of telephonic transmissions to one every 30 days. The codes 93268-93272 are divided on the basis of the component(s) that were provided.

A **cardiovascular stress test** is used to evaluate and diagnose chest pain, to screen for heart disease, to evaluate irregular heart rhythms, and to investigate many other cardiovascular abnormalities. The patient is placed on a treadmill or a stationary bicycle and ECG leads are attached. The patient then exercises until he or she reaches maximal (220 minus age) or submaximal (85% of maximal) heart rate. During certain intervals, recordings are taken by means of ECG, heart rate, and blood pressure of the patient.

The codes for stress tests (93015-93018) are divided on the basis of the components provided. Code 93015 reports the global outpatient service, and 93016-93018 reports components (parts) of the service. The ECG is bundled into the stress test, so do not unbundle and report an ECG or any reading separately. Medication can be administered to mimic the stressing of the heart and is used when factors are present that limit a patient's ability to exercise, such as arthritis, morbid obesity, or stroke. Stress test codes are used for both stress-induced (exercise) and pharmacologically induced (drug) studies. Medications and radiology services may be reported separately.

Implantable and Wearable Cardiac Device Evaluations

Cardiovascular monitoring is a diagnostic service that may be performed in person or using technology to access cardiovascular data, and these services are reported with codes in the 93279-93299 range. Codes 93279-93285 are reported per procedure, such as a single, dual, or multiple lead pacemaker or implantable defibrillator programming device evaluation. There are extensive notes before the subheading that are must reading before you begin to assign these codes.

Codes 93286 and 93287 report periprocedural (shortly before or shortly after) evaluation of a device based on if the device is a pacemaker or an implantable defibrillator. The codes may be reported once before and once after surgery because they are the testing of the device to ensure it functions correctly.

Codes in the 93288-93292 range are reported per procedure and are in-person evaluations of a pacemaker or an implantable defibrillator system based on the type of device and the type of analysis performed.

Evaluation of a pacemaker by means of a telephone is reported once in a 90-day period with 93293. The service includes the written report of the data analysis. Face-to-face evaluations of the device are referred to as interrogation device evaluations and are reported with 93294-93299. These codes are divided based on the type of device (pacemaker or implantable defibrillator) and the time period. For example, 93297 reports remote interrogation evaluation(s) up to 30 days and 93294 reports remote interrogation evaluation(s) up to 90 days.

Echocardiography

Echocardiography (93303-93355) is a noninvasive diagnostic method that uses ultrasonographic images to detect the presence of heart disease or valvular disease. A sliced image is used to detail the various walls of the heart. A **transducer** is placed on the outside of the chest wall, and it sends sound waves through the chest (Fig. 21-27).

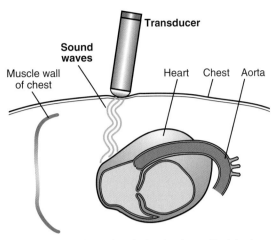

FIGURE 21–27 Echocardiography. A transducer is placed on the outside of the chest wall, and it sends sound waves through the chest. When the heart is in systole, the heart is contracting and the dots on the echocardiogram appear farther apart. When the heart is in diastole, it is relaxing and the dots on the echocardiogram appear closer together.

As the sound reflects back from each organ wall, dots are recorded, indicating the point of reflection. When the heart is in systole, it is contracting, and the dots on the recording appear farther apart. When the heart is in diastole, it is relaxing, and the dots on the recording appear closer together.

Bundled into the complete echocardiography procedures (93303-93355) are the obtaining of the signal from the heart and great arteries by means of two-dimensional imaging and/or Doppler ultrasound, the interpretation, and the report. Modifiers -26, professional service only, and -TC, technical component, may be applied to these codes if only one component is provided. The codes are divided on the basis of whether it was a complete echocardiogram or a follow-up/limited study, the type of echocardiogram, and the approach used.

EXERCISE 21-7 *Therapeutic Services, Cardiography, and Echocardiography*

Using the CPT, ICD-10-CM and/or ICD-9-CM manuals, code the following:

1 A physician provides CPR to a patient in cardiac arrest.

CPT Code: _____

2 Cardiovascular stress test performed in the physician's office, using submaximal bicycle exercise with continuous ECG; physician was in attendance for supervision and provided the interpretation and report.

CPT Code: _____

3 Percutaneous transluminal coronary balloon angioplasty of the right coronary artery and two vessels of the left anterior descending.

CPT Codes: _____, _____

4 SAECG with ECG, interpretation and report only. Diagnosis of unsustained ventricular tachycardia.

CPT Code: _____

ICD-10-CM Code: _____ (ICD-9-CM Code: _____)

(Answers are located in Appendix B)

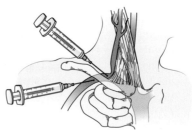

FIGURE 21-28   Percutaneous method of catheterization (Seldinger technique).

Cardiac Catheterization

Catheterization (93451-93572) is an invasive diagnostic medical procedure in which the physician percutaneously inserts a catheter and manipulates the catheter into coronary vessels and/or the heart. Fig. 21-28 illustrates a percutaneous method of catheterization called the Seldinger technique, after the inventor of the method. This catheterization is at the right subclavian artery. Following insertion of the fine-gauge needle, a guidewire and then a catheter are inserted. The cardiac catheter measures pressure, oxygen, and blood gases, takes blood samples, and measures the output of the heart. A cardiac catheterization is a study of both the circulation and the movement of the blood of the heart; the physician may inject a dye into the vessel or heart and observe the movement of the dye by means of angiography. When injection of contrast material is used to improve visualization, the injection is bundled into the Cardiac Catheterization code.

Component coding requires you to examine services that were provided to the patient, identify each component, or part, of that service, identify who performed each component, and code each service provided. The three cardiac catheterization components of catheter placement, injection, and imaging are reported in one combination code. For example, 93456 includes catheterization, injection, and imaging. However, some cardiac catheterization codes require multiple codes. For example, 93531 reports catheterization for congenital cardiac anomalies, but the injection/imagining code (93563/93564) must be added to completely describe the service provided. Only careful reading of the code descriptions in the cardiac catheterization codes will result in correct coding.

If the private physician (such as the clinic physician) performs the catheterization procedure in the catheterization laboratory at the hospital, you would add modifier -26 to the cardiac catheterization code. The hospital would submit charges for the technical component of the procedure.

Access for cardiac catheterization can be made in several locations, depending on the patient's condition and the physician's preference—for example, the right femoral artery (access site).

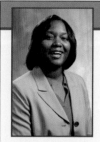

From the Trenches

"Teamwork is important in this environment. . . . As a profession, we must be a resource to each other and the health care community as a whole."

LETITIA

Cardiac catheterization can indicate valve disorders, abnormal flow of blood, and a variety of cardiac output abnormalities. Often, a cardiac catheterization leads to a more definite treatment, such as a valvoplasty, stent placement, angioplasty, or bypass.

Bundled into the cardiac catheterization codes are the introduction, positioning, and repositioning of the catheter(s); the recording of pressures inside the heart or vessels; the taking of blood samples; rest/exercise studies; final evaluation; and final report.

Injection codes 93563 and 93564 are only reported with cardiac catheterization codes 93530-93533, which are codes for cardiac catheterization for congenital abnormalities. These two injection codes are divided based on if the procedure was for "coronary angiography" (93563) or "aortocoronary venous or arterial bypass graft(s)" (93564). Both codes also include the imaging service. The codes are listed in addition to the primary cardiac catheter procedure.

There are also other injection codes (93565-93568) and these codes also include the imaging service. These injection codes are assigned with cardiac catheterization codes when additional injections are performed. For example, 93456 reports right heart catheterization with injections/imaging/angiography. If the physician also performed an aortography, the code reported for this additional service would be 93567.

There are several codes (93561-93572) in the category. These codes are for the **indicator dilution studies,** which are already bundled into the cardiac catheterization codes and are to be reported only when the complete cardiac catheterization procedure was not performed. For example, if only the dye or thermal dilution study was performed, without a cardiac catheterization, an indicator dilution study code would be assigned to report the service.

EXERCISE 21-8 | *Cardiac Catheterization*

Code the following using the CPT, ICD-10-CM and/or ICD-9-CM manuals:

1 Right heart catheterization was performed by means of the introduction of a cardiac catheter into the venous system, with further manipulation into the right atrium, including injection into the right atrium of contrast material, multiple measurements, and sampling; image supervision was provided by the physician.

   CPT Code: _____

2 Left heart catheterization of left ventricle was performed, with cutdown entry into the brachiocephalic artery, and contrast medium was injected for left ventricular angiography, including supervision, interpretation, and report. Diagnosis of coronary artery disease, native and unstable angina.

   CPT Code: _____

   ICD-10-CM Code: _____

   (ICD-9-CM Codes: _____, _____)

3 Indicator dilution studies when done with a cardiac catheterization are to be billed separately.

   True   False

4 Bundled into the cardiac catheterization codes are the positioning and repositioning of the catheter(s).

   True   False

5 Modifier -51 can be added to all codes in the Cardiac Catheterization subheading.

   True   False

(Answers are located in Appendix B)

Intracoronary Brachytherapy

Intracoronary brachytherapy is the use of radioactive substances as a therapy for in-stent restenosis of a coronary vessel, as illustrated in Fig. 21-29. For example, a patient has a coronary artery stent placed to open a vessel that is blocked with plaque (stenosis). The stent reopens the vessel so blood can once again flow without obstruction. However, the stent can also become occluded with plaque and when this happens, the physician may use intracoronary brachytherapy in which a radioactive strip of material is inserted by means of a catheter into the area of blockage, where it is left for up to 45 minutes and then removed.

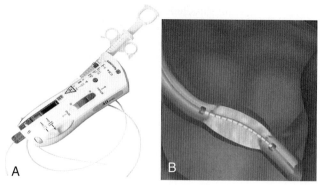

FIGURE 21–29 Brachytherapy delivery systems for coronary artery stent restenosis. **A,** The Novoste Transfer Device uses a saline-filled syringe to advance the radiation seeds to the treatment site. The same device is used to remove the seeds at the end of the brachytherapy treatment. **B,** The Novoste delivery catheter advances seeds to the site of angioplasty.

The procedure would usually be performed by an interventional cardiologist and a radiation oncologist. The interventional cardiologist would place the radioactive-element guidewire and report that service with 92974 (add-on code), which is the catheter placement code. The radiation oncologist would then place the radioactive elements and report the services with codes 77785-77787.

Intracardiac Electrophysiologic Procedures/Studies

As you learned earlier in this chapter, surgical electrophysiologic procedures (33250-33261) are those that repair the electrical system of the heart using invasive surgical procedures. In the Medicine section, the Intracardiac Electrophysiological Procedures/Studies category (93600-93662) contains codes that describe services that diagnose and treat the electrical system of the heart using less invasive procedures. Although the Medicine section procedures are invasive, they are percutaneous procedures, not open procedures.

Fig. 21-30 illustrates the electrical conduction system of the heart, which begins with the sinoatrial node (SA), known as the heart's pacemaker. The sinoatrial node sends impulses to the atrioventricular (AV) node, which in turn passes the impulses to the bundle of His, and finally on to the Purkinje fibers to stimulate the muscle tissues of the ventricles of the heart to contract. Lesions or diseases involving these structures along the electrical conduction pathway underlie many of the disturbances of cardiac rhythm.

To diagnose the origin of an electrophysiologic abnormality, the physician takes recordings at various sites along the pathway. The physician may also stimulate the heart to induce arrhythmia by means of a catheter attached to a pacing device that sends electrical impulses

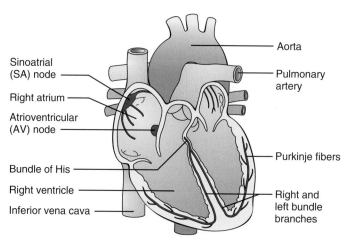

FIGURE 21–30 Electrical conduction system of the heart.

to various sites within the heart. A protocol (a set order) for the placement of the catheter is a **programmed stimulation.**

Pacing is the regulation of the heart rate. A cardiac pacemaker is a permanent pacer; but the pacing referred to in the EP codes is a temporary pacing done in an attempt to stabilize the beating of the heart. **Recording** is a record of the electrical activity of the heart taken by means of an ECG. Recording services are reported with codes in the range of 93600-93603, and pacing services are reported with codes 93610 and 93612. Combination codes that indicate both recording and pacing begin with 93619. These codes are not used as much as they used to be when EP was a new technique and readings were commonly taken at just one site. Today, more complex EP studies are usually done, including multiple pacings and recordings in combinations based on established protocols using three or more catheters. These complex services are reported with codes in the 93619-93622 range. Carefully read the notes in parentheses following several of the combination codes, as the notes indicate when the use of the combination code is appropriate and even indicate the codes that are bundled into the one combination code.

Bundle of His recording is a reading taken inside the heart (intracardiac) at the tip of the bundle of His. The bundle of His is also known as the atrioventricular bundle or AV bundle and is the bundle of cardiac muscle fibers that conducts electrical impulses that regulate heartbeats. The physician percutaneously inserts into a vessel a special catheter that can sense electrical impulses. The catheter is advanced to the right heart. The femoral vein is the usual site of entry, and fluoroscopic guidance is usually used for placement of the catheter into the heart.

Codes 93602 and 93603 describe a single **recording** based on the location—intra-arterial or right ventricle. Codes 93610 and 93612 describe single intra-arterial or intraventricular **pacing** in an atrial or a ventricular location.

Code 93631 reports **pacing** and **mapping** done during an open surgical procedure in which the surgeon opens the chest and exposes the heart. The EP physician performs the mapping (locating the origin of the arrhythmia and defining the pathway), and the surgeon then destroys the source of the arrhythmia. When reporting the services of both physicians for this procedure, use 93631 to report the mapping service and a surgery code from the range 33250-33261 to report the arrhythmia ablation. Make a notation next to the mapping code 93631 to report any surgical ablation (33250-33261) to remind yourself to code both procedures if required. If the mapping is not done intraoperatively (during surgery), report the service with 93609 or 93613.

Ablation can also be performed by using a catheter with a tip that emits electric current. When the tip is placed on tissue and activated, the tissue is destroyed. Sometimes physicians destroy certain sites along the conduction pathway as a treatment for slow (bradycardia) or fast (tachycardia) heart rhythms. Ablation procedures are reported according to whether they were at the AV node (93650), a separate (93655) or an additional treatment (93657).

There are two ways ablation can be performed. The first way does not require open heart surgery. An area of the patient's upper thigh is numbed, but the patient is awake. Then the physician inserts a thin tube through a blood vessel (usually the femoral vein) and all the way up to the heart. At the tip of the tube is a small wire that can deliver **radiofrequency** energy to burn away the abnormal areas of the heart. Then the heart can beat normally again.

The second way ablation can be performed is by means of open heart surgery. In the Maze procedure, the surgeon makes small **cuts** in the heart to direct healthy electrical rhythms. In **cryoablation,** a very cold substance is used to freeze the cells that are creating problems. In **endocardial resection,** the surgeon removes a section of the thin layer of the heart where the abnormal rhythms originate.

> **CAUTION** *Most of the EP codes have many items bundled into them, so read the description of each code completely so as to avoid unbundling the services.*

Peripheral Arterial Disease Rehabilitation

Peripheral arterial disease (PAD) rehabilitation sessions (93668) last 45 to 60 minutes; these are rehabilitative physical exercises done either on a motorized treadmill or on a track to build the patient's cardiovascular endurance. An exercise physiologist or nurse supervises the sessions. If a session produces symptoms of angina or other negative symptoms, the physician reviews the information and may determine to re-evaluate the patient. The physician services are not included in the PAD codes, rather the physician services are reported with an additional Evaluation and Management (E/M) code.

Noninvasive Physiologic Studies and Procedures

If a patient has a pacemaker or defibrillator in place, periodic monitoring must occur to ensure that the device is functioning properly. Codes from the Noninvasive Physiologic Studies and Procedures (93701-93790) category and the Implantable and Wearable Cardiac Device Evaluations (93279-93299) category reflect these services. Codes are assigned according to the type of pacemaker (single- or dual-chamber) or implantable defibrillator and whether reprogramming of an existing pacemaker or defibrillator was done.

Ambulatory blood pressure monitoring (93784-93790) is an outpatient procedure that is conducted over a 24-hour period by means of a portable device worn by the patient. There is a code for the total procedure—including recording, analysis, and interpretation/report—and there are codes for each of the individual components—recording only, analysis only, and interpretation/report only.

Other Procedures

The Other Procedures codes (93797-93799) report physician services that are provided for cardiac rehabilitation of outpatients, either with or without electrocardiographic monitoring.

EXERCISE 21-9 *EP and Vascular Studies*

Using the CPT, ICD-10-CM and/or ICD-9-CM manuals, code the following physician services:

1 Bundle of His recording

  CPT Code: _____

2 Comprehensive electrophysiologic evaluation was performed, including recording and pacing of the right atrium and right ventricle. Three electrodes were repositioned. Left ventricular recordings were also made, with pacing and induction of arrhythmia. Diagnosis of vasovagal syncope.

  CPT Codes: _____, _____

  ICD-10-CM Code: _____ (ICD-9-CM Code: _____)

(Answers are located in Appendix B)

CARDIOVASCULAR CODING IN THE RADIOLOGY SECTION

The Radiology section of the CPT manual used to contain combination codes that included both the **professional** and **technical components** in one code. For example, 75659 existed to report the services of both the angiography (technical component) and the injection procedure (professional component) in a brachial angiography procedure. When the complete procedure code, 75659, was deleted, the injection procedure (professional component) was moved to the Surgery section and a code to report the technical component (angiography) remained in the Radiology section. Now, to report both the injection procedure and the angiography services (the complete procedure), the coder assigns a Surgery code to report the professional component and a Radiology code to report the technical component. The division of the technical and professional components makes it possible to specify the various parts of a procedure, which is important because some cardiologists perform both components of these cardiovascular procedures, and some cardiologists perform only the injection procedure and have a radiologist do the angiography portion of the procedure. Component coding allows for the flexibility necessary to report these various situations. Component coding also makes it easier to identify the various diagnostic tests used in cardiovascular conditions. For example, one cardiologist may prefer to use an ultrasonic procedure in the diagnosis of arterial stenosis and another may prefer angiography. Both procedures require the insertion of a catheter and, as such, the insertion code remains the same, but the diagnostic tools may change.

Radiology codes often contain the statement "supervision and interpretation." **Supervision** is the radiologist's overseeing of the technician who is performing the procedure or indicates that the radiologist is performing the procedure himself/herself. **Interpretation** is the summary of the findings, also known as the final report, and the radiologist or cardiologist may do this portion of the service. There are actually two components (parts) in a code with supervision and interpretation in the description—the professional and technical components. The technical component is the equipment and the technician who actually provides the service. The professional component is the interpretation of the results and the writing of a report about the results, as illustrated in Fig. 21-31. Both components are not necessarily done by the same organization. Let's take an x-ray as an example of a service and see how you report the components.

If a clinic owns its own x-ray equipment and employs a radiologist to interpret the x-rays and write the reports, and also employs the technician who, under the supervision of the radiologist, takes the x-rays, the clinic could report the x-ray service using the appropriate radiology code, with supervision and interpretation in the description and no modifier. The clinic provides the total service, also known as the **global service.**

Another clinic owns the equipment and employs the technician who takes the x-ray, but then the clinic sends the x-ray out to a radiologist at another clinic who reads the x-ray and writes the report. The radiologist would report the service with the appropriate radiology code and modifier -26 to indicate that he or she provided only the professional component of the service. The clinic that employs the technician and owns the equipment would report the same radiology code but would attach the HCPCS modifier -TC (technical component) to indicate that only the technical component of the service was provided.

A third clinic has no x-ray equipment, so the physicians in the clinic send patients to an outside radiologist who hires the technician who takes x-rays on equipment owned by the radiologist, the radiologist interprets the results, and writes the report. The outside radiologist would report the service using the global radiology code with no modifier, because both the professional component and the technical component were provided.

Examination:	Chest
Clinical symptoms:	Aortic stenosis, abnormal cardiac stress test
Date ordered:	Today's date
Date Completed:	Today's date
Ordering Dr.:	Timothy Swenson, MD
Attending Dr.:	Timothy Swenson, MD
Date of Birth:	04/13/65 Record #: 456980
PA & Lateral chest:	Radiographic examination reveals no abnormality of the lungs, heart, mediastinum, or visualized bony structures.
Impression:	Radiographically normal chest.

Ronald A. Potts, MD

Ronald A. Potts, MD

Radiologist

RAP/rnf

FIGURE 21–31 The final radiology report contains the radiologist's interpretation of findings.

Contrast material is commonly used with radiology procedures to enhance the image. If the Radiology section code states "with contrast" or "with or without contrast," you will know that the injection of contrast material and the contrast material itself (the substance used for contrasting) are bundled into the code; therefore, you would not report the contrast material or injection separately. If, however, there is no indication of contrast in the code description, and the physician used contrast, you would code both the injection of the contrast material and the contrast material itself. Injection of contrast is usually included in the radiology code. If guidelines state that you should report injections separately, report with the appropriate code from the Surgery section—for example, 47500, Injection procedure for percutaneous transhepatic cholangiography, and 74320 for the radiology portion of the service. The contrast material is reported separately using code 99070 from the Medicine section or with a HCPCS code.

CODING SHOT

Not all contrast material can be reported separately! Oral or rectal contrast is considered a part of the procedure and is not reported separately. Intravenous, intra-arterial, or intrathecal (fluid-filled space between the layers of tissue covering the brain and spinal cord) injection of contrast material can be reported separately if the code description does not refer to inclusion of contrast material.

■ **STOP** *Now, don't get discouraged with all of these codes from all of these sections! Remember that only with repeated use of these codes can you master them. At first, it sounds so confusing that you might wonder if you can ever absorb all of this information and the variations. You can! But you must be patient with the process. To be a coder is to be able to concentrate on details and commit yourself to the process of learning the details through repeated use. Everyone starts at the same place. Now, let's get back to learning about component coding.*

Two physicians, a cardiologist and a radiologist from the same facility, perform an angiography of the brachiocephalic artery (first order) using contrast material. Access was the right femoral artery. The coding is as follows:
■ Cardiologist placing the catheter: 36215, Surgery section
■ Radiologist performing the angiography: 75710, Radiology section
■ Supply of the contrast material: 99070, Medicine section, or HCPCS Level II code (such as A4641, Radiopharmaceutical, diagnostic)

Two physicians, a cardiologist and a radiologist from different facilities, perform an angiography of the brachiocephalic artery (first order) using contrast material. The coding for the cardiologist is as follows:
■ Cardiologist placing the catheter: 36215, Surgery section

The coding for the radiologist is as follows:
■ Radiologist performing the angiography: 75710, Radiology section
■ Supply of the contrast material: 99070, Medicine section, or a HCPCS Level II code (such as A4641, Radiopharmaceutical, diagnostic)

CODING SHOT

If the radiologist is at the same facility as the equipment, you report 75710 (angiography). If the angiography was performed at the hospital and the radiologist from a clinic read the angiography, the radiologist would report 75710-26 and the hospital would report 75710-TC.

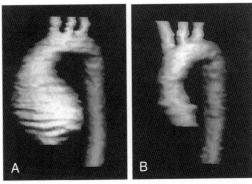

FIGURE 21–32 **A,** Preoperative MRI of a patient with an ascending aortic aneurysm. **B,** Postoperative MRI of the same ascending aortic area.

Heart

The Heart subsection (75557-75574) of the Radiology section contains codes that report cardiac magnetic resonance imaging (MRI) of the heart. An **MRI**, as illustrated in Fig. 21-32, *A* and *B,* is the use of radiation to show the body in a cross-sectional view. MRI may include the use of injectable dyes (radiographic contrast) to aid in imaging. Other MRI codes are located throughout the Radiology section according to the body part being imaged, but the codes in the Heart subsection are just for cardiac MRIs.

Aorta and Arteries

In Radiology, the Aorta and Arteries subsection (75600-75791) includes codes for aortography excluding the heart—thoracic, abdominal, cervicocerebral, brachial, external carotid, carotid, vertebral, spinal, extremity, renal, visceral, adrenal, pelvic, pulmonary, and internal mammary.

The Aorta and Arteries subsection codes are reported with coding components of cardiovascular services.

TOOLBOX

Denise is a busy medical administrator at the local hospital. She has a very stressful job and has been having heart palpitations, especially in the late afternoon and evening. Her physician has implanted a patient-activated event recorder.

QUESTIONS
1. The electrodes for this monitor are _____ the body.
2. When Denise feels an irregular heartbeat, what is she to do? _____
3. Two other names for this test: _____ _____ or _____.

▼ **ANSWERS**

1. inside, 2. press a button, 3. cardiac event recorder or loop recorder

EXERCISE 21-10 *Heart, Aorta, and Arteries*

Using the CPT, ICD-10-CM and/or ICD-9-CM manuals, code the following:

1 Code a selective catheter placement in the first-order brachiocephalic artery from the right common femoral artery access point, with angiography, including contrast done at the clinic catheterization laboratory.

CPT Codes: _____, _____, _____

2 Bilateral angiography of the arteries of the legs, with radiological supervision and interpretation.

CPT Code: _____

3 CT scan of the heart performed for evaluation of cardiac structure and morphology, which included assessment of the cardiac function and evaluation of the venous structures, with contrast material.

CPT Code: _____

4 Complete cardiac MRI for morphology and function without contrast followed by contrast along with four additional sequences and stress imaging. Diagnosis of congestive heart failure and premature ventricular contractions.

CPT Code: _____

ICD-10-CM Codes: _____, _____

(ICD-9-CM Codes: _____, _____)

(Answers are located in Appendix B)

CHAPTER REVIEW

CHAPTER 21, PART I, THEORY

Without the use of reference material, complete the following:

1 What are the two subheadings within the Cardiovascular System subsection? _____,
   _____

2 The subspecialty of internal medicine that is concerned with the diagnosis and treatment of the heart is _____.

3 In Chapter 21 you learned about coding from which three sections of the CPT? _____,
   _____, and _____

4 Procedures that break the skin for correction or examination are known as _____ procedures.

5 Procedures that do not break the skin are known as _____ procedures.

6 The study of the heart's electrical system is known as _____.

7 The use of radioactive radiologic procedures to aid in the diagnosis of cardiologic conditions is termed
   _____ _____ cardiology.

8 A catheter that is inserted into an artery and manipulated to a further order is termed
   _____ placement.

9 A catheter that is inserted into an artery and not manipulated to a further order is termed
   _____ placement.

10 Surgical procedures in the Heart and Pericardium subheading contain procedures that are performed through both open
   surgical sites and _____.

CHAPTER 21, PART II, PRACTICAL

Code the following cases for the surgical procedures, the office visits, and the cardiology-related Radiology and Medicine section codes and the diagnoses codes. Do not code the laboratory work.

11 Dennis Smith, a 42-year-old railroad employee (established patient), has a history of severe mitral stenosis with regurgitation, rheumatic. He is now symptomatic and his physician recommends a mitral valve replacement be performed immediately. Dennis agrees to the surgery, and the physician does a comprehensive history and physical in preparation for surgery. The physician orders a general health panel blood workup and a urinalysis (automated). On the next day, the physician performs a mitral valve replacement. Dennis recovers uneventfully and is discharged from the hospital 5 days later.

CPT Codes: _____, _____

ICD-10-CM Code: _____

(ICD-9-CM Code: _____)

12 Thrombectomy of arterial graft

CPT Code: _____

13 Direct repair of aneurysm and graft insertion for occlusive disease of the common femoral artery

CPT Code: _____

14 A surgical assistant (MD) assists in performing five venous grafts in a coronary artery bypass procedure for arteriosclerosis of native arteries.

CPT Code: _____

ICD-10-CM Code: _____

(ICD-9-CM Code: _____)

15 Open-heart repair of mitral valve with use of cardiopulmonary bypass

CPT Code: _____

16 Removal of a single-lead implantable defibrillator pulse generator

CPT Code: _____

17 Pericardiotomy for removal of clot

CPT Code: _____

18 Complete repair of tetralogy of Fallot is made with closure of a ventricular septal defect, and a conduit from the pulmonary artery to the right ventricle is constructed. A pulmonary graft valve is then secured.

CPT Code: _____

19 Shunting from subclavian to pulmonary artery using the Blalock-Taussig operation for Fallot's tetralogy

CPT Code: _____

ICD-10-CM Code: _____

(ICD-9-CM Code: _____)

20 Pulmonary endarterectomy with embolectomy requiring cardiopulmonary bypass

CPT Code: _____

21 Direct repair of aneurysm associated with occlusion of the vertebral artery

CPT Code: _____

ICD-10-CM Codes: _____, _____

(ICD-9-CM Codes: _____, _____)

22 Thromboendarterectomy with patch graft of iliac artery

CPT Code: _____

ICD-10-CM Code: _____

(ICD-9-CM Code: _____)

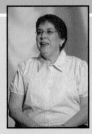

"One of the benefits of working in medical coding is to know you're making a positive impact on the health care industry.... I consider myself as taking care of the patient by looking out for their best interest, especially with accuracy in diagnostic coding."

Sharon J. Oliver, CPC, CPC-I, CPMA
Senior Inpatient Coder
East Tennessee State University Physicians &
Associates
Johnson City, Tennessee

Hemic, Lymphatic, Mediastinum, and Diaphragm

Chapter Topics

Hemic and Lymphatic Systems

Mediastinum and Diaphragm

Chapter Review

Learning Objectives

After completing this chapter you should be able to

1 Review the Hemic and Lymphatic Systems subsection format.

2 Understand the Hemic and Lymphatic Systems subheadings.

3 Demonstrate the ability to code Hemic and Lymphatic System services.

4 Review the format of the Mediastinum and Diaphragm subsection codes.

5 Understand the Mediastinum and Diaphragm information.

6 Demonstrate the ability to code Mediastinum and Diaphragm services.

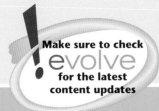

Make sure to check
evolve
for the latest
content updates

HEMIC AND LYMPHATIC SYSTEMS

Format

The Hemic and Lymphatic Systems subsection (38100-38999) is divided into subheadings: Spleen, General, and Lymph Nodes and Lymphatic Channels (Fig. 22-1). Further division is based on type of procedure (i.e., excision, incision, repair). The codes for spleen and lymph nodes are located in the CPT manual index under main terms such as "Spleen," "Lymph Nodes," or "Bone Marrow."

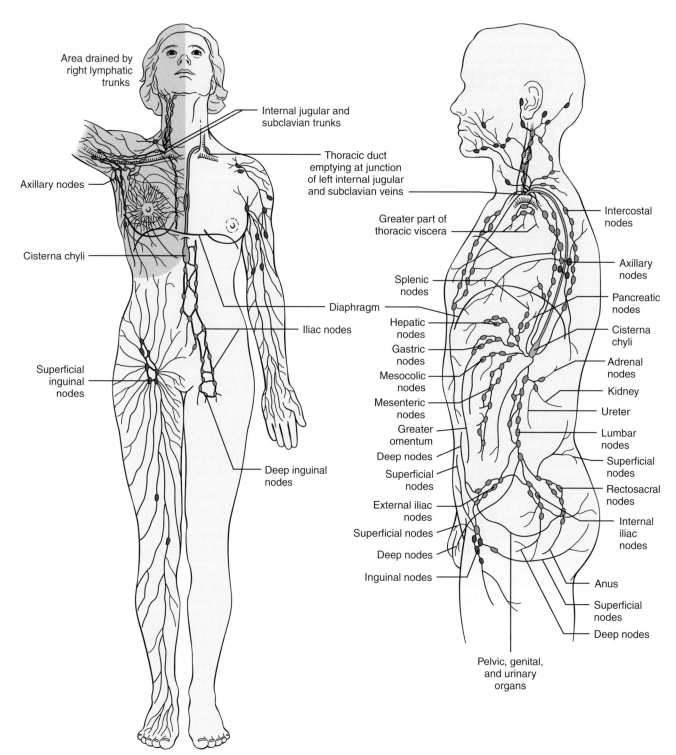

Area drained by right lymphatic trunks

Internal jugular and subclavian trunks

Thoracic duct emptying at junction of left internal jugular and subclavian veins

Axillary nodes

Cisterna chyli

Diaphragm

Iliac nodes

Superficial inguinal nodes

Deep inguinal nodes

Greater part of thoracic viscera

Intercostal nodes

Splenic nodes

Axillary nodes

Pancreatic nodes

Hepatic nodes

Cisterna chyli

Gastric nodes

Adrenal nodes

Mesocolic nodes

Kidney

Mesenteric nodes

Ureter

Greater omentum

Lumbar nodes

Deep nodes

Superficial nodes

Superficial nodes

Rectosacral nodes

External iliac nodes

Internal iliac nodes

Superficial nodes

Deep nodes

Anus

Inguinal nodes

Superficial nodes

Deep nodes

Pelvic, genital, and urinary organs

FIGURE 22–1 Lymph nodes and lymph channels.

Spleen. The spleen is composed of lymph tissue and is located in the left upper quadrant of the abdomen. The spleen is easily ruptured and may result in massive hemorrhage. The spleen initiates an immune response, filters, removes bacteria from the bloodstream, and destroys worn out blood cells. A person can live without a spleen because the bone marrow, liver, and lymph nodes take over the work of the spleen after a total removal (splenectomy).

Codes in the subheading Spleen (38100-38200) are further divided into categories of excision, repair, laparoscopy, and introduction. Codes in the Excision category are based on the type of splenectomy: total, partial, or total for extensive disease. The splenectomy (total and partial) carries the designation "(separate procedure)" behind the code description (38100, 38101). This means that if the splenectomy is an integral part of another procedure, it is bundled into the primary procedure code and not reported separately.

CODING SHOT

If a repair of a ruptured spleen was performed and the surgeon removed only a portion of the spleen, you would report only the repair code (38115) because removal is bundled into the primary repair code.

Laparoscopy. The surgical laparoscopy codes (38120, 38129) always include a diagnostic laparoscopy if one is performed. Report a diagnostic laparoscopy with 49320, Laparoscopy, abdomen, peritoneum, and omentum, diagnostic, with or without collection of specimen(s) by brushing or washing (separate procedure).

Introduction. A splenoportography is an x-ray of the portal and circulatory vessels of the spleen. Code 38200 reports the injection portion of the procedure. The physician makes an incision in the left axilla area and inserts a catheter into the spleen. Radiopaque dye is inserted and x-rays are taken. The physician then removes the catheter and closes the area. The radiological supervision and interpretation portion of the service is reported with 75810.

General. A bone marrow or blood cell transplant is a treatment for some blood diseases, such as leukemia or lymphoma. During the procedure, the patient's bone marrow or blood cells are replaced with healthy marrow or blood cells from a donor. There are three sources for blood cell formation: bone marrow, bloodstream, and umbilical cord. Bone marrow is the inner core of bones that manufactures most blood cells. Immature blood cells, called stem cells, originate in the marrow of bones. Leukemia is a malignant disease of the bone marrow in which excessive white blood cells are produced. Treatment often includes total-body irradiation or aggressive chemotherapy followed by transplantation of normal bone marrow. **Bone marrow aspiration** (38220) is a procedure in which a sample of the bone marrow is taken by means of a needle that is inserted into the marrow cavity. Marrow is then aspirated (pulled) through the needle and into the syringe. Usually the marrow is taken from the iliac crest, pelvic bone, or sternum. **Bone marrow biopsy** (38221) is a procedure in which small pieces of the marrow are obtained by means of a needle or trocar. These small chips are then processed in the laboratory by dissolving the pieces in a decalcification solution. The resulting substance is then analyzed and the service is reported with a Pathology/Laboratory code (88305). **Bone marrow harvesting** (38230) is a procedure in which a larger amount of bone marrow is aspirated from a donor by means of a large aspiration needle. The marrow is then transplanted into the recipient patient.

Transplantation and cellular infusions, 38240-38243, are procedures in which hematopoietic cells, obtained from bone marrow, peripheral blood apheresis, or umbilical cord blood, are infused into the patient. Code 38242 represents allogenic infusion. The preparation and storage of the cells prior to transplantation or infusion are reported with 38207-38215. **Allogenic** is from the same species (human), such as a cadaver, a close relative, or a non-related donor. **Autologous** bone marrow is collected from the patient, processed, and later transplanted or reinfused into the patient. **Stem cell harvesting** is the collection of stem cells from the blood system through a process termed apheresis. A needle is placed into a vein in one arm of the donor and the blood is removed. The blood is then filtered to remove the stem cells. The blood, with the stem cells removed, is returned to the donor through the other arm. Usually this process takes 4-6 hours and is usually completed in two sessions. The harvesting and return of the blood to the donor (replantation) is reported with codes 38205-38206.

QUICK CHECK 22-1

1. According to the notes in the CPT, the Bone Marrow/Stem Cell Services/Procedures (38207-38215) may be reported only once per day.

   True or False?

(Answers are located in Appendix C)

Lymph Nodes and Lymphatic Channels

The lymphatic system is a transportation system that takes interstitial fluids, proteins, and fats through the lymphatic channels and back to the bloodstream. Stations along the lymphatic system are called lymph nodes. The nodes fight disease when lymphocytes from the nodes produce antibodies. The subheading of Lymph Nodes and Lymphatic Channels is divided on the basis of the various procedures (i.e., incision, excision, resection, and introduction). The majority of the Excision codes (38500-38555) are for biopsy or excision based on the method (open or needle) and the location (e.g., axillary or cervical). For the open procedures, the choice of codes depends on whether the procedure was superficial (38500), deep (38510-38525), or internal mammary (38530).

Within the Lymph Node and Lymphatic Channels subheading are two categories of codes for lymphadenectomies that are based on whether the lymphadenectomy is limited or radical. A **limited** lymphadenectomy (38562-38564) is the removal of the lymph nodes only; a **radical** lymphadenectomy (38700-38780) is the removal of the lymph nodes, gland(s), and surrounding tissue. Sometimes, a limited lymphadenectomy will be bundled into a more major procedure, such as prostatectomy. If this is the case, you would not report the lymphadenectomy separately. Rather, you would report only the more major procedure.

The codes to report a laparoscopic lymph node biopsy or removal are located in the 38570-38589 range. The codes are divided based on the extent of the procedure:

■ 38570 reports retroperitoneal lymph node biopsy, single or multiple.

■ 38571 reports a bilateral total pelvic lymphadenectomy.

■ 38572 also reports a bilateral total pelvic lymphadenectomy and includes the single or multiple biopsy of the periaortic lymph node.

A surgical laparoscopy always includes a diagnostic laparoscopy and is, therefore, not unbundled and reported separately. If only a diagnostic laparoscopy is performed, you would report the Digestive System code 49320.

QUICK CHECK 22-2

1. Review the Radical Lymphadenectomy codes (38700-38780). According to the parenthetical statements, what modifier may be used under appropriate circumstances? _____

(Answers are located in Appendix C)

Regions of Neck Lymph Nodes. The lymph nodes of the neck are named based on the anatomical location:

- Submental and submandibular nodes are located at the chin area and beneath the body of the mandible.
- Upper jugular nodes are divided in two groups and are located at the mandibular angle and the front of the sternocleidomastoid muscle.
- Middle jugular nodes are located between the hyoid bone and the cricoid cartilage.
- Lower jugular nodes are located between the cricoid cartilage and the clavicle.
- Posterior triangle nodes are divided into two groups.
- Upper visceral nodes are located by the hyoid bone.
- Superior mediastinal nodes are located between the left and right common carotid arteries.

Refer to Fig. 22-2 for the lymph vessels and nodes of the head and neck.

The term "complete neck dissection" in code 38720 is the same as radical neck dissection. During a complete or radical neck dissection, the lymph nodes in all five regions are resected (removed). In addition, the internal jugular vein, spinal accessory nerve, and sternocleidomastoid muscle are removed. The code is a unilateral code, so modifier -50 is required if a bilateral procedure is reported. A modified radical neck dissection as reported with 38724 is the removal of all lymph nodes that are routinely removed by radical neck dissection; however, the internal jugular vein, spinal accessory nerve, and sternocleidomastoid muscle are preserved rather than removed. The code is a unilateral code, so modifier -50 is required if a bilateral procedure is reported. The **suprahyoid neck dissection** is a variation of the modified radical neck dissection and is reported with 38700.

A lymphangiogram (38790) is a procedure in which contrast medium is injected into lymph vessels in the foot, and x-rays are taken to image the lymph flow. This procedure is often performed for staging and diagnosis of lymphoma. **Staging** is determining the grade or level of a neoplasm based on a common grading system, such as the TNM (tumors, nodes, and metastases). A unilateral procedure is reported with 38790. The radiological supervision and interpretation portion of the service is reported with codes 75801-75807.

CMS RULES

Sentinel node biopsy may be indicated in breast carcinoma and is eligible for Medicare reimbursement when the following conditions are met:

1. Clinical Stage I and II carcinoma of the breast with no palpable lymph nodes in the axilla, and
2. If a second sentinel node is excised from a different lymphatic chain through a separate incision at the same operative session, report the appropriate CPT code for the second incision and append the -59 modifier.

Examples of payable diagnosis codes: C50.-/174.0-174.9, C50.029-C50.929/175.0-175.9

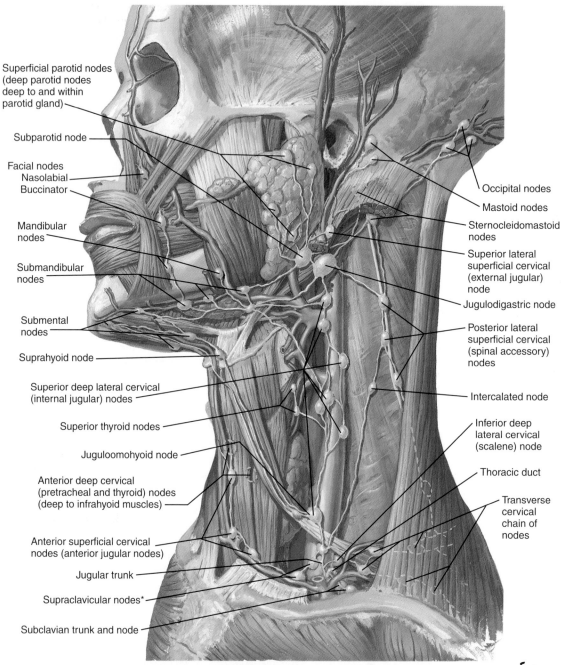

Superficial parotid nodes (deep parotid nodes deep to and within parotid gland)

Subparotid node

Facial nodes
Nasolabial
Buccinator

Mandibular nodes

Submandibular nodes

Submental nodes

Suprahyoid node

Superior deep lateral cervical (internal jugular) nodes

Superior thyroid nodes

Juguloomohyoid node

Anterior deep cervical (pretracheal and thyroid) nodes (deep to infrahyoid muscles)

Anterior superficial cervical nodes (anterior jugular nodes)

Jugular trunk

Supraclavicular nodes*

Subclavian trunk and node

Occipital nodes

Mastoid nodes

Sternocleidomastoid nodes

Superior lateral superficial cervical (external jugular) node

Jugulodigastric node

Posterior lateral superficial cervical (spinal accessory) nodes

Intercalated node

Inferior deep lateral cervical (scalene) node

Thoracic duct

Transverse cervical chain of nodes

*The supraclavicular group of nodes (also known as the lower deep cervical group), especially on the left, are also sometimes referred to as the signal or sentinel lymph nodes of Virchow or Troisier, especially when sufficiently enlarged and palpable. These nodes (or a single node) are so termed because they may be the first recognized presumptive evidence of malignant disease in the viscera.

FIGURE 22–2 Lymph vessels and nodes of the head and neck. (Modified from Netter FH: *Atlas of Human Anatomy*, ed 4, Philadelphia, 2006, Saunders).

A sentinel lymph node biopsy is bundled into a planned lymphadenectomy and not paid separately. The injection of dye to visualize the sentinel node should be reported by the surgeon/physician who performs the injection with 38792 or 38900 if the surgeon who is performing the surgical procedure also provided the injection procedure intraoperatively. This code is reported only once for the injection of the dye regardless of the number of injections made around the lesion.

EXERCISE 22-1 | *Hemic and Lymphatic Systems*

Using the CPT, ICD-10-CM and/or ICD-9-CM manuals, code the following:

1 Excision of an axillary cystic hygroma, which the patient medical record indicates involved no deep neurovascular dissection

CPT Code: _____

ICD-10-CM Code: _____ (ICD-9-CM Code: _____)

2 Total removal of the spleen due to Gaucher's splenomegaly

CPT Code: _____

ICD-10-CM Code: _____ (ICD-9-CM Code: _____)

3 Injection procedure for a radiographic view of the portal vein of the spleen

CPT Code: _____

4 Bone marrow transplant, autologous

CPT Code: _____

(Answers are located in Appendix B)

MEDIASTINUM AND DIAPHRAGM

Mediastinum

The mediastinum is the area between the lungs (Fig. 22-3). The Mediastinum subheading of the Mediastinum and Diaphragm subsection (39000-39599) of the CPT manual is divided by procedures and includes incision, excision, and endoscopy.

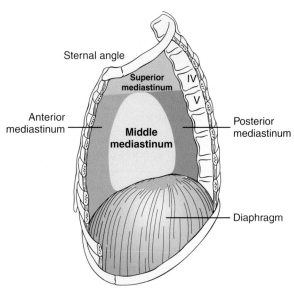

FIGURE 22-3 Mediastinum and diaphragm.

Incision. The difference between the mediastinotomy codes (39000, 39010) is the surgical approach. The approach can be either cervical (neck area), across the thoracic area (transthoracic), or sternum. A mediastinotomy is performed by making an incision next to the breastbone for the purposes of exploration, drainage, removal of a foreign body, or biopsy. You may think removal of a foreign body would be in the Excision codes, but the Excision codes are only reported for cysts or tumors.

Excision. Excision codes 39200 and 39220 are based on whether a cyst or tumor was excised. The surgical approach is one in which the surgeon makes the incision just below the nipple line and retracts the rib cage and muscles to expose the thoracic cavity. The cyst or tumor is removed and the incision closed.

If the thyroid gland is removed using an excision into the mediastinum, the procedure is reported with 60270 from the Endocrine System subsection and not with an excision code from the Mediastinum subcategory. Also, if the thymus gland is removed using a mediastinum approach, you would report the procedure with 60520.

Endoscopy. There is only one mediastinoscopy code (39400), and the procedure includes any biopsy performed during the procedure. The procedure is performed by making a small incision above the sternum. The scope is inserted through the incision for exploration (and/or biopsy).

Diaphragm

The diaphragm is the wall of muscle that separates the thoracic and abdominal cavities. The codes in the Diaphragm subheading (39501-39599) are repair codes. Repairs are usually for a hernia or laceration. Diaphragm codes are located in the CPT manual index under "Diaphragm."

There is one code for imbrication of the diaphragm. An imbrication of the diaphragm may be performed for eventration, which is when the diaphragm moves up, usually because of the paralysis of the diaphragmatic nerve (phrenic nerve). In this case the surgeon sutures the diaphragm back into place.

EXERCISE 22-2   *Mediastinum and Diaphragm*

Using the CPT, ICD-10-CM and/or ICD-9-CM manuals, code the following:

1 Exploratory mediastinotomy with biopsy of mediastinal lesion accomplished with approach through the neck. Pathology report later indicated primary, malignant neoplasm.

   CPT Code: _____

   ICD-10-CM Code: _____ (ICD-9-CM Code: _____)

2 Resection of benign tumor of the mediastinum

   CPT Code: _____

   ICD-10-CM Code: _____ (ICD-9-CM Code: _____)

(Answers are located in Appendix B)

CHAPTER REVIEW

CHAPTER 22, PART I, THEORY

Complete the following:

1 The difference between the mediastinum incision codes is the surgical _____.

2 The spleen initiates an immune response, filters and removes _____ from the bloodstream and destroys worn out blood cells.

3 Total or partial splenectomy codes are designated in the CPT manual as _____ procedures.

4 A marrow or _____ _____ transplant is a treatment for patients with blood diseases, such as leukemia or lymphoma.

5 A bone marrow _____ is a procedure in which a sample of bone marrow is taken by means of a needle that is inserted into the marrow cavity.

6 A(n) _____ bone marrow comes from a close relative.

7 A(n) _____ bone marrow comes from the patient, is processed, and later transplanted or reinfused.

8 A(n) _____ lymphadenectomy is the removal of the lymph nodes only.

9 The Mediastinum category of codes is based on the _____ _____ taken to perform the mediastinotomy.

10 Another name for the diaphragmatic nerve is the _____ nerve.

CHAPTER 22, PART II, PRACTICAL

Code the following cases:

11 Using a cervical approach, ligation of the thoracic duct was accomplished.

   CPT Code: _____

12 Surgical laparoscopy with bilateral total pelvic lymphadenectomy

   CPT Code: _____

13 Superficial inguinofemoral lymphadenectomy with pelvic lymphadenectomy, including the external iliac, hypogastric, and obturator nodes

   CPT Code: _____

14 Diaphragmatic resection of a secondary, malignant lesion that included extensive use of prosthetic material. The primary malignancy was located in the uterus, which has been previously removed, followed by a course of radiation and chemotherapy with no further evidence of existence.

   CPT Code: _____

   ICD-10-CM Codes: _____, _____

   (ICD-9-CM Codes: _____, _____)

15 Excisional biopsy of superficial lymph nodes of the neck by means of an open procedure for non-Hodgkin lymphoma

   CPT Code: _____

   ICD-10-CM Code: _____

   (ICD-9-CM Code: _____)

Chapter Review answers are only available in the TEACH Instructor Resources on Evolve

16 Dissection of the deep jugular nodes, diagnosis of thyroid gland primary cancer

CPT Code: _____

ICD-10-CM Code: _____

(ICD-9-CM Code: _____)

17 Excision of congenital cervical cystic hygroma with dissection of deep neurovascularity

CPT Code: _____

ICD-10-CM Code: _____

(ICD-9-CM Code: _____)

18 Limited lymphadenectomy for staging of para-aortic lymph nodes in malignant primary prostate cancer

CPT Code: _____

ICD-10-CM Code: _____

(ICD-9-CM Code: _____)

19 Bilateral injection procedure for lymphangiography of axillary node enlargement, left side

CPT Code: _____

ICD-10-CM Code: _____

(ICD-9-CM Code: _____)

20 Mediastinoscopy with biopsy for mass

CPT Code: _____

ICD-10-CM Code: _____

(ICD-9-CM Code: _____)

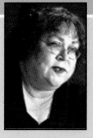

"I love not doing the same thing each day, and I love looking at different things and mastering them. And that's what coding is!"

Belinda D. Inabinet, CPC, CCC, CMC
Coding Coordinator SC Heart Center
Columbia, South Carolina

Digestive System

Chapter Topics

Format

Lips

Vestibule of Mouth

Tongue and Floor of Mouth

Dentoalveolar Structures

Palate and Uvula

Salivary Gland and Ducts

Pharynx, Adenoids, and Tonsils

Esophagus

Stomach

Intestines (Except Rectum)

Meckel's Diverticulum and the Mesentery

Appendix

Colon and Rectum

Anus

Liver

Learning Objectives

After completing this chapter you should be able to

1 Understand the format of the Digestive System subsection.

2 Report procedures of the lips.

3 Report procedures of the vestibule of the mouth.

4 Report procedures of the tongue and floor of the mouth.

5 Report procedures of the dentoalveolar structures.

6 Report procedures of the palate and uvula.

7 Report procedures of the salivary gland and ducts.

8 Report procedures of the pharynx, adenoids, and tonsils.

9 Report procedures of the esophagus.

10 Report procedures of the stomach.

11 Report procedures of the intestines (except rectum).

12 Report procedures of the Meckel's diverticulum and mesentery.

13 Report procedures of the appendix.

14 Report procedures of the colon and rectum.

15 Report procedures of the anus.

16 Report procedures of the liver.

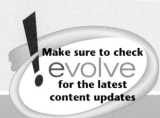

Make sure to check **evolve** for the latest content updates

FORMAT

The format of the Digestive System subsection (40490-49999) is divided according to anatomic site (Fig. 23-1) and procedure. Included in this subsection are codes for sites beginning with the mouth and ending with the anus. Also included are those internal organs that aid in the digestive process, including the pancreas, liver, and gallbladder.

This subsection includes codes for procedures of the abdomen, peritoneum, omentum, and hernia repairs. Endoscopic codes are located throughout the subsection on the basis of the anatomic site.

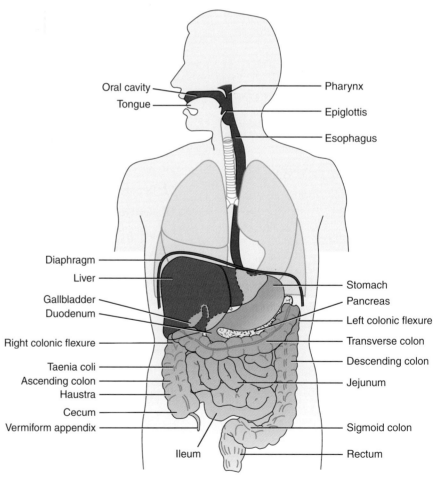

FIGURE 23-1 Digestive system.

LIPS

Codes in the Lips subheading (40490-40799) include the categories of Excision, Repair (Cheiloplasty), and Other Procedures. If the procedure was performed on the skin of the lips, assign a code from the Integumentary System, not a Digestive System code.

A **vermilionectomy** (40500) is shaving of the lip. The vermilion zone is the red part of the lips (Fig. 23-2). The surgeon removes an area of tissue and repairs the defect by moving the mucosal surface to reconnect the lip, thereby forming a new vermilion border. If the area of defect is larger, a more extensive excisional procedure may be necessary (40510-40527). For example, during a **transverse wedge excision** (40510), a wedge of lip tissue is removed and tissue flaps are placed to repair the defect. Code 40525 describes a full-thickness lip excision with reconstruction with local flap. There are many services bundled into 40525, such as:

- 11440-11444 and 11446 (benign lesion excision)
- 11640-11644 and 11646 (malignant lesion excision)
- 40500 (vermilionectomy with mucosal advancement)
- 40510 and 40520 (excision of lip)

The **Abbe-Estlander** (40527, also known as Abbe flap or cross flap) is a reconstructive procedure in which a graft is taken from a portion of the lip and the non-defective area above the lip is used to repair the area of defect. For example, a patient had cancer of the lower lip due to smoking, as illustrated in Fig. 23-3, *A*. The surgeon removed the area of defect from the lower lip and identified a superior (above lip) flap. In Fig. 23-3, *B*, the superior flap was moved to cover the area of defect. Fig. 23-3, *C*, illustrates the results of the **reconstruction**. If more than one-fourth of the lip surface is removed, the procedure is considered a **resection** and is reported with 40530. If reconstruction of the lip is required to repair the defect that remains after the resection, the procedure is reported separately with a code from 13131-13153 (complex repair of lip and face). The reconstruction code is assigned based on location and size of the defect.

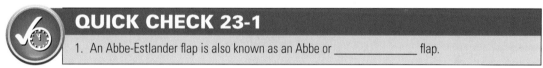

QUICK CHECK 23-1

1. An Abbe-Estlander flap is also known as an Abbe or _____ flap.

(Answers are located in Appendix C)

The codes for **cheiloplasty** (lip repair) are located in the Repair category. There are two types of Repair codes: those that report full-thickness repair of the lip (40650-40654) and those that report cleft lip repair (40700-40761). The full-thickness repairs are based on the extent of the repair, for example, vermilion only (40650), up to half of the vertical height of the lip (40652), and over one-half of the vertical height of the lip (40654, complex repair).

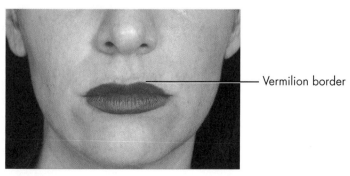

Vermilion border

FIGURE 23-2 Vermilion border.

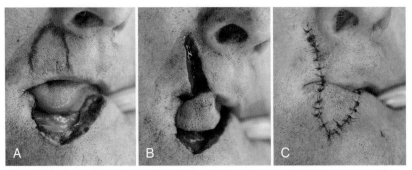

FIGURE 23–3 **A,** Abbe-Estlander flap for lip reconstruction with defective area excised and flap area outlined. **B,** Abbe-Estlander flap for lip reconstruction with flap moved down and positioned in defect area. **C,** Completed Abbe-Estlander flap.

A **cleft lip** is a congenital defect in which the muscle and tissue of the lip did not close properly. Fig. 23-4, *B,* illustrates a unilateral defect and Fig. 23-4, *C,* illustrates a bilateral defect. Some of the cleft lip Repair codes report bilateral procedures (40701, 40702) and other codes report unilateral procedures (40700, 40720). If a bilateral procedure was performed and the code description does not indicate a bilateral procedure, add modifier -50.

A **rhinoplasty** may be required if a nasal deformity has occurred with the cleft lip defect. These defects occur when the muscle, rather than encircling the mouth, attaches to the nose and pulls the nose out of normal position. If a rhinoplasty is performed with a cleft lip repair, the rhinoplasty is reported separately with 30460 or 30462. **A cleft** palate (Fig. 23-4, *A*) may also be present with a cleft lip, and if repair of the palate is performed at the time of the lip repair, the palate repair is reported separately with codes from the 42200 series. For example, 42205 reports a palatoplasty for a cleft palate with closure of the soft tissue of the alveolar ridge.

VESTIBULE OF MOUTH

The vestibule of the mouth is also known as the buccal cavity and is part of the oral cavity. Codes for the Vestibule of Mouth (40800-40899) do not include codes for services of the Tongue and Floor of Mouth (41000-41599) or Dentoalveolar Structures (41800-41899). The categories included within the Vestibule of Mouth subheading are incisions (e.g., abscess, cyst, or hematoma), excision/destruction (e.g., biopsy or lesion excision), and repair (e.g., closure or vestibuloplasty). The procedures are based on the complexity of the procedure (e.g., simple or complex) and whether the procedure is bilateral or unilateral.

TONGUE AND FLOOR OF MOUTH

The Tongue and Floor of Mouth subheading (41000-41599) includes codes to report the incision and drainage of abscess, cyst, or hematoma of the tongue or floor of the mouth. These

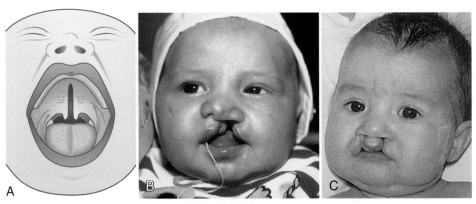

FIGURE 23–4 **A,** Cleft palate. **B,** Unilateral cleft lip. Note the nasal deformity in which the nose is out of normal position. **C,** Bilateral cleft lip.

incision and drainage codes (41000-41009) are based on the location of the abscess, cyst, or hematoma, such as under the tongue (**sublingual**), under the mandible (**submandibular**), or within the space from the floor of the mouth to the hyoid bone (**masticator space**). The sublingual codes are further based on whether the abscess, cyst, or hematoma is superficial or deep.

The **lingual frenum** is the flap of skin under the tongue. **Ankyloglossia** (tongue tie) is illustrated in Fig. 23-5 and is due to a tight lingual frenum. This condition is often diagnosed by the pediatrician during a newborn examination. Ankyloglossia occurs in 4.8% of the population and may interfere with feeding. The procedure in which an incision is made in this flap is a frenotomy. The incision procedure (41010) frees the tongue to allow greater motion. During a frenotomy, the lingual frenum is only incised, not excised. If a frenectomy (excision of the lingual frenum) is performed, the service is reported with 41115 from the Excision category. If the lingual frenum is surgically repaired (frenoplasty), the procedure is reported with 41520 from the Other Procedures category.

Extraoral incision and drainage (I&D) is performed on an abscess, cyst, or hematoma located outside the mouth or on the floor of the mouth. Code range 41015-41018 reports extraoral (outside the mouth) incision and drainage based on the location of sublingual, submental (under the chin), submandibular, or masticator space. The masticator space is a deep facial space, bounded by the superficial layer of deep cervical fascia and containing the four muscles of mastication, ramus, and posterior body of the mandible.

Excision codes (41100-41155) report oral biopsies, excision of oral lesions, and removal of all or part of the tongue (glossectomy). The biopsy codes (41100-41108) are reported based on the location from which the biopsy was obtained. The codes for excision of a lesion are also based on the location (such as floor of mouth, tongue, or lingual frenum). If a local tongue flap is required to repair the excisional defect, report the repair with 41114 in addition to the code for the primary excision procedure.

Repair (41250-41252) of the tongue is reported based on the size of the repair:
- 2.5 cm or less
- Over 2.6 cm

In addition to the size, the tongue repair codes are also based on the location of the repair:
- Floor of the mouth and/or anterior two thirds of tongue
- Posterior one third of tongue

If the length of the repair is stated in inches, the measurement must be converted to centimeters. One inch equals 2.54 cm, and the formula for conversion is:
- Centimeters × 0.3937008 = inches
- Inches × 2.54 = centimeters

If the repair is stated in millimeters (mm) the conversion to centimeters is:
- 1 millimeter = 0.1 centimeters

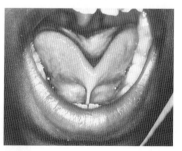

FIGURE 23–5 Ankyloglossia.

For example, if the medical record indicated 15 millimeters, the calculation would be 15 × 0.1 = 1.5 centimeters.

DENTOALVEOLAR STRUCTURES

The dentoalveolar structures are the bone (osseous) and soft structures of the mouth that anchor the teeth (Fig. 23-6). Codes 41800-41899 report incision, excision/destruction, and other types of procedures performed on the dentoalveolar structures. Examples of these procedures include drainage of an abscess, cyst, or hematoma (41800) or excision of a lesion with simple repair (41826). Some of the codes are based on the quadrant in which the procedure is performed, such as excision of the gingiva (gingivectomy), reported with 41820 for each quadrant or, as another example, excision of the alveolar mucosa, reported with 41828 for each quadrant.

The American Dental Association (ADA) publishes a dental claim form that is most often used to report dental services.

> ### CMS RULES
>
> For current information on the dental coverage for Medicare patients, refer to the Internet Only Manuals (IOM) (www.cms.gov/Regulations-and-Guidance/Guidance/Manuals/Internet-Only-Manuals-IOMs.html) 100-01, Chapter 5, Section 70.2 and 100-02, Chapter 15, Section 150.

PALATE AND UVULA

Services to the palate (roof of mouth) and uvula (pendulous structure at the back of the throat) are reported with codes 42000-42299. This subheading contains the usual codes for incision, excision/destruction, and repair. If grafting is required to repair the area of defect after excision of a lesion, the grafting service is reported in addition to the excision code. The choice of grafting codes is based on whether a skin graft (14040-14302) or an oral mucosal graft (40818) was used for repair. Within the Repair codes you will also locate the codes to report repair procedures for cleft palate (42200-42225), as discussed previously.

Code 42145 describes a palatopharyngoplasty (palate and pharynx repair) procedure and has limited medically indicated reasons for the surgical procedure. One medically indicated reason for the procedure is obstructive sleep apnea (OSA) that is documented to be unresponsive to conservative measures, such as continuous positive airway pressure (CPAP), positional therapy, dental devices, and weight loss. OSA is characterized by frequent episodes of hypopnea (shallow breathing) or apnea during sleep.

SALIVARY GLAND AND DUCTS

There are three salivary glands as illustrated in Fig. 23-7 (parotid, submandibular, and sublingual). It is important to note the technique for performing biopsy procedures of the salivary glands. Code 42400 states the biopsy of the salivary gland using a needle technique, and

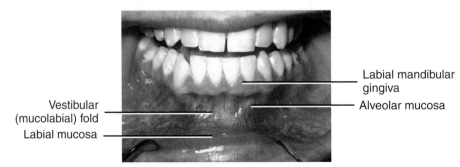

FIGURE 23-6 Alveolar mucosa.

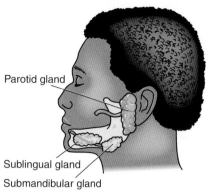

FIGURE 23-7 Salivary glands.

42405 uses an incisional approach. There is an injection procedure that is reported with 42550 for a sialography (x-ray of salivary gland), and the radiological component of the procedure is reported with 70390. It is important to read all notes before or after a code description because the parenthetical statement in the CPT manual located after 42550 directs the coder to report the radiological supervision and interpretation with 70390. Imaging guidance may be used for salivary gland biopsy (42400) and is reported in addition to the biopsy service depending on the guidance type—77002 (fluoroscopic), 77012 (CT), 77021 (MRI), or 76942 (ultrasound).

The codes in this subheading (42300-42699) are often divided based on the gland. For example, excision of a tumor of the parotid gland is reported with 42410; of the submandibular gland, 42440; and of the sublingual gland, 42450. Other services are reported based on the number of glands involved. The parotid duct is a duct opening from the cheek into the vestibule of the mouth opposite the neck of the upper second molar tooth as illustrated in Fig. 23-8. The parotid duct is also known as the Steno's or Stensen's duct. When a gland is excised with the parotid duct diversion, the service for both the diversion and excision of two submandibular glands are reported with 42509.

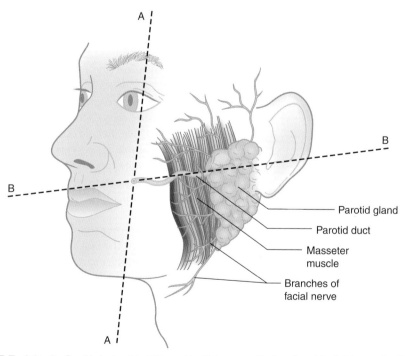

FIGURE 23-8 Parotid gland and duct (Stensen's) with the surrounding branches of the facial nerve. Line B approximates the course of the duct, which enters the mouth at the junction of lines A and B.

EXERCISE 23-1 — Lips, Vestibule of Mouth, Tongue and Floor of Mouth, Dentoalveolar Structures, Palate and Uvula, and Salivary Gland and Ducts

Using the CPT, ICD-10-CM and/or ICD-9-CM manuals, complete the following:

1 A _____ is shaving of the lip.

2 In addition to the sites from the mouth to the anus, the Digestive System codes include codes for the pancreas, liver, and

_____ .

3 How many centimeters are there in 4 inches (round to the nearest tenth)? _____

4 An Abbe-Estlander reconstruction for cleft lip

CPT Code: _____

ICD-10-CM Code: _____ (ICD-9-CM Code: _____)

5 A complex, full-thickness repair of the vermilion after resection of buccal-mucosal squamous cell carcinoma of upper lip

CPT Code: _____

ICD-10-CM Code: _____ (ICD-9-CM Code: _____)

6 Simple drainage of a hematoma of the vestibule of the mouth

CPT Code: _____

7 Repair of a laceration of the tongue, measuring 1.5 inches

CPT Code: _____

(Answers are located in Appendix B)

PHARYNX, ADENOIDS, AND TONSILS

It is within the 42700-42999 range of codes that you will locate the often reported codes for tonsillectomy and adenoidectomy. In addition there are codes for incisions, biopsies, excisions, and repair procedures.

The Incision category (42700-42725) codes report the drainage of an abscess. The codes are assigned based on the **location** (peritonsillar [around the tonsil], retropharyngeal [behind the pharynx], parapharyngeal [adjacent to the pharynx]) of the abscess and the **approach** utilized (intraoral or external). Careful reading of the operative report is necessary to identify the location and approach to ensure correct code assignment.

Biopsy codes 42800-42806 include obtaining the biopsy sample but do not include the use of a scope to obtain the sample. If a laryngoscopic biopsy is performed, the service is reported with a code from the Respiratory System, not with a code from the Digestive System. For example, 31510 (indirect diagnostic, views through reflection with a mirror), 31535 (direct operative, views with a scope), or 31536 (direct operative, views direct with scope, plus operating microscope assistance).

A **branchial cleft** cyst is a congenital defect that appears as a gill located on the neck. Branchia is Greek for gills, which the cyst resembles. Reporting an excision of the branchial cleft cyst is based on the extent of the procedure. If the extent of the defect was confined to the skin and subcutaneous tissue, report the service with 42810. If the defect extended beneath the subcutaneous tissue and perhaps into the pharynx, report the service with 42815.

Tonsillectomy and **adenoidectomy** are commonly reported surgical procedures (42820-42836). The tonsils are two glands located at the back of the throat (Fig. 23-9, *A*), and the adenoids (Fig. 23-9, *B*) are located behind the nose and above the soft palate

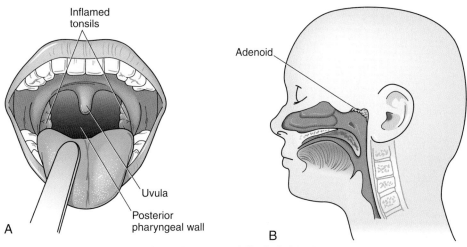

FIGURE 23-9 **A,** Tonsils. **B,** Adenoid.

(roof of mouth) and cannot be visualized without a mirror or scope. The selection of the correct code is based on if:

■ Only the tonsils are removed
■ Only the adenoids are removed
■ Both the tonsils and adenoids are removed
■ The patient is under 12 years of age, or age 12 or over

Many codes contain age descriptors or primary (initial removal) or secondary (subsequent removal of tissue that has grown back).

CODING SHOT

The codes for tonsillectomy and/or adenoidectomy in the range 42820-42836 are performed bilaterally. If a procedure is reported with the -50 modifier, or with modifiers -RT and -LT, the third-party payer will usually not recognize the modifier(s) and will pay based on the amount for a single procedure. If only one side is removed, modifier -52 (Reduced service) must be appended to the CPT code.

A **pharyngoplasty** (42950) is the surgical repair of the pharynx and includes the use of flaps fashioned from the skin, tongue, and/or tissue located near the area of defect (regional cutaneous flaps) used in the repair procedure. If a pharyngeal flap is used, report the service with 42225, as directed in the parenthetical note.

A **pharyngostomy** (42955) is a procedure to create an opening for insertion of a long-term feeding tube. An incision is made below the jaw line on the skin and the incision is carried down to the pharynx. The opening is reinforced with sutures, and a long-term feeding tube is inserted through the opening into the pharynx. A nasogastric feeding tube (NGT, nose to stomach) is a more well-known method, but in some patients (i.e., severe facial trauma), pharyngostomy is the necessary approach.

Codes to report the control of oropharyngeal (between the soft palate and the epiglottis) or nasopharyngeal (above the soft palate) hemorrhage are located in the Other Procedures subheading (42955-42999). Codes 42960-42972 (esophagotomy or myotomy) are reported based on whether the procedure is a primary or secondary procedure and the level of complexity.

ESOPHAGUS

Procedures of the esophagus are reported with codes in the 43020-43499 range and are performed by incision, excision, endoscopy, repair, and manipulation. The **approach** is the first step to determine selection of the correct code. For example, 43100 describes the excision of lesion, esophagus, with primary repair; cervical approach, and 43101 describes the same procedure but with a thoracic or abdominal approach. Codes 43180-43233 report endoscopic services limited to the esophagus. The scope may be advanced into the stomach but does not advance to the pylorus (stricture at end of stomach).

The types of esophagus procedures are diagnostic endoscopy, injection, biopsy, removal of foreign body, insertion of plastic tube/stent, dilation, and hemorrhage control. Some codes, such as 43220 (balloon dilation), do not include imaging guidance (74360), whereas other codes include the guidance, such as 43231 (diagnostic esophagoscopy with endoscopic ultrasound examination). Note that many codes include conscious sedation as a part of the service as indicated by the bullseye symbol to the left of the code.

The Incision codes include both cervical approach (43020) and thoracic approach (43045) for removal of a foreign body as illustrated in Fig. 23-10. It is important to confirm the approach used when coding removal of a foreign body from the esophagus. The Excision codes (43100-43135) also include various approaches in the code description, such as cervical, thoracic, and abdominal.

If a lesion is removed from the esophagus, report the service with 43100 (cervical) or 43101 (thoracic or abdominal), depending on the approach used. If a partial, near total, or total removal (wide excision) of the esophagus is performed with total removal of the larynx, the service may or may not include extensive (radical) neck dissection. These removal services are reported with 43107, 43116 (with graft), 43124, or 31360 (total laryngectomy from the Respiratory System). Note that some of these codes also specify the approach. For example, 43116 indicates a cervical approach.

Code 43191 is a transoral esophagoscopy by means of a rigid scope and 43200 is by means of a flexible scope. Both are diagnostic and include the collection of specimen(s) by brushing or washing. Both are categorized as separate procedures and only reported if no more major esophageal procedure was performed. Both are bundled into the surgical services. The scope type—rigid or flexible—is the only difference between these codes. The same procedure using a transnasal approach is reported with 43197.

Medical necessity for a diagnostic procedure must be documented in the medical record. For example, the signs and/or symptoms demonstrate the medical necessity of the service. If the service has 0 global days, this means the procedure includes all preoperative and postoperative care related to performing the procedure on the day of the procedure; but before or after the day of the procedure, any services related to the procedure are reported separately. The diagnostic esophagoscopy is bundled into all endoscopy procedures reported with 43180-43233 and 43235-43259.

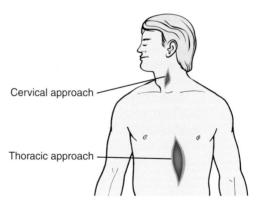

FIGURE 23–10   Cervical and thoracic approaches for removal of a foreign body from the esophagus.

Codes 43180-43233 describe therapeutic procedures on the esophagus. Codes 43192 and 43201 describe transoral esophagoscopy with submucosal injections of any substance. You must report the substance injected; for example, botulinum toxin (J0585) to treat esophageal spasms.

Codes 43193, 43198, and 43202 describe single or multiple biopsy procedures based on the approach—transoral or transnasal—and the type of scope—flexible or rigid. As with all codes, the diagnosis must support the medical necessity of the esophagoscopy. For example, some diagnoses that would support the medical necessity of the esophagoscopy would be K22.8/530.83, esophageal leukoplakia, K21.9, esophageal reflux, or R13.10, unspecified dysphagia.

Codes 43194 or 43215 report a transoral esophagoscopy for removal of foreign body(s). The medical necessity of this procedure would be demonstrated by a diagnosis code such as T18.1/935.1 (foreign body in esophagus). If radiology is used during the procedure, report the radiology service with 74235 (Removal of foreign body(s), esophageal, with use of balloon catheter, radiological supervision, and interpretation).

The removal or ablation of esophageal polyp(s), tumor(s), or other lesion(s) are reported with 43216 or 43217. Hot biopsy forceps use high frequency electrical current to remove and cauterize in one maneuver. The forceps may be monopolar (single electrode) or bipolar (two electrodes).

The following dilation procedures may use fluoroscopy (74360) but do not include endoscopy:

■ 43450, dilation of the esophagus, by unguided sound or bougie (cylinder), single or multiple passes
■ 43453, dilation of the esophagus, over guidewire
■ 43460, esophagogastric tamponade, with balloon (Sengstaken type) (A balloon is placed into the esophagus and inflated to stop bleeding.)

If an endoscopy is performed in addition to any of these dilation procedures, report a code that bundles the dilation and the endoscopic guidance, such as 43213.

A submucosal injection is one that is performed to ease the removal of polyps. Fluid, usually saline, is injected around the polyp and the fluid elevates the polyp to allow for easier excision. When a submucosal injection is performed, report the service based on the delivery method. For example, submucosal injection by means of:

■ Esophagoscopy, 43192, 43201
■ EGD, 43236
■ Sigmoidoscopy, 45335
■ Colonoscopy, 45381

An **EGD** (esophagogastroduodenoscopy) is a procedure performed to examine the esophagus, stomach, duodenum, and sometimes the jejunum for signs of bleeding, tumors, erosion, ulcers, or other abnormalities. The EGD is often performed in conjunction with another procedure. For example, code 43405 reports an EGD with suturing of the esophagogastric junction. During this procedure, a special suturing system is inserted through the scope, the physician then places a series of stitches in the esophagogastric junction, essentially pleating the sphincter to prevent the backflow of stomach acid into the esophagus. The medical necessity of the procedure would be demonstrated with a diagnosis code, such as K21.9/530.81.

CODING SHOT

EGD code 43259 is assigned when an endoscopic **ultrasound** examination is performed. As stated in the parenthetical note immediately following CPT code 43259, the radiological supervision and interpretation is **NOT** reported separately with 76975.

More than one procedure may be performed during the same operative session, for example, a transoral with flexible scope EGD performed with **biopsy** and **dilation** of gastric outlet due to obstruction. The services are performed during the same endoscopic session and are reported as:

■ **43245** (Esophagogastroduodenoscopy, flexible, transoral; with **dilation** of gastric/duodenal stricture(s) [e.g., balloon, bougie])

■ **43239** (Esophagogastroduodenoscopy, flexible, transoral; with **biopsy**, single or multiple)

TOOLBOX

Karla has complaints of a tightening sensation in her throat when she swallows and feels as if she is choking when she eats. She has lost 10 pounds in the last 4 months because she is hesitant to eat for fear of choking. The physician performs a procedure that is reported with 43213.

QUESTIONS

1. What is the diagnostic term that describes Karla's chief complaint? _____

2. What is the code description term that means "against the flow"? _____ _____

3. Does 43213 include fluoroscopic guidance? _____

▼ ANSWERS

1. dysphagia, 2. retrograde, 3. yes

An endoscopic retrograde cholangiopancreatography (**ERCP,** 43260-43278) is an endoscopic procedure of the pancreatic ducts, hepatic ducts, common bile ducts, duodenal papilla, and/or gallbladder (hepatobiliary system) and is performed primarily to diagnose and treat conditions of the bile ducts, including gallstones, inflammatory strictures (scars), leaks (due to trauma or surgery), and cancer. ERCP combines the use of x-rays and endoscope. Through the endoscope, the physician can visualize the inside of the stomach and duodenum, and injects dye into the ducts of the biliary tree and pancreas to be viewed on x-ray. The scope is advanced through the esophagus, into the stomach, to the duodenal papilla (papilla of Vater), and contrast is then injected to visualize the bile ducts and biliary tract, including the gallbladder. Assignment of these codes is based on purpose of the procedure as diagnostic or therapeutic. The codes do not include the radiological supervision and interpretation, so when performed, report:

■ 74328 (biliary ductal system)

■ 74329 (pancreatic ductal system)

■ 74330 (biliary and pancreatic ductal systems)

When an ERCP is performed for a **diagnostic** purpose by means of an endoscopy, report the service with 43260. During the procedure, the physician may view the common bile duct or the entire biliary tract. The procedure may be with or without the collection of specimen(s) by brushing or washing, which is not reported separately because collection is included in the code description. If there is no definitive diagnosis documented in the medical record, assign code(s) for the documented signs and symptoms.

CODING SHOT

There are times when the insertion for visualization cannot be accomplished, due to a variety of factors. A failed ERCP is reported with 43235-43259.

Laparoscopy (43279-43289). Surgical laparoscopy is a procedure to examine the organs of the abdominal cavity and always includes diagnostic laparoscopy. A laparoscope is a thin flexible tube containing a camera. The scope is placed through a small incision in the abdomen (Fig. 23-11) and produces images that can be viewed on a computer screen. A similar procedure is utilized to view the organs of the pelvis (gynecologic laparoscopy or pelviscopy).

EXERCISE 23-2 *Pharynx, Adenoids, Tonsils, and Esophagus*

Using the CPT, ICD-10-CM and/or ICD-9-CM manuals, code the following:

1 Tonsillectomy of an 18-year-old with chronic hypertrophic tonsillitis

  CPT Code: _____

  ICD-10-CM Code: _____ (ICD-9-CM Code: _____)

2 Suture of pharynx after injury

  CPT Code: _____

3 Esophagotomy using a thoracic approach for removal of a penny that was lodged in the child's throat

  CPT Code: _____

4 Thoracic approach was employed for excision of a lesion from the esophagus. The procedure included primary repair.

  CPT Code: _____

5 Dilation of the esophagus by means of a bougie with multiple passes.

  CPT Code: _____

(Answers are located in Appendix B)

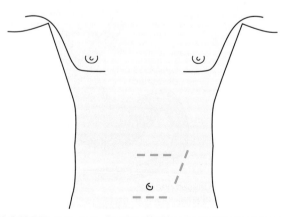

FIGURE 23–11 Location of incisions for insertion of laparoscope.

STOMACH

The Stomach codes 43500-43999 include incisional procedures in which the stomach is exposed to the view of the surgeon, such as 43500 (gastrotomy with exploration or foreign body removal). Other procedures are performed by means of a scope, such as 43653 (laparoscopic gastrostomy). Be certain to identify the method used to perform the procedure before assigning a code.

Gastric bypass surgery is performed on patients who are morbidly obese with the outcome of decreasing the size of the stomach and/or intestines to aid with weight loss. There are many techniques used for gastric bypass procedures. A **Roux-en-Y** (RNY) is a Y-shaped surgical connection in which the intestine is detached from its original origin and reattached so as to bypass a part of the stomach and the entire duodenum (first part of the small intestine) as illustrated in Fig. 23-12. The Roux-en-Y term is used in several code descriptions, such as 43621 (total gastrectomy with Roux-en-Y reconstruction) and 43644 (laparoscopic gastric restriction, with gastric bypass and Roux-en-Y gastroenterostomy). For an open procedure, a 6- to 9-inch incision is made in the abdomen to gain access to the stomach and intestines. For a laparoscopic procedure about six access ports are established measuring about ¼ to ½ inch each in diameter through which the surgical instruments are inserted. The laparoscopic procedures are much less invasive and decrease the time the patient spends in the hospital, recovery time, and complications.

Bariatric Surgery codes 43770-43775 also report procedures performed for gastric restrictive procedures that are accomplished by placing a restrictive device around the stomach to decrease its functional size. Code 43770 reports "placement of adjustable gastric restrictive device (e.g., gastric band and subcutaneous port components)" (Fig. 23-13). The band is adjustable because the band is hollow and contains a tube that can be inflated with fluid. After surgery, fluid is gradually inserted into the tube through a subcutaneous port (just beneath the skin) with a syringe. The physician can adjust the amount of fluid in the tube and thereby adjust the amount of food that can pass through the banded area. The procedure may be performed on an outpatient basis and is reversible by removal of the banding apparatus.

Medicare released its new policy for bariatric surgery in February, 2009, which covers open and laparoscopic Roux-en-Y gastric bypass, laparoscopic adjustable gastric banding, and open and laparoscopic biliopancreatic diversion with duodenal switch. CMS will not require that candidates for bariatric surgery first attempt a dietary weight-loss program. Bariatric surgery is available for any Medicare beneficiary with a body mass index of 35 or greater with at least one comorbidity related to obesity. Coverage is provided only if the bariatric surgery is performed at a medical center designated as a Center of Excellence by the American Society for Bariatric Surgery (ASBS) or certified as a Level 1 Bariatric Surgery Center by the American College of Surgeons.

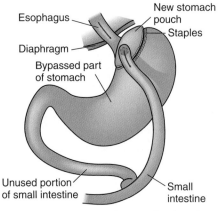

FIGURE 23-12 Roux-en-Y (RNY) gastric bypass.

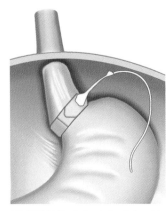

FIGURE 23-13 Adjustable gastric restrictive device.

INTESTINES (EXCEPT RECTUM)

The large intestine is about 5 feet long with a wider diameter than the small intestine. The small intestine is about 30 feet long. The Intestine codes 44005-44799 exclude codes to report services for the anus and rectum.

Separate procedures are common in this subheading. Colostomies (creation of an artificial opening) are always bundled into a more major procedure unless the code specifically states to report the colostomy separately. For example, code 44141 is a partial colectomy and includes establishment of a colostomy.

Many intestinal procedures are performed through endoscopes (such as the gastroscopy in Fig. 23-14). Endoscope codes are available for procedures depending on how far down (through the mouth) or up (through the anus) the scope is passed. The code selection varies according to the procedure performed and includes the sites the scope passed through to accomplish the procedure. To choose the proper code, the extent of the procedure must be determined. For example, if a flexible scope is passed to the esophagus only, the code would be chosen from the endoscopy codes 43180-43233. If the scoping is continued through the esophagus to the stomach, duodenum, and/or jejunum, the code selection would be from the endoscopy codes 43235-43259 (upper GI). Once the anatomic site of the endoscope procedure is correctly identified, the surgical procedure(s) performed guides the selection of the code. A surgical endoscopy always includes a diagnostic endoscopy. Assign modifier -51 if more than one procedure is performed.

CODING SHOT

To choose the correct endoscopy, identify the farthest **extent** to which the scope was passed and then the procedure(s) performed.

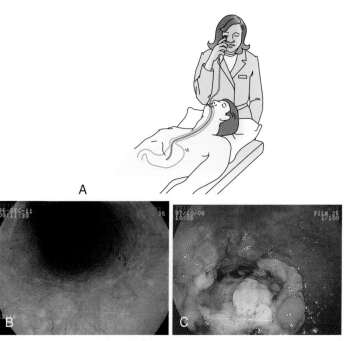

FIGURE 23–14 Illustration of endoscopy and endoscopic images of the gastroesophageal junction. **A,** Endoscopy. **B,** Normal. **C,** Esophageal cancer at the gastroesophageal junction.

Resection of the intestine means taking out a portion of the intestine and either joining the remaining ends (anastomosis) directly or developing an artificial opening (exteriorizing) through the abdominal wall. Fig. 23-15 illustrates three types of anastomoses. The artificial opening (stoma) allows for the removal of body waste products (Fig. 23-16), as with the colostomy. The type of anastomosis or exteriorization depends on the medical condition of the patient and on the amount of intestine (large or small) that has to be removed. Some patients have temporary exteriorization for the length of time it takes the remaining intestine to heal and begin to perform the necessary functions. Other patients have permanent exteriorization because too much of the intestine has been removed to allow for adequate functioning. Openings to the outside of the body are named for the part of the intestine from which they are formed—colostomy is an artificial opening from the colon, ileostomy from the ileum, gastrostomy from the stomach, and so forth (Fig. 23-17). To assign the correct code, identify the correct anatomic site from which the ostomy originated, as well as the procedure used to establish the ostomy.

QUICK CHECK 23-2

1. The first step to choosing the correct GI endoscopic code is to determine the
_____ to which the scope was passed.

(Answers are located in Appendix C)

Sometimes, a laparotomy is used as the approach in digestive system surgeries, and the approach is never coded separately. An exploratory laparotomy may be performed to investigate the cause of a patient's illness. If only the exploratory laparotomy is performed, it is appropriate to report the service with an exploratory laparotomy code, such as 49000. However, if the exploratory procedure progressed to a more definitive surgical treatment (such as an appendectomy), only the definitive treatment (appendectomy) is reported.

Anastomoses

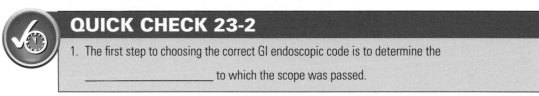

End to end

End to side

Side to side

FIGURE 23–15   Three types of anastomoses.

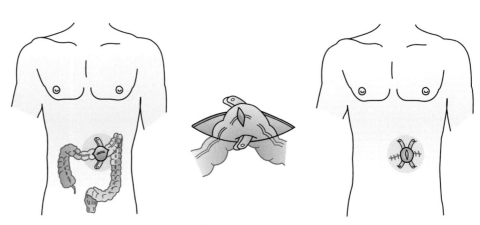

FIGURE 23–16   Stoma.

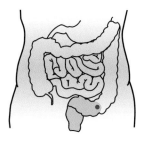

Sigmoid colostomy

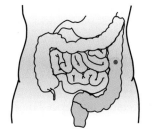

Descending colostomy

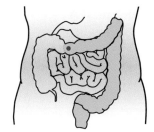

Transverse (single B) colostomy

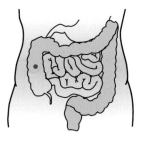

Ascending colostomy

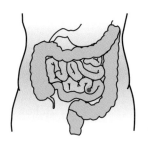

Ileostomy

FIGURE 23–17 Various ostomies.

MECKEL'S DIVERTICULUM AND THE MESENTERY

A Meckel's diverticulum is a fairly common congenital pouch on the wall of the small bowel that may contain pancreatic or stomach tissue and may require surgical removal (44800). Removal of the omphalomesenteric duct refers to the embryonic passage that connects an egg sac to the intestine and is included in the code description of 44800.

| EXERCISE 23-3 | *Stomach and Intestines (Except Rectum)* |

Using your knowledge of medical terminology, identify the following surgical communications:

1 Coloproctostomy: from the _____ to the _____

2 Ileostomy: from the _____ to the _____ surface

3 Colostomy: from the _____ intestine to the _____ surface

4 Enteroenterostomy: between _____ of intestine

Using the CPT, ICD-10-CM and/or ICD-9-CM manuals, code the following:

5 Partial bowel resection with colostomy for primary, malignant neoplasm

　　CPT Code: _____

　　ICD-10-CM Code: _____ (ICD-9-CM Code: _____)

6 Resection of small intestine, single resection, with anastomosis

　　CPT Code: _____

(Answers are located in Appendix B)

APPENDIX

Surgical procedures of the appendix may be accomplished by means of

Open procedures:
- 44900, open I&D of abscess
- 44950, open surgical appendectomy

Percutaneous procedures:
- 49406, percutaneous image-guided I&D of abscess

Laparoscopic procedures:
- 44970, laparoscopic appendectomy

There are two other codes to report appendectomy procedures.
- 44955, appendectomy performed at the time of a major procedure for an indicated purpose
- 44960, appendectomy when appendix has ruptured or there is generalized peritonitis

The reporting of 44950 and 44955 needs special attention because there are times when a surgeon will remove a healthy appendix during the course of another abdominal procedure. Because the abdomen is already open to the view of the surgeon, the incidental appendectomy (44950) does not add to the complexity of the procedure and is not reported separately. If, however, during another major abdominal procedure, the surgeon removes the appendix due to a medically necessary reason, the service is reported with 44955.

COLON AND RECTUM

Colon and Rectum procedures are reported with codes from the 45000-45999 range. These procedures involve the colon and rectum and employ techniques such as incision, excision, and destruction. Many of the codes are very complex. For example:
- 45126, Pelvic exenteration for colorectal malignancy, with proctectomy (with or without colostomy), with removal of bladder and ureteral transplantations, and/or hysterectomy, or cervicectomy, with or without removal of tube(s), with or without removal of ovary(s), or any combination thereof

This complex code description contains many procedures that may or may not have been performed as indicated by the "with or without." For example, with or without colostomy or with or without removal of tubes and ovaries. If any of the listed procedures were performed, they are bundled in the main code (45126) and not reported separately. Complex codes such as 45126 increase the potential for unintentional unbundling.

Endoscopy (Proctosigmoidoscopy, Sigmoidoscopy, and Colonoscopy)

Rectal endoscopic procedures are frequently performed and include proctosigmoidoscopy, sigmoidoscopy, and colonoscopy (Fig. 23-18).

Proctosigmoidoscopy. Endoscopic examination of the rectum (proct/o = rectum) and the sigmoid colon (45300-45327). The scope is advanced 6-25 cm (2.4-9.8 in). Code 45300 describes a rigid proctosigmoidoscopy, diagnostic, with or without collection of specimen(s) by brushing or washing (separate procedure). Do not assign 45300 when reported with codes 45303-45327, because these codes report surgical procedures, so the diagnostic service of 45300 is bundled into the surgical procedure. If no definitive diagnosis is documented, report the documented signs/symptoms.

Sigmoidoscopy. Endoscopic examination of the sigmoid colon may include the descending colon (45330-45350). The scope is advanced 26-60 cm (10.2-23.6 in). A sigmoidoscopy is the examination of the entire rectum and sigmoid colon and may include examination of a portion of the descending colon but stops before reaching the splenic flexure (the turn beneath the spleen that connects the descending to the transverse colon). Code 45330 describes a flexible diagnostic sigmoidoscopy that includes the collection of specimen(s) by brushing or washing

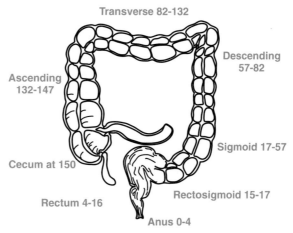

Transverse 82-132

Descending 57-82

Ascending 132-147

Sigmoid 17-57

Cecum at 150

Rectosigmoid 15-17

Rectum 4-16

Anus 0-4

FIGURE 23-18 Colonoscopy measurements (cm).

(separate procedure). Do not code 45330 when also reporting 45331-45350 because they are surgical procedures and the diagnostic procedure (45330) is always included in the surgical procedure. If a definitive diagnosis has not been documented, report the documented signs/symptoms.

Diagnostic Colonoscopy. Endoscopic examination of the colon from rectum to cecum is reported with codes from the 45378-45398 range. The scope is advanced more than 60 cm (more than 23.6 in).

The diagnostic colonoscopy codes are divided based on the extent and the purpose of the procedure. The diagnostic stand-alone codes 45300, 45330, and 45378 each have a list of indented procedure codes based on the purpose of the procedure (such as biopsy, foreign body removal, ablation, control of bleeding, etc.). Take a moment to locate these codes in the CPT manual and familiarize yourself with the types of procedures reported with the codes.

If the patient is fully prepared for the endoscopic procedure, and the procedure has begun but is not completed because of extenuating circumstances, use modifier -53 (Discontinued Procedure) appended to the endoscopic code. Some payers, such as Medicare, require the coder to report -53 for a procedure that could not be completed. These extenuating circumstances could be that the patient has become unstable, the bowel preparation for the surgery was not sufficient to continue the procedure, or an equipment failure occurred. Use either -52 or -53 and provide supporting documentation as to why the procedure was discontinued.

Colonoscopy. Codes 45378-45398 describe procedures in which the endoscope is advanced to the proximal colon (past the splenic flexure) to the cecum or into a portion of the terminal ileum (most distant part of the small intestine).

To report colonoscopy procedures, first determine how the procedure was performed:
- Through a colostomy (44380-44408)
- Through a colotomy (45399)
- Through the rectum (45378-45398)

When the colon is examined through a colostomy (surgically created opening in the abdominal wall), the diagnostic or therapeutic service is reported with codes 44388-44397.

Report 45380 (colonoscopy with biopsy(ies)) when a "**cold biopsy**" is performed. A cold biopsy is generally accepted to mean the use of forceps to grasp and remove a small piece of tissue without the application of cautery. For example, one polyp was snared and three polyps were biopsied with cold biopsy forceps. The service would be reported with 45385 (colonoscopy with removal of tumor/polyp/lesion by snare technique) and 45380 (colonoscopy with biopsy(ies)). During a snare procedure, a wire loop is placed around the lesion and the wire is then heated to shave off the lesion. Larger lesions may be removed with a single application of the snare or with several applications (called piecemeal). Remnants may also be cauterized or ablated to completely destroy the lesion. The assignment of the code is not dependent on the histology of the tissue obtained for analysis. Report only one technique for each lesion or polyp.

Colonoscopy with removal by snare technique (45385) should not be reported when describing the removal of a small polyp by biopsy or cold forceps technique.

A colonoscopy with biopsy and polypectomy in separate sites are reported with two codes. The biopsy may require modifier -59 to identify the service as a separate procedure from the polyp procedure.

Code 45378 describes a flexible diagnostic colonoscopy up to the splenic flexure and is bundled into the colonoscopy procedure codes 45379-45398. If no definitive diagnosis is documented, assign diagnosis code(s) for signs/symptoms.

CMS RULES

When a covered colonoscopy is attempted but cannot be completed due to extenuating circumstances (e.g., the inability to extend beyond the splenic flexure), Medicare will usually pay for the interrupted colonoscopy at the rate of a flexible sigmoidoscopy.

Here are some endoscopic biopsy highlights:
- If a single lesion is biopsied, but not entirely removed, only a biopsy code would be assigned.
- If a biopsy is obtained and the lesion is also excised, only the excision of a lesion code would be reported.
- If a biopsy and excision were performed, it would be appropriate to report the biopsy if taken from a lesion other than the lesion that was excised. The CPT code for the excision will sometimes state "with or without biopsy," in which case you would not report the biopsy separately. If multiple biopsy specimens are obtained, whether from the same or different sites, and none of the lesions are excised, only one unit ($\times 1$) of the biopsy code is assigned.

Evaluation and Management Services Reported with a Diagnostic Colonoscopy. Reporting a minor procedure (10-day global period) with an office visit service can be problematic. The E/M service must be medically necessary and include work above and beyond what is required for the minor procedure. If the E/M service is medically necessary, the E/M code will require modifier -25, which reports a significantly separate E/M service that occurs on the same day as the procedure or service by the same individual. Check the documentation to determine if the E/M service was prompted by a complaint, symptom, condition, problem, or circumstance that was or was not related to the procedure or other service provided.

CMS RULES

HCPCS Level II Codes for Colorectal Cancer Screening The following are the guidelines to report screening services for colorectal cancer for patients who are beneficiaries under the Medicare program. Screening means no presenting symptoms or disease is present.

A therapeutic procedure is reported when a disease is identified or additional procedures are performed via the scope (biopsy, ablation, etc.). The examination may begin as screening and changes to a therapeutic service if pathology is found or if additional procedures (biopsy, etc.) were performed. According to MLN Matters, Number SE0746, the diagnosis code(s) assigned would be the code for the screening exam, Z12.11/V76.51, followed by the abnormal findings, such as polyp of colon, K63.5/211.3. This rule is synonymous with the *Official Guidelines for Coding and Reporting,* which states, "Should a condition be discovered during the screening then the code for the condition may be assigned as an additional diagnosis." Medicare waives the Part B deductible for colorectal cancer screening under the Affordable Care Act. When a screening

Continued

scope is converted to a diagnostic or therapeutic procedure (i.e., when a defect is found and when a found defect is corrected), the procedure is still covered, if it began as a screening exam. To alert CMS that a screening exam has been converted to a diagnostic or therapeutic procedure, append modifier –PT to the screening code. The deductible will be waived for the patient.

HCPCS code G0328 (immunoassay) reports fecal-occult blood tests, which examine the stool for blood. When the patient returns the fecal sample cards, the laboratory performs one to three simultaneous determinations. This means that one to three of the cards will be tested for the presence of blood. Occult blood is that which cannot be seen but is present microscopically. The order for and the results of the test must be documented in the medical record. Usually this service is provided to patients 50 years of age and older once every year as a screening for colorectal cancer.

Coverage of G0104, a screening flexible sigmoidoscopy, is provided to patients who are at least 50 years of age and is covered once every 4 years. If a lesion is identified, removed, or biopsied during a screening flexible sigmoidoscopy, the procedure is reported as a diagnostic flexible sigmoidoscopy with biopsy or removal of lesion using 45331, 45332, 45333, 45338, 45346 (sigmoidoscopy with biopsy, removal or ablation). The first-listed diagnosis code would report the screening, Z12.11/V76.51, followed by the lesion (the finding).

Code G0105 reports a screening colonoscopy on a patient at high risk; which means the patient has a:

■ Personal history of colorectal cancer (Z85.038, Z85.048/V10.05, V10.06)
■ Personal history of adenomatous polyps (Z86.010/V12.72)
■ Inflammatory bowel disease, including Crohn's disease, and ulcerative colitis
■ A close relative (sibling, parent, or child) who has had colorectal cancer or an adenomatous polyposis (Z80.0, Z83.71/V16.0, V18.5X)
■ Family history of adenomatous polyposis (Z83.71/V18.5X)
■ Family history of nonpolyposis colorectal cancer (Z80.0/V16.0)

If during a screening colonoscopy, a lesion or growth is detected that results in a biopsy or removal of the growth, the appropriate therapeutic procedure is reported with modifier –PT.

Code 45378 describes a diagnostic, flexible colonoscopy of the colon from the anus to the cecum or terminal ileum. An appropriate screening diagnosis for this procedure would be Z12.11/V76.51 (Special screening for malignant neoplasms, colon). This code is reported when there are no additional procedures performed by means of the scope.

These are the HCPCS colorectal screening codes:

■ G0104 flexible sigmoidoscopy
■ G0105 colonoscopy on individual at high risk
■ G0106 alternative to G0104, screening sigmoidoscopy, barium enema
■ G0120 alternative to G0105, screening colonoscopy, barium enema
■ G0121 colonoscopy on individual not meeting criteria for high risk
■ G0122 colorectal cancer screening, barium enema

A barium enema is a series of x-rays of the colon and rectum taken after the patient drinks a white, chalky solution that contains barium (a metallic element). The barium outlines the intestines on the x-rays. The barium enema (G0106, screening sigmoidoscopy, barium enema) may be performed as an alternative to a screening sigmoidoscopy (G0104, flexible sigmoidoscopy) based on documentation that the physician determined that the barium enema would be as good as or better than a flexible sigmoidoscopy or screening colonoscopy due to the patient's specific medical problem. G0104 may also be assigned as an alternative to G0106 for patients who are:

■ At least 50 years old
■ Not at high risk for colorectal cancer
■ It has been at least 48 months since the last screening was performed

Code G0120 reports a colorectal screening with barium enema that is performed as an alternative to G0105 (colonoscopy on individual at high risk for colorectal cancer).

If the patient does not meet the criteria for a high-risk patient, G0121 is reported once every 10 years for patients over 50 years of age. The diagnosis code Z12.11/V76.51 is reported with submission of G0121.

(CMS Transmittal 684, issued March 2, 2011)

Colonoscopy Injection. The injection service described in 45381 may be performed when the polyp is injected with saline to lift the polyp prior to removal by another technique. Other injection services include the placement of a tattoo with India ink for later identification of the area during a surgical procedure. When the purpose of an injection is to control spontaneous bleeding from conditions such as diverticulosis and angiodysplasia (AVM), report the service with 45382 (colonoscopy with control of bleeding, including injection) rather than 45381 (colonoscopy with submucosal injection). Code 45381 is reported as an additional service to another therapeutic service procedure, but it is not an add-on code. Bleeding caused by the procedure and controlled by any method is considered part of the therapeutic procedure and is not reported separately with codes 45382 or 45381.

Multiple Procedures. If multiple lesions are removed from the colon using the same technique (snare), use only one code to report the services because the colon is considered one anatomical location. If the procedure is prolonged or unusually extensive, report modifier -22 and include the time the procedure extended beyond the time usual for the procedure. The submission of modifier -22 requires documentation sent with the claim form that supports the assignment of the modifier.

Virtual Colonoscopy. A virtual colonoscopy (VC) utilizes x-rays and computer to produce a two- and three-dimensional image of the colon. The procedure is used to diagnose colon and bowel disease, including polyps, cancer, and diverticulosis (91110 and 91111). The VC can also be performed using computed tomography (CT) or magnetic resonance imagining (MRI), as illustrated in Fig. 23-19. The procedure is performed in a radiology department and does not require sedation. A tube is inserted into the rectum and air is pumped into the colon thereby inflating the colon, which allows for better visualization. The patient lies on a table that is moved into a scanner that produces the images by means of the computer. This process is repeated with the patient lying on his/her back and again, on the stomach.

Virtual colonoscopy may be performed when a colonoscopy cannot be successfully completed and is used as a technique for screening. Because colonoscopy can more accurately detect colon cancer, virtual colonoscopy may be medically necessary only when colonoscopy cannot be successfully performed or extended to the cecum, to evaluate submucosal abnormalities detected by other imaging studies, or immediately following a failed standard colonoscopy.

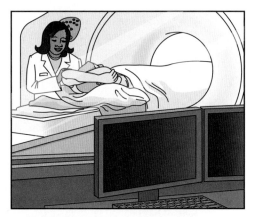

FIGURE 23-19 The virtual colonoscopy.

CMS RULES

When reporting the CT colonography service for Medicare patients, report:

■ **74261-74262** (Computed tomographic [CT] colonography, diagnostic, including image postprocessing; without contrast and with contrast material(s), including non-contrast images, if performed)

NOTE: **74263** (Computed tomographic [CT] colonography, screening, including imagine postprocessing) is not a covered Medicare service (Pub 100-03, Transmittal 105, August 7, 2009).

EXERCISE 23-4 | *Appendix, Colon, and Rectum*

Using the CPT, ICD-10-CM and/or ICD-9-CM manuals, code the following:

1 Appendectomy on a patient with acute ruptured appendix, with generalized peritonitis

CPT Code: _____

ICD-10-CM Code: _____ (ICD-9-CM Code: _____)

2 Flexible sigmoidoscopy with three biopsies

CPT Code: _____

3 Colonoscopy with removal of polyp by a snare

CPT Code: _____

4 The patient presents for removal of sigmoid and rectal polyps. The Pentax video sigmoidoscope was inserted and four polyps were seen scattered between the rectum and proximal sigmoid colon. The largest measured about 1.5 cm in diameter. The others were diminutive, about 4 or 5 mm in diameter. Biopsies were taken of two of these polyps. The pathology report indicated benign polyps.

CPT Code: _____

(Answers are located in Appendix B)

ANUS

Abscess is a common anal condition that is usually treated with incision and drainage (I&D); however, when I&D fails to satisfactorily treat the abscess, other methods may be used. Procedures on the anus are reported with 46020-46999 and include incision, excision, introduction, endoscopy, repair, destruction, and other procedures.

Several of the codes in the Anus subheading refer to a seton, such as 46020 (seton placement) or 46030 (seton removal). A seton is a treatment for anal fistula (abnormal passage between anus and skin), which is usually the result of a previous abscess that has drained but not completely healed. A nonabsorbable suture is threaded through the fistula, out through the anus, and the two ends of the suture are tied together, as illustrated in Fig. 23-20. The seton is left in place until healing has occurred. Scar tissue forms around the suture and the ends of the seton are eventually cut away. Usually the seton can be placed during an office procedure that does not require anesthesia. If the fistula is more complex and requires opening of the fistula track, the service would be reported with a code from the 46270-46285 range.

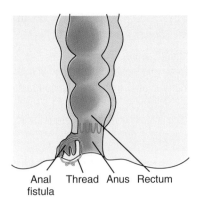

Anal   Thread   Anus   Rectum
fistula

FIGURE 23-20   Suture threaded
through the fistula.

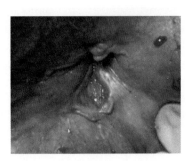

FIGURE 23-21   Anal fissure.

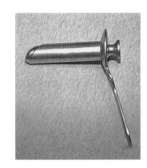

FIGURE 23-22   Stainless steel anoscope.

A **fissure** is a cleft or a groove, normal or otherwise, as illustrated in Fig. 23-21. An anal fissure is a painful ulcer usually located at the margin of the anus. Code 46200 reports a fissurectomy, which is the excision of the fissure. Sphincterotomy is a surgical incision of a sphincter and if it is performed in conjunction with a fissurectomy, it is bundled into 46200 and not reported separately.

A more complex type of anal repair procedure is the closure of an anal fistula with rectal advancement flap. This procedure is reported with 46288, and often third-party payers bundle many other procedures into the closure procedure. So read the payer guidelines carefully before submitting.

CMS RULES

When reporting 46288 for a Medicare patient, the NCCI edits indicate the following codes are bundled into 46288: 43752, 45900, 45905, 45910, 45915, 45990, 46040, 46080, 46200, 46220, 46221, 46230, 46250, 46257, 46258, 46260-46262, 46270, 46275, 46280, 46285, 46600, 46706, 46707, 46940, and 46942. These component codes cannot be reported to Medicare when performed at the same session as code 46288. The edits are posted on the CMS website at www.cms.gov/NationalCorrectCodInitEd/.

An anoscope is an instrument that is inserted a short distance into the anal canal (Fig. 23-22). Once inserted, various procedures may be performed, such as dilation, biopsy, removal of a foreign body or lesion, and control of hemorrhage. Procedures that utilize an anoscope are reported with endoscopy codes 46600-46615.

Code 46600 describes a **diagnostic anoscopy** (up to 5 cm [2 in]) with dilation and includes collection of specimens. This code is designated as a "separate procedure," which means it cannot be reported if performed with another related service during the same session.

The remaining Endoscopy codes describe procedures for foreign body removal, removal of tumor or polyp by different techniques, and control of bleeding.

Destruction of anal lesions can be accomplished by various methods, such as chemical, electrodesiccation, cryosurgery, laser surgery, and surgical excision. Destruction of anal lesions is reported with codes 46900-46942, often based on the type of destruction utilized. For example, 46900 reports chemical destruction, 46910 reports electrodesiccation, and 46916 reports cryosurgery. The method of destruction will be documented in the medical record.

Hemorrhoids are a frequent condition of the anus. Hemorrhoids (piles) arise from an inflammation of the venous plexuses (congregation of vessels) around the anus and may be inside or outside of the anal canal. Hemorrhoids are classified into four degrees depending on severity:

■ First degree may bleed but do not protrude outside of the anal canal.
■ Second degree protrudes outside of the anal canal occasionally but retracts spontaneously.
■ Third degree protrudes outside the anal canal more often and must be manually placed back into the anal canal.
■ Fourth degree protrudes outside the anal canal but cannot be manually placed back into the anal canal. Fourth degree hemorrhoid may be strangulated or thrombosed as illustrated in Fig. 23-23.

The surgical treatment is determined by the type of hemorrhoid. For example, 46250 reports an external hemorrhoidectomy, whereas 46260 reports a hemorrhoidectomy of both internal and external hemorrhoids.

Sometimes, as an alternative to surgery, hemorrhoids are treated by injection of a sclerosing (caustic) solution, which causes irritation of the tissue that results in increased healing. The sclerosing solution injection is reported with 46500.

CODING SHOT

The dentate line is the line where the anal mucosal lining meets the skin (mucocutaneous junction or anal verge). An internal hemorrhoid is one that is 1-1.5 cm above this line. The internal hemorrhoid is the one most often treated by a gastroenterologist. An external hemorrhoid is one that is located below the dentate line.

LIVER

Biopsy of the liver may be performed percutaneously (47000) using imaging guidance that is reported separately. If the biopsy is performed at the time of a more major procedure, the biopsy is reported with add-on code 47001. A liver biopsy may also be performed as a wedge biopsy (47100) that involves removal, through an incision, of a small fan-shaped section of tissue for examination.

A liver **transplant** is a complex procedure that usually involves the surgical expertise of several physicians and a trained surgical team. The transplant procedure involves obtaining the graft to be transplanted (from a cadaver or living donor), backbench work (special preparation of the graft before transplantation), and transplantation into the recipient. Each component of the transplant is reported separately. There are extensive notes preceding the transplant codes 47133-47147 that must be carefully read before assigning codes to these complex procedures.

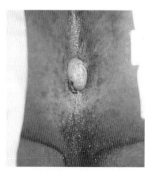

FIGURE 23-23 Large thrombosed external hemorrhoid.

BILIARY TRACT

The gallbladder is connected to the liver and the small intestine by the biliary tract. The tract can be the site of conditions such as calculi and tumor that may obstruct the flow of bile. An incisional procedure (hepaticotomy or hepaticostomy) with exploration of the tract may be performed to determine the cause of obstruction (47400) and may include removal of calculus or drainage of bile from the tract.

A **choledochotomy** is an incision into the biliary tract, and a cholecystostomy is the formation of a stoma between the abdominal wall and the gallbladder. You locate the codes for these procedures in the Incision category of the Biliary Tract subheading (47400-47490).

An **injection** procedure may be necessary to determine if the biliary tract is obstructed. The assignment of a code is based on if the injection is performed percutaneously (47500) or through an existing catheter (47505). The biliary tract may become obstructed due to disease, such as neoplasm. **Stents** may be placed in the obstructed biliary tract to open the area (47511). Drainage catheters may also be changed (47525) or revised/reinserted (47530).

Laparoscopic cholecystectomy involves the placement of ports through the abdominal wall into which the laparoscope and instrumentation are inserted to remove the gallbladder. The codes are located in the Laparoscopy category (47560-47579). The operative report will indicate the method used for the removal of the gallbladder, which determines the assignment of the code. For example, 47562 reports a laparoscopic removal of the gallbladder, and 47600 reports an incisional removal of the gallbladder.

Occasionally, the surgeon will begin the procedure using one technique and due to a difficulty, convert the procedure to another technique, for example, a procedure that is begun as a laparoscopic procedure (47563) and is converted to an open procedure during the same operative session (47605). Only the successful approach is reported, which in this case is the open procedure (47605). Reporting both a laparoscopic and an open surgical approach to accomplish the same outcome is duplication of services.

PANCREAS

The pancreas is located behind (posterior to) the stomach and produces enzymes and hormones. The pancreas may become inflamed (pancreatitis) and require the placement of drains to remove the excess fluid. If the drain is placed by means of an incision, report 48000, but if the procedure also included cholecystostomy, gastrostomy, and jejunostomy, report the service with 48001.

The pancreas can also be the site of a calculus that may be removed through an incision (48020).

Biopsies of the pancreas may be performed by means of an open (48100) or percutaneous (48102) procedure. Guidance is not included in the percutaneous biopsy code, so guidance is reported separately depending on the type of guidance used. If there was an injection portion to the intraoperative pancreatogram (radiography of pancreas during the procedure), the injection is reported separately with add-on code 48400 (Injection procedure, intraoperative pancreatography).

The pancreas can be totally or partially removed and codes for the pancreatectomies (48140-48160) are divided based on the extent of removal and other procedures that may be performed during the same operative session.

The pancreas may be transplanted (48550-48554) and includes harvesting the pancreas graft from a cadaver, backbench work in preparation for transplantation, and transplantation of the graft into the recipient.

ABDOMEN, PERITONEUM, AND OMENTUM

Laparoscopy code 49320 reports a diagnostic laparoscopic procedure. If the procedure was a surgical procedure, the diagnostic laparoscopy is included in the surgical procedure and not reported separately, for example, if the procedure began as a diagnostic laparoscopy but a lymphocele of the peritoneal cavity was identified and drained. The diagnostic laparoscopy converted to a surgical laparoscopy and would be reported with the surgical laparoscopy code 49323.

Hernia codes are listed according to type of hernia (see Repair 49491-49611 and Laparoscopy 49650-49659). Fig. 23-24 is an illustration of an inguinal hernia that would usually be surgically repaired by a herniorrhaphy. The defect would be closed with sutures. Other factors in coding hernias are whether the hernia is **strangulated** (the blood supply is cut off) or **incarcerated** (cannot be returned to the abdominal cavity); the repair is an initial or subsequent repair; the hernia is reducible (can be returned to the abdominal cavity); and the age of the patient.

QUICK CHECK 23-3

1. Name two hernia types (locations) that affect code selection for hernia repair:

   _____ and _____

(Answers are located in Appendix C)

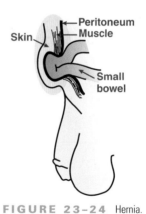

FIGURE 23-24 Hernia.

EXERCISE 23-5 *Anus, Liver, Biliary Tract, Pancreas, Abdomen, Peritoneum, and Omentum*

Using the CPT manual, code the following:

1 Exploratory laparotomy with a cholecystectomy

CPT Code: _____

2 Cholecystotomy with exploration and removal of calculus by means of an open procedure

CPT Code: _____

3 Repair of recurrent reducible incisional hernia, with implantation of a mesh graft, abdominal approach

CPT Codes: _____, _____

4 Repair of an initial incarcerated inguinal hernia in a 5½-year-old

CPT Code: _____

5 Total pancreatectomy

CPT Code: _____

6 Sphincterotomy and one quadrant hemorrhoidectomy for an anal fissure is performed. During the procedure an enlarged hemorrhoid/sentinel tag was noted at the 10 o'clock position and a fissure right at the base of this. Anoscope and a Kelly clamp were placed, and a sentinel tag excised. The defect was closed with sutures.

CPT Code: _____

(Answers are located in Appendix B)

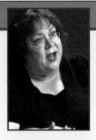

From the Trenches

What advice would you give an entry-level coder?

"Network. Find people who are doing what you are doing now or what you are getting ready to start doing . . . Pick up the phone and give him or her a call!"

BELINDA

CHAPTER REVIEW

CHAPTER 23, PART I, THEORY

Without the use of reference material, complete the following:

1 The codes in the Digestive System subsection begin with this anatomic part: _____, and end with this anatomic part: _____.

2 In the Digestive System, many of the procedures performed to view the esophagus and stomach are performed with this instrument: _____

3 What type of endoscopy is always included in a surgical endoscopy and would therefore never be reported separately? _____

4 What is the term that describes a surgical opening into the abdomen? _____

5 When a hernia can be returned to the abdominal cavity, it is said to be _____.

CHAPTER 23, PART II, PRACTICAL

Code the following cases using the CPT, ICD-10-CM and/or ICD-9-CM:

6 Repair of recurrent, reducible incisional hernia

   CPT Code: _____

7 Repair of an incarcerated umbilical hernia for a 4-year-old patient

   CPT Code: _____

8 Excision of full thickness lip lesion with Abbe-Estlander flap reconstruction

   CPT Code: _____

9 Thoracic approach used in a diverticulectomy of hypopharynx

   CPT Code: _____

10 Total open abdominal colectomy with ileostomy

   CPT Code: _____

11 Multiple biopsies of the small intestine by means of endoscopy with progression past the second portion of the duodenum

   CPT Code: _____

12 Proctosigmoidoscopy using rigid endoscope with collection of multiple specimens by brushing

   CPT Code: _____

13 A sigmoidoscopy with endoscopic biopsy is performed on a Medicare patient who has an area of ulceration in the rectosigmoid region. The excision of the tissue specimen causes bleeding that is controlled endoscopically.

   ❀ CPT Code(s): _____

   ❀ ICD-10-CM Code(s): _____

   (❀ ICD-9-CM Code(s): _____)

Chapter Review is only available in the TEACH Instructor Resources on Evolve

14 A Medicare patient presents for a flexible EGD with biopsy and dilation of gastric outlet for obstruction both performed during the same endoscopic session. What would the physician report?

    ⊛ CPT Code(s): _____

    ⊛ ICD-10-CM Code(s): _____

    (⊛ ICD-9-CM Code(s): _____)

15 During a colonoscopy, a mucosal lesion was removed from the mid right colon with snare electrocautery; a colon polyp in the left colon was removed with snare electrocautery; an excrescence 35 cm from the anal verge was removed with biopsy forceps; additional colon polyps were removed by snare electrocautery at 30 and 25 cm from the anal verge; and a hyperplastic lesion was removed with piecemeal polypectomy using hot biopsy forceps.

    ⊛ CPT Code(s): _____

16 This Medicare patient undergoes a flexible EGD with biopsies and dilation of an esophageal stricture. The EGD was placed into the esophagus where stricture and esophagitis was noted. This area was biopsied. The scope was taken to the second portion of the duodenum and slowly withdrawn to the stomach where further biopsies were taken. The scope was withdrawn to the esophagus where a 20-mm balloon was inserted and the esophageal stricture was dilated. The scope and dilator were then withdrawn.

    ⊛ CPT Code(s): _____

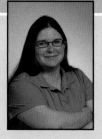

"If someone expresses an interest in becoming a medical coder, I'd advise them to take a position in a physician's office or billing area first, so that they can get a feel for the field. Any experience in the field helps."

Ellen Dooley, BA, CPC-A
Compliance Analyst
University of Missouri Health Care
Columbia, Missouri

Urinary and Male Genital Systems

Chapter Topics

Urinary System

Male Genital System

Chapter Review

Learning Objectives

After completing this chapter you should be able to

1   Understand the format and codes of the Urinary System subsection.

2   Review the subheadings and categories of the Urinary System subsection.

3   Report services with Urinary System codes.

4   Understand the format and codes of the Male Genital System subsection.

5   Review the subheadings and categories of the Male Genital System subsection.

6   Report services with Male Genital System codes.

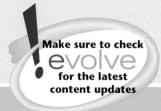

Make sure to check
evolve
for the latest
content updates

URINARY SYSTEM

The Urinary System subsection (50010-53899) of the CPT manual is arranged anatomically by the subheadings of kidney, ureter, bladder, and urethra (Fig. 24-1), with category codes arranged by procedure (i.e., incision, excision, introduction, repair). A wide range of terminology is used in the subsection. The Glossary at the back of this book includes many of the terms that you will encounter in the CPT manual. Always be certain you know the meaning of all the words in the code description before you assign a code.

Kidney

The first subheading in the Urinary subsection is Kidney (50010-50593).

Incision. The Incision codes (50010-50135) are assigned to report exploration, nephrostomy, drainage, nephrolithotomy, and pyelotomy services.

Renal exploration is a procedure performed if the cause of a patient's condition is unknown. For example, surgical exploration of an injured kidney when the patient is clinically unstable and appears to be having renal blood loss. Access for the exploration procedure is from the side (flank). Note that a parenthetical statement preceding 50010 indicates "For retroperitoneal exploration, abscess, tumor, or cyst, see 49010, 49060, 49203-49205," which are Digestive System codes. Code 49010 reports an exploration of the retroperitoneum. The term **retroperitoneal** refers to that area located behind (retro to) the peritoneum (lines the abdominal walls and covers most of the organs) that is located in the abdominal cavity. The retroperitoneal space may be accessed by means of an abdominal incision. When coding an exploration of the retroperitoneal space, be careful to determine the exact anatomical location(s) explored to report the correct services because there are many organ systems located in the abdominal cavity. For example, the kidney is located in the retroperitoneal space. If only the kidney was explored, report the service with the Urinary System code 50010; if the retroperitoneal area was explored, report the service with the Digestive System code 49010, exploration of retroperitoneal area.

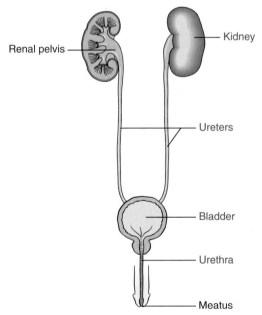

FIGURE 24–1 The four subheadings of the Urinary System subsection in the CPT manual are: Kidney, Ureter, Bladder, and Urethra.

If a procedure begins as an exploratory procedure but becomes a definitive or corrective procedure, such as repair of a lacerated kidney, only the definitive procedure is reported. The exploration is considered a diagnostic procedure that is bundled into the definitive procedure when both are performed during the same operative session.

Open drainage of a perirenal or renal abscess (50020) reports the drainage of a **kidney abscess** or the surrounding kidney tissue. If the drainage was of a retroperitoneal abscess, the service would be reported with the Digestive System code 49060 that reports an open drainage of a retroperitoneal abscess. Again, the exact location of the abscess is the critical factor when assigning the abscess drainage code. The renal abscess can also be accessed percutaneously, in which case the service would be reported with 49405. When performing a percutaneous access to the kidney, image guidance may be used for the needle placement and is bundled into 49405.

CODING SHOT

Code 49405 has the symbol next to it to indicate that conscious (moderate) sedation is included with the procedure and not reported separately.

A **nephrostomy** is a procedure used to decompress the renal system by means of the insertion of a catheter into the kidney while leaving the other end of the catheter outside the body to temporarily drain the kidney. The renal collecting system may be obstructed by a calculus or a defect of the renal pelvis or ureter. Code 50040 reports incisional placement of a drainage tube that involves incision into the renal pelvis (pyelotomy). The physician then inserts a catheter into the kidney with the other end carried to the skin surface and sutured in place on the flank.

A **nephrotomy** is exploration of the inside of the kidney. During this exploration (50045), no definitive procedure is performed. If a definitive procedure is performed the exploration is bundled into the definitive procedure. For example, if the surgeon began a procedure as an exploration to determine the cause of urinary obstruction and identified a renal calculus (kidney stone) and removed the calculus, the procedure no longer would be an exploration. The procedure would be reported with 50060, kidney stone removal (nephrolithotomy). The surgeon may also perform a renal endoscopy at the same time as the nephrotomy (such as, to place stents or perform some other type of repair procedure), and the endoscopy is reported separately with a code from range 50570-50580 (Endoscopy, kidney).

Nephrolithotomy procedures include removal of calculus (50060), secondary surgical operation for calculus (50065), procedures complicated by congenital kidney abnormality (50070), and removal of a staghorn calculus (50075). The staghorn calculus (Fig. 24-2) is shaped like a deer antler and can become large and create extensive obstruction. If the calculus involves the renal pelvis and at least two calyces, it is classified as a staghorn calculus. These types of stones account for about 30% of stones reported and are usually associated with urinary infections. With a staghorn, a nephrolithotomy may be performed after extracorporeal shock wave lithotripsy (ESWL), which fragments the stones (50590).

ESWL used to be performed with a machine in which the patient was submersed in a fluid. Newer machines do not require submersion, rather the patient is placed on an x-ray table, and a water-filled cushion is placed under the patient's back (Fig. 24-3). The procedure is performed under general anesthesia in an operating room with a built-in ESWL machine.

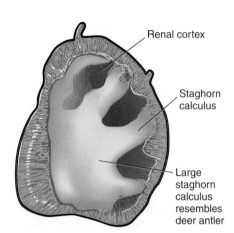

Renal cortex

Staghorn calculus

Large staghorn calculus resembles deer antler

FIGURE 24-2 Large staghorn calculus inside the kidney filling the pelvis and calyceal system.

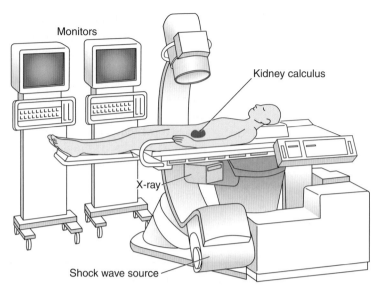

Monitors

Kidney calculus

X-ray

Shock wave source

FIGURE 24-3 Extracorporeal shock wave lithotripsy (ESWL).

The shock waves are targeted to the stones by means of x-ray and pulverize the stones with repeated shocks. Usually, the particles subsequently pass through the urinary tract.

Percutaneous nephrolithotomy (nephrolithotripsy) is a more invasive method of treating kidney stones and usually is performed with ultrasound. An incision is made over the kidney, a probe is inserted, and shock waves pulverize the stone. Electrohydraulic or mechanical lithotripsy may be used instead of shock waves, but the use of shock waves is the most common method. A tiny basket may also be attached to a probe that is passed into the kidney and the stones removed. Because the stone fragments of a staghorn are so large, they may not pass through the urinary system spontaneously, and an open or percutaneous procedure may need to be performed to remove the fragments. The lithotripsy is reported separately (50590 lithotripsy or 52353 cystourethroscope with lithotripsy).

QUICK CHECK 24-1

1. When lithotripsy is performed to fragment kidney stones, the particles always pass out of the body through the urinary system.

   True or False?

(Answers are located in Appendix C)

Percutaneous **nephrostolithotomy** (PCNL) or a **pyelostolithotomy** is a procedure to remove kidney stones. In this procedure, entry is through the patient's back. The procedure is reported based on the size of the stone removed (50080, to 2 cm; 50081, >2 cm). Internal lithotripsy is included in 50080 and 50081 and is not reported separately. External lithotripsy is not included in the codes and can be reported in addition to 50080 and 50081; but remember to attach modifier -51 to the lesser procedure. The procedure is performed with fluoroscopic guidance that is reported separately with 76000 for the radiologist or 76001 for the radiologist who assists a nonradiological physician.

Excision. There are Excision codes in the Kidney subheading for biopsy, nephrectomy (removal of the kidney), and removal of a cyst. The biopsy codes (50200, 50205) are based on the approach, either percutaneous (through the skin) or by surgical exposure of the kidney.

A **nephrectomy** is the removal of a kidney, either partial or radical (total). A radical nephrectomy includes removal of the fascia and surrounding fatty tissue, regional lymph nodes, and the adrenal gland. The nephrectomy codes (50220-50240) are based on the complexity and extent of the procedure. Nephrectomies can also be performed by means of a laparoscope (50543, 50545-50548), based on whether the procedure was partial, radical, or donor, and whether the procedure included a partial or total ureterectomy.

Ablation is the cutting away or erosion of tissue. Code 50250 reports ablation of a kidney lesion by means of cryosurgery (use of subfreezing temperatures) and is usually performed with ultrasonic guidance. If used, the ultrasonic guidance is not reported separately because it is included in the code description. Monitoring is also included in the code. The surgeon accesses the kidney through an incision and inserts a cryosurgical probe into the lesion. The cryosurgical machine is turned on, and subfreezing temperature is delivered to the lesion (Fig. 24-4). The area is brought back to above freezing, and the treatment is applied again. At times, more than two cycles are applied to ensure the lesion is ablated. This procedure can also be performed percutaneously (50593) or by use of a laparoscope (50542).

Renal Transplantation. Allotransplantation is the transfer of tissue or an organ between two people who are not related (genetically different). Autotransplantation is transfer of tissue from one part of a person's body to another part of that person's body, also known as autograft or autotransplant. A surgeon may perform a renal autotransplant to reposition the kidney, which may be necessary when the kidney has been severely damaged from trauma or disease. A renal autotransplantation is reported with 50380. Backbench work is the work involved in preparation for the transplant surgery and includes:

- Open organ **retrieval** from a deceased (50300) or living (50320) donor; laparoscopic organ retrieval from a living (50547) donor.
- Standard **preparation** based on deceased (50323) or living (50325) donor. As a part of this preparation the surgeon may perform additional surgery on the organ, such as venous, arterial, or ureteral anastomosis (50327-50329).
- **Allotransplantation** service reported with 50360 (without nephrectomy) or 50365 (with nephrectomy) with modifier -50 added for a bilateral procedure.

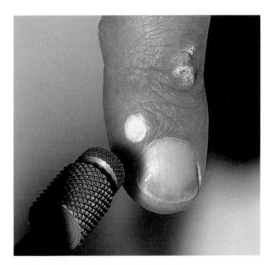

FIGURE 24-4 Liquid nitrogen spray.

If backbench procedures were performed, those services would be reported in addition to the transplantation service with modifier -51 added to indicate multiple procedures.

CODING SHOT

If the recipient requires a nephrectomy, the procedure is reported separately with 50340 and with modifier -50 for a bilateral procedure.

Introduction. Introduction category codes in the Kidney subheading are for aspiration, catheters, injections for radiography, guides, and tube changes. There are also extensive notes within the category.

Codes in the range 50382-50389 are percutaneous, transurethral, or externally accessible procedures that report removal and/or replacement of renal stents and tubes. These stents are not renal artery stents but are ureteral stents that are placed through the renal pelvis. The codes only report a unilateral procedure, so if a bilateral procedure was performed, add modifier -50.

Imaging guidance is used for the codes in this range and is included in the code description, so do not report the guidance separately. If imaging guidance was not used for removal without replacement of an externally accessible ureteral stent, you would report the removal with an E/M code.

QUICK CHECK 24-2

1. An Evaluation and Management (E/M) code is used to report removal of an _____ accessible stent when imaging guidance is not used.

(Answers are located in Appendix C)

Approximately half of the population over age 50 has renal cysts that are asymptomatic (no symptoms) and are often only discovered as an incidental finding on ultrasound or computed tomography. When these cysts are symptomatic, percutaneous aspiration or injection may be performed. The procedure is performed by use of local anesthetic and on an outpatient basis. A sclerosing agent (such as alcohol) may be injected into the cyst. The code description for 50390 indicates "aspiration and/or injection," which means if both an aspiration and injection are performed during the same operative session, 50390 is reported only one time. Image guidance is not included in the code description, so any guidance used is reported separately.

Repair. Repair category codes (50400-50540) include plastic surgery (pyeloplasty), suturing (nephrorrhaphy), and closure of fistula.

Pyeloplasty is a surgical procedure for an obstruction of the ureteropelvic junction (UPJ), which connects the renal pelvis to the ureter (Fig. 24-5). Usually, this is a congenital condition, but it may also be an acquired condition. If an obstruction occurs the urine will not drain, which results in dilatation of the collecting system and enlargement of the renal pelvis (hydronephrosis). The goal of a pyeloplasty is to remove the obstruction and repair the renal pelvis (Fig. 24-6). As a part of the repair, a nephropexy (surgical fixation of mobile kidney), nephrostomy (a passageway from the kidney to exterior of the body), pyelostomy (a passageway between the renal pelvis and the exterior of the body), and ureteral splinting are included in the codes for a **simple** pyeloplasty (50400). A **complicated** pyeloplasty (50405) includes all of the procedures in the simple pyeloplasty, as indicated by the placement of the semicolon in 50400. (Note that the semicolon is after the term "splinting," which means that all

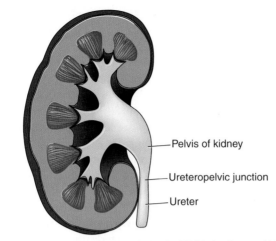

FIGURE 24–5 Ureteropelvic junction (UPJ) is the place at which the ureter joins the kidney at the renal pelvis.

- Pelvis of kidney
- Ureteropelvic junction
- Ureter

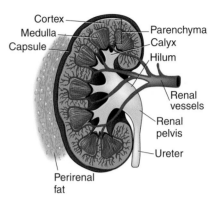

FIGURE 24–6 Structure of kidney.

- Cortex
- Medulla
- Capsule
- Parenchyma
- Calyx
- Hilum
- Renal vessels
- Renal pelvis
- Ureter
- Perirenal fat

the terms that precede the semicolon are included in the code description for the indented code 50405.) In addition to all the procedures in the simple pyeloplasty, the complicated pyeloplasty is more difficult, because the procedure may include repair of a congenital kidney abnormality (which can be an extensive procedure), further plastic repair of the pelvis of the kidney, repair of a solitary kidney (patient only has one kidney), or a calycoplasty. A calycoplasty is repair of the calyx (the cup-shaped structure) of the kidney.

TOOLBOX

John, a 43-year-old male patient, presents to his family physician, Dr. Marsh, with complaints of dull groin pain, an ache on the lower left side of his back, and a decrease in urinary output. A pyelogram was ordered and the final diagnosis was hydronephrosis. Antibiotics were prescribed and John is to return for a follow-up in 30 days.

QUESTIONS

1. For this diagnosis, would you expect the renal pelvis, renal column, or renal papilla to be enlarged?_____

2. When you reference "Pyelogram" in the CPT index, what is the "See" direction?

_____

_____

▼ ANSWERS

1. Renal pelvis, 2. See Urography, Intravenous; Urography, Retrograde

Closures of nephrocutaneous, pyelocutaneous, or nephrovisceral fistulas (abnormal openings) are reported with codes from the 50520-50526 range. Code 50520 reports the closure of a fistula between the renal pelvis and the exterior of the body or of the kidney and the exterior. Codes 50525 and 50526 report closure of a fistula between the kidney and another organ, such as the kidney and the bladder. The approach to close the fistula may be abdominal (50525) or thoracic (50526).

Laparoscopy. The Laparoscopy codes (50541-50549) report ablation of renal cysts (50541) or lesions (50542). Open cryosurgical ablation of renal tumors is reported with 50250, and percutaneous ablation is reported with 50593.

Laparoscopic nephrectomies and pyeloplasty are also reported with codes from the Laparoscopy category and are based on the extent of the procedure.

Endoscopy. Endoscopy codes (50551-50580) are frequently reported for kidney procedures, because these types of procedures are less invasive than the open procedures and are often performed in an outpatient setting. Renal endoscopies may be performed by means of an established connection between the kidney and the exterior of the body. The codes in the Endoscopy category are divided into those procedures performed through an established nephrostomy or pyelostomy and those that are not. For example, 50555 reports a renal endoscopy through an established nephrostomy/pyelostomy, and 50574 reports the same endoscopic biopsy but not through a nephrostomy/pyelostomy. The codes are further divided based on the reason for the procedure: ureteral catheterization, biopsy, fulguration, or foreign body/calculus removal or tumor resection.

The code descriptions in the Endoscopy category code descriptions state "exclusive of radiologic service," which means that the radiologic services are reported in addition to the endoscopic procedures. If, for example, a biopsy (50555) is performed with ultrasound, you would report the biopsy procedure in addition to the ultrasound.

QUICK CHECK 24-3

1. Renal Endoscopy codes 50551-50562 are reported when the scope is inserted through an established _____ or _____ opening.

(Answers are located in Appendix C)

Kidney Index Locations. You will locate the kidney codes in the CPT manual index under "Kidney"; they are subtermed primarily by category (e.g., insertion, excision, or repair). Another method of locating kidney codes in the CPT manual index is to reference the medical term for the procedure (e.g., nephrostomy or nephrotomy). Again, there are other index location methods; these are just a couple to help you get started locating the codes.

The following kidney codes or code ranges are unilateral and require modifier -50 if the procedure was performed bilaterally:

50080-50081, 50120-50135	Incision
50200-50230	Excision
50320, 50340, 50360, 50365	Renal Transplantation
50382-50390, 50392-50398	Introduction
50545-50547, 50549	Laparoscopy
50551-50561, 50570-50580	Endoscopy
50590, 50592	Other Procedures

The third-party payer may require the use of -RT and -LT rather than modifier -50.

EXERCISE 24-1 *Kidney*

Using the CPT manual, code the following:

1 Repeat nephrolithotomy

CPT Code: _____

2 The patient presents for a nephrostomy tube exchange. The patient was placed prone on the angiographic table and has pre-existing left nephrostomy tube. The patient did not receive conscious sedation. The back was prepped and draped in the usual sterile fashion. A guidewire was advanced through the nephrostomy tube. The tube was exchanged, and the tube was secured to the skin with suture.

CPT Code: _____

3 The patient presents with right renal calculus with stent for a right ESWL, cystoscopy, and stent removal. The patient was placed on the lithotripsy table and administered a general anesthetic. The stone was targeted, shock head engaged. Total of 2400 shocks at maximum kV of 24 were administered to the stone. Good fragmentation was noted. The patient was then prepped and draped in the supine position. The urethra was anesthetized with 2% Xylocaine jelly. The patient was cystoscoped with the flexible instrument; stent was visualized, grasped, and removed intact.

CPT Codes: _____ , _____

(Answers are located in Appendix B)

Ureter

The next subheading (50600-50980) in the Urinary System subsection is Ureter. The codes are based on the procedure (i.e., incision, excision, introduction, repairs, laparoscopy, or endoscopy). The ureter is the tube that leads from the kidney to the bladder and may be the site of an assortment of conditions, such as obstruction by calculus, cysts, or lesions in addition to reflux, congenital abnormalities, and fistulas.

Incision. The Incision codes (50600-50630) report open procedures to explore or drain (50600), insert indwelling stent (50605), and removal of calculus (ureterolithotomy) based on the location of the calculus as upper third, middle third, or lower third of the ureter (50610-50630). The incisional procedures also have laparoscopic, endoscopic, and/or transvesical counterparts. For example, to report a laparoscopic ureterolithotomy of the upper third of the ureter, report 50945, and for an incisional ureterolithotomy, report 50610. It is very important to check the documentation for the method utilized for the procedure to ensure selection of the correct code.

QUICK CHECK 24-4

1. Laparoscopic ureterolithotomy is reported with code _____ , regardless of which portion of the ureter is involved.

(Answers are located in Appendix C)

Excision. The codes in the Excision category (50650, 50660) report ureterectomy either with bladder cuff or a total excision. The **bladder cuff** is the tissue that connects the ureter to the bladder, and the excision of the bladder cuff is only reported if it is the only procedure performed during the surgical session. A total ureterectomy may be performed by means of an abdominal, vaginal, or perineal approach or a combination of the three approaches. Code 50660 includes all three approaches or a combination of approaches. This means that if two or three approaches were utilized, you still only report 50660 one time.

Introduction. The Introduction codes (50684-50690) include injection procedures, manometric studies (see paragraph below), and change of tubes and/or stents. Code 50684 reports an **injection** procedure performed through an indwelling catheter to determine the status of the renal collecting system. The physician injects a contrast agent through the catheter and an x-ray is taken. The radiological supervision and interpretation is reported separately with 74425.

Manometric studies (50686) are tests to measure kidney and ureter flow and pressure. The study is conducted by means of a machine (manometer) through an access site, which is connected to an ureterostomy or ureteral catheter filled with fluid. A tube carrying sterile fluid is inserted through the access site and into the kidney or bladder and the area is flooded. The pressures and flow are then measured and recorded.

> ✋ **CAUTION** *Watch the Repair codes for use of modifier -50! Unless stated, the procedure is unilateral and requires modifier -50 for bilateral procedures.*

Repair. Repair procedures (50700-50940) includes ureteroplasty (plastic repair of the ureter), ureterolysis (freeing of fibrous tissue), ureteropyelostomy (connection of upper ureter to renal pelvis), ureterocalicostomy (connection of upper ureter to renal calyx), and ureteroureterostomy (bypass of obstructed ureter), in addition to numerous other procedures to repair the ureter.

Laparoscopy. Laparoscopic ureter codes 50947 and 50948 report the placement of a ureteral stent, which may be performed in conjunction with or without cystoscopy. The stent is placed because of an obstruction of the ureterovesical junction (UVJ). The surgeon laparoscopically repositions the ureter on the bladder and then by means of the cystoscope places the ureteral stent.

Endoscopy. The Endoscopy codes (50951-50980) report procedures that are performed through an established stoma (ureterostomy, 50951-50961) or through an incision into the ureter (ureterotomy, 50970-50980). The procedures conducted through a ureterostomy are similar to the types of procedures conducted through a nephrostomy (e.g., 50551-50562, biopsy, catheterization, irrigation, and instillation). Excellent medical terminology skills are essential for working within this subheading, because the words can be intimidating. Keep your medical dictionary close by to look up any words you are not absolutely sure about. You can also refer to the Glossary at the back of the book. The time you spend now increasing the depth and breadth of your medical terminology is an excellent investment and will greatly increase your coding accuracy.

The endoscopy procedures are for irrigation, instillation, catheterization, biopsy, fulguration, and foreign body or calculus removal. The procedures often utilize radiological services, but these services are reported separately. Note that the stand-alone code descriptions in the category (50951, 50970) indicate that the service is "exclusive of radiologic service," meaning that you report those services in addition to the procedure. This also means that all indented codes that follow 50951 and 50970 do not include radiologic services.

When a ureterocystography is performed, the physician injects a radioactive contrast material through a catheter inserted into the bladder via the urethra or through a previously established stoma. The injection procedure is reported in addition to the primary procedure. For example, if the procedure was an endoscopic biopsy of the right ureter through an established stoma, you would report 50955-RT and the injection procedure would be reported with 50684-RT. In addition to the primary and injection procedures, you also report the radiological supervision and interpretation with a Radiology code. For example, 74425 reports retrograde urography. Retrograde urography is performed by injecting contrast directly into the lower end of the system, and the contrast flows backwards through the system allowing for visualization of the tract.

CMS RULES

According to CMS, 50955 and 50684 cannot be reported together as CMS bundles these codes. Only if 50684 is a uniquely distinct procedure could you report it with 50955. You must add modifier -59 to the 50684 code. Refer to Fig. 24-7 for an example of the codes that are bundled into 50955. This figure illustrates that 50684 is bundled into 50955. In the far right column, the number 1 indicates that the code can be reported separately with modifier -59 (distinct procedure) added, and the 0 indicates that the code cannot be reported with -59 and is always bundled with the primary code.

The following ureter codes or code ranges are unilateral and require modifier -50 if the procedure was performed bilaterally:

50601-50630	Incision
50684	Introduction
50715	Repair
50780-50800, 50815, 50820	Repair
50840, 50860, 50940	Repair
50945-50980	Laparoscopy/Endoscopy

The third-party payer may require the use of -RT and/or -LT rather than modifier -50.

Code	Bundled	Modifier -59
50955	J2001	1
50955	00910	0
50955	0213T	0
50955	0216T	0
50955	36000	1
50955	36400	1
50955	36405	1
50955	36406	1
50955	36410	1
50955	36420	1
50955	36425	1
50955	36430	1
50955	36440	1
50955	36600	1
50955	36640	1
50955	37202	1
50955	43752	1
50955	50684	1
50955	50715	1
50955	50951	1
50955	51701	1
50955	51702	1
50955	51703	1
50955	76000	1
50955	76001	1
50955	93000	1
50955	93005	1
50955	93010	1
50955	93040	1
50955	93041	1
50955	93042	1
50955	93318	1
50955	94002	1
50955	94200	1
50955	94250	1
50955	94680	1
50955	94681	1
50955	94690	1
50955	94770	1
50955	95812	1
50955	95813	1
50955	95816	1
50955	95819	1
50955	95822	1
50955	95829	1
50955	95955	1
50955	96360	1
50955	96365	1
50955	96372	1
50955	96374	1
50955	96375	1
50955	96376	1

FIGURE 24–7 Codes bundled into 50955.

EXERCISE 24-2 *Ureter*

Using the CPT manual, code the following:

1 Ureterolithotomy of the lower one-third of the left ureter

CPT Code: _____

2 Bilateral ureteroneocystostomy

CPT Code: _____

3 Ureteral endoscopic biopsy through an established right ureterostomy with injection of contrast

CPT Codes: _____, _____, _____

(Answers are located in Appendix B)

Bladder

The Bladder subheading (51020-52700) contains codes not only for the usual services, such as incision and excision, but also for some unique services such as urodynamics and procedures performed on the prostate. Review the anatomy of the bladder in Fig. 24-8.

Incision. **Cystotomy** (51020-51045) is often performed to fulgurate (use of electric current), insert radioactive material, or cryosurgically to destroy a lesion. In addition, the procedure is used for drainage, placement of catheter/stent, or a cystolithotomy (removal of calculus).

A cystolithotomy reported with 51050 is one in which an incision is made in the skin and into the bladder. The physician removes the calculus through the incision but does not excise the bladder neck. A transvesical ureterolithotomy described in 51060 is a similar procedure to 51050, but the calculus is removed through an incision in the bladder and the ureter. The ureter calculus is removed by basket extract through an incision in 51065, and in some cases the calculus is first fragmented by ultrasound or electrohydraulic means. Electrohydraulic fragmentation is the use of a probe containing two electrodes that are applied, one on each side of the calculus. Electrical current is then directed through the electrodes, which fragments the calculus.

Removal. **Aspiration** of urine from the bladder may be accomplished by means of needle, trocar (a sharply pointed surgical instrument), or intracatheter (plastic tube with a needle on the end). A suprapubic (above the pubic bone) catheter may also be inserted during the aspiration service (51102). Aspirations are often performed by means of imaging guidance, which is reported separately. If imaging guidance is used, report the guidance separately with 76942, 77002, or 77012.

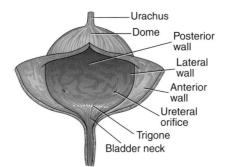

FIGURE 24–8 Bladder anatomy.

Excision. A **urachal cyst** is between the umbilicus and bladder dome and is often diagnosed in young children when the cyst becomes infected. Because of the proximity to the abdominal cavity and potential to rupture, a urachal cyst is a condition that warrants prompt medical attention. A urachal sinus is a congential abnormality in which prenatal tissue remains, causes drainage to the umbilicus, and results in infection. The excision of a urachal cyst or sinus is reported with 51500 and may or may not include umbilical hernia repair.

Cystotomies and cystectomies (51520-51596) are performed for a variety of reasons, such as excision of a portion of or all of the bladder, repair of a ureterocele, or to replant a ureter into the bladder. The codes are divided based on the extent of the procedure. If the procedure is performed transurethrally, such as a bladder resection, codes from the Transurethral Surgery category (52204-52318) would be reported.

Pelvic exenteration (51597) is also known as total pelvic exenteration (TPE) and is the removal of the pelvic organs and adjacent structures due to malignancy. If TPE is performed due to gynecologic malignancy, report the service with the Female Genital system code 58240. A hysterectomy may be performed with 51597, but the initial and primary reason the procedure is being performed is for other than a gynecological malignancy.

QUICK CHECK 24-5

1. Pelvic exenteration is reported with 51597, unless the diagnosis is a gynecologic malignancy, then code _____ should be reported.

(Answers are located in Appendix C)

Introduction. The **injection** procedures reported with codes 51600-51610 are for urethrocystography (x-ray of lower urinary tract, also known as a cystourethroscopy). The radiological supervision and interpretation are reported in addition to the injection procedure. Note that the parenthetical statements after each of the injection codes direct the coder to the correct radiology code(s).

Insertion of bladder catheters may be non-indwelling (51701) or temporary indwelling (51702, 51703). The non-indwelling catheter is the type that is inserted into the urethra and manipulated into the bladder to drain residual urine. The temporary indwelling procedure can be a simple catheterization (such as with a Foley) or a complicated catheterization due to an anatomical anomaly.

Catheter fracturing may occur, for example, when a patient pulls the catheter out while the balloon is still inflated. This is a rare complication and does not describe the insertion but rather why it was necessary to reinsert another catheter.

Instillation is a procedure that is performed for bladder cancer. An anticarcinogenic agent is introduced into the bladder by means of a catheter. For example, immunotherapy is the instillation of a nonactive tuberculosis agent into the bladder. The agent is retained in the bladder for a period of time (such as 1 hour) with the patient in a supine position. The agent is then drained and the treatment is concluded. A series of these instillations is performed in a course of treatment. Code 51720 reports the instillation as well as the retention time and drainage.

Urodynamics.   Urodynamics pertains to the motion and flow of urine. Urinary tract flow can be obstructed by renal calculi, narrowing (stricture) of the ureter, cysts, and so forth. The procedures in the Urodynamics subheading (51725-51798) are to be conducted by or under the direct supervision of a physician, and all the instruments, equipment, supplies, and technical assistance necessary to conduct the procedure are bundled into the codes. If the physician performs only the professional service (e.g., interpretation of the results), modifier -26 (professional component) is reported with the code to indicate that the technical portion of the service (performance of test or tests) was provided elsewhere. For example, if a physician provides only the interpretation (-26) of a complex urethral pressure profile (UPP) (51727), report only the professional component of the service as 51727-26.

Repair and Laparoscopy.   Repair procedures (51800-51980) include procedures such as cystoplasty (bladder repair), cystourethroplasty (bladder and urethra), vesicourethropexy/urethropexy (repair for urinary incontinence), and closure of fistulas.

Stress incontinence may be surgically repaired by a colposuspension procedure in which a urethral sling is placed to support and elevate the urethra. There are several types of these sling procedures, such as the Marshall-Marchetti-Krantz (MMK), Burch, paravaginal repair, anterior vesicourethropexy, or urethropexy. These procedures are reported with 51840 for a simple procedure and 51841 for a complicated repair, which would include a secondary repair of the bladder. The urethral suspension and sling operation are also performed by means of laparoscopy (51990, 51992). A sling operation for stress incontinence is also reported with 57288 when vaginal and abdominal incisions are used. A Pereyra procedure (57289) is also known as a needle bladder neck suspension in which sutures are used to support and anchor the bladder. The codes (57287-57289) are in the Female Genital System subsection, Vagina subheading, because the procedure includes repair of the vagina. There are also codes in the Urethra subsection (53431-53442) that refer to the creation, removal, or revision of a sling operation for male urinary incontinence and plastic repair of the bladder for incontinence.

Endoscopy.   There are codes (52000-52010) for bundled endoscopy procedures (i.e., cystoscopy, urethroscopy, and cystourethroscopy). The codes contain the primary procedure of a cystourethroscopy (endoscopic procedure to view the bladder and urethra) and minor related procedures performed at the same time. For example, if a cystourethroscopy is performed for the biopsy of the ureter with radiography, bundled into the code for the procedure (52007) are the catheterization, endoscopic procedure, and biopsy(ies). To unbundle the code and report the individual components of the procedure separately would not be correct. If the secondary procedure(s) required significant additional time or effort that is documented in the medical record, the procedure can be identified using modifier -22 (increased procedure). There are combination codes that include many components of a procedure bundled into one code. For example, 52005 reports a cystourethroscopy with ureteral catheterization, with/without irrigation, instillation, or ureteropyelography with the one code. Be careful to read each description in this category before assigning a code to be certain you have identified each component included in the code before you assign additional codes. For example, you cannot report a cystourethroscopy (52005) with a catheterization (51701) because a catheterization is included in the code description for 52005. Many third-party payers, such as CMS, have lists of codes (edits) that cannot be reported with other codes. For example, 52000 (cystourethroscopy) cannot be reported with 51701 (catheterization), even though catheterization is not stated in the code description. You need to know not only the limitations set by the notes and codes in the CPT manual but also the limitations set by the third-party payer.

CODING SHOT

For a complete list of the CMS Correct Coding Initiative (CCI) edits, check out www.cms.gov/NationalCorrectCodInitEd/.

A cystourethroscopy is a diagnostic procedure to assess lower urinary tract symptoms (LUTS), such as incontinence or benign prostate hypertrophy (BPH). The procedure is reported only if it is performed as the only procedure during the operative session, because it is designated a separate procedure.

CODING SHOT

Usually, third-party payers will not reimburse for more than two cystourethroscopic procedures per episode of illness unless bladder or urethral malignancies are being treated.

QUICK CHECK 24-6

1. To locate endoscopy codes in the CPT index, use the main terms _____,
_____, or cystourethroscopy.

(Answers are located in Appendix C)

Transurethral Surgery. Transurethral Surgery codes (52204-52355) are for the urethra/bladder (52204-52318) and ureter/pelvis (52320-52355).

Code 52204 reports a cystourethroscopy with biopsy and 52000 is also a cystourethroscopy. The difference is that 52000 is a diagnostic procedure only. No additional procedure was performed when reporting 52000. When reporting 52204, a biopsy was performed, so the procedure was not only diagnostic but also a surgical procedure. The procedure may have begun as a diagnostic procedure, but it progressed to a biopsy on identification of a lesion. The diagnostic procedure is then bundled into the surgical procedure and not reported separately.

CODING SHOT

Many third-party payers will bundle 52204 (cystourethroscopy) into many major procedures. For example, Medicare bundles the cystourethroscopy into the transurethral resection of a bladder tumor (52234-52240).

A **transurethral resection of a bladder tumor** (TURBT) is a procedure in which a bladder tumor is removed by fulguration (electric current) or excision. Note that the code descriptions 52234-52240 contain multiple methods of removal of the bladder tumor, that is, "with fulguration (including cryosurgery or laser surgery) and/or resection." If any, or a combination of, these methods has been used to eradicate the tumor, you can assign a code based on the **size** of the bladder tumor. The code description indicates the size as small (0.5-2.0 cm), medium (2.0-5.0 cm), and large (>5 cm). Code 52224 is a cystoure-throscopy with fulguration or treatment of a minor (<0.5 cm) lesion(s). The lesion(s) are treated with fulguration (electrocautery), cryosurgery or a laser. This procedure may or may not include a biopsy prior to eradication.

Many of the code descriptions require the coder to be familiar with the anatomy of the bladder and surrounding structures, for example, 52214 (cystourethroscopy) with fulgu-ration (including cryosurgery or laser surgery) of trigone, bladder neck, prostatic fossa, urethra, or periurethral glands. Refer to Fig. 24-8 for bladder anatomy and location of the trigone and bladder neck. To code correctly the coder also needs to know the anatomy surrounding the bladder, such as the prostatic fossa, which is the depression or cavity (prostatic bed) in which the prostate is located.

The codes in the Ureter and Pelvis subsection (52320-52355) all include insertion and removal of temporary stents during the procedure, even though the code descrip-tions may not all state that fact. You know this only when you read the notes preced-ing code 52320. That does not mean that insertion and/or removal of temporary stents cannot be reported with other procedures, such as ESWL (50590), only that temporary stents are not reported separately with the codes in the 52320-52355 range. Make a note in your CPT manual next to this range of codes stating "includes insertion/removal of temporary stents" as a reminder of this important point or highlight the paragraph in the notes preceding code 52320 ("The insertion and removal of a temporary ureteral catheter. . . ."). Insertion of indwelling stents is reported separately with 52332-51 in addition to the primary procedure. Code 52332 reports **insertion** of unilateral stents, so modifiers to indicate bilateral procedures were performed would also be needed; for example, 52332-51-50. To report **removal** of indwelling stents, use 52310 (simple re-moval) or 52315 (complicated removal) with modifier -58 (staged or related procedure or service by same individual during the postoperative period). It is a good idea to place a bracket next to codes 52310 and 52315 and write "-58" as a reminder of how to report these codes, because the direction for the use of this modifier is located in notes before code 52320.

Vesical Neck and Prostate. The Vesical Neck and Prostate codes 52400-52700 contain codes to report cystourethroscopy and transurethral procedures. Many of these codes are reviewed in the Male Genital System information because many of these procedures are of the prostate with access through the urethra, such as 52450, transurethral incision of the prostate.

When the procedure is a transurethral **resection** of the bladder neck, report 52500. If a transurethral **incision** of the bladder neck is performed, report 52276 (Bladder, Urethrotomy).

The following bladder codes or code ranges are unilateral and require modifier -50 if the procedure was performed bilaterally:

52007	Endoscopy/Cystoscopy, Urethroscopy and Cystourethroscopy
52320-52344, 52352-52355	Ureter and Pelvis

The third-party payer may require the use of -RT and/or -LT rather than modifier -50.

EXERCISE 24-3 *Bladder*

Using the CPT manual, code the following:

1 Needle aspiration of bladder

  CPT Code: _____

2 Endoscopy for establishment of a right Gibbons ureteral stent

  CPT Code: _____

3 Cystoscopy, left retrograde pyelogram using contrast, under fluoroscopic control, insertion of left ureteral stent

  CPT Codes: _____, _____

4 The patient has been diagnosed with incontinence and presents for an urethropexy. The patient was brought to the operating room and placed on the operating table in the supine position, prepped, and draped. A small horizontal incision is made in the abdomen just above the symphysis pubis. The bladder was then suspended by placing sutures bilaterally at the mid-portion of the urethra 1 cm lateral and at the bladder neck 2 cm lateral. The sutures were then suspended to the Cooper's ligament bilaterally. The urethra was then elevated to the horizontal position.

  CPT Code: _____

5 The 33-year-old patient has postoperative diagnosis of left ureteral calculus and presents for a cystoscopy, bilateral retrograde pyelograms, left ureteroscopy, and stone extraction. The patient was cystoscoped using a 21-French instrument. There was no evidence of urethral or bladder abnormality. Bilateral retrograde pyelograms were performed that indicated normal collecting system of the right-hand side. There was only a minimal suggestion of a filling defect in the distal ureter on the left. A guidewire was advanced up the ureter under fluoroscopic control and then a rigid short ureteroscope followed this. A stone was visualized and was entrapped in a basket and withdrawn under visual guidance.

  CPT Codes: _____, _____

(Answers are located in Appendix B)

Urethra

The subheading Urethra contains codes (53000-53899) for the usual procedures of incision, excision, and repair. For endoscopic procedures of the urethra, refer to codes 52000-52700, which contain cystoscopy, urethroscopy, and cystourethroscopy procedures.

If the physician performs the injection procedure for radiology studies for examination of the urethra, report 51600-51610 based on the type of study being performed. The radiological supervision and interpretation is reported separately with 74430 (cystography), 74450 (retrograde urethrocystography), or 74455 (voiding urethrocystography).

Incision. A meatotomy is surgical incision of the meatus, which is the opening of the urethra to the outside of the body (urethral meatus). This procedure is often bundled into other more major procedures. Codes 53020 (except infant) and 53025 (infant) report a meatotomy if it is performed as a separate procedure. Because 53025 is specifically for infants, do not append modifier -63 (Procedure performed on infants less than 4 kg).

The **Skene's glands** are also known as the paraurethral or the lesser vestibular glands and are located on either side of the urethra. These glands drain into the urethra near the meatus (urethral opening). When infected, the gland will become enlarged and tender and may require drainage or excision. **Drainage** of an abscess or cyst of the Skene's glands is reported with 53060. **Excision** of the Skene's glands is reported with code 53270.

Excision. The Excision category of codes (53200-53275) includes services such as biopsy, urethrectomy, lesion excision, fulguration, and marsupialization (creating a pouch).

When the urethra is totally surgically removed (urethrectomy), the service is reported with 53210 for a female and 53215 for a male. A urethrectomy involves removal of the urethra and creation of an opening from the bladder to the skin that is then used to drain urine. The procedure would include removal of any tumors of the urethra. If the urethra was not removed and only the tumor was removed, report with 53220.

The bulbourethral gland is also known as the Cowper's gland and is a pair of glands about the size of a pea located beneath the prostate. These glands secrete a fluid that forms part of the semen and drains directly into the urethra. Excision of the bulbourethral gland is reported with 53250.

Repair. A urethroplasty may be completed in one stage or two stages (53400-53431). The choice of codes to report a urethroplasty is based on the number of stages and type of repair. Codes 53420 (first stage) and 53425 (second stage) report the two stages of an urethroplasty, and 53415 reports a one-stage urethroplasty.

A tandem cuff or dual cuff is an artificial urinary sphincter (AUS) that is placed due to atrophy, disease, or defect of the urinary sphincter and reported with 53444. An artificial sphincter is inflatable and includes a pump, reservoir, and cuff, is inserted through a subpubic incision, and is illustrated in Fig. 24-9. The small switch in the scrotum can be manipulated to activate the pump and control urinary continence. Codes 53446-53448 report the removal and/or replacement of an AUS system, and 53449 reports repair of a previously placed system.

Urethromeatoplasty is repair of the meatus and the urethra (53450, 53460) and is performed to open and/or reconstruct the urethra.

Manipulation. The Manipulation category codes (53600-53665) are a bit different from those you have encountered previously. Manipulation is performed on the urethra (e.g., dilation or catheterization). Dilation stretches or dilates a passage that has narrowed. The Dilation codes are based on initial or subsequent dilation of a male or female patient.

EXERCISE 24-4   *Urethra*

Using the CPT manual, code the following:

1 Closure of a urethrostomy in a 54-year-old man
   CPT Code: _____

2 Second stage, surgical reconstruction of the urethra, with urinary diversion
   CPT Code: _____

(Answers are located in Appendix B)

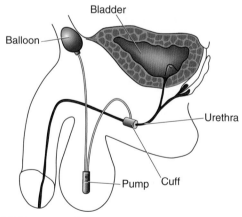

FIGURE 24-9   The cuff on the urethra squeezes the urethra closed.

MALE GENITAL SYSTEM

Format

The Male Genital System subsection (54000-55899) of the CPT manual is divided into anatomic subheadings (penis, testis, epididymis, tunica vaginalis, scrotum, vas deferens, spermatic cord, seminal vesicles, and prostate) (Fig. 24-10). The category codes are divided according to procedure. The greatest number of category codes are under the subheading Penis because there are many repair codes in this subheading. The other subheadings are primarily for incision and excision, with only a few repair codes for the remaining subheadings.

Penis

Incisions. Under the Incision category (54000-54015) of the subheading Penis, there is an incision and drainage code (54015). Recall that under the Integumentary System section there are incision and drainage codes. The code from the Penis subheading is for a deep incision, not just an abscess of the skin. For the deep abscess described in 54015, the area is anesthetized, the abscess is opened and cleaned, and often a drain is placed to maintain adequate drainage.

QUICK CHECK 24-7

1. For a superficial incision and drainage of the penis, you would select a code from the _____ System subsection of the CPT manual.

(Answers are located in Appendix C)

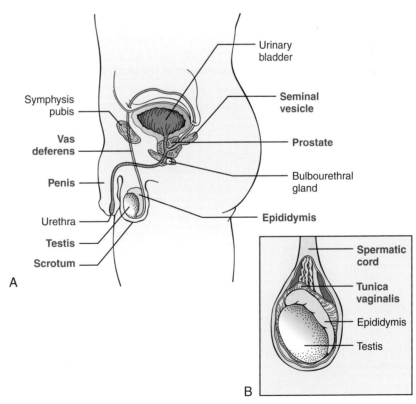

FIGURE 24-10 **A,** Male genital system. **B,** Testis.

Destruction. Under the Destruction category (54050-54065) of the subheading Penis there are also destruction codes for lesions of the penis. These lesion destruction codes are divided on the basis of whether the destruction is simple or extensive. Simple destruction is further divided according to the method of destruction (e.g., chemical, cryosurgery, laser). The code for extensive lesion destruction can be reported no matter which method was employed to accomplish the extensive destruction.

Excision. Excision codes (54100-54164) include codes to report biopsy of the penis (54100, 54105). Note that 54100 has a designation of "separate procedure," which means that the code is reported when the biopsy was the only procedure performed during the operative session. To accomplish the biopsy, the physician removes a portion of a lesion by excision of a small section of the lesion (scalpel or scissors) or by a punch biopsy. A punch biopsy is commonly used with skin lesions and is performed with an instrument that is pencil-shaped (Fig. 24-11) that removes a round disk of tissue. The opening left by the punch may require simple closure (suture) depending on the size of the skin defect created by the biopsy. A more complex biopsy (54105) of the penis involves the deeper layers of the penis and may require layered closure, which is reported separately.

Peyronie's disease is a curvature of the penis that results from plaque formation on the cavernous sheaths of the penis as illustrated in Fig. 24-12. The plaque develops on the lower and upper side of the penis where the erectile tissue is located. Inflammation results and leads to the formation of scar tissue. Over time, this fibrous plaque bends the penis. In severe cases, the penis arches during erection, causing pain. Surgical correction of the curvature involves removal of the penile plaque (54110-54112). Grafting of the defect may be necessary, depending on the extent of the removal. Code 54110 reports the excision of penile plaque when no grafting is required and 54111/54112 report excision when grafting is required.

Penile amputation can occur as a result of trauma or as a surgical procedure for penile cancer. If the procedure is the removal of only the penis (partial or complete), report the service with 54120 or 54125. If the procedure includes removal of the inguinofemoral lymph nodes, report the service based on the extent of the removal (54130, 54135).

Circumcision codes 54150-54161 are divided based on whether the circumcision was accomplished by means of a clamp/other device or surgical excision and whether the procedure was performed on a neonate or non-neonate. A clamp is a device that is used to restrain the foreskin of the penis while the skin is trimmed. Report newborn circumcisions

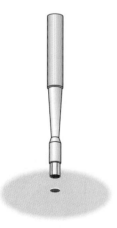

FIGUREE 24-11 A punch biopsy is used for deeper lesions and the area may require closure.

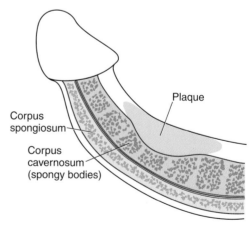

Plaque

Corpus spongiosum

Corpus cavernosum (spongy bodies)

FIGURE 24-12 Curvature of penis due to Peyronie's disease.

that utilize a clamp or other device with 54150. Surgical excision of the foreskin is a procedure in which a clamp or other device is not used, and the surgeon directly excises the skin from the penis. Once the skin has been removed, the incision is closed with sutures. Report the surgical excision without the use of a clamp or other device with 54160 (neonate) or 54161 (except neonate).

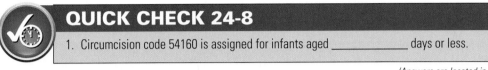

QUICK CHECK 24-8

1. Circumcision code 54160 is assigned for infants aged _____ days or less.

(Answers are located in Appendix C)

Introduction. Introduction codes (54200-54250) report various injection procedures, irrigations, plethysmography, and other tests. An example would be an injection procedure for Peyronie's disease in which steroids are injected into the fibrous tissue of the penis to decrease pain, deformity, and fibrous tissue size. There are two ways the fibrous tissue can be injected: the first way is to inject steroids directly into the area of the lump formed by the fibrous tissue (54200), and the second way is to expose the fibrous tissue through an incision and then inject steroids into the fibrous tissue (54205).

Priapism is a state of prolonged erection that can last from hours to days because of the inability of the blood to flow from the penis, which returns the penis to a flaccid state. The condition may be caused by medications used to treat impotence, such as sildenafil citrate (Viagra) or medical conditions, such as leukemia, multiple myeloma, or tumor infiltrate. If medical intervention is necessary, the surgeon introduces a large needle into the corpus cavernosum and aspirates blood, which is keeping the penis erect. The corpus cavernosum is then irrigated with a saline solution. The entire procedure is reported with 54220.

Repair. Repair category (54300-54440) codes are for various repairs made to the penis. The code descriptions often state the condition for which the procedure is being performed. For example, 54304 is plastic repair for correction of chordee or a first-stage hypospadias (defined in next paragraph) repair, and 54380 is plastic repair for epispadias. Many other codes also indicate the stage of the procedure.

Many of the Repair codes refer to repair of chordee and hypospadias. **Chordee** is a condition in which the penis has a ventral (downward) curve and is a congenital deformity. **Hypospadias** is a congenital abnormality in which the urethral meatus (opening) is abnormally placed, usually along the ventral aspect (underside) of the shaft. Degrees of hypospadias are classified according to location: anterior, middle, or posterior. Hypospadias may lead to chordee. The farther from the glans penis the opening is, the greater the chordee. Read the code descriptions for Repair codes carefully as many of the descriptions have only slight differences.

Codes in the range 54400-54417 report insertion, repair, or removal of various types of penile prostheses. The codes are divided based on the type of service and often on the circumstances of the service. Erectile dysfunction (impotence) is a condition in which the penis does not become erect. Impotence may be caused by a variety of conditions, such as obesity, chronic illness, or as a result of medication. One surgical solution to impotence is insertion of a **penile implant**. There are various types of penile implants, but mainly there are two broad categories: non-inflatable (malleable or semi-rigid, 54400) and inflatable (54401). These implants are inserted deep within the penile tissue. If the implant is subsequently removed, the removal procedure is reported with 54406 (inflatable) or 54115 (non-inflatable).

On occasion, removal and replacement are accomplished during the same operative session. Removal of a previously placed prosthesis with insertion of a new prosthesis during the same operative session is reported with 54410, 54411 (inflatable), or 54416/54417 (non-inflatable).

QUICK CHECK 24-9

1. When coding for penile prostheses the code selection is determined by the type of implant, which may be _____ or _____, and the type of service insertion, repair, removal, and/or replacement.

(Answers are located in Appendix C)

EXERCISE 24-5 *Penis*

Using the CPT, ICD-10-CM and/or ICD-9-CM manuals, code the following:

1 Extensive electrodesiccation of a condyloma on the penis

CPT Code: _____

ICD-10-CM Code: _____ (ICD-9-CM Code: _____)

2 Patient presents for removal of a previously implanted semi-rigid penile implant

CPT Code: _____

(Answers are located in Appendix B)

Testis

Excision. The Excision category (54500-54535) codes report services such as biopsy, excision, orchiectomy, and exploration of the testis. Biopsies may be percutaneous (54500) or incisional (54505). If an incisional biopsy of the testis is performed bilaterally, report modifier -50 with 54505.

Extraparenchymal is defined as unrelated to the essential elements of an organ. Removal of an extraparenchymal lesion of the testis is reported with 54512. An incision is made on the scrotum, and the testicle is pulled out through the incision where the tunica vaginalis is opened and the lesion is removed. The testicle is returned to the scrotum and the area is sutured closed.

An **orchiectomy** is the removal of a testis. CPT codes 54520-54535 report orchiectomies based on if the procedure was simple/radical, unilateral/bilateral, with/without testicular prosthesis insertion, and the approach used to gain access to the site. Watch for codes that specify unilateral or bilateral. For example, a simple orchiectomy with or without testicular prosthesis insertion (54520) reports a unilateral procedure. When the procedure is bilateral, modifier -50 must be added to correctly report the procedure.

Exploration, Repair, and Laparoscopy. Undescended testis (cryptorchidism) is a congenital condition in which the testis(es) did not descend into the scrotal sac. The condition may be unilateral or bilateral. The testis(es) may remain in the abdominal, inguinal, or prescrotal areas or may move back and forth between areas. Often, undescended testis is associated with a hernia, and if this was the case, during the hernia repair procedure, the undescended testis is brought down into the scrotum and anchored with sutures (orchiopexy). An exploration may be necessary to locate the undescended testis(es), and the choice of codes (54550, 54560) is determined based on the approach used (inguinal/scrotal or abdominal) to gain access to the area. The exploration codes report a unilateral procedure, so if a bilateral procedure was performed, add modifier -50. During an exploration, when no more definitive procedure is performed, it is only reported as an exploration. If the testis was located during the exploration and the surgeon moved the testis into the scrotal sac, the procedure is no longer an exploration but a corrective procedure (orchiopexy). An orchiopexy is reported with codes from the Repair category or the Laparoscopy category, depending on the technique used.

An orchiopexy in which the operative site is opened to the surgeon's view is reported with 54640 or 54650, depending on whether the approach was inguinal or abdominal. If the orchiopexy is performed laparoscopically, report the procedure with 54692.

QUICK CHECK 24-10

1. If during an exploratory procedure the testis is located and moved to the scrotal sac, the procedure becomes this corrective procedure: _____.

(Answers are located in Appendix C)

The following testes code ranges are unilateral and require modifier -50 if the procedure was performed bilaterally:

54500-54535	Excision
54550-54560	Exploration
54640-54680	Repair
54690-54692	Laparoscopy

The third-party payer may require the use of -RT and/or -LT rather than modifier -50.

EXERCISE 24-6   *Testis*

Using the CPT manual, code the following:

1 Simple bilateral orchiectomy with insertion of prosthesis using scrotal approach

CPT Code: _____

2 The diagnosis is azoospermia and the procedure bilateral testicular biopsies. The patient was given a general mask anesthetic, prepped and draped in supine position. Bilateral testicular cord blocks were performed. Beginning on the right side, a scrotal incision was made. The tunica vaginalis was identified, opened, and a stay stitch placed in the testis. A small incision was made, tubules delivered, resected, and sent for permanent section. The testis, vaginalis, and skin were closed with 3-0 chromic. The procedure was repeated in identical fashion on the contralateral side.

CPT Code: _____

(Answers are located in Appendix B)

Epididymis

The **epididymis** is a narrow, coiled tube located on the top of the testes that connects the efferent ducts at the back of each testicle to the vas deferens. The epididymis is divided into the caput (head), corpus (body), and cauda (tail). The epididymis can become infected, inflamed, or obstructed. When an abscess or hematoma forms in the epididymis, the surgeon may incise and drain the area (54700). At times, the testis, scrotal space, and epididymis are the site of abscess or hematoma. When any or all of these areas are incised and drained, the service is reported with 54700. For example, if the surgeon incised and drained the scrotal space, the service is reported with 54700. Or, if the surgeon incised and drained the testis, scrotal space, and epididymis, the service is reported with 54700. The one code reports incision and drainage of each or all of the areas.

QUICK CHECK 24-11

1. Code _____ is used to report incision and drainage of abscess or hematoma of the testis, scrotal space, and/or epididymis.

(Answers are located in Appendix C)

Excision. The Excision category (54800-54861) of the Epididymis codes reports biopsy, exploration (with/without biopsy), lesion or spermatocele excision, and unilateral or bilateral removal. A spermatocele is a cyst that contains sperm, and during the excision of the cyst the epididymis may or may not be removed depending on the damage to the area caused by the presence of the cyst. Code 54840 reports the excision of a spermatocele with or without an epididymectomy.

Repair. Repair to the epididymis is an **epididymovasostomy**. During epididymovasostomy, the epididymis is connected to the vas deferens. The surgical procedure is reported with 54900 or 54901, depending if the procedure was unilateral or bilateral. An operating microscope is often used during this procedure and reported separately with 69990.

The following epididymis codes or code ranges are unilateral and require modifier -50 if the procedure was performed bilaterally:

54700	Incision
54800-54840	Excision
54865	Exploration

The third-party payer may require the use of -RT and/or -LT rather than modifier -50.

Tunica Vaginalis

Incision and Excision. The **tunica vaginalis** is a serous sheath of the testis, which can be the site of a hydrocele (fluid collection). The physician may aspirate the fluid or inject a substance such as a sclerosing agent (55000) to help prevent further accumulation of fluid. Another method of management of a hydrocele is excision (unilateral, 55040 or bilateral, 55041), which may be accompanied by a hernia repair that is reported separately (49495-49501).

Repair. A Bottle type repair (55060) is a surgical procedure performed to remedy a hydrocele of the tunica vaginalis. An incision is made in the inguinal or scrotal area, and the hydrocele is drained and repositioned. A catheter may be left in place to ensure continued drainage of the area and to prevent further fluid accumulation.

Scrotum

Incision. The scrotum is the sac that contains the testes. If a lesion of the skin of the scrotum is removed, assign codes from the Integumentary System to report the service. However, if the abscess is in the scrotal wall and requires drainage, report the procedure with 55100 (Drainage of scrotal wall abscess). If the abscess is of the epididymis, testis, and/or scrotal space, report the service with 54700 because the code reports procedures to any of the three areas.

Repair. Scrotoplasty (also known as oscheoplasty) is repair of a congenital abnormality or traumatic defect of the scrotum. Skin flaps may be utilized during a simple repair (55175) and in the more complex repair (55180) rotational pedicle grafts and/or free skin grafts may be used. Simple skin flaps are included in the scrotoplasty and not reported separately, but the more complex grafts are reported in addition to the scrotoplasty.

Vas Deferens

Incision. The vas deferens is the tube that carries sperm from the testes to the ejaculatory duct and the urethra. A vasotomy (55200) is cutting into the vas deferens. Usually the procedure is performed to obtain a semen sample or to determine if there is obstruction. Code 55200 includes cannulization of the vas deferens. The code describes a unilateral or bilateral procedure, so there is no need to report modifier -50 with this code.

Excision. A vasectomy (55250) is a procedure in which a section of the vas deferens is removed for purposes of sterilization. A small incision is made on the scrotum, and the vas deferens is identified and brought out through the incision. A section of the vas deferens tube is cut and tied, stitched or sealed, and the vas deferens is returned to its natural position. The procedure includes a unilateral or bilateral procedure and postoperative semen examination(s). The semen is examined at intervals after sterilization to ensure the procedure was a success.

Introduction. A vasotomy (55300) may also be performed for a vasogram, seminal vesiculogram, or epididymogram in which colored dye is traced through the vas deferens to visualize any obstruction. The radiological supervision/interpretation is reported separately with 74440. When a vastomy is combined with a testis biopsy, report 54505-51.

Repair. A vasovasostomy or vasovasorrhaphy is a procedure to remove obstruction from the vas deferens or for a vasectomy reversal. Injection of dye is used during the procedure to identify the area of blockage. Once the area is identified, it is removed, and the ends of the vas deferens are anastomosed (reconnected end to end). Semen sampling may be conducted to ensure the removal of the blockage. Code 55400 reports a unilateral procedure; modifier -50 should be added to indicate a bilateral procedure. An operating microscope is often used during the procedure and is reported separately with 69990.

EXERCISE 24-7 | *Epididymis, Tunica Vaginalis, and Vas Deferens*

Using the CPT, ICD-10-CM and/or ICD-9-CM manuals, code the following:

1 Epididymis exploration without biopsy due to pain in epididymis

CPT Code: _____

ICD-10-CM Code: _____ (ICD-9-CM Code: _____)

2 Aspiration of fluid sac on the testicular covering

CPT Code: _____

3 Reversal of previously completed vasectomy, bilateral, using an operating microscope

CPT Code: _____

(Answers are located in Appendix B)

Spermatic Cord

Excision and Laparoscopy. The spermatic cord is a collection of structures that suspends the testes in the scrotum as illustrated in Fig. 24-13. The spermatic cord may be the site of formation of a hydrocele, lesion, or varicocele. Unilateral excision of a spermatic cord hydrocele is reported with 55500 with modifier -50 added to report a bilateral procedure. A **varicocele** is a mass of enlarged vessels that occurs when the valves that control blood flow in and out of the vessel become defective, and the blood is not able to circulate out of the vessel. The trapped blood causes the vessel to swell. Excision of a varicocele by means of a scrotal

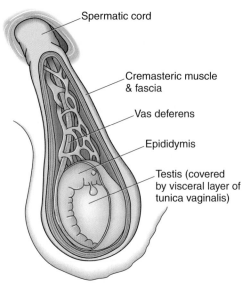

FIGURE 24–13 Spermatic cord.

approach is reported with 55530, and an abdominal approach with 55535. A hernia repair may be performed during the same operative session, and with other procedures in this subsection have been reported separately. However, the single code 55540 reports both the varicocele excision and a hernia repair. If the varicocele is repaired using surgical laparoscopy, report the procedure with 55550.

The following spermatic cord code range is unilateral and requires modifier -50 if the procedure was performed bilaterally:

55500-55550   Spermatic cord (Excision and Laparoscopy categories)

The third-party payer may require the use of -RT and/or -LT rather than modifier -50.

Seminal Vesicles

The seminal vesicles are a pair of glands located posterior to (behind) the bladder. The glands provide the majority of the fluid that becomes semen and empties into the ejaculatory ducts and the urethra. Seminal vesicles codes are located in the 55600-55680 range.

Incision. A vesiculotomy is surgical cutting into the seminal vesicles. The approach can be by an incision into the lower abdomen or the perineum (between the anus and scrotum). Frequently, the procedure is performed to relieve pressure due to inflammation. There are two codes to report a vesiculotomy based on the extent of the dissection required to accomplish the procedure. If the procedure required **simple** dissection, report 55600, and if **complicated** dissection was required, report 55605. The codes are unilateral, so a bilateral procedure requires modifier -50.

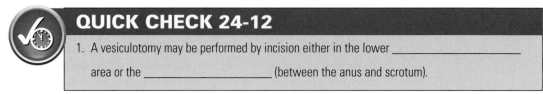

QUICK CHECK 24-12

1. A vesiculotomy may be performed by incision either in the lower _____

   area or the _____ (between the anus and scrotum).

(Answers are located in Appendix C)

Excision. A vesiculectomy is the removal of one of the seminal vesicles. The procedure is performed to remove a tumor, calculus (stone), or other obstruction. The approach may be through the lower abdomen or perineum, but the choice of codes is the same (55650) because the code description indicates "vesiculectomy, any approach." The code reports a unilateral procedure, so modifier -50 is required for a bilateral procedure.

The **Mullerian ducts** develop prenatally in females, and the Wolffian ducts degenerate. In males it is the opposite, the Wolffian ducts develop, and the Mullerian ducts degenerate. The Mullerian system develops into oviduct, uterus, and upper vagina. The Wolffian ducts develop into epididymis, vas deferens, and seminal vesicles. In some males a remnant of the Mullerian duct remains and a cyst may form at that site. The cyst may be excised using a lower abdominal or perineal approach and reported with 55680.

Prostate

The most common conditions involving the prostate are inflammation (prostatitis), benign enlargement (BPH, benign prostatic hypertrophy), and cancer. Prostate cancer is the most common type of cancer in men.

Benign Prostatic Hyperplasia and Prostatectomy. The symptoms of BPH are urinary frequency, nocturia, urgency, decreased force of urine stream, and the feeling that the bladder has not completely emptied. These symptoms are a result of the excess prostate tissue pressing against the urethra and bladder. Treatment for BPH is based on the degree of prostate enlargement and severity of symptoms. Minimally invasive treatments include balloon dilation, prostatic stents, and thermal-based therapies. If these treatments are not successful, surgical intervention may be necessary, such as coagulation, transurethral resection, laser vaporization, or open surgical procedure.

BPH treatment and prostatectomy procedures are reported with codes from both the Urinary System and/or the Male Genital System.

Prostatic **stents** (52282 [permanent], 53855 [temporary]) are flexible metal mesh tubes designed to be inserted into the urethra at the level of the prostate and expanded after placement. The stent keeps the urethra open. Over time, the urothelial tissue grows over the stent and the stent becomes incorporated into the urethral wall.

Transurethral microwave heat treatment (**TUMT**, 53850) is the use of microwaves that are sent through a catheter and introduced into the urethra to coagulate excess prostate tissue and allow the urethra to be less constricted.

Transurethral needle ablation (**TUNA**, 53852) is a procedure that utilizes radiofrequency to create heat that is applied to the prostate to destroy excess prostate tissue. During this procedure the urethra is punctured to allow the needles to be placed directly into the prostate. The needles are insulated, so the urethra is not damaged when pierced.

For some patients these less radical treatments are not effective or advisable. For example, for patients with renal insufficiency, recurrent gross hematuria, or bladder stones because of BPH, a surgical procedure is the recommended treatment option. Surgical therapies include transurethral prostate incision, electrovaporization, and laser ablation/coagulation. Let's take a closer look at each of these surgical options:

Transurethral resection of the prostate (**TURP**, 52601, 52630) is the gold-standard of surgical procedures for removal of tumor or prostatic tissue. A special type of cystoscope is inserted through the urethra. The scope has lights, valves for controlling irrigation fluids, and an electrical loop to remove tissue and/or obstructions and cauterize blood vessels.

Transurethral incision of the prostate (**TUIP**, 52450) is used when the prostate is only slightly enlarged. Two incisions are made in the prostate to relieve the pressure on the urethra without removing tissue.

When a laser is used to accomplish the prostatectomy, the choice of codes is first based on whether the procedure was a coagulation (52647) or vaporization (52648). Code 52648 includes with or without transurethral resection of the prostate.

LASER COAGULATION (52647)

- Transurethral ultrasound-guided laser induced prostatectomy (**TULIP,** non-contact) is a procedure in which a laser is used to coagulate prostate tissue. There is no direct visualization of the prostate using this method, and the penetration is not as deep as with other more commonly performed methods.
- Visual laser of the prostate (**VLAP,** non-contact) is under the direct vision of the surgeon, but the laser fiber does not come in direct contact with the prostate. This method coagulates the tissue rather than vaporizing it. Once coagulated, the tissue dies and is sloughed off, which relieves the pressure.
- Interstitial laser coagulation of prostate (**ILCP,** contact) uses several laser fibers that are placed directly into the prostate to coagulate the tissue. There is no direct visualization with the ILCP.

QUICK CHECK 24-13

1. Code 52647, laser coagulation of the prostate, may be accomplished by one of three techniques:

TULIP (non-contact, no direct visualization), _____ (non-contact, direct visualization), or

_____ (contact, no direct visualization).

(Answers are located in Appendix C)

LASER VAPORIZATION (52648)

- Transurethral vaporization of the prostate (**TUVP** or **TVP,** contact) uses electrical current to vaporize tissue of the prostate by means of a ball that is rolled over the tissue. The ball contains a current that vaporizes the tissue. This procedure is a modification of a TURP.

LASER VAPORIZATION WITH/WITHOUT RESECTION (52648)

- Holmium laser enucleation of the prostate (**HoLEP,** contact), also known as transurethral holmium laser resection (**THLR),** is a procedure used to resect prostate tissue by means of a holmium laser fiber. There is less intraoperative bleeding with this procedure than with a TURP.

There are many different techniques used to remove the prostate (prostatectomy). Codes in the Excision category (55801-55865) represent open surgical procedures. Determination of the correct code to report a prostatectomy (removal of the prostate) is based first on the **approach** (perineal, suprapubic, or retropubic).

- Perineal approach is through the space between the rectum and the base of the scrotum and is used to gain access to a prostate that is located closer to the perineal area.
- Suprapubic approach is through the lower abdominal region, and it is used to gain access to the front (anterior) surface of the bladder. The access to the prostate is gained by an opening in the bladder neck.
- Retropubic approach is also through the lower abdominal region and is used to gain access to the front (anterior) of the prostate.

Once the correct approach has been identified, the **extent** of the procedure will determine code selection. The term "subtotal" used in many of the code descriptions means anything less than the total removal of the prostate, and the term "radical" means total removal of the prostate.

QUICK CHECK 24-14

There are different approaches to an open prostatectomy. Match the approach with the definition.
1. Perineal _____
2. Suprapubic _____
3. Retropubic _____

a. Through the lower abdominal region to gain access to the anterior prostate
b. Through the space between the rectum and the base of the scrotum
c. Through the lower abdominal region to gain access to the anterior surface of the bladder, opening the bladder neck to access the prostate

(Answers are located in Appendix C)

Codes 55812-55815 and 55842-55845 include code selection based on the lymph node biopsy/removal performed. If lymph node biopsy (single or multiple) and limited removal of pelvic lymph node(s) was performed, report 55812 (perineal approach) or 55842 (retropubic approach). If lymph nodes were removed bilaterally and include the external iliac, hypogastric and obturator nodes, report 55815 (perineal approach) or 55845 (retropubic approach).

A laparoscopic retropubic prostatectomy (**LRP,** 55866) is a minimally invasive procedure that may be utilized instead of an open procedure. Robotic assisted prostatectomy (**RAP**) is a new instrumentation used with LRP and is designed to assist in the performance of some surgical tasks. Several small incisions are made through which robotic instrumentation is inserted. The surgeon operates the instrumentation from a console. The use of RAP necessitates an assistant during surgery. Surgeons who use a RAP system are extensively trained by the manufacturer of the system before using the system during surgery. The new robotic systems enhance the precision with which the procedure can be performed.

CHECK THIS OUT ☞ One such robotic system is the da Vinci® prostatectomy system and a video about the procedure can be viewed at www.davinciprostatectomy.com/da-vinci-prostatectomy/.

Now that you have reviewed BPH treatment and prostatectomies, let's review the remaining codes in the Prostate category.

Biopsy. Biopsy of the prostate may be performed with a needle, punch, or by incision. Report a prostate biopsy with 55700 (needle, punch), 55705 (incisional), or 55706 (transperineal, stereotactic). Do not report these codes during the same procedure. For example, if, during the same operative session, a needle or punch biopsy of the prostate (55700) is undertaken, and it is followed by an incisional biopsy (55705) either to supplement or to obtain adequate tissue, the appropriate CPT code to report is 55705, not both codes. Do not confuse a prostate biopsy with a fine needle aspiration (FNA). During an FNA, fluid is withdrawn for analysis and is reported with 10021 or 10022.

QUICK CHECK 24-15

1. Biopsy of the prostate may be accomplished by one of three methods: incision,

_____, or _____.

(Answers are located in Appendix C)

A **prostatotomy** is an incision into the prostate. Codes 55720 (simple) and 55725 (complicated) describe prostatotomies performed to drain an abscess. The surgeon inserts a needle into the prostate via the perineum or through the rectum. Reporting of the procedure is based on if the procedure was simple or complicated. A complicated prostatotomy would document excess bleeding or other factors that increase time and effort necessary to complete the service.

Brachytherapy. Brachytherapy (55860-55865) is a type of radiation treatment for prostate cancer and utilizes high dose rate (HDR, temporary method) or low dose (permanent seeds) and may be used in combination with biopsy/removal of lymph nodes (Fig. 24-14). The placement of the brachytherapy element(s) can be accomplished by transperineal placement (through the area between scrotum and anus) or with open exposure of the prostate. The transperineal placement involves the fastening of a template to the perineal area. The template contains a pattern of holes that indicate where the catheters or needles are to be placed to correctly access the area around the prostate. Approximately 100 permanent seeds are placed for the low-dose method.

For the high-dose method of temporary delivery, small catheters are placed into the prostate, and a series of radiation treatments are delivered. For example, a patient would present to an outpatient department of the hospital where a template would be fastened to the perineal area. The catheters would be inserted through the holes in the template into the prostate. The treatment plan is established by the radiation oncologist, and the computer that is attached to the catheters is set to deliver the prescribed dose of radiation. If the prescribed dose cannot be administered in one session, the catheters remain in place, and the patient remains in the hospital overnight. The next day, the patient would receive another radiation treatment. The catheters would be removed, and the patient would be discharged from the hospital. An advantage of the HDR is that the physician can regulate the radiation dosage more precisely than with the low-dose method.

The transperineal placement is reported by the surgeon or urologist with 55875 and includes the use of a cystoscope if applicable. The placement of the radioelements is reported separately by the radiation oncologist with 77776-77778. If ultrasound guidance is used during the placement, the guidance is reported separately with 76965, ultrasonic guidance for interstitial radioelement application.

Another approach for placement of radioactive substances is the open approach in which the prostate is viewed by the surgeon. The exposure procedure is reported by the surgeon or urologist with 55860, and the application of the radioelements is reported by the radiation oncologist with 77776-77778, based on the number of sources placed: simple (1-4), intermediate (5-10), complex (>10). During the same operative session in which the radioelements are placed, the surgeon may biopsy lymph nodes and/or may perform a lymphadenectomy

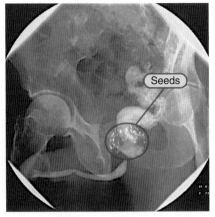

FIGURE 24-14   Brachytherapy for prostate cancer.

(55862). If a bilateral pelvic lymphadenectomy is performed and includes the external iliac, hypogastric, and obturator nodes, the procedure is reported with 55865.

Transrectal ultrasound (**TRU**, 76872) is guidance that is often used when reporting biopsy, evaluation and staging for prostate cancer, delivery of brachytherapy, evaluation or aspiration of prostate abscess, evaluation of infertility, diagnosis of prostate abnormalities, and monitoring of treatment response.

EXERCISE 24-8 | *Spermatic Cord and Prostate*

Using the CPT, ICD-10-CM and/or ICD-9-CM manuals, code the following:

1 A 75-year-old male patient presents with a PSA of 8.1. He has a 100-gram prostate, and 1 out of 10 cores were positive for adenocarcinoma. The patient was placed in the supine position and a number 20 French Foley catheter was inserted into the bladder. A lower abdominal midline incision was made and the retropubic space was entered. Bilateral pelvic lymphadenectomy was performed in the usual manner and included the external iliac, obturator, and hypogastric nodes. Lymph nodes were small and were sent for permanent section to pathology. The prostate was extremely large. The prostate was mobilized using blunt dissection technique. The area was closed in the usual manner. Pathology report later indicated primary malignant neoplasm of the prostate.

   CPT Code: _____

   ICD-10-CM Code: _____ (ICD-9-CM Code: _____)

2 The 68-year-old male patient presents with BPH. Two 18-gauge needles were affixed to the catheter, and by means of a rigid cystoscope, the needles were transurethrally inserted into the prostate. Radiofrequency waves were set at 490 kHz and 99ºC was obtained. Ablation of the area was completed and the cystoscope withdrawn.

   CPT Code: _____

(Answers are located in Appendix B)

CHAPTER REVIEW

CHAPTER 24, PART I, THEORY

Without the use of reference material, complete the following:

1 The greatest number of category codes in the Male Genital System fall under the _____ subheading because of the numerous repairs made to this anatomic area.

2 In what section of the CPT manual would you find a code for a superficial abscess of the skin of the penis? _____

3 What is the term that pertains to the motion and flow of urine? _____

4 What is the modifier that indicates that only the professional portion of the service was performed? _____

5 The Urinary System subsection is arranged _____ by the subheadings.

6 The _____ area is located behind the abdominal cavity and during surgical procedures is often accessed by an abdominal incision.

7 A(n) _____ is a procedure that is used to decompress the renal system by means of inserting a catheter into the kidney while leaving the other end of the catheter outside the body to temporarily drain the kidney.

8 A(n) _____ calculus involves at least two calyces and the renal pelvis and accounts for about 30% of the stones reported.

9 You report the removal of an accessible stent of kidney when imaging guidance is not indicated using a(n)

   _____ code.

10 If an obstruction occurs, the urine will not drain and may result in dilatation of the collecting system and enlargement of

   the renal pelvis, also known as _____.

11 A transvesical ureterolithotomy is one that is performed through the bladder for the removal of _____.

12 A urethroplasty may be one stage or two stages, and the choice of codes is based on the number of stages, type of repair,

   and for some codes the _____ of the patient.

CHAPTER 24, PART II, PRACTICAL

Code the following cases with CPT, ICD-10-CM and/or ICD-9-CM codes:

13 Incision and drainage of deep penis abscess

CPT Code: _____

ICD-10-CM Code: _____

(ICD-9-CM Code: _____)

14 Extensive destruction of penile herpetic vesicle lesions using cryosurgery

CPT Code: _____

ICD-10-CM Code: _____

(ICD-9-CM Code: _____)

15 Biopsy of kidney with percutaneous incision by trocar for a patient with a diagnosis of microalbuminuria

CPT Code: _____

ICD-10-CM Code: _____

(ICD-9-CM Code: _____)

16 Physician providing the technical and professional component of a cystography with contrast and four views for a patient with hematuria

CPT Codes: _____, _____

ICD-10-CM Code: _____

(ICD-9-CM Code: _____)

17 A one-stage distal hypospadias repair with circumcision and a V-flap for meatal advancement

CPT Code: _____

ICD-10-CM Code: _____

(ICD-9-CM Code: _____)

18 Needle biopsy with ultrasound guidance of the prostate of an 87-year-old male with an elevated PSA. The pathology results of the biopsy are negative for malignancy.

CPT Codes: _____, _____

ICD-10-CM Code: _____

(ICD-9-CM Code: _____)

19 Dilation with urethral dilator of a urethral stricture of male due to syphilis

CPT Code: _____

ICD-10-CM Code: _____

(ICD-9-CM Codes: _____, _____)

20 Injection procedure for Peyronie's disease

CPT Code: _____

ICD-10-CM Code: _____

(ICD-9-CM Code: _____)

Chapter Review answers are only available in the TEACH Instructor Resources on Evolve

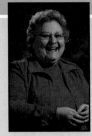

Patricia Sommerfeld, CPC
Senior Client Manager
HealthMed Inc.
Adjunct Instructor
Mercy College of Health Sciences
Des Moines, Iowa

"My motto for my billing and coding students is, 'Persist until you succeed.'"

Reproductive, Intersex Surgery, Female Genital System, and Maternity Care and Delivery

Chapter Topics

Reproductive System Procedures

Intersex Surgery

Female Genital System

Maternity Care and Delivery

Chapter Review

Learning Objectives

After completing this chapter you should be able to

1 Describe reproductive services.

2 Report reproductive services.

3 Report intersex surgery services.

4 Understand the format of the Female Genital System subsection.

5 Identify elements of component coding with Female Genital System codes.

6 Define the critical terms in maternity and delivery services.

7 Define services in the global maternity and delivery package.

8 Understand the format of the Maternity Care and Delivery subsection services.

9 Demonstrate the ability to code the Female Genital and Maternity Care and Delivery subsection.

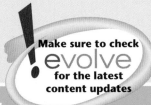

Make sure to check
evolve
for the latest
content updates

REPRODUCTIVE SYSTEM PROCEDURES

The Reproductive System Procedures subsection (55920) is located after the Male Genital System subsection and consists of only one code. Code 55920 reports the placement of needles or catheters into the pelvic organs and/or genitalia (except prostate) for the subsequent interstitial radioelement application (brachytherapy). This procedure is performed with the patient anesthetized. The surgeon examines the diseased areas to determine the area(s) that require treatment. A template device is inserted into the vagina and positioned over the areas to receive the radioelement insertions. The number and depth of the needles or catheters varies depending on the area to be treated, but typically 32 flexiguide catheters are inserted.

This code is not used to report radioelement application for the prostate, which is reported with 55875. Insertion of a vaginal ovoid brachytherapy system is a common type used to treat cervical cancer and is reported with 57155. A Heyman capsule indicated in the parenthetical statement following 55920 directs the coder to 58346 when reporting Heyman capsule insertion. A Heyman capsule was a method of manual loading that was used in the early days of brachytherapy. The physician would manually insert the capsule into the treatment area, which necessitated the physician being in contact with the radioactive source. The newer methods of brachytherapy are safer as the radioelements are inserted via catheters, thus reducing the exposure of health care providers.

INTERSEX SURGERY

The Intersex Surgery subsection (55970, 55980) is located before the Female Genital Surgery subsection and contains only two codes: one for a surgical procedure to change the sex organs of a male into those of a female and one to change the sex organs of a female into those of a male. These specialized procedures include a series of procedures that take place over an extended period of time. The procedures are performed by physicians who have special skills and training.

The procedure for changing male genitalia into female genitalia involves removing the penis but preserving the nerves and vessels intact. These tissues are used to form a clitoris and a vagina. The urethral opening is shifted to be in the position of that of a female.

The surgical procedure for changing the female genitalia into male genitalia involves a series of procedures that use the genitalia and surrounding skin to form a penis and testicle structures into which prostheses are inserted.

QUICK CHECK 25-1

1. How many codes are there in the Intersex Surgery subsection? _____

(Answers are located in Appendix C)

FEMALE GENITAL SYSTEM

Format

The Female Genital System subsection (56405-58999) is divided according to anatomic site, from the vulva up to the ovaries (Fig. 25-1). The anatomic sites are then divided on the basis of category of procedure (i.e., incision, excision, destruction). Codes for in vitro fertilization are located at the end of the subsection.

The subsection has a wide variety of codes for minor procedures that are performed in a physician's office as well as for major procedures that are performed in a hospital setting. It

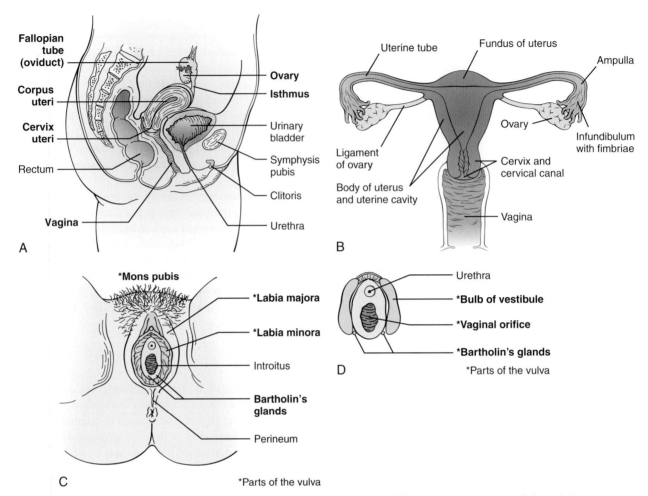

FIGURE 25–1 **A,** Female genital system. **B,** Anterior view, female genital system. **C,** External female genital system. **D,** Parts of vulva.

is important to read the descriptions of the codes as well as the notes to avoid unbundling in this subsection. For example, if a total abdominal hysterectomy was performed as well as a bilateral oophorectomy (removal of ovaries), only 58150 would be reported because the code description includes the statement "with or without removal of ovary(s)." Bundled into the code are both the abdominal hysterectomy and a bilateral oophorectomy.

There are many screening (well woman) services provided, such as screening mammography, Pap tests, and pelvic examination, in addition to colorectal cancer screening and bone mass measurements. In this text, these services are reviewed in the chapter that refers to the codes that would be submitted for the services. For example, mammography is in Chapter 28, Radiology.

Vulva, Perineum, and Introitus

There is a repeated note in the Vulva, Perineum, and Introitus subheading (56405-56821) indicating procedures performed on the Skene's glands are not reported using codes in the Female Genital System subsection but instead are coded using Surgery section, Urinary System subsection codes. That is because Skene's glands, also known as **para-urethral ducts,** are a group of small mucous glands located near the lower end of the urethra and are part of the urinary system. Procedures involving Skene's glands are, therefore, reported using Urinary System codes (53060 or 53270).

Incision. The vulva includes the following parts: mons pubis, labia majora, labia minora, bulb of vestibule, vaginal orifice or vestibule of the vagina, and the greater (Bartholin's gland) and lesser vestibule glands (see Fig. 25-1, *C* and *D*). When the code description indicates the incision and drainage of an abscess of the vulva, the code reports an abscess of any of those anatomic areas. For example, if a medical record indicates "an incision and drainage of an abscess of Bartholin's gland," you must know that Bartholin's gland is considered a part of the vulva, so the code will be located in that subheading.

Destruction. Destruction of lesions of the vulva, perineum, or introitus can be accomplished using a variety of methods—laser surgery, cryosurgery, electrosurgery, or chemical destruction. Destruction codes are divided on the basis of whether the destruction is simple or extensive, although the code description does not define simple or extensive. Complexity is based on the physician's judgment of complexity, and the complexity will be stated in the medical record.

Excision. The first two codes (56605 and 56606) in the Excision category are for biopsies in which the physician takes a tissue sample by removing a piece of tissue with a scalpel or punch. The area to be biopsied is anesthetized with local anesthetic before the biopsy is performed. The physician may suture the area or use clips for closure. The local anesthesia and closure are included in the package of an excision code, so be careful not to unbundle and report these separately. The codes are also divided on the number of lesions, one and each additional lesion. When using the additional lesions code, be certain to specify the number of lesions biopsied by listing the number of units on the CMS-1500 form in Block 24-G.

> **CAUTION** *Destruction is not excision. Destruction is obliteration or eradication. Excision is removal. With destruction no tissue is removed, as the tissue is destroyed. There is no pathology report after a lesion has been destroyed because there is nothing for the pathologist to analyze.*

CODING SHOT

If the excision is of a lesion of the skin of the genitalia, report the service with 11420-11426 (Excision of benign lesion) or 11620-11626 (Excision of malignant lesion).

Vulvectomy is the surgical removal of a portion of the vulva. Usually a vulvectomy is performed to treat a malignant or premalignant lesion. The following definitions apply to the vulvectomy codes (56620-56640) and describe the extent and size of the vulvar area removed during the procedure.

EXTENT

Simple	skin and superficial subcutaneous tissue
Radical	skin and deep subcutaneous tissue

SIZE

Partial	less than 80%
Complete	greater than 80%

The vulvectomy codes are divided on the basis of these definitions of extent and size. The extent and size are stated in combination. For example, simple partial vulvectomy describes a superficial subcutaneous tissue **(extent)** removal of 78% **(size)** of the vulvar area. Bundled into the codes is usual closure, but if plastic repair is required, you would report the repair in addition to the procedure. The operative report will indicate the extent of the procedure and the closure.

CODING SHOT

There are two labia: labia minora and labia majora (Fig. 25-2). A partial vulvectomy (less than 80%) pertains to leaving at least 20% of the vulvar area.

The more radical procedures involving the vulva are usually performed because of a demonstrated malignancy, and more extensive removal takes place. This radical removal can include the removal of deep lymph nodes, saphenous veins, ligaments, or large amounts of tissue from the lower abdomen or even from the thigh. The procedure may also be performed bilaterally, so don't forget to add modifier -50 when reporting a bilateral procedure.

CODING SHOT

Most payers do not make a reimbursement adjustment for bilateral procedures of the vulva. For example, Medicare does not make an adjustment. You must review each payer's guidelines to determine how to submit this code.

Repair. The procedure codes in the Repair category (56800-56810) describe plastic repair of the vulva, perineum, or introitus. Plastic repair of the **introitus** is surgical repair of the opening of the vagina. The extent and nature of the procedure are determined by the defect being repaired and varies greatly from patient to patient.

Clitoroplasty is surgical reduction of a clitoris (Fig. 25-3) that has become enlarged due to an adrenal gland imbalance.

Perineoplasty is plastic repair of the perineum, usually to provide additional support to the perineal area.

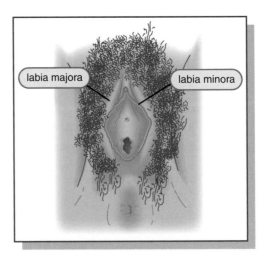

F I G U R E 2 5 – 2   Labia majora and labia minora.

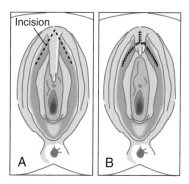

FIGURE 25-3 Reduction clitoroplasty.

Vagina

The Vagina subheading includes the code range 57000-57426. **Colpotomy** (57000-57010) is cutting into the vagina to gain access to the pelvic cavity. The procedure is performed to explore the pelvic cavity or to drain a pelvic abscess. **Colpocentesis** (57020) is the insertion of a long needle (puncture) attached to a syringe through the back wall of the vagina to gain access to the peritoneal cul-de-sac—the area between the uterus and the rectum—to drain fluid. If the colpocentesis is a part of a more major procedure, you do not report it separately, as it is considered to be bundled into the more major procedure. Note that 57020 has "(separate procedure)" after it to designate colpocentesis as a minor procedure that is reported only if it is the only procedure performed of the area.

Destruction. As with the destruction codes for the vulva, the destruction codes (57061, 57065) for the Vagina subsection are divided on the basis of whether the destruction was simple or extensive, in the judgment of the physician. Any method of destruction is acceptable for assignment of these codes.

Excision. The Excision category of the Vagina subsection contains codes (57100-57135) for reporting the services of biopsy, vaginectomy (removal of part or all of the vagina), colpocleisis (closure of the vaginal canal), and cyst/lesion removal. The vaginectomy codes are divided according to the extent of the procedure—**partial** or **total**—and the extent to which tissue and adjacent structure(s) are removed.

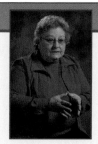

From the Trenches

"Be willing to learn everything there is to know. Medical terminology and anatomy/physiology are a must for the successful coder."

PATRICIA

Introduction. The Introduction category (57150-57180) contains codes for vaginal irrigation. Also included is the insertion of a tandem and/or vaginal ovoids for brachytherapy. The tandems and/or vaginal ovoids are internal implants that contain a radioactive substance and are often used in the treatment of cervical cancer, as illustrated in Fig. 25-4. A tandem is a small, hollow metal tube that is inserted through the vagina into the uterus (intrauterine tandem). Vaginal ovoids are small metal cylinders that are placed into the vagina and

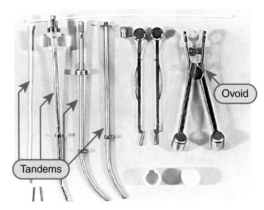

FIGURE 25-4 Tandem and ovoid.

positioned against the cervix (intravaginal ovoid). The implants then deliver a concentrated dose of radiation to the site of the tumor.

Other codes in the Introduction category report the insertion of a support device (pessary, Fig. 25-5), diaphragm, or cervical cap (to prevent pregnancy); and packing of the vagina (for vaginal hemorrhage). Pessaries are used for vaginal prolapse. The pessary and diaphragm/cervical cap are not included in these Introduction codes. The supply of these devices would be reported using code 99070, supplies, or a HCPCS code (e.g., A4561).

Repair. The Repair category (57200-57335) is rather extensive, as the possible forms of repair of the vagina are many. A note in parentheses, "(nonobstetrical)," sometimes follows the code description in the Female Genital System subsection because if the procedure was performed as a part of an obstetric procedure, you would use a code from the Maternity Care and Delivery subsection.

A surgeon performs a **colporrhaphy** to strengthen an area on the wall of the vagina that is weak by pulling together the weakened vaginal area with sutures. Excess tissue can also be removed to tighten the area. The reinforcement might be performed for several reasons,

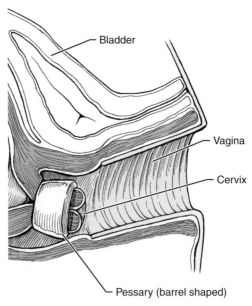

FIGURE 25-5 Vaginal pessary (Arabin type).

but it is commonly done to prevent the bladder from protruding into the weakened vaginal wall (cystocele) or the rectum from protruding into the vagina (rectocele).

In this Repair category, the codes are often divided on the basis of the approach used. For example, an abdominal approach (open, 57270) to the repair of an enterocele (herniation of intestines through intact vaginal mucosa) has a different code than a vaginal approach (57268) to the same repair; and an anterior colporrhaphy (vaginal repair) (57240) differs from a posterior colporrhaphy (57250). Pay particular attention to the **approach** used. You will find the approach documented in the operative report.

One method of vaginal repair that is not in the Repair category is the laparoscopic repair. Codes for repair of the vagina using a colposcope (microscope) are located in the Vagina subheading, Endoscopy category. The colposcope enables the physician to directly view changes in the vagina and cervix.

Notes throughout the Repair category will frequently direct you to the correct code or code range in the Urinary System subsection. Often, the only difference between surgical procedures reported with Female Genital System codes and those reported with the Urinary System codes is the **approach**. For example, Female Genital System code 57330 describes the closure of a vesicovaginal fistula (abnormal channel between bladder and vagina) using a vaginal approach, whereas Urinary System code 51900 describes the same procedure using an abdominal approach. The approach would be documented in the operative report.

> ✋ **CAUTION** *Coders need to pay close attention to the **method** as well as to the **approach**. For example, a surgeon might perform an open procedure as opposed to a laparoscopic procedure.*

Manipulation. **Manipulation** of the vagina includes dilation (stretching), pelvic examination, and removal of foreign material. What these three different procedures have in common is that they are all performed under **general anesthesia** because a patient cannot tolerate the procedure while awake. If a local anesthetic or no anesthetic was used, which is the usual case, you would not use a Manipulation code (57400-57415); instead, the service would be included in the Evaluation and Management (E/M) service. For example, if a physician removed an impacted tampon from the vagina and used no anesthetic during the procedure, only the office visit at which the removal took place would be reported.

Endoscopy. As discussed earlier in this chapter, the endoscopic procedure codes (57420-57426) in the Endoscopy category of the Vagina subheading are for colposcopic procedures. The colposcopic procedures are often bundled into other, more major procedures. Fig. 25-6 illustrates an endocervical polyp protruding through the external os (mouth of the cervix) as seen by the physician using a colposcope. Only when a colposcopic procedure is performed as the only procedure or is unrelated to another procedure(s) being performed is the colposcopy reported.

If a biopsy of the vagina or cervix is performed with colposcopy, the code to report the service is 57421. The code specifies "biopsy(s)," so whether one or multiple biopsies were taken, 57421 represents the total service.

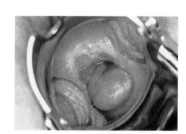

FIGURE 25-6 Endocervical polyp protruding through the mouth of the cervix as seen through a colposcope.

Cervix Uteri

The Cervix Uteri subheading contains codes (57452-57800) for endoscopy, excision, repair, and manipulation.

Endoscopy. Similar to the vaginal endoscopic codes, the colposcopy codes report procedures of the cervix uteri (57452-57461). A loop electrode excision procedure is referred to as LEEP, LETZ, or cervical loop diathermy and is an office procedure that uses heated wire (Fig. 25-7) to remove cervical tissue. The device is attached to an electric generator that heats the wire. The procedure has a lower risk level and is less expensive than other methods. A LEEP would usually be performed after an abnormal Pap smear result or an abnormal examination. The cervix is moistened, and the loop is positioned over the cervix and drawn across the area. The resulting slice is examined by a pathologist. The device is also used to cauterize the area at the end of the procedure by means of a different attachment.

Excision. The codes in the Excision category often specify "(separate procedure)" because many times the procedures are bundled into a more major procedure. For example, the excision procedure of a biopsy is often incidental to a more major surgical procedure, such as a hysterectomy, and the biopsy would not be reported separately.

Codes for **conization** of the cervix are divided on the basis of the method used to obtain the tissue (Fig. 25-8). In conization, a cone of tissue is removed from the cervix for a biopsy or treatment of a lesion by means of excision of the lesion. Although a laser is a frequently used method of conization, LEEP technology is also widely used. The code for a LEEP procedure with **cervical biopsy** in the Cervix Uteri subheading, Endoscopy category, is 57460, and the code for a LEEP procedure with **cervical conization** is 57461. The difference between the codes is that the cervical biopsy procedure only removes a sample with return in the future if the lesion is to be completely removed. The conization procedure removes a cone-shaped tissue of the cervix after application of iodine to highlight the abnormal tissue. Also, the cervical biopsy is performed with the use of a colposcope (endoscopy), and the conization is performed using a speculum (Fig. 25-9) (an instrument inserted into a cavity to stretch the opening). Be certain, when coding cervical biopsy and conization, that the information in the medical record provides sufficient detail to allow you to distinguish between a biopsy and a conization. If the record is not complete enough to make the determination, obtain the information from the physician before assigning a code.

Repair. Nonobstetric **cerclage** (repair of the cervix) involves extensive suturing of the cervix to decrease the size of the opening into the vagina (reported with 57700). **Trachelorrhaphy** (57720) is a complex cervical repair in which plastic methods are used to repair a laceration of the cervix. Both Repair codes use a vaginal approach.

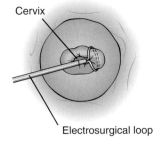

Cervix

Electrosurgical loop

FIGURE 25-7 The loop used in the electrosurgical excision procedure.

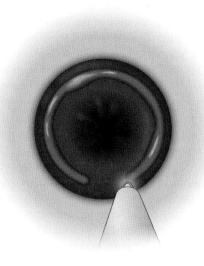

FIGURE 25-8 Conization.

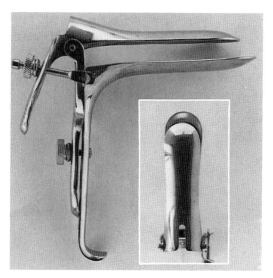

FIGURE 25-9 Graves specula.

Manipulation. Dilation of the cervix is coded separately only if it is the only procedure performed (57800). Dilation of the cervix, like dilation of the vagina, is usually bundled into a more major procedure.

Corpus Uteri

The corpus uteri (58100-58579) is the anatomic area above the isthmus and below the opening for the fallopian tubes. The subheading contains the categories of excision, introduction, repair, and laparoscopy/hysteroscopy procedures. Many of the procedures in the category are very complex, and some of them have several variations. Let's review some of the highlights of corpus uteri coding.

Excision. Endometrial **sampling** is a biopsy of the mucous lining of the uterus. The physician inserts a curet (spoon-shaped instrument) into the endocervical canal to extract tissue samples for pathologic examination. If the sampling is the only procedure performed, it is reported (58100, 58110), but if it is performed as part of a more major procedure involving the cervix, it is considered incidental to the more major procedure and is bundled into the surgical package.

Dilation and curettage (D&C; 58120) can be a diagnostic or therapeutic procedure performed when an endometrial biopsy has failed or was inconclusive or to determine the cause of abnormal bleeding or locate a neoplasm. Clamps are used to manipulate the cervix, a curet is inserted into the uterus, and fragments are removed from the endometrium. The tissue is sent to pathology for analysis. D&C in the Corpus Uteri subheading is for nonobstetric patients only. If a D&C is performed because of postpartum hemorrhage, a code from the subsection Maternity Care and Delivery would be assigned to report the service (59160).

CODING SHOT

Many third-party payers will not reimburse for a dilation and curettage if it is performed with any other pelvic surgery because it is thought to be integral to or a part of the procedure. The CPT manual does not list a D&C as a "(separate procedure)"; therefore, you need to be familiar with the specific reimbursement policies of the payer.

Hysterectomy codes (58150-58294) represent the majority of the codes in the Corpus Uteri subheading. A **hysterectomy** is the removal of the uterus, but in the CPT manual there are many variations of this procedure. The division of the hysterectomy codes is based first on the **approach** (abdominal or vaginal), then on the secondary procedures **(extent)** that were performed (removal of tubes, biopsy, bladder, etc.). You have to read the code descriptions carefully to determine what is bundled into each code. Because so many procedures are bundled into some of the codes, you also have to be careful not to unbundle and code for items already covered in the main procedure. For example, a total abdominal hysterectomy can include the removal of the ovaries and/or the fallopian tubes; therefore, billing separately for the removal of the ovaries or tubes would be unbundling.

Within the Excision category there are codes for abdominal approaches for hysterectomies. An **abdominal approach** is one in which the surgeon opens the abdomen to view by means of an incision. Review the codes in the range 58150-58240 and underline "abdominal" in each of the codes as a reminder of the approach used in these codes. The other type of surgical approach for hysterectomies listed in the Excision category is the vaginal approach. Using the **vaginal approach,** the surgeon makes an incision in the vagina around the cervix and removes the uterus and/or ovaries/fallopian tubes (salpingo-oophorectomy) through the incision. The cuff of the vagina is then closed with sutures. Review the codes in the range 58260-58294 and underline "vaginal" as a reminder of the approach used in these codes.

QUICK CHECK 25-2

1. What is the difference between codes 58260 and 58290?

   _____

2. Locate the myomectomy codes 58140, 58145, 58545, and 58546 in the CPT manual. Review the codes and identify the determining factors when selecting a code.
   a. approach, location, number
   b. approach, number, weight
   c. location, weight, pathological outcome
   d. weight, number, age of patient

(Answers are located in Appendix C)

Introduction. It is in the Introduction category (58300-58356) that you will locate the codes for some very common procedures such as the insertion and removal of an **intrauterine device** (IUD), as illustrated in Fig. 25-10, for birth control and for some not-so-common procedures such as artificial insemination. There are also several codes that have radiology components—your component coding skills will again be used.

Because intrauterine device (IUD) insertion is reported using Introduction category code 58300, you might think IUD removal would be in a removal category, but it is in the Introduction category (58301).

CODING SHOT

The cost of the IUD is not included in the code for the insertion of the IUD. You report the cost of the device separately, using 99070 or a HCPCS code (J7300 or S4989).

Don't confuse the insertion of an IUD with the placement of an implantable contraceptive such as Norplant, as described in the Integumentary subsection.

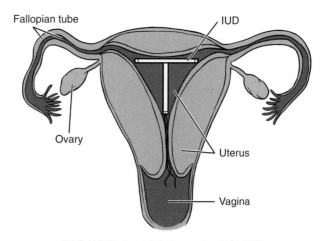

FIGURE 25-10 Intrauterine device (IUD).

The specialized fertility procedure of **artificial insemination** (58321-58323) and the preparation of the sperm for insemination are reported with Introduction category codes. During the insemination procedure, sperm is injected into the cervix and often a cervical cap is inserted to keep the sperm in the cervical area. **In vitro fertilization** is a different procedure in which an egg from the female is withdrawn and fertilized with sperm in a laboratory for 2 to 3 days with subsequent implantation into the uterus. There is an In Vitro Fertilization subheading containing codes 58970-58976 to report these services, located at the end of the Female Genital System subsection.

Catheterization and introduction (58340) of saline or contrast material through the cervix and uterus and into the fallopian tubes (hysterosalpingography) is performed by a physician to identify blockage or abnormalities of the fallopian tubes. Ultrasound can also be used for the same procedure (hysterosonography). You need to remember your component coding and report the radiology or ultrasound portion of the procedure with a code from the Radiology section. A note following 58340 in the CPT manual directs you to the correct component code. For the radiographic supervision and interpretation, the component code is 74740; for the ultrasound (sonohysterography), the code is 76831.

A **hysterosalpingography** is a diagnostic procedure to test the patency (unblocked) of the fallopian tubes. Saline or contrast material is injected into a tube (58340). A catheter may be introduced (58345) and passed through the fallopian tube using x-ray to show where the catheter encounters an obstruction or a narrowing of the tube. A code from the Radiology section, Gynecological and Obstetrical subsection, would report the radiology portion of the service (74742). **Chromotubation** (58350) is a surgical procedure to open an obstructed or narrowed tube.

Laparoscopy/Hysteroscopy. An increasing number of procedures are being performed by using an endoscope instead of opening the area to complete view. With an endoscopic procedure, usually two or three small incisions are made through which lights, cameras, and instruments may be passed. The surgeon first inserts an instrument into the vagina to grasp the cervix. The laparoscope is then inserted into the abdomen and the uterus and/or ovaries/fallopian tubes are excised. An incision is made in the vagina and the surgically excised material is removed through the vaginal incision. The vagina is then repaired by means of sutures. Review the codes in the range 58541-58579 and underline "Laparoscopy" or "Hysteroscopy" as a reminder of the approach used in these codes. It is very important to read the full code description to identify the approach. Because endoscopic procedures are less invasive, patients are more accepting of the procedures, and recovery times and risks are reduced. Fig. 25-11 illustrates a laparoscopy procedure and Fig. 25-12 illustrates a laparoscopy/hysteroscopy procedure.

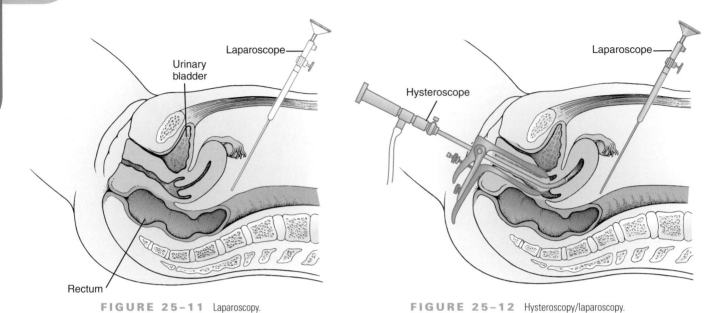

FIGURE 25-11 Laparoscopy.

FIGURE 25-12 Hysteroscopy/laparoscopy.

 CAUTION *If the laparoscopy is of the peritoneum, you assign a code (49320) from the laparoscopy category of the Digestive System, Abdomen, Peritoneum, and Omentum subheading.*

The first rule of a laparoscopy or hysteroscopy is that all surgical procedures include a **diagnostic** procedure. You never unbundle a surgical laparoscopic procedure by also reporting a diagnostic procedure. If a procedure started out as a diagnostic laparoscopic procedure and ended up being a surgical laparoscopic procedure, you report only for the surgical laparoscopy.

The codes in the Laparoscopy/Hysteroscopy category are divided on the basis of approach—laparoscopy or hysteroscopy—and further divided by other procedures that might have been performed.

Oviduct/Ovary

The Oviduct/Ovary subheading (58600-58770) is divided into incision, laparoscopy, excision, and repair. Fallopian tube procedures are located in this subheading.

Incision. The Incision category is where you will locate the codes for tubal ligation, which is a permanent, highly effective method of birth control. The codes are divided according to the type of ligation performed and the circumstances at the time of the ligation. The types of ligation are as follows: **tying** off the tube with suture material (ligation), **removing** a portion of the tube (transection), and **blocking** the tube with a device, such as a clip, ring, or band (occlusion). The circumstance under which the procedure is performed affects the choice of codes. For example, a procedure can be performed either on one side (unilateral) or on both sides (bilateral). The procedure can be performed at different times, such as during the same hospitalization period as the period of delivery, during the postpartum period, or during another surgical procedure and these circumstances affect code assignment.

CODING SHOT

Do not use a bilateral procedure modifier (-50) with codes in the Incision category because the code descriptions indicate "tube(s)" or "unilateral or bilateral." Also, do not code tubal ligations performed by means of a laparoscopic procedure using the Incision category codes. There are codes for laparoscopic tubal ligation procedures in the Laparoscopy category of subheading Oviduct/Ovary (58660-58679).

A ligation can be performed by an abdominal or a vaginal approach. If a ligation or transection of the fallopian tube(s) is performed during the same operative procedure as a cesarean delivery or other intra-abdominal surgery, you report the ligation/transection using 58611. Code 58611 only reports the tubal ligation as a component of the more major surgical procedure and is listed in addition to the primary code.

Often at the time of an abdominal tubal ligation, lysis (loosening) of adhesions will be performed. Lysis is not bundled into the ligation code. You report the lysis of adhesions separately, using a Repair category code such as 58660, if allowed by the third-party payer.

CODING SHOT

58740, lysis of adhesions, is performed for restoration of fertility, not for lysis of adhesions at the time of tubal ligation (such as 58660).

Laparoscopy. The procedures described in the Oviduct/Ovary subheading, Laparoscopy category (58660-58679) are surgical laparoscopy and always include a diagnostic laparoscopy. If only a diagnostic laparoscopy was performed, you report 49320 from the Digestive System subsection, Abdomen, Peritoneum, and Omentum category, because the scope is being passed into the abdomen for examination only. Once a definitive procedure such as a tubal ligation has begun, the examination/diagnostic laparoscopic procedure is bundled into the surgical procedure. For example, if a diagnostic laparoscopy was performed and did not lead to a definitive procedure, the diagnostic laparoscopic code 49320 from the Digestive System subsection would be reported to describe the procedure of examining the abdomen using an endoscope. But if a diagnostic laparoscopy was performed and did lead to a fulguration of the oviducts, code 58670 from the Female Genital System subsection would be assigned. The terminal (end or final) procedure dictates the code choice.

The laparoscopy codes are divided on the basis of the procedure performed, for example, lysis of adhesions, oophorectomy, and lesion excision.

Excision. The Excision category codes report salpingectomy (removal of uterine tube) or salpingo-oophorectomy (removal of uterine tube and ovary) and describe unilateral or bilateral procedures that are either complete or partial. An unbundling issue presents itself with the assignment of these codes. If either a salpingectomy or salpingo-oophorectomy is performed with a more major procedure such as a hysterectomy, each is considered bundled into the more major procedure and not reported separately.

Repair. Within the Repair category are codes for lysis of adhesions and various repairs to the fallopian tubes. All of the repairs are performed for the purpose of restoring fertility. Often the repairs are made through small incisions above the pubic hairline, but they can also be performed through a laparoscope, so note the approach used for repairs to the fallopian tubes.

Lysis of adhesions performed on the fallopian tubes (**salpingolysis**) or the ovaries (**ovariolysis**) uses a small incision to insert instrumentation to complete the repairs. Lysis is a procedure that is often performed at the time of another, more major procedure and is usually bundled into the more major procedure. If the lysis takes an extensive amount of time, you can report the service separately with supportive documentation indicating the additional time and effort required to perform the lysis. Another option is to report modifier -22 to indicate that the procedure required more time than normal. The time to complete the lysis portion of the procedure must be clearly documented in the operative report.

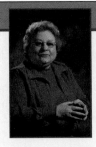

From the Trenches

"Teamwork with other coders gives you support with the 'problem' codes. It is extremely important with the physicians because services must be presented accurately and correctly to the insurance companies."

PATRICIA

Ovary

The subheading Ovary (58800-58960) contains the two categories Incision and Excision. The Incision codes report ovarian incision and drainage. The Excision codes report ovarian biopsy, cystectomy, and oophorectomy procedures.

QUICK CHECK 25-3

1. Review code range 58950-58956. Which codes include the statement "total abdominal hysterectomy"? _____

(Answers are located in Appendix C)

In Vitro Fertilization

In vitro fertilization means to fertilize an egg outside the body. The codes in the In Vitro Fertilization category describe several methods that are used in modern fertility practice. Third-party payers often do not pay for the fertility treatments. You will have to be certain that you know the policy of the payer regarding fertility treatments.

Code 58970, aspiration of the ova, is often performed with ultrasonic guidance and when it is, assign 76948 (Radiology section, Ultrasonic Guidance Procedures) to report the service.

EXERCISE 25-1   *Female Genital System*

Using the CPT manual, code the following:

1 Simple destruction of one lesion of the vaginal vestibule

CPT Code: _____

2 Biopsy of three lesions of the vulva

CPT Codes: _____, _____ × _____

3 Closure of rectovaginal fistula, abdominal approach

CPT Code: _____

4 Cone biopsy (laser) of cervix with dilation and curettage

CPT Code: _____

5 Unilateral, right, laparoscopic, ovarian cystectomy

CPT Code: _____

(Continued)

Using the vulvectomy notes in the CPT manual, match each of the following procedures with its correct definition:

PROCEDURE	THE REMOVAL OF:
6 simple _____	**a** greater than 80% of the vulvar area
7 radical _____	**b** skin and deep subcutaneous tissues
8 partial _____	**c** skin and superficial subcutaneous tissues
9 complete _____	**d** less than 80% of the vulvar area

(Answers are located in Appendix B)

MATERNITY CARE AND DELIVERY

Format

The Maternity Care and Delivery subsection (59000-59899) is divided according to type of procedure. As a general rule, the subsection progresses from antepartum procedures through delivery procedures. The guidelines are very detailed as to the services included in antepartum and delivery care, not only to facilitate coding but also to help guard against unbundling. Notes at the beginning of this subsection describe, in depth, the services listed in obstetric care. Be certain to read these notes.

Abortion codes, whether for spontaneous abortion, missed abortion, or induction of abortion, are at the end of the subsection. Abortion codes indicate treatment of a spontaneous abortion or missed abortion, including additional division on the basis of **trimester** and induction of abortion by **method**. You must be aware of the gestational age of the fetus to determine the correct code.

Treatment for ectopic pregnancies is based on the site of the pregnancy, the extent of the surgery, and whether the approach was by means of laparoscopy or laparotomy (incision through abdominal wall).

Maternity and Delivery

The gestation of a fetus takes approximately 266 days; but when the estimated date of delivery (**EDD**) is calculated, 280 days are often used, counting the time from the last menstrual period (**LMP**). The gestation is divided into three time periods, called trimesters. The trimesters are as follows:

- First   LMP to week 12
- Second   Weeks 13-27
- Third   Weeks 28-EDD

When a maternity case is uncomplicated, the service codes normally include the antepartum care, delivery, and postpartum care in the global package. **Antepartum care** is considered to include both the initial and subsequent history and physical examinations, blood pressures, patient's weight, routine urinalysis, fetal heart tones, and monthly visits to 28 weeks of gestation, biweekly visits from gestation weeks 29 through 36, and weekly visits from week 37 to delivery when these services are provided by the same physician. If the patient is seen by the same physician for a service other than those identified as part of antepartum care, you would report that service separately. For example, if a patient in week 32 came to the office with a chief complaint of cold symptoms, an E/M service code would be reported for the service and the diagnosis code would further indicate that the service was provided due to a cold not pregnancy.

Admission to the hospital is bundled into the **delivery** codes and includes the admitting history and examination, management of an uncomplicated labor, and delivery that is either vaginal or by cesarean section (including any episiotomy, illustrated in Fig. 25-13, and use of forceps, as illustrated in Fig. 25-14). Included in **postpartum care** are the hospital visits and/or office visits for 6 weeks after a delivery. If the postpartum care is complicated or if services

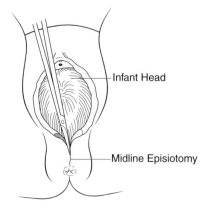

FIGURE 25-13   Midline (median) episiotomy.

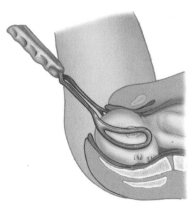

FIGURE 25-14   Use of forceps.

provided to the patient during the postpartum period are not generally part of the postpartum care, you would report those additional services separately.

Routine Obstetric Care

There are four codes that describe the global routine obstetric care that includes the antepartum care, delivery, and postpartum care, based on the type of delivery:

- 59400   Vaginal delivery
- 59510   Cesarean delivery
- 59610   Vaginal delivery after a previous cesarean delivery
- 59618   Cesarean delivery following attempted vaginal delivery after previous cesarean delivery

Two abbreviations commonly found on the delivery record are VBAC (vaginal birth after cesarean) and VBACS (vaginal birth after cesarean section), which assist in assigning the correct code.

CODING SHOT

Bundled into the vaginal delivery codes are an episiotomy (cutting of the perineum) and/or the use of forceps during delivery and, therefore, neither is reported separately.

If the physician provided only a portion of the global routine obstetric care, the service is reported with codes that describe that portion of the service as delivery only or postpartum care only, based on the delivery method. For example, if a physician provided only the delivery portion of the service, you would report the service with:

- 59409   Vaginal delivery only
- 59514   Cesarean delivery only
- 59612   Vaginal delivery only, after previous cesarean delivery
- 59620   Cesarean delivery only, following attempted vaginal delivery after previous cesarean delivery

If the global obstetric care is provided and twins are delivered, the same codes are reported but, depending on the third-party payer, modifier -22 (Increased Procedural Services) or -51 (Multiple Procedures) is added. Usually, if both twins are delivered vaginally, report 59400 for Twin A and 59409-51 for Twin B. If one is delivered vaginally and one is delivered cesarean, report 59510 for Twin B and 59409-51 for Twin A. If both are delivered via cesarean, report only 59510 (because only one cesarean was performed).

Delivery Method	Code for TWIN A	Code for TWIN B
Both twins delivered vaginally	59400	59409-51
One twin delivered vaginally Other twin delivered cesarian	59409-51	59510
Both twins delivered cesarian	59510	

Some payers, such as Medicaid in Illinois and Texas, require 59409 (vaginal delivery) or 59410 (cesarean delivery) to be reported since they do not recognize the global obstetric care codes. Each prenatal visit and the delivery is billed separately. Just another reminder that knowledge of the payers' rules will ensure prompt and proper payments.

TOOLBOX

This is Sally's first pregnancy and she goes into labor. The baby is in a breech position but her physician, who has provided all her maternity care, is able to manipulate the baby to correct cephalic presentation. An episiotomy is performed during the course of the vaginal delivery.

QUESTIONS

1. Does the fact that this is Sally's first pregnancy affect the choice of CPT codes? _____
2. Is the episiotomy reported separately? _____
3. Does the manipulation to correct presentation indicate the addition of modifier -22? _____

▼ **ANSWERS**

1. no, 2. no, 3. no

Antepartum Services

Amniocentesis (59000, 59001) is a procedure in which the physician inserts a needle into the pregnant uterus to withdraw amniotic fluid and is only performed after the first 14 weeks of pregnancy. In this procedure, ultrasound is used to guide the needle, and the supervision and interpretation (S&I) service is reported using 76946 from the Radiology section, Ultrasonic Guidance Procedures subsection.

CODING SHOT

Radiological procedures require a separate medical document before you can submit for reimbursement. Modifier -26 may be required depending on where the service was performed and who owned the radiology equipment.

Several of the antepartum services require component coding in order to fully report the services provided. Attention to the code descriptions and parenthetic statements is necessary to ensure that all services are reported.

Cordocentesis (59012) is a procedure in which fetal blood is drawn. This procedure is performed under ultrasonic guidance to assess the status of the fetus. Cordocentesis is not included in normal antepartum care and should be reported separately. The ultrasonic guidance (76941) would also be reported separately.

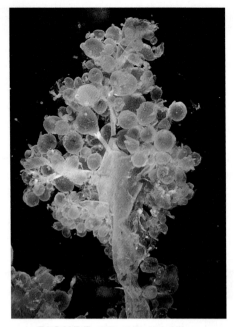

FIGURE 25–15 Hydatidiform.

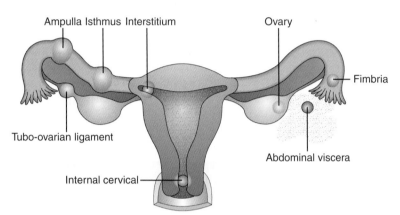

FIGURE 25–16 Implantation sites of ectopic pregnancy.

Excision. Abdominal **hysterotomy** (59100) may be performed to remove a hydatidiform mole (cystlike structure) (Fig. 25-15) or an embryo. If a tubal ligation is performed at the same time as a hysterotomy, be certain to report 58611 to indicate the ligation.

An **ectopic pregnancy** is one in which the fertilized ovum has become implanted outside of the uterus, as illustrated in Fig. 25-16. The surgical treatment for this condition can use either an abdominal or a vaginal approach (59120-59150); most often, the abdominal approach is used. If the area has not ruptured, the pregnancy is removed. If a rupture has occurred, a more extensive procedure is required. You have to identify the location of the ectopic pregnancy, the extent of the necessary repair, and the approach to the repair—vaginal, abdominal, or laparoscopic—to correctly code the procedure.

Postpartum curettage is performed within the first 6 weeks after delivery to remove remaining pieces of the placenta or clotted blood. Code 59160 is only for use with postpartum curettage. If the curettage is nonobstetric, report 58120.

Introduction. A cervical dilator (such as laminaria, which is a compound on a stick that swells from surrounding moisture) may be inserted prior to a procedure in which the cervix is to be dilated; it prepares the cervix for an abortive procedure or a delivery. The dilator initiates uterine contractions, which in turn cause cervical dilatation. Induction can be elective—at the convenience of the patient or the physician—or required, based on a medical risk factor to the mother or fetus. Physicians use a scoring system to measure the stage of cervical ripening, as illustrated in Fig. 25-17.

To induce cervical ripening (softening and dilation), a preparation such as Prepidil gel is introduced intracervically using a catheter. The cervical ripening takes place in the delivery ward.

Score	Dilation (cm)	Effacement (%)	Station	Consistency	Cervical Position
0	Closed	0-30	–3	Firm	Posterior
1	1-2	40-50	–2	Medium	Midposition
2	3-4	60-70	–1, 0	Soft	Anterior
3	>4	>70	+1, +2	—	—

FIGURE 25–17 The Bishop Scoring System of cervical ripening.

CODING SHOT

You can report 59200 (cervical ripening) with an induced abortion (59840 or 59841) but not with an abortion induced by means of vaginal suppositories (59855-59857). Also, do not report an induction procedure using a code that describes a manual dilation as a part of the procedure, such as D&C.

Many third-party payers will not pay separately for an induction procedure, as it is considered to be part of the package for obstetric care. You will have to check with your payers to determine their policies regarding the induction procedure.

Repair. The obstetric repairs can be to the vulva, vagina, cervix, or uterus. All of these repairs are also located in the Female Genital subsection, but here in the Maternity Care and Delivery subsection, the codes are reported only for repairs made during pregnancy. Repairs made during delivery or after pregnancy are included in the delivery codes 59400-59622.

CODING SHOT

Vaginal repairs can be reported separately only by a physician other than the attending physician. When the attending physician performs a procedure such as an episiotomy, it is considered part of the package for obstetric care. Each third-party payer determines what is included in the obstetric package.

Abortion Services. The abortion codes (59812-59857) include services for treatment for several types of procedures. A **spontaneous** abortion (miscarriage) is one that happens naturally. If the uterus is completely emptied during the miscarriage and the physician manages the postmiscarriage, the services are reported with E/M codes. Sometimes the abortion is **incomplete** and requires intervention to remove the remaining fetal material (59812). A **missed** abortion is one in which the fetus has died naturally sometime during the first half of the pregnancy but remains in the uterus. The physician removes the fetal material from the uterus and reports the service based on the trimester in which the service was provided (59820-59821). A **septic** abortion, whether induced or missed, has the added complication of infection. The physician removes the fetal material from the uterus and vigorously treats the infection (59830).

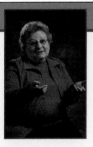

From the Trenches

"Certification means that the coder has been exposed to a lot more knowledge about coding than simply what is used in a particular workplace. It also means more money for the coder."

PATRICIA

The induced abortions are those in which the death of the fetus is brought about by medical intervention (59840-59857). One of three methods is used: dilation with either curettage (scraping) or evacuation (removal by means of suction), intra-amniotic injections, or vaginal suppositories. The selection of the code depends on which of the three methods was used to accomplish the abortion. Dilation and curettage is a procedure in which the cervix is dilated and the fetal material is scraped out by means of a curet. When the dilation and evacuation method is used, the cervix is dilated and the contents are suctioned out by means of a vacuum aspirator. The intra-amniotic injections are of urea or saline, which induces an abortion. Vaginal suppositories (such as prostaglandin) can be inserted into the cervix, with or without cervical dilation, to induce an abortion. A hysterotomy (cutting into the uterus, 59857) may be performed if the medical intervention by injection or vaginal suppositories fails.

EXERCISE 25-2   *Maternity Care and Delivery*

Using the CPT manual, code the following:

1 Laparoscopic salpingectomy for tubal ectopic pregnancy

     CPT Code: _____

2 Version of breech presentation, successfully converted to cephalic presentation, with normal spontaneous delivery

     CPT Codes: _____, _____

3 Thirty-year-old woman, 20 weeks' gestation, with cervical cerclage by vaginal approach

     CPT Code: _____

(Answers are located in Appendix B)

CHAPTER REVIEW

CHAPTER 25, PART I, THEORY

Without the use of reference material, complete the following:

1 The Female Genital System subsection is divided by _____ site from the vulva to the ovaries.

2 Skene's glands procedures are reported using codes from which subsection? _____

3 The vulva includes the following:

mons _____,

labia _____,

labia _____,

bulb of _____,

vaginal orifice or vestibule, greater and _____ glands.

4 Who is responsible for determining the complexity of destruction of lesions of the vulva? _____

5 Destruction of a lesion is also known as excision.

True   False

6 Would you expect a pathology report to be available for a lesion that was removed by destruction?

Yes   No

7 The term that describes the removal of a portion of the vulva is a(n) _____.

8 The removal of the vulvar area is reported with which two measures? _____ and _____

9 Vulvar area tissue removal that involves the skin and superficial subcutaneous tissues is termed _____.

10 Vulvar area tissue removal that involves the skin and deep subcutaneous tissues is termed _____.

11 A(n) _____ vulvectomy involves less than 80% of the vulva and a(n) _____ vulvectomy involves more than 80% of the vulva.

CHAPTER 25, PART II, PRACTICAL

Using the CPT, ICD-10-CM and/or ICD-9-CM manuals, code the following:

12 Sue Lind, age 29, has a Pap test. The pathology report comes back positive for malignancy. Her physician recommends and performs a diagnostic colposcopy. Evidence of further primary malignancy of the uterus is seen and the physician does a laparoscopically assisted vaginal hysterectomy 20 days later of a 236-gram uterus. Report only the hysterectomy and diagnosis code that indicates the medical necessity of the procedure.

CPT Code: _____

ICD-10-CM Code: _____

(ICD-9-CM Code: _____)

13 Laparoscopy with fulguration of obstructed oviducts

CPT Code: _____

ICD-10-CM Code: _____

(ICD-9-CM Code: _____)

14 Oocyte retrieval for in vitro fertilization from a donor by means of a follicle puncture

CPT Code: _____

ICD-10-CM Code: _____

(ICD-9-CM Code: _____)

15 The attending physician, who has provided Sally Fisher's obstetric care, performed a cesarean delivery, due to breech presentation, and ligation of the fallopian tubes (sterilization at the request of the patient) and routinely followed up with Sally in the postpartum period. The newborn was an 8 lb 2 oz male.

CPT Codes: _____ (Cesarean delivery, routine care); _____ (Cesarean delivery, tubal ligation)

ICD-10-CM Codes: _____ (Cesarean delivery), _____ (outcome of delivery), _____ (sterilization)

(ICD-9-CM Codes: _____ (Cesarean delivery), _____ (outcome of delivery), _____ (sterilization))

16 Colpopexy for displaced uterus using an abdominal approach

CPT Code: _____

ICD-10-CM Code: _____

(ICD-9-CM Code: _____)

17 Biopsy of three lesions of the vulva. Pathology report later indicated primary squamous cell carcinoma.

❧ CPT Code(s): _____

❧ ICD-10-CM Code(s): _____

(❧ ICD-9-CM Code(s): _____)

18 Fitting and supply of a diaphragm with instructions for use

    ✆ CPT Code(s): _____

19 Extensive biopsy of mucosa of vagina, requiring closure

    CPT Code: _____

20 Using instrumentation, the cervical canal was dilated and examination was completed.

    CPT Code: _____

21 Simple incision and drainage of an abscess of the vulva

    CPT Code: _____

22 Colpocentesis

    CPT Code: _____

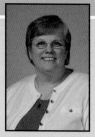
"The benefit to working in medical coding is job security, because the field is constantly expanding."

Christine A. Patterson
Coder and Biller
Reinhart Family Healthcare
Monticello, Arkansas

Endocrine and Nervous Systems

Chapter Topics

Endocrine System

Nervous System

Chapter Review

Learning Objectives

After completing this chapter you should be able to

1   Review the Endocrine System subsection format.

2   Understand the Endocrine System subheadings.

3   Demonstrate the ability to code Endocrine System services.

4   Review the Nervous System subsection format.

5   Understand the Nervous System subheadings.

6   Demonstrate the ability to code Nervous System services.

Make sure to check evolve **for the latest content updates**

ENDOCRINE SYSTEM

Format

There are nine glands in the endocrine system (Fig. 26-1), but only **four** are included in the Endocrine subsection (60000-60699) of the CPT manual. The four glands in the Endocrine subsection are:

■ Thyroid (60000-60300)
■ Parathyroid (60500-60512)
■ Thymus (60520-60522)
■ Adrenal (60540-60545, 60650)

The pituitary and pineal gland codes are in the Nervous System subsection of the CPT manual, the pancreas codes are in the Digestive System subsection, and the ovaries and testes codes are in the respective Female or Male Genital System subsections.

Coding Highlights

The Endocrine System subsection (60000-60699) includes two subheadings of:

■ Thyroid Gland
■ Parathyroid, Thymus, Adrenal Glands, Pancreas, and Carotid Body (see Fig. 26-2)

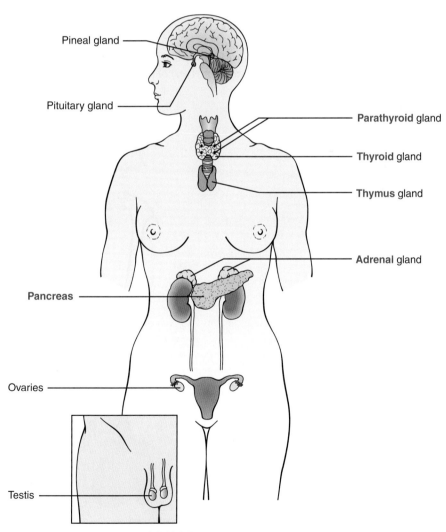

FIGURE 26-1 Endocrine system.

The **thyroid** gland is composed of a right and left lobe on either side of the trachea, just below a large piece of cartilage (thyroid cartilage). Two of the hormones secreted by the thyroid gland are T3 (triiodothyronine) and T4 (thyroxine). The thyroid gland normally produces 80% T4 and 20% T3. These hormones are necessary to maintain the normal level of metabolism in the cells of the body. Thyroid Function Tests (TFTs) assess the levels of hormones produced by the thyroid gland. Within the Thyroid Gland subheading in the CPT manual (60000-60300) there are the categories of Incision, Excision, and Removal.

Parathyroid glands are four small oval bodies located on the dorsal aspect (back) of the thyroid gland. These glands secrete parathyroid hormone (PTH). That mobilizes calcium from bones into the bloodstream, which is necessary for the proper functioning of body tissues, especially muscles. Within the Parathyroid, Thymus, Adrenal Glands, Pancreas, and Carotid Body subsection (60500-60699) there are categories Excision, Laparoscopy, and Other Procedures.

Adrenal glands (suprarenal) are two small glands situated one on top of each kidney. There are two parts to each gland, the cortex (outer portion) and the medulla (inner portion). The cortex secretes the hormones corticosteroids, and the medulla secretes the hormones catecholamines.

The **thymus** gland is located behind the breast bone, in front of the heart, and is involved in maturation (development) of the immune system. Thymectomy is removal of the thymus and is usually performed by cutting through the breast bone, similar to heart surgery.

The **pancreas** is an organ that is located behind the stomach, and the head of the organ is attached to the duodenum (first section of the small intestine). Although the organ is listed in the heading (Parathyroid, Thymus, Adrenal Glands, Pancreas, and Carotid Body), the codes for procedures involving the pancreas are located in the Digestive System subsection (48000-48999).

The **carotid body** is tissue rich in capillaries that act as receptors located near the bifurcation (splitting into two) of the carotid arteries as illustrated in Fig. 26-2. The receptors monitor

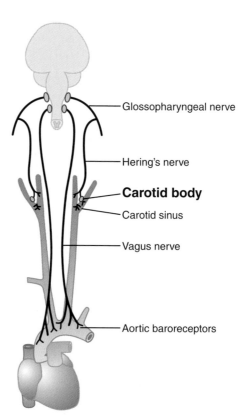

FIGURE 26–2 The baroreceptor system for controlling arterial pressure.

arterial oxygen content and pressure. Tumors that develop in the carotid body may be excised and the service reported with 60600 or 60605.

All **endocrine** glands are ductless, which means they secrete hormones directly into the bloodstream rather than through ducts leading to the exterior of the body. Exocrine glands send their chemical substances into ducts and then out of the body. Examples of **exocrine** glands are sweat, mammary, mucous, salivary, and lacrimal (tear ducts).

From the Trenches

"I think coders automatically network because no one person can know it all. We just help each other as best we can. Teamwork is the difference between a clean, accurate claim for optimum value or a denial."

CHRISTINE

Thyroid Gland Incision and Excision. A thyroidectomy is the removal of all or part of the thyroid gland. The thyroid gland consists of two lobes, one on each side of the throat, connected by a narrow band of thyroid tissue (isthmus). The term "thyroidectomy" can apply to a total removal of the gland (total thyroidectomy), removal of one or part of one of the lobes (lobectomy), or the isthmus (isthmusectomy).

A thyroidectomy is performed to assist in treatment of various thyroid diseases, such as thyroid nodules, hyperthyroidism (overactive thyroid gland), cancer of the thyroid gland, or enlargement of the thyroid (goiter) that may cause breathing or swallowing difficulties.

The amount of thyroid tissue removed is determined prior to the surgical procedure. The surgeon works closely with an endocrinologist (a physician specializing in gland tissue disorders) to determine the thyroid gland function and the amount of tissue to remove. Usually thyroid function tests (blood tests) and thyroid scanning are performed before the procedure. For cases in which thyroid cancer is suspected, a biopsy may also be performed.

A partial thyroid lobectomy is reported with 60210 or 60212 and is not performed often. For this to be the technique of choice, the lesion must be located in the upper or lower portion of only one lobe.

Total thyroid lobectomy (60220 or 60225) is typically the least complex operation performed on the thyroid gland. It is performed for solitary nodules that are suspected to be cancerous or those that are indeterminate following biopsy, such as follicular adenomas, solitary nodules, or goiters that are isolated to one lobe (not common). The procedure may or may not include an isthmusectomy (removal of the part that connects the two thyroid lobes) because the code description states "with or without isthmusectomy." An isthmusectomy removes more thyroid tissue than a simple lobectomy and is performed when a larger margin of tissue is needed to assure that all suspect tissue has been removed. Subtotal thyroidectomy (60210, 60212, 60252, 60254) is performed to excise all questionable tissue on the side of the gland as well as the isthmus and the majority of the opposite lobe. This operation is typical for small, non-aggressive thyroid neoplasms. It is also a common operation for goiters that result in problems in the neck or those that extend into the chest (substernal goiters).

Total thyroidectomy (60240, 60252) removes all of the thyroid gland and is often the procedure of choice for thyroid neoplasms that are larger and/or aggressive. Many surgeons prefer the complete removal of thyroid tissue in those patients with thyroid neoplasms regardless of the type of neoplasm.

The technique for a thyroidectomy utilizes a standard neck incision typically measuring about 4-5 inches in length. Many surgeons perform this procedure through an incision as small as 3 inches. The incision is made in the lower part of the central neck and typically involves the removal of that part of the thyroid that contains the suspect tissue. The surgeon must be careful of the laryngeal nerves that are very close to the back side of the thyroid and are responsible for movement of the vocal cords. Damage to a nerve will cause hoarseness of the voice, which although it is usually temporary, may be permanent, although this is an uncommon complication (about 1% to 2%).

A cyst may form on the thyroid and a surgeon may aspirate and/or inject the cyst. The service is reported with 60300. As with other aspiration/injection codes, if the surgeon provides an aspiration and injection, both procedures are reported with one unit of the code (60300), not two units (60300 × 2).

Parathyroid Excision. Parathyroidectomy is performed through an incision made above the collar bone that is approximately 4 inches in length. The four parathyroid glands are located by the surgeon and removed, a drain is inserted at either end of the incision, and sutures or surgical clips are applied.

EXERCISE 26-1 *Endocrine System*

Using the CPT manual, code the following. You do not need to assign -RT or -LT to the codes for this exercise.

1 Excision of an adenoma from posterior aspect of the thyroid gland

CPT Code: _____

2 Surgical removal of a thyroglossal duct cyst

CPT Code: _____

3 Thymectomy using the transthoracic approach, with radical mediastinal dissection

CPT Code: _____

4 Removal of tumor affixed to the carotid body

CPT Code: _____

5 Partial unilateral thyroid lobectomy, with isthmusectomy

CPT Code: _____

6 Surgical laparoscopy, with partial adrenalectomy, with biopsy, transabdominal approach

CPT Code: _____

7 Parathyroidectomy, with mediastinal exploration, and sternal split, with parathyroid autotransplantation

CPT Codes: _____, _____

8 Re-exploration of parathyroids, with partial thymectomy, transcervical approach

CPT Code: _____

9 Excision of carotid body tumor with excision of the carotid artery

CPT Code: _____

(Answers are located in Appendix B)

NERVOUS SYSTEM

Structure and Function of the Nervous System

Central Nervous and Peripheral Nervous Systems. The central nervous system includes the brain and spinal cord. The peripheral nervous system contains 12 pairs of cranial nerves and 31 pairs of spinal nerves as illustrated in Fig. 26-3. The peripheral nervous system is divided into the somatic nervous system, autonomic nervous system, and the enteric

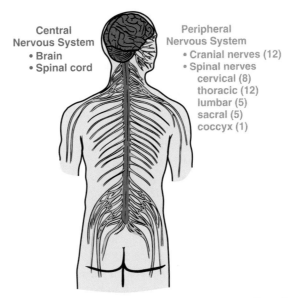

Central
Nervous System
• Brain
• Spinal cord

Peripheral
Nervous System
• Cranial nerves (12)
• Spinal nerves
   cervical (8)
   thoracic (12)
   lumbar (5)
   sacral (5)
   coccyx (1)

FIGURE 26–3   The central nervous system consists of the brain and spinal cord. The peripheral nervous system consists of nerves that lie outside the skull and spinal cord.

nervous system. The somatic nervous system coordinates body movements and receives external stimuli and is under conscious control. The autonomic nervous system is divided into the sympathetic (responds to stress), parasympathetic (constricts pupils, slows heartbeat, dilates blood vessels, stimulates digestion), and enteric divisions (manages digestion) and is not under conscious control.

Brain

- Cerebrum—largest part of the brain.
- Cerebral hemispheres—paired halves of the cerebrum. Each hemisphere is subdivided into four major lobes named for the cranial (skull) bones they overlie:
   Frontal
   Parietal
   Occipital
   Temporal
- Cerebellum—posterior part of the brain that coordinates the voluntary muscle movements and maintains balance.
- Cerebral cortex—outer region of the cerebrum (gray matter).
- Fissure—groove in the surface of the cerebral cortex.
- Medulla oblongata—part of the brain located just above the spinal cord that controls breathing, heartbeat, and blood vessel size.
- Ventricles—reservoirs in the interior of the brain filled with cerebrospinal fluid.

The following structures connect the cerebrum with the spinal cord:

- Cerebellum
- Pons (part of brain stem)
- Medulla oblongata (part of brain stem)

These terms are important as they relate to correct code assignment.

Spinal Cord.   The spinal cord is a column of nerve tissue extending from the medulla oblongata to the second lumbar vertebra. Located at the end of the spinal cord is the cauda equina (a group of nerve fibers found below the second lumbar vertebra of the spinal column). The cauda equina carries all the nerves that affect the lower part and limbs of the body and serves as the pathway for impulses going to and from the brain.

Meninges. The meninges consists of three layers of connective membranes that surround the brain and spinal cord. The outermost membrane of the meninges is the dura mater, which is a thick, tough membrane that contains channels by which blood enters the brain tissue. The subdural space is located below the dural membrane and contains multiple blood vessels. The second layer around the brain and spinal cord is the arachnoid membrane. The third layer of the meninges and the one closest to the brain and spinal cord is the pia mater.

Neurological diseases of this area are classified as:

- Congenital
- Degenerative, movement, and seizure
- Infectious
- Neoplastic
- Traumatic
- Vascular

Code Assignment

The Nervous System subsection (61000-64999) codes report procedures performed on the brain, spinal cord, nerves, and all associated parts. The subheadings are divided according to anatomic site—whether it is a part of the brain or spinal column or a type of nerve. The subheadings are further divided by **type** of procedure. The codes report services on both the central nervous system and the peripheral nervous system.

To assign the correct code, the coder must first know the **purpose** of the procedure, because many of the code descriptions indicate the condition responsible for the procedure. Examples include abscess, cyst, hematoma, foreign body, tumor, seizure, aneurysm, vascular malformation, rhinorrhea, hydrocephalus, spondylolisthesis, herniated disc, meningocele, nerve pain, spasm, neuroma, neurofibroma, in addition to the technique used for the procedure. Many of the procedures require radiological supervision and interpretation. Next, the coder must know the **location** of the procedure within the skull, meninges, or brain.

Skull, Meninges, and Brain

Punctures, Twists, or Burr Holes. The first two categories of codes are Injection, Drainage, or Aspiration (61000-61070) and Twist Drill, Burr Hole(s), or Trephine (61105-61253) that deal with conditions that may require holes or openings be made into the brain to relieve pressure, insertion of monitoring devices, placement of tubing, injection of contrast material, or to drain a hemorrhage. A **ventricular** puncture (61020-61026) requires a puncture through the top portion of the skull, while a **cisternal** puncture (61050, 61055) is an approach at the base of the skull. To accomplish many of these procedures, twist or burr holes are made through the skull, which leaves the skull intact except for the small openings (holes).

Craniectomy/Craniotomy. Codes in the category Craniectomy or Craniotomy (61304-61576) describe procedures that deal with incision into the skull with possible removal of a portion of the skull to open the operative site to the surgeon. Assignment of these codes is based on the site and condition (e.g., evacuation of hematoma, supratentorial, subdural, 61312).

As in other subsections, many procedures are bundled into one craniectomy/craniotomy code. Only by careful attention to code description can you prevent unbundling surgical procedures and incorrectly report bundled components separately. Carefully review the descriptions of these codes before assigning a code.

When craniectomies are performed, it is not uncommon that additional grafting is required to repair the surgical defect caused by opening the skull. These grafting procedures are reported separately, in addition to the major surgical procedure.

Surgery of Skull Base. The **skull base** is the area at the base of the cranium where the lobes of the brain rest. When lesions are located within the skull base, it often takes the skill of several surgeons working together to perform surgery dealing with these conditions.

The procedures located in the category Surgery of Skull Base (61580-61619) are very involved, taking many hours to complete. The procedures are divided on the approach procedure, the definitive procedure, and the reconstruction/repair procedure.

The **approach procedure** (61580-61598) is the method used to obtain exposure of the lesion (e.g., anterior cranial fossa, middle cranial fossa, posterior cranial fossa). The approach procedure is the anatomical location. The **definitive procedure** (61600-61616) is what was done to the lesion (e.g., biopsy, excision, repair, resection). If one physician did both the approach and the definitive procedures, both would be reported. For example, a neoplasm is excised at the base of the anterior cranial fossa, extradural using a craniofacial approach to the anterior skull base. This would be reported with 61600 for the procedure (definitive procedure, extradural excision of a neoplasm) and 61580 for the approach (approach procedure, craniofacial). Because two procedures (approach and definitive) were performed by the same surgeon, both codes would be reported for the physician—61600 and 61580. The most resource-intensive procedure would be listed first without a modifier (definitive), and the lesser procedure (approach) would be listed second with modifier -51 appended.

Code 61613 describes the obliteration (total destruction) of a carotid aneurysm, arteriovenous malformation, or carotid fistula and does not include the approach. Codes 61615 and 61616 report services at the base of the posterior cranial fossa and describe the resection or excision of extradural (outside the dura) or intradural (inside the dura) vascular or infectious lesions with or without graft. The approach for the resection is reported separately.

Codes in the Repair and/or Reconstruction of Surgical Defects of the Skull Base (61618, 61619) are performed to rebuild the area used for entry into the skull. This type of repair is the last step of reconstruction and is reported separately, only if the service was documented in the medical record as extensive.

At any point, one or more surgeons may be performing distinctly different portions of these complex procedures. When one surgeon performs the approach procedure, another surgeon performs the definitive procedure, and another surgeon performs the reconstruction/repair procedure, each surgeon's services would be reported with the code for the specific procedure he or she individually performed. Again, if one surgeon performs more than one procedure (e.g., the approach procedure, the definitive procedure, and the reconstruction/repair procedure), each procedure is reported separately, adding modifier -51 to the secondary procedures. For example, one surgeon performs the approach procedure (61580), definitive procedure (61600), and reconstruction/repair (61619). The services are reported as 61600 (the most resource intense), 61619-51, and 61580-51.

Aneurysm, Arteriovenous Malformation, or Vascular Disease. Aneurysms may develop within the brain and require surgical repair. An arteriovenous malformation is a condition in which the arteries and veins are not in the correct anatomic position, usually congenital. Codes to indicate the definitive procedure or repair of these conditions are located in the category Surgery for Aneurysm, Arteriovenous Malformation, or Vascular Disease (61680-61711). These codes are divided on the basis of the **approach** and **method** of procedure.

CODING SHOT

An electroencephalograph (EEG) is used to monitor currents emanating from the brain and is usually utilized any time a procedure on the brain is performed. Report the EEG service separately with 95950.

Cerebrospinal Fluid (CSF) Shunts. A **shunt** can be considered a draining device that enables fluids to flow from one area to another. A shunt is necessary when the body is not able to perform the drainage function on its own. In the case of cerebrospinal fluid shunts (62180-62258), the fluid is produced in the ventricles of the brain but does not drain properly and may continue to accumulate in the brain, building pressure and causing brain damage.

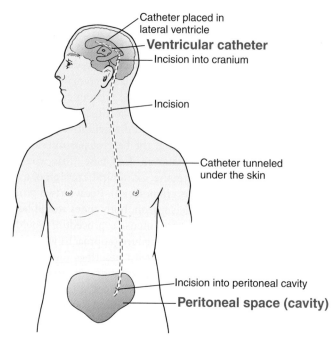

FIGURE 26-4 Ventriculoperitoneal shunt placed for chronic hydrocephalus.

Drains or shunts are placed from the area of collection to a drainage area to keep the fluid level within a normal range. For instance, code 62223 describes the creation of a shunt from the ventricle to the peritoneal space (ventriculoperitoneal), as illustrated in Fig. 26-4. This means that the shunt originates in the ventricle of the brain and terminates in the peritoneum. Codes in the CSF Shunt category describe all the various types of shunting procedures, including placement of shunting devices and subsequent repair, replacement, and removal. Shunt systems may also be placed to drain obstructed CSF from the spine.

Spine and Spinal Cord

The subheading Spine and Spinal Cord (62263-63746) includes codes for injections, laminectomies, excisions, repairs, and shunting. You should be familiar with the terminology for parts of the spinal column (Fig. 26-5). A medical dictionary will help you become familiar with the other parts of the vertebral column, including the lamina, foramina, vertebral bodies, discs, facets, and nerve roots. The basic distinction among the codes in these ranges is the **condition**

TOOLBOX

Jason requires insertion of a shunt from the ventricle to the peritoneal space due to a buildup of fluid caused by a congenital malformation in his brain. The shunt is to move the fluid from the brain to the abdomen where his body can absorb the excess fluid.

QUESTIONS

1. When you reference "Shunt, Cerebrospinal Fluid" in the index of the CPT manual, what direction do you find located there?

   _____

2. Within what ranges of codes in the CPT manual would you locate the code to report the shunt Jason received? _____

3. Which CSF code includes the use of a stereotactic neuroendoscopic method?

   _____

▼ **ANSWERS**

1. *See Cerebrospinal Fluid Shunt,* 2. 62180-62192, 62200-62223, 3. 62201

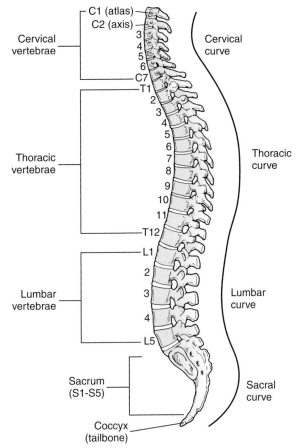

FIGURE 26–5 Vertebral column.

(such as a herniated intervertebral disc versus a neoplastic lesion of the spinal cord) as well as the **approach** (e.g., anterior, posterior, costovertebral).

The complexity of the procedure is determined by the condition and approach. For example, a patient with a herniated disc at L5-S1 would require less time in surgery for the removal of the disc and decompression of the nerve root than would a patient with a neoplastic growth intertwined in the same area, because removal of a piece of disc would not be as involved as separating a lesion from multiple components of the spinal column. The approaches differ in the amount of expertise and time required. A posterior approach means a surgical opening was formed from the back. An anterior approach means a surgical opening was formed from the front.

When reporting spinal procedures, you must determine the condition, the approach, whether the procedure was unilateral or bilateral, and whether multiple procedures were performed.

Often when a laminectomy (removal of a lamina) (Fig. 26-6) is performed, an arthrodesis (surgical fusion of joints) is also performed. In some cases spinal instrumentation procedures (the use of rods, wires, and screws to create fusions) are also performed. When multiple procedures are performed, you must review the operative report and confirm all procedures are reported.

QUICK CHECK 26-1

1. This term describes an approach that is from the front: _____, and this term describes an approach that is from the back: _____.

(Answers are located in Appendix C)

ANTERIOR

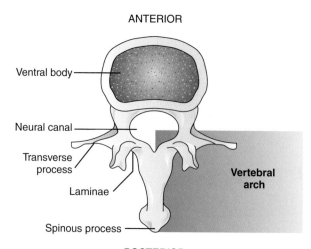

Ventral body

Neural canal

Transverse
process

Laminae

Vertebral
arch

Spinous process

POSTERIOR

FIGURE 26-6 Vertebra viewed from above.

A **lumbar puncture** (62270), or spinal tap, obtains cerebrospinal fluid by insertion of a needle into the subarachnoid space in the lumbar region, as illustrated in Fig. 26-7. The fluid is analyzed to diagnose various conditions. For example, if the fluid is pinkish in color and contains erythrocytes, there may be a hemorrhage. A yellowish, cloudy fluid with numerous white blood cells (WBCs) may indicate an infection.

Notes throughout the Spine and Spinal Cord subsection refer you to other code ranges for commonly performed additional procedures (e.g., arthrodesis codes are in the Musculoskeletal subsection). Remember to use the modifier -51 for multiple procedures if more than one procedure is performed during the operative session.

CODING SHOT

A sensory evoked study, which monitors the central nervous system, is usually performed with spinal surgery and reported separately with 95925 (upper limbs) or 95926 (lower limbs).

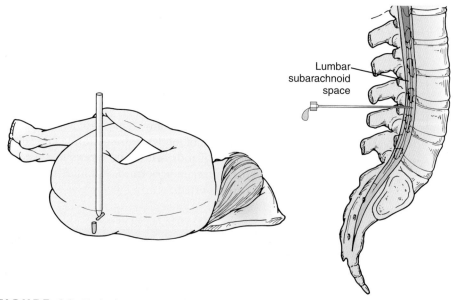

Lumbar
subarachnoid
space

FIGURE 26-7 Lumbar puncture, or spinal tap, in which the cerebrospinal fluid is obtained by inserting a needle into the subarachnoid space. The patient lies laterally with knees drawn up to increase the spaces between the vertebrae.

Destruction by a **neurolytic agent** includes chemical denervation (alcohol or glycerol by injection), radiofrequency (passes a current through an electrode carefully positioned using fluoroscopy), or cryogenic surgery (inserting a probe into tissue, with fluoroscopy guidance, and freezing a region of tissue). Codes 62280-62282 describe neurolytic substances that are injected/infused at specific anatomic sites (e.g., subarachnoid and epidural). Code 62280 reports a subarachnoid injection/infusion of a neurolytic substance. Codes 62281 and 62282 report epidural injection/infusion of a neurolytic substance based on the location as into the cervical or thoracic region (62281) or the lumbar, sacral region (62282).

CODING SHOT

Codes 62280-62282 include the injection of contrast material; therefore, the injection of contrast during fluoroscopic guidance and localization is bundled into the codes and is not reported separately.

Codes 62318 and 62319 include the setup and start of the infusion of the therapeutic substance(s). When providing the daily maintenance of the epidural or subarachnoid catheter drug administration, report the service separately with 01996.

Codes in the 62310-62319 range report injection services based on the route of administration (not type of substance administered). These codes exclude injection of a neurolytic substance (nerve destroying) that are usually reported with codes 62280-62282.

CODING SHOT

During fluoroscopic guidance (77003) for localization, the injection of contrast material is bundled into the 62310-62319 code range and not separately reported.

Extracranial Nerves, Peripheral Nerves, and Autonomic Nervous System. Nerves are our sensing devices, and they carry stimuli to and from all parts of the body. Some common procedures performed on nerves include injection, destruction, decompression, and suture/repair and are reported with codes from the Extracranial Nerves, Peripheral Nerves, and Autonomic Nervous System subheading (64400-64999).

The space around the nerves can be injected with anesthetic agents to cause a temporary loss of feeling (64400-64530). The code is assigned according to the type of nerve being injected. Nerves may also be injected to cause destruction of the nerve and permanent loss of feeling in a specific area of the body (64600-64647, 64680-64681). Persons with debilitating pain may undergo this type of procedure, and the diagnoses codes must support the medical necessity of the procedure. For example, reporting of 64612 (destruction by neurolytic agent; muscles innervated [supplied] by facial nerve) is supported by diagnosis codes such as G24.5/333.81(blepharospasm), G24.4/333.82 (oral mandibular dystonia), or G51.3/351.8 (hemifacial spasm nerve).

When reporting Introduction/Injection of Anesthetic Agent (Nerve Block), Diagnostic or Therapeutic codes in the 64400-64530 range, the coder must know the nerves, nerve groupings, and the interaction of the nerve with the body system(s). It is also important to identify the substance injected and the specific nerve the substance was injected into. Let's take a closer look at the origin of these nerves and the interaction each has with the body system(s):

■ Trigeminal nerve (5th cranial) emerges from the lateral surface of the pons. The trigeminal nerve is a sensory nerve that supplies the face, teeth, mouth and nasal cavity, and a motor nerve that supplies the muscles of mastication (chewing).

■ Facial nerve (7th cranial) consists of the large motor root (supplies the muscles of facial expression) and a smaller root (nervus intermedius) that contains the sensory and parasympathetic fibers of the facial nerve.

■ Greater occipital nerve is a spinal nerve originating from the cervical spinal nerve C2. It supplies stimuli to the scalp, over the ears, and the parotid gland.

- Vagus nerve (10th cranial) has its origin in the lateral side of medulla oblongata and supplies sensory fibers to the ear, tongue, pharynx, and larynx and motor fibers to the pharynx, larynx, and esophagus.
- Phrenic nerve affects the pleura, pericardium, diaphragm, peritoneum, and sympathetic plexuses. A plexus is a collection (aggregate) of nerves and ganglia.
- Cervical plexus (posterior) is a plexus in the posterior cervical region that is formed by the dorsal rami of the first three or four cervical spinal nerves.
- Axillary nerve originates from the brachial plexus at the axilla (armpit) level and is responsible for sensory information from the shoulder joint and the inferior region of the deltoid muscle.
- Suprascapular nerve has its origin in the brachial plexus at the C5-C6 level that descends through suprascapular and spinoglenoid notches and supplies acromioclavicular and shoulder joints, and supraspinatus muscles.
- Pudendal originates in the sacral plexus at the S2-S4, and sometimes S5. Divides into the perineal nerve and the dorsal nerve of the penis (clitoris) distributed to the muscles, skin, and erectile tissue of perineum.

Injection of anesthetic onto or around these nerves may be performed to block the pain sensation and provide relief from various pain, such as neck, lower back, myofascial pain syndrome, or cancer pain. There are many types of blocks, such as:

- Brachial plexus block for upper extremity pain.
- Celiac plexus (sympathetic nerve) block for pain in the abdomen.
- Ilioinguinal block for pain from the pelvis area (groin, inguinal, or femoral).
- Intercostal nerve block is for any of the 12 sets of nerves that travel between the spine and the rib cage.
- Sympathetic blocks the nerves that are located along both sides of the spine and supplies the limbs and the abdomen.
- Stellate ganglion block is performed for relief of sympathetic pain of the head or neck. The stellate ganglion is a group of nerves located on each side of the neck and help control blood vessels, sweat glands, and indirectly the temperature of the face, arms, and hands.
- Paravertebral nerve block is performed for pain in the cervical, thoracic, or lumbar regions.
- Somatic or sympathetic nerve injection is a rhizotomy. The agent injected may be chemical, thermal electrical, or radiofrequency.

CODING SHOT

Blocks are considered unilateral; modifier -50 should be used for bilateral procedures. When more than one level is involved, use the appropriate add-on code.

Blocks may also be performed when confirming a diagnosis. For example, a lumbar-sacral paravertebral facet joint block (64490-64495) is one method utilized to document or confirm pain of the back. The patient with this condition usually has localized back pain aggravated by motion of the spine. During the procedure, a needle is placed in the facet joint or near the facet joint nerve under fluoroscopic guidance and a local anesthetic agent is injected. After control of the pain has been obtained, the patient is asked to perform activities that usually aggravate the pain. If the patient has decreased pain or absence of pain, the facet joint is identified as the source of the pain and appropriate treatment may be prescribed.

QUICK CHECK 26-2

1. Nerve blocks to cause temporary loss of feeling are reported with this range of codes:

   _____

2. Nerve blocks to cause permanent loss of feeling are reported with this range of codes:

   _____

(Answers are located in Appendix C)

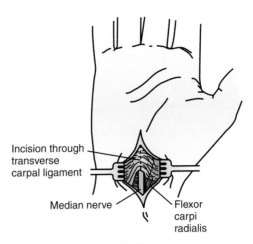

FIGURE 26–8 Carpal tunnel release.

Neuroplasty is the decompression (freeing) of intact nerves (e.g., from scar tissue). If nerves receive excessive pressure from a source, such as scar tissue or displacement of intervertebral disc material, pain may occur. Movement or freeing of nerves is reported with codes from the Neuroplasty (Exploration, Neurolysis, or Nerve Decompression) category (64702-64727). Perhaps the most commonly known neuroplasty procedure is a carpal tunnel release, reported with 64721, during which the median nerve and the transverse carpal ligament of the wrist are surgically released (Fig. 26-8).

Nerves can also be removed or they can be repaired (sutured). The codes in the Neurorrhaphy (64831-64876) and the Neurorrhaphy with Nerve Graft (64885-64911) categories describe nerve repairs on the basis of the specific nerve being repaired. This category also includes codes that describe grafting on the basis of the size of the graft.

EXERCISE 26-2 *Nervous System*

Using the CPT, ICD-10-CM and/or ICD-9-CM manuals, code the following:

1 Drainage of a nontraumatic subdural hematoma using burr holes

CPT Code: _____

ICD-10-CM Code: _____ (ICD-9-CM Code: _____)

2 Drainage of traumatic subdural hematoma with craniectomy, supratentorial

CPT Code: _____

ICD-10-CM Code: _____ (ICD-9-CM Code: _____)

3 Resection of primary, malignant neoplasm, midline skull base, extradural, using infratemporal post-auricular approach to middle cranial fossa

CPT Codes: _____, _____

ICD-10-CM Code: _____ (ICD-9-CM Code: _____)

4 Removal of complete cerebrospinal fluid shunt system, with replacement due to congenital hydrocephalus

CPT Code: _____

ICD-10-CM Code: _____ (ICD-9-CM Code: _____)

(Answers are located in Appendix B)

CHAPTER REVIEW

CHAPTER 26, PART I, THEORY

Complete the following:

1 How many endocrine glands are included in the Endocrine subsection of the CPT manual?

_____

2 The pituitary and pineal gland procedure codes are in what subsection of the Surgery section?

_____

3 The codes for pancreatic procedures are located in what subsection of the Surgery section?

_____

4 Both subtotal and partial mean something less than _____.

5 Twist or _____ holes are made through the skull to accomplish procedures of the brain.

6 The _____ procedure is the method used to obtain exposure to a lesion of the skull base, and the

_____ procedure is what is done to the lesion.

7 CSF means _____.

8 The most commonly known neuroplasty procedure is a(n) _____ _____ release.

9 This term describes the location of the bifurcation of the carotid artery in the neck: _____

_____

10 Would you report separately the additional grafting required to repair the surgical defect caused by a craniectomy?

Yes No

Chapter Review answers are only available in the TEACH Instructor Resources on Evolve

CHAPTER 26, PART II, PRACTICAL

Code the following cases using the CPT manual:

11 Total thyroidectomy

CPT Code: _____

12 Surgical laparoscopy with partial adrenalectomy using a transabdominal approach

CPT Code: _____

13 Parathyroidectomy with mediastinal exploration

CPT Code: _____

14 Stereotactic creation of a thalamus lesion with multiple staging

CPT Code: _____

15 Torkildsen type operation with CSF shunt insertion

CPT Code: _____

16 Implantation of a tunneled epidural catheter for long-term administration of medication

CPT Code: _____

17 Partial resection of a single segment of a vertebral (cervical) body using an anterior approach with decompression of the spinal cord and nerve roots

CPT Code: _____

18 Therapeutic injection of the greater occipital nerve with an anesthetic agent

CPT Code: _____

19 Complete transection of the facial nerve

CPT Code: _____

20 Nerve graft of a single strand of nerve, 5 cm in length, to the foot, procedure included procurement of graft

CPT Code: _____

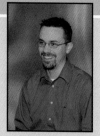

"Most will struggle with terminology, but asking questions will save and often benefit your career. Take my word for it, the best thing you can do is keep asking questions until you understand."

Thomas Mobley, CPC, COC, CEDC, CIRCC, CPC-I
Healthcare Coding Consultants, LLC
Gilbert, Arizona

Eye, Ocular Adnexa, Auditory, and Operating Microscope

Chapter Topics

Eye and Ocular Adnexa

Auditory System

Operating Microscope

Chapter Review

Learning Objectives

After completing this chapter you should be able to

1 Review the Eye and Ocular Adnexa subsection.

2 Understand the Eye and Ocular Adnexa subheadings.

3 Demonstrate the ability to code Eye and Ocular Adnexa services.

4 Review the Auditory System subsection format.

5 Understand Auditory System subheadings.

6 Demonstrate the ability to code Auditory System services.

7 Review reporting use of an operating microscope.

8 Demonstrate the ability to report the use of an operating microscope.

Make sure to check
evolve
for the latest
content updates

EYE AND OCULAR ADNEXA

Format

The Eye and Ocular Adnexa subsection (65091-68899) includes the subheadings Eyeball, Anterior Segment, Posterior Segment, Ocular Adnexa, and Conjunctiva. There are the typical incision, excision, repair, and destruction categories but also some that are unique. For example, the subheading Eyeball includes categories for both Removal of Eye (65091-65114) and Removal of Foreign Body (65205-65265), although you would expect to find all removal codes in a removal category.

From the Trenches

"The keys to long-term success are flexibility and a lust for knowledge. This field is ever evolving and growing, for to remain relevant you must embrace that change."

TOM

CODING SHOT

Remember to use modifier -50 (bilateral procedure) when the procedure is performed on both eyes. Modifiers -RT and -LT may be assigned for bilateral procedures of anatomic sites that are in pairs; i.e., eyes, breasts, legs, arms, etc.

In this section are codes that include previous surgery to the eye. For example, in the subheading Ocular Adnexa, 67331 is reported for patients undergoing strabismus surgery who have had previous eye surgery or injury. Also, the category Prophylaxis (preventive treatment) (67141, 67145), under the subheading Posterior Segment, has notes regarding the assignment of these codes. The Prophylaxis codes include all the sessions in a treatment period. The Destruction codes in this subcategory include "one or more sessions." Read the code descriptions carefully so you know which elements are included in the code because what is or is not included in the code descriptions varies greatly.

As in all sections of the CPT manual, there are directional notes throughout that will help you think about what defines a particular code. For example, code 67850 is for the "Destruction of lesion of lid margin (up to 1 cm)." This description includes a note in parentheses: "(For Mohs micrographic surgery, see 17311-17315)." This helpful note gives you the category of codes to refer to if the lesion destruction was performed using Mohs micrographic surgery.

Refer to Figs. 27-1 through 27-4 as you prepare to code services to the eye and ocular adnexa.

Eyeball

Removal of Eye. The Removal of Eye category contains codes to report **evisceration**, which is removal of the contents of the globe while leaving the extraocular muscles and sclera intact (65091, 65093); **enucleation**, which is removal of the eye while leaving

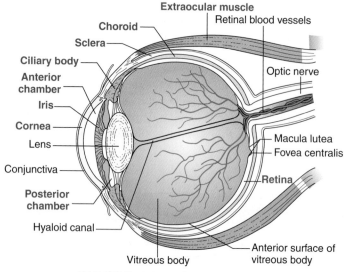

Extraocular muscle
Retinal blood vessels
Choroid
Sclera
Ciliary body
Optic nerve
Anterior chamber
Iris
Cornea
Macula lutea
Lens
Fovea centralis
Conjunctiva
Retina
Posterior chamber
Hyaloid canal
Anterior surface of vitreous body
Vitreous body

FIGURE 27–1 Eye and ocular adnexa.

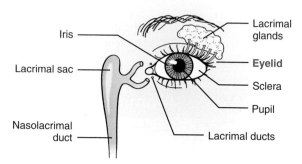

Iris
Lacrimal glands
Lacrimal sac
Eyelid
Sclera
Nasolacrimal duct
Pupil
Lacrimal ducts

FIGURE 27–2 Lacrimal apparatus.

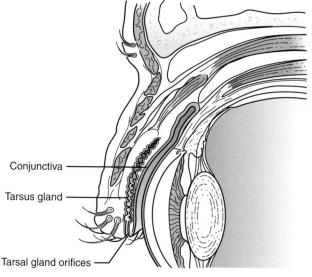

Conjunctiva
Tarsus gland
Tarsal gland orifices

FIGURE 27–3 Eyelid.

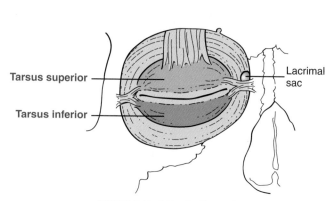

Tarsus superior
Lacrimal sac
Tarsus inferior

FIGURE 27–4 Two tarsi.

the orbital structures intact, (65101-65105); and **exenteration**, which is removal of the eye, adnexa, and part of the bony orbit (65110-65114). The codes in the Removal of Eye category are divided based on which of these procedures was performed, if an implant was inserted, and in the case of the exenteration, if the bony orbit was removed or a muscle or myocutaneous flap was performed. These codes do not report skin grafting to the orbit. When the operative report indicates skin grafting, report the service separately with codes from the Integumentary System (15120/15121 or 15260/15261). If the eyelid was repaired deeper than skin level, refer to the reconstruction codes 67930/67935 (partial or full thickness repair).

Secondary Implant(s) Procedures. Implants may be placed inside the muscular cone (ocular implant or fake eye) or outside the muscular cone (orbital implant) as illustrated in Fig. 27-5. The ocular implant is the artificial eye, and the orbital implant replaces the orbit that was occupied by the eyeball before removal. With some implants, the muscles are attached to the implant to enable the artificial eye to move and thus appear more natural. The codes in the 65125-65155 range report a subsequent implantation of ocular implants based on the type of service provided with the implant, such as grafting or attachment of muscles to implant. Removal of an ocular implant is reported with 65175. An orbital implant is a cosmetic device that covers the outer portion of the eye and is also known as a scleral shell prosthesis. Orbital implant insertion is reported with 67550 and removal with 67560.

Removal of Foreign Body. Note the extensive list of parenthetical notes preceding 65205. Take time now to read these notes as they list important concepts that you need to know. The removal codes are for foreign bodies that are located in the external eye or the intraocular eye. A **slit lamp** is a low-powered microscope with a high-intensity light source that focuses the light as a long narrow beam (slit) and is used to examine eyes (Fig. 27-6). Note that the only difference between 65220 and 65222 is whether a slit lamp is or is not utilized.

Repair of Laceration. The repair codes are assigned to report laceration repair based on where the laceration is located (conjunctiva, cornea, and/or sclera). Code 65286 reports the application of tissue glue for a perforation of the eyeball.

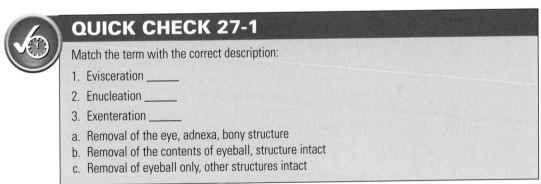

QUICK CHECK 27-1

Match the term with the correct description:

1. Evisceration _____
2. Enucleation _____
3. Exenteration _____

a. Removal of the eye, adnexa, bony structure
b. Removal of the contents of eyeball, structure intact
c. Removal of eyeball only, other structures intact

(Answers are located in Appendix C)

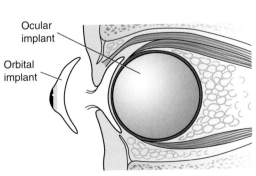

FIGURE 27-5   Ocular and orbital implants.

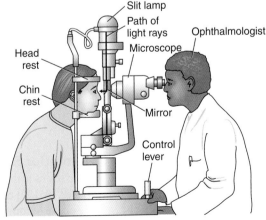

FIGURE 27-6   A slit lamp is a microscope with a light attached. The name is derived from the adjustable light beam.

Anterior Segment

The anterior segment includes the cornea, anterior chamber, anterior sclera, iris, ciliary body, and lens.

Cornea. The cornea is the transparent part of the eye. The cornea may be the site of a superficial lesion that is completely removed and reported with 65400. If only a portion of the corneal lesion was removed for pathology analysis, report the service as a biopsy with 65410.

A **keratoplasty** is repair of the cornea. Codes 65710-65756 report keratoplasty based on the type of procedure performed and include grafts and preparation of donor material. A penetrating keratoplasty (65730-65755) is the removal of the full thickness of the cornea and replacement with donor cornea. A lamellar keratoplasty (65710) is a procedure in which only a thin layer of the cornea is removed and replaced with donor cornea. **Aphakia** is absence of the lens of the eye, and **pseudophakia** is the presence of an artificial lens after cataract surgery. These terms are in three of the keratoplasty code descriptions.

Anterior Chamber. The anterior chamber of the eye is a fluid-filled (aqueous humor) space, located behind the cornea and in front of the iris. The categories of Incision (65800-65880), Removal (65900-65930), and Introduction (66020-66030) are for procedures performed on the anterior chamber of the eye.

Paracentesis is the removal of fluid. When a physician performs paracentesis of the anterior chamber of the eye, a needle is inserted into the anterior chamber and fluid is withdrawn. The fluid may be withdrawn for diagnostic purposes (65800) or for therapeutic purposes (65810-65815). If an injection procedure is also performed, report 66020 or 66030.

Goniotomy (65820) is a surgical procedure that utilizes an instrument called a goniolens. This procedure may be performed for congenital glaucoma, a condition in which the optic nerve at the back of the eye may be damaged and cause a loss of vision, especially peripheral vision. A note following code 65820 directs the coder not to use modifier -63 (procedure performed on infants less than 4 kg) with the code.

Codes for severing adhesions or scar tissue from the anterior chamber of the eye are based on the location of the adhesion or scar tissue (65860-65880). **Posterior synechiae** are adhesions of the iris to the lens of the eye, and **anterior synechiae** are adhesions of the iris to the cornea. Severing of the adhesions is performed using either laser (66821) or incisional technique.

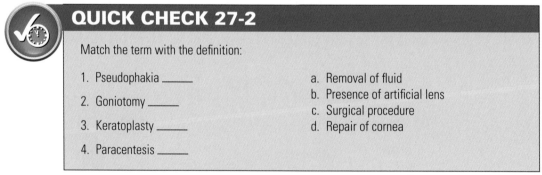

QUICK CHECK 27-2

Match the term with the definition:

1. Pseudophakia _____
2. Goniotomy _____
3. Keratoplasty _____
4. Paracentesis _____

a. Removal of fluid
b. Presence of artificial lens
c. Surgical procedure
d. Repair of cornea

(Answers are located in Appendix C)

Anterior Sclera. The sclera is the white, fibrous outer layer of the eyeball and the anterior sclera is the front part of the eye. The anterior sclera may be the site of lesions that are excised (66130) by incision of the conjunctiva to gain access to the lesion. Depending on the size of the lesion, the area of the sclera may not require sutures.

Sometimes, the flow of the aqueous humor is not absorbed or too much fluid is produced, and a surgeon may perform a fistulization (creation of a passage) of the sclera to decrease the pressure. The fistulization can be created by means of removal of a portion of the sclera and iris (e.g., 66150), thermocauterization (e.g., hot probe, 66155), or punch or scissor removal (e.g., 66160). A trabeculotomy ab externo or trabeculectomy ab externo (e.g., 65850, 66170, 66172) is a surgical procedure in which the trabecular meshwork (iris-scleral junction, drains aqueous humor) is reshaped or punctured. This procedure may be performed as a treatment for glaucoma.

Iris, Ciliary Body. The ciliary body is located behind the iris (colored part of the eye) and produces aqueous humor. The smooth muscle of the ciliary body attaches to the lens. An iridectomy is usually performed for removal of a lesion (66600) or as a treatment for glaucoma (66625, 66630) by creation of an opening to drain aqueous humor. If the iridotomy/iridectomy is performed by means of laser, report the procedure with 66761. If an iridoplasty is performed by means of photocoagulation, report the procedure with 66762.

Lens. A common procedure performed on the lens of the eye is cataract removal. Cataract removal and lens replacements (66830-66990) utilize one of two different approaches or techniques:
■ Extracapsular cataract extraction (66984) (ECCE) is partial removal of the capsule and is the most common method. It removes the hard nucleus of the lens in one piece and the soft cortex in multiple pieces. The posterior lens capsule is left in place.
■ Intracapsular cataract extraction (66983) (ICCE) is the removal of the lens and surrounding lens capsule, which removes the cataract in one piece.
Today, most cataract surgery is performed using phacoemulsification, which dissolves the hard nucleus by ultrasound, then removes the soft cortex in multiple pieces.

Extraocular Muscles. Under the subheading of Ocular Adnexa are codes for strabismus surgery, which corrects muscle misalignment. The codes are divided based on repair of vertical (67314, 67316) or horizontal (67311, 67312) muscles and are reported by the number of muscles repaired. Vertical muscles move the eye up and down, while the horizontal muscles move the eye side to side.

Orbit. Under the subheading Orbit are codes for orbitotomy and fine needle aspiration. The orbitotomy codes are divided based on the approach and if a bone flap was or was not placed. Orbitotomy that is performed without a bone flap and with either a frontal or transconjunctival approach (illustrated in Fig. 27-7) is reported with codes 67400-67414. Orbitotomy performed with a bone flap and with a lateral approach is reported with codes 67420-67450. The codes for a transcranial orbitotomy are located in the Nervous System subsection (61330-61333). Within the Orbit subheading there is also a code (67415) for fine needle aspiration of the orbital contents, and it is usually performed as a biopsy method for an orbital mass.

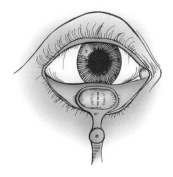

FIGURE 27-7 Transconjunctival approach.

Eyelids. The Eyelids subheading includes procedures performed by incision, excision, destruction, and tarsorrhaphy (suturing the eyelids together). There are also codes to report eyelid repair and reconstruction. Eyelid repairs include ectropion (outward sagging/turning, 67914-67917) as illustrated in Fig. 27-8 and entropion (inward turning, 67921-67924) illustrated in Fig. 27-9.

HCPCS modifiers are added to the procedure code to indicate the specific eyelid:

- ■ -E1 upper left eyelid
- ■ -E2 lower left eyelid
- ■ -E3 upper right eyelid
- ■ -E4 lower right eyelid

Conjunctiva. The Conjunctiva subheading includes Incision and Drainage (68020, 68040), Excision and/or Destruction (68100-68135), Injection (68200), Conjunctivoplasty (68320-68340), and the Lacrimal System (68400-68850). Conjunctivoplasty (68326-68328) involves reconstruction of the cul-de-sac with a conjunctival graft or rearrangement. Lacrimal System (see Fig. 27-2) procedures includes incision, excision, repair, and probing. The most common procedure performed is nasolacrimal duct probing generally due to an obstruction and reported with 68810 or 68811.

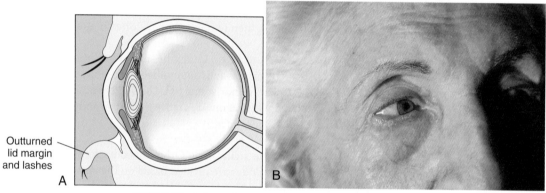

FIGURE 27–8 Ectropion is an outward sagging of the eyelid.

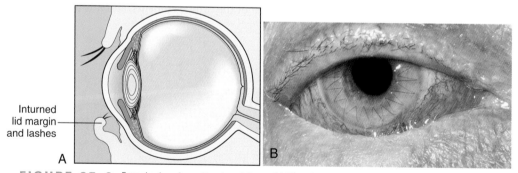

FIGURE 27–9 Entropion is an inward turning of the eyelid. (Note that the patient in **B** has undergone corneal transplantation.)

EXERCISE 27-1 *Eye and Ocular Adnexa*

Using the CPT manual, code the following:

1 Blood clot removal from anterior segment of the left eye

CPT Code: _____

2 New patient strabismus surgery involving the superior oblique muscle of the right eye

CPT Code: _____

3 Xenon arc used in three sessions to prevent retinal detachment of left eye

CPT Code: _____

4 Corneal incision for revision of earlier procedure that resulted in astigmatism of right eye

CPT Code: _____

5 Removal of left eye, with implant, muscles attached to implant

CPT Code: _____

(Answers are located in Appendix B)

AUDITORY SYSTEM

Format

The Auditory System subsection (69000-69979) is divided into the subheadings External Ear, Middle Ear, Inner Ear, and Temporal Bone, Middle Fossa Approach. The first three subheadings represent the anatomic divisions of the auditory system: external, middle, and inner ear (Fig. 27-10). The categories listed under each subheading include introduction, incision, excision, removal, repair, and other procedures, depending on the particular subheading. The subheading Temporal Bone, Middle Fossa Approach (69950-69979) contains codes that describe

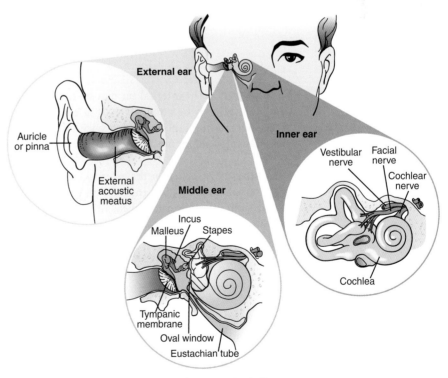

FIGURE 27-10 Auditory system.

various surgical procedures in which the surgeon makes an incision anterior to the auricle and extends superiorly, exposing the temporalis muscle. Through this incision, the surgeon performs a craniotomy and exposes the brain. The surgeon then repairs the nerve, removes a tumor, or otherwise treats the area.

OPERATING MICROSCOPE

The code for reporting the use of an operating microscope, 69990, is in a subsection of a single code following the Auditory System subsection. This code is an add-on code and is never reported alone; rather, it is reported with the procedure in which the operating microscope was used. Code 69990 is assigned with codes from any subsection within the Surgery section. Read the extensive notes preceding the code to better understand when this code should or should not be reported.

EXERCISE 27-2 *Auditory System*

Using the CPT manual, code the following:

1 Left labyrinthotomy with cryosurgery with multiple perfusions, transcanal

CPT Code: _____

2 Bilateral insertion of pressure equalization tubes, using general anesthesia

CPT Codes: _____, _____

3 Transcranial approach with sectioning of the left vestibular nerve

CPT Code: _____

4 Reconstruction of the right external auditory canal, due to injury

CPT Code: _____

5 Establishment of an opening in the inner wall of the right inner ear, semicircular canal

CPT Code: _____

(Answers are located in Appendix B)

External Ear

Incision. The external ear may be the site of an abscess or hematoma, and the incision and drainage may be simple (69000) or complicated (69005). If the abscess drained is within the auditory canal, report the service with 69020. Be careful when reporting 69020 as it can be bundled into a major procedure and not reported separately.

Excision. Codes for the external ear include biopsy by location of external ear (69100) or external auditory canal (69105), excision of the external ear, either partially or complete (69110, 69120). If the external ear was reconstructed after the excision, report the repair with split thickness autograft codes (15120, 15121) from the Integumentary System based on the square centimeters used in the repair.

Exostosis is a bony growth and when present in the external auditory canal, it is termed "surfer's ear," because it is associated with chronic cold water exposure. An incision is made behind the ear to gain access to the canal, and the bony growth is excised (69140).

Removal of Foreign Body. With the shape of the ear, it is easy to see how foreign bodies and cerumen (earwax) can become lodged in the external ear. When a foreign body is removed from the ear, the code reported is based on whether general anesthesia was or was not used (69200, 69205). Removal of impacted cerumen (69210) by means of instrumentation is reported with modifier -50 if the procedure was bilateral.

Repair.   An **otoplasty** is a procedure performed for a protruding ear that may or may not include a decrease in the size of the ear. This procedure is usually performed with the use of conscious sedation, which is included in 69300. When an otoplasty is performed bilaterally, modifier -50 is added to code.

Reconstruction of the external auditory canal (canalplasty/canaloplasty) may be performed for conditions such as stenosis due to injury or infection (69310) or for a congenital defect (69320). Canaloplasty is bundled into some middle ear repair codes, such as 69631-69646 and not reported separately.

Middle Ear

Myringotomy and Tympanostomy.   The eustachian tube connects the middle ear to the back of the throat and allows for drainage of fluid. When a eustachian tube dysfunctions, fluid collects in the middle ear. The tube can also become inflamed from allergies or infection. Eustachian tube dysfunction is a fairly common condition in children, because the tube does not always mature to the level of normal function and therefore does not function properly. The fluid or inflammation prevents air from entering the middle ear, resulting in a pressure increase in the middle ear. Surgical intervention is an inflation of the eustachian tube with access through the nose (transnasal). **Myringotomy** is the incision into the tympanic membrane (69420, 69421) and reinflation of the eustachian tube. **Tympanostomy** is the insertion of a small plastic or metal tube (PE [pressure equalization] tube) that allows the fluid to drain (69433, 69436). The tubes may later be removed, fall out naturally, or sometimes be left in place. Surgical removal of a ventilation tube is reported with 69424, which is a procedure that requires general anesthesia. Ventilation tube removal is bundled into many major procedures, in which case the removal is not reported separately.

CODING SHOT

Code 69424 is unilateral, so if the tubes were removed bilaterally, add modifier -50.

TOOLBOX

PE tubes are often recommended for children with repeated ear infections (acute otitis media) or those who have hearing loss due to constant middle ear fluid (otitis media with effusion). In fact, PE tubes are the most common childhood surgery.

QUESTIONS
1. The surgical procedure in which PE tubes are inserted is a(n) _____.
2. If an ear tube was not inserted, the incision into the tympanic membrane would do what in just a few days? _____
3. The tiny PE tubes allow what to enter the middle ear? _____

▼ **ANSWERS**

1. tympanostomy, 2. heal or close up, 3. air

Excision.   Middle ear excision procedures include antrotomy (simple mastoidectomy, 69501), mastoidectomy (complete, modified radical, or radical, 69502-69511), polyp removal (69540), and tumor removal (69550-69554).

Also included in the Excision category is a petrous apicectomy. The petrous apex (Fig. 27-11) of the temporal bone may be the site of infection (petrous apicitis) that can lead to more complicated infection, such as brain abscess or meningitis. Sometimes, to remove the infected bone, a mastoidectomy is performed and is included in the petrous apicectomy code 69530.

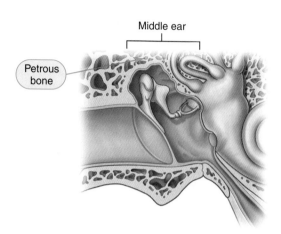

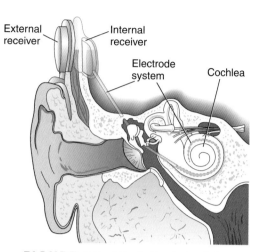

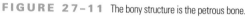

FIGURE 27–11 The bony structure is the petrous bone.

FIGURE 27–12 Cochlear implant device.

Repair. Middle ear repair procedures include revision mastoidectomies based on the extent of the procedure. For example, a simple mastoidectomy is performed on a patient with cholesteatoma of the middle ear. A **cholesteatoma** is a benign growth of skin in an abnormal location, in this case in the middle ear. The growth may reoccur and the surgeon may perform a complete mastoidectomy (69601). If the disease has progressed to the point where the tympanic membrane is damaged and requires repair, the procedure is reported with 69604.

The two major divisions in the tympanoplasty codes are with or without removal of the mastoid bone (mastoidectomy). When no mastoidectomy is performed, choose the code from the 69631-69633 range, based on the extent of the procedure. When a mastoidectomy is performed, report the service with codes from the 69641-69646 range, based on the extent of the procedure. The **ossicular chain** is the bones of the ear that include the malleus (hammer), incus (anvil), and stapes (stirrup). The chain may be eroded and repaired as a part of a tympanoplasty (69632 or 69642). The repair may be so extensive that it may require the use of prosthesis, such as a partial ossicular replacement prosthesis (PORP, incus and malleus are absent or damaged) or total ossicular replacement prosthesis (TORP, incus and arch of the stapes are damaged, or the malleus, incus and arch of the stapes are absent). PORP and TORP are reported with 69633 or 69637, depending upon other repairs performed during the tympanoplasty.

Inner Ear

Incision and/or Destruction. A **labyrinth** is a cavelike structure, located in the inner ear. The labyrinth is dominated by two fluid-filled spaces that contain endolymph and perilymph. These spaces contain the nerve tissue responsible for hearing and balance. When the pressure within the space is altered, vertigo, ringing in the ears, and hearing loss may occur. A **labyrinthotomy** is a procedure in which the labyrinth is surgically incised and various procedures performed to return the labyrinth to functional condition. Code 69801 is reported for a labyrinthotomy.

Excision. A **labyrinthectomy** is a procedure in which the incus and stapes are removed. If a transcanal approach is used, report 69905. If a postauricular incision (behind the ear) is used as the approach, report 69910.

Introduction. A **cochlear device implant** (Fig. 27-12) is a computerized device that restores partial hearing in those who are profoundly hearing impaired. A receiver on the outside of the skin behind the ear picks up sound waves. The receiver is placed over the transmitter, which is surgically implanted under the skin behind the ear. A sound processor is connected to an electrode implanted between the processor and the cochlea, and it receives a signal from the transmitter and transfers the signal to the cochlear nerve. The implantation of the cochlear device is reported with 69930.

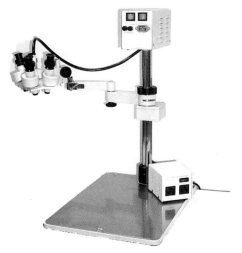

FIGURE 27–13 The operating microscope allows for visualization of minute structures, such as nerve fibers and blood vessels.

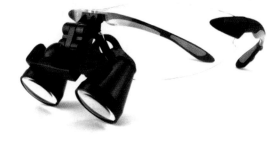

FIGURE 27–14 Magnifying loupes are produced in a range of powers.

Temporal Bone, Middle Fossa Approach. The middle fossa approach is used by surgeons to excise acoustic neuromas, to decompress the facial nerve (proximal temporal), and repair nerves in the vestibular labyrinth. The codes in the Temporal Bone, Middle Fossa Approach subheading report removal of the vestibular nerve (69950), relief of pressure (decompression) of the facial nerve and/or repair (69955), decompression of the internal auditory canal (69960), and removal of tumors of the temporal bone (69970).

Operating Microscope. An operating microscope (Fig. 27-13) is used in microsurgical procedures and is reported separately with add-on code 69990, unless the code indicates the inclusion of use of an operating microscope. This does not include magnifying loupes (Fig. 27-14) that are used to enlarge the area being viewed.

QUICK CHECK 27-3

1. The operating microscope code is used only with procedures on the ear.
   True or False?

(Answers are located in Appendix C)

EXERCISE 27-3   *Ear and Operating Microscope*

Complete the following:

1 This is a bony growth that is also known as surfer's ear: _____

2 For a protruding ear, the surgeon may perform this procedure: _____

3 This is a benign growth of the skin in an abnormal location, such as the middle ear: _____

4 The code to report the use of an operating microscope in addition to the procedure is _____.

(Answers are located in Appendix B)

CHAPTER REVIEW

CHAPTER 27, PART I, THEORY

Complete the following:

Match the terms for the ossicular chain:

1 hammer _____   a. Incus

2 anvil _____   b. Stapes

3 stirrup _____   c. Malleus

4 This is a benign growth of skin in an abnormal location.
   a cholesteatoma
   b glucogonomas
   c TSH-oma
   d schwannoma

5 This is the removal of the eye, adnexa, and part of the bony orbit.
   a evisceration
   b enucleation
   c exenteration
   d none of the above

6 This is a low-powered microscope with a high-intensity light source that focuses the light as a long narrow beam and is used to examine the eyes.
   a goniolens
   b otoscope
   c ophthalmoscope
   d slit lamp

7 This is a cosmetic implant that covers the outer portion of the eye and is also known as a scleral shell prosthesis.
   a ocular
   b orbital
   c conjunctival
   d intraocular

8 This is a bony growth that is also known as surfer's ear because it is associated with chronic cold water exposure.
   a vestibular
   b mastoiditis
   c exostosis
   d labyrinthitis

9 During this procedure, small plastic or metal tubes are inserted through the tympanic membrane to allow for the drainage of fluid. Later the tubes may be removed, fall out naturally, or be left in place.
   a myringotomy
   b antrotomy
   c tympanostomy
   d mastoidectomy

10 This is a cavelike structure that is dominated by two fluid-filled spaces.
   a labyrinth
   b auricle
   c external acoustic meatus
   d malleus

Chapter Review answers are only available in the TEACH Instructor Resources on Evolve

CHAPTER 27, PART II, PRACTICAL

Code the following cases using the CPT, ICD-10-CM and/or ICD-9-CM manuals:

11 Excision of corneal lesion of right eye

CPT Code: _____

12 Iridectomy with corneal section for removal of lesion from left eye

CPT Code: _____

13 Left lamellar keratoplasty with replacement of a thin layer of the cornea with donor cornea

CPT Code(s): _____

14 Corneal biopsy of the right eye

CPT Code(s): _____

15 Diagnostic paracentesis of aqueous in the anterior chamber of the left eye

CPT Code: _____

16 A one stage, right eye ECCE with insertion of intraocular lens prosthesis using a manual technique

CPT Code: _____

17 A one stage ICCE of the left eye with insertion of intraocular lens prosthesis

CPT Code: _____

18 Iridotomy for removal of a primary lesion by means of corneal section, right

CPT Code: _____

19 A male patient, age 69, with type 2 diabetes and progressive diabetic retinopathy resulting in retinal hemorrhage. The physician provides three sessions of photocoagulation to his right eye over the course of 2 weeks

CPT Code: _____

ICD-10-CM Codes: _____, _____

(ICD-9-CM Codes: _____, _____)

20 Repair of a detached right retina by means of an encircling procedure and including scleral dissection, implant, cryotherapy, and drainage of subretinal fluid

CPT Code: _____

ICD-10-CM Code: _____

(ICD-9-CM Code: _____)

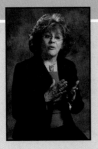

"Try not to stay in just one specialty. Become educated and learn other specialties so you can grow in all types of coding."

Patricia Champion, CPC
Licensed PMCC Instructor, Educator/Trainer
AAPC National Advisory Board
Nashville, Tennessee

Radiology

Chapter Topics

Learning Objectives

After completing this chapter you should be able to

1 Demonstrate an understanding of Radiology terminology.

2 Analyze the elements of component coding in reporting radiology services.

3 Identify elements of the global procedure.

4 State the appropriate coding of contrast material.

5 Explain the format of the Radiology section.

6 Demonstrate the ability to code Radiology services and procedures.

Make sure to check **evolve** for the latest content updates

FORMAT

Radiology is the branch of medicine that uses radiant energy to diagnose and treat patients. The term originally referred to the use of x-rays to produce radiographs but is now commonly applied to all types of medical imaging. A physician who specializes in radiology is a **radiologist.** Radiologists can provide services to patients independent of or in conjunction with another physician of a different specialty. The Radiology section of the CPT manual is divided into subsections:

- Diagnostic Radiology (Diagnostic Imaging)
- Diagnostic Ultrasound
- Radiologic Guidance
- Breast, Mammography
- Bone/Joint Studies
- Radiation Oncology
- Nuclear Medicine

RADIOLOGY TERMINOLOGY

The suffix *-graphy* means "making of a film" using a variety of methods. **Radiography** is a broad term used to indicate any number of methods used by radiologists to do diagnostic testing. The following exercise will familiarize you with some of the numerous radiographic procedures in the CPT manual.

EXERCISE 28-1 *Radiology Terminology*

The following words end in "-graphy," meaning "making of a film." For example, in angiocardiography, "angio" means vessels and "cardio" means heart, so angiocardiography is the making of a film of the heart and vessels. What do the other "-graphy" words mean?

angiocardiography _____ heart and vessels _____

1 aortography _____

2 arthrography _____

3 cholangiopancreatography _____

4 cholangiography _____

5 cystography _____

6 dacryocystography _____

7 duodenography _____

8 echocardiography _____

9 encephalography _____

10 epididymography _____

11 hepatography _____

12 hysterosalpingography _____

13 laryngography _____

14 lymphangiography _____

15 myelography _____

16 pyelography _____

Continued

17 sialography _____

18 sinography _____

19 splenography _____

20 urography _____

21 venography _____

22 vesiculography _____

(Answers are located in Appendix B)

TERMS

Here are just a few more radiographic terms for your review:

1. **Fluoroscopy** is an x-ray procedure that allows the visualization of internal organs in motion. It uses real-time video images. After x-rays pass through the patient, instead of using film, the images are captured by a device called an image intensifier and converted into light. The light is then captured by a camera and displayed on a video monitor. Fluoroscopy allows the study of the function of the organ (physiology) as well as the structure of the organ (anatomy).

2. **Magnetic resonance imaging (MRI)** is a radiology technique that uses magnetism, radio waves, and a computer to produce images of body structures. The MRI scanner is a tube surrounded by a giant circular magnet. The patient is placed on a moveable bed that is inserted into the magnet. The magnet creates a strong magnetic field that aligns the protons of hydrogen atoms, which are then exposed to a beam of radio waves. This spins the various protons of the body and produces a faint signal that is detected by the receiver portion of the MRI scanner. The received information is processed by a computer, and an image is then produced.

3. **Tomography** is the process of producing a tomogram, a two-dimensional image of a slice or section, through a three-dimensional object. Tomography achieves this result by simply moving an x-ray source in one direction as the x-ray film is moved in the opposite direction. The tomogram is the picture, tomograph is the apparatus, and tomography is the process.

4. **Biometry** is the application of a statistical method to a biologic fact. For example, the application of this science in radiology has resulted in analysis of data, for example, of the effectiveness of radiation used in the treatment of brain tumors—science applied to biology.

PLANES

Terminology referring to planes of the body and the positioning of the body is often used in the Radiology section. A **position** is how the patient is placed during the x-ray examination (such as lying down or standing up), and a **projection** is the path of the x-ray beam. An example of a projection is anteroposterior, which denotes that the x-ray beam enters the patient's body at the front (anterior) and exits from the back (posterior). An example of a position is **prone,** which means the patient is lying on his or her anterior (front), but the entrance and exit of the x-ray beam are not specified. Familiarity with this terminology will aid you as you review the Radiology section and begin to choose the correct codes for physician services. Fig. 28-1 illustrates the major planes and the surfaces of the body that can be accessed by positioning the body.

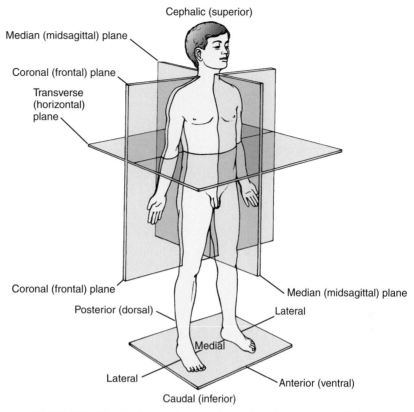

FIGURE 28-1 Planes of the body and terms of location and position of the body.

Fig. 28-2 shows proximal and distal body references. **Proximal** and **distal** are directional body references that mean closest to (proximal) or farthest from (distal) the trunk of the body. These terms are relative, meaning they are used to describe the position of the part as compared with another part. Therefore, the term "proximal" describes a part as being closer to the body trunk than another part, and the term "distal" describes a part as being farther away from the body than another part. The knee would be described as being proximal to the ankle, and it would also be described as being distal to the thigh or hip. Fig. 28-3 illustrates the **anteroposterior (AP)** (front to back) position, in which the patient has his or her front (anterior) closest to the x-ray machine, and the x-ray travels through the patient from the front to the back. In Fig. 28-4, the **posteroanterior (PA)** position, the patient has his or her back (posterior) located closest to the machine, and the beam travels through the patient from back to front.

Lateral positions are side positions. When the patient's right side is closest to the film, it is called *right lateral*. When the patient's left side is closest to the film, it is called *left lateral*. For

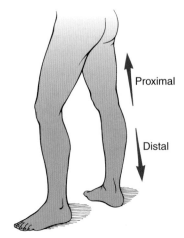

FIGURE 28–2   Proximal and distal.

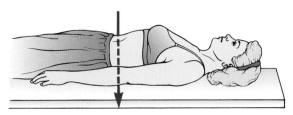

FIGURE 28–3   Anteroposterior (AP) projection.

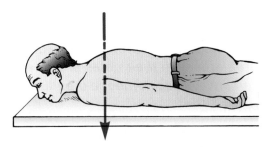

FIGURE 28–4   Posteroanterior (PA) projection.

example, Fig. 28-5 shows a left lateral position, and Fig. 28-6 shows a right lateral position. The use of these various positions allows the physician to view the body from a variety of angles. Fig. 28-7, *A and B* shows posteroanterior and lateral positions used to view a patient's lung with emphysema.

Dorsal (more commonly refers to the "back" but may be stated to mean "supine") means lying on the back; **ventral** (more commonly refers to the "anterior" but may be stated as "prone") means lying on the stomach; and **lateral** means lying on the side.

Decubitus positions are recumbent (lying) positions; the x-ray beam is placed horizontally. Ventral decubitus (prone) is the act of lying on the stomach (Fig. 28-8, *A*), and dorsal decubitus (supine) is the act of lying on the back (Fig. 28-8, *B*). The term "decubitus,"

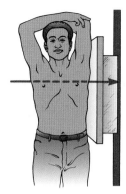

FIGURE 28-5   Left lateral projection.

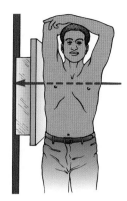

FIGURE 28-6   Right lateral projection.

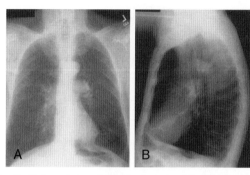

FIGURE 28-7   Posteroanterior and lateral radiographs of the thorax in a patient with emphysema.

generally shortened to "decub," has a special meaning in radiology. The simple act of lying on one's back would be referred to as lying supine, but if a horizontal x-ray beam is used, the position becomes decubitus. The type of decubitus is determined by the body surface the patient is lying on.

Recumbent means lying down. Thus, right lateral recumbent means the patient is lying on the right side (Fig. 28-8, *C*), and left lateral recumbent means the patient is lying on the left side (Fig. 28-8, *D*). In the ventral decubitus position, the patient is positioned prone and the x-ray beam comes into the patient from the right side and exits on the left (Fig. 28-8, *E*).

In the left lateral decubitus position, the patient is lying on the left side with the beam coming from the front and passing through to the back (anteroposterior) (Fig. 28-8, *F*).

When the patient is positioned on his or her back (dorsal decubitus) and the x-ray beam comes into the left side of the patient, the positioning is dorsal decubitus, but the view obtained is a right lateral (because the right side is closest to the film) (Fig. 28-8, *G*).

Oblique views refer to those obtained while the body is rotated so it is not in a full anteroposterior or posteroanterior position but somewhat diagonal. Oblique views are termed according to the body surface on which the patient is lying. The left anterior oblique (LAO) position is depicted in Fig. 28-8, *H* with the patient's left side rotated forward toward the table. The patient is lying on the left anterior aspect of his or her body. The right anterior oblique (RAO) position has the patient on his or her right side rotated forward toward the table, as in Fig. 28-8, *I*.

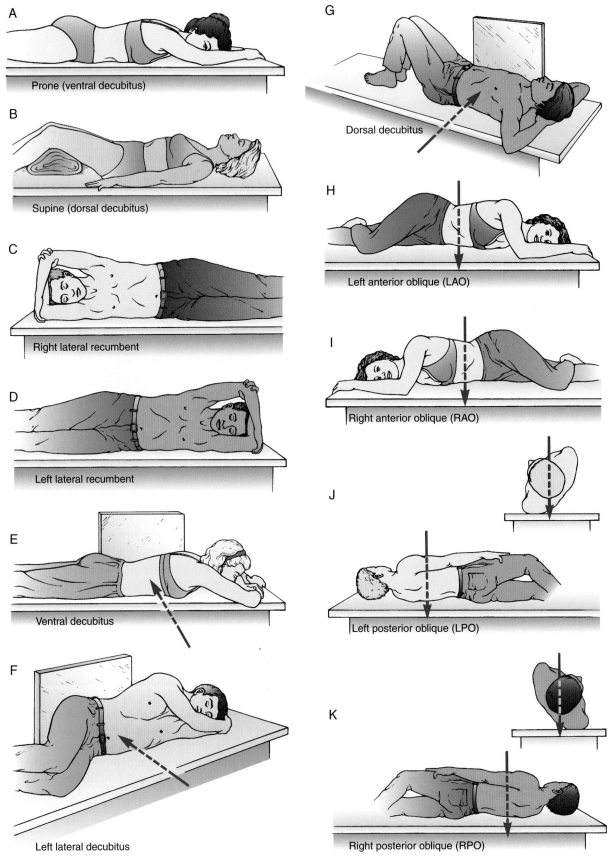

FIGURE 28–8 Radiographic positions. **A,** Prone (ventral decubitus). **B,** Supine (dorsal decubitus). **C,** Right lateral recumbent. **D,** Left lateral recumbent. **E,** Ventral decubitus. **F,** Left lateral decubitus. **G,** Dorsal decubitus. **H,** Left anterior oblique (LAO). **I,** Right anterior oblique (RAO). **J,** Left posterior oblique (LPO). **K,** Right posterior oblique (RPO).

Two more oblique views are left posterior oblique and right posterior oblique. In the left posterior oblique (LPO) view, the patient is rotated so that the left posterior aspect of his or her body is against the table, as in Fig. 28-8, *J*. The right posterior oblique (RPO) view has the patient with the right side rotated back, as in Fig. 28-8, *K*.

The last two terms that describe projections are tangential and axial. **Tangential** is the position that allows the beam to skim the body part, which produces a profile of the structure of the body (Fig. 28-9, *A*). Fig. 28-9, *B* illustrates the **axial** projection, which is any projection that allows the beam to pass through the body part lengthwise.

EXERCISE 28-2   *Planes*

Fill in the blanks with the correct words:

1 What is the word that indicates how the patient is placed during the x-ray examination? _____

2 What is the term that indicates the path the x-ray beam travels? _____

What do the following abbreviations mean?

3 AP _____

4 PA _____

5 RAO _____

6 LPO _____

7 What term indicates that a patient is lying supine, or on his or her back? _____

8 What term indicates that a patient is lying prone, or on his or her stomach? _____

9 What term indicates that a patient is lying on his or her right side? _____

10 What is the term that indicates when a patient is on his or her back and the x-ray beam comes into the right side of the patient?

_____

(Answers are located in Appendix B)

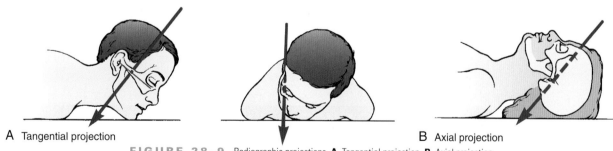

A Tangential projection   B Axial projection

FIGURE 28-9 Radiographic projections. **A,** Tangential projection. **B,** Axial projection.

GUIDELINES

As with all Guidelines, the Radiology Guidelines should be read carefully before radiologic procedures or services are reported. The Guidelines contain the unique instructions used within the section and the indications for multiple procedures, separate procedures, unlisted radiology procedure codes, and applicable modifiers.

Guidelines that are used more commonly in this section than in others are those explaining the professional, technical, and global components of a procedure. These components are as follows:

1. **Professional:** describes the services of the physician, including the supervision of the taking of the x-ray film and the interpretation with report of the x-ray films.
2. **Technical:** describes the services of the technologist, as well as the use of the equipment, film, and other supplies.
3. **Global:** describes the combination of the professional and technical components (1 and 2).

For example, if a patient undergoes a radiology procedure in a clinic that owns its own equipment, employs its own technologist(s), and also employs the radiologist who supervises, interprets, and reports on the radiologic results, the global procedure is reported. But if the radiologist is reading and interpreting films that were taken at another facility, only the professional component would be reported for physician services.

CODING SHOT

Third-party payment is generally 40% for the professional component, 60% for the technical component, and 100% for the global service.

When only the professional component of the service is provided, modifier -26 is placed after the CPT code. Modifier -26 alerts the third-party payer to the fact that only the professional component was provided. If, for example, an independent radiology facility takes a complete chest x-ray (71030) and sends the x-rays to an independent radiologist who reads the x-rays and writes a report of the findings in the x-rays, the coding for the independent radiologist would be the professional component only:

71030-26   Complete chest x-ray, four views

There is no CPT modifier to indicate the technical component of radiologic services. The modifier most commonly used is the HCPCS Level II modifier -TC, which reports the technical component. When submitting claims for radiologic services in which only the technical component was provided, use a code followed by -TC. For example, if you were the coder for the independent radiology facility that took the chest x-ray (71030) but sent it elsewhere to be interpreted, you would report the technical component only:

71030-TC   Complete chest x-ray, four views

CODING SHOT

-TC (Technical Component) and -26 (Professional Component) are terms used by third-party payers. When contacting a payer regarding payment of a service, first determine if there is a separate allowance for the -TC and -26.

Supervision and Interpretation

The other coding practice most commonly used in the Radiology section is called **component** or **combination coding,** which means that a code from the Radiology section as well as a code from one of the other sections must be reported to fully describe the procedure. For example, interventional radiologists may inject contrast material; place stents, catheters, or guidewires; or perform any number of procedures found throughout the CPT manual. Many times, before radiology procedures can be performed, a contrast material must be injected into the patient to make certain organs or vessels stand out more clearly on the radiographic image. When this contrast material is injected into the patient by the radiologist, a CPT code from the Surgery section must be used to indicate the injection procedure, and a HCPCS Level II code is reported for the contrast substance, such as A4641.

CODING SHOT

Codes in the Radiology section describe only the radiology procedures, not the injections or placement of other material necessary to perform the procedure.

Suppose, for example, a voiding urethrocystography with contrast medium enhancement is performed. In this procedure, a physician injects a radioactive material into the bladder. An x-ray of the bladder (cystography) is then obtained; the x-rays show filling, voiding, and post-voiding. The injection portion of the procedure is reported with a surgery code (51600: Injection procedure for cystography or voiding urethrocystography); the cystography is reported with a radiology code (74455: Urethrocystography, voiding, radiologic supervision and interpretation).

As a new coder, you will need to pay special attention to the information in parentheses below the codes in the Radiology section. This parenthetic material gives you information about other components of procedures and other codes to consider. Previous editions of the CPT manual had combination codes that were used when the physician did both components of some procedures. Using the combination code replaced the use of one code from surgery and one code from radiology; but many of these combination codes have been deleted to allow the physicians to more specifically indicate the services provided. There are many parenthetic phrases throughout the Radiology section, and you will want to refer to them when coding component procedures.

TOOLBOX

Doris is sent to the local Radiology Associates by her family practice physician because she has had a chronic cough that has not responded to any conservative treatment. The radiologist takes a 2-view chest x-ray, interprets the results, and writes a report.

QUESTIONS

1. Would you add a modifier to the CPT code for the chest x-ray? _____

2. What is your reason for your answer to Question 1? _____
_____

3. What would the radiologist send to the family practice physician regarding Doris? _____

▼ **ANSWERS**

1. No, 2. Because the radiologist provided the professional and the technical portions of the service, 3. written report

Odds and Ends

Many of the code descriptions state "radiologic supervision and interpretation" and alert you to component coding, letting you know that -26 or -TC may be appropriate. Always read the parenthetic information that follows these component codes.

Some codes are divided based on the extent of the radiologic examination, such as procedures that specify "with KUB" (kidney, ureter, and bladder). You must read the radiologist's report or the details in the medical record to understand the extent of the procedure.

CMS RULES

The NCCI Version 18.1 bundles some x-rays into a main x-ray procedure. For example, code 74241 (radiologic examination, gastrointestinal tract, upper; with or without delayed films, with KUB). According to the CCI edits, all the following codes are bundled into 74241:

- 74000 – x-ray of the abdomen, single anteroposterior
- 74010 – x-ray of abdomen, anteroposterior and additional oblique and cone views
- 74210 – x-ray exam, pharynx and/or cervical esophagus
- 74220 – x-ray exam of the esophagus
- 74240 – x-ray exam, gastrointestinal tract, upper, with or without delayed films, without KUB

Some of these codes may be reported if a modifier (e.g., -59) is added to indicate the service was separate and distinct from the main service reported with 74241.

Codes are also often divided on the basis of whether contrast material was or was not used. The phrase "with contrast" in the CPT manual means contrast that was administered intravascularly, intra-articularly, or intrathecally (into the subarachnoid space). If the procedure indicates that contrast was administered orally or rectally, the service is reported as "without contrast."

CODING SHOT

Report the supply of contrast material with Medicine section code 99070, supplies, or a HCPCS code. The injection of the contrast material is included in the "with contrast" radiology procedure code, unless guidelines state that a surgical code should also be listed to report the injection procedure. Avoid reporting 99070 if there is a more definite HCPCS code available.

There are new guidelines issued by CMS that were originally titled Medically Unbelievable Edits (MUEs). CMS changed the name to Medically Unlikely Edits. This information is included in a software system that allows Medicare to reduce the number of claims that contain medically improbable information, such as a hysterectomy on a male patient. There are approximately 3000 edits in the software, and 60 of those directly relate to radiology service. One type of edit is the maximum number of units that can be reported. If the MUE indicated that the maximum number of units for a particular radiology service was two for a particular service and you submitted three units, the claim would be automatically edited (kicked out). Unlike some edits, you cannot override the MUEs by appending a modifier.

Denied claims must be appealed with supporting documentation that indicates the service was medically necessary, was administered in a separate session, or was a repeat procedure by the same physician.

Radiographic procedures are located in the CPT manual index under the main term "X-ray," with subterms for the anatomic part (e.g., hand, spine).

EXERCISE 28-3 *Guidelines*

Fill in the blanks using the Radiology Guidelines of your CPT manual:

1 What procedure is one that is "performed independently of, and is not immediately related to, other services"?

_____

2 What is the name of the Medicare edit software? _____

3 Using your CPT manual, list at least four of the subsections of the Radiology section.

_____

_____

_____

_____

(Answers are located in Appendix B)

DIAGNOSTIC RADIOLOGY

The most standard radiographic procedures are contained in the Diagnostic Radiology subsection (70010-76499) of the Radiology section. This subsection describes diagnostic imaging, including plain x-ray films, the use of computed axial tomography (CAT or CT) scanning, magnetic resonance imaging (MRI), magnetic resonance angiography (MRA), and angiography. CT scanning uses an x-ray beam that rotates around the patient, as illustrated in Fig. 28-10. Fig. 28-11 shows the detail that can be obtained with MRI and CT scans. Special computer software is used with CT scanners to produce three-dimensional images that enable the study of internal structures. Tomography, CT scanning, and MRI may include the use of injectable dyes (radiographic contrast) to aid in imaging, and the codes are divided on the basis of whether or not contrast was used. For example, under the subheading Spine and Pelvis (72010-72295), the codes for CAT, MRI, and MRA are divided as follows:

72192   Computerized tomography, pelvis; without contrast material
72195   Magnetic resonance (e.g., proton) imaging, pelvis; without contrast material(s)
72198   Magnetic resonance angiography, pelvis, with or without contrast material(s)

Note one of these codes is for CAT, one code for the MRI, and one code for the MRA. The codes are divided by CAT, MRI, and MRA throughout the Diagnostic Radiology subsection. So you must read carefully to ensure that you report the correct type of imaging. Fig. 28-12 is an example of a magnetic resonance image of the brain.

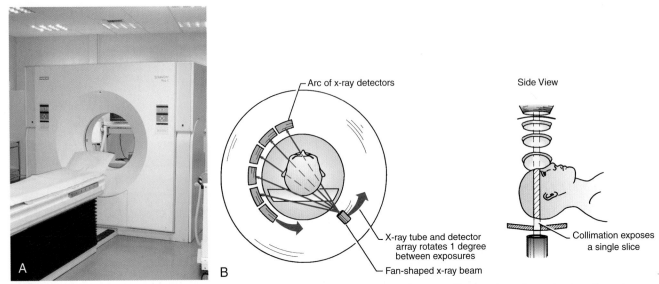

Arc of x-ray detectors

Side View

X-ray tube and detector array rotates 1 degree between exposures

Fan-shaped x-ray beam

Collimation exposes a single slice

FIGURE 28-10 **A,** Computed tomography scanner. **B,** Principles of computed tomographic (CT) scanning. The x-ray tube produces a fan-shaped beam that passes through a section (slice) of the patient. This fan-shaped beam is received by a circular array of detectors at the opposite side. These detectors receive x-rays along the path through the patient's body. The detector and x-ray source rotate around the axis, producing exposures at 1-degree intervals of rotation.

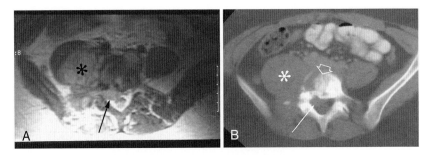

FIGURE 28-11 Axial MRI frame. *Arrows* highlight the descending aorta.

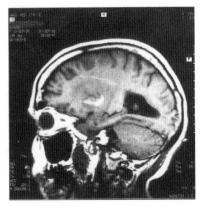

FIGURE 28-12 Magnetic resonance imaging (MRI) scan slice in the axial, coronal, and sagittal planes from a patient with subcortical aphasia. The lesion is an infarction involving the anterior caudate, putamen, and anterior limb of the left internal capsule.

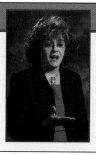

In **angiography,** dyes are injected into the vessels to add contrast that facilitates the visualization of vessels' lumen size and condition. The lumen is the cavity or channel within the vessel. Angiography is performed to view blood vessels after injecting them with a radio-opaque dye that outlines the vessels on x-ray. Angiography is used to identify abnormalities inside the vessels. Fig. 28-13 shows an angiogram of the aortic arch and brachiocephalic vessels. The radiologist studies the vessels using angiography to detect conditions such as malformations, strokes, or myocardial infarctions.

There are some combination codes in the angiography codes; so you must carefully read the complete procedure descriptor and parenthetical information to assure correct coding.

Codes in the Diagnostic Radiology subsection are divided according to anatomic site, from the head down. Some of the codes indicate a specific number of views, such as a minimum of three views or a single view. You should pay special attention to the description in each code and understand clearly how many views are specified in the code.

CODING SHOT

If fewer than the total number of views specified in the code are taken, modifier -52 would be used to indicate to the third-party payer that less of the procedure was performed than is described by the code, unless a code already exists for the smaller number of views.

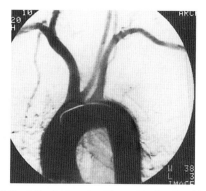

FIGURE 28–13   Angiography of the aortic arch and brachiocephalic vessels.

BREAST, MAMMOGRAPHY

Mammography (77051-77063) is the use of diagnostic radiology to detect breast tumors or other abnormal breast conditions, such as these codes used to report mammography services:

77055	Mammography; unilateral
77056	bilateral
77057	Screening mammography, bilateral (2-view film study of each breast)

Codes 77055 and 77056 report mammography performed to detect a suspected tumor. For example, a patient who upon examination has demonstrated an abnormality in a breast would appropriately have the service reported with 77055. If, however, a patient has presented for the usual screening mammography, report the service with 77057. Note that the description for the usual screening mammography indicates "bilateral," because screening mammography is performed on both breasts.

When new codes are published, their submission requires special attention. Under Radiology Guidelines, if a service is rarely provided, unusual, variable, or new, when submitting for reimbursement of the service a special report may be necessary. The report would include the complexity of symptoms, final diagnosis, pertinent physical findings, diagnostic/therapeutic procedures, concurrent problems, and follow-up care.

EXERCISE 28-4 *Diagnostic Radiology and Breast Mammography*

Code the radiology portion of the procedures unless otherwise directed:

1 What is the code for a diagnostic mammography, bilateral?

CPT Code: _____

2 What is the code for an unlisted diagnostic radiologic procedure?

CPT Code: _____

3 What is the code for the supervision and interpretation of an aortography, thoracic, by serialography?

CPT Code: _____

(Answers are located in Appendix B)

DIAGNOSTIC ULTRASOUND

Another subsection in Radiology is Diagnostic Ultrasound (76506-76999). **Diagnostic ultrasound** is the use of high-frequency sound waves to image anatomic structures and to detect the cause of illness and disease. It is used by the physician in the diagnostic process. Ultrasound moves at different speeds through tissue, depending on the density of the tissue. Forms and outlines of organs can be identified by ultrasound as the sound waves move through or bounce back (echo) from the tissues.

QUICK CHECK 28-1

1. According to the information in Diagnostic Ultrasound, Pelvis codes 76805 and _____ include determination of the number of fetuses.

(Answers are located in Appendix C)

There are many uses for ultrasound in medicine, such as showing a gallstone (Fig. 28-14) or showing twins (Fig. 28-15). You may think that these ultrasound procedures do not produce a picture clear enough to be of use to the physician in the diagnostic process, but a professional trained in the interpretation of ultrasound images is able to read them clearly.

Codes for ultrasound procedures are found in three locations:

■ Radiology section, Diagnostic Ultrasound subsection, 76506-76999, is usually divided on the basis of the anatomic location of the procedure (chest, pelvis)

■ Medicine section, Non-Invasive Vascular Diagnostic Studies subsection, 93880-93998, divided on the basis of the anatomic location of the procedure (cerebrovascular, extremity)

■ Medicine section, Echocardiography (ultrasound of the heart and great arteries), 93303-93355

An **interventional radiologist** is a physician who is skilled in both the surgical procedure and the radiology portion of an interventional radiologic service. The interventional radiologist is a board-certified physician who specializes in minimally invasive treatments performed using image guidance. These procedures have less risk, pain, and recovery time compared with open surgery. For example, an interventional radiologist who performed a liver biopsy using CT guidance to locate the lesion would report the services with a surgery code (47000) and a radiology code (77012-26). The interventional radiologist provided the surgical portion of the service, reported with a surgery code, and provided the professional portion of the CT guidance service, reported with a code from the Radiology section with modifier -26.

Most of the services in the Diagnostic Ultrasound subsection are located in the index of the CPT manual under the main term "Ultrasound." These terms are subdivided anatomically and by procedure (e.g., guidance or drainage).

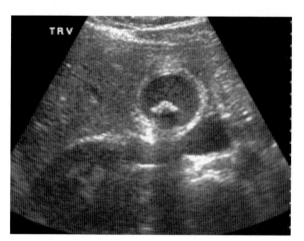

FIGURE 28-14 Ultrasound showing a gallstone.

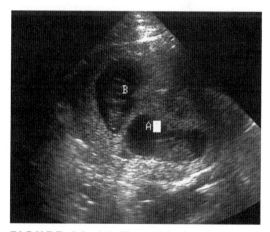

FIGURE 28-15 Ultrasound showing twins in separate sacs.

EXERCISE 28-5   *Diagnostic Ultrasound*

In the CPT manual, Diagnostic Ultrasound is usually divided into subheadings.

Locate and list the subheadings:

1 _____

2 _____

3 _____

4 _____

5 _____

6 _____

7 _____

8 _____

9 _____

(Answers are located in Appendix B)

The ultrasound sound waves are sent through body tissues with a device called a **transducer.** The transducer is placed directly on the skin to which a gel has been applied. The sound waves that are sent by the transducer through the body are then reflected by internal structures that return an echo to the transducer. The echoes are then transmitted electronically to the viewing monitor. The echo images are recorded on film or video tape. The technical term for ultrasound testing and recording is sonography. Ultrasound testing is painless and involves no radiation and produces no harmful side effects.

Ultrasound examinations can be utilized in various areas of the body for a multitude of purposes. These purposes can include examination of the chest, abdomen, and blood vessels (such as to detect blood clots in veins). Ultrasound can obtain detailed images of the size and function of the heart and detect abnormalities of the valves (such as mitral valve prolapse and aortic stenosis) and endocarditis (infection of the heart). Ultrasound is commonly used to guide fluid withdrawal (aspiration) from the chest, lung, or heart. Other uses of ultrasound include gallstone detection and viewing of the ureter, liver, spleen, pancreas, and aorta within the abdomen. Ultrasound can detect fluid, cysts, tumors, or abscesses in the abdomen or liver, aortic aneurysms, evaluate the structure of the thyroid gland in the neck, arteriosclerosis in the legs, and evaluate the size, gender, movement, and position of the growing baby during pregnancy.

Modes and Scans

There are four different types of ultrasound listed in the CPT manual: A-mode, M-mode, B-scan, and real-time scan.

A-mode: one-dimensional display reflecting the time it takes the sound wave to reach a structure and reflect back. This process maps the outline of the structure. "A" is for amplitude of sound return (echo).

M-mode: one-dimensional display of the movement of structures. "M" stands for motion.

B-scan: two-dimensional display of the movement of tissues and organs. "B" stands for brightness. The sound waves bounce off tissue or organs and are projected onto a black and white television screen. The strong signals display as black and the weaker signals display as lighter shades of gray. B-scan is also called gray-scale ultrasound.

Real-time scan: two-dimensional display of both the structure and the motion of tissues and organs that indicates the size, shape, and movement of the tissue or organ.

Codes are often divided on the basis of the scan or mode that was used and the medical record will indicate the scan or mode used.

Several codes within the subsection include the use of Doppler ultrasound. **Doppler ultrasound** is the use of sound that can be transmitted only through solids or liquids and is a specific version of ultrasonography, or ultrasound. Doppler ultrasound is named for an Austrian physicist, Johann Doppler, who discovered a relationship between sound and light waves—a relationship upon which ultrasound technology was built. Doppler ultrasound is used to measure moving objects and as such is ideal for measuring bloodflow. Codes often state "with or without Doppler." Doppler ultrasound can be standard black and white or color. Color Doppler translates the standard black and white into colored images. Just imagine how much easier it is to see a leak in a vessel when the vessel is yellow and the blood is red. The code descriptions will specifically state "color-flow Doppler."

There is some component coding necessary, but it occurs mostly under the subheading of Ultrasonic Guidance Procedures (76930-76999). The parenthetic information will refer you to the surgical procedure code. For example, 76945 is for the radiologic supervision and interpretation of ultrasonic guidance for chorionic villus sampling, which is an aspiration of cells for analysis to determine any cell abnormalities. The physician guides the insertion of a needle to withdraw the sample. If the physician performed both the radiologic portion of the procedure and the surgical procedure, you would report 59015 from the Surgery section and 76945 from the Radiology section. The radiology service reported with 76945 is not bundled into the surgical service (59015) and would be separately reimbursed. Modifier -26 would be reported with 76945, unless the radiologist owned the equipment.

EXERCISE 28-6 *Modes and Scans*

Assign codes using the CPT, ICD-10-CM and/or ICD-9-CM manuals for the following:

1 An ultrasound of the spinal canal

CPT Code: _____

2 An ultrasound of the chest and mediastinum, real time

CPT Code: _____

3 A complete abdominal ultrasound in real time with image documentation

CPT Code: _____

4 A repeat uterine ultrasound in real time with image documentation of a 32-week pregnant female with twins

CPT Code: _____

ICD-10-CM Code: _____ (pregnancy)

(ICD-9-CM Codes: _____ (pregnancy) _____ (multiple gestation V Code))

5 A fetal profile, biophysical, with nonstress testing in a mother with Type 1 Diabetes mellitus

CPT Code: _____

ICD-10-CM Code: _____ (pregnancy)

(ICD-9-CM Codes: _____ (pregnancy), _____ (diabetes))

(Answers are located in Appendix B)

RADIATION ONCOLOGY

The Radiation Oncology subsection (77261-77799) of the Radiology section reports both professional and technical treatments utilizing radiation to destroy tumors, and special attention must be given to reporting the components. The subsection is divided on the basis of treatment. Read all of the definitions carefully to make certain you know what is bundled into the code. Many third-party payers have developed strict guidelines determining the number of times some procedures are allowed within each treatment course. You should work closely with third-party payers to understand their preferred reporting.

From the Trenches

"There are so many opportunities and not enough skilled coders to fill the positions for physician's offices, clinics, hospitals, as health care consultants, and also in colleges to teach coding at a college level."

PATRICIA

The codes within this subheading include codes for the initial consultation through management of the patient during the course of treatment. When the initial consultation occurs, the code for the service would be an E/M code. For example, the patient might be an inpatient when the therapeutic radiologist first sees the patient for evaluation of treatment options and before a decision for treatment is made. You would report this consultation service with an Inpatient Consultation code from the E/M section.

Clinical Treatment Planning

Clinical Treatment Planning (77261-77263) reflects professional services by the physician. It includes interpretation of special testing, tumor localization, treatment volume determination, treatment time/dosage determination, choice of treatment modality (method), determination of number and size of treatment ports, selection of appropriate treatment devices, and any other procedures necessary to adequately develop a course of treatment. A treatment plan is established for all patients requiring radiation therapy.

There are three types of clinical treatment plans: simple, intermediate, and complex.

Simple planning requires that there be a single treatment area that is encompassed by a single port or by simple parallel opposed ports with simple or no blocking.

Intermediate planning requires that there be three or more converging ports, two separate treatment areas, multiple blocks, or special time/dose constraints.

Complex planning requires that there be highly complex blocking, custom shielding blocks, tangential ports, special wedges or compensators, three or more separate treatment areas, rotational or special beam consideration, or a combination of therapeutic modalities.

Simulation

Simulation (77280-77299) is the service of determining treatment areas and the placement of the ports for radiation treatment but does not include the administration of the radiation. A simulation can be performed on a simulator designated for use only in simulations in a radiation therapy treatment unit, or on a diagnostic x-ray machine. Codes are divided into four levels of service:

Simple simulation of a single treatment area, with either a single port or parallel opposed ports and simple or no blocking

Intermediate simulation of three or more converging ports, with two separate treatment areas and multiple blocks

Complex simulation of tangential ports, with three or more treatment areas, rotation or arc therapy, complex blocking, custom shielding blocks, brachytherapy source verification, hyperthermia probe verification, and any use of contrast material

Three-dimensional (3D) computer-generated reconstruction of tumor volume and surrounding critical normal tissue structures based on direct CT scan and/or MRI data in preparation for non-coplanar or coplanar therapy. This is a simulation that utilizes documented three-dimensional beam's-eye view volume dose displays of multiple or moving beams. Documentation of three-dimensional volume reconstruction and dose distribution is required.

After the initial simulation and treatment plans have been established for a patient, if any change is made in the field of treatment, a new simulation billing is required. When coding for a treatment period, you will have codes for planning, simulation, the isodose plan, devices, treatment management (the number of treatments determines the number of times billed), and the radiation delivery.

The codes in Clinical Treatment Planning are located in the index of the CPT manual under the main term "Radiation Therapy." Codes can also be located under the main term of the specific service, such as "Field Set-up."

EXERCISE 28-7 *Clinical Treatment Planning*

Using the CPT manual, code the following:

1 Complex therapeutic radiology simulation-aided field setting

    CPT Code: _____

2 Therapeutic radiology treatment planning; simple

    CPT Code: _____

(Answers are located in Appendix B)

Medical Radiation Physics, Dosimetry, Treatment Devices, and Special Services

Medical Radiation Physics, Dosimetry, Treatment Devices, and Special Services (77300-77370, 77399) reports the decision making of the physician as to the type of treatment (modality), dose, and development of treatment devices. It is common to have several dosimetry or device changes during a treatment course. **Dosimetry** is the calculation of the radiation dose and placement.

Codes in this subheading are divided mostly on the basis of the level of treatment (simple, intermediate, complex). The codes are located in the index of the CPT manual under the main term "Radiation Therapy" and the subterm of the specific service, such as Dose Plan or Treatment Delivery.

EXERCISE 28-8   *Medical Radiation Physics, Dosimetry, Treatment Devices, and Special Services*

Using the CPT, ICD-10-CM and/or ICD-9-CM manuals, code the following:

1 Design and construction of a bite block, intermediate

CPT Code: _____

2 Calculation of an isodose plan for brachytherapy, single plane, two sources, simple

CPT Code: _____

3 Teletherapy, isodose plan, to one area, simple, for cancer of the prostate, primary malignant

CPT Code: _____

ICD-10-CM Code: _____ (ICD-9-CM Code: _____)

(Answers are located in Appendix B)

Radiation Treatment Delivery

Stereotactic Radiation Treatment Delivery (77371-77373) and Radiation Treatment Delivery (77401-77423) reflect **technical components** only. These codes report the actual delivery of the radiation. Radiation treatment is delivered in units called megaelectron volts (MeV). A megaelectron volt is a unit of energy. The radiation energy **delivered** by the machine is measured in megaelectron volts; the energy that is **deposited** in the patient's tissue is measured in Gray (one Gray = 100 rads; 1 centigray [cGy] = 1 rad). A rad is a radiation-absorbed dose. The therapy dose in a cancer treatment would typically be in the thousands of rads.

To report Radiation Treatment Delivery services, you need to know the amount of radiation delivered (6-10 MeV, 11-19 MeV) and the number of the following:

■ **Areas** treated (single, two, three or more)
■ **Ports** involved (single, three or more, tangential)
■ **Blocks** used (none, multiple, custom)

EXERCISE 28-9   *Radiation Treatment Delivery*

Using the CPT, ICD-10-CM and/or ICD-9-CM manuals, code the following:

The patient receives radiation treatment delivery:

1 To a single area at 4 MeV, simple

CPT Code: _____

2 With superficial voltage only

CPT Code: _____

3 To four separate areas with a rotational beam at 4 MeV, complex

CPT Code: _____

4 For two separate areas, using three or more ports with multiple blocks at 5 MeV, intermediate

CPT Code: _____

5 For three or more separate areas using custom blocks, wedges, rotation beams, up to 5 MeV (complex) for bone metastasis of the thoracic and lumbar spine (unknown primary)

CPT Code: _____

ICD-10-CM Codes: _____, _____

(ICD-9-CM Codes: _____, _____)

(Answers are located in Appendix B)

Radiation Treatment Management

Radiation Treatment Management codes (77427-77499) report the **professional component** of radiation treatment management. The codes report management of radiation therapy. The notes under the heading Radiation Treatment Management state that clinical management is based on five fractions or treatment sessions regardless of the time interval separating the delivery of treatment. This means that code 77427 may be reported if the patient receives at least five treatments, no matter the length of time between the treatments. Multiple fractions furnished on the same day may be reported separately as long as there was a break between fractions and the fractions represent the characteristics of those typically delivered may still be reported.

If the patient receives five treatments and then receives an additional one or two fractions, you do not report the additional fractions. Only if three or more fractions beyond the original five are delivered would you report 77427 to indicate the additional treatment management.

Bundled into the Radiation Treatment Management codes are the following physician services:

- Review of port films
- Review of dosimetry, dose delivery, and treatment parameters
- Review of patient treatment setup
- Examination of the patient for medical evaluation and management (e.g., assessment of the patient's response to treatment, coordination of care and treatment, review of imaging and/or lab test results)

CODING SHOT

Services related to and covered under Radiation Treatment Management are based on the third-party payer.

The following can be reported in addition to 77427 (treatment management) because none of the following are bundled into the treatment management:

- 77417 Port films, two per week per treatment course
- 77300 Basic plan calculation at the onset of treatment
- 77263 Complex planning reported at the beginning of treatment
- E/M code: Usually on the first day of treatment as either an office visit or a consultation service

CODING SHOT

Code 77427 is reported once per each unit of five fractions or treatment sessions. All five sessions/treatments must be completed to report code 77427. The continuing medical physics consultation code 77336 is reported by the physicist once per every fifth fraction. This is a facility/technical service code and is not reported by the radiation oncologist.

It would be inappropriate to report these items individually. For example, the physician sees the patient in the office to evaluate the patient's response to treatment. You might think you should use an E/M code to report the office visit, but that would be incorrect because the management codes already include the office visit service.

Proton Beam Treatment Delivery

The delivery of radiation treatment (77520-77525) using a proton beam utilizes particles that are positively charged with electricity. The use of the proton beam is an alternative delivery method for radiation in which proton (electromagnetic) radiation would be used. The codes in the subheading are divided according to whether the delivery was simple, intermediate, or complex.

Hyperthermia

Hyperthermia (77600-77615) is an increase in body temperature and is used as an adjunct to radiation therapy or chemotherapy for the treatment of cancer. The heat source can be ultrasound, microwave, or another means of increasing the temperature in an area. When the temperature of an area is increased, metabolism increases, which boosts the ability of the body to eradicate the cancer cells. The location of the heat source can be external (to a depth of greater or less than 4 cm), interstitial (within the tissues), or intracavitary (inside the body). External treatment would be the application to the skin of a heat source. Interstitial treatment is the insertion of a probe that delivers heat directly to the treatment area. Codes 77600-77615 report external or interstitial treatment delivery.

Intracavitary hyperthermia treatment delivery requires the insertion of a heat-producing probe into a body orifice, such as the rectum or vagina. Code 77620 reports intracavitary treatment and is the only code listed under the heading Clinical Intracavitary Hyperthermia.

QUICK CHECK 28-2

1. Hyperthermia is used as an independent treatment modality.
   True or False?

(Answers are located in Appendix C)

EXERCISE 28-10   *Clinical Treatment Management*

Using the CPT manual, code the following management services:

1 Five radiation treatments

   CPT Code: _____

2 Unlisted procedure code for therapeutic radiation clinical treatment management (Submission of this unlisted procedure code would necessitate a special report and assumes that no Category III code exists for the procedure.)

   CPT Code: _____

(Answers are located in Appendix B)

Clinical Brachytherapy

Clinical **brachytherapy** (77750-77799) is the placement of radioactive material directly into or surrounding the site of the tumor as discussed earlier in this text. Placement may be intracavitary or interstitial, and material may be placed permanently or temporarily.

The terms "source" and "ribbon" are used in the Clinical Brachytherapy codes. A **source** is a container holding a radioactive element that can be inserted directly into the body where it delivers the radiation dose over time. Sources come in various forms, such as seeds or capsules, and are placed in a cavity (intracavitary) or permanently placed within the tissue (interstitial). Fig. 28-16 illustrates the results of a single permanent seed implanted into the

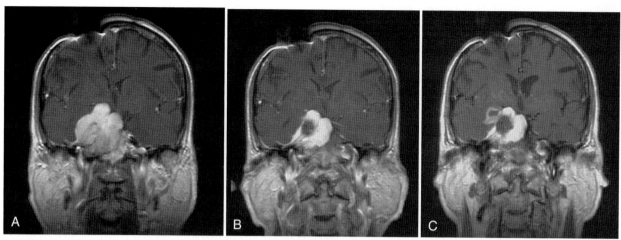

FIGURE 28–16 A, MR image scan of 80-year-old man with large petroclival meningioma previously treated with radiosurgery 6 years earlier. **B,** Results 3 months after placement of single permanent I-125 seed. **C,** Results 9 months after placement of single seed.

cranial posterior fossa of a patient with a meningioma. A ribbon is another source and ribbons are seeds embedded on a tape. The ribbon is cut to the desired length to control the amount of radiation the patient receives. Ribbons are inserted temporarily into the tissue.

Codes are divided on the basis of the number of sources or ribbons used in an application:

- Simple   1-4
- Intermediate   5-10
- Complex   11 or more

The Clinical Brachytherapy codes include the physician's work related to the patient's admission to the hospital as well as the daily hospital visits.

EXERCISE 28-11 *Clinical Brachytherapy*

Using the CPT, ICD-10-CM and/or ICD-9-CM manuals, code the following:

1 A simple application of a radioactive source, intracavitary

   CPT Code: _____

2 A simple application of a radioactive source, interstitial

   CPT Code: _____

3 Surface application of a radiation source for ovarian cancer, primary

   CPT Code: _____

   ICD-10-CM Code: _____ (ICD-9-CM Code: _____)

(Answers are located in Appendix B)

NUCLEAR MEDICINE

Nuclear medicine (78012-79999) reports placement of radionuclides within the body and the monitoring of emissions from the radioactive elements. Nuclear medicine is used not only for diagnostic studies but also for therapeutic treatment, such as treatment of thyroid conditions.

Stress tests are an example of nuclear medicine techniques. Radioactive material may be used during stress tests to monitor coronary artery bloodflow. Radioactive material (called a tracer) adheres to red blood cells (such as thallium or technetium sestamibi [Cardiolite]). The radioactive materials on the red blood cells allow an image of the heart to be seen and indicate areas where blood is flowing. The radioactive materials are injected 1 minute before the end of a stress test and then again 24 hours later for a comparison study. If the bloodflow is decreased or absent, the image will show a blank area. If the coronary arteries are clear and allow blood to flow to the heart muscle, the image will show blood dispersement to all areas. If the arteries are partially blocked, the flow may be decreased but would be adequate during rest. During exercise, however, the necessary amount of oxygenated blood may not be adequate to keep the heart functioning properly, and that is when chest pain may occur. During a stress test, if radionuclide dispersement is absent during exercise (showing inadequate blood supply to the area during peak demand) but is present during resting periods (showing adequate flow at rest), this is called **reversible ischemia,** meaning that heart muscle death has not occurred. With intervention, arteries may be opened or bypassed to increase the supply of blood to the muscle before heart muscle death does occur. If the radionuclide is absent during rest and exercise, the ischemia is considered **irreversible,** meaning that heart muscle death has already occurred. A stress test is one of the many uses of nuclear medicine for diagnostic purposes. As you code, you will become familiar with these various diagnostic tests and how they are reported.

CODING SHOT

None of the codes in the subsection includes the radiopharmaceutical(s) used for diagnosis or therapy services. When radiopharmaceutical(s) are supplied for diagnostic purposes, report 79005 (oral), 79101 (intravenous), 79440 (intra-articular) or 79445 (intra-arterial), or use the specific Level II HCPCS code. The oral and intravenous administration codes include the administration service. For intra-arterial, intra-cavity, and intra-articular administration, also report the appropriate injection/procedure codes in addition to the imaging guidance and radiological supervision/interpretation when appropriate.

Two other subheadings within the Nuclear Medicine subsection are Diagnostic (78012-78999) and Therapeutic (79005-79999). The subheading Diagnostic is further divided into category codes based on system, such as the endocrine system and the cardiovascular system.

EXERCISE 28-12   *Nuclear Medicine*

Which category in the Nuclear Medicine subsection would you reference to locate codes for the following?

1 Liver _____

2 Thyroid _____

3 Spleen _____

4 Bone _____

5 Brain _____

(Answers are located in Appendix B)

CHAPTER REVIEW

CHAPTER 28, PART I, THEORY

Without the use of the CPT manual, complete the following:

1 What is a branch of medicine that uses radiant energy to diagnose and treat patients?

_____

2 The CPT manual divides the Radiology section into subsections of Radiologic Guidance, Breast Mammography, Bone/Joint Studies, Diagnostic Radiology, _____, _____ _____, and Nuclear Medicine.

3 What type of procedure is "performed independently of, and is not immediately related to, other services"?

_____

4 One Gray equals how many rads? _____

5 The modifier used to indicate the Professional Component is _____.

6 The two words that mean supervising the taking of the x-rays and reading/reporting the results of the films are

_____ and _____.

7 The name for the use of high-frequency sound waves in an imaging process that is used to diagnose patient illness is

_____

8 The Radiation Oncology section of the CPT manual is divided into subsections based on the _____ of service provided to the patient.

9 The scientific study of energy is _____.

10 The scientific calculation of the radiation emitted from various radioactive sources is

_____

11 Radiation treatment delivery codes are based on the treatment area involved and further divided based on levels of what?

_____

12 MeV stands for _____.

13 Radiation Treatment Management is reported in units of _____ fractions.

14 Nuclear Medicine uses these to image organs for diagnosis and treatment: _____

Identify the planes of the body on the figure on the next page:

15 _____

16 _____

17 _____

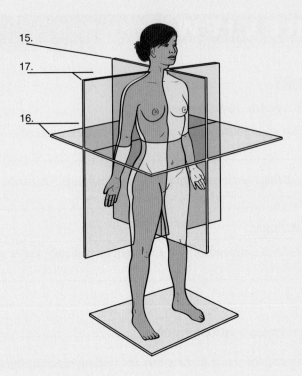

15.

17.

16.

CHAPTER 28, PART II, PRACTICAL

The coding exercise that follows uses codes from a variety of CPT sections.

Using the CPT, ICD-10-CM and/or ICD-9-CM manuals, code the following:

18 An established patient is seen in the physician's office with the chief complaint of a persistent cough. Otherwise, the patient claims to be in good health. The physician collects a history, including the chief complaint and the history of the present illness. The physical examination performed focuses on the respiratory tract. The decision making is straightforward because the physician wants to evaluate the patient for a possible case of bronchitis.

CPT Code: _____

The patient is sent to the clinic's radiology department for a two-view chest x-ray study, frontal and lateral.

CPT Code: _____

The radiologist sends the x-ray results to the physician, who reviews them and decides to order a consultation with a pulmonologist from another clinic. The patient sees the other clinic's pulmonologist, who performs a comprehensive history and a comprehensive examination with moderate complexity.

CPT Code: _____

The pulmonologist orders a CT of the chest, without contrast, and the radiologist supervises and interprets the results.

CPT Code: _____

A bronchoscopy with transbronchial lung biopsy is performed in the ambulatory surgery center.

CPT Code: _____

19 A new patient is seen in the office for unilateral ear pain. In the expanded problem focused history and the physical examination, the physician focuses his attention on the head, ears, nose, and throat. The physician's provisional diagnoses include otalgia and possible ear infections. The decision making is straightforward for the physician.

CPT Code: _____

The patient is sent to the clinic's radiologist for an x-ray of the ear.

CPT Code: _____

The patient is then sent to the clinic's ear specialist, who inserts a ventilation tube (tympanostomy) using local anesthesia.

CPT Code: _____

ICD-10-CM Code: _____

(ICD-9-CM Code: _____)

20   A new patient is seen in the office for a variety of complaints, but in particular a swelling and heaviness of his right leg. The physician documents the patient's complaints, collects a comprehensive history of the present illness, performs a comprehensive review of systems, and inquires about the patient's past, family, and social history. A complete multisystem physical examination is performed. The physician's working diagnosis is edema of the lower extremity, cause to be determined. Given the nature of the problem, the physician considers the decision-making process to be highly complex.

CPT Code: _____

ICD-10-CM Code: _____

(ICD-9-CM Code: _____)

21A   The patient is sent to radiology for a unilateral lymphangiography of one extremity due to swelling of the arm. The patient has a history of breast cancer.

CPT Code: _____

ICD-10-CM Codes: _____, _____

(ICD-9-CM Codes: _____, _____)

21B   Another physician performs the injection procedure for the lymphangiography.

CPT Code: _____

ICD-10-CM Codes: _____, _____

(ICD-9-CM Codes: _____, _____)

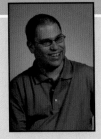

"Coding is a diverse field, so there are a lot of opportunities in many areas. . . . Find an area of interest and become an expert in it; make yourself valuable."

Keith Russell, CPC, COC
Senior Compliance Analyst
Baylor College of Medicine
Houston, Texas

Pathology/Laboratory

<table>
<tr><td>

Chapter Topics

Format

Organ or Disease-Oriented Panels

Drug Assay

Therapeutic Drug Assays

Evocative/Suppression Testing

Consultations (Clinical Pathology)

Urinalysis, Molecular Pathology, and Chemistry

Molecular Pathology

Hematology and Coagulation

Immunology

Transfusion Medicine

Microbiology

Anatomic Pathology

Cytopathology and Cytogenic Studies

Surgical Pathology

Other Procedures

Chapter Review

</td><td>

Learning Objectives

After completing this chapter you should be able to

1 Explain the format of the Pathology and Laboratory section.

2 Understand the information in the Pathology and Laboratory Guidelines.

3 Demonstrate an understanding of Pathology and Laboratory terminology.

4 Differentiate amongst the Organ or Disease Oriented Panels codes.

5 Recognize Drug Assay codes.

6 Identify Therapeutic Drug Assays codes.

7 Classify Evocative/Suppression Testing codes.

8 Explain Consultations (Clinical Pathology) codes.

9 Interpret Urinalysis, Molecular Pathology, and Chemistry codes.

10 Evaluate Hematology and Coagulation codes.

11 Describe Immunology codes.

12 Discriminate amongst Transfusion Medicine codes.

13 Interpret Microbiology codes.

14 Evaluate Anatomic Pathology codes.

15 Summarize Cytopathology and Cytogenic Studies codes.

16 Explain Surgical Pathology codes.

17 Choose Other Procedures codes.

18 Demonstrate the ability to code Pathology and Laboratory services.

</td></tr>
</table>

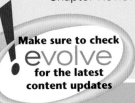

Make sure to check *evolve* for the latest content updates

FORMAT

The Pathology and Laboratory section of the CPT manual is formatted according to type of test performed—automated multichannel, panels, assays, and so forth. To familiarize yourself with the content of the Pathology and Laboratory section, review the subsections in the CPT manual. This will help you get a broad overview of the contents of this important section as you prepare to learn the specifics.

Laboratories have built-in **indicators** that allow additional tests to be performed without a written order from the physician. These standards are set by the medical facility and imply that when a certain test is positive, it is assumed that the physician would want further information on the condition and specific additional tests performed. For example, if a routine urinalysis is performed, a culture is performed if the test is positive for bacteria. If a culture is performed to identify the organism, a sensitivity test is performed if the bacteria are of a certain type or count, as predetermined by the medical facility to warrant the additional laboratory studies. You will code only after the tests are performed, because an order for a laboratory test does not ensure that the test will be performed. This standard ensures that all laboratory tests performed are reported. Remember that what the physician ordered may not be all the laboratory work performed, depending on the facility's policy concerning indicators.

The services in the Pathology and Laboratory section include the laboratory **tests** only. The **collection** of the specimen is reported separately from the analysis of the test. For example, if a technician in a clinic laboratory withdraws blood by means of a venipuncture from the arm, and the blood sample was then analyzed in the laboratory, you would report 36415 for the venipuncture as shown in Fig. 29-1 in addition to a code to report the test performed on the blood in the laboratory.

Most Pathology and Laboratory subsections contain notes. Whenever notes are available, be sure to read them before assigning codes from the subsection because specific information pertinent to the codes is contained in these notes.

ORGAN OR DISEASE-ORIENTED PANELS

The codes in the Organ or Disease-Oriented Panels subsection (80047-80076) are grouped according to the usual laboratory work ordered by a physician for the diagnosis of or screening for various diseases or conditions. Groups of tests may be performed together using automated equipment, depending on the situation or disease. For example, during the first obstetric visit, a mother is commonly asked to have baseline laboratory tests performed to ensure that appropriate antepartum care is provided. CPT code 80055 describes an obstetric panel that would typically be performed during the first obstetric visit.

To assign a panel code, each test listed in the panel description must be performed. Additional tests are reported separately. The development of panels saves the facility from having to report each test separately, and it is often more economical for the patient. You cannot assign modifier -52 (reduced service) with a panel. For example, if all of the tests in

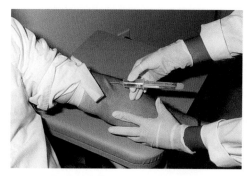

FIGURE 29-1 Venipuncture.

the obstetric panel were done except the syphilis test, you could not report 80055 (Obstetrical Panel) with modifier -52. You would instead list each of the tests separately.

CODING SHOT

Be careful when coding multiple panels on the same day for the same patient. Sometimes several panels include some of the same tests. For example, a hepatitis B surface antigen test is included in both the obstetric panel and the acute hepatitis panel. It would be inappropriate to report the same test twice.

The laboratory and pathology reports in the patient medical record will describe the method by which the test was performed. There are many different methods of performing the same test. For example, a urinalysis can be automated or nonautomated and can include or exclude microscopy. It is necessary to know these details if you are to assign the correct urinalysis code. If the details you need are not in the medical record, ask the laboratory staff or physician for further clarification.

EXERCISE 29-1   *Organ or Disease-Oriented Panels*

Complete the following:

1 Hepatic function panel code in a patient with hepatitis B serum virus, chronic

CPT Code: _____

ICD-10-CM Code: _____ (ICD-9-CM Code: _____)

2 How many laboratory tests must be included in a hepatic function panel? _____

3 Does an obstetric panel include a rubella antibody test? _____

4 Is blood typing ABO included in an obstetric panel? _____

(Answers are located in Appendix B)

DRUG ASSAY

Laboratory Presumptive Drug Class Screening (80300-80304) is performed to identify the presence or absence of a drug. Testing that determines the presence or absence of a drug is **qualitative** (the drug is either present or not present in the specimen).

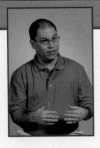

From the Trenches

Why should a coder consider getting certified?

"Certification indicates a level of competence and many employers now require applicants to be certified. Plus, salary surveys have shown that certified coders command higher salaries than non-certified coders."

KEITH

The screening of drug classes is divided by class, Drug Class List A and Drug Class List B, both found in the CPT, and also divided based on whether the screening is presumptive. Codes 80300, 80301 report drug screening of any number of drug classes from List A. Code 80302 reports presumptive drug screening of any number of drug classes from List B. Presumptive drug screen codes 80303, 80304 report the drug screening of any number of drug classes, single or multiple. The Drug Screen codes are further divided based on date of service or each procedure.

An example of a Drug Class List B screen is a patient who has been on tramadol for a long time for treatment of pain and needs to undergo testing to determine whether the drug level is at the correct therapeutic level.

QUICK CHECK 29-1

1. What is the repeat clinical laboratory test modifier? _____

(Answers are located in Appendix C)

TOOLBOX

Jason has been sent to the clinic to have a drug test, as are all employees of the company for which he works. The company requests all employees be screened for barbiturates and antidepressants.

QUESTIONS

1. Your clinic uses a multiple drug classes chromatograph method to determine two drug classes. How would you report the service chromatographic determination of two drugs? _____
2. If your clinic did not use chromatography but rather did a test for each of the two tests, how would you report the tests? _____

▼ **ANSWERS**

1. 80100, chromatographic determination, 2. 80101 3 2, single drug class method

THERAPEUTIC DRUG ASSAYS

Drug assays (80150-80299) test for a specific drug and for the amount of that drug. Many types of drugs are listed in this subsection. If the drug is not listed, it is possible that quantitative analysis may be listed under the methodology (e.g., immunoassay, radioassay).

Therapeutic drug assays are performed to help the physician monitor the level of medication in the patient's system or to monitor the patient's compliance. For example, levels may be measured to make certain the patient is getting the correct level of antibiotics. Blood specimens for drug monitoring are usually taken during the drug's highest therapeutic concentration (peak level) and at the drug's lowest therapeutic concentration (trough or residual level). Peak and trough levels should be within the therapeutic range directed by the physician.

The drugs are listed by their generic names, not their brand names. A *Physician's Desk Reference* that lists pharmaceuticals by the generic and brand name will be helpful as you code drug testing and assays.

One location of Drug Testing codes in the index of the CPT manual is under the main term "Drug," subtermed by the reason for the tests—analysis or confirmation. Therapeutic Drug Assay subsection codes can be found under the main term "Drug Assay" and subterms of the material examined, for example, amikacin, digoxin.

EXERCISE 29-2   *Therapeutic Drug Testing and Drug Assays*

Assign the correct CPT, ICD-10-CM and/or ICD-9-CM codes for the following drug tests:

1 Drug screen of cocaine, single drug class method

    CPT Code: _____

2 Identify the amount of total digoxin in the blood (quantitative)

    CPT Code: _____

3 Quantitative examination of blood for amikacin in a patient with fever and immune neutropenia

    CPT Code: _____

    ICD-10-CM Codes: _____, _____

    (ICD-9-CM Codes: _____, _____, _____)

4 Examination of blood, quantitative for lithium in a patient with manic depression syndrome

    CPT Code: _____

    ICD-10-CM Code: _____

    (ICD-9-CM Code: _____)

(Answers are located in Appendix B)

EVOCATIVE/SUPPRESSION TESTING

🖐 **CAUTION**   *Remember that the codes from the Pathology and Laboratory section are only for the tests performed and do not reflect the complete service provided to the patient.*

Evocative/Suppression (80400-80439) testing is performed to measure the effect of evocative or suppressive agents on chemical constituents. For example, 80400 is reported when a patient undergoes testing to determine whether adrenocorticotropic hormone (ACTH) is being produced in the body. The patient may have adrenal gland insufficiency. Note that following each of the code descriptions is a statement of the services that must have been provided for the code to be reported. For example, the requirement to report 80400 ACTH stimulation panel is "Cortisol (82533 × 2)" or two cortisol tests were performed. Code 80400 bundles two units of 82533 into one code. Before you can assign 80400, however, you must read the code description for 82533 to ensure that the code reports the correct test.

To code the components of Evocative/Suppression Testing consider the following:

- If the physician **supplied** the agent, report the supply using 99070 from the Medicine section or a HCPCS code.
- If the physician **administered** the agent, report the infusion or injection with codes 96365-96379 from the Medicine section.
- If the test involved **prolonged attendance** by the physician, report the service with the appropriate E/M code.

CONSULTATIONS (CLINICAL PATHOLOGY)

A clinical pathologist, upon request from a primary care physician, will perform a consultation to render additional medical interpretation of test results. For example, a primary care physician reviews lab test results and requests a clinical pathologist to review, interpret, and prepare a written report on the findings, which represents a clinical pathology consultation.

There are two codes under the subsection Consultations (80500, 80502). These consultations are based on whether the consultation was limited or comprehensive. A **limited consultation** is one that was done without the pathologist's review of the medical record of the patient, and a **comprehensive consultation** is one in which the medical record was reviewed as a part of the consultative services. When either of these consultation codes is submitted to a third-party payer, the submission is accompanied by a written report.

These are not the only consultation codes in the Pathology and Laboratory section of the CPT manual. There are also consultation codes toward the end of the section in the Surgical

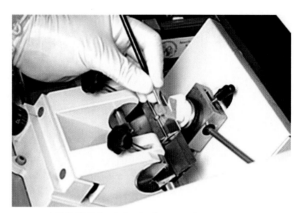

FIGURE 29-2 Frozen section preparation.

Pathology subsection (88321-88334) that report the services of a pathologist who reviews and gives an opinion or advice concerning pathology slides, specimens, material, or records that were prepared elsewhere or for pathology consultation during surgery. Pathology consultations during surgery are provided to examine tissue removed from a patient during a surgical procedure. If the pathologist did not use a microscope to examine the tissue, report 88329. If a microscope was used to examine the tissue, report 88331 or 88332, depending on the number of specimens that were examined.

A **specimen** is a sample of tissue from a suspect area; a **block** is a frozen piece of a specimen; and a **section** is a slice of a frozen block. A pathologist prepares a specimen by cutting it into blocks and taking sections from the blocks. The preparation of a frozen section is illustrated in Fig. 29-2. The number of sections taken depends on the judgment of the pathologist as to the number of areas of the specimen that need to be examined. The frozen section is placed (mounted) on a slide or held by other means that allow the pathologist to view the tissue under a microscope.

CODING SHOT

Each specimen may be reported separately, but each slide from that specimen may not.

When one block is sectioned and examined, the service of examining that first section is reported using 88331. The second and subsequent sections of the same block are included in the reporting of 88331. If another block from another area (a second block) was sectioned, the first section would be reported using 88331, and subsequent sections from the second block using 88332. You cannot use 88332 without first reporting 88331. Although 88332 is not marked as an add-on code (one that is used only with another code), its function is that of an add-on code because it is for subsequent sections that were examined.

CMS RULES

The edits bundle **88329** (pathology consultation during surgery) with **88331** (first tissue block) and **88332** (each additional tissue block). By issuing this guideline, CMS includes the frozen sections in the consultation bundle, which would usually be reported separately.

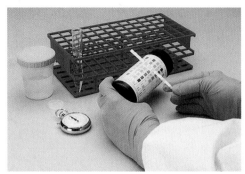

FIGURE 29-3 Urinalysis with chemical reagent strips.

URINALYSIS, MOLECULAR PATHOLOGY, AND CHEMISTRY

Many types of tests are located under the Urinalysis and Chemistry subsections (81000-84999). Urinalysis codes are for **nonspecific** tests performed on urine. Chemistry codes are for **specific** tests performed on material from any source (e.g., urine, blood, breath, feces, sputum) (Fig. 29-3). For example, a urinalysis using a dipstick (81000-81003) would report the presence and quantity of the following constituents: bilirubin, glucose, hemoglobin, ketones, leukocytes, nitrite, pH, protein, specific gravity, and urobilinogen. Any number of these constituents may be analyzed and reported using a code from the Urinalysis subsection (81000-81099). However, if the physician ordered an analysis of the urine specifically to determine the presence of urobilinogen (reduced bilirubin) and the exact amount of urobilinogen present (quantitative analysis), you would choose a code (84580) from the Chemistry subsection. The main things to remember when coding from these two subsections are:

1. Identify specific tests
2. Determine if the test was automated (by machine) or nonautomated (manual)
3. Number of tests performed
4. Identify combination codes for similar types of tests
5. Whether the results are qualitative or quantitative
6. Method of testing

MOLECULAR PATHOLOGY

The Molecular Pathology codes are divided into Tier 1 and Tier 2 codes. Tier 1 codes (81161, 81200-81383) report services for molecular assays that are more commonly performed. For example, 81211 is an essay to determine the presence of a breast cancer gene—BRCA1 (breast cancer 1) and BRCA2 (breast cancer 2). There are many conditions in which a genetic predisposition can be predicted, such as cystic fibrosis and colon cancer. Tier 2 codes 81400-81479 involve less commonly performed analyses and are arranged by the required level of technical resources and the level of physician interpretation or other qualified health professional.

EXERCISE 29-3 *Urinalysis, Molecular Pathology, and Chemistry*

Code the following:

1 An automated urinalysis without microscopy

CPT Code: _____

2 Urinalysis, microscopic only

CPT Code: _____

3 Albumin, serum

CPT Code: _____

4 Total bilirubin

CPT Code: _____

5 Gases, blood pH only, in a patient with respiratory failure

CPT Code: _____

ICD-10-CM Code: _____ (ICD-9-CM Code: _____)

6 Sodium, urine, in a patient with congestive heart failure

CPT Code: _____

ICD-10-CM Code: _____ (ICD-9-CM Code: _____)

7 Uric acid, blood in a patient with acute gouty arthritis

CPT Code: _____

ICD-10-CM Code: _____ (ICD-9-CM Code: _____)

(Answers are located in Appendix B)

HEMATOLOGY AND COAGULATION

The Hematology and Coagulation subsection contains codes (85002-85999) based on the various blood-drawing methods and tests. The method used to perform the test is often what determines code assignment. A blood count is used to measure the kind and number of cells in the blood, such as red and white blood cells. It is a commonly used test to detect various abnormalities in the blood. Blood counts can be manual or automated (Fig. 29-4), with many variations of the tests. For example, codes in the range 85004-85049 are blood count codes divided by method (manual or automated) and type of count, such as white blood count (WBC, 85004-85009) or a complete blood count (CBC, 85025, 85027). To accurately code a blood count, the method and the type of the count must be documented.

There are codes within the Hematology and Coagulation subsection for blood smear and bone marrow smear interpretations (85060, 85097). When a physician procures the bone marrow by means of aspiration, the service is reported with a code from the Surgery section (38220); but that is only part of the service. The other part of the service is the pathology analysis of the aspirated specimen. As the coder in a clinic setting, you may be reporting only the surgical services or only the pathology/laboratory services or a combination of both. When reporting the surgical services, always review the pathology report as a part of the code assignment, and when reporting the pathology services, always review the operative report.

There are many blood coagulation tests located in the Hematology and Coagulation subsection. The codes are divided based on the particular factor being tested. Great care must be taken to ensure that the correct coagulation factor has been reported based on the information in the medical record. Coagulation factor tests analyze the level of certain proteins in the blood that enable the blood to congeal properly. Low levels of a factor may result in excessive bleeding and high levels may lead to clot formation (thrombosis). For example, 85610 reports

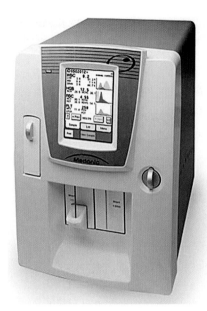

FIGURE 29-4 Hematology analyzer.

a test to assess the level of factor II (also known as a prothrombin). This test is often performed when a patient is on a blood thinning medication and the physician wants to determine if the factor is at the optimal level.

Most of the tests in the Hematology and Coagulation subsection can be located in the index of the CPT manual under the name of the test, such as prothrombin time, coagulation time, or hemogram.

EXERCISE 29-4   *Hematology and Coagulation*

Code the following:

1 Blood count by an automated hemogram (RBC, WBC, Hgb, Hct, and platelet count)

CPT Code: _____

2 Blood count by an automated hemogram and platelet count with complete differential white blood cell count in a patient with anemia due to acute blood loss

CPT Code: _____

ICD-10-CM Code: _____ (ICD-9-CM Code: _____)

3 Automated RBC

CPT Code: _____

4 Interpretation of a bone marrow smear in a patient with acute leukemia, in remission

CPT Code: _____

ICD-10-CM Code: _____ (ICD-9-CM Code: _____)

(Answers are located in Appendix B)

As you can see, there are many variations of just a blood count test! Read the medical record and code descriptions carefully before assigning the codes.

IMMUNOLOGY

Immunology codes (86000-86804) report identification of conditions of the immune system caused by the action of antibodies (e.g., hypersensitivity, allergic reactions, immunity, and alterations of body tissue).

EXERCISE 29-5 *Immunology*

Code the following:

1 ANA (antinuclear antibody) titer

    CPT Code: _____

2 ASO (antistreptolysin O) screen

    CPT Code: _____

3 Cold agglutinin screen in a patient with acute upper respiratory infections

    CPT Code: _____

    ICD-10-CM Code: _____ (ICD-9-CM Code: _____)

(Answers are located in Appendix B)

TRANSFUSION MEDICINE

The Transfusion Medicine subsection codes (86850-86999) report tests performed on blood or blood products. Tests include screening of blood (Fig. 29-5) for antibodies, Coombs testing, autologous blood collection and processing, blood typing, compatibility testing, and preparation of and treatments performed on blood and blood products.

Transfusion of blood and blood components is reported with codes from a variety of locations. For example, to report the actual blood transfusion, assign 36430 from the Surgery section of the CPT manual. You must also report the substance being transfused, such as whole blood, HCPCS code P9010 per unit or red blood cells, P9021 per unit. The blood bank would provide and report the collection, processing, and storing of the autologous blood with 86890.

EXERCISE 29-6 *Transfusion Medicine*

Code the following:

1 ABO and Rh blood typing, serologic

    CPT Codes: _____, _____

2 Irradiation of blood product, 3 units

    CPT Code: _____

(Answers are located in Appendix B)

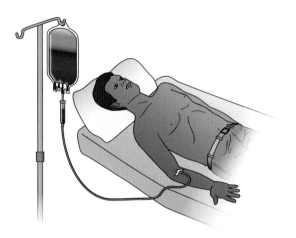

FIGURE 29–5   Blood transfusion.

MICROBIOLOGY

Microbiology codes (87001-87999) report the study of microorganisms and include bacteriology (study of bacteria), mycology (study of fungi), parasitology (study of parasites), and virology (study of viruses). For example, Fig. 29-6 illustrates a Petri dish used to culture microbes. Culture codes for the identification of organisms as well as the identification of sensitivities of the organism to antibiotics (called culture and sensitivity) are located in this subsection. Culture codes must be read carefully because some codes report screening only to detect the presence of an organism; some codes indicate the identification of specific organisms; and others indicate additional sensitivity testing to determine which antibiotic would be best for treatment of the specified bacteria. You report all tests performed on the basis of whether they are quantitative or qualitative and/or a sensitivity study.

QUICK CHECK 29-2

1. According to the Microbiology Guidelines, how do you report multiple procedures rendered on the same day? _____

(Answers are located in Appendix C)

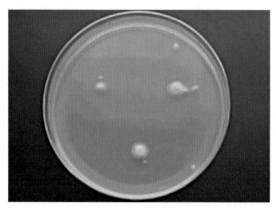

FIGURE 29–6   Mold growing in Petri dish.

EXERCISE 29-7 *Microbiology*

Code the following:

1 HIV-1, quantification

CPT Code: _____

2 Streptococcus, group A, using an amplified probe method in a patient with headache and fever

CPT Code: _____

ICD-10-CM Codes: _____, _____

(ICD-9-CM Codes: _____, _____)

3 Quantification of *Gardnerella vaginalis,* herpes simplex, and *Candida* species, in a patient with bacterial vaginosis

CPT Codes: _____, _____, _____

ICD-10-CM Code: _____ (ICD-9-CM Code: _____)

4 Direct probe method of mycobacterial tuberculosis, herpes simplex virus, and *Chlamydia trachomatis*

CPT Codes: _____, _____, _____

5 Bacterial culture of urine, quantitative with colony count for urination frequency

⊛ CPT Code(s): _____

⊛ ICD-10-CM Code(s): _____ (⊛ ICD-9-CM Code(s): _____)

(Answers are located in Appendix B)

ANATOMIC PATHOLOGY

Anatomic Pathology codes (88000-88099) report examination of body fluids or tissues in postmortem (after death) examination. Postmortem examination involves the completion of gross, microscopic, and limited autopsies. Codes are divided according to the extent of the examination. This subsection also contains codes for forensic examination and coroner's call. For example, some codes report an examination without the central nervous system (88000, 88020), with the brain (88005, 88025), with the brain and the spinal cord (88007, 88027), etc. There are two codes for each extent because one is a gross examination and one is a microscopic examination.

CYTOPATHOLOGY AND CYTOGENIC STUDIES

The Cytopathology subsection codes (88104-88199) report the laboratory work performed to determine whether cellular changes are present. For example, a very common cytopathology procedure is the Papanicolaou smear (Pap smear). Cytopathology may also be performed on fluids that have been aspirated from a site to identify cellular changes. Cytogenetic Studies (88230-88299) include tests performed for genetic and chromosomal studies.

QUICK CHECK 29-3

1. Which codes report conventional Pap smears examined using non-Bethesda reporting?

_____

(Answers are located in Appendix C)

SURGICAL PATHOLOGY

Surgical Pathology codes (88300-88399) describe the evaluation of specimens to determine the pathology of disease processes. When choosing the correct code for pathology, identify the source of the specimen and the reason for the surgical procedure. The Surgical Pathology subsection codes are divided into six levels (Levels I through VI) based on the specimen examined and the level of work required by the pathologist. Pathology testing is performed on all tissue removed from the body. The surgical pathology classification level is determined by the complexity of the pathologic examination.

From the Trenches

"Being certified opens many doors, but it also gives a level of credibility and confidence to your work, which makes a difference when dealing with other professions."

KEITH

Level I pathology code 88300 identifies specimens that normally do not need to be viewed under a microscope for pathologic diagnosis (e.g., a tooth)—those for which the probability of disease or malignancy is minimal.

Level II pathology code 88302 deals with those tissues that are usually considered normal tissue and have been removed not because of the probability of the presence of disease or malignancy, but for some other reason (e.g., a fallopian tube for sterilization, foreskin of a newborn).

Level III pathology code 88304 is assigned for specimens with a low probability of disease or malignancy. For example, a gallbladder may be neoplastic (benign or malignant), but when the gallbladder is removed for cholecystitis (inflammation of the gallbladder), it is usually inflamed from chronic disease and not because of cancerous changes.

Level IV pathology code 88305 designates a higher probability of malignancy or decision making for disease pathology. For example, a uterus is removed because of a diagnosis of prolapse. There is a possibility that the uterus is malignant or that there are other causes of disease pathology.

Level V pathology code 88307 classifies more complex pathology evaluations (e.g., examination of a uterus that was removed for reasons other than prolapse or neoplasm).

Level VI pathology code 88309 includes examination of neoplastic tissue or very involved specimens, such as a total resection of a colon.

For example, 88305 reports examination of tissue from a breast biopsy that does not require microscopic evaluation of the margins or tissue from a breast reduction; 88307 reports examination of tissue from the excision of a breast lesion that does require microscopic evaluation of the margins and a partial/simple mastectomy; and 88309 reports examination of tissue from a mastectomy with regional lymph node. The probability of cancer increases with each code.

CODING SHOT

A specimen is defined as tissue submitted for examination. If two specimens of the same area are received and examined, each specimen is reported. For example, if two separately identified anus tags are received and each is examined, report 88304 × 2. If one anus tag is received and two different areas of the tag are examined, report 88304 only once.

The remaining codes at the end of the subsection classify specialized procedures, utilization of stains, consultations performed, preparations used, and/or instrumentation needed to complete testing.

The surgical pathology codes are located in the index under the main term "Pathology" and subterms "Surgical" and "Gross and Micro Exam."

EXERCISE 29-8   *Surgical Pathology*

Code the following using one of the six surgical pathology codes in the CPT manual:

1 The specimen is a uterus, tubes, and ovaries. The procedure was an abdominal hysterectomy for ovarian cancer.

CPT Code: _____

2 The specimen is a portion of a lung. The procedure was a left lower lobe segmental resection.

CPT Code: _____

3 The specimen is the prostate. The procedure was a transurethral resection of the prostate.

CPT Code: _____

4 What is the surgical pathology code for the following pathology report?

CPT Code: _____

PATHOLOGY DEPARTMENT

Patient:	Alice C. Fisher	**Date Collected:**	02/09/XX
DOB:	12/06/37	**Date Received:**	02/09/XX
Sex:	F	**Date Examined:**	02/10/XX
Record Number:	5909890	**Access Number:**	P4218
Account:	MP8352	**Surgeon:**	Dr. White

CLINICAL HISTORY: UMBILICAL HERNIA, INFLAMED

TISSUE RECEIVED: UMBILICAL HERNIA

GROSS DESCRIPTION: The specimen is labeled with the patient's name and "umbilical hernia" and consists of yellow-white fibrofatty tissue approximately 3.5 × 2 × 1 cm. Representative sections are processed in two slides.

MICROSCOPIC DIAGNOSIS: Mature adipose tissue with fibrovascular and fibrotendinous tissue with focal reactive fibrous tissue consistent with umbilical hernia.

Alberto Matusa, MD
_____
Alberto Matusa, MD
Head, Pathology Department
Merry Brook Hospital

(Answers are located in Appendix B)

OTHER PROCEDURES

Other Procedures includes miscellaneous testing on body fluids, the use of special instrumentation, and testing performed on oocytes and sperm.

CHAPTER REVIEW

CHAPTER 29, PART I, THEORY

Without the use of the CPT manual, complete the following:

1 The Pathology and Laboratory section of the CPT manual is formatted according to the type of _____ performed.

2 Laboratories have built-in _____ that allow additional tests to be performed without the written order of the physician.

3 Codes that are grouped according to the usual laboratory work ordered by a physician for diagnosis or screening of various diseases or conditions are _____.

4 Can you use a reduced service modifier with pathology or laboratory codes?

    Yes   No

5 Will the medical record contain the method used to perform the test?

    Yes   No

CHAPTER 29, PART II, PRACTICAL

Answer the following:

6 The Hematology and Coagulation subsections contain codes based on the various testing methods and tests. The method used to do the test is often the code determiner. Blood cell counts can be manual or automated, with many variations of the tests. What would the code be for an automated blood count (hemogram) with automated differential WBC count? A manual blood count (hemogram) with manual cell count?

    Automated CPT Code: _____

    Manual CPT Code: _____ × _____

Code the following three cases with the correct pathology code from the CPT:

7 The specimen is tonsils and adenoids. The procedure is a tonsillectomy with adenoidectomy.

    🔴 CPT Code(s): _____

8 The specimen is an appendix. The procedure is an incidental appendectomy.

    🔴 CPT Code(s): _____

9 The specimen is a tooth. The procedure is an odontectomy, gross examination only.

    🔴 CPT Code(s): _____

Code the following:

10 Western Blot of blood, with interpretation and report

    🔴 CPT Code(s): _____

11 Vitamin K analysis of blood

    🔴 CPT Code(s): _____

12 Quantitative analysis of urine for alkaloids

    🔴 CPT Code(s): _____

13 Three specimens of gastric secretions for total gastric acid

    🔴 CPT Code(s): _____

Chapter Review answers are only available in the TEACH Instructor Resources on Evolve

14 Blood analysis for HGH

    CPT Code(s): _____

15 Total insulin

    CPT Code(s): _____

16 LDL cholesterol using direct measurements

    CPT Code(s): _____

17 Blood count (leukocyte only): one manual cell count

    CPT Code(s): _____

18 Blood smear interpretation

    CPT Code(s): _____

19 PTT of whole blood

    CPT Code(s): _____

20 Sedimentation rate, automated for fever and swelling in hand

    CPT Code(s): _____

    ICD-10-CM Code(s): _____

    (ICD-9-CM Code(s): _____)

21 Lee and White coagulation time

    CPT Code(s): _____

22 Clotting factor XII (Hageman factor) for excessive bleeding menopausal onset

    CPT Code(s): _____

    ICD-10-CM Code(s): _____

    (ICD-9-CM Code(s): _____)

23 Blood typing for paternity test, ABO, Rh, and MN

    CPT Code(s): _____

24 Culture of urine for bacteria with colony count for pain on urination

    CPT Code(s): _____

    ICD-10-CM Code(s): _____

    (ICD-9-CM Code(s): _____)

25 Schlichter test for complaints of leg pain and fever

    CPT Code(s): _____

    ICD-10-CM Code(s): _____

    (ICD-9-CM Code(s): _____)

26 Postmortem examination, gross only, with brain and spinal cord

    CPT Code(s): _____

27 Therapeutic drug assay for total digoxin and vancomycin, patient has chronic sinus bradycardia

    CPT Code(s): _____

    ICD-10-CM Code(s): _____

    (ICD-9-CM Code(s): _____)

28 Pathology consultation during surgery

    CPT Code(s): _____

Chapter Review answers are only available in the TEACH Instructor Resources on Evolve

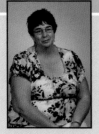

"Teamwork is so important! You have to be able to work with other people, and keep your mind open at all times. . . . Coding can be subjective; there is no one who knows everything."

Stephanie A. Lewis, CPC, ACS-EM, CCP
Compliance Analyst
University of Missouri Health Care
Columbia, Missouri

Medicine

Chapter Topics

Format

Introduction to Immunizations

Psychiatry

Biofeedback

Dialysis

Gastroenterology

Ophthalmology

Special Otorhinolaryngologic Services

Cardiovascular

Pulmonary

Allergy and Clinical Immunology

Endocrinology

Neurology and Neuromuscular Procedures

Central Nervous System Assessments/Tests

Health and Behavior Assessment/Intervention

Learning Objectives

After completing this chapter you should be able to

1 Analyze the format of the Medicine section.

2 Report psychiatric services.

3 Identify biofeedback services.

4 List components of dialysis reporting.

5 Demonstrate ability to report gastrointestinal services.

6 Understand ophthalmology and otorhinolaryngologic reporting.

7 Report cardiovascular services.

8 Identify services reported with pulmonary codes.

9 List the important elements of coding allergy and clinical immunology services.

10 Report endocrine services.

11 Define neurology and neuromuscular services.

12 Demonstrate an understanding of central nervous system assessment and intervention.

13 Analyze chemotherapy services.

14 Report special services and dermatologic procedures.

15 Code physical medicine and rehabilitation services.

16 Report active wound management.

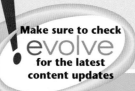

Make sure to check **evolve** for the latest content updates

17 Define osteopathic and chiropractic services.

18 Understand non-face-to-face services.

19 Code special services, procedures, and reports.

20 Report medical services using Medicine section codes.

The Medicine section (90281-99607) reports diagnostic and therapeutic services that are generally **noninvasive** (not entering a body cavity), but there are also **invasive** (entering a body cavity) procedures in the section, such as cardiac catheterization. The section begins with Subsection Information and Guidelines applicable to all of the Medicine section codes, such as Add-on Codes, Separate Procedures, Unlisted Service/Procedure, Special Report, and Supplied Materials.

The various subsections of Medicine contain many specific notes to be applied with a certain group of codes, so be certain to read all notes that pertain to the group of codes with which you are working.

FORMAT

Take a moment now to review the Medicine section in the CPT manual to have an overview of the subsections.

Many specialized types of tests are located in the Medicine section (e.g., biofeedback, audiologic function tests, electrocardiograms). Codes in this section do not usually include the supplies used in the testing, therapy, or diagnostic treatments unless specifically stated in the code description or guidelines. You report supplies, including drugs, separately unless otherwise instructed in the code information. CPT code 99070 is the supplies and materials code used to identify the supplying of drugs, trays, supplies, or materials needed to provide

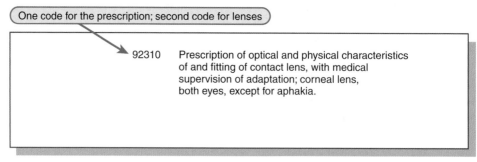

FIGURE 30–1 Some codes are for the supply only.

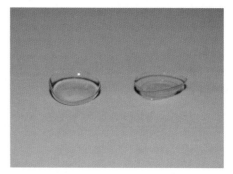

FIGURE 30–2 Contact lenses.

the service or the specific HCPCS supply code, which is usually what the payer will require. For example, Fig. 30-1 illustrates the code for the service of a prescription for corneal contact lenses (also known as contacts, see Fig. 30-2) for both eyes (92310). When the lenses and the prescription services are provided, both the lenses and the prescription service are reported. The supply of contact lenses may be reported as part of the service of fitting or reported separately using the appropriate HCPCS Level II supply code (V2500-V2599). Reporting the supply of the lens depends on the third-party payer guidelines.

INTRODUCTION TO IMMUNIZATIONS

There are two types of immunization—active and passive. **Active immunization** is the type given when it is anticipated that the person will be in contact with the disease. Active immunization agents can be toxoids or vaccines. Toxoids are bacteria that have been made nontoxic and when injected, produce an immune response that builds protection against a disease. Vaccines are viruses that are given in small doses and cause an immune response. **Passive immunization** does not cause an immune response; rather, the injected material contains a high level of antibodies against a disease (e.g., rabies, hepatitis B, tetanus), called immune globulins.

The first three subsections in the Medicine section are:

- Immune Globulins, Serum or Recombinant Products
- Immunization Administration for Vaccines/Toxoids
- Vaccines, Toxoids

Immune Globulins

The immune globulins (90281-90399) are passive immunization agents obtained from pooled human plasma that is immune to a particular disease.

The codes in this subsection identify only the immune globulin **product** and must be reported with the appropriate **administration** code (96365-96368, 96372, 96374, or 96375 as appropriate).

QUICK CHECK 30-1

1. Immune globulins are _____ injections.
   a. Active
   b. Passive
   c. Both a and b
   d. Neither a nor b

(Answers are located in Appendix C)

Codes in the Immune Globulins subsection are categorized according to the:
■ Type of immune globulin (rabies, hepatitis B, etc.)
■ Method of injection (IM, IV, SC, etc.)
■ Type of dose (full dose, mini-dose, etc.)

Immunization Administration for Vaccines/Toxoids

The Immunization Administration subsection codes (90460-90474) are reported in conjunction with the Vaccines, Toxoids subsection codes (90476-90749). Immunization reporting requires two codes: one to report the **administration** and one to report the **substance** administered. A variety of administration methods are utilized to deliver the vaccine/toxoid: percutaneous, intradermal, subcutaneous, intramuscular, intranasal, or oral. The administration codes are divided based on the **method** of administration and in some codes, the patient **age, when administered with physician counseling.** Report each dose administered—single or combination with the appropriate administration code.

■ Codes 90460-90461 report immunization administration for patients through age 18 and for which counseling has been provided to the patient's family regarding the vaccine/toxoid. Report 90460 for each vaccine administered. For vaccines with multiple components (combined vaccines), report 90460 in conjunction with 90461 for each additional component in the vaccine.

■ Codes 90471-90474 report immunizations at which the physician did NOT provide counseling for patients of **any age,** including patients through age 18.

For example, you can report multiple administrations by reporting 90471 for the first administration and then reporting 90472 for each administration after the first.

Example without counseling

90471	**Administration** service for tetanus
90703	Tetanus toxoid (substance injected, IM)
90472	**Administration** service for rubella
90706	Rubella virus (substance injected, SC)
90472	**Administration** service for diphtheria (may require modifier -59, based on payer guidelines)
90719	Diphtheria toxoid (substance injected, IM)

Or you can report the first administration with 90471, as you would usually do, and then report 90472 times the number of injections after the first one.

Example—Administration

90471	Administration service for tetanus
90472 × 2	Administration service, rubella and diphtheria

If several vaccines were administered, report the service as:

Example—Multiple Vaccines

90471	Administration service for tetanus and diphtheria
90702	Tetanus and diphtheria toxoids (substances injected, IM)
90472	Administration service for rubella
90706	Rubella virus (substance injected, SC)

CMS RULES

Medicare reimburses for tetanus injections (90703 [tetanus, age 7>, IM]) when given for an acute injury to a person who is incompletely immunized. When a tetanus booster is given to a patient in the absence of an injury, the injection (90703) is not covered by Medicare.

Vaccines, Toxoids

The Vaccines, Toxoids subsection codes (90476-90749) report vaccine products for immunizations. The subsection contains many codes for a single disease (e.g., 90703 for tetanus toxoid) as well as codes for a combination of diseases (e.g., 90700 for diphtheria, tetanus, and acellular pertussis [DTaP]). In many of the code descriptions, specific ages are identified. For example, 90658, trivalent (3 viruses) influenza virus vaccine, specifies age 3 and above, whereas code 90657, trivalent influenza virus vaccine, specifies ages 6 to 35 months. Vaccines have pediatric or adult listed on the label of the vial. You must carefully review the description of the vaccine product to determine which disease is specified in the code you are assigning. When one code is available to describe multiple products given, the combination code must be assigned. If each vaccine were to be listed separately when a combination vaccine was administered, it would be considered unbundling.

CMS RULES

When reporting an adult dose of a pneumococcal vaccine (90732) to Medicare, the pneumococcal administration code is **G0009** with a diagnosis code of **Z23/V03.02** (prophylactic vaccination, streptococcus pneumoniae). Once Medicare has assigned a HCPCS Level II administration code for a vaccine, the CPT administration code is not accepted.

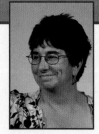

From the Trenches

"I often tell coders and auditors I work with that they are detectives and should think and act like a detective, never giving up until they have dug up all the information that they can to back up what they are telling a physician or non-physician practitioner."

STEPHANIE

✋ **CAUTION** *There are often multiple codes available for variations of the product. For example, there are eight codes with combinations of diphtheria. Read all descriptions carefully before assigning a code.*

There are codes with schedules for a vaccine, such as a three-dose or four-dose schedule. For example, 90634 is a two-dose hepatitis A vaccine that is intended to be administered on a two-dose schedule. Each time the vaccine is administered, 90634 is reported along with the date of the injection. The term "schedule" refers to the number of doses provided and the timing of the administration. The doses and timing must be exactly as specified in the code.

The CPT Guidelines state that modifier -51 (multiple procedures) should not be reported for the vaccines/toxoids when performed with administration procedures. Most payers want you to report the administration codes multiple times or use the "times" symbol (×) to indicate the number of injections given.

If a patient is given a vaccine in the course of an E/M service, the administration and Vaccines/Toxoids codes are assigned in addition to the E/M code. Some third-party payers require a -25 modifier on the E/M code, so be certain to check with your local payer on how to submit the E/M code.

CODING SHOT

If the only service is administration of a vaccine and no other service was provided, do not report an E/M service.

CPT Influenza Vaccine Codes:

CPT	90657	Influenza virus vaccine, trivalent, split virus, when administered to children **6-35 months of age,** for intramuscular use
	90658	Influenza virus vaccine, trivalent, split virus, when administered to individuals **3 years of age and older,** for intramuscular use

Report Administration of Influenza Vaccine:

HCPCS	G0008	Administration of influenza vaccine (Medicare only)
CPT	90471	Immunization administration, one vaccine
	90472	Immunization administration, each additional vaccine

CPT Pneumococcal Vaccine Code:

	90732	Pneumococcal polysaccharide **vaccine,** 23-valent, 2 years of age and older, for subcutaneous or intramuscular use

Report Administration of Pneumococcal Vaccine:

HCPCS	G0009	Administration of pneumococcal vaccine (Medicare only)
CPT	90471	Immunization administration, one vaccine
	90472	Immunization administration, each additional vaccine

CMS RULES

If a Medicare patient receives reasonable and necessary services constituting an office visit level of service, the physician may bill for the office visit, the vaccine and the administration of the vaccine. Do not report 99211 instead of the administration service when only the administration is performed.

Hepatitis B vaccines and the administration are available to Medicare beneficiaries who are at high or intermediate risk of contracting hepatitis B. Diagnosis code Z23/V05.3 (prophylactic vaccination against viral hepatitis) must be submitted to demonstrate the medical necessity. The administration code for Medicare is G0010 (administration of hepatitis B vaccine) and for other payers the administration is 90471.

CODING SHOT

The diagnosis codes Z23/V03-V06 report the need for a prophylactic (preventative) vaccination or inoculation. These codes can be located in the Index of the ICD-10-CM/ICD-9-CM manual under the main term "Vaccination."

EXERCISE 30-1 | *Immunizations*

To report an E/M service with a vaccine service, a separate identifiable E/M service must have been provided and documented in the medical record. The following vaccines were administered to a variety of patients. If they have a brief history and examination performed to assess vaccine needs and general health status no E/M service will be reported except if the question indicates there was a "separate service" provided.

1 A parent takes a 9-year-old child to the child's physician for an oral poliomyelitis vaccine. The physician's assistant evaluates the child (established patient) and administers the vaccine orally to the child.

   CPT Codes: _____ (poliovirus vaccine), _____ (administration)

   ICD-10-CM Code: _____ (ICD-9-CM Code: _____)

2 An established patient (10 years old); the only service for the visit is an injection of DTP (diphtheria, tetanus toxoid, pertussis) and oral poliovirus. Services were provided by the nurse, at the direction of the physician.

   CPT Codes: _____ (DTP vaccine), _____ (poliovirus vaccine), _____
   _____ (administrations)

   ICD-10-CM Code: _____ (ICD-9-CM Codes: _____, _____)

3 An established patient, a 1-year-old, is brought in for a well-baby checkup (separate service) by the physician, and the following are given: DT and IM injectable poliomyelitis. The physician counseled the parent on the vaccines. A comprehensive preventative medicine evaluation was provided by the physician.

   CPT Codes: _____ (E/M), _____ (vaccine), _____
   (vaccine), _____ _____ (administrations)

   ICD-10-CM Codes: _____ (child examination), _____ (immunization encounter),
   _____ (counseling)

   (ICD-9-CM Codes: _____ (child examination), _____ (vaccination) _____
   (vaccination))

4 A 64-year-old established patient comes in for a trivalent influenza virus (not preservative-free) vaccine that is administered intramuscularly by the nurse. The vaccine is the only service provided at that visit.

   CPT Codes: _____ (vaccination), _____ (administration)

   ICD-10-CM Code: _____ (ICD-9-CM Code: _____)

5 A new patient, 30 years old, comes for an office visit to evaluate her hypothyroid status at which time the physician does an expanded problem focused history and physical examination (separate service) and also administers a DTP and *Haemophilus influenzae* B (Hib) vaccine.

   CPT Codes: _____ (E/M), _____ (vaccine), _____ (administration)

   ICD-10-CM Codes: _____, _____

   (ICD-9-CM Codes: _____, _____, _____)

6 A parent brings an 18-month-old infant (established patient) for a well-baby examination (separate service) at which the physician administers a vaccine intramuscularly for diphtheria and tetanus toxoid (DT) after counseling the parent on the vaccines.

   CPT Codes: _____ (E/M), _____ (vaccine), _____,
   _____ (administration)

   ICD-10-CM Codes: _____, _____, _____

   (ICD-9-CM Codes: _____, _____)

7 A 50-year-old established patient presents to the nurse for a trivalent flu shot.

   CPT Codes: _____, _____

   ICD-10-CM Code: _____ (ICD-9-CM Code: _____)

(Answers are located in Appendix B)

PSYCHIATRY

The Psychiatry subsection (90785-90899) has a lengthy note under the heading detailing the use of psychiatric codes. If psychiatric treatments are rendered on the same day as E/M services, both the E/M service and the psychiatric treatment are reported with one code from the Psychiatry subsection. For example, if a patient is admitted to the hospital with a drug overdose secondary to depression, and the physician spends 60 minutes in crisis psychotherapy with the patient several hours after he was admitted to the hospital, services are reported with 90839 (Other Psychotherapy) for the psychiatric treatment and medical evaluation/management on the same day. Code 90839 includes the development of orders, the review and interpretation of laboratory work or other diagnostic studies, and the review of therapy reports and other information from the medical record. If the psychiatric treatment is provided on a different day than the E/M service, a code from the E/M section would be reported in addition to the psychiatry code. You will work closely with third-party payers to determine any specific regional instructions for coding psychiatric services.

Partial hospitalization refers to a hospital setting in which the patients are in the hospital during the day and return to their homes in the evenings and on weekends. The facilities may be open only during the day, 5 days a week, although there are also facilities that are open 7 days a week. When a physician admits a patient to a partial hospital facility, the physician is responsible for preparing all of the admission paperwork that is prepared for admission to an acute care hospital. E/M Initial Hospital Care and Subsequent Hospital Care codes (99221-99233) report inpatient stays. The psychiatric services the physician provides to the patient are listed separately unless the E/M service and psychiatric service are provided on the same day. These same-day services are reported with codes from the Psychiatry subsection.

Specific descriptions of services included in each of the codes appear in the Psychiatry subsection. Some codes reflect evaluation or diagnostic services, such as CPT code 90791 (diagnostic evaluation); some reflect therapeutic procedures, such as 90832 (psychotherapy); and still others, located in the Central Nervous System Assessments/Tests, report psychological testing, such as code 96101 (psychological testing, per hour).

A **psychiatrist** is a physician who specializes in psychiatry, the practice of diagnosing and treating mental disorders. A **psychologist** is not a physician but is a qualified specialist in psychiatry. States have varying regulations about how a psychologist reports services provided, and some states require a psychologist to provide and report services only under the supervision of a psychiatrist. Third-party payers may also restrict the types of service a psychologist may report for reimbursement.

Time is the major billing factor in the Psychiatry subsection. Diagnostic and therapeutic time must be documented in the patient's record to provide accurate billing.

Codes 90791 and 90792, psychiatric diagnostic evaluation and comprehensive psychiatric service, are described as the elicitation (gathering) of a complete medical (including past, family, social) and psychiatric history, establishment of a tentative diagnosis, and an evaluation of the patient's ability and willingness to work to solve the mental problem. This service includes a complete mental status exam. Information may be obtained from the patient, other physicians, and/or family. There may be overlapping of the medical and psychiatric history depending on the problem. An E/M service may be substituted for the initial interview procedure, including consultation codes (99241-99245), provided the required elements of the E/M service are provided. Consultation services require, in addition to the history and examination, a written report of the consultation's opinion or advice. Consultation does not include psychiatric treatment.

Psychotherapy is the therapeutic treatment of a psychological disorder or behavior and is reported with codes 90832-90838. The codes are time-based (30, 45, or 60 minutes) and subdivided based on if the psychotherapy was provided in addition to another primary procedure. The medical record must identify the time spent providing the psychotherapy service. If the time spent providing the service is not recorded on the medical record, the physician should be queried. If no time can be identified, report the service with an E/M code, not a Psychotherapy code. The psychotherapy service may be provided to a patient and/or the patient's family member.

Crisis psychotherapy (90839, 90840) provides treatment to a patient experiencing a reaction to a more specific event or situation; for example, a drug overdose, attempted suicide, or an episode of severe depression. Crisis psychotherapy focuses on the immediate assessment and treatment of the patient in a crisis and is not intended to treat chronic psychological conditions.

Some patients receive psychotherapy only and others receive psychotherapy and medical E/M services. E/M services involve a variety of responsibilities unique to the medical management of psychiatric patients, such as medical diagnostic evaluation, drug management when indicated, physician orders, interpretation of laboratory or other medical diagnostic studies and observations, review of activity therapy reports, the supervision of nursing and ancillary personnel, and scheduling of hospital resources for diagnosis and treatment, and leadership or direction of a treatment team.

The medical record must indicate the **time** spent in the psychotherapy encounter and the therapeutic maneuvers, such as behavior modification, supportive interactions, and interpretation of unconscious motivation, that were applied to produce the therapeutic change.

The medical record should document the symptoms, the goals of therapy, and the methods of monitoring the outcome. It should also document why the chosen therapy is the appropriate treatment modality either instead of or in addition to another form of psychiatric treatment.

EXERCISE 30-2   *Psychiatry*

Using the CPT, ICD-10-CM and/or ICD-9-CM manuals, code the following:

1 Diagnostic psychotherapy evaluation in office for 30 minutes. The patient was diagnosed with chronic paranoid psychosis.

    CPT Code: _____

    ICD-10-CM Code: _____ (ICD-9-CM Code: _____)

2 Psychological testing, 2 hours, administered by a physician. The patient presents with moderate undersocialized aggressive outburst conduct disorder.

    CPT Code: _____ × _____

    ICD-10-CM Code: _____ (ICD-9-CM Code: _____)

3 Psychiatric evaluation of tests, medical records, or hospital data to make appropriate diagnosis for a 16-year-old male. Documentation supports an overanxious disorder.

    CPT Code: _____

    ICD-10-CM Code: _____ (ICD-9-CM Code: _____)

4 A 70 minute psychotherapy session for a patient who presents in a depressive state with tremors.

    CPT Code: _____

    ICD-10-CM Codes: _____ , _____

    (ICD-9-CM Codes: _____ , _____)

(Answers are located in Appendix B)

BIOFEEDBACK

Biofeedback is the process of giving a person self-information. The information can be used by patients to gain control over physiologic processes, such as blood pressure, heart rate, or pain. Patients are trained to use biofeedback by a professional and then continue the use of the therapy on their own. Biofeedback training is often incorporated in individual psychophysiologic therapy. When biofeedback is part of the individual psychophysiologic therapy, one code is reported for both the biofeedback training and the individual psychophysiologic therapy (90875-90876).

Biofeedback codes (90901, 90911) are located in the CPT manual index under the main terms "Training" and "Biofeedback."

EXERCISE 30-3 *Biofeedback*

Using the CPT, ICD-10-CM and/or ICD-9-CM manuals, code the following:

1 A 40-year-old woman has been seen by the physician for several individual psychiatric sessions as the patient attempts to give up a two-pack-a-day cigarette **addiction** of 15 years' continuous duration. The patient is experiencing increased **anxiety** and **insomnia**, which is the reason for this visit. As a part of the last 30-minute psychiatric session, the physician teaches the patient to use biofeedback in an attempt to help her alleviate the generalized anxiety and idiopathic insomnia. The patient is instructed to use the biofeedback techniques three times a day until the next session.

CPT Code: _____

ICD-10-CM Codes: _____, _____, _____

(ICD-9-CM Codes: _____, _____, _____)

2 A 52-year-old man is referred to the physician by his primary care physician for biofeedback to help regulate his blood pressure. The patient was diagnosed with hypertensive heart disease. There is no evidence of heart failure. The physician conducts a 60-minute session during which the patient is trained in the use of biofeedback.

CPT Code: _____

ICD-10-CM Code: _____ (ICD-9-CM Code: _____)

(Answers are located in Appendix B)

DIALYSIS

Dialysis is the cleansing of the blood of waste products when it is not possible for the body to perform the cleansing function adequately on its own. Dialysis may be temporary, as in the case of a patient who has acute renal failure from which he or she recovers, or permanent, as in the case of a patient with end-stage renal disease (ESRD) who will not recover without a kidney transplant.

The Dialysis subsection of the Medicine section (90935-90999) is divided into types of dialysis (see Table 30-1).

Hemodialysis

Hemodialysis is the routing of blood and its waste products to the outside of the body where it is filtered. After the blood is cleansed, it is returned to the body. Hemodialysis codes (90935 and 90937) are reported for each day the service is provided. The codes in the hemodialysis category are based on the number of times the physician evaluates the patient during the procedure.

Peritoneal Dialysis

Peritoneal dialysis (90945, 90947) involves using the peritoneal cavity as a filter. Dialysis fluid is introduced into the cavity and left there for several hours so cleansing can take place (Fig. 30-3). The dialysis fluid is then drained from the peritoneal cavity. Peritoneal dialysis is reported on the basis of each day the service is provided. Some patients learn how to perform dialysis for themselves. Dialysis teaching codes are located under Other Dialysis Procedures.

TABLE 30–1

TYPES OF DIALYSIS

The codes to report physician services for patients with end-stage renal disease are located in the 90951-90970 range. Codes 90951-90962 report a full month of physician service that includes monitoring the nutritional needs of the patient, assessing the status of the patient, and counseling. The monthly services are reported based on the age of the patient and number of face-to-face visits that occurred during the month.

Age	Visits per Month	Code
≤2	4+	90951
	2-3	90952
	1	90953
2-11	4+	90954
	2-3	90955
	1	90956
12-19	4+	90957
	2-3	90958
	1	90959
20+	4+	90960
	2-3	90961
	1	90962

If the physician provides the same evaluation and management to a patient receiving home dialysis, the monthly service is reported based on the age of the patient.

Age	Code
≤2	90963
2-11	90964
12-19	90965
20+	90966

If the physician provides these same services for less than a total month, the services are also reported based on the age of the patient.

Age	Code
≤2	90967
2-11	90968
12-19	90969
20+	90970

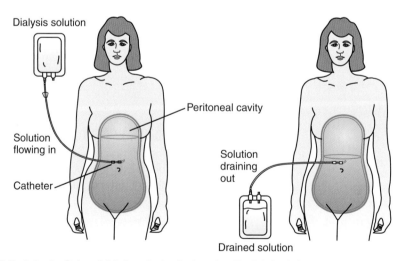

Dialysis solution

Solution flowing in

Catheter

Peritoneal cavity

Solution draining out

Drained solution

FIGURE 30–3 Peritoneal dialysis can be done by the patient. The dialysis solution enters the peritoneal cavity by a catheter. After the solution has been inside the patient for several hours, it is drained out through the catheter.

End Stage Renal Disease

The subheading (End Stage Renal Disease Services) deals with dialysis of an ongoing nature. The 90951-90966 codes reflect all services included in treating a patient with ESRD and are listed according to patient age (e.g., younger than 2 years of age, 2-11 years of age) and number of visits (1, 2-3, 4+) per month. Dialysis services are reported as a monthly fee. For those cases in which a patient may be, for example, visiting the area and will not require a full month of dialysis, daily fees may be reported using codes 90967-90970 in the ESRD category. Few third-party payers allow E/M codes to be reported in addition to dialysis service codes. Most payers consider the dialysis codes to be bundled to include all the treatment necessary for a patient with renal disease, including the E/M services. To report a separate E/M service, the condition would have to be unrelated to the renal condition, and modifier -25 must be added to the E/M code. The diagnosis code reported would also indicate that the E/M service was unrelated to the ESRD service.

Dialysis is usually performed in an outpatient setting at a hospital or other outpatient dialysis facility (Fig. 30-4). The physician services are reported based on the **type** of dialysis the patient is receiving, the **complexity** of the service, and the **number** of visits the physician provides to the patient. The reporting of just one code covers all physician visits to the dialysis laboratory during that month. During a physician's visit to the dialysis laboratory, the physician assesses the patient while the patient is receiving dialysis. The monthly services also include nutrition assessment and telephone calls.

CODING SHOT

If a patient is admitted to the hospital and requires management of his/her dialysis while in the hospital, the physician can report those services but then cannot report the monthly service for the time period the patient is in the hospital. The monthly service for services provided when the patient was not in the hospital is then reported with 90967-90970, which are per day codes.

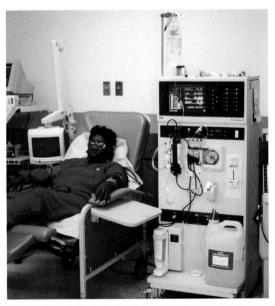

FIGURE 30-4 Patient receiving hemodialysis.

Dialysis patients must sometimes be admitted to the hospital and while in the hospital must continue to receive dialysis treatments. When the physician assesses the inpatient while the patient is undergoing dialysis, report 90935 (single visit) or 90937 (multiple visits). Code 90937 may include a significant revision of the dialysis prescription. If a hospitalized patient receiving peritoneal dialysis is assessed by the physician, the physician services are reported with 90945 (single visit) and 90947 (multiple visits). Code 90947 may also include a significant revision of the dialysis prescription. Modifier -26 is not used on these codes, as the code descriptions describe only the physician service to the dialysis patient.

When a patient does not receive a full month of dialysis in the outpatient setting because of a kidney transplant, relocation, or death, report the number of days the patient had dialysis. For example, a 50-year-old patient receives peritoneal dialysis from March 1 through 10. On March 11, the patient receives a kidney transplant. The 10 days of service are reported with 90970 × 10.

"Dialysis" is the main term to be referenced in the CPT manual index.

EXERCISE 30-4 *Dialysis*

Using the CPT, ICD-10-CM and/or ICD-9-CM manuals, code the following dialysis services:

1 A 10-year-old patient with end-stage renal disease has 3 encounters during a full month of hemodialysis treatment.

CPT Code: _____

ICD-10-CM Codes: _____, _____

(ICD-9-CM Codes: _____, _____)

2 Hemodialysis for an inpatient with a single physician evaluation for acute renal failure

CPT Code: _____

ICD-10-CM Code: _____ (ICD-9-CM Code: _____)

3 Peritoneal dialysis provided for an inpatient with repeated physician evaluations. The patient has acute renal failure with tubular necrosis.

CPT Code: _____

ICD-10-CM Code: _____ (ICD-9-CM Code: _____)

Define the following terms or abbreviations:

4 peritoneal _____

5 hemofiltration _____

6 ESRD _____

(Answers are located in Appendix B)

GASTROENTEROLOGY

The Gastroenterology subsection (91013-91299) contains many types of tests and treatments that are performed on the esophagus, stomach, and intestine. Several intubation codes are listed in the Gastroenterology subsection. You must carefully review the code descriptions to determine which services are bundled into the code.

EXERCISE 30-5 *Gastroenterology*

Using the CPT, ICD-10-CM and/or ICD-9-CM manuals, code the following:

1 A 2-hour gastroesophageal reflux test with nasal catheter intraluminal impedance electrode for detection of reflux. The patient was diagnosed with gastroesophageal reflux.

    CPT Code: _____

    ICD-10-CM Code: _____ (ICD-9-CM Code: _____)

2 Colon motility study of 7 hours with continuous recordings and interpretation and report.

    CPT Code: _____

3 Gastric intubation with aspiration and slide preparation for cytology. The patient has persistent abdominal pain and loss of appetite.

    CPT Code: _____ (Surgery code)

    ICD-10-CM Codes: _____, _____

    (ICD-9-CM Codes: _____, _____)

Define the following terms:

4 motility study _____

5 manometric studies _____

(Answers are located in Appendix B)

OPHTHALMOLOGY

The notes located at the beginning of the Ophthalmology subsection (92002-92499) describe the services included in the various types of ophthalmologic services. Ophthalmology is a very specialized field and ophthalmologists treat patients for a variety of diseases and injuries. Often the services provided and documented do not adequately fall into an E/M definition. Therefore, the AMA developed specialized codes that deal specifically with ophthalmology services. There are extensive subsection notes that are required reading before you code in the subsection. The notes explain the levels of service and present excellent examples to clarify the assignment of the codes.

The general ophthalmologic services (e.g., routine yearly eye examinations) are located in the subheading General Ophthalmological Services. The codes in this subsection are based on whether the patient is a new or an established patient and on the complexity of service provided. There are two levels of service (intermediate and comprehensive). Of special note are the definitions of new and established patients.

The definitions of the terms "new" and "established" patient are the same as those used in the E/M section. You will recall that those definitions are as follows:

New patient: One who has not received professional service from the physician, or another physician of the exact same specialty and subspecialty who belongs to the same group practice, within the past 3 years.

Established patient: One who has received professional services from the physician, or another physician of the exact same specialty and subspecialty who belongs to the same group practice, within the past 3 years.

The subheading Special Ophthalmological Services contains **bilateral** codes. Each service in this subheading is performed on both eyes, and the codes do not require a modifier to indicate that two eyes were examined or tested. In fact, should you need to report only one eye from these codes, you add modifier -52 to indicate a reduced service. It is a good idea to make a note next to the codes that are bilateral in the CPT manual and also to make a note of modifier -52, to reduce the service if it was performed for only one eye.

Special Ophthalmological Service codes are those services that are not normally performed in a general eye examination. Services in this group are performed for medically indicated reasons. For example, an ophthalmological examination under general anesthesia with manipulation of the globe of the eye to determine the range of motion (92018). The definitions of the codes are very comprehensive in detailing the services involved with each code.

Other codes that are located in the Ophthalmology subsection under the subheading Spectacle Services report the provision of materials to the patient (e.g., spectacles, contact lenses, or ocular prostheses). The refraction that is performed to determine the lens prescription may be reported separately, depending on the policies set by third-party payers.

The decision to assign an ophthalmology code or an E/M code is determined by the service provided. The ophthalmology codes have specific notes prior to code 92002 that serve as a guideline for an intermediate or comprehensive service. Documentation should include the chief complaint, history, and general medical examination. Testing may include the following types of measures:

- External examination, ophthalmoscopy, and biomicroscopy
- Visual acuity (clarity of vision)
- Basic sensorimotor examination (tests sensory and motor coordination)
- Confrontation visual fields (peripheral vision)
- Tonometry (intraocular pressure)
- Evaluation of complete visual system
- May include mydriasis (excess dilation of pupil) for ophthalmoscopy
- Initiation of diagnosis and treatment programs

An **intermediate** ophthalmological service (92002, 92012) describes an evaluation of a new or existing condition complicated with a new diagnosis or management problem not necessarily relating to the primary diagnosis.

A **comprehensive** service (92004, 92014) describes a general evaluation of the complete visual system (Fig. 30-5). The comprehensive services constitute a single service that may be performed at different sessions but is reported only once.

The initiation of a diagnostic and treatment program includes the prescription of medication and arranging for special ophthalmological diagnostic or treatment services, consultations, laboratory procedures, and radiological services.

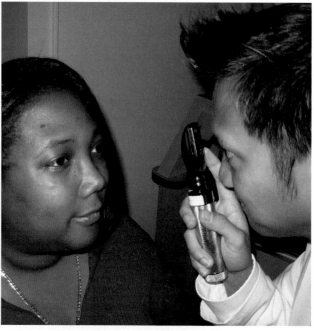

FIGURE 30-5 Examination of the eye.

From the Trenches

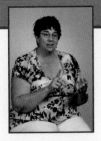

"Coding is an evolving science; in order to be successful a coder needs to be willing to use every day to the fullest by continuing their education and learning something new and useful."

STEPHANIE

QUICK CHECK 30-2

1. Many of the codes for Contact Lens and Spectacle services are selected based on the diagnosis of aphakia. Define aphakia.

_____

(Answers are located in Appendix C)

EXERCISE 30-6   *Ophthalmology*

Using the CPT, ICD-10-CM and/or ICD-9-CM manuals, code the following:

1 Established patient, comprehensive ophthalmologic examination

CPT Code: _____

2 Fitting of contact lens for treatment of ocular surface disease

CPT Code: _____

3 Serial tonography with multiple measurements of intraocular pressure. The patient presented with preglaucoma.

CPT Code: _____

ICD-10-CM Code: _____ (ICD-9-CM Code: _____)

4 New patient, comprehensive ophthalmologic examination. The patient presented with proliferative diabetic retinopathy. The patient has Type 2 diabetes mellitus under good control.

CPT Code: _____

ICD-10-CM Codes: _____, _____

(ICD-9-CM Codes: _____, _____)

(Answers are located in Appendix B)

SPECIAL OTORHINOLARYNGOLOGIC SERVICES

The services in this subsection (92502-92700) are special tests or studies of the ears, nose, and larynx. Audiology (hearing) testing is also located in the Special Otorhinolaryngologic Services subsection. An audiology test may be performed by a physician or an audiologist trained in this area.

Otorhinolaryngologic diagnostic and treatment services are usually reported using codes from the Surgery section. Special services are reported using the otorhinolaryngologic codes from the Medicine section. For example, a nasopharyngoscopy with endoscopy provided during an office visit would be reported with 92511 (nasopharyngoscopy with endoscopy, the procedure) and a code from the E/M section for the office visit (with modifier -25).

EXERCISE 30-7　*Special Otorhinolaryngologic Services*

Using the CPT, ICD-10-CM and/or ICD-9-CM manuals, code the following:

1 Monaural hearing aid check in ear (monaural: "mon," one and "aural," ear)

　　CPT Code: _____

2 Screening test, pure tone, air only

　　CPT Code: _____

3 A nasopharyngoscopy with endoscope due to recent bloody sputum

　　CPT Code: _____

　　ICD-10-CM Code: _____　(ICD-9-CM Code: _____)

4 Nasal function study due to inadequate respiratory air flow

　　CPT Code: _____

　　ICD-10-CM Code: _____　(ICD-9-CM Code: _____)

(Answers are located in Appendix B)

CONGRATULATIONS! Keep up the hard work; you will soon be finished with the entire CPT manual!

CARDIOVASCULAR

The Cardiovascular subsection is discussed in Chapter 21, but there are also some services that are reported with Medicine codes that you have not reviewed yet. Let's take a closer look at these services.

Coronary Therapeutic Services and Procedures

Under this heading you will find invasive and noninvasive cardiovascular service codes (92920-92998), such as cardiopulmonary resuscitation (CPR) and cardioversion (changing [converting] an abnormal heart rhythm to a normal one). Percutaneous transluminal coronary angioplasty (PTCA) codes 92920 and 92921 are also located here. The femoral or brachial artery is usually accessed and a catheter with a balloon tip is threaded up to the heart, into the coronary artery. The balloon is inflated in the area of occlusion and the occlusive material is pressed back, thereby widening the vessel.

Cardiography (93000-93278), Implantable and Wearable Cardiac Device Evaluations (93279-93299), and Echocardiography (93303-93355) were reviewed in Chapter 21 of this text.

Cardiac Catheterization

Codes 93451-93572 report cardiac catheterization, which is a diagnostic medical procedure performed on the heart. Cardiac Catheterization codes were also reviewed in Chapter 21 of this text.

The right side of the heart may be accessed by entering the right femoral vein and advancing through the inferior vena cava or entering the basilic vein in the arm and advancing through the superior vena cava. Right heart catheters are used to measure and record right atrial, right ventricular, pulmonary artery, and pulmonary capillary wedge pressures. Right-sided pressure measurements help diagnose congestive heart failure and right-sided valve disease.

The left side of the heart is approached through the arterial system. Access is commonly through the right femoral artery and advancing through the ascending aorta, the aortic valve, and into the left ventricle. A left heart catheterization will help to diagnose coronary artery disease, left ventricular dysfunction, and valve disease.

Fig. 30-6 shows examples of both right and left cardiac catheterizations.

Noninvasive Vascular Diagnostic Studies

The codes in this subsection (93880-93998) report procedures that are conducted to study veins and arteries other than the heart and great vessels. These studies use the same devices as are used in heart and great-vessel echocardiography, except that the divisions are based on the location of the vein or artery being studied.

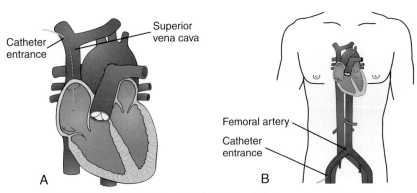

FIGURE 30–6 Cardiac catheterization through **A,** the superior vena cava, or **B,** the femoral artery.

EXERCISE 30-8   *Noninvasive Vascular Diagnostic Studies*

Using the CPT, ICD-10-CM and/or ICD-9-CM manuals, code the following:

1 A patient is referred for a single-level, bilateral venous occlusion plethysmography of the legs. The patient has complained of intermittent leg claudication.

    CPT Code: _____

    ICD-10-CM Code: _____ (ICD-9-CM Code: _____)

2 A 34-year-old patient presents with a history of inability to sustain an erection due to organic impotence. The physician uses a duplex scan to conduct a complete study of the arterial and venous flow of the penis.

    CPT Code: _____

    ICD-10-CM Code: _____ (ICD-9-CM Code: _____)

(Answers are located in Appendix B)

PULMONARY

Codes in the Pulmonary subsection (94002-94799) report therapies, such as nebulizer treatments, incentive spirometry (illustrated in Fig. 30-7), and diagnostic tests, such as pulmonary function tests. A nebulizer (Figs. 30-8, 30-9) is a device that produces a spray, which is inhaled; it is used to treat patients with, for example, asthma. Pulmonary function tests monitor the function of the pulmonary system and examine the lung capacity of patients with, for example, emphysema. In most cases, several pulmonary function tests are performed together. The data are then compiled, and a diagnosis is made. Several indicators

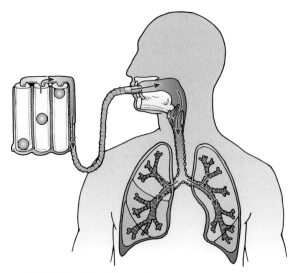

FIGURE 30-7 Incentive spirometry is used to promote alveolar inflation and lung capacity.

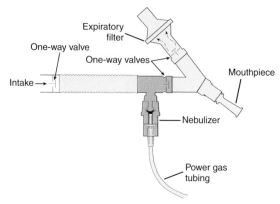

FIGURE 30-8 Diagrammatic illustration of Respirgard II nebulizer system.

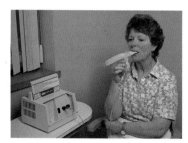

FIGURE 30-9 Patient receiving a nebulizer treatment.

must be present from a variety of tests, and those tests must be performed many times and produce the same result each time for the results to be considered conclusive. In most cases, each type of test is reported separately, unless it is specifically stated otherwise in the code description.

CODING SHOT

Add -26 to the code when reporting only the physician interpretation of the test if the physician does not own the testing equipment.

EXERCISE 30-9   *Pulmonary*

Using the CPT, ICD-10-CM and/or ICD-9-CM manuals, code the following:

1 Pulmonary stress test, simple

   CPT Code: _____

2 Vital capacity, total

   CPT Code: _____

3 Bronchodilation responsiveness evaluation in the office with spirometry before and after bronchodilator treatment. The patient has a cough and a 20-year smoking dependence.

   CPT Code: _____

   ICD-10-CM Codes: _____, _____

   (ICD-9-CM Codes: _____, _____)

(Answers are located in Appendix B)

ALLERGY AND CLINICAL IMMUNOLOGY

Read the notes that appear at the beginning of the Allergy and Clinical Immunology subsection (95004-95199). The subsection is divided into three parts. The **first** is Allergy Testing, which describes allergy testing by various methods (percutaneous, intracutaneous, inhalation) and the type of tests (allergenic extracts, venoms, biologicals, food). The number of tests must always be specified for reporting purposes because for most of these codes, payment is made per test.

Allergy testing consists of the performance, evaluation, and interpretation of allergens. The testing should be based on a complete history and physical examination of the patient and correlated with signs and symptoms related to the presence of possible allergy diagnoses during allergy testing (95004-95071).

The **second** subheading is Ingestion Challenge Testing (95076, 95079). Code 95076 reports the initial 120 minutes of testing time and 95079 reports each additional 60 minutes.

The **third** subheading is Allergen Immunotherapy and the codes specify three types of services: Injection only, prescription and injection, provision of antigen only.

All the codes in Allergen Immunotherapy have specific notes that you must read to know whether the code is for injection, prescription and injection, or antigen only. For example, code 95115 reports the injection of antigen only and does not include the extract, but code 95120 reports the prescription, extract, and injection. Careful reading of the descriptions is a necessity.

The professional service necessary to provide the immunotherapy is bundled into the code, so an office visit code would not usually be reported. If the physician provided another identifiable service at the time of the immunotherapy, an office visit may be reported. But for the patient who has only the injection, prescription, antigen, or any combination of these three, the codes already contain the professional service.

Allergen Immunotherapy is the repeated administration of allergens to patients for the purpose of providing protection against the allergic symptoms and reactions associated with exposure to these allergens. Immunotherapy (hyposensitization) may extend over a period of months, usually on an increasing dosage scale. This is followed by a build-up of tolerance to the antigen (as evidenced by the higher doses that can be administered) and a decline in the symptoms and medication requirements.

EXERCISE 30-10   *Allergy and Clinical Immunology*

Using the CPT, ICD-10-CM and/or ICD-9-CM manuals, code the following:

1 Direct nasal mucous membrane allergy test

    CPT Code: _____

2 Percutaneous test using allergen extracts, immediate type reaction, 10 tests

    CPT Code: _____ × _____

3 Single injection of allergen using extract provided by the patient. Patient has documented allergy to ragweed.

    CPT Code: _____

    ICD-10-CM Code: _____ (ICD-9-CM Code: _____)

4 Physician prepares a 10-dose multi-vial allergenic extract for a patient. At the same encounter, one dose from this vial is administered by one injection to the patient.

    CPT Codes: _____ × _____, _____

(Answers are located in Appendix B)

Indications for allergen immunotherapy are determined by diagnostic testing appropriate to the individual needs of each patient and his/her clinical history of allergic diseases.

ENDOCRINOLOGY

This subsection contains only codes used to report glucose monitoring (95250, 95251). Continuous glucose monitoring is a procedure in which a probe is inserted subcutaneously and attached to a monitor that is worn by the patient. The monitor records the glucose level for a 72-hour period at which time the probe is removed and the data are downloaded from the monitor. The patient records his or her insulin administration, meals, exercise, and any hypoglycemic events during the monitoring period, in addition to performing the usual finger stick glucose four times a day during the 3-day period. The service includes the initial hookup, calibration of the monitor, patient training, removal of sensor, printout of recording, and interpretation and report (95251).

NEUROLOGY AND NEUROMUSCULAR PROCEDURES

There are codes in the Neurology and Neuromuscular Procedures (95782-96020) subsection for sleep testing, muscle testing (electromyography), range of motion measurements (Fig. 30-10), cerebral seizure monitoring, and a variety of neurologic function tests. The codes in this subsection are usually reported by physicians who specialize in neurology (neurologists). Sleep studies in newborns are performed by pediatric pulmonologists. A neurologist usually is a consultant to a physician who is seeking the advice and input of another physician concerning a patient with suspected neurologic problems.

One of the specialized tests conducted in the neurology specialty area is sleep studies (95800-95811). **Sleep studies** are the monitoring of a patient's sleep for 6 or more hours. The studies include the tracing (technical component) and the physician's review, interpretation, and report (professional component). If a physician performs only the professional component, modifier -26 is reported.

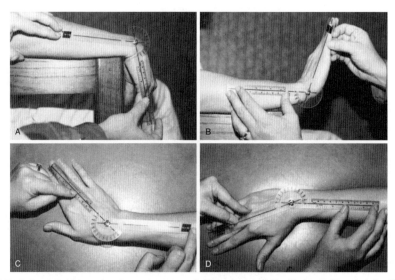

FIGURE 30-10   Range-of-motion measurements. **A,** Palmar flexion. **B,** Dorsiflexion. **C,** Ulnar deviation. **D,** Radial deviation.

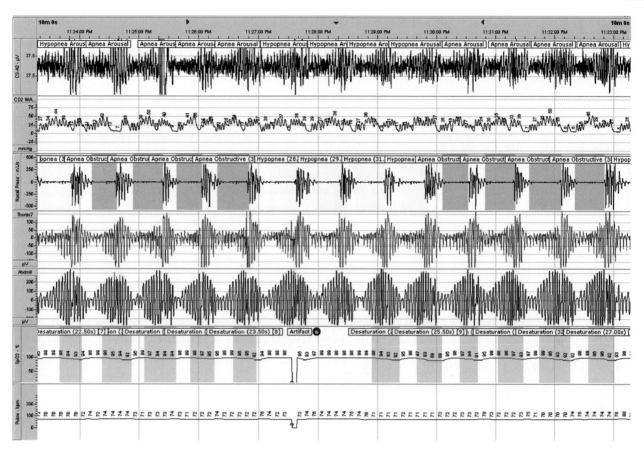

FIGURE 30–11 Continuous 10-minute polysomnographic tracing in a patient with severe obstructive sleep apnea.

Sleep studies diagnose various sleep disorders and measure a patient's response to therapy. An electroencephalogram (EEG) is a procedure that records changes in brain waves. **Polysomnography** (Fig. 30-11) is the measurement of the brain waves during sleep but with the added feature of recording the various stages of sleep (i.e., excited, relaxed, drowsy, asleep, or deep sleep). During each of these stages, the rate and amplitude (height) of the brain waves are measured and compared with normal ranges. Certain neurologic conditions may be identified by the degree to which brain waves vary from normal ranges.

Nerve conduction tests (95905-95913) are usually performed in conjunction with conventional motor nerve conduction studies of the same nerve and may include F-wave studies. **F-wave** studies assess motor nerve function along the entire extent of that nerve. An impulse generated at the stimulating electrode travels up the motor nerves to the motor neuron cell bodies in the spinal cord. The impulse then travels down the same motor nerves to the neuromuscular junction, and then to the muscle. Codes 95907-95913 are to be reported for each nerve tested, regardless of the number of stimulation sites along the sensory or motor nerve being tested. For a given patient, multiple motor or sensory nerve conduction codes may be assigned if multiple motor or sensory nerves are tested. Appendix J of the CPT manual lists the specific nerves tested for codes 95905-95913.

Codes 95905-95913 report both sensory and motor nerve conduction studies with or without F-wave study and includes the interpretation and report.

Code 95905 reports motor and/or sensory nerve conduction using preconfigured electrodes that have been customized to specific anatomic sites.

Parameters are what are being measured during a sleep test. For example, parameters include the measurement of snoring or blood pressure. The number of parameters measured is listed in the code description. The patient's medical record will contain the parameters, or measurements, recorded during the test. To report sleep tests accurately, you must know the parameters and stages of testing. Additionally, many codes include a time component (such as 95803); so it is important to have the duration of the test stated in the medical record.

Electromyographic (EMG) studies use needles and electric current to stimulate nerves and record the results. Assessments of dysphasia, developmental testing, neurobehavior status, and neuropsychological test codes are also located in this subsection.

QUICK CHECK 30-3

1. According to the Sleep Testing Guidelines, polysomnography includes sleep staging with:
   a. EEG, EOG, EMG, ECG
   b. Monitoring snoring, continuous blood pressures, and body positions
   c. ECG, Extended EEG, NCPAP
   d. EEG, EOG, EMG

(Answers are located in Appendix C)

EXERCISE 30-11   *Neurology and Neuromuscular Procedures*

Using the notes under the Sleep Testing subheading and the code descriptions following the notes, identify the following abbreviations:

1 NCPAP _____

2 EEG _____

3 EMG _____

4 EOG _____

Using the CPT, ICD-10-CM and/or ICD-9-CM manuals, code the following:

5 Awake and drowsy EEG and photic stimulation in clinic. The patient presents with episodes of sleep apnea.

   CPT Code: _____

   ICD-10-CM Code: _____ (ICD-9-CM Code: _____)

6 Needle electromyography, three extremities and related paraspinal areas. The patient complains of numbness in arms and legs.

   CPT Code: _____

   ICD-10-CM Code: _____ (ICD-9-CM Code: _____)

7 Range-of-motion measurement and report on both legs. The patient is experiencing muscular incoordination.

   CPT Code: _____ × _____

   ICD-10-CM Code: _____ (ICD-9-CM Code: _____)

(Answers are located in Appendix B)

CENTRAL NERVOUS SYSTEM ASSESSMENTS/TESTS

The Central Nervous System Assessments/Tests codes (96101-96127) identify psychological testing, speech/language (aphasia) assessment, developmental progress assessments, and thinking/reasoning status examination (neurobehavioral). Except for the basic developmental testing, the codes are defined on a per-hour basis. The results of all the tests are to be developed into a report that is included in the patient record.

EXERCISE 30-12   *Central Nervous System Assessments/Tests*

Using the CPT, ICD-10-CM and/or ICD-9-CM manuals, code the following (code all cases at 60 minutes in length):

1 A mother presented to the office of a psychiatrist with a 10-year-old who had been referred by the child's pediatrician for his nonconformist conduct disturbance. At the psychiatric office visit, the mother expressed great concern about the child's inability to behave as she and the child's father believed appropriate. One week later the psychiatrist conducted Developmental Screening Test II for this patient. The psychiatrist then discussed the results of the test with the mother. Code only the developmental screening.

   CPT Code: _____

   ICD-10-CM Code: _____ (ICD-9-CM Code: _____)

2 A young executive is referred for an 80-minute psychologist-administered Minnesota Multiphasic Personality Inventory (MMPI) test by his employer. The employer requests the testing for all newly hired executives who will be working with highly sensitive government documents.

   CPT Code: _____

   ICD-10-CM Code: _____ (ICD-9-CM Code: _____)

3 A 14-year-old is seen in the office for a 70-minute assessment of the child's attention span. The child is experiencing increasingly severe episodes of lethargy. The physician conducts a clinical assessment of the child's cognitive function.

   CPT Code: _____

   ICD-10-CM Code: _____ (ICD-9-CM Code: _____)

(Answers are located in Appendix B)

HEALTH AND BEHAVIOR ASSESSMENT/INTERVENTION

The codes in this subsection (96150-96155) do not report preventive medicine services, nor do they report psychiatric treatments. Instead, these codes report assessment and/or intervention for behavioral, emotional, social, psychological, or knowledge factors that are affecting the patient's health. Examples of **assessments** are clinical interview, behavior observation, and questionnaires. Examples of **interventions** are individual, group, or family sessions. All services are based on 15-minute increments. These services are not performed by a physician. If these services are performed by a physician they are reported with E/M codes.

HYDRATION

Codes 96360 and 96361 report hydration services. The physician's work related to these services usually involves oversight of the treatment plan and staff supervision. When the physician provides a significant separately identifiable E/M service, report the service with an appropriate E/M service reporting modifier -25. Modifier -25 must be added to the E/M code or the service will be assumed to be related to the physician's service for the hydration, injection, or infusion service.

Bundled into the hydration services are local anesthesia, placing the intravenous line, accessing an indwelling access line/catheter/port, flushing at the end of the infusion, and all standard supplies.

Codes 96360 and 96361 report intravenous hydration infusions that include the **prepackaged** fluid and electrolytes. If other than a prepackaged substance is used, that substance would be reported separately. Saline is not reported separately unless given alone for hydration. If the drugs are mixed into the saline, then only the drug is reported and the saline is bundled into the cost of the drug and not reported separately. Included in these hydration codes are the physician supervision and oversight of the staff providing the service. Code 96360 reports 31 minutes to 1 hour of intravenous infusion hydration service and 96361, the add-on code, reports each additional hour. You can only report 96361 if the service is at least 31 minutes over the 1 hour that was reported with 96360. Time under 31 minutes is not reported.

TOOLBOX

Your physician provided direct supervision of an IV infusion of a 500-cc bag of common saline solution to Carol/Carl (depending on female or male patient). It is documented that the infusion administration occurred from 3:20-4:00 PM (40 minutes).

QUESTION

1. Because the IV infusion lasted less than 1 hour but was greater than 31 minutes, you report the service with what code(s)?

   _____

▼ **ANSWER**

1. 96360

Therapeutic, Prophylactic, and Diagnostic Injections and Infusions

Codes 96365-96379 report the administration of therapeutic, prophylactic, or diagnostic intravenous infusion or injection. Intravenous **infusions** are reported with 96365-96368 and are divided based on the time and type of infusion. The initial infusion is reported with 96365 (up to 1 hour), and each additional hour (over 30 minutes) is reported with 96366. Sometimes one infusion is provided followed by another infusion with a different medication (sequential infusions), in which case the initial infusion is listed first and the **sequential** infusion (add-on code 96367) is listed second. There are times when more than one infusion is provided at the same time, which is a concurrent infusion. A **concurrent** infusion is when there is one site and two lines infusing at the same time. Report the initial infusion first and then the concurrent infusion (96368).

Subcutaneous infusions are reported with codes 96369-96371. Initial set up and first hour are reported with 96369. Each additional hour is reported with 96370. Additional set up for a new infusion site is reported with 96371.

To report therapeutic, prophylactic, and diagnostic **injections** (96372-96376), the physician must be present. Note that add-on code 96376 can only be reported when the service is provided in a facility. Therapeutic, prophylactic, and diagnostic injections are divided based on the method used for the administration (Fig. 30-12). **Subcutaneous** and **intramuscular** injections are reported with 96372 in addition to a code to report the substance injected. For example, if the injection was a subcutaneous human rabies immune globulin, report 90375 for the substance and 96372 for the administration. The administration codes for vaccines/toxoids are reported with 90460/90461 or 90471-90474. Code 96372 is not used to report

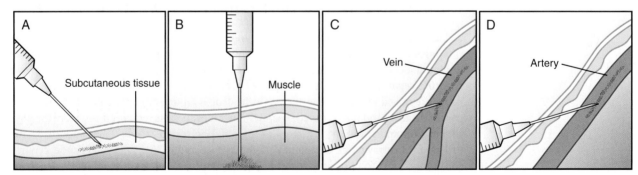

FIGURE 30–12 Injection methods. **A,** Subcutaneous (SC). **B,** Intramuscular (IM). **C,** Intravenous (IV). **D,** Intra-arterial.

chemotherapy administration (see 96401-96549). Injections for allergen immunotherapy are reported with 95115/95117, not with therapeutic, prophylactic, or diagnostic injection codes. **Intra-arterial** (96373) and **intravenous push** (96374/96375/96376) are reported with therapeutic, prophylactic, and diagnostic injection codes.

CHEMOTHERAPY ADMINISTRATION

Chemotherapy codes 96401-96549 report a variety of chemotherapy services. The Injection and Intravenous Infusion Chemotherapy codes (96401-96417) report subcutaneous/intramuscular, intralesional, and intravenous chemotherapy. Intra-Arterial Chemotherapy codes (96420-96425) report various forms of chemotherapy administered via the arteries. Other Injection and Infusion Services codes (96440-96549) report other types of chemotherapy, such as pleural (96440), peritoneal via an indwelling port (96446), and central nervous system (96450), in addition to refilling/maintenance of portable or implantable pumps or reservoirs (96521, 96522).

There are two other sets of codes used to report chemotherapy services: Hydration (96360-96361) and Therapeutic, Prophylactic, and Diagnostic Injections and Infusions (96365-96379), which you learned about earlier in this chapter. In addition to these CPT codes, Level II HCPCS "J" codes report the substances injected or infused.

Included (not reported separately) with chemotherapy infusion or injection codes 96401-96549 are the following:
1. Use of local anesthesia
2. IV start
3. Access to indwelling intravenous, subcutaneous catheter, or port
4. Flush at the conclusion of infusion
5. Standard tubing, syringes, and supplies
6. Preparation of the chemotherapy agent(s)

If other services are provided, they may be reported separately.

The initial intravenous infusion (the treatment) is reported with 96365 and each additional hour of infusion, up to 8 hours, is reported with 96366. If a sequential (one after another) intravenous therapy is provided, the service is reported with 96367. When a concurrent (at the same time as another) intravenous therapy is provided the service is reported with 96368. A concurrent infusion is one in which multiple infusions are provided through the same intravenous line. A concurrent infusion can be billed only once per patient encounter.

If more than one substance is placed in the **one** bag, it is considered **one** infusate and **one** infusion. You would report **one** administration code and a Level II HCPCS J code for each substance or drug.

Any administration that is 15 minutes or less is considered a push, not an infusion. The administration of an initial or single intravenous push is reported with 96374 and each additional push is reported with 96375. Report only one push per drug. For example, if a patient is given a push of morphine 2 mg at the beginning of a service and morphine 2 mg later in the service, bill one administration code for the two IV pushes of morphine. The appropriate units of the J code (J2270—morphine up to 10 mg × 1) would also be billed for the total dose.

If two drugs are mixed in the same bag and administered for 15 minutes or less, the service is reported with the appropriate push CPT code (initial or subsequent) × 1 unit. The drug(s) or substance would be separately reported with the appropriate J code based on the amount and type.

A patient will often receive hydration and ancillary medications before or after chemotherapy. Only one initial administration code can be reported for each encounter; other services are reported with secondary or subsequent codes.

> ### Example
>
> A patient presents for a chemotherapy intravenous infusion session and is given a 40-minute hydration prior to chemotherapy reported with 96361. If the patient receives hydration before and after chemotherapy, calculate the entire time of hydration infusion and code the appropriate number of units for 96361. For example, a patient received 1 hour of hydration before chemotherapy infusion and 40 minutes of hydration after chemotherapy. The total hydration time is 100 minutes. Code 96361 × 2 units.

Modifier -59 should be reported to indicate that hydration was provided prior to or following chemotherapy. Hydration provided at the same time as chemotherapy to facilitate drug delivery is not reported separately. All infusions must have a documented start and stop time.

The patient may also receive medications before and/or after chemotherapy, such as anti-nausea medications. These medications are reported in addition to the chemotherapy because chemotherapy is always the primary service. When the patient receives multiple intravenous infusions of medications and these medications are administered individually, each is reported separately; but if the medications are mixed together and given in one infusion, they are reported as one infusion.

Code 96375 is an add-on code and is only reported with another code, such as 96413, Chemotherapy administration. The charges for the patients in the examples that follow would list the chemotherapy administration first, followed by the other service codes since the chemotherapy is the primary service.

> ### Example
>
> After chemotherapy, a patient received Aloxi (J2469), Benadryl (J1200), and Decadron (J1100) in three separate infusions of less than 15 minutes (pushes). The J codes are reported along with 96375 × 3.

If the medications are all mixed together and administered in one infusion of less than 15 minutes, the J codes are reported along with 96375 × 1.

> ### Example
>
> A patient presents for chemotherapy and receives two pushes, one of Aloxi, 0.25 mg, and one of Benadryl, 50 mg. Chemotherapy with Rituximab, 100 mg, is administered for 3 hours by means of an intravenous infusion. After therapy, the patient is administered Decadron, 1 mg, by intravenous push. The services are reported as follows:
>
> Pre- and post-medications: 96375 × 3 (three total IV pushes); J2469 (Aloxi) × 10 units; J1200 (Benadryl) × 1 unit; and J1100 (Decadron) × 1 unit. NOTE: 1 unit of Aloxi = 25 mcg; therefore, 0.25 mg = 250 mcg = 10 units.
>
> Chemotherapy: 96413 (initial hour); 96415 × 2 (2 additional hours); J9310 × 1 (Rituximab). Chemotherapy is the initial infusion and the hydration and pushes are secondary/subsequent.

If a significant identifiable office visit service was provided in addition to the chemotherapy administration, report that service with an E/M code, adding -25 to indicate the service was separate and significant.

CODING SHOT

Chemotherapy administration codes (96401-96459) include the use of local anesthesia, initiating the intravenous therapy, access to an indwelling port, flush at conclusion, tubing/supplies/syringes, and preparation of the chemotherapy agent(s). These services are not reported separately.

EXERCISE 30-13 *Chemotherapy Administration*

Using the CPT, ICD-10-CM and/or ICD-9-CM manuals, code only the chemotherapy administration:

1 Chemotherapy injected into the pleural cavity with thoracentesis. The patient has documented primary cancer of the lungs.

CPT Code: _____

ICD-10-CM Code: _____ (ICD-9-CM Code: _____)

2 Refilling and maintenance of a patient's portable pump. The patient has primary adenocarcinoma of the colon.

CPT Code: _____

ICD-10-CM Code: _____ (ICD-9-CM Code: _____)

3 Chemotherapy administered subcutaneously with local anesthesia. The patient has melanoma of the chest wall.

CPT Code: _____

ICD-10-CM Code: _____ (ICD-9-CM Code: _____)

4 Chemotherapy administered intravenously using the infusion technique for 50 minutes. The patient has breast cancer with metastasis (secondary site) to the bone of the spinal column.

CPT Code: _____

ICD-10-CM Codes: _____, _____

(ICD-9-CM Codes: _____, _____)

5 Chemotherapy injected into the central nervous system using a lumbar puncture. Patient has cancer of the brain, primary.

CPT Code: _____

ICD-10-CM Code: _____ (ICD-9-CM Code: _____)

6 An established patient is seen in the office for pernicious anemia. The nurse administers an injection of vitamin B_{12}, 900 mcg with direct physician supervision. Report the substance with a HCPCS Level II code. The service was not significant enough to report a separate E/M code for the office visit.

CPT Codes: _____ (therapeutic injection), _____ (substance HCPCS code)

(Answers are located in Appendix B)

PHOTODYNAMIC THERAPY

The photodynamic therapy services (96570-96571) are add-on codes reported in conjunction with the bronchoscopy or endoscopy services. An agent is injected into the patient that remains in cancerous cells longer than in the normal cells. After the agent has dissipated from the normal cells, the patient is exposed to laser light. The agent absorbs the light and the light produces oxygen, destroying the cancerous cells.

Codes for endoscopic application are divided on the basis of time—the first 30 minutes and each additional 15 minutes. External application of light (96567) is based on each exposure session.

SPECIAL DERMATOLOGICAL PROCEDURES

The dermatology codes (96900-96999) are usually reported by a dermatologist who provides services to a patient in an office on a consultation basis. The dermatology codes for special procedures would typically be reported in addition to an E/M code, for example, if a patient is referred by his family physician to a dermatologist for treatment of acne. The dermatologist conducts a history and examination and treats the patient with ultraviolet light (actinotherapy). The reporting would be an Office or Other Outpatient code, depending on the level of service provided, and 96900 to report the actinotherapy.

EXERCISE 30-14 *Special Dermatological Procedures*

Using the CPT, ICD-10-CM and/or ICD-9-CM manuals, code the following:

1 A 16-year-old patient sees a dermatologist in consultation, at which time the physician does a problem focused history and physical examination regarding the patient's acne vulgaris. The physician prescribes and provides a treatment of ultraviolet light therapy.

  CPT Codes: _____, _____

  ICD-10-CM Code: _____ (ICD-9-CM Code: _____)

2 Photochemotherapy is provided for a 34-year-old consultative patient with severe bullous dermatosis. The patient receives 8 hours of treatment. The physician provides a comprehensive history and physical examination with moderately complex medical decision making.

  CPT Codes: _____, _____

  ICD-10-CM Code: _____ (ICD-9-CM Code: _____)

(Answers are located in Appendix B)

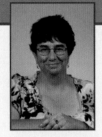

From the Trenches

"Having good working relationships with physicians is the #1 priority. You need to be confident that what you are telling them is correct, and when they realize that you know what you are talking about, they will respect you."

STEPHANIE

PHYSICAL MEDICINE AND REHABILITATION

The codes in the Physical Medicine and Rehabilitation subsection (97001-97799) are reported by a physician or therapist. The subsection includes codes for different modalities of treatments (e.g., traction, whirlpool, electrical stimulation) as well as various types of patient training (e.g., functional activities, gait training, massage). The codes are reported on the basis of time or treatment area, as stated in the description of the code. Codes are divided by supervision or constant attendance. Unit coding (i.e., ×2, ×3) is necessary if the time spent administering the treatment exceeds the time listed in the code.

Example

Reporting for patient's prosthetic training of 60 minutes would be:

  97761 × 4   Prosthetic training, each 15 minutes

CODING SHOT

An **orthotic** is a support, splint, or brace used to align a body part, such as an elbow brace (L3700-L3766). A **prosthetic** is a replacement, such as a breast prosthesis (L8000-L8039).

All services provided by independent physical therapists and occupational therapists require a written referral from a physician that includes documentation of the disease or injury being treated and the diagnosis.

The services are rendered according to a written treatment plan determined by the provider after an appropriate assessment of the illness or injury. All providers rendering therapy must document the appropriate history, examination, diagnosis, related physician orders, therapy goals and potential for achievement, any contraindications, functional assessment, type of treatment, the body areas to be treated, the date that therapy initiated, and expected frequency and duration of treatments. This documentation must be maintained in the patient's medical record.

Documentation should indicate the prognosis for restoration of function and the medical necessity of the treatment.

Physical therapy test and measurement codes are listed by the type of testing and the time the testing requires. The type of test would be such as functional capacity. Note the use of type and time in the following CPT code.

Example

97750   Physical performance test or measurement (e.g., musculoskeletal, functional capacity, with written report, each 15 minutes)

CODING SHOT

For all codes that are time based, the time must be documented in the patient's medical record.

The codes in Physical Medicine and Rehabilitation are reported for physical medicine and therapy as well as for other rehabilitation, for example, community/work reintegration (97537).

Active Wound Care Management

Nonphysician personnel perform the procedures described in Active Wound Care Management codes (97597-97610). Codes 97597 and 97598 report debridement services by means of high pressure waterjets, scissors, scalpels, or forceps based on the first 20 sq cm or less (97597) and each additional 20 sq cm or part thereof (97598). The codes are not reported with or to replace the surgical debridement represented by 11042-11047. If a physician performed the procedures, the services would be reported with the 11042-11047 codes.

Wound management codes are based on nonselective or negative pressure procedures. **Nonselective** debridement is that in which healthy tissue is removed along with necrotic tissue. The tissue is gradually loosened with water (hydrotherapy). Loosened tissue may be cut away with sharp instruments. Nonselective debridement is usually done over the course of several visits.

Negative Pressure Wound Therapy (NPWT, 97605, 97606), as illustrated in Figs. 30-13 and 30-14, may include vacuuming the drainage and tissue from the wound area, application of topical medications or ointments, assessment of the wound, and directions to the patient for continued care of the wound. Choice of codes is dependent on the square centimeters treated.

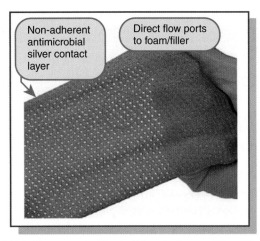

FIGURE 30–13 Silverlon® Negative Pressure Wound Therapy dressing.

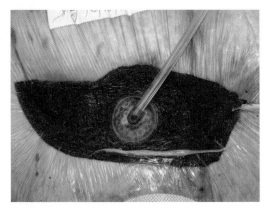

FIGURE 30–14 Negative pressure-assisted wound closure sponge in place on patient's abdomen.

EXERCISE 30-15   *Physical Medicine and Rehabilitation*

Using the CPT, ICD-10-CM and/or ICD-9-CM manuals, code the following:

1 Application of cold packs to one area (modality)

CPT Code: _____

2 Initial prosthetic training, 30 minutes

CPT Code: _____ × _____

3 Physical medicine treatment procedure, gait training, 30 minutes. Patient status is post-acute Cerebrovascular Accident.

CPT Code: _____

ICD-10-CM Code: _____ (ICD-9-CM Code: _____)

(Answers are located in Appendix B)

MEDICAL NUTRITION THERAPY

These codes (97802-97804) are reported by non-physician personnel for medical nutritional therapy assessment (NTA) or intervention. If a physician provides the service, the service is reported using E/M codes or Preventive Medicine codes.

The codes report face-to-face services with the patient based on time of 15 minutes for initial or re-assessments and 30 minutes for group assessments. The provider would review the patient's medical record, including the history of present illness and past medical history, along with pertinent laboratory data. The nutritional history would be obtained from the patient and an appropriate examination would be conducted. Documentation would indicate the nutritional assessment and prescription recommended to the patient and this information would be communicated to the health care provider.

OSTEOPATHIC MANIPULATIVE TREATMENT (OMT)

Osteopathic manipulative treatment (98925-98929) is a form of manual treatment applied by a physician to eliminate or alleviate somatic (body) dysfunction and related disorders. The codes are listed according to body regions. These body regions are the head; cervical, thoracic, lumbar, sacral, and pelvic regions; lower extremities; upper extremities; rib cage; abdomen and viscera region. Codes are separated on the basis of the number of body regions treated. These codes are usually reported by osteopathic physicians (doctors of osteopathy, DO).

CHIROPRACTIC MANIPULATIVE TREATMENT (CMT)

The Chiropractic Manipulative Treatment subsection (98940-98943) is divided by the number of regions manipulated. For this subsection, the **spine** is divided into five regions (cervical, thoracic, lumbar, sacral, and pelvic), and the **extraspinal** regions are divided into five regions (head, lower extremities, upper extremities, rib cage, and abdomen). Chiropractic manipulation is the manipulation of the spinal column and other structures. Each of the codes in the Chiropractic Manipulative Treatment subsection has a professional assessment bundled into the code. An office visit code is reported only if the patient had a significant separately identifiable service provided; otherwise, the service of the office visit is bundled into the code.

EXERCISE 30-16 *Manipulative Treatment*

Using the CPT, ICD-10-CM and/or ICD-9-CM manuals, code the following therapies:

1 Sally, a 43-year-old woman, presents with the complaint of a seizing pain in the area of her lower left hip. The chiropractor conducts an assessment of the patient and provides a chiropractic alignment to two spinal regions.

CPT Code: _____

ICD-10-CM Code: _____ (ICD-9-CM Code: _____)

2 Osteopathic lumbar manipulation (OMT), one region. Patient has chronic low back pain.

CPT Code: _____

ICD-10-CM Code: _____ (ICD-9-CM Code: _____)

(Answers are located in Appendix B)

NON-FACE-TO-FACE NONPHYSICIAN SERVICES

This subsection is divided into Telephone Services (98966-98968) and On-Line Medical Evaluation (98969) services provided by qualified health care professionals. The notes and the code descriptions for these codes indicate that the telephone or online service cannot originate from a related assessment that was provided within the previous 7 days or result in an appointment within the next 24 hours or the soonest available appointment. The telephone services are reported based on the documented time, and the online service is per incident.

SPECIAL SERVICES, PROCEDURES, AND REPORTS

Special Services, Procedures, and Reports (99000-99091) is a miscellaneous subsection that includes codes for services that are not reported with codes from other sections. The codes report services that are, for example, rendered at unusual hours of the day or on holidays. These codes are considered adjunct codes and are to be reported in addition to the codes for the major service. For example, if a physician goes to the office on a Sunday to meet an established patient and provide urgent, but not emergency, service, the E/M service code for the office visit would be reported in addition to 99050 to indicate the unusual time at which the service was provided.

An often reported code is 99024 for an office visit provided during a global period. Third-party payers do not reimburse for the submission of this code; however, it communicates that the service was provided to the patient during the follow-period of a previous surgical procedure.

You have assigned 99070, supplies, from this subsection before. One of the big advantages of the HCPCS coding system is that you specifically identify the supply reported rather than the more general 99070. For example, you may report 99070 for a body sock for a patient. With the HCPCS coding system, you can specify the body sock with a code L0984. It is best to use HCPCS codes when reporting supplies since most third-party payers will request additional information when 99070 is submitted.

The subsection also contains codes for medical testimony, the completion of complicated reports, education services, unusual travel, and supplies. Although this subsection is small, it contains codes that are reported often. Take a few minutes to become familiar with the codes listed within Special Services, Procedures, and Reports and mark the subsection for future use.

The codes for Special Services are located in the CPT manual index under the main term "Special Services."

EXERCISE 30-17 *Special Services, Procedures, and Reports*

Using the CPT manual, code the following:

1 What medicine code is reported in addition to the basic service code when a service is provided after hours on Monday?

CPT Code: _____

2 Conveyance of a specimen from the physician's office to a laboratory

CPT Code: _____

3 Supplies provided for an office visit exceeding those usually used

CPT Code: _____

(Answers are located in Appendix B)

Qualifying Circumstances for Anesthesia. Anesthesia is discussed in Chapter 16.

Moderate Sedation. Sedation reported with 99143-99150 is discussed in Chapter 16.

OTHER SERVICES AND PROCEDURES

A wide variety of codes (99170-99199) is located in this subsection of the Medicine section. For example, you will find codes for anogenital examination with a colposcope of a child in a case of suspected trauma, visual function screenings, pumping poison from the stomach, and therapeutic phlebotomy treatments. Because the codes are so varied, the way in which they are divided is also varied. For example, the code range 99190-99192 is divided on the basis of time, whereas other codes are divided according to the extent of the service.

HOME HEALTH PROCEDURES/SERVICES

These codes (99500-99602) report non-physician services provided at the patient's residence. The residence may be an assisted living apartment, custodial care facility, group home, or other nontraditional residence. The codes are divided based on the reason for the service (e.g., injection, hemodialysis).

Home Infusion Procedures Services

The codes 99601 and 99602 represent services of administration of a variety of therapies (e.g., nutrition, chemotherapy, pain management). The services are provided by non-physician allied health professionals. Codes are divided based on the time spent providing the infusion.

MEDICATION THERAPY MANAGEMENT SERVICES

These codes (99605-99607) are for patient assessments and interventions by a pharmacist, upon request. These codes do not describe the product-specific information that a pharmacist would ordinarily provide to a patient regarding a medication; but rather to assist in the management of treatment-related medication complications or interactions. The codes are reported by the pharmacist based on the patient status (new or established) and the time spent in assessment and intervention.

CHAPTER REVIEW

CHAPTER 30, PART I, THEORY

Without the use of the CPT manual, answer the following questions:

1 There are two types of services in the Medicine section. One is diagnostic and the other is

_____.

2 What do the following abbreviations mean?

a IV _____

b IM _____

c SC _____

3 The routing of blood, including the waste products, outside of the body for cleansing is _____.

4 The dialysis that involves using a cavity as a filter is known as what kind of dialysis? _____

5 What is the name of the test that checks the intraocular pressure of the eye? _____

6 What is the name of the scope that is used to examine color vision? _____

7 What is the word that means the body of knowledge about the ear, nose, and larynx?

_____

8 In what subsection of the Medicine section would you find CPR, coronary atherectomies, and heart valvuloplasties?

_____

9 What kind of scanning uses ultrasonic technology with a display of both structure and motion with time?

_____

10 What is the name of the ultrasonic documentation that records velocity mapping and imaging? _____

11 In what Medicine subsection would you find therapies such as nebulizer treatments? _____

12 Percutaneous, intracutaneous, and inhalation are examples of what from the Allergy subsection? _____

13 Allergenic extracts, venoms, biologicals, and food are examples of what from the Allergy subsection?

_____

14 If you were looking for the code number to indicate the circumstance in which a physician sees a patient between the hours of 10 PM and 8 AM, in what subsection of the Medicine section would you find that code?

_____

Chapter Review answers are only available in the TEACH Instructor Resources on Evolve

CHAPTER 30, PART II, PRACTICAL

Using the CPT, ICD-10-CM and/or ICD-9-CM manuals, code the following:

15 An 18-month-old established patient receives a DT that is administered intramuscularly by the physician, after the physician counseled the parents on the vaccine.

CPT Codes: _____, _____, _____

ICD-10-CM Codes: _____, _____

(ICD-9-CM Codes: _____, _____)

16 A 30-year-old established patient receives a tetanus toxoid that is administered intramuscularly by the physician's assistant.

CPT Codes: _____, _____

ICD-10-CM Code: _____

(ICD-9-CM Code: _____)

17 A DTaP and an oral poliomyelitis vaccine (live) are administered to a new 5-year-old patient. A problem focused history and examination are performed for an acute URI, and the medical decision making is straightforward (separate identifiable service).

CPT Codes: _____, _____, _____, _____,
_____

ICD-10-CM Codes: _____, _____

(ICD-9-CM Codes: _____, _____)

18 An established, 70-year-old Medicare patient presents to the nurse for a pneumonia (Polysaccharide 23-Valent) and a trivalent flu immunization (2 injections).

🌐 CPT Code(s): _____

🌐 ICD-10-CM Code(s): _____

(🌐 ICD-9-CM Code(s): _____)

19 A patient brings his allergy medication into the office, and a single injection service is provided by the nurse. The patient is allergic to primrose.

CPT Code: _____

ICD-10-CM Code: _____

(ICD-9-CM Code: _____)

20 A patient receives the initial 30-minute training for her prosthetic arm. Patient has a congenital absence of forearm and hand.

CPT Code: _____ × _____

ICD-10-CM Code: _____

(ICD-9-CM Code: _____)

21 The patient presents for a bronchospasm evaluation before and after a spirometry that is administered to monitor his lung capacity. The patient has episodes of shortness of breath.

CPT Codes: _____, _____

ICD-10-CM Code: _____

(ICD-9-CM Code: _____)

22 Nasopharyngoscopy with endoscope. The patient has persistent nosebleeds.

    CPT Code: _____

    ICD-10-CM Code: _____

    (ICD-9-CM Code: _____)

23 A 30-year-old with end-stage renal disease receives a full month of dialysis with eight encounters.

    CPT Code: _____

    ICD-10-CM Code: _____

    (ICD-9-CM Code: _____)

24 Ophthalmology Clinic Progress Note

Today, I saw a new patient who is a 46-year-old white female who was diagnosed with Graves', toxic diffuse goiter, early last year. She had some swelling of the eyes and was originally told she had an allergy; then the same person, after he found out she had Graves', put her on prednisone. It was unknown what the dose was, but the patient showed me her bottles and it is obvious that she was on 20 mg a day, taken at suppertime. She has now come down from this. She was also on prednisone acetate eye drops. The patient denies any history of any problems except that she became quite depressed and her head felt funny on the steroids. The patient had a history of an ulcer problem in the past, which was treated with diet. The patient allegedly had a positive Mantoux test years ago, but her chest x-rays have always been negative.

    Today when I saw her, she was 20/80 in the right and 20/40 in the left with her refraction. The lids are markedly swollen, and she has marked inferior ptosis from the sagging lids, the water collection, and the redness. There is marked chemosis of the conjunctivae and thickening of the lids. The patient has full extraocular motility, except she cannot converge. There is marked swelling of the globes on the retropulsion exam. The pressures are 21 and 20 in primary gaze and 30 and 24 in up gaze. The discs are flat. The patient has pseudoexfoliation in the right eye and nuclear sclerotic cataracts in both eyes, right greater than left.

    I counseled the patient about the treatment of this and offered her radiation therapy along with the proper dose of steroids of 100 mg a day for a week and then taper down from the 100 mg. I will send her to see Dr. Zapata for consultation radiation therapy, and then I think we would see her weekly as we get this problem under control. I did not feel she needed any topical medication, and she definitely does not need surgery now since there is no proptosis at this time. We will see her again in 1 week. I counseled her about the side effects of the high dose of steroids and how to take them.

    CPT Code: _____

    ICD-10-CM Codes: _____, _____, _____, _____, _____

    (ICD-9-CM Codes: _____, _____, _____, _____, _____)

Chapter Review answers are only available in the TEACH Instructor Resources on Evolve

"A good coder has to be able to work independently and like to solve puzzles, while sometimes a coder will have to figure out which parts of the puzzle are missing and clarify with the physician. Coding is even more rewarding when you know that you can positively impact a facility's bottom line by doing a great job."

Karla R. Lovaasen, RHIA, CCS, CCS-P
Coding and Consulting Services
Abingdon, Maryland

Inpatient Coding

Karla R. Lovaasen, RHIA, CCS, CCS-P
Co-author: ICD-10-CM/PCS Coding: Theory and Practice, 2015 Edition *(St. Louis, 2015, Saunders); and* ICD-9-CM Coding: Theory and Practice with ICD-10, 2013/2014 Edition *(St. Louis, 2013, Saunders)*

Chapter Topics

Differences between Inpatient and Outpatient Coding

Selection of Principal Diagnosis

Reporting Additional Diagnoses

Present on Admission (POA)

Development of the ICD-10-PCS

Chapter Review

Learning Objectives

After completing this chapter you should be able to

1 Explain the differences between inpatient and outpatient coding.

2 Define principal diagnosis and procedure.

3 Examine the *Official Guidelines for Coding and Reporting*.

4 Review the Guidelines for Selection of a Principal Diagnosis.

5 Determine when a condition should be reported as an additional diagnosis.

6 Explain the purpose of the present on admission indicators.

7 Examine the ICD-10-PCS system.

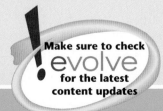
Make sure to check
evolve
for the latest
content updates

DIFFERENCES BETWEEN INPATIENT AND OUTPATIENT CODING

Our studies until now have focused on physician services and how to report these services. This chapter will review coding for hospital services.

For physicians, payment is based on specific services and supplies reported with CPT and HCPCS codes. The medical necessity of the services and supplies is reported with diagnostic codes. As a result, many coders and physicians call CPT and HCPCS codes the "money codes." Physician services are often referred to as "professional" services because they are performed by individuals. Physician services can be performed in many places, including hospitals.

Because the services provided by hospitals are broader than those provided by physicians, hospitals are reimbursed differently than physicians. The hospital is paid for its "hospitality," ensuring the patient is housed, fed, and nurtured back to health until the patient is discharged. The length of stay and intensity of services provided to the patient in a hospital vary according to the patient's condition. For example, a young woman admitted to the hospital for a normal, uncomplicated birth usually requires much less nursing care and recovery time than an elderly patient admitted for multiple organ failure in sepsis. The physicians are still paid using CPT/HCPCS codes to report services. Hospitals, however, are paid for their "hospitality" using a complex formula (MS-DRG) based on the severity of the patient's illness, the patient's other health conditions, patient age, and whether the patient required an operating room during the stay. For hospitals, the diagnosis is the key in determining the resources required by a patient. For hospitals, diagnostic codes are the "money codes."

The accuracy of the MS-DRG (Medical Severity Diagnosis Related Group) is dependent on coders following the Guidelines for inpatient coding very precisely. For physicians, the first-listed diagnostic code indicates the reason for the encounter and the diagnostic code has a support role because CPT/HCPCS provides the "money code." For inpatient coding, the reason for the hospitalization, termed the **principal diagnosis,** is crucial to the MS-DRG formula. The principal diagnosis is the first-listed code.

Sequencing of diagnostic codes is more crucial to reimbursement for hospitals, and the rules for diagnostic coding also differ. For example, a patient is admitted to the hospital experiencing severe chest pain and sweating, to rule out myocardial infarction. The patient requires 36 hours in the hospital to undergo intense diagnostics to determine the cause of the chest pain. Ultimately the patient is diagnosed with anxiety and heartburn. During the hospitalization, resources expended on this patient are identical to resources for a patient with a myocardial infarct. Therefore, the hospital would report the "rule-out" diagnosis, MI, as the principal diagnosis.

In an inpatient setting, you must be familiar with the inpatient Guidelines so that the coding leads to the correct MS-DRG. Coders do not need to know the formulas for MS-DRGs. A computer program, a grouper, assigns the MS-DRG based on the ICD-9 codes.

Many hospitalizations are medical in nature (uncontrolled diabetes, pneumonia) while others are surgical in nature (mastectomy, total hip replacement). Procedure codes are used to report operating room utilization. Procedure codes contribute to the MS-DRG formula.

Volume 3 of ICD-9 and ICD-10-PCS are inpatient procedural coding systems.

ICD-9-CM OFFICIAL GUIDELINES FOR CODING AND REPORTING

Introduction (Paragraph 3)

These guidelines are based on the coding and sequencing instructions in Volume I, II and III of ICD-9-CM, but provide additional instruction. Adherence to these guidelines when assigning ICD-9-CM diagnosis and procedure codes is required under the Health Insurance Portability and Accountability Act (HIPAA). The diagnosis codes (Volumes 1-2) have been adopted under HIPAA for all healthcare settings. Volume 3 procedure codes have been adopted for inpatient procedures reported by hospitals.

In the inpatient setting, ICD-9-CM procedure codes (Volume 3) are assigned instead of CPT or HCPCS codes. Procedure codes need to be sequenced properly with the principal procedure as the first-listed procedure. The **principal procedure** is one that is performed for definitive treatment rather than for diagnostic or exploratory purposes, or one necessary for a complication. If two procedures appear to meet this definition, then the one most closely related to the principal diagnosis should be assigned as the principal procedure. A procedure is considered to be significant if it:

■ Is surgical in nature
■ Carries a procedural risk
■ Carries an anesthetic risk
■ Requires specialized training to perform

For a procedure to be significant it does not have to be performed in the operating room. Many procedures are performed in the emergency department, at a patient's bedside, treatment room, or in an interventional radiology department. Any procedure that affects reimbursement should be coded and reported. Most facilities will have a policy regarding what procedures should be coded.

SELECTION OF PRINCIPAL DIAGNOSIS

> ### ICD-9-CM OFFICIAL GUIDELINES FOR CODING AND REPORTING
>
> **SECTION II. Selection of Principal Diagnosis**
>
> The circumstances of inpatient admission always govern the selection of principal diagnosis. The principal diagnosis is defined in the Uniform Hospital Discharge Data Set (UHDDS) as "that condition established after study to be chiefly responsible for occasioning the admission of the patient to the hospital for care."
>
> The UHDDS definitions are used by hospitals to report inpatient data elements in a standardized manner. These data elements and their definitions can be found in the July 31, 1985, Federal Register (Vol. 50, No. 147), pp. 31038-40.
>
> Since that time the application of the UHDDS definitions has been expanded to include all non-outpatient settings (acute care, short term, long term care and psychiatric hospitals; home health agencies; rehab facilities; nursing homes, etc).
>
> In determining principal diagnosis the coding conventions in the ICD-9-CM, Volumes I and II take precedence over these official coding guidelines. *(See Section I. A., Conventions for the ICD-9-CM)*
>
> The importance of consistent, complete documentation in the medical record cannot be overemphasized. Without such documentation the application of all coding guidelines is a difficult, if not impossible, task.

The **principal** diagnosis is sequenced **first** in inpatient coding. In an outpatient setting, the term first-listed condition is used in lieu of the term principal diagnosis and is used to indicate the main reason for the visit. Additional diagnoses may be necessary in order to substantiate adjunct services (such as laboratory and radiology). The terminology "principal diagnosis" refers only to an acute care setting and is used in conjunction with the MS-DRG payment scheme; "first-listed diagnosis" refers only to outpatient settings. There are specific guidelines that assist with the selection of the principal diagnosis.

Symptoms, Signs, and Ill-Defined Conditions

> ### ICD-9-CM OFFICIAL GUIDELINES FOR CODING AND REPORTING
>
> **SECTION II.**
> **A. Codes for symptoms, signs, and ill-defined conditions**
>
> Codes for symptoms, signs, and ill-defined conditions from Chapter 16 are not to be used as a principal diagnosis when a related definitive diagnosis has been established.

EXERCISE 31-1 *Symptoms, Signs, and Ill-Defined Conditions*

1 A 63-year-old male is admitted with chest pain. Cardiac enzyme levels are elevated and the ECG indicates an acute myocardial infarction. The principal diagnosis is acute myocardial infarction. Chest pain is not coded, because it is a symptom of the definitive diagnosis of acute myocardial infarction.

Let's code this case together.

   a For an acute myocardial infarction, infarction is the **manifestation.** "Acute" indicates the **episode** of care and "myocardial" indicates the general **site** of the infarction.

   b Locate the term "Infarct, infarction" in the Index.

   c Under the term "Infarct, infarction" locate the subterm "myocardium." Note after "myocardium, myocardial" you find "(acute…)" and are directed to code 410.9. You can never stop at the Index. You must always refer to the Tabular; otherwise you will miss important notes, such as "a fifth digit is required."

   d Now turn to 410.9 in the Tabular, Volume 1.

   e Under "410.9 Unspecified site" you are presented with a notation that a fifth digit is required.

   f Go back to the three-digit category code 410 where the fifth digits are listed. The fifth digit 0 is for an unspecified episode of care; the fifth digit 1 is for the initial episode of care; and the fifth digit 2 is for a subsequent episode of care. The myocardial infarction was diagnosed during this visit, so that would be the initial episode of care as defined in the ICD-9-CM. The correct fifth digit is 1.

   g The complete, correct code is 410.91.

Now you try one.

2 A patient is admitted to the hospital with severe flank pain and hematuria. A urinalysis is done and it is positive for *Escherichia coli*. The discharge summary states acute pyelonephritis due to *E. coli.*

   a What is the principal diagnosis? _____

   b Locate the principal diagnosis in the Index. What code does the Index direct you to locate?

      ICD-10-CM Code: _____ (ICD-9-CM Code: _____)

   c Locate the code in the Tabular. What is the three-digit category code and the title of the category you were directed to?

      ICD-9-CM Code and title: _____

   d Was there a mention of a lesion in the case above? _____

   e What is the correct principal code for this case?

      ICD-10-CM Code: _____ (ICD-9-CM Code: _____)

   f Why do you think "severe flank pain and hematuria" are noted on this patient's case? _____

(Answers are located in Appendix B)

Two or More Interrelated Conditions

ICD-9-CM OFFICIAL GUIDELINES FOR CODING AND REPORTING

SECTION II.

B. Two or more interrelated conditions, each potentially meeting the definition for principal diagnosis

When there are two or more interrelated conditions (such as diseases in the same ICD-9-CM chapter or manifestations characteristically associated with a certain disease) potentially meeting the definition of principal diagnosis, either condition may be sequenced first, unless the circumstances of the admission, the therapy provided, the Tabular List, or the Alphabetic Index indicate otherwise.

EXERCISE 31-2   *Two or More Interrelated Conditions*

1 A patient is admitted with chest pain, shortness of breath, and a heart murmur. The patient undergoes a diagnostic cardiac catheterization, which shows two-vessel coronary artery disease (native coronary arteries) and severe mitral (valve) stenosis. It is recommended that bypass surgery with mitral valve replacement be performed as soon as possible.

The patient has two conditions, each of which has the potential to be the principal diagnosis: mitral valve stenosis and coronary artery disease.

a Locate stenosis in the Index: both "mitral" and "valve" indicate the site of the stenosis the patient has—the condition is stenosis. Under the main term "Stenosis," locate the subterm "mitral." The words in parentheses indicate the kinds of mitral stenosis, such as valve, chronic, or inactive. You are looking for valve, so the correct four-digit subcategory code for the mitral valve stenosis is likely to be 394.0.

b Locate coronary artery disease by locating the main term "Disease" and the subterms "artery" and "coronary." The entry directs you to "*see* Arteriosclerosis, coronary." Under the main term "Arteriosclerosis" and the subterm "coronary (native artery)" you will be directed to code 414.01. If the Tabular validates codes 394.0 (mitral valve stenosis) and 414.01 (coronary artery disease, native artery), either code could be sequenced first because none of the information indicates one condition warranted more care than the other.

Now you do one.

2 A patient is involved in a car accident and is admitted with an open fracture of the right humerus and an open fracture of the right distal femur. Both fractures require open reduction, which means that the fracture will be repaired using an open incision into the fracture site.

a What are the two diagnoses? _____

Either of these diagnoses may be principal, because both are addressed and plans are made to treat both surgically. They were equally the reason for admission to the hospital.

b Under what main term in the Index would you locate both diagnoses? _____

c After the main term "Fracture," what would be the first applicable subterm for the fracture of the right humerus? _____
_____

d What is the word that appears in parentheses after humerus? _____

Because the patient's case states "open," you know that 812.20 is not the correct code because 812.20 specifies "closed." Go farther down the list of subterms to "Fracture, humerus, open." What is the code for "open"?

ICD-10-CM Code: _____ (ICD-9-CM Code: _____)

e In the Tabular, does the code you chose in the Index match the description and if it does, why? _____
_____

Continued

You still have to locate the code for the open fracture of the distal femur.

f After looking in the Index using the main term "Fracture," what is the subterm you would locate?

_____

g What is the word in parentheses after the first subterm? _____

h What is the next subterm? _____

i What does this subterm direct you to do? _____

j When you take the subterm direction, what is the next subterm that you must use to locate the correct code?

_____

Note: If "open" or "closed" fracture is not stated, assume it is a "closed" fracture.

k What is the code that you are directed to look up under "Fracture, femur, lower end, open"?

ICD-10-CM Code: _____ (ICD-9-CM Code: _____)

l After checking the code in the Tabular, is the code correct? _____

(Answers are located in Appendix B)

Two or More Diagnoses

If two or more diagnoses are equally responsible for the outpatient visit, either can be sequenced as the principal diagnosis. The same is applicable in the inpatient setting.

ICD-9-CM OFFICIAL GUIDELINES FOR CODING AND REPORTING

SECTION II.

C. Two or more diagnoses that equally meet the definition for principal diagnosis

In the unusual instance when two or more diagnoses equally meet the criteria for principal diagnosis as determined by the circumstances of admission, diagnostic workup and/or therapy provided, and the Alphabetic Index, Tabular List, or another coding guideline does not provide sequencing direction, any one of the diagnoses may be sequenced first.

EXERCISE 31-3 *Two or More Diagnoses*

1 A patient is admitted with weakness, diarrhea of 2 days' duration, diaphoresis, and abdominal pain. The attending physician lists the diagnoses as viral gastroenteritis and dehydration. Intravenous fluids with electrolyte supplements are ordered.

a Locate "Gastroenteritis" as the main term in the Index and then the subterm "viral." When you do this you will be directed to code 008.8 (unspecified) because the record does not specify the organism type.

b After you have located code 008.8 in the Tabular and made sure it is the correct code, look for any notes under the three-digit category code to see if there are any fifth digits that need to be assigned.

c The correct code is 008.8 and there is no fifth digit to assign. Now you need to code the other diagnosis of dehydration. It seems almost too good to be true: There is only one word in the diagnosis. "Dehydration" is the main term. Dehydration appears in the Index, and it points to only one code. Check out the code 276.51 in the Tabular.

d The Tabular confirms that 276.51 is for dehydration and there is no note regarding any *Excludes* that concern this case. The correct code is 276.51.

Continued

e Remember, when two equally important diagnoses are indicated, it does not matter which code is sequenced first. So, the two codes for this case can be stated as 008.8 and 276.51 *or* 276.51 and 008.8. The order of the codes may not seem too earth-shattering right now, but the order of the codes is significant. One of these diagnoses may be reimbursed at a higher rate than the other; therefore, selection of the principal diagnosis is critically important.

Now you have the opportunity to do the next case.

2 A patient was admitted with heavy menstrual bleeding of 2 days' duration, severe abdominal pain, and anemia due to acute blood loss. The patient was given medication intravenously to control the pain and bleeding. She also received two units of packed cells for the anemia. Investigations were performed to determine a cause of the heavy bleeding.

   a What is the medical term for heavy menstrual/uterine bleeding? _____

   b The medical term from the question above is one of the diagnoses that you will need to locate. What code does the Index indicate and the Tabular of the text confirm as a code for the first diagnosis?

       ICD-10-CM Code: _____ (ICD-9-CM Code: _____)

   c What is the second diagnosis? _____

   d Locate the second diagnosis code and confirm your finding in the Tabular. (Hint: The subterms for the second code are "blood loss" and "acute.") What is the code?

       ICD-10-CM Code: _____ (ICD-9-CM Code: _____)

(Answers are located in Appendix B)

Comparative or Contrasting Conditions

ICD-9-CM OFFICIAL GUIDELINES FOR CODING AND REPORTING

SECTION II.

D. Two or more comparative or contrasting conditions.

In those rare instances when two or more contrasting or comparative diagnoses are documented as "either/or" (or similar terminology), they are coded as if the diagnoses were confirmed and the diagnoses are sequenced according to the circumstances of the admission. If no further determination can be made as to which diagnosis should be principal, either diagnosis may be sequenced first.

EXERCISE 31-4   *Comparative or Contrasting Conditions*

1 A patient is admitted to the hospital with chest pain, nausea, and dyspnea. The patient has a history of a prior myocardial infarction 2 years earlier. The pain is atypical (irregular). An ECG and cardiac enzyme study (creatine phosphokinase) are ordered, as well as an upper gastrointestinal series to rule out esophageal reflux. The admitting diagnosis by the attending physician is unstable angina or esophageal reflux.

   a Angina is located by the main term "Angina" and the subterm "unstable." The correct code is 411.1.

   b The second diagnosis is reflux, esophageal, located in the Index under the main term "Reflux" and the subterm "esophageal." You are directed to code 530.81. After checking this in the Tabular to be sure this is the correct code and that it has no exclusions or additions, you have the second of the two contrasting conditions, 530.81. Only further evaluation by the physician will finally determine what the principal diagnosis is; but for now, the case has been coded to the greatest specificity possible with the information available in the patient record as 530.81 and 411.1 or 411.1 and 530.81. Either diagnosis may be selected as the principal diagnosis. Also code the history of MI (412) secondarily.

Continued

Here's a case for you to code.

2 A 75-year-old man is admitted with severe low back pain. He is known to have prostate cancer as well as severe spondylosis. Spine x-ray films and a bone scan are ordered. Differential diagnoses are compression fracture versus bone metastases from prostate cancer. (Note: The physician would have to be consulted to determine whether prostate cancer is "current" prostate cancer or "history of" prostate cancer.)

a What is the main term for compression fracture? _____

b Using "Fracture" as the main term and "compression" as the subterm, what are you directed to do?

_____

Before you continue to look up other possible subterms, you need to consider why the patient has severe low back pain. You may need to query the physician or review the record to determine whether or not the compression fracture was due to trauma. The term "idiopathic" means of unknown cause; the term "pathologic" means due to a disease or accompanying a disease. Let us assume that the patient record substantiates a diagnosis of a fracture due to a disease (pathologic). Locate Fracture, pathological and then the subterm "vertebra." You are then forwarded to 733.13, which is the correct code according to the Tabular.

c The second diagnosis in the differential diagnoses is metastasis from prostate cancer. Locating cancer in the Index, you find: "*see also* Neoplasm, by site, malignant." The potential neoplasm is of the bone. "Neoplasm" is the main term and "bone" is a subterm. Secondary is the type of malignancy because the record states that this patient has prostate cancer (primary) and now has the potential to have bone (secondary) cancer. Under the "Secondary" column, what is the correct code for "Neoplasm, bone" for this patient?

ICD-10-CM Code: _____ (ICD-9-CM Code: _____)

An additional code would be assigned for the prostate cancer.

(Answers are located in Appendix B)

🛑 **STOP** *The difference between Guidelines Section II, D (Two or More Comparative or Contrasting Conditions), and Section II, E (Symptom[s] Followed by Contrasting/Comparative Diagnosis) is the way the physician states the final diagnosis. In the Guideline Section II, D, symptoms are documented but the physician states "X versus Y" instead of listing the symptoms. In Guideline Section II, E, the physician states the diagnosis as "symptoms due to X versus Y."*

Symptom(s) Followed by Contrasting/Comparative Diagnoses

ICD-9-CM OFFICIAL GUIDELINES FOR CODING AND REPORTING

SECTION II.
E. A symptom(s) followed by contrasting/comparative diagnoses

When a symptom(s) is followed by contrasting/comparative diagnoses, the symptom code is sequenced first. All the contrasting/comparative diagnoses should be coded as additional diagnoses.

EXERCISE 31-5 *Symptom(s) Followed by Contrasting/Comparative Diagnoses*

1 The patient presents with knee pain of 3 months' duration, with no known trauma, either bucket-handle tear of medial meniscus or loose body in the knee joint. The final diagnosis is knee pain due to bucket-handle tear of medial meniscus versus loose body in the knee joint.

There will be three codes for this case: one for the **pain** in the knee joint, one for the **tear** in the meniscus, and one for the **loose body** in the knee joint.

a Using "Pain, joint, knee" for the first condition, what is the correct code?

ICD-10-CM Code: _____ (ICD-9-CM Code: _____)

b Using "Tear, meniscus, bucket handle, old," what is the correct second code?

ICD-10-CM Code: _____ (ICD-9-CM Code: _____)

c Using "Loose, body, joint, knee," what is the correct third code?

ICD-10-CM Code: _____ (ICD-9-CM Code: _____)

(Answers are located in Appendix B)

Original Treatment Plan Not Carried Out

ICD-9-CM OFFICIAL GUIDELINES FOR CODING AND REPORTING

SECTION II.
F. Original treatment plan not carried out

Sequence as the principal diagnosis the condition, which after study occasioned the admission to the hospital, even though treatment may not have been carried out due to unforeseen circumstances.

EXERCISE 31-6 *Original Treatment Plan Not Carried Out*

1 A patient is admitted to the hospital for an elective cholecystectomy. The patient has chronic cholecystitis, and gallstones were visualized on x-ray films. After admission, it is noticed that the patient has a fever, is coughing, and shows some patchy infiltrates on the chest x-ray film. Surgery is canceled because the patient may have pneumonia.

This case will have three codes: the cholecystitis with gallstones (cholelithiasis), pneumonia, and surgery not done.

a Cholelithiasis with cholecystitis, without mention of obstruction. What is the code?

ICD-10-CM Code: _____ (ICD-9-CM Code: _____)

b What is the pneumonia code?

ICD-10-CM Code: _____ (ICD-9-CM Code: _____)

c The surgery that was not done is located in the Index under "Surgery, not done because of." Why was the surgery not done?

_____

d What is the code for the surgery not done?

ICD-10-CM Code: _____ (ICD-9-CM Code: _____)

Continued

No procedure code is submitted because no procedure was done.

2 A patient is admitted for elective sterilization by tubal ligation. The patient and her husband decide not to go through with the surgery, and the surgery is canceled.

   a How many codes will there be for this case, and what are the main terms for each? _____

_____

   b What is the Z/V code for the sterilization?

      ICD-10-CM Code: _____ (ICD-9-CM Code: _____)

   c What is the code for the surgery not done?

      ICD-10-CM Code: _____ (ICD-9-CM Code: _____)

(Answers are located in Appendix B)

Complications

ICD-9-CM OFFICIAL GUIDELINES FOR CODING AND REPORTING

SECTION II.
G. Complications of surgery and other medical care

When the admission is for treatment of a complication resulting from surgery or other medical care, the complication code is sequenced as the principal diagnosis. If the complication is classified to the 996-999 series and the code lacks the necessary specificity in describing the complication, an additional code for the specific complication should be assigned.

EXERCISE 31-7 *Complications of Surgery and Other Medical Care*

1 A patient is admitted to the hospital because of a postoperative ileus. The patient had a colectomy for colon cancer at another facility last week. On admission patient has abdominal pain with distension and nausea and vomiting.

Patient has not had a bowel movement for 3 days. Patient is scheduled to see an oncologist regarding adjunctive treatment for colon cancer.

   a Patient was admitted for a complication due to surgery. What is the complication? _____

   b What code is assigned as the principal diagnosis?

      ICD-10-CM Code: _____ (ICD-9-CM Code: _____)

   c Is there an additional code that should be assigned to indicate the exact nature of the complication? _____

   d What is the additional code?

      ICD-10-CM Code: _____ (ICD-9-CM Code: _____)

   e Are there any secondary diagnosis codes that should be assigned? _____ If so, what are those codes? _____

_____

2 A patient is admitted because of a malfunction of insulin pump. The patient is a type 1 diabetic and the pump has not been delivering an accurate dose of insulin.

   a What is the principal diagnosis and code for this case? _____

   b What is the Z/V code for long-term use of insulin?

      ICD-10-CM Code: _____ (ICD-9-CM Code: _____)

   c What additional codes should be assigned in this case? _____

_____

No ICD-9-CM procedure code is submitted because no procedure was done.

(Answers are located in Appendix B)

Uncertain Diagnosis

> ### ICD-9-CM OFFICIAL GUIDELINES FOR CODING AND REPORTING
>
> **SECTION II.**
> **H. Uncertain Diagnosis**
>
> If the diagnosis documented at the time of discharge is qualified as "probable", "suspected", "likely", "questionable", "possible", or "still to be ruled out", or other similar terms indicating uncertainty, code the condition as if it existed or was established. The bases for these guidelines are the diagnostic workup, arrangements for further workup or observation, and initial therapeutic approach that correspond most closely with the established diagnosis.
>
> **Note:** This guideline is applicable only to inpatient admissions to short-term, acute, long-term care and psychiatric hospitals.

The basis for this guideline is that the diagnostic workup and arrangements for further work-up, observation, or therapies are the same whether treating the confirmed condition or ruling the condition out.

Because hospitals are reimbursed a set payment (Medicare Severity Diagnosis-Related Groups amount) for each hospitalization for Medicare patients, the facility resources used are averaged across the entire patient stay in the hospital. In an outpatient setting, only confirmed diagnoses may be reported, and rule-out, possible, or probable diagnoses are not reported if there is a chief complaint, sign, or symptom that occasioned the visit. In an outpatient setting, each visit in the process of confirming a diagnosis is reported.

Examples

Uncertain Diagnosis

Hospital Inpatient

Diagnosis:	Probable bronchitis (code as bronchitis)
Index:	**Bronchitis** 490
Tabular:	**490 Bronchitis**

Hospital Inpatient

Diagnosis:	Rule out Graves' disease (code as Graves' disease)
Index:	**Graves' Disease** 242.0
Tabular:	**242.00 Toxic diffuse goiter** (Graves' disease)

Clinic Outpatient

Diagnosis:	Chest pain, rule out myocardial infarction (code as chest pain)
Index:	**Pain(s),** chest 786.50
Tabular:	**786.50 Chest pain, unspecified**

Clinic Outpatient

Diagnosis:	Cough and fever, probably pneumonia (code as cough and fever)
Index:	**Cough** 786.2
Index:	**Fever** 780.60
Tabular:	**786.2 Cough**
	780.60 Pyrexia of unknown origin (fever)

There are two exceptions to this guideline that are identified in the chapter-specific guidelines. The exceptions are:

■ Code 042, AIDS should only be assigned for confirmed cases.
■ Code 488.0X, Avian influenza should only be assigned for confirmed cases.

EXERCISE 31-8   *Uncertain Diagnoses*

1 Patient was admitted from the nursing home with fever, cough, and shortness of breath. Patient has a history of previous cerebrovascular accident with resultant dysphagia. Patient is being treated for hypertension. The physician documents the discharge diagnosis as probable aspiration pneumonia.

   a What is the principal diagnosis? _____

   b How do you code probable aspiration pneumonia?

      ICD-10-CM Code: _____ (ICD-9-CM Code: _____)

   c Are there any additional diagnosis codes that should be assigned in this case?

      ICD-10-CM Codes: _____, _____

      (ICD-9-CM Codes: _____, _____, _____)

2 Patient is admitted with hematuria. Investigations show that the patient likely has a malignant neoplasm of the right kidney. The patient refused any further interventions or workup. The physician's final diagnosis is suspected malignancy right kidney.

   a What is the principal diagnosis? _____

   b How do you code suspected malignancy right kidney?

      ICD-10-CM Code: _____ (ICD-9-CM Code: _____)

   c Are there additional diagnosis codes that should be assigned in this case?

      ICD-10-CM Code: _____ (ICD-9-CM Code: _____)

(Answers are located in Appendix B)

ICD-9-CM OFFICIAL GUIDELINES FOR CODING AND REPORTING

SECTION II.
I. Admission from Observation Unit

   1. Admission Following Medical Observation

      When a patient is admitted to an observation unit for a medical condition, which either worsens or does not improve, and is subsequently admitted as an inpatient of the same hospital for this same medical condition, the principal diagnosis would be the medical condition which led to the hospital admission.

   2. Admission Following Post-Operative Observation

      When a patient is admitted to an observation unit to monitor a condition (or complication) that develops following outpatient surgery, and then is subsequently admitted as an inpatient of the same hospital, hospitals should apply the Uniform Hospital Discharge Data Set (UHDDS) definition of principal diagnosis as "that condition established after study to be chiefly responsible for occasioning the admission of the patient to the hospital for care."

ICD-9-CM OFFICIAL GUIDELINES FOR CODING AND REPORTING

SECTION II.

J. Admission from Outpatient Surgery

When a patient receives surgery in the hospital's outpatient surgery department and is subsequently admitted for continuing inpatient care at the same hospital, the following guidelines should be followed in selecting the principal diagnosis for the inpatient admission:

- If the reason for the inpatient admission is a complication, assign the complication as the principal diagnosis.
- If no complication, or other condition, is documented as the reason for the inpatient admission, assign the reason for the outpatient surgery as the principal diagnosis.
- If the reason for the inpatient admission is another condition unrelated to the surgery, assign the unrelated condition as the principal diagnosis.

EXERCISE 31-9   *Admission from Observation Unit or Outpatient Surgery*

1 Patient is admitted after outpatient percutaneous needle biopsy of the kidney. Patient developed atrial fibrillation in the recovery room and decision was made to admit to ICU. Patient was treated and monitored on telemetry. The atrial fibrillation resolved and the patient's biopsy showed that the patient had lupus nephritis.

a What is the principal diagnosis? _____

b What code is assigned to the principal diagnosis?

ICD-10-CM Code: _____ (ICD-9-CM Code: _____)

c What secondary diagnosis codes are assigned?

ICD-10-CM Codes: _____, _____

(ICD-9-CM Codes: _____, _____, _____)

d Should a procedure code be assigned? _____

If so, what ICD-9-CM procedure code is assigned? _____

e What External Cause codes would be assigned?

ICD-10-CM Code: _____ Complication of other surgical operation

ICD-10-CM Code: _____ Place of occurrence, facility

(ICD-9-CM Code: _____ Complication of other surgical operation

ICD-9-CM Code: _____ Place of occurrence, facility)

(Answers are located in Appendix B)

REPORTING ADDITIONAL DIAGNOSES

After determining and coding the principal diagnosis and any procedures that were performed, a thorough review of the record is necessary to determine if any additional diagnoses should be coded and reported. These additional diagnoses have the potential to affect reimbursement so it is important to capture these conditions.

ICD-9-CM OFFICIAL GUIDELINES FOR CODING AND REPORTING

SECTION III. Reporting Additional Diagnoses
GENERAL RULES FOR OTHER (ADDITIONAL) DIAGNOSES

For reporting purposes the definition for "other diagnoses" is interpreted as additional conditions that affect patient care in terms of requiring:

> clinical evaluation; or
> therapeutic treatment; or
> diagnostic procedures; or
> extended length of hospital stay; or
> increased nursing care and/or monitoring.

The UHDDS item #11-b defines Other Diagnoses as "all conditions that coexist at the time of admission, that develop subsequently, or that affect the treatment received and/or the length of stay. Diagnoses that relate to an earlier episode which have no bearing on the current hospital stay are to be excluded." UHDDS definitions apply to inpatients in acute care, short-term, long term care and psychiatric hospital setting. The UHDDS definitions are used by acute care short-term hospitals to report inpatient data elements in a standardized manner. These data elements and their definitions can be found in the July 31, 1985, Federal Register (Vol. 50, No. 147), pp. 31038-40.

Since that time the application of the UHDDS definitions has been expanded to include all non-outpatient settings (acute care, short term, long term care and psychiatric hospitals; home health agencies; rehab facilities; nursing homes, etc).

The general rule is that for reporting purposes, the term "other diagnoses" is interpreted to refer to additional conditions that affect patient care in terms of requiring:

- Clinical evaluation; or
- Therapeutic treatment; or
- Diagnostic procedures; or
- Extended length of hospital stay, or
- Increased nursing care and/or monitoring

ICD-9-CM OFFICIAL GUIDELINES FOR CODING AND REPORTING

SECTION III. Reporting Additional Diagnoses (Paragraph 4)

The following guidelines are to be applied in designating "other diagnoses" when neither the Alphabetic Index nor the Tabular List in ICD-9-CM provide direction. The listing of the diagnoses in the patient record is the responsibility of the attending provider.

A. Previous conditions

If the provider has included a diagnosis in the final diagnostic statement, such as the discharge summary or the face sheet, it should ordinarily be coded. Some providers include in the diagnostic statement resolved conditions or diagnoses and status-post procedures from previous admission that have no bearing on the current stay. Such conditions are not to be reported and are coded only if required by hospital policy.

However, history codes (V10-V19) may be used as secondary codes if the historical condition or family history has an impact on current care or influences treatment.

EXERCISE 31-10   *Previous Conditions*

Circle the conditions in the following diagnostic lists that would NOT be coded:

1 Herpes zoster

History of hysterectomy

Diabetes

2 Influenza

Hypertension (currently controlled by medication)

History of peptic ulcer disease

3 Congestive heart failure

Remote history of appendectomy

Previous arthroscopic surgery to left knee

(Answers are located in Appendix B)

ICD-9-CM OFFICIAL GUIDELINES FOR CODING AND REPORTING

SECTION III.

B. Abnormal findings

Abnormal findings (laboratory, x-ray, pathologic, and other diagnostic results) are not coded and reported unless the provider indicates their clinical significance. If the findings are outside the normal range and the attending provider has ordered other tests to evaluate the condition or prescribed treatment, it is appropriate to ask the provider whether the abnormal finding should be added.

Please note: This differs from the coding practices in the outpatient setting for coding encounters for diagnostic tests that have been interpreted by a provider.

EXERCISE 31-11   *Abnormal Findings*

1 If the physician documents that a patient's potassium level is 2.5 and orders potassium supplements with a repeat potassium lab test, is it acceptable to query the physician about the 2.5 potassium level? _____

2 On review of the record the coder notices that the patient's sodium level is slightly below normal. There is no documentation of any treatment, evaluation, or monitoring. Is it acceptable to query the physician about the abnormal sodium level? _____

(Answers are located in Appendix B)

The Guideline for uncertain diagnoses is repeated in Section III, Reporting Additional Diagnoses. Sometimes a physician will document "rule out" as a final diagnostic statement, but upon review of the record it is apparent that the diagnosis was actually ruled out. A diagnosis that has been ruled out should not be coded as if it exists.

ICD-9-CM OFFICIAL GUIDELINES FOR CODING AND REPORTING

SECTION III.

C. Uncertain Diagnosis

If the diagnosis documented at the time of discharge is qualified as "probable", "suspected", "likely", "questionable", "possible", or "still to be ruled out" or other similar terms indicating uncertainty, code the condition as if it existed or was established. The bases for these guidelines are the diagnostic workup, arrangements for further workup or observation, and initial therapeutic approach that correspond most closely with the established diagnosis.

Note: This guideline is applicable only to inpatient admissions to short-term, acute, long-term care and psychiatric hospitals.

PRESENT ON ADMISSION (POA)

The Deficit Reduction Act (DRA) mandated that all acute-care facilities that are reimbursed under MS-DRGs identify and report diagnoses that were present at the time of a patient's admission. This policy was implemented October 1, 2007, and expected to save lives and health care dollars by no longer paying for the treatment of preventable errors, injuries, and infections that can occur in the hospital setting. CMS will not pay for conditions considered preventable, such as pressure ulcers, falls resulting in injury, infections due to genitourinary or central line catheters, or other complications that occur during hospitalization.

The Present on Admission (POA) indicator distinguishes between conditions that develop during a particular hospital stay and those conditions present at the time of admission. Hospitals were allowed a 1-year grace time and after October 1, 2008, a hospital's reimbursement may be affected if certain complications develop after admission to the hospital. Coding staff will have to assign the POA indicators to the ICD-9-CM codes that are assigned. This requirement makes it even more important to have accurate and complete documentation in the health record. In some instances, it may be necessary to query the physician if a condition was present at the time of admission. The Cooperating Parties have developed POA guidelines that are supplemental to the ICD-9-CM *Official Guidelines for Coding and Reporting* to assist with the application of the POA requirement.

DEVELOPMENT OF THE ICD-10-PCS

ICD-10-PCS will allow more expansion than was possible with Volume 3 of the ICD-9-CM because I-9 lacks specificity (exactness) and does not provide for sufficient expansion to support government payment systems and data needs. CMS contracted with 3M Health Information Systems to develop the ICD-10-PCS to replace the ICD-9-CM procedure codes (Volume 3) for reporting **inpatient** procedures.

Four major objectives guided the development of ICD-10-PCS:

1. **Completeness.** There is a unique code for all substantially different procedures. Currently, procedures performed on different body parts, using different approaches or of different types, are sometimes assigned the same code.
2. **Expandability.** As new procedures are developed, the structure of the ICD-10-PCS should allow for incorporation of these new procedures as unique codes.
3. **Multiaxial** (more than one part). ICD-10-PCS should have a structure such that each code character has, as much as possible, the same meaning, both within the specific procedure section and across procedure sections.
4. **Standardized terminology.** Although the meaning of a specific word may vary in common usage, ICD-10-PCS should not include multiple meanings for the same term; each term should be assigned a specific meaning, and ICD-10-PCS should include definitions of the terminology.

A complete, expandable, multiaxial ICD-10-PCS with standardized terminology allows coding specialists to determine the accurate code with minimal effort.

The Seven Characters of the ICD-10-PCS

The ICD-10-PCS has a seven-character alphanumeric code structure. Each character has as many as 34 different values: 10 digits (0-9) and 24 letters (A-H, J-N, and P-Z) may be assigned to each character. The letters O and I are not used in order to avoid confusion with the digits 0 and 1. In the ICD-10-PCS, the term "procedure" refers to the complete designation of the seven characters. Procedures are divided into sections according to the type of procedure.

Character 1 Identifies the Section. The first character of the procedure code identifies the section. To assign an ICD-10-PCS code, the section where the procedure is coded must be identified. For example, a chest x-ray is in the Imaging section, a breast biopsy is in the Medical and Surgical section, and crisis intervention is in the Mental Health section. Each section is identified by a specific character—number or letter. Section titles and numbers/letters are shown in Fig. 31-1.

EXERCISE 31-12 | *ICD-10-PCS First Character*

Using Fig. 31-1, identify the first section character that would be assigned to the following procedures. For example, chiropractic would be "9."

1 _____ Gait training (Physical Rehabilitation)

2 _____ Cesarean section (Obstetrics)

3 _____ Computerized tomography, spine (Imaging)

4 _____ Cholecystectomy (Medical and Surgical)

5 _____ Insertion of radium into cervix (brachytherapy) (Radiation Oncology)

6 _____ Cranioplasty (Medical and Surgical)

(Answers are located in Appendix B)

SECTIONS

0	Medical and Surgical
1	Obstetrics
2	Placement
3	Administration
4	Measurement and Monitoring
5	Extracorporeal Assistance and Performance
6	Extracorporeal Therapies
7	Osteopathic
8	Other Procedures
9	Chiropractic
B	Imaging
C	Nuclear Medicine
D	Radiation Therapy
F	Physical Rehabilitation and Diagnostic Audiology
G	Mental Health
H	Substance Abuse Treatment

FIGURE 31–1 Sections of ICD-10-PCS.

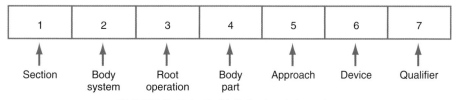

FIGURE 31-2 Medical and surgical procedures.

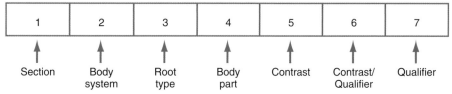

FIGURE 31-3 Imaging procedures.

Changing Characters. Characters 2 through 7 have a standard meaning within each section but may have different meanings across sections. The meanings for each character are described in each section. For example, Fig. 31-2 shows the meanings of the seven characters for the Medical and Surgical sections, and Fig. 31-3 shows the meanings for the Imaging section. Notice that several characters have different meanings across these sections. For instance, the third character in medical and surgical procedures (see Fig. 31-2) is used to define the root *operation* (extraction, insertion, removal, etc.), whereas the third character in imaging procedures (see Fig. 31-3) is used to define the root *type* (fluoroscopy, MRI, CT, ultrasonography, etc.).

STOP   *Each code must include seven characters. If a character is not applicable to a specific procedure, the letter Z is assigned.*

Character 2 Is the Body System. The second character identifies the body system in all sections except Rehabilitation and Mental Health. In these two sections, the second character identifies the type of procedure performed.

Character 3 Is the Root Operation. The third character identifies the root operation in all sections except Radiation Therapy, Rehabilitation, and Mental Health. In many sections, only a few root operations are performed, and these operations are defined in that section. The Medical and Surgical section uses an extensive list of root operations. The Obstetrics and Placement sections use some of these same root operations as well as section-specific root operations. See Table 31-1 (pp. 869-872) for a list of the Medical and Surgical root operations definitions, explanations, and examples.

EXERCISE 31-13 *Root Operation*

Using Table 31-1, place the character for the root operation term before its definition:

1 _____ Taking or letting out fluids and/or gases from a body part

2 _____ Freeing a body part from an abnormal physical constraint

3 _____ Taking out or off a device from a body part

4 _____ Visually and/or manually exploring a body part

5 _____ Restoring, to the extent possible, a body part to its normal anatomic structure and function

6 _____ Altering the route of passage of the contents of a tubular body part

7 _____ Cutting out or off, without replacement, all of a body part

8 _____ Physical eradication of all or a portion of a body part by direct use of energy, force, or a destructive agent

9 _____ Correcting, to the extent possible, a portion of a malfunctioning device or the position of a displaced device

10 _____ Cutting out or off, without replacement, a portion of a body part of device in

1 Bypass

5 Destruction

7 Drainage

8 Excision

L Release

M Removal of Device

N Repair

R Resection

G Inspection

T Revision

(Answers are located in Appendix B)

A Closer Look at Root Operations. The root operation is described by one of the main terms, as outlined on page 872 in Table 31-1 (e.g., Alteration, Change, Bypass). These root operations can be grouped into types of operations, such as operations that always involve devices: insertion, replacement, removal, change. Table 31-2 (pp. 872–874) shows the root operations grouped by types.

EXERCISE 31-14 *Root Operation Terms*

Using Table 31-2, identify the root operation term for each example:

1 _____ Tendon transfer

2 _____ Sigmoid polypectomy

3 _____ Diagnostic arthroscopy

4 _____ Heart transplant

5 _____ Pacemaker insertion

6 _____ Cardiac pacemaker removal

7 _____ Lithotripsy, gallstones

8 _____ Fallopian tube ligation

9 _____ Hip prosthesis adjustment

10 _____ Peritoneal adhesiolysis

(Answers are located in Appendix B)

The Index

ICD-10-PCS codes are described in both the Index and the Tabular List. The Index is used to locate codes by means of an alphabetic lookup. The Index is arranged according to root operation terms and has subentries based on:

- Body System
- Body Part
- Operation (for Revision)
- Device (for Change)

The Index may also be consulted for a specific operation term such as "Hysterectomy," where a cross-reference directs you to "*see* Resection, Female Reproductive System, OUT." Although you need to become very familiar with the root operations, you may be able to locate a code for a specific operation such as an appendectomy more rapidly by looking under the term "Appendectomy" than by consulting the root operation term "Resection," subterms "by Body Part," and "Appendix." See Fig. 31-4 for an example of the Index of the ICD-10-PCS.

Codes may also be located in the Index by specific procedures such as X-ray—*see* Imaging. The Index refers you to a specific entry in the Tabular List by providing the first three or four digits of the procedure code. It is always necessary to refer to the Tabular List to obtain the complete code because the Index contains only the first few numbers and letters.

The Tabular List Completes the Code

The Tabular List provides the remaining characters needed to complete the code listed in the Index. The Tabular List is arranged by sections, and most sections are subdivided by body systems. For each body system, the Tabular List begins with a list of the operations performed, that is, the root operations. When a procedure involves distinct parts, multiple codes are

Flexor hallucis longus muscle
    use Muscle, Lower Leg, Right
    use Muscle, Lower Leg, Left
Flexor pollicis longus muscle
    use Muscle, Lower Arm and Wrist, Left
    use Muscle, Lower Arm and Wrist, Right
Fluoroscopy
    Abdomen and Pelvis BW11
    Airway, Upper BB1DZZZ
    Ankle
        Left BQ1H
        Right BQ1G
    Aorta
        Abdominal B410
            Laser, Intraoperative B410
        Thoracic B310
            Laser, Intraoperative B310
        Thoraco-Abdominal B31P
            Laser, Intraoperative B31P
    Aorta and Bilateral Lower Extremity Arteries B41D
        Laser, Intraoperative B41D
    Arm
        Left BP1FZZZ
        Right BP1EZZZ
    Artery
        Brachiocephalic-Subclavian Right B311
            Laser, Intraoperative B311
        Bronchial B31L
            Laser, Intraoperative B31L
        Bypass Graft, Other B21F

FIGURE 31–4 ICD-10-PCS Index.

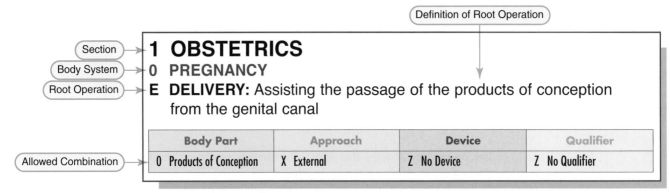

FIGURE 31–5 ICD-10-PCS Tabular.

provided. For example, a section of the listing of operations performed in respect to the central nervous system is as follows:

■ Bypass
■ Change
■ Destruction
■ Division
■ Drainage
■ Excision

The Tabular List for each body system also includes a list of the body parts, approaches, devices, and qualifiers for that system. These lists are followed by tables for each root operation in that body system. At the top of each of the tables is the name of the section, body system, and root operation as well as the definition of the root operation. The list is formatted as a grid, with rows and columns. The four columns in the grid represent the last four characters of the code (which are labeled Body Part, Approach, Device, and Qualifier in the Obstetrics and Medical and Surgical sections). Each row in the grid specifies the allowable combinations of the last four characters. For example, referring to the grid in Fig. 31-5, you see that the code for delivery of products of conception is 10E0XZZ:

1 Obstetrics (Section)
0 Pregnancy (Body System)
E Delivery (Root Operation)
0 Products of Conception (Body Part, Character 4)
X External (Approach, Character 5)
Z None (Device, Character 6)
Z None (Qualifier, Character 7)

Code 10E0XZZ would be the only allowable code for Products of Conception, using an external approach with no devices, because you may not complete a code by choosing entries from different rows (a row may consist of multiple entries in a box). Thus the code 10E0XZ6 is not permitted because the qualifier 6 is not an option. If you choose the character 0, Products of Conception, you must continue to choose from the available numbers or letters in that same line.

From the Trenches

"Don't stress over learning ICD-10. If you've been using ICD-9 for several years and are comfortable with it, ICD-10 will not be difficult to learn."

LORI

EXERCISE 31-15   *ICD-10-PCS Format*

Complete the following:

Achievement of the four major objectives guiding the development of the ICD-10-PCS will result in a classification system that is

1 _____

2 _____

3 _____

4 _____

Provide the requested information about the ICD-10-PCS code structure:

5 The ICD-10-PCS has a _____ character code structure.

6 The characters in ICD-10-PCS are _____.

7 Each character has up to _____ different values.

8 The letters _____ are not used as character values.

9 The complete specification of seven characters describes a _____ in the ICD-10-PCS.

(Answers are located in Appendix B)

TABLE 31–1

MEDICAL AND SURGICAL ROOT OPERATION DEFINITIONS (SELECT)

Alteration	Definition:	Modifying the anatomic structure of a body part without affecting the function of the body part
	Explanation:	Principal purpose is to improve appearance
	Includes/ Examples:	Face lift, breast augmentation
Bypass	Definition:	Altering the route of passage of the contents of a tubular body part
	Explanation:	Rerouting contents of a body part to a downstream area of the normal route, to a similar route and body part, or to an abnormal route and dissimilar body part. It includes one or more anastomosis, with or without the use of a device
	Includes/ Examples:	Coronary artery bypass, colostomy formation
Change	Definition:	Taking out or off a device from a body part and putting back an identical or similar device in or on the same body part without cutting or puncturing the skin or a mucous membrane
	Explanation:	ALL CHANGE procedures are coded using the approach EXTERNAL
	Includes/ Examples:	Urinary catheter change, gastrostomy tube change
Control	Definition:	Stopping, or attempting to stop, postprocedural bleeding
	Explanation:	The site of the bleeding is coded as an anatomical region and not to a specific body part
	Includes/ Examples:	Control of post-prostatectomy hemorrhage, control of post-tonsillectomy hemorrhage
Creation	Definition:	Making a new genital structure that does not physically take the place of a body part
	Explanation:	Used only for sex change operations
	Includes/ Examples:	Creation of vagina in a male, creation of penis in a female

Continued

TABLE 31–1

MEDICAL AND SURGICAL ROOT OPERATION DEFINITIONS (SELECT)—cont'd

Destruction	**Definition:**	Physical eradication of all or a portion of a body part by the direct use of energy, force or a destructive agent
	Explanation:	None of the body part is physically taken out
	Includes/ Examples:	Fulguration of rectal polyp, cautery of skin lesion
Detachment	**Definition:**	Cutting off all or a portion of the upper or lower extremities
	Explanation:	The body part value is the site of the detachment, with a qualifier if applicable to further specify the level where the extremity was detached
	Includes/ Examples:	Below knee amputation, disarticulation of shoulder
Dilation	**Definition:**	Expanding an orifice or the lumen of a tubular body part
	Explanation:	The orifice can be a natural orifice or an artificially created orifice. Accomplished by stretching a tubular body part using intraluminal pressure or by cutting part of the orifice or wall of the tubular body part
	Includes/ Examples:	Percutaneous transluminal angioplasty, pyloromyotomy
Division	**Definition:**	Cutting into a body part, without draining fluids and/or gases from the body part, in order to separate or transect a body part
	Explanation:	All or a portion of the body part is separated into two or more portions.
	Includes/ Examples:	Spinal cordotomy, osteotomy
Drainage	**Definition:**	Taking or letting out fluids and/or gases from a body part
	Explanation:	The qualifier DIAGNOSTIC is used to identify drainage procedures that are biopsies.
	Includes/ Examples:	Thoracentesis, incision and drainage
Excision	**Definition:**	Cutting out or off, without replacement, a portion of a body part
	Explanation:	The qualifier DIAGNOSTIC is used to identify excision procedures that are biopsies
	Includes/ Examples:	Partial nephrectomy, liver biopsy
Extirpation	**Definition:**	Taking or cutting out solid matter from a body part
	Explanation:	The solid matter may be an abnormal byproduct of a biological function or a foreign body; it may be imbedded in a body part in the lumen of a tubular body part. The solid matter may or may not have been previously broken into pieces
	Includes/ Examples:	Thrombectomy, choledocholithotomy
Extraction	**Definition:**	Pulling or stripping out or off all or a portion of a body part by the use of force
	Explanation:	The qualifier DIAGNOSTIC is used to identify extraction procedures that are biopsies
	Includes/ Examples:	Dilation and curettage, vein stripping
Fragmentation	**Definition:**	Breaking solid matter in a body part into pieces
	Explanation:	Physical force (e.g., manual, ultrasonic) applied directly or indirectly is used to break the solid matter into pieces. The solid matter may be an abnormal byproduct of a biological function or a foreign body. The pieces of solid matter are not taken out
	Includes/ Examples:	Extracorporeal shockwave lithotripsy, transurethral lithotripsy
Fusion	**Definition:**	Joining together portions of an articular body part rendering the articular body part immobile
	Explanation:	The body part is joined together by fixation device, bone graft, or other means
	Includes/ Examples:	Spinal fusion, ankle arthrodesis

Continued

TABLE 31–1

MEDICAL AND SURGICAL ROOT OPERATION DEFINITIONS (SELECT)—cont'd

Insertion	Definition:	Putting in a nonbiological appliance that monitors, assists, performs, or prevents a physiological function but does not physically take the place of a body part
	Explanation:	N/A
	Includes/Examples:	Insertion of radioactive implant, insertion of central venous catheter
Inspection	Definition:	Visually and/or manually exploring a body part
	Explanation:	Visual exploration may be performed with or without optical instrumentation. Manual exploration may be performed directly or through intervening body layers
	Includes/Examples:	Diagnostic arthroscopy, exploratory laparotomy
Map	Definition:	Locating the route of passage of electrical impulses and/or locating functional areas in a body part
	Explanation:	Applicable only to the cardiac conduction mechanism and the central nervous system
	Includes/Examples:	Cardiac mapping, cortical mapping
Occlusion	Definition:	Completely closing an orifice or lumen of a tubular body part
	Explanation:	The orifice can be a natural orifice or an artificially created orifice
	Includes/Examples:	Fallopian tube ligation, ligation of inferior vena cava
Reattachment	Definition:	Putting back in or on all or a portion of a separated body part to its normal location or other suitable location
	Explanation:	Vascular circulation and nervous pathways may or may not be re-established
	Includes/Examples:	Reattachment of hand, reattachment of avulsed kidney
Release	Definition:	Freeing a body part from an abnormal physical constraint
	Explanation:	Some of the restraining tissue may be taken out but none of the body part is taken out
	Includes/Examples:	Adhesiolysis, carpal tunnel release
Removal of device from	Definition:	Taking out or off a device from a body part
	Explanation:	If the device is taken out and a similar device is put in without cutting or puncturing the skin or mucous membrane, the procedure is coded to the root operation CHANGE. Otherwise, the procedure for taking out the device is coded to the root operation REMOVAL
	Includes/Examples:	Drainage tube removal, cardiac pacemaker removal
Repair	Definition:	Restoring, to the extent possible, a body part to its normal anatomic structure and function
	Explanation:	Used only when the method to accomplish the repair is not one of the other root operations
	Includes/Examples:	Colostomy takedown, suture of laceration
Replacement	Definition:	Putting in or on biological or synthetic material that physically takes the place and/or function of all or a portion of a body part
	Explanation:	The body part may have been taken out or replaced, or may be taken out, physically eradicated, or rendered nonfunctional during the Replacement procedure. A Removal procedure is coded for taking out the device used in a previous replacement procedure
	Includes/Examples:	Total hip replacement, bone graft, free skin graft
Reposition	Definition:	Moving to its normal location or other suitable location, all or a portion of a body part
	Explanation:	The body part is moved to a new location from an abnormal location, or from a normal location where it is not functioning correctly. The body part may or may not be cut out or off to be moved to the new location
	Includes/Examples:	Reposition of undescended testicle, fracture reduction

Continued

TABLE 31–1

MEDICAL AND SURGICAL ROOT OPERATION DEFINITIONS (SELECT)—cont'd

Resection	Definition:	Cutting out or off, without replacement, all of a body part
	Explanation:	N/A
	Includes/Examples:	Total nephrectomy, total lobectomy of lung
Restriction	Definition:	Partially closing the orifice or lumen of a tubular body part
	Explanation:	The orifice can be a natural orifice or an artificially created orifice
	Includes/Examples:	Esophagogastric fundoplication, cervical cerclage
Revision	Definition:	Correcting, to the extent possible, a portion of a malfunctioning or the position of a displaced device
	Explanation:	Revision can include correcting a malfunctioning or displaced device by taking out and/or putting in a part of the device
	Includes/Examples:	Adjustment of position of pacemaker lead, recementing of hip prosthesis
Supplement	Definition:	Putting in or on biologic or synthetic material that physically reinforces and/or augments the function of a portion of a body part
	Explanation:	The biological material is non-living, or is living and from the same individual. The body part may have been previously replaced, and the Supplement procedure is performed to physically reinforce and/or augment the function of the replaced body part
	Includes/Examples:	Herniorrhaphy using mesh, free nerve graft, mitral valve ring annuloplasty, put a new acetabular liner in a previous hip replacement
Transfer	Definition:	Moving, without taking out, all or a portion of a body part to another location to take over the function of all or a portion of a body part
	Explanation:	The body part transferred remains connected to its vascular and nervous supply
	Includes/Examples:	Tendon transfer, skin pedicle flap transfer
Transplantation	Definition:	Putting in or on all or a portion of a living body part taken from another individual or animal to physically take the place and/or function of all or a portion of a similar body part
	Explanation:	The native body part may or may not be taken out, and the transplanted body part may take over all or a portion of its function
	Includes/Examples:	Kidney transplant, heart transplant

TABLE 31–2

COMPARISON OF MEDICAL AND SURGICAL ROOT OPERATIONS (SELECT)

Operation	Action	Target	Clarification	Example
		Procedures that take out or eliminate all or a portion of a body part:		
Excision	Cutting out or off	Portion of a body part	Without replacing body part	Sigmoid polypectomy
Resection	Cutting out or off	All of a body part	Without replacing body part	Total nephrectomy
Extraction	Pulling out or off by physical force	All or a portion of a body part	Without replacing body part	Toenail extraction
Destruction	Eradicating	All or a portion of a body part	Without taking out or replacing body part	Rectal polyp fulguration
Detachment	Cutting off	All or a portion of an extremity	Without replacing extremity	Below knee amputation

Continued

TABLE 31–2

COMPARISON OF MEDICAL AND SURGICAL ROOT OPERATIONS (SELECT)—cont'd

Operation	Action	Target	Clarification	Example
Procedures that involve putting in or on, putting back, or moving living body parts:				
Transplantation	Putting in or on	All or a portion of a living body part from other individual or animal	Physically takes the place and/or function of all or a portion of a body part	Heart transplant
Reattachment	Putting back in or on	All or a portion of a separated body part	Put in its normal or other suitable location	Finger reattachment
Reposition	Moving	All or a portion of a body part	Put in its normal or other suitable location. Body part may or may not be cut out or off	Reposition undescended testicle
Transfer	Moving	All or a portion of a body part	Without taking out body part; assumes function of similar body part and remains connected to its vascular and nervous supply	Tendon transfer
Procedures that take out or eliminate solid matter, fluids, or gases from a body part:				
Drainage	Taking or letting out	Fluids and/or gases from a body part	Without taking out any of the body part	Incision and drainage
Extirpation	Taking or cutting out	Solid matter in a body part	Without taking out any of the body part	Thrombectomy
Fragmentation	Breaking down	Solid matter in a body part	Without taking out any of the body part or any solid matter	Lithotripsy of gallstones
Procedures that only involve examination of body parts and regions:				
Inspection	Visual and/or manual exploration	A body part	Performed with or without optical instrumentation, directly or through body layers	Diagnostic arthroscopy
Map	Locating	Route of passage of electrical impulses or functional areas in a body part	Applicable only to cardiac conduction mechanism and central nervous system	Cardiac mapping
Procedures that can be performed only on tubular body parts:				
Bypass	Altering the route of passage	Contents of tubular body part	May include use of living tissue, non-living biological material or synthetic material which does not take the place of the body part	Gastrojejunal bypass
Dilation	Expanding	Orifice or lumen of tubular body part	By application of intraluminal pressure or by cutting the wall or orifice	Anal sphincter dilation
Occlusion	Completely closing	Orifice or lumen of tubular body part	N/A	Fallopian tube ligation
Restriction	Partially closing	Orifice or lumen of tubular body part	N/A	Cervical cerclage
Procedures that always involve devices:				
Insertion	Putting in	Device in or on a body part	Does not physically take the place of a body part	Pacemaker insertion
Replacement	Putting in or on	Biological or synthetic material; living tissue taken from same individual	Physically takes the place of all or a portion of a body part	Total hip replacement
Supplement	Putting in or on	Biological or synthetic material; living tissue taken from same individual	Physically reinforces or augments a portion of a body part	Herniorrhaphy using mesh

Continued

TABLE 31–2

COMPARISON OF MEDICAL AND SURGICAL ROOT OPERATIONS (SELECT)—cont'd

Operation	Action	Target	Clarification	Example
Removal	Taking out or off	Device from a body part	N/A	Cardiac pacemaker removal
Change	Taking out or off and putting back	Identical or similar device in or on a body part	Without cutting or puncturing skin or mucous membrane	Drainage tube change
Revision	Correcting	Malfunctioning or displaced device in or on a body part	To the extent possible	Hip prosthesis adjustment
Procedures involving cutting or separation only:				
Division	Separating	A body part	Without taking out any of the body part	Osteotomy
Release	Freeing	A body part	Eliminating abnormal constraint without taking out any of the body part	Peritoneal adhesiolysis
Procedures involving other repairs:				
Control	Stopping or attempting to stop	Postprocedural bleeding	Limited to anatomic regions and extremities	Control of postprostatectomy bleeding
Repair	Restoring	A body part to its normal structure	To the extent possible	Hernia repair
Procedures with other objectives:				
Alteration	Modifying	Anatomic structure of a body part	Without affecting function of body part, performed for cosmetic purposes	Face lift
Creation	Making	New genital structure	Does not physically take the place of a body part, used for sex change operations	Artificial vagina creation
Fusion	Joining together	An articular body part	Rendering body part immobile	Spinal fusion

CHECK THIS OUT ☞ Third-party companies typically employ **Clinical Documentation Improvement (CDI)** specialists, who are then hired by medical providers to advise and implement programs that improve documentation practices. The use of CDI is especially important to ensure documentation is specific enough to support the level of detail required from ICD-10-CM/ICD-10-PCS. Ultimately, it's the coders' responsibility to follow up with the provider in order to ensure proper documentation that meets the quality of coding, medical necessity, and denial standards of ICD-10-CM/ICD-10-PCS.

CHAPTER REVIEW

1 Codes can be assigned to diagnoses that are documented as being "probable," "suspected," or "likely" in which setting?

Inpatient   Outpatient

2 In which setting can any confirmed or definitive diagnoses be coded from the interpretation of a diagnostic test result?

Inpatient   Outpatient

3 In which setting would a CPT code be assigned for a herniorrhaphy?

Inpatient   Outpatient

4 Which statement about a significant procedure is NOT true?
  a Requires specialized training
  b Carries an anesthetic risk
  c Is surgical in nature
  d Must be performed in an operating room

5 The physician documents flank pain due to renal stone. The flank pain is the principal diagnosis.

True   False

6 In the inpatient setting, the physician documents suspected cholelithiasis in the discharge summary. The cholelithiasis is coded as if it exists.

True   False

7 If the coder doesn't know if a diagnosis is present on admission, a POA indicator is not assigned.

True   False

8 A patient is admitted with low-grade fever and right upper quadrant pain. The physician documents that the patient's right upper quadrant pain is due to chronic cholecystitis versus peptic ulcer disease. Which diagnoses should be reported?
  a Chronic cholecystitis
  b Peptic ulcer disease
  c Chronic cholecystitis, peptic ulcer disease
  d Right upper quadrant pain, chronic cholecystitis, peptic ulcer disease

9 Patient is admitted with hyperglycemia due to new-onset diabetes, type 2. Patient has had polydipsia, polyuria, and unexplained weight loss. Which diagnoses should be reported?
  a Hyperglycemia, diabetes, type 2
  b Diabetes, type 2
  c Diabetes, type 2, polydipsia, polyuria, weight loss
  d Hyperglycemia, diabetes, type 2, weight loss

10 Patient is admitted with heartburn due to gastroesophageal reflux disease (GERD). Which diagnoses should be reported?
  a Heartburn
  b Heartburn and GERD
  c GERD and heartburn
  d GERD

11 The American Medical Association is responsible for the development of ICD-10-PCS.

True   False

Chapter Review answers are only available in the TEACH Instructor Resources on Evolve

12 In ICD-10-PCS, if a character is not applicable, the letter X is used.

True   False

13 The term "fusion" means the freeing of a body part.

True   False

14 An example of a procedure that involves inspection is:
   a gastrojejunal bypass
   b control of postprocedural bleeding
   c diagnostic arthroscopy
   d incision and drainage of abscess

15 Altering the route of passage of the contents of a tubular body part is a _____.
   a resection
   b bypass
   c revision
   d drainage

CHAPTER 31, PART II, PRACTICAL

Assign and sequence codes to the following inpatient diagnoses.

16 Headache due to malignant neoplasm of the brain

ICD-10-CM Code: _____

(ICD-9-CM Code: _____)

17 Patient was admitted with shortness of breath. Patient was found to have both pneumonia and decompensated congestive heart failure. The pneumonia was treated with IV antibiotics and the congestive heart failure with IV Lasix. Both were present on admission.

ICD-10-CM Codes: _____, _____

(ICD-9-CM Codes: _____, _____)

18 Acute cholecystitis versus acute pancreatitis

ICD-10-CM Codes: _____, _____

(ICD-9-CM Codes: _____, _____)

19 Epigastric pain due to acute cholecystitis versus acute pancreatitis

ICD-10-CM Codes: _____, _____

(ICD-9-CM Codes: _____, _____)

20 Patient was admitted for elective D&C because of post-menopausal bleeding. The surgery was cancelled because the surgeon became ill. The patient's surgery was rescheduled for next week.

ICD-10-CM Codes: _____, _____

(ICD-9-CM Codes: _____, _____)

21 Patient was admitted for dehiscence of abdominal incision.

ICD-10-CM Code(s): _____

(ICD-9-CM Code(s): _____)

22 Patient was admitted for medical observation for chest pain. After the patient was determined to have suffered a NSTEMI (Non-ST Elevation Myocardial Infarction), the patient was admitted to acute care.

ICD-10-CM Code(s): _____

(ICD-9-CM Code(s): _____)

23 Patient was admitted for suspected avian influenza. Avian influenza was ruled out and it was determined that the patient's symptoms were due to viral pneumonia.

⊛ ICD-10-CM Code(s): _____

(⊛ ICD-9-CM Code(s): _____)

24 Patient was admitted to the observation unit for exacerbation of COPD. The patient did not improve and was admitted for continued care and treatment.

⊛ ICD-10-CM Code(s): _____

(⊛ ICD-9-CM Code(s): _____)

25 Patient was admitted following an outpatient esophagogastroduodenoscopy for dilatation of an esophageal stricture. The patient was unable to void and was admitted because of urinary retention.

⊛ ICD-10-CM Code(s): _____

(⊛ ICD-9-CM Code(s): _____)

Online Resources

The Evolve Learning Resources offer helpful material that will extend your studies beyond the classroom. Encoder practice exercises provide added practice and help you understand how to utilize an Encoder product. *Official Guidelines for Coding and Reporting,* Code Updates, and Chapter WebLinks offer you the opportunity to expand your knowledge base and stay current with this ever changing field. Extra Coding Cases, ICD GEMs files, and Coding Tips are also available to check your understanding.

Once registered for your free Evolve resources at http://evolve.elsevier.com/Buck/step, go to the *Course Documents* section and click *Resources* to reference the following:

Coding Updates, Tips, and Links
- GEMS Files
- *ICD-10-CM Official Guidelines for Coding and Reporting*
- *ICD-10-PCS Official Guidelines for Coding and Reporting*
- *ICD-9-CM Official Guidelines for Coding and Reporting*
- 1995 Guidelines for E/M Services
- 1997 Documentation Guidelines for Evaluation and Management Services
- CPT Updates
- ICD-10-CM Updates
- ICD-9-CM Updates
- HCPCS Updates
- Study Tips
- WebLinks

Content Updates – Student

To access the **Online Activities,** go to the *Course Documents* section and click *Assessments.*
To access the **Encoder Exercises,** go to the *Course Documents* section and click on the encoder asset.

Exercise Answers

CHAPTER 1

Exercise 1-1
1. the government
2. 1965
3. A
4. B

Exercise 1-2
1. October
2. November or December
3. Department of Health and Human Services
4. January 2, 2014
5. technical error
6. John Kane

Exercise 1-3
1. Resource-Based Relative Value Scale
2. *Federal Register*
3. OBRA

Exercise 1-4
1. fraud
2. Office of the Inspector General or OIG
3. gatekeeper
4. Program for All-Inclusive Care of the Elderly

CHAPTER 2

Exercise 2-1
1. d
2. c
3. morbidity, mortality
4. clinical modification
5. Any four of the following six (or similar wording):
   a. facilitate payment for health services
   b. evaluate patients' use of health care facilities (utilization patterns)
   c. study health care costs
   d. research the quality of health care
   e. predict health care trends
   f. plan for future health care needs
6. verbal, narrative
7. d

Exercise 2-2
1. c 10. a
2. e 11. e
3. a 12. d
4. b 13. b
5. f 14. c
6. d 15. a
7. c 16. b
8. f 17. a
9. b

Exercise 2-3
1. c 3. b
2. a 4. d

Exercise 2-4
1. e 4. c
2. b 5. a
3. d

CHAPTER 3

Exercise 3-1
1. urinary tract infection
2. Crohn's disease
3. sprained knee
4. COPD or CHF (either could be first-listed)
5. pneumonia

Exercise 3-2
1. **R10.9** (Pain, abdominal); **K92.1** (Blood, in, feces). Either diagnosis could be listed first
2. **K51.90** (Colitis, ulcerative (chronic))
3. **R53.83** (Fatigue); **R17** (Jaundice (yellow)). Either diagnosis could be listed first
4. **B19.20** (Hepatitis C (viral))

Exercise 3-3
1. admission for elective sterilization
2. benign prostatic hypertrophy
3. hematuria

Exercise 3-4

1. **Y92.815** (Place of Occurrence, train)
2. **V48.5XXA** (Accident, transport, car occupant, driver, noncollision accident [traffic])
3. **V86.59XA** (Accident, transport, all-terrain vehicle occupant, driver)
4. **V80.790A** (Accident, transport, animal-rider, collision with, non-motor vehicle)
5. **V91.89XA** (Accident, watercraft, causing, injury NEC)

Exercise 3-5

1. Contact, smallpox (laboratory); **Z20.89**
2. Immunization, encounter for; **Z23**
3. History, personal, malignant neoplasm (of), oral cavity, specified site; **Z85.818**
4. **Z45.018** (Admission for, adjustment (of), device, implanted, cardiac, pacemaker)
5. **Z30.019** (Contraception, initial prescription, subdermal implantable)
6. **Z85.46** (History, personal, malignant neoplasm [of], prostate)
7. **Z23** (Immunization, encounter for)
8. **Z12.31** (Mammogram, routine)
9. **Z02.1** (Encounter, administrative purposes only, examination for, employment)

Exercise 3-6

1. a. **Z04.1**; b. **S40.811A**
2. **Z04.41**
3. Pelvic pain
4. Biliary duct stricture
5. Post-menopausal bleeding

Exercise 3-7

1. Palpitations **R00.2**, Arthritis, rheumatoid, **M06.9**
2. Memory loss **R41.3,** diabetes mellitus, type II **E11.9,** long-term (current) use of insulin **Z79.4**
3. Urinary tract infection **N39.0**, psoriasis **L40.9**

Exercise 3-8

1. Pain, joint, knee **M25.561**, Stiffness, knee **M25.661**. Osteoarthritis is not reported because it has not been confirmed and is a "rule out" diagnosis.
2. Pain, wrist **M25.532**, numbness **R20.0**. Carpal tunnel syndrome is not reported because the condition has not been confirmed, rather it is a "probable" condition.
3. Amenorrhea **N91.2,** Galactorrhea not associated with childbirth, **N64.3**. Pituitary tumor is not coded because it has not been confirmed.
4. Breast lump **N63**. Breast cancer is not reported because the condition has not been confirmed.

Exercise 3-9

1. **J44.0** (Bronchitis, acute or subacute, with, chronic obstructive pulmonary disease), **F17.210** (Dependence, nicotine, cigarettes)

2. **J44.9** (Disease, airway, obstructive, chronic), **F17.210** (Dependence, nicotine, cigarettes)

Exercise 3-10

1. **Z01.83** (Encounter, blood typing)
2. **Z00.00** (Examination, annual)

Exercise 3-11

1. **Z51.11** (Chemotherapy, neoplasm); **C56.2** (Table of Neoplasms, Neoplasm, ovary, Malignant Primary)
2. **D52.0** (Anemia, deficiency, folate, dietary)
3. **Z01.82** (Examination, allergy)

Exercise 3-12

1. a
2. b
3. c

CHAPTER 4

Exercise 4-1

1. **K46.9, K40.90, K40.3, K40.31**
2. **I10**

Exercise 4-2

1. Abdominal pain, nausea and sometimes vomiting, loss of appetite, low-grade fever, constipation, diarrhea, inability to pass gas, abdominal swelling (any two of these)
2. chest pain
3. False
4. False
5. chest pain, shortness of breath
6. hip pain, contusion of hip

Exercise 4-3

1. **N41.1** (Prostatitis, chronic); **B95.5** (Infection, bacterial, as cause of disease classified elsewhere, Streptococcus) [in this order]
2. **J20.8** (Bronchitis, due to, specified organism NEC); **B96.5** (Infection, bacterial, as cause of disease classified elsewhere, Pseudomonas) [in this order]
3. **E10.52** (Diabetes, Type 1, with, gangrene). It would be incorrect to report E10.59 and I96 when a combination code is available.
4. **N39.0** (Infection, urinary [tract]); **B96.20** (Infection, bacterial, as cause of disease classified elsewhere, Escherichia coli) [in this order]
5. **E85.4** (Cardiomyopathy, amyloid); **I43** (Cardiomyopathy, amyloid). When referencing Cardiomyopathy as the main term and amyloid as the subterm in the Index of the I-10, the coder is directed to report I43 by the placement of I43 in brackets following E85.4. The codes must also be reported in the order directed in the Index—code E85.4 is reported first followed by I43.

Exercise 4-4

1. **J14** (Pneumonia, Hemophilus influenzae)
2. **B37.0** (Candidiasis, mouth)
3. **A04.7** (Enteritis, Clostridium, difficile)
4. **A02.0** (Gastroenteritis, Salmonella)

Exercise 4-5

1. Residual: scars, face
   Cause: third-degree burns
2. Residual: constrictive pericarditis
   Cause: tuberculosis infection
3. Residual: foreign body, femur
   Cause: gunshot injury, femur
4. Residual: intellectual disabilities
   Cause: poliomyelitis
5. Residual: leg pain
   Cause: fracture, femur
6. Residual: arthritis
   Cause: pathological fracture
   Code: **M12.851** (Arthropathy, specified, hip); **M84.451S** (Fracture, pathologic, femur)
7. Residual: sensorineural deafness
   Cause: meningitis
   Codes: **H90.5** (Deafness, sensorineural); **G09** (Sequela [of], meningitis, other or unspecified cause)

CHAPTER 5

Exercise 5-1

1. **A08.4** (Gastroenteritis, viral NEC)
2. **A41.52** (Sepsis, Gram-negative[organism]); **R65.21** (Shock, septic [due to severe sepsis])
3. **A80.9** (Poliomyelitis)

Exercise 5-2

1. **B37.3** (Candidiasis, vagina)
2. **B01.12** (Myelitis, postchickenpox)
3. **B34.3** (Infection, parvovirus NEC)
4. **B37.0** (Thrush, oral)
5. **B85.1** (Infestation, Pediculus, body)

Exercise 5-3

1. **Z51.11** (Chemotherapy, [session] [for], cancer); **C56.9** (Neoplasm, ovary, Malignant Primary)
2. **Z51.0** (Admission [for], radiation therapy [antineoplastic]); **C79.51** (Neoplasm, bone, Malignant Secondary); **Z85.3** (History, personal [of], malignant neoplasm, breast)
3. a. metastatic carcinoma of bronchus
   b. primary, unknown
   c. secondary
   d. **C78.00** (Neoplasm, bronchus, Malignant Secondary); **C80.1** (Neoplasm, unknown site or unspecified, Malignant Primary)
4. a. Three
   b. Nausea with vomiting; **R11.2** (Nausea, with vomiting)

c. Adverse affect code; **T88.7XXA** (Complication(s), chemotherapy NEC)
d. Lung cancer; **C34.90** (Neoplasm, lung, unspecified site, Malignant Primary)
5. **C16.9** (Neoplasm, stomach, Malignant Primary), **D63.0** (Anemia, in neoplastic disease)

Exercise 5-4

1. **C90.00** (Myeloma, [multiple])
2. **D06.9** (Neoplasm, cervix, Ca in situ)
3. **C18.7** (Neoplasm, intestine, intestinal, large, colon, sigmoid, Malignant Primary); **C78.6** (Neoplasm, peritoneum [cavity], Malignant Secondary)
4. **C61** (Neoplasm, prostate [gland], Malignant Primary); **C79.51** (Neoplasm, bone, Malignant Secondary)
5. **C79.31** (Neoplasm, brain NEC, Malignant Secondary); **C80.1** (Neoplasm, unknown site or unspecified, Malignant Primary)
6. **C78.00** (Neoplasm, lung, unspecified site, Malignant Secondary); **Z85.3** (History, personal (of), malignant neoplasm (of), breast). Note: This is personal history, not family history, Z80.3
7. **Z51.11** (Encounter, chemotherapy, for neoplasm); **C18.7** (Neoplasm, intestine, large, colon, sigmoid, Malignant Primary)

Exercise 5-5

1. **D51.0** (Anemia, pernicious)
2. **D65** (Afibrinogenemia, acquired)
3. **D66** (Hemophilia, A)
4. **D62** (Anemia, blood loss, acute)
5. **D75.0** (Polycythemia, benign [familial])

Exercise 5-6

1. **E27.1** (Addison's, disease [bronze] or syndrome)
2. **E86.0** (Dehydration)
3. **E11.641** (Diabetes, type 2, with, hypoglycemia, with coma)
4. **E05.01** (Hyperthyroidism, with goiter [diffuse], with thyroid storm)
5. **E10.59** (Diabetes, type 1, with circulatory complication NEC); **E10.621** (Diabetes, type I, with foot ulcer); **L97.509** (Ulcer, lower limb, foot specified NEC); **E11.65** (Diabetes, diabetic, with, hyperglycemia)
6. **E46** (Malnutrition)

Exercise 5-7

1. **G30.9** (Disease, Alzheimer's); **F02.81** (Disease, Alzheimer's, with behavioral disturbance) [in this order]
2. **F41.8** (Depression, anxiety)
3. **F73** (Disability, intellectual, profound [IQ under 20])
4. **F50.00** (Anorexia, nervosa)
5. **F10.231** (Dependence [on], alcohol, with, withdrawal, with, delirium)
6. **F11.23** (Dependence, drug, opioid, with, withdrawal)

Exercise 5-8

1. **G00.8** (Meningitis, bacterial, specified organism NEC); **B96.4** (Infection, bacterial NOS, as cause of disease classified elsewhere, Proteus [mirabilis] [morganii])
2. **G35** (Sclerosis, multiple)
3. **G51.0** (Palsy, facial)
4. **G40.901** (Seizure, febrile, complex, with status epilepticus)

Exercise 5-9

1. **H40.11X0** (Glaucoma, open angle, primary)
2. **H04.571** (Stenosis, lacrimal, sac)

Exercise 5-10

1. **H66.91** (Otitis, media, acute)
2. **H60.332** (Swimmer's ear)
3. **H65.03** (Otitis, media, nonsuppurative, acute or subacute, serous)

Exercise 5-11

1. **I50.9** (Failure, heart, congestive)
2. **I21.4** (Infarction, subendocardial)
3. **M30.0** (Periarteritis nodosa); **I15.8** (Hypertension, secondary, specified NEC)
4. **I63.30** (Infarct, cerebral, due to, thrombosis, cerebral artery)
5. **I60.9** (Hemorrhage, intracranial [nontraumatic], subarachnoid)
6. **N17.9** (Failure, kidney, acute); **I10** (Hypertension)

Exercise 5-12

1. **J05.0** (Croup)
2. **I50.9** (Failure, heart, congestive); **J96.90** (Failure, respiratory)
3. **J44.9** (Disease, lung, obstructive [chronic], with, bronchitis)
4. **J11.1** (Influenza, with, respiratory manifestations NEC)
5. **J14** (Pneumonia, due to, Hemophilus influenzae)
6. **J44.9** (Disease, lung, obstructive, with emphysema)
7. **J69.0** (Pneumonia, aspiration)

CHAPTER 6

Exercise 6-1

1. **K35.2** (Appendicitis, with, peritonitis, generalized)
2. **K26.0** (Ulcer, duodenum, acute, with, hemorrhage)
3. **K80.12** (Calculus, gallbladder, with, cholecystitis, acute, with, chronic cholecystitis)
4. **K52.9** (Gastroenteritis)
5. **K21.9** (Reflux, gastroesophageal)

Exercise 6-2

1. **L29.2** (Pruritus, vulva, vulvae)
2. **L74.0** (Rash, heat)
3. **L40.1** (Psoriasis, pustular [generalized])
4. **L89.309** (Ulcer, pressure, buttock)
5. **L23.7** (Dermatitis, contact, allergic, due to, plants, non-food)
6. **L03.039** (Cellulitis, toe)
7. **L05.01** (Cyst, pilonidal, with abscess)

Exercise 6-3

1. **M06.9** (Arthritis, rheumatoid)
2. **M54.2** (Pain, neck NEC)
3. **M24.411** (Dislocation, recurrent, shoulder)
4. **M84.522A** (Fracture, pathological, due to, neoplastic disease, humerus); **C79.51** (Neoplasm, bone, Malignant Secondary); **Z85.3** (History, personal (of), malignant neoplasm, breast)

CHAPTER 7

Exercise 7-1

1. **O02.0** (Blighted ovum)
2. **O03.4** (Abortion, incomplete [spontaneous])
3. **O47.1** (False, labor [pains], at or after 37 completed weeks of gestation)
4. **O70.3** (Laceration, perineum, female, during delivery, fourth degree); **Z37.0** (Outcome of delivery, single NEC, liveborn)
5. **O65.4** (Delivery, complicated by, obstructed labor, due to, fetopelvic disproportion); **Z37.0** (Outcome of delivery, single NEC, liveborn)

Exercise 7-2

1. **Q17.8** (Absence [of], ear, congenital, lobe)
2. **Z38.00** (Newborn [infant] [liveborn] [singleton], born in hospital); **Q53.20** (Cryptorchid, bilateral)
3. **Q99.2** (Syndrome, fragile X)
4. **Q65.01** (Dislocation, hip, congenital, unilateral)

Exercise 7-3

1. **R68.12** (Fussy baby)
2. **R07.1** (Pain[s], chest, on breathing)
3. **R92.8** (Abnormal, mammogram NEC)
4. **R87.619** (Abnormal, Papanicolaou (smear), cervix)
5. **R03.0** (Blood, pressure, high, incidental reading, without diagnosis of hypertension)
6. **R10.9** (Pain[s], abdominal); **R50.9** (Fever); **R30.0** (Dysuria). Urosepsis is not coded because it was ruled out.
7. **R07.9** (Pain[s], chest); **R10.13** (Pain[s], epigastric). Myocardial infarction would not be reported as it is being "ruled out."

Exercise 7-4

1. **T21.32XA** (Burn, abdomen, third degree); **T24.219A** (Burn, thigh, second degree); **T31.11**—15% with 10% third degree (Burn, extent); **X12.XXXA** (External Cause Index: Burning, hot, fluid)
2. **T24.312D** (Burn, thigh, left, third degree); **B99.9** (Infection); **T31.0**—4½% (Burn, extent) (No X code is required for subsequent treatment.)
3. **T25.221A** (Burn, foot, right, second degree) (Note that only the highest-level burn is coded when burns are in the same area.); **T31.0**—2¼% (Burn, extent); **X03.0XXA** (External Cause Index: Fire, controlled, not in building or structure) Note when referencing Exposure, bonfire,

the External Cause Index directs the coder to reference Exposure, fire, controlled, not in building.

4. **T23.301D** (Burn, hand, right, third degree); **T31.0**—2¼% (Burn, extent) (No X code is required for subsequent treatment.)
5. **T21.31XD** (Burn, chest wall, third degree); **T22.211D** (Burn, forearm, second degree); **T23.101D** (Burn, hand, right, first degree); **T31.10**—11% (Burn, extent) with 0-9% third degree [in this order] (No X code is required for subsequent treatment.)

Exercise 7-5
1. **T51.0X4D** (Alcohol, ethyl, Poisoning, Undetermined)
2. **T60.3X1D** (Herbicide NEC, Poisoning, Accidental)
3. **T42.4X1A** (Valium, Poisoning, Accidental)

Exercise 7-6
1. **S72.92XM** (Fracture, traumatic, femur); **D62** (Anemia, post-hemorrhagic, acute)

Exercise 7-7
1. **T85.79XA** (Complications, breast implants, infection or inflammation)
2. **T86.01** (Rejection, transplant, bone, marrow)
3. **T81.4XXD** (Abscess, operative wound); **B99.9** (Infection, infected, infective [opportunistic])
4. **T82.118D** (Complications, cardiovascular device, graft, or implant, electronic, mechanical, breakdown)

CHAPTER 8

Exercise 8-1
1. morbidity or sickness (also acceptable for morbidity is mortality or death rate)
2. ICD-9
3. Clinical Modification
4. Any four of the following six (or similar wording):
   a. facilitate payment for health services
   b. evaluate patients' use of health care facilities (utilization patterns)
   c. study health care costs
   d. research the quality of health care
   e. predict health care trends
   f. plan for future health care needs
5. verbal, narrative

Exercise 8-2
1. Endocrine, Nutritional and Metabolic Diseases, and Immunity Disorders (240-279)
2. Disorders of Thyroid Gland (240-246)
3. 240 Simple and unspecified goiter
4. 240.0 Goiter, specified as simple

Exercise 8-3
1. **711.06**
2. No
3. By adding fourth and fifth digits to the codes

Exercise 8-4
1. a. Appendix B
   b. Appendix D
   c. Appendix A
   d. Appendix E
   e. Appendix C
2. Appendix D: Industrial Accidents

Exercise 8-5
1. Normocytic anemia
2. Acute prostatitis
3. Severe protein calorie malnutrition
4. Granuloma lung
5. Pain in neck

Exercise 8-6
1. essential
2. nonessential
3. essential
4. nonessential
5. nonessential

Exercise 8-7
1. No, 205.10 per Excludes note and remember to assign the fifth digit
2. Yes
3. No, 754.51, which specifically describes congenital talipes equinovarus
4. Yes
5. No. Per Excludes note see category 532

Exercise 8-8
1. No answer required
2. a. **710.0** *[424.91]*
   b. **710.0**
   c. Diffuse diseases of connective tissue
   d. all collagen diseases whose effects are not mainly confined to a single system
   e. **424.91**
   f. **710.0**
   g. **710.0, 424.91**

Exercise 8-9
1. *see* Human immunodeficiency virus
2. No cross-reference is listed
3. *see also* Pruritus
4. *see also* Adenitis
5. *see* condition

Exercise 8-10
1. **331.11, 294.11**
2. **117.3, 484.6**
3. **440.23, 707.13**
4. **600.01, 788.20**
5. **695.10, 713.3**

Exercise 8-11

1. f
2. b
3. c
4. d
5. a
6. e
7. g

Exercise 8-12

1. f
2. g
3. a
4. h
5. k
6. i
7. e
8. d
9. j
10. b
11. c
12. false
13. true

Exercise 8-13

1. Obstetrical Procedures
2. Miscellaneous Diagnostic and Therapeutic Procedures
3. Procedures and Interventions, Not Elsewhere Classified

Exercise 8-14

1. referring to vena cava
2. pertaining to the lungs or pulmonary artery
3. joining together of two openings
4. pertaining to the heart and lungs
5. circulation that occurs outside of the body
6. a surgical procedure that joins the superior vena cava and pulmonary artery
7. manages the heart and lung functions of a patient during a surgical procedure

Exercise 8-15

1. **45.24** (Sigmoidoscopy flexible)
2. **63.73** (Vasectomy)
3. **76.73** (Reduction, fracture, maxilla)
4. **99.04** (Transfusion, packed cells)
5. **21.03** (Cauterization, nose, for epistaxis (with packing))

CHAPTER 9

Exercise 9-1

1. Urinary tract infection
2. Crohn's disease
3. Sprain knee
4. COPD and CHF (either could be first-listed)
5. Pneumonia

Exercise 9-2

1. **789.00** (Pain, abdominal, unspecified), **787.91** (Diarrhea) Either diagnosis could be listed first
2. **556.9** (Colitis, ulcerative, unspecified)
3. **780.79** (Fatigue), **782.4** (Jaundice, unspecified) Either diagnosis could be listed first
4. **070.70** (Hepatitis C, unspecified)

Exercise 9-3

1. Admission for elective sterilization
2. Benign prostatic hypertrophy
3. Hematuria

Exercise 9-4

1. Pelvic pain
2. Biliary duct stricture
3. Post-menopausal bleeding

Exercise 9-5

1. Contact, smallpox; **V01.3**
2. Vaccination, prophylactic, smallpox; **V04.1**
3. History, malignant neoplasm, tongue; **V10.01**
4. **V53.31** (Cardiac, device, pacemaker, cardiac, fitting or adjustment)
5. **V25.5** (Insertion, subdermal implantable contraceptive)
6. **V10.46** (History (personal), malignant neoplasm, prostate)
7. **V06.4** (Vaccination, mumps, with measles and rubella [MMR])
8. **V76.12** (Screening, mammogram)
9. **V70.5** (Examination, medical, pre-employment)

Exercise 9-6

1. a. **V71.4**
   b. **913.0**
2. **V71.5** (Rape)

Exercise 9-7

1. Palpitations **785.1** (Palpitations), rheumatoid arthritis **714.0** (Arthritis, arthritic, rheumatoid)
2. Memory loss **780.93** (Memory disturbance, loss or lack), diabetes mellitus, type II **250.00** (Diabetes, diabetic [mellitus])
3. Urinary tract infection **599.0** (Infection, urinary [tract] NEC), psoriasis **696.1** (Psoriasis)

Exercise 9-8

1. Pain, knee **719.46** (Pain, joint, knee), Stiffness, knee **719.56** (Stiffness, joint, knee). Osteoarthritis is not coded because it has not been confirmed.
2. Pain, wrist **719.43** (Pain, joint, wrist), numbness **782.0** (Numbness). Carpal tunnel syndrome is not coded because it has not been confirmed.
3. Amenorrhea **626.0** (Amenorrhea [primary] [secondary]), galactorrhea **611.6** (Galactorrhea, not associated with child birth). Pituitary tumor is not coded because it has not been confirmed.
4. Breast lump **611.72** (Breast, lump). Breast cancer is not coded because it has not been confirmed.

Exercise 9-9

1. a, c (asthma, systemic lupus erythematous)
2. e, f, d, l (diabetes, atherosclerosis, status post op CABG, insulin use)

3. i, j (contact dermatitis, colostomy)
4. k (eye exam)
5. b, g, h (follow-up vaginal pap smear, status post hysterectomy for malignant condition, acquired absence of both cervix and uterus, personal history of primary malignancy of cervix uteri)

CHAPTER 10

Exercise 10-1

1. category code, subcategory code, subclassification code
2. category code, subcategory code, subclassification code

Exercise 10-2

1. Abdominal pain, nausea and sometimes vomiting, loss of appetite, low-grade fever, constipation, diarrhea, inability to pass gas, abdominal swelling (any two of these)
2. chest pain
3. False
4. False
5. chest pain, shortness of breath
6. hip pain, contusion of hip

Exercise 10-3

1. **601.1** (Prostatitis, chronic); **041.00** (Infection, streptococcal) [in this order]
2. **466.0** (Bronchitis, with acute or subacute); **041.7** (Infection, *Pseudomonas* NEC) [in this order]
3. **250.71** (Diabetes, with gangrene); **785.4** (Gangrene) [in this order]
4. **599.0** (Infection, urinary [tract] NEC); **041.49** (Infection, *Escherichia coli* (E. coli)) [in this order]
5. **277.39** (Cardiomyopathy, amyloid); **425.7** (Cardiomyopathy, metabolic NEC, amyloid)

Exercise 10-4

1. **482.2** (Pneumonia, due to, *Haemophilus influenzae*)
2. **112.0** (Thrush)
3. **008.45** (Enteritis, *Clostridium difficile*)
4. **003.0** (Gastroenteritis, *salmonella*)
5. **823.82** (Fracture, tibia (closed), with fibula)

Exercise 10-5

1. Residual: scars, face
   Cause: third-degree burns
2. Residual: constrictive pericarditis
   Cause: tuberculosis infection
3. Residual: foreign body, femur
   Cause: gunshot injury, femur
4. Residual: intellectual disabilities
   Cause: poliomyelitis
5. Residual: leg pain
   Cause: fracture, femur

Exercise 10-6

1. Residual: arthritis, ankle, traumatic
   Code: **716.17** (Arthritis, traumatic)
   Cause: fracture, ankle
   Code: **905.4** (Late effect, fracture, extremity, lower)
2. Residual: dysphasia
   Code: There is no code for the residual because there is one combination code that reports both the residual and the cause.
   Cause: cerebrovascular accident
   Code: **438.12** (Late effect, cerebrovascular disease with dysphasia)
3. Residual: deafness, sensorineural
   Code: **389.10** (Deafness, sensorineural)
   Cause: meningitis
   Code: **326** (Late effect, meningitis, unspecified cause)

Exercise 10-7

1. **434.91** (Stroke, in evolution)
2. **291.0** (Impending, delirium tremens)
3. **640.00** (Threatened, miscarriage, unspecified)
4. **644.10** (Labor, threatened unspecified)
5. **411.1** (Impending, coronary, syndrome)

CHAPTER 11

Exercise 11-1

1. **008.8** (Gastroenteritis, viral NEC)
2. **038.43** (Septicemia, *Pseudomonas*); **995.92** (Sepsis, severe); **785.52** (Septic, shock)
3. **045.90** (Poliomyelitis, unspecified type)
4. **112.1** (Candidiasis, vagina)

Exercise 11-2

1. i
2. c
3. h
4. g
5. a
6. b
7. e
8. f
9. d

Exercise 11-3

1. **V58.11** (Chemotherapy, encounter for); **183.0** (Neoplasm, ovary, primary)
2. **V58.0** (Admission, radiation management); **198.5** (Neoplasm, bone, secondary); **V10.3** (History, malignant neoplasm, breast)
3. a. metastatic carcinoma of bronchus
   b. primary, unknown
   c. secondary
   d. **197.0** (Neoplasm, lung, main bronchus, secondary); **199.1** (Neoplasm, unknown site or unspecified, primary)
4. a. Two
   b. Uncontrolled nausea and vomiting
   c. Lung cancer
   d. **787.01** (Nausea, with vomiting)

e. **162.9** (Neoplasm, lung, Malignant, Primary); **E933.1** (Table of Drugs and Chemicals, Antineoplastic Agents, Therapeutic Use)

Exercise 11-4

1. **203.00** (Myeloma, multiple)
2. **233.1** (Neoplasm, cervix, Malignant, Ca in situ)
3. **153.3** (Neoplasm, intestinal, colon, sigmoid, Malignant, Primary); **197.6** (Neoplasm, peritoneum, secondary)
4. **185** (Neoplasm, prostate, Malignant, Primary); **198.5** (Neoplasm, bone, Malignant, Secondary)
5. **198.3** (Neoplasm, brain, Malignant, Secondary); **199.1** (Neoplasm, unknown, Malignant, Primary)
6. **197.0** (Neoplasm, lung, Malignant, Secondary); **V10.3** (History (of), malignant neoplasm (of), breast). Note: This is personal history, not family history, V16.3.

Exercise 11-5

1. **255.41** (Disease, Addison's)
2. **276.51** (Dehydration)
3. **250.30** (Diabetes, coma, hypoglycemic)
4. **242.01** (Goiter, toxic, with mention of thyrotoxic crisis or storm)

Exercise 11-6

1. **281.0** (Anemia, pernicious)
2. **286.6** (Coagulation, intravascular)
3. **286.0** (Hemophilia)
4. **285.1** (Anemia, blood loss, acute)
5. **289.6** (Polycythemia, familial)

Exercise 11-7

1. **331.0** (Alzheimer's, disease or sclerosis); **294.11** (Alzheimer's, dementia, with behavior disturbance) [in this order]
2. **300.4** (Depression, anxiety)
3. **318.2** (Disabilities, intellectual, profound, IQ under 20)
4. **307.1** (Anorexia, nervosa)
5. **291.0** (Delirium, withdrawal, alcoholic, acute); **303.91** (Dependence, alcohol, alcoholic)

Exercise 11-8

1. **320.82** (Meningitis, *Proteus morganii*)
2. **340** (Sclerosis, multiple)
3. **382.9** (Otitis, media, acute)
4. **365.11** (Glaucoma, chronic, open angle); **365.72** (Glaucoma, stage, moderate)
5. **351.0** (Palsy, Bell's)

Exercise 11-9

1. **428.0** (Failure, heart, congestive)
2. **410.71** (Infarction, subendocardial)
3. **446.0** (Periarteritis); **405.99** (Hypertension, due to, periarteritis nodosa)
4. **434.01** (Infarction, brain, thrombotic)
5. **430** (Hemorrhage, subarachnoid)

Exercise 11-10

1. **464.4** (Croup)
2. **518.81** (Respiratory, failure); **428.0** (Disease, heart, congestive)
3. **491.20** (Disease, lung, obstructive with, bronchitis)
4. **487.1** (Influenza, with, bronchitis)
5. **482.2** (Pneumonia, due to, Hemophilus influenzae)

CHAPTER 12

Exercise 12-1

1. **540.0** (Appendicitis, with perforation, peritonitis or rupture)
2. **532.00** (Ulcer, duodenum, acute, with hemorrhage)
3. **574.00** (Cholelithiasis, with cholecystitis, acute); **574.10** (Cholelithiasis, with cholecystitis, chronic). Note acute before chronic.
4. **558.9** (Gastroenteritis)
5. **530.81** (Reflux, gastroesophageal)

Exercise 12-2

1. **614.9** (Disease, pelvis, inflammatory)
2. **599.70** (Hematuria)
3. **590.10** (Pyelonephritis, acute); **590.00** (Pyelonephritis, chronic). Note acute before chronic.
4. **600.00** (Hypertrophy, prostate, benign)
5. **610.1** (Disease, breast, fibrocystic)

Exercise 12-3

1. **631.8** (Blighted ovum)
2. **634.91** (Abortion, spontaneous)
3. **644.13** (Labor, false)
4. **664.31** (Laceration, perineum, complicating delivery, fourth degree); **V27.0** (Outcome of delivery, single, liveborn)
5. **660.11** (Delivery, complicated [by], cephalopelvic disproportion [normally formed fetus], causing obstructed labor), **653.41** (Fetopelvic, disproportion); **V27.0** (Outcome of delivery, single, liveborn)

Exercise 12-4

1. **698.9** (Pruritus)
2. **705.1** (Rash, heat)
3. **696.1** (Psoriasis)
4. **707.05** (Ulcer, decubitus buttock); **707.20** (Ulcer, pressure, unspecified [healing])
5. **692.6** (Dermatitis, due to, poison ivy)

Exercise 12-5

1. **714.0** (Arthritis, rheumatoid)
2. **723.1** (Pain, neck)
3. **718.31** (Dislocation, shoulder, recurrent)
4. **733.11** (Fracture, pathologic, humerus); **198.5** (Neoplasm, bone, secondary); **V10.3** (History (of), malignant neoplasm, breast)

Exercise 12-6

1. **744.21** (Absence, ear, lobe)
2. **V30.00** (Newborn, single, born in hospital, without mention of cesarean delivery or section); **752.51** (Undescended, testis)
3. **759.83** (Syndrome, fragile X)
4. **754.30** (Dislocation, hip, congenital)

Exercise 12-7

1. **780.91** (Fussy infant)
2. **786.52** (Pain, chest, wall)
3. **793.80** (Abnormal, mammogram)
4. **780.39** (Seizures)
5. **796.2** (Blood, pressure, high, incidental reading, without diagnosis of hypertension)

Exercise 12-8

1. Derailment, railway; **E802.0**
2. Accident, motor vehicle, not involving collision; **E816.0**
3. Collision, off-road vehicle and other object, fixed; **E821.0**
4. Collision, animal being ridden; **E828.2**
5. Collision, watercraft, causing, injury; **E831.1**

Exercise 12-9

1. **980.0** (Alcohol, grain, beverage, Poisoning), **E980.9** (Poisoning, Alcohol, grain, beverage, Undetermined)
2. **989.89** (Antifreeze, Poisoning), **E980.9** (Poisoning, antifreeze, Undetermined)
3. **969.4** (Valium, Poisoning), **E853.2** (Poisoning, Valium, Accidental)
4. Due to drugs and medicines

Exercise 12-10

1. **942.33** (Burn, abdomen, third degree); **945.26** (Burn, thigh, second degree); **E924.0** (Burning, hot, liquid); **948.11**—15% with 10% third degree (Burn, extent)
2. **945.36** (Burn, thigh, third degree); **958.3** (Burn, infected); **948.00**—4½% (Burn, extent) (No E code is required for subsequent treatment.)
3. **945.22** (Burn, foot, second degree) (Note that only the highest-level burn is coded when burns are in the same area.); **948.00**—2¼% (Burn, extent); **E897** (Fire, controlled, bonfire)
4. **944.30** (Burn, hand, third degree); **948.00**—2¼% (Burn, extent) (No E code is required for subsequent treatment.)
5. **942.32** (Burn, chest wall, third degree); **943.21** (Burn, forearm, second degree); **944.10** (Burn, hand, first degree); **948.10**—11% (Burn, extent) [in this order] (No E code is required for subsequent treatment.)

Exercise 12-11

1. **996.69** (Complications, breast implants, infection or inflammation)
2. **996.85** (Rejection, transplant, bone marrow)
3. **998.59** (Complications, surgical procedure, stitch abscess)
4. **996.01** (Complications, mechanical, device NEC, cardiac)

CHAPTER 13

Exercise 13-1

1. American Medical Association or AMA
2. Current Procedural Terminology
3. services
4. 1966
5. 1983

Exercise 13-2

1. c
2. a
3. g
4. b
5. d
6. e
7. f
8. Appendix B
9. Appendix E
10. Appendix D

Exercise 13-3

1. Surgery
2. Respiratory System
3. Nose
4. Excision

Exercise 13-4

1. A concise statement describing the symptom, problem, condition, diagnosis, or other factor that is the reason for the encounter, usually stated in the patient's words
2. different
3. interpreting physician
4. a physician
5. 99070

Exercise 13-5

1. those codes that have full description (or similar wording)
2. those codes that include their own description as well as that portion of the stand-alone code description found before the semicolon in a preceding code (or similar wording)
3. alternative anatomic site, alternative procedure, or description of the extent of service (in any order and similar wording)

Exercise 13-6

1. -62
2. 43820-62
3. -50
4. -78
5. -57
6. -51
7. -66
8. -80

Exercise 13-7

1. 69799, 29999, 43499
2. 88299, 81099, 84999
3. 99199
4. 77799, 78999

Exercise 13-8
1. 49900
2. 27303
3. 27786-27814

Exercise 13-9
1. a. Emergency
   b. 99288 (Emergency Department Services, Physician Direction of Advanced Life Support)
2. a. Fracture
   b. 27238 (Fracture, Femur, Intertrochanteric, Closed Treatment)
3. a. Gallbladder
   b. 47480 (Calculus, Removal, Biliary Tract)
4. a. Lung
   b. 32141 (Bulla, Lung, Resection)

Exercise 13-10
1. *See* Dialysis
2. *See* Antinuclear Antibodies (ANA)
3. *See* Radius; Ulna; Wrist

Exercise 13-11
1. into the subarachnoid space
2. into a vein
3. into a muscle
4. under the skin
5. through the respiratory system

Exercise 13-12
1. a. Current Procedural Terminology or CPT, Level I
   b. National Codes, Level II
2. K, G, Q, S (in any order)
3. No
4. J codes
5. oral
6. E codes
7. a. -NU
   b. -E2
   c. -AM
8. IM
9. up to 5 mg
10. J1730
11. A4918

CHAPTER 14

Exercise 14-1
1. 57270-22
2. 54535-22
   ICD-10-CM: **C62.12** (Neoplasm, testis, testes, descended, Malignant Primary), **N99.61** (Complications, intraoperative, hemorrhage, genitourinary organ or structure, during procedure on genitourinary organ or structure)
   ICD-9-CM: **186.9** (Neoplasm, testis, testes, Malignant, Primary), **998.11** (Complications, hemorrhage)

3. -23
   ICD-10-CM: **K92.0** (Hematemesis); **G30.9** (Disease, Alzheimer's), **G30.9 [F02.81]** (Disease, Alzheimer's, with behavioral disturbance)
   ICD-9-CM: **578.0** (Hematemesis), **331.0, 294.11** (Alzheimer's, dementia, with behavioral disturbance) Suspected peptic ulcer is not reported since it has not been confirmed.
4. -24
   ICD-10-CM: **G30.9, F02.80** (Disease, Alzheimer's)
   ICD-9-CM: **331.0, 294.10** (Alzheimer's, dementia (senile), without behavioral disturbance)
5. -25
6. -26

Exercise 14-2
1. -32
   ICD-10-CM: **Z02.6** (Encounter, administrative purpose only, examination for, insurance)
   ICD-9-CM: **V70.3** (Examination, medical, insurance certification)
2. -47
3. -50
   ICD-10-CM: **G56.01** (Syndrome, carpal tunnel), **G56.02** (Syndrome, carpal tunnel)
   ICD-9-CM: **354.0** (Carpal tunnel syndrome)
4. 17274 and 17264-51
   ICD-10-CM: **C44.00** (Neoplasm, skin, neck, Malignant Primary); **C44.601** (Neoplasm, skin, limb, upper Malignant Primary)
   ICD-9-CM: **173.40** (Neoplasm, neck, skin, Malignant, Primary), **173.60** (Neoplasm, skin, arm, Malignant, Primary)
   (Code 17274 is more resource-intensive and listed first without the modifier.)
5. 61154 and 61154-50 or 61154-50
   ICD-10-CM: **I62.03** (Hemorrhage, intracranial, subdural, chronic)
   ICD-9-CM: **432.1** (Hematoma, subdural)
6. 28450 and 28450-51
7. 27447 and 27447-50 (Arthroplasty, Knee)
8. -52
9. 24006 and 24006-50 or 24006-50 or 24006-RT and 24006-LT
10. 19305 and 19305-50 or 19305-50 and 19305-RT and 19305-LT

Exercise 14-3
1. -58
   ICD-10-CM: **C77.9** (Neoplasm, lymph, gland, Malignant Secondary); **C80.1** (Neoplasm, unknown site, Malignant Primary)
   ICD-9-CM: **196.0** (Neoplasm, lymph, gland, cervical, Malignant, Secondary), **199.1** Neoplasm, unknown site, Malignant, Primary)
2. 43124-54

3. 19306-55
4. 19306-56

Exercise 14-4

1. -62
2. -66
   ICD-10-CM: **B18.2** (Hepatitis, C [viral], chronic);
   K74.60 (Cirrhosis)
   ICD-9-CM: **070.54** (Hepatitis, viral type C, chronic),
   571.5 (Cirrhosis)
3. -80
4. -81
5. -78
6. -79
7. -77

Exercise 14-5

1. -99
2. -90
3. -91

CHAPTER 15

Exercise 15-1

1. office or in an outpatient or other ambulatory facility
2. office visit or other outpatient service
3. new
4. 99201
5. five
6. five

Exercise 15-2

1. problem focused
2. expanded problem focused
3. detailed
4. comprehensive
5. comprehensive

Exercise 15-3

1. problem focused
2. expanded problem focused
3. detailed
4. comprehensive
5. comprehensive

Exercise 15-4

1. OS	11. OS
2. BA	12. OS
3. OS	13. BA
4. OS	14. OS
5. OS	15. OS
6. OS	16. BA
7. OS	17. OS
8. BA	18. OS
9. BA	19. OS
10. BA	20. OS

Note: Some terms—thorax, lungs, heart, vagina, blood vessels, neurologic—are specifically presented in the text as being a body area or an organ system. For other terms, you have to make the connection; for example, the thorax is examined as a body area but the lungs are examined as an organ system.

21. a. expanded problem focused (CC, brief HPI, problem pertinent ROS, and no PFSH required)
    b. expanded problem focused (the constitutional and one organ system, equals 2 for an expanded problem focused examination)

22.

CC:	Cold
HPI:	Quality (dry, hacking)
	Location (nasal)
	Duration (9 days)
	Associated Signs and Symptoms (sleeplessness)
	HPI ELEMENTS (4) = COMPREHENSIVE
PFSH:	Personal
	Family
	PFSH ELEMENTS (2) = COMPREHENSIVE
ROS:	Constitutional (fever, aching)
	Respiratory (coughing)
	ROS ELEMENTS (2) = DETAILED

a. detailed (Level 3)
   General survey: Minor distress
   Vital signs: Temperature, BP, pulse
   CONSTITUTIONAL (no matter how many elements checked off it only counts as 1) = 1
   BODY AREAS: Head = 1
   ORGAN SYSTEMS: Respiratory (mucous membranes, lungs clear to percussion and auscultation), Otolaryngologic (ears, nose) 5 2
b. Expanded Problem Focused
   Detailed history
   EPF Exam

Exercise 15-5

1. limited (Some chart audit forms classify a new problem with no further follow-up planned as multiple.)
2. limited (The data could be moderate if the patient has brought records that the physician would have to review.)
3. moderate
4. low
5. 99203
   ICD-10-CM: **M51.06** (Disorder, disc, with, myelopathy, lumbosacral region)
   ICD-9-CM: **722.73** (Myelopathy, due to or with, intervertebral disc disorder, lumbar, lumbosacral)
6. straightforward or low
   ICD-10-CM: **H65.01** (Otitis, media, nonsuppurative, acute, serous)
   ICD-9-CM: **381.01** (Otitis, media, acute, serous)
7. low (risks are increased for the elderly)
   ICD-10-CM: **J01.90** (Sinusitis, acute)
   ICD-9-CM: **461.9** (Sinusitis)

Exercise 15-6

1. b or c
   ICD-10-CM: **H65.191** (Otitis, media, nonsuppurative, acute or subacute NEC)
   ICD-9-CM: **381.00** (Otitis, media, acute, exudative)
2. d or e
   ICD-10-CM: **J44.1** (Disease, lung, obstructive, with, acute, exacerbation NEC), **Z99.81** (Dependence, on, oxygen)
   ICD-9-CM: **491.21** (Disease, lung, obstructive, with, acute, exacerbation NEC), **V46.2** (Dependence, on, supplemental oxygen)
3. e
   ICD-10-CM: **R06.02** (Shortness, breath), **I42.0** (Cardiomyopathy, congestive)
   ICD-9-CM: **786.05** (Short, breath); **425.4** (Cardiomyopathy, congestive)
4. c
   ICD-10-CM: **S63.602A** (Sprain, thumb), **V00.138A** (External Cause Index, Accident, transport, pedestrian, conveyance occupant, skateboard), **Y93.51** (External Cause Index, Activity, skateboarding)
   ICD-9-CM: **842.10** (Sprain, thumb), **E885.2** (Index to External Causes, Fall, from, off, skateboard), **E006.0** (Index to External Causes, Activity, skateboarding)
5. a
   ICD-10-CM: **I10** (Hypertension, hypertensive)
   ICD-9-CM: **401.0** (Hypertension, Malignant)
6. b
   ICD-10-CM: **J30.1** (Allergy, grass [pollen])
   ICD-9-CM: **477.0** (Allergy, grass [pollen])

Exercise 15-7

1. detailed, detailed, low
2. comprehensive, comprehensive, moderate
3. comprehensive, comprehensive, high
4. 99203 (Office and/or Other Outpatient Services, Office Visit, New Patient)
   ICD-10-CM: **Z30.09** (Counseling, contraceptive)
   ICD-9-CM: **V25.09** (Counseling, contraceptive management)
5. 99201 (Office and/or Other Outpatient Services, Office Visit, New Patient)
   ICD-10-CM: **Z48.02** (Suture, removal)
   ICD-9-CM: **V58.32** (Suture, removal)
6. 99205 (Office and/or Other Outpatient Services, Office Visit, New Patient)
   ICD-10-CM: **F32.9** (Depression), **R45.851** (Ideation, suicidal), **G47.00** (Insomnia), **F17.210** (Dependence, drug, nicotine, cigarettes)
   ICD-9-CM: **311** (Depression), **V62.84** (Ideation, suicidal), **780.52** (Sleeplessness); **305.1** (Dependence, with, nicotine)
7. 99203 (Office and/or Other Outpatient Services, Office Visit, New Patient)
   ICD-10-CM: **S83.411A** (Sprain, knee, [tibial] medial collateral ligament), **Y93.22** (External Cause Index, Activity, ice, hockey)

ICD-9-CM: **844.1** (Sprain, strain; medial collateral, knee), **E003.1** (External Cause Index, Activity, involving, hockey [ice])

8. 99202 (Office and/or Other Outpatient Services, Office Visit, New Patient)
   ICD-10-CM: **J30.1** (Allergy, grass, [pollen])
   ICD-9-CM: **477.0** (Allergy, grass, pollen)

Exercise 15-8

1. yes
2. 99212 (Office and/or Other Outpatient Services, Office Visit, Established Patient) (Note: Some chart audit forms would assign 99213 because of the antibiotic prescription.)
3. 99211 (Office and/or Other Outpatient Services, Office Visit, Established Patient)
   ICD-10-CM: **S83.512D** (Sprain, knee, cruciate ligament, anterior)
   ICD-9-CM: **717.83** (Sprain, knee, old, cruciate, anterior)
4. 99215 (Office and/or Other Outpatient Services, Office Visit, Established Patient)
   ICD-10-CM: **R55** (Fainting)
   ICD-9-CM: **780.2** (Fainting)
5. 99213 (Office and/or Other Outpatient Services, Office Visit, Established Patient)
   ICD-10-CM: **R53.81** (Malaise), **R53.83** (Fatigue), **T46.5X5A** (Table of Drugs and Chemicals, Antihypertensive drug NEC, Adverse Effect), **I10** (Hypertension, Unspecified)
   ICD-9-CM: **780.79** (Malaise), **E942.6** (Table of Drugs and Chemicals, Antihypertensive agents NEC, Therapeutic Use), **995.20** (Effect, adverse, drug/medicinals, correct substance properly administered); **401.9** (Hypertension, Unspecified)
   (Note: Although the MDM complexity is at the level of code 99214, the history and examination were at the level of code 99213; because two of the three key components must be documented in order to use 99214, you must assign the lower level, 99213.)
6. 99212 (Office and/or Other Outpatient Services, Office Visit, Established Patient)
   ICD-10-CM: **L91.8** (Tag, skin)
   ICD-9-CM: **701.9** (Tag, skin)
7. 99213 (Office and/or Other Outpatient Services, Office Visit, Established Patient)
   ICD-10-CM: **R19.7** (Diarrhea)
   ICD-9-CM: **787.91** (Diarrhea)

Exercise 15-9

1. 99219 (Hospital Services, Observation, Initial Care)
   ICD-10-CM: **S06.0X1A** (Concussion), **V49.9** (External Cause Index, Accident, transport, car, occupant)
   ICD-9-CM: **850.11** (Concussion, with, loss of consciousness, brief, 30 minutes or less), **E819.9** (Index to External Causes, Accident, motor vehicle)

Exercise 15-10

1. 99221 (Hospital Services, Inpatient Services, Initial Hospital Care)
2. 99223 (Hospital Services, Inpatient Services, Initial Hospital Care)
3. comprehensive, moderate
4. 99221 (Hospital Services, Inpatient Services, Initial Hospital Care)
   ICD-10-CM: **N30.01** (Cystitis, acute, with hematuria), **N10** (Pyelitis, acute)
   ICD-9-CM: **595.0** (Cystitis, acute); **590.10** (Pyelitis, acute)

Exercise 15-11

1. 30 minutes or less, more than 30 minutes
2. no

Exercise 15-12

1. 99244 (Consultation, Office and/or Other Outpatient)
   ICD-10-CM: **M84.48XA** (Fracture, pathological, due to, specified disease NEC, vertebrae), **Z85.3** (History, personal, malignant neoplasm, breast)
   ICD-9-CM: **733.13** (Fracture, pathologic, vertebrae), **V10.3** (History, personal, malignant neoplasm, breast)
2. 99241 (Consultation, Office and/or Other Outpatient)
   ICD-10-CM: **M77.8** (Enthesopathy, elbow region), **M70.31** (Bursitis, elbow)
   ICD-9-CM: **726.90** (Tendinitis), **726.33** (Bursitis, elbow)
3. 99242 (Consultation, Office and/or Other Outpatient)
   ICD-10-CM: **Z01.810** (Examination, pre-procedural, cardiovascular), **M17.11** (Osteoarthrosis, localized, primary, knee), **I10** (Hypertension), **I25.10** (Arteriosclerosis, coronary [artery])
   ICD-9-CM: **V72.81** (Examination, preoperative, cardiovascular), **715.16** (Osteoarthrosis, localized, primary) **401.9** (Hypertension, benign), **414.01** (Arteriosclerosis, coronary [artery], native)
4. 99241 (Consultation, Office and/or Other Outpatient)
   ICD-10-CM: **K64.8** (Hemorrhoids, internal)
   ICD-9-CM: **455.2** (Hemorrhoids, internal, bleeding)
5. 99244 (Consultation, Office and/or Other Outpatient)
   ICD-10-CM: **R06.00** (Dyspnea), **R53.83** (Fatigue), **R42** (Dizziness), **I34.0** (Insufficiency, mitral [valve]), **Z95.0** (Status, pacemaker, cardiac)
   ICD-9-CM: **786.09** (Dyspnea), **780.79** (Fatigue), **780.4** (Dizziness), **424.0** (Insufficiency, mitral [valve]), **V45.01** (Status, cardiac, device, pacemaker)
6. 99252 (Consultation, Inpatient)
   ICD-10-CM: **I48.91** (Fibrillation, atrial)
   ICD-9-CM: **427.31** (Fibrillation, atrial)
7. 99255-57 (Consultation, Inpatient) (Modifier -57 indicates the decision to perform surgery.)
8. 99252 (Consultation, Inpatient)
9. 99255 (Consultation, Inpatient)
   ICD-10-CM: **R56.00** (Convulsions, febrile)
   ICD-9-CM: **780.31** (Febrile, convulsion)
10. 99233 (Hospital Inpatient Services, Subsequent Hospital Care)
    ICD-10-CM: **I23.7** (Angina, following acute myocardial infarction), **I47.2** (Tachycardia, ventricular)
    ICD-9-CM: **410.11** (Infarct, infarction, myocardial, anterior [wall])
    (Note that angina and tachycardia are not reported as both of these are symptoms of myocardial infarction.)
11. 99233 (Hospital Inpatient Services, Subsequent Hospital Care)
    ICD-10-CM: **R56.00** (Seizures, febrile)
    ICD-9-CM: **780.39** (Febrile, convulsion)
12. 99244 (Consultation, Office
    ICD-10-CM: **Q21.3** (Tetralogy of Fallot)
    ICD-9-CM: **745.2** (Tetralogy of Fallot)
13. 99242-32 (Consultation, Office) (Modifier -32, insurance company requested)
14. 99244-32 (Consultation, Office and/or Other Outpatient) (Modifier -32 indicates a mandatory consultation.)

Exercise 15-13

1. self-limited or minor
2. high
3. moderate
4. low to moderate
5. 99285 (Evaluation and Management, Emergency Department)
   ICD-10-CM: **I46.9** (Arrest, cardiac)
   ICD-9-CM: **427.5** (Arrest, cardiac)
6. 99285 (Emergency Department Services)
   ICD-10-CM: **J80** (Distress, respiratory, adult)
   ICD-9-CM: **518.82** (Distress, respiratory, acute [adult])
7. 99283 (Evaluation and Management, Emergency Department)
8. 99288 (Emergency Department Services, Physician Direction of Advanced Life Support)

Exercise 15-14

1. 99291 (Evaluation and Management, Critical Care Services)
2. no
3. 99291 and 99292 × 4 (180 minutes of care) (Critical Care Services)
   ICD-10-CM: **T31.50** (Burn, unspecified site)
   ICD-9-CM: **948.50** (Burn, unspecified site, multiple, 50-59 percent)

Exercise 15-15

1. moderate
2. 99306 (Nursing Facility Services, Initial Care)
   ICD-10-CM: **I69.352** (Sequelae, infarction, cerebral, hemiplegia), **E11.9** (Diabetes), **I10** (Hypertension, Unspecified)
   ICD-9-CM: **438.21** (Late effect, cerebrovascular disease), **250.00** (Diabetes), **401.9** (Hypertension, Unspecified)
3. c

4. b
5. a
6. 99308 (Nursing Facility Services, Subsequent Care)
   ICD-10-CM: **J06.9** (Infection, respiratory, upper [acute]
   NOS), **R40.20** (Coma), **S06.9X6S** (Injury, brain [traumatic])
   ICD-9-CM: **465.9** (Infection, respiratory, upper NEC),
   780.01 (Coma) **907.0** (Late effect[s], injury, intracranial)

Exercise 15-16
1. 99347 (Home Services, Established Patient)

Exercise 15-17
1. no
2. no, in addition to another E/M code
3. no, the physician has to spend at least 30 minutes
4. whether the patient is an inpatient or an outpatient
5. no, by time
6. no

Exercise 15-18
1. 30 minutes or more
2. 99366, 99367, 99368

Exercise 15-19
1. age
2. -25

Exercise 15-20
1. Basic Life and/or Disability Evaluation Services
2. Work-Related or Medical Disability Evaluation Services
3. whether the treating physician or a physician other than
   the treating physician conducted the evaluation
4. 99455 (Insurance, Disability Examination, Disability)
   ICD-10-CM: **Z02.71** (Encounter [with health service]
   [for], administrative purpose only, examination for, disability determination), **J44.9** (Disease, lung, obstructive,
   with, emphysema)
   ICD-9-CM: **V68.01** (Encounter for, disability exam),
   492.8 (Disease, lung, obstructive, with, emphysema NEC)

Exercise 15-21
1. very low birth weight
2. 99466 (Critical Care Services, Interfacility Transport)
3. 99463 (Newborn Care, History and Examination)
4. 99476 (Critical Care Services, Pediatric, Subsequent)
5. 99478 (Critical Care Services, Neonatal, Low Birth
   Weight Infant)

Exercise 15-22
1. 99201 (Office and/or Other Outpatient Services, Office
   Visits, New Patient)
   ICD-10-CM: **H70.009** (Mastoiditis, acute)
   ICD-9-CM: **383.00** (Mastoiditis, acute)
2. 99212 (Office and Other Outpatient Visits, Office Visits,
   Established Patient)
   ICD-10-CM: **H66.90** (Otitis, media, acute)
   ICD-9-CM: **382.9** (Otitis, media, acute)

3. 99211 (Office and/or Other Outpatient Services, Office
   Visits, Established Patient)
4. 99306 (Nursing Facility Services, Initial Care)
5. 99202 (Office and/or Other Outpatient Services, Office
   Visits, New Patient)
   ICD-10-CM: **L70.0** (Acne, pustular)
   ICD-9-CM: **706.1** (Acne)
6. 99211 (Office and/or Other Outpatient Services,
   Office Visits, Established Patient)
7. 99285 (Evaluation and Management, Emergency
   Department)
   ICD-10-CM: **I47.1** (Tachycardia, paroxysmal, nodal)
   ICD-9-CM: **427.0** (Tachycardia, paroxysmal, nodal)
8. 99291 (Evaluation and Management, Critical Care)
9. 99291 (Evaluation and Management, Critical Care) and
   99292 (Evaluation and Management, Critical Care)
10. 99214 (Office and/or Other Outpatient Services,
    Established Patient)
11. 99254 (Evaluation and Management, Consultation)

CHAPTER 16

Exercise 16-1
1. Radiologic Procedures, Burn Excisions or Debridement,
   Obstetrics, and Other Procedures
2. absence of pain
3. induction or administration of a drug to obtain partial
   or complete loss of sensation (or similar wording)
4. general, regional, local, sacral, caudal, lumbar, endotracheal, epidural, and analgesia (pain controlled)
5. moderate or conscious sedation
6. Medicine

Exercise 16-2
1. P2
2. P3
3. 99116
4. actual
5. Stop
6. start

Exercise 16-3
1. -22
2. -23
3. -AD
4. -QS
5. -QX

Exercise 16-4
1. 01999 (Anesthesia, Unlisted Services and Procedures)
2. Anesthesia, Thyroid, 00322
3. Anesthesia, Cesarean Delivery, 01961
4. Anesthesia, Prostate, or Anesthesia, Transurethral Procedures, 00914
5. Anesthesia, Cleft Palate Repair, 00172
6. Anesthesia, Achilles Tendon Repair, 01472

7. **$109.00** (B = 3, T = 1, M = 1; total 5; 5 $21.80)
8. a. **$226.89** (B = 5, T = 4, M = 0; total 9; 9 $25.21)
   b. **$197.37** (B = 5, T = 4, M = 0; total 9; 9 $21.93)
9. a. **$218.40** (B = 7, T = 2, M = 1; total 10; 10 $21.84)
   b. **$240.24** (B = 7, T = 3, M = 1; total 11; 11 $21.84)

CHAPTER 17

Exercise 17-1
1. 20999
2. 69949
3. 17999
4. 27899
5. 64999
6. 67999

Exercise 17-2
1. pre-, intra-, and postoperative services, or similar wording
2. no
3. no

Exercise 17-3
1. 10021 (Fine Needle Aspiration, Diagnostic)
2. 10022 (Fine Needle Aspiration, Diagnostic), 76942 (Ultrasound, Guidance, Needle Biopsy)

CHAPTER 18

Exercise 18-1
1. 11056 (Lesion, Skin, Paring/Curettement)
   ICD-10-CM: **B07.8** (Wart, common)
   ICD-9-CM: **078.19** (Wart, common)
2. 11200 (Lesion, Skin Tags, Removal)
   ICD-10-CM: **L91.8** (Tag, skin)
   ICD-9-CM: **701.9** (Tag, skin)
3. 11311 (Lesion, Skin, Shaving)
   ICD-10-CM: **L98.9** (Lesion, skin)
   ICD-9-CM: **709.9** (Lesion, dermal)

Exercise 18-2
1. 13132 (Repair, Wound, Complex)
   ICD-10-CM: **S61.401A** (Wound, open, hand)
   ICD-9-CM: **882.0** (Wound, open, hand)
2. 13101 for complex repair of abdomen (Repair, Wound, Complex); 12004-59 for 12-cm simple repair of back, forearm, and neck added together (Repair, Wound, Simple). (Note that the same types of repair are combined—back (trunk), forearm (extremities), and neck are all included in the code description for 12004.)
3. 13121 for the 5.6 cm complex forearm repair (Wound, Repair, Arm, Complex); 12032-59 for the 5.1 cm intermediate forearm repair (Wound, Repair, Arm, Intermediate); 12002-59 for the 3.1 cm simple scalp repair (Repair, Wound, Simple)
4. Cheek graft: 15120 (Skin Grafts and Flaps, Split Grafts)
   Upper chest: 15100-51, 15101 (Skin Grafts and Flaps, Split Grafts) [no modifier on add-on code 15101]
   Site prep, cheek, 100 cm²: 15004-51 (Skin Grafts and Flaps, Recipient Site Preparation)
   Site prep, chest, 200 cm²: 15002-51, 15003 (Skin Grafts and Flaps, Recipient Site Preparation) [no modifier on add-on code 15003]
   Note: If this claim were submitted to Medicare, modifier -51 would not be appended on the site preparation codes.
5. 14041 (Skin, Adjacent Tissue Transfer)
6. 14040 (Skin, Adjacent Tissue Transfer) (Note that a Z-plasty is a form of adjacent tissue transfer. The excision is included in the adjacent tissue transfer code.)
7. 15732 (Skin, Myocutaneous Flaps) (Note that modifier -58 may also be used if the procedure was a staged procedure.)
8. Week 1: 16025 × 5 (Burns, Debridement/Dressing)
   Weeks 2 and 3: 16025 × 6 (Burns, Debridement/Dressing)
   (Some payers would allow you to submit all treatments together with 16025 × 11.)

Exercise 18-3
1. 17110 (Destruction, Lesion, Skin, Benign) (If a specific anatomic area was indicated, you could report the destruction with a more specific code. For example, 56501 for destruction of a lesion of the vulva.)
2. 17000 (Destruction, Lesion, Skin, Premalignant), 17003 × 13 (Destruction, Lesion, Skin, Premalignant)
   ICD-10-CM: **L57.0** (Keratosis, actinic)
   ICD-9-CM: **702.0** (Keratosis, actinic)
3. 17311 (Mohs Micrographic Surgery)

Exercise 18-4
1. 19000 (Breast, Cyst, Puncture Aspiration)
2. 19303 and 19303-50 or 19303-50 or 19303-RT and 19303-LT (Breast, Removal, Simple, Complete)
3. 19307-RT (Breast, Removal, Modified Radical)
4. 19287-LT (Placement, Needle Wire, Breast)
5. 19350-RT (Breast, Reconstruction, Nipple, Areola)

CHAPTER 19

Exercise 19-1
1. 21310 (Nasal Bone, Fracture, Closed Treatment)
2. 21820 (Sternum, Fracture, Closed Treatment)
3. 28675 (Dislocation, Interphalangeal Joint, Toe, Open Treatment)
4. 27792 (Fracture, Fibula, Open Treatment)
5. 27500 (Fracture, Femur, Closed Treatment)
6. 27235 (Fracture, Femur, Percutaneous Fixation)
7. 23670 (Fracture, Humerus, with Dislocation, Open Treatment)
   ICD-10-CM: **S42.256A** (Fracture, humerus, upper end, great tuberosity)
   ICD-9-CM: **812.03** (Fracture, humerus, great tuberosity)
   According to Coding Clinic, 3rd Quarter 1990, p. 13: "For purposes of classification, ICD-9-CM assigns only the fracture code to fracture-dislocations of the same site. It is incorrect to also code the dislocation."

8. 21453 (Fracture, Mandible, Closed Treatment, Interdental Fixation)
   ICD-10-CM: **S02.609A** (Fracture, mandible [lower jaw] [bone])
   ICD-9-CM: **802.20** (Fracture, mandible [closed])
9. 25606 (Fracture, Radius, Percutaneous Fixation)
   ICD-10-CM: **S52.509A** (Fracture, radius, lower end)
   ICD-9-CM: **813.42** (Fracture, radius, lower end or extremity [distal end])
10. 27840 (Ankle, Dislocation, Closed Treatment)
    ICD-10-CM: **S93.06XA** (Dislocation, ankle)
    ICD-9-CM: **837.0** (Dislocation, ankle [closed])

Exercise 19-2

1. 20103 (Wound, Exploration, Penetrating Extremity)
2. 20838 (Replantation, Foot)
3. 21015 (Radial Resection, Tumor, Face)
4. 20974 (Electrical Stimulation, Bone Healing, Noninvasive)
5. 20206 (Biopsy, Muscle)
   ICD-10-CM: **G71.11** (Dystrophy, muscular, congenital, myotonic)
   ICD-9-CM: **359.22** (Dystrophy, muscular, congenital, myotonic)
6. 20600 (Aspiration, Joint)
   ICD-10-CM: **M19.049** (Osteoarthritis, primary, hand joint)
   ICD-9-CM: **716.94** (Arthritis, hand)

Exercise 19-3

1. 29065-58 (Cast, Long Arm); 99070 or A4580-A4590 or O4005-O4008 (Supply, Materials)
2. 29425 (Cast, Ambulatory, Walking)
3. 29705 (Cast, Removal)
4. 29530 (Strapping, Knee)
5. 29345 (Cast, Thigh to Toes); 99070 or A4580-A4590 or O4005-O4008 (Supply, Materials)

Exercise 19-4

1. 29898 (Arthroscopy, Surgical, Ankle)
2. 29870 (Arthroscopy, Diagnostic, Knee)
3. 29805 (Arthroscopy, Shoulder)
4. 29850 (Fracture, Knee, Arthroscopic Treatment)
5. 29891 (Arthroscopy, Surgical, Ankle)

CHAPTER 20

Exercise 20-1

1. 31256 (Antrostomy, Sinus, Maxillary)
2. 31530 (Laryngoscopy, Direct, Operative)
3. 31628 (Bronchoscopy, Biopsy)
4. 32601 (Thoracoscopy, Diagnostic)
5. 32663 (Thoracoscopy, Surgical, with Lobectomy)

Exercise 20-2

1. 30100 (Biopsy, Nose, Intranasal)
   ICD-10-CM: **J34.89** (Lesion, nose [internal])
   ICD-9-CM: **478.19** (Lesions, nose [internal])
2. 30420 (Rhinoplasty, Primary)
   ICD-10-CM: **J34.2** (Deviation [in], nasal septum)
   ICD-9-CM: **470** (Deviation, septum [acquired] [nasal])
3. 30901 (Hemorrhage, Control, Nasal, Simple)
   ICD-10-CM: **R04.0** (Hemorrhage, nose)
   ICD-9-CM: **784.7** (Hemorrhage, nose)
4. 30520 (Septoplasty)
5. 30300 (Removal, Foreign Body, Nose)

Exercise 20-3

1. 31000 and 31000-50 (Sinuses, Maxillary, Irrigation)
2. 31070-LT (Sinusotomy, Frontal Sinus, Exploratory)
3. 31090 (Sinusotomy, Combined)
4. 31030-RT (Sinusotomy, Maxillary)
5. 31040 (Ptergomaxillary Fossa, Incision)
   ICD-10-CM: **J01.01** (Sinusitis, maxillary, recurrent)
   ICD-9-CM: **473.0** (Sinusitis, chronic, maxillary)

Exercise 20-4

1. 31320 (Laryngotomy, Diagnostic)
2. 31580 (Laryngoplasty, Laryngeal Web)
3. 31500 (Endotracheal Tube, Intubation)
4. 31368 (Laryngectomy, Subtotal)
   ICD-10-CM: **C10.1** (Neoplasm, glosso-epiglottic fold[s], Malignant Primary)
   ICD-9-CM: **146.4** (Neoplasm, glossoepiglottic folds, Malignant, Primary)
5. 31390 (Pharyngolaryngectomy)
   ICD-10-CM: **C14.0** (Neoplasm, pharynx region, Malignant Primary)
   ICD-9-CM: **149.0** (Neoplasm, pharynx, region, Malignant, Primary)

Exercise 20-5

1. 31605 (Tracheostomy, Emergency)
2. 31785 (Excision, Tumor, Trachea)
3. 31717 (Bronchial Brush Biopsy)
4. 31600 (Tracheostomy, Planned)
   ICD-10-CM: **J96.00** (Failure, respiration, acute)
   ICD-9-CM: **518.81** (Failure, respiration, respiratory, acute)
5. 31717 (Bronchial Brush Biopsy, with Catheterization)
   ICD-10-CM: **J21.9** (Bronchiolitis [acute])
   ICD-9-CM: **466.19** (Bronchiolitis, acute)

Exercise 20-6

1. 32100 (Lung, Exploration)
2. 32405 (Biopsy, Lung, Needle)
3. 32480 (Lobectomy, Lung), 32501 (Bronchoplasty) (Note that code 32501 is an add-on code and does not require modifier -51.)
4. 32503 (Lung, Tumor, Resection)
   ICD-10-CM: **C34.10** (Neoplasm, lung, upper lobe [unspecified side], Malignant Primary)
   ICD-9-CM: **162.3** (Neoplasm, lung, upper lobe, Malignant, Primary)

5. 32200 (Pneumonostomy)
   ICD-10-CM: **J85.2** (Abscess, lung)
   ICD-9-CM: **513.0** (Abscess, lung)

CHAPTER 21

Exercise 21-1

1. invasive
2. internal
3. Medicine, Surgery, Radiology (any order)
4. interventional
5. electrophysiology
6. nuclear

Exercise 21-2

1. 33207 (Pacemaker, Heart, Insertion)
2. 33216-78 (Pacemaker, Heart, Insertion, Electrode). Note that -78 is appended because the patient is in a postoperative period. The patient had a single-lead pacemaker implanted. The replacement of the lead wire is reported as insertion of a new electrode, the removal of the defective electrode is not separately reported.
3. 33214 (Pacemaker, Conversion) also known as an upgrade
4. 33010 (Pericardiocentesis)
   ICD-10-CM: **J81.0** (Edema, lung, acute), **I30.0** (Pericarditis, acute, nonspecific)
   ICD-9-CM: **518.4** (Edema, pulmonary, lung, acute), **420.90** (Effusion, pericardium, acute)
5. 33120 (Tumor, Heart, Excision)
   ICD-10-CM: **C38.0** (Neoplasm, heart, Malignant Primary)
   ICD-9-CM: **164.1** (Neoplasm, heart, endocardium, Malignant, Primary)

Exercise 21-3

1. 33430 (Mitral Valve, Replacement)
2. 33405 (Aorta, Valve, Replacement, with Prosthesis) (Note that a prosthetic valve, and not a homograft valve, is used.)
3. 33261 (Arrhythmogenic Focus, Heart, Ablation)
   ICD-10-CM: **I49.8** (Arrhythmia, specified NEC)
   ICD-9-CM: **427.89** (Arrhythmia, bigeminal rhythm)
4. 33282 (Implantation, Cardiac Event Recorder)
   ICD-10-CM: **R00.2** (Palpitations [heart]), **R42** (Dizziness)
   ICD-9-CM: **785.1** (Palpitation [heart]), **780.4** (Dizziness)

Exercise 21-4

1. 33511 (Bypass Graft, Venous, Coronary)
2A. 33534 (Coronary Artery Bypass Graft, Arterial)
2B. 33519 (Coronary Artery Bypass Graft, Arterial-Venous)
   ICD-10-CM: **I25.10** (Disease, heart, ischemic, atherosclerotic)
   ICD-9-CM: **414.01** (Arteriosclerosis, coronary artery native artery)
3. 33533 (Bypass Graft, Arterial, Coronary) and 33519 (Bypass Graft, Arterial-Venous, Coronary)

ICD-10-CM: **I25.10** (Disease, heart, ischemic, atherosclerotic), **I11.9** (Hypertensive, heart, due to, hypertension)
ICD-9-CM: **414.01** (Arteriosclerosis, coronary artery native artery), **402.10** (Hypertension, with heart disease, benign)

Exercise 21-5

1. 34201 (Thrombectomy, Aortoiliac Artery)
2. 34001 (Embolectomy, Carotid Artery)
3. 35875 (Thrombectomy, Bypass Graft, Other than Hemodialysis Graft or Fistula)
   ICD-10-CM: **T82.868A** (Complication[s], graft, vascular, thrombosis)
   ICD-9-CM: **996.74** (Complication, vascular device, implant, or graft NEC)

Exercise 21-6

1. 35506 (Artery, Carotid, Bypass Graft)
2. 35556 (Bypass Graft, Venous, Femoral-Popliteal)
3. 35650 (Bypass Graft, Venous, Axillary-Axillary)
4. 35141 (Aneurysm Repair, Femoral Artery)
   ICD-10-CM: **I72.4** (Aneurysm, femoral [artery])
   ICD-9-CM: **442.3** (Aneurysm, femoral artery)
5. 36246-LT or 36246-59-LT (Catheterization, Legs), 75716-26 (Angiography, Leg Artery)
   ICD-10-CM: **I73.9** (Disease, peripheral, vascular NOS)
   ICD-9-CM: **443.9** (Disease, peripheral, vascular)

Exercise 21-7

1. 92950 (CPR [Cardiopulmonary Resuscitation])
2. 93015 (Stress Tests, Cardiovascular)
3. 92920-RC, 92921-LD (Angioplasty, Percutaneous Transluminal, Coronary)
4. 93278-26 (Electrocardiography, Signal-Averaged)
   ICD-10-CM: **I47.2** (Tachycardia, ventricular)
   ICD-9-CM: **427.1** (Tachycardia, ventricular)

Exercise 21-8

1. 93451-26 (Cardiac, Catheterization, Right Heart)
2. 93458-26 (Cardiac, Catheterization, Left Heart)
   ICD-10-CM: **I25.110** (Arteriosclerosis, coronary [artery], native vessel, with, angina pectoris, unstable)
   ICD-9-CM: **414.01** (Arteriosclerosis, coronary (artery), native artery), **411.1** (Angina, unstable)
3. False; they are already bundled into the codes.
4. True
5. False; some codes are modifier -51-exempt.

Exercise 21-9

1. 93600-26 (Electrophysiology Procedure)
2. 93620-26, 93622-26 (Electrophysiology Procedure)
   ICD-10-CM: **R55** (Syncope, vasovagal)
   ICD-9-CM: **780.2** (Syncope, vasovagal)

Exercise 21-10

1. Injection procedure for angiography 36215-RT (Catheterization, Brachiocephalic Artery), angiography 75710 (Angiography, Brachial Artery); contrast material 99070 (Supply, Materials)
2. 75716-26 (Angiography, Leg Artery)
3. 75572-26 (CT Scan, Heart, Evaluation, for Structure and Morphology)
4. 75563-26 (Magnetic Resonance Imaging [MRI], Heart)
   ICD-10-CM: **I50.9** (Failure, heart, congestive), **I49.3** (Premature, contraction, ventricular)
   ICD-9-CM: **428.0** (Failure, heart, congestive); **427.69** (Premature beats, ventricular)

CHAPTER 22

Exercise 22-1

1. 38550 (Lymph Nodes, Hygroma Cystic Axillary/Cervical, Excision)
   ICD-10-CM: **D18.1** (Hygroma)
   ICD-9-CM: **228.1** (Hygroma)
2. 38100 (Splenectomy, Total)
   ICD-10-CM: **E75.22** (Splenomegaly, Gaucher's)
   ICD-9-CM: **272.7** (Gaucher's splenomegaly)
3. 38200 (Splenoportography, Injection Procedures)
4. 38241 (Transplantation, Bone Marrow)

Exercise 22-2

1. 39000 (Mediastinum, Exploration)
   ICD-10-CM: **C38.3** (Neoplasm, mediastinum, mediastinal, Malignant, Primary)
   ICD-9-CM: **164.9** (Neoplasm, mediastinum, mediastinal, Malignant, Primary)
2. 39220 (Mediastinum, Resection, Tumor, Excision)
   ICD-10-CM: **D15.2** (Neoplasm, mediastinum, mediastinal, Benign)
   ICD-9-CM: **212.5** (Neoplasm, mediastinum, mediastinal, Benign)

CHAPTER 23

Exercise 23-1

1. vermilionectomy
2. gallbladder
3. 10.2 (4 × 2.54)
4. 40527 (Repair, Cleft Lip)
   ICD-10-CM: **Q36.9** (Cleft, lip)
   ICD-9-CM: **749.10** (Cleft, lip)
5. 40650 (Repair, Lip)
   ICD-10-CM: **C00.3** (Neoplasm, lip, internal, upper, Malignant Primary)
   ICD-9-CM: **140.5** (Neoplasm, lip, Malignant, Primary)
6. 40800 (Mouth, Hematoma, Incision and Drainage)
7. 41252 (Tongue, Repair, Laceration). Note that the measurement of the laceration was stated in inches and must be converted to centimeters (1.5 in × 2.54 = 3.8 cm).

Exercise 23-2

1. 42826 (Tonsillectomy)
   ICD-10-CM: **J35.01** (Tonsillitis, hypertrophic)
   ICD-9-CM: **474.00** (Tonsillitis, hypertrophic)
2. 42900 (Suture, Pharynx, Wound)
3. 43045 (Esophagotomy)
4. 43101 (Esophagus, Lesion, Excision)
5. 43450 (Dilation, Esophagus)

Exercise 23-3

1. surgical communication from the colon to the rectum
2. surgical communication from the ileum to the body surface
3. surgical communication from the large intestine to the body surface
4. surgical communication between segments of intestine
5. 44141 (Colon, Excision, Partial)
   ICD-10-CM: **C18.9** (Neoplasm, intestine, large, colon, Malignant Primary)
   ICD-9-CM: **153.9** (Neoplasm, intestine, colon, Malignant, Primary)
6. 44120 (Enterectomy, Small Intestine)

Exercise 23-4

1. 44960 (Excision, Appendix)
   ICD-10-CM: **K35.2** (Appendicitis, with, peritonitis, generalized [perforation, or rupture])
   ICD-9-CM: **540.0** (Appendicitis, acute, with, perforation, or rupture)
2. 45331 (Sigmoidoscopy, Biopsy). The description states biopsy, single or multiple, so only one code is used for multiple (three) biopsies.
3. 45385 (Colonoscopy, Flexible, Removal, Polyp)
4. 45331 (Endoscopy, Colon-Sigmoid, Biopsy)

Exercise 23-5

1. 47600 (Cholecystectomy, Excision). Note that the exploratory laparotomy is not coded, as it turns into the surgical approach once the cholecystectomy is performed.
2. 47480 (Cholecystotomy, Open)
3. 49565 (Hernia Repair, Incisional, Recurrent), 49568 (Implantation, Mesh, Hernia Repair). Note that the mesh code can be used only with incisional hernias, and it is stated to "list separately," so a -51 modifier is not necessary.
4. 49507 (Hernia Repair, Inguinal, Incarcerated)
5. 48155 (Pancreatectomy, Total)
6. 46257 (Hemorrhoidectomy, Simple, with Fissurectomy). Note that 46220 (Papillectomy) and 46080 (Sphincterotomy, Anal) are not reported as they are both bundled into code 46257.

CHAPTER 24

Exercise 24-1

1. 50065 (Nephrolithotomy). Note that the term "secondary" means that the procedure is being repeated. Some may

code this 50060-76, but this would not be correct because there is a more accurate code to assign.

2. 50398-LT (Nephrostomy, Change Tube)
3. 50590-RT (Lithotripsy, Kidney), 52310-RT (Cystoure-throscopy, Removal, Urethral Stent)

Exercise 24-2

1. 50630-LT (Ureterolithotomy)
2. 50780-50 (Ureteroneocystostomy) Modifier -50 indicates a bilateral procedure.
3. 50955-RT (Ureter, Endoscopy, Biopsy), 50684-RT (Ureter, Injection, Radiologic), 74425 (X-Ray, Urinary Tract)

Exercise 24-3

1. 51100 (Aspiration, Bladder)
2. 52332-RT (Cystourethroscopy, Insertion, Indwelling Ureteral Stent)
3. 52332-LT (Ureter, Endoscopy, Insertion, Stent), 74420-26 (Urography, Retrograde)
4. 51840 (Urethropexy)
5. 52320-LT (Ureter, Endoscopy, Removal, Calculus), 74420-26 (Urography, Retrograde)

Exercise 24-4

1. 53520 (Urethra, Repair, Fistula)
2. 53405 (Urethra, Repair, Fistula)

Exercise 24-5

1. 54065 (Penis, Lesion, Destruction, Extensive)
   ICD-10-CM: A63.0 (Condyloma)
   ICD-9-CM: 078.11 (Condyloma)
2. 54415 (Removal, Prosthesis, Penis)

Exercise 24-6

1. 54520-50 (Orchiectomy, Simple) (Note that the terms "simple" and "radical" are based on the interpretation of the physician.)
2. 54505-50 (Biopsy, Testes)

Exercise 24-7

1. 54865 (Epididymis, Exploration, Biopsy)
   ICD-10-CM: N50.8 (Pain, scrotum)
   ICD-9-CM: 608.9 (Pain[s], genital, organ, male)
   (Note that even though the question states without biopsy, the CPT code states with or without biopsy, so this would be the correct code to assign.)
2. 55000 (Tunica Vaginalis, Hydrocele, Aspiration)
3. 55400-50 (Vas Deferens, Repair, Suture), 69990 (Operating Microscope)

Exercise 24-8

1. 55845 (Prostatectomy, Retropubic, Radical)
   ICD-10-CM: C61 (Neoplasm, prostate, Malignant Primary)
   ICD-9-CM: 185 (Neoplasm, prostate Malignant, Primary)
2. 53852 (Transurethral Procedure, Prostate, Thermotherapy, Radiofrequency)

CHAPTER 25

Exercise 25-1

1. 57061 (Destruction, Lesion, Vagina, Simple)
2. 56605, 56606 × 2 (Vulva, Perineum, Biopsy) (Note that the code 56605 is for the first lesion, and 56606 is for *each* additional lesion.)
3. 57305 (Vagina, Repair, Fistula, Rectovaginal)
4. 57520 (Cervix, Conization) (Note that dilation and curettage is not coded separately because it is included in the description of the conization.)
5. 58661-RT (Cystectomy, Ovarian, Laparoscopic)
6. c
7. b
8. d
9. a

Exercise 25-2

1. 59151 (Laparoscopy, Ectopic Pregnancy with Salpingec-tomy and/or Oophorectomy)
2. 59409 (Vaginal Delivery, Delivery only); 59412 (External Cephalic Version) (Note that the version is stated "list in addition"; therefore, modifier -51 is not necessary.)
3. 59320 (Cerclage, Cervix, Vaginal)

CHAPTER 26

Exercise 26-1

1. 60200 (Thyroid Gland, Cyst, Excision)
2. 60280 (Thyroglossal Duct, Cyst, Excision)
3. 60522 (Thymectomy, Sternal Split/Transthoracic Approach)
4. 60600 (Carotid Body, Lesion, Excision)
5. 60210 (Thyroid Gland, Excision, Partial)
6. 60650 (Laparoscopy, Adrenal Gland)
7. 60505 (Parathyroidectomy, Excision), 60512 (Parathy-roid Gland, Autotransplant)
8. 60502 (Parathyroid, Exploration). The partial thymectomy is listed as a separate procedure and is not reported.
9. 60605 (Carotid Body, Tumor, Excision)

Exercise 26-2

1. 61154 (Burr Hole, for, Drainage, Hematoma)
   ICD-10-CM: I62.00 (Hematoma, subdural, nontraumatic)
   ICD-9-CM: 432.1 (Hematoma, subdural, nontraumatic)
2. 61312 (Craniectomy, Surgical)
   ICD-10-CM: S06.5X9A (Injury, intracranial, subdural hemorrhage, traumatic)
   ICD-9-CM: 852.20 (Hematoma, brain, subdural)
3. 61607 Definitive Procedure: (Skull Base Surgery, Middle Cranial Fossa, Extradural), 61591-51 Approach Procedure: (Skull Base Surgery, Middle Cranial Fossa, Infratemporal Post-Auricular Approach)
   ICD-10-CM: C71.9 (Neoplasm, brain, Malignant Primary)
   ICD-9-CM: 191.9 (Neoplasm, fossa, cranial, Malignant, Primary)

4. 62258 (Shunt, Brain, Replacement)
   ICD-10-CM: **Q03.9** (Hydrocephalus, congenital)
   ICD-9-CM: **742.3** (Hydrocephalus, congenital)

CHAPTER 27

Exercise 27-1

1. 65930-LT (Eye, Removal, Blood Clot)
2. 67318-RT (Strabismus, Repair, Superior Oblique Muscle)
3. 67145-LT (Retina, Repair, Prophylaxis, Detachment)
4. 65772-RT (Cornea, Relaxing, Incision, Astigmatism)
5. 65105-LT (Removal, Eye, with Implant, Muscles Attached)

Exercise 27-2

1. 69801-LT (Labyrinthotomy, Transcranial)
2. 69436 and 69436-50 (Tympanostomy, General Anesthesia)
3. 69950-LT (Vestibular Nerve, Section, Transcranial Approach)
4. 69310-RT (Reconstruction, Auditory Canal, External)
5. 69820-RT (Ear, Inner, Incision, Semicircular Canal)

Exercise 27-3

1. exostosis
2. otoplasty
3. cholesteatoma
4. 69990

CHAPTER 28

Exercise 28-1

1. aorta
2. joint
3. biliary system and pancreas
4. bile ducts
5. urinary bladder
6. lacrimal sac or tear duct sac
7. duodenum or first part of the small intestine
8. heart or heart walls or neighboring tissues
9. subarachnoid space and ventricles of the brain
10. epididymis with contrast material
11. liver
12. uterine cavity and fallopian tubes
13. larynx
14. lymphatic vessels and node
15. spinal cord
16. ureter and renal pelvis
17. salivary duct and branches
18. sinus or sinus tract
19. spleen
20. any part of the urinary system
21. vein and tributaries
22. seminal vesicles

Exercise 28-2

1. position
2. projection
3. anteroposterior
4. posteroanterior
5. right anterior oblique
6. left posterior oblique
7. dorsal
8. ventral
9. right lateral recumbent
10. dorsal decubitus, left lateral

Exercise 28-3

1. separate
2. MUE or Medically Unlikely Edits, or Medically Unbelievable Edits
3. Diagnostic Radiology; Diagnostic Ultrasound; Breast, Mammography; Bone/Joint Studies; Radiation Oncology; or Nuclear Medicine (in any order)

Exercise 28-4

1. 77056 (Mammography)
2. 76499 (Radiology, Unlisted Services and Procedures, Radiographic)
3. 75605 (Aortography, Aorta Imaging)

Exercise 28-5

1. Head and Neck
2. Chest
3. Abdomen and Retroperitoneum
4. Spinal Canal
5. Pelvis
6. Genitalia
7. Extremities
8. Ultrasonic Guidance Procedures
9. Other Procedures

Exercise 28-6

1. 76800 (Ultrasound, Spine)
2. 76604 (Ultrasound, Chest)
3. 76700 (Ultrasound, Abdomen)
4. 76816 × 2 (Ultrasound, Pregnant Uterus)
   ICD-10-CM: **O30.003** (Pregnancy, twin)
   ICD-9-CM: **651.03** (Pregnancy, twin, antepartum), **V91.00** (Gestation, multiple)
5. 76818 (Ultrasound, Fetus)
   ICD-10-CM: **O24.019** (Pregnancy, complicated by diabetes (mellitus), pre-exiting, type 1)
   ICD-9-CM: **648.03** (Pregnancy, complicated by, diabetes), **250.01** (Diabetes)

Exercise 28-7

1. 77290 (Radiation Therapy, Field Set-Up)
2. 77261 (Radiation Therapy, Planning)

Exercise 28-8

1. 77333 (Radiation Therapy, Treatment Device)
2. 77316 (Radiation Therapy, Dose Plan, Brachytherapy)
3. 77306 (Radiation Therapy, Dose Plan, Teletherapy)

ICD-10-CM: **C61** (Neoplasm, prostate, Malignant Primary)

ICD-9-CM: **185** (Neoplasm, prostate, Malignant, Primary)

Exercise 28-9

1. 77402 (Radiation Therapy, Treatment Delivery)
2. 77401 (Radiation Therapy, Treatment Delivery)
3. 77412 (Radiation Therapy, Treatment Delivery)
4. 77407 (Radiation Therapy, Treatment Delivery)
5. 77412 (Radiation Therapy, Treatment Delivery)
   ICD-10-CM: **C79.51** (Neoplasm, bone, spine, Malignant Secondary), **C80.1** (Neoplasm, unknown site or unspecified, Malignant Primary)
   ICD-9-CM: **198.5** (Neoplasm, bone, spine, Malignant, Secondary), **199.1** (Neoplasm, unknown site or unspecified, Malignant, Primary)

Exercise 28-10

1. 77427 (Radiation Therapy, Treatment Delivery, Weekly)
2. 77499 (Radiation Therapy, Treatment Management, Unlisted Services and Procedures)

Exercise 28-11

1. 77761 (Brachytherapy, Intracavity Application)
2. 77776 (Brachytherapy, Application)
3. 77789 (Brachytherapy, Surface Application)
   ICD-10-CM: **C56.9** (Neoplasm, ovary, Malignant Primary)
   ICD-9-CM: **183.0** (Neoplasm, ovary, Malignant, Primary)

Exercise 28-12

1. Gastrointestinal System
2. Endocrine System
3. Hematopoietic, Reticuloendothelial, and Lymphatic System
4. Musculoskeletal System
5. Nervous System

CHAPTER 29

Exercise 29-1

1. 80076 (Organ or Disease Oriented Panel, Hepatic Function Panel)
   ICD-10-CM: **B18.1** (Hepatitis, type, B, chronic)
   ICD-9-CM: **070.32** (Hepatitis, type B, chronic)
2. seven
3. yes
4. yes

Exercise 29-2

1. 80300 (Drug Assay, Cocaine)
2. 80162 (Drug Assay, Digoxin)
3. 80150 (Drug Assay, Amikacin
   ICD-10-CM: **D70.9** (Neutropenia, [immune]), **R50.81** (Fever, due to, conditions classified elsewhere)

ICD-9-CM: **780.60** (Fever); **288.09** (Neutropenia, immune), **780.61** (Fever, in conditions classified elsewhere).

The notes in the Tabular after D70 state to "Use additional code" for any associated fever (R50.81).

The notes in the Tabular after 288.0 state to "Use additional code" for any associated fever (780.61).

4. 80178 (Drug Assay, Lithium)
   ICD-10-CM: **F31.9** (Manic-depressive)
   ICD-9-CM: **296.80** (Depression, manic)

Exercise 29-3

1. 81003 (Urinalysis, Automated)
2. 81015 (Urinalysis, Microscopic)
3. 82040 (Albumin, Serum)
4. 82247 (Bilirubin, Total, Direct)
5. 82800 (Blood Gases, pH)
   ICD-10-CM: **J96.90** (Failure, respiratory)
   ICD-9-CM: **518.81** (Failure, respiratory)
6. 84300 (Sodium, Urine)
   ICD-10-CM: **I50.9** (Failure, heart, congestive)
   ICD-9-CM: **428.0** (Failure, heart, congestive)
7. 84550 (Uric Acid, Blood)
   ICD-10-CM: **M10.00** (Gout, idiopathic)
   ICD-9-CM: **274.01** (Gout, arthritis, acute)

Exercise 29-4

1. 85027 (Hemogram, Automated)
2. 85025 (Hemogram, Automated)
   ICD-10-CM: **D62** (Anemia, blood loss, acute)
   ICD-9-CM: **285.1** (Anemia, blood loss, acute)
3. 85041 (Red Blood Cell, Count)
4. 85097 (Bone Marrow, Smear)
   ICD-10-CM: **C95.01** (Leukemia, unspecified cell type, acute)
   ICD-9-CM: **208.01** (Leukemia, acute, in remission)

Exercise 29-5

1. 86039 (Antibody, Antinuclear)
2. 86063 (Antibody, Antistreptolysin O)
3. 86156 (Cold Agglutinin)
   ICD-10-CM: **J06.9** (Infection, respiratory, upper)
   ICD-9-CM: **465.9** (Infection, respiratory, upper [acute])

Exercise 29-6

1. 86900 (Blood Typing, gerologic, ABO only); 86901 (Blood Typing, gerologic, Rh)
2. 86945 × 3 (Blood Products, Irradiation)

Exercise 29-7

1. 87536 (Microbiology)
2. 87651 (Microbiology)
   ICD-10-CM: **R51** (Headache), **R50.9** (Fever)
   ICD-9-CM: **784.0** (Headache), **780.60** (Fever)

3. 87512 (Microbiology); 87530 (Microbiology); 87482 (Microbiology)
   ICD-10-CM: **N76.0** (Vaginitis, bacterial)
   ICD-9-CM: **616.10** (Vaginitis, bacterial)
4. 87555 (Microbiology); 87528 (Microbiology); 87490 (Microbiology)
5. 87086 (Culture, Bacteria, Urine)
   ICD-10-CM: **R35.0** (Frequency, micturition)
   ICD-9-CM: **788.41** (Frequency [urinary])

Exercise 29-8

1. 88309 (Pathology, Surgical, Gross and Micro Exam Level VI)
2. 88309 (Pathology, Surgical, Gross and Micro Exam Level VI)
3. 88305 (Pathology, Surgical, Gross and Micro Exam Level IV)
4. 88302 (Pathology, Surgical, Gross and Micro Exam Level II)

CHAPTER 30

Exercise 30-1

1. 90712 (Vaccines, Poliovirus, Live, Oral); 90473 (Immunization Administration, One Vaccine/Toxoid)
   ICD-10-CM: **Z23** (Immunization, encounter for)
   ICD-9-CM: **V04.0** (Vaccination, prophylactic, poliomyelitis)
2. 90715 (Vaccines, Tetanus, Diphtheria, Acellular Pertussis); 90712 (Vaccines, Polio Virus, Live, Oral); 90471 for first injection; and 90474 for the administration service (Immunization Administration)
   ICD-10-CM: **Z23** (Immunization, encounter for)
   ICD-9-CM: **V06.1** (Vaccination, prophylactic, diphtheria, with, tetanus, pertussis combined [DTP]), **V04.0** (Vaccination, prophylactic, poliomyelitis)
3. 99392-25 (Preventive Medicine, Established Patient); 90713 (Vaccines, Poliovirus, Inactivated, Intramuscular or Subcutaneous); 90702 (Vaccines, Diphtheria, Tetanus [DT]); 90460 (Immunization Administration, One Vaccine/Toxoid, with Counseling), 90461 (Immunization Administration, Each Additional Vaccine/Toxoid, with Counseling)
   ICD-10-CM: **Z00.129** (Examination, child), **Z23** (Immunization, encounter for), **Z71.89** (Counseling, medical [for], specified reason NEC)
   ICD-9-CM: **V20.2** (Examination, child care, routine), **V06.5** (Vaccination, tetanus toxoid, with diphtheria), **V04.0** (Vaccination, prophylactic, poliomyelitis) (Admission for: well baby and child care; and, admission for vaccination)
   Note that E/M code 99392 is used here because the well-baby checkup service provided is significant and separate from the injection service.
4. 90658 (Vaccines, Influenza); 90471 (Immunization Administration, One Vaccine/Toxoid)
   ICD-10-CM: **Z23** (Immunization, encounter for)
   ICD-9-CM: **V04.81** (Vaccination, prophylactic, influenza)

5. 99202-25 (Office and/or Other Outpatient Services, New Patient); 90720, combination code for DTP and Hib (Vaccines, Diphtheria, Tetanus, Whole Cell Pertussis and Hemophilus Influenza B); 90471 (Immunization Administration, One Vaccine/Toxoid)
   ICD-10-CM: **E03.9** (Hypothyroidism [acquired]), **Z23** (Immunization, encounter for)
   ICD-9-CM: **244.9** (Hypothyroidism), **V06.1** (Vaccination, prophylactic, diphtheria, tetanus, pertussis combined), **V03.81** (Vaccination, prophylactic, Haemophilus influenzae, type B [HIB])
   Note: E/M code 99202 is assigned here because the E/M service provided was significant and separate from the injection service.
6. 99392-25 (Preventive Medicine, Established Patient); 90702 (Vaccines, Diphtheria, Tetanus [DT]); 90460 (Immunization Administration, One Vaccine/Toxoid, with Counseling), 90461 (Immunization Administration, Each Additional Vaccine/Toxoid, with Counseling)
   ICD-10-CM: **Z00.129** (Examination, child), **Z23** (Immunization, encounter for), **Z71.89** (Counseling, medical [for], specified reason NEC)
   ICD-9-CM: **V20.2** (Examination, child care, routine), **V06.5** (Vaccination, prophylactic, diphtheria, with tetanus)
   Note that an E/M code, 99392, is used here because the E/M service provided was significant and was separate from the injection service.
7. 90658 (Vaccines, Influenza, Trivalent), 90471 (Immunization Administration, One Vaccine/Toxoid)
   ICD-10-CM: **Z23** (Immunization, encounter for)
   ICD-9-CM: **V04.81** (Vaccination, prophylactic, influenza)

Exercise 30-2

1. 90791 (Psychiatric Evaluation)
   ICD-10-CM: **F22** (Psychosis, paranoid)
   ICD-9-CM: **297.1** (Psychosis, paranoid, chronic)
2. 96101 × 2 (Psychiatric Diagnosis, Psychological Testing)
   ICD-10-CM: **F91.1** (Disturbance, conduct, undersocialized)
   ICD-9-CM: **312.02** (Disturbance, conduct, undersocialized, aggressive)
3. 90885 (Psychiatric Diagnosis, Evaluation of Records or Reports)
   ICD-10-CM: **F93.8** (Disturbance, emotions specific to childhood and adolescence, with anxiety and fearfulness)
   ICD-9-CM: **313.0** (Disorder, overanxious, of childhood and adolescence)
4. 90837 (Psychotherapy, Individual Patient/Family Member)
   ICD-10-CM: **F32.9** (Depression), **R25.1** (Tremor)
   ICD-9-CM: **311** (Depression), **781.0** (Tremor)

Exercise 30-3

1. 90875 (Biofeedback, Psychophysiological)
   ICD-10-CM: **F41.1** (Anxiety, generalized), **F51.01** (Insomnia, idiopathic), **F17.218** (Dependence, nicotine, cigarettes)

ICD-9-CM: **300.02** (Anxiety, generalized), **307.42** (Insomnia, idiopathic), **305.1** (Dependence, nicotine)
2. 90901 (Training, Biofeedback)
ICD-10-CM: **I11.9** (Hypertension, heart)
ICD-9-CM: **402.90** (Hypertension, with heart involvement)

Exercise 30-4

1. 90955 (Dialysis, End-Stage Renal Disease)
ICD-10-CM: **N18.6** (Disease, renal, end-stage [failure]), **Z99.2** (Status, dialysis)
ICD-9-CM: **585.6** (Disease, kidney, chronic, requiring chronic dialysis), **V45.11** (Status, renal dialysis)
2. 90935 (Dialysis, Hemodialysis)
ICD-10-CM: **N17.9** (Failure, renal, acute)
ICD-9-CM: **584.9** (Failure, renal, acute)
3. 90947 (Dialysis, Peritoneal)
ICD-10-CM: **N17.0** (Failure, renal, with, tubular necrosis)
ICD-9-CM: **584.5** (Failure, renal, with lesion of necrosis, tubular)
4. within the lining of the abdominal cavity
5. filtration of blood and waste products through a filter outside the body
6. end-stage renal disease

Exercise 30-5

1. 91038 (Esophagus, Acid Reflux Tests)
ICD-10-CM: **K21.9** (Reflux, gastroesophageal)
ICD-9-CM: **530.81** (Reflux, gastroesophageal)
2. 91117 (Motility Study, Colon)
3. 43754 (Intubation, Specimen Collection, Gastric)
ICD-10-CM: **R10.9** (Pain, abdominal), **R63.0** (Appetite, lack or loss)
ICD-9-CM: **789.00** (Pain, abdominal), **783.0** (Appetite, loss)
4. spontaneous movement study
5. pressure measurements

Exercise 30-6

1. 92014 (Ophthalmology, Diagnostic, Eye Exam, Established Patient)
2. 92071 (Contact Lens Services, Fittings and Prescription)
3. 92100 (Ophthalmology, Diagnostic, Tonometry, Serial)
ICD-10-CM: **H40.009** (Glaucoma, borderline)
ICD-9-CM: **365.00** (Glaucoma, borderline) (the stage of glaucoma is not reported as the documentation stated "preglaucoma")
4. 92004 (Ophthalmology, Diagnostic, Eye Exam, New Patient)
ICD-10-CM: **E11.359** (Diabetes, type 2, with, retinopathy, proliferative)
ICD-9-CM: **250.51, 362.02** (Diabetes, with ophthalmic manifestations)

Exercise 30-7

1. 92592 (Hearing Aid Check)
2. 92551 (Audiologic Function Tests, Screening)
3. 92511 (Nasopharyngoscopy)

ICD-10-CM: **R04.2** (Sputum, blood stained)
ICD-9-CM: **786.30** (Sputum, bloody)
4. 92512 (Nasal Function Study)
ICD-10-CM: **R06.89** (Hypoventilation)
ICD-9-CM: **786.09** (Inadequate, respiration)

Exercise 30-8

1. 93965 (Plethysmography, Extremities, Veins)
ICD-10-CM: **I73.9** (Claudication, intermittent)
ICD-9-CM: **443.9** (Claudication, intermittent)
2. 93980 (Vascular Studies, Penile Vessels)
ICD-10-CM: **N52.9** (Impotence, organic origin)
ICD-9-CM: **607.84** (Impotence, organic)

Exercise 30-9

1. 94620 (Pulmonology, Diagnostic, Stress Test, Pulmonary)
2. 94150 (Vital Capacity Measurement)
3. 94060 (Pulmonology, Diagnostic, Spirometry); **99070** (Supply, materials)
ICD-10-CM: **R05** (Cough), **F17.200** (Dependence, nicotine)
ICD-9-CM: **786.2** (Cough), **305.1** (Dependence, nicotine)

Exercise 30-10

1. 95065 (Allergy Tests, Nose Allergy)
2. 95004 × 10 (Allergy Tests, Skin Tests, Allergen Extract) (Note that one unit is used for each test.)
3. 95115 (Allergen Immunotherapy, Allergen, Injection)
ICD-10-CM: **J30.1** (Allergy, ragweed)
ICD-9-CM: **477.0** (Allergy, ragweed)
4. 95165 × 10 (Allergen Immunotherapy, Antigens, Preparation and Provision), 95115 (Allergen Immunotherapy, Allergenic Extracts, Injection)

Exercise 30-11

1. nasal continuous positive airway pressure
2. electroencephalogram
3. electromyogram
4. electro-oculogram
5. 95816 (Electroencephalography)
ICD-10-CM: **G47.30** (Apnea, sleep)
ICD-9-CM: **780.57** (Apnea, sleep)
6. 95863 (Electromyography, Needle, Extremities)
ICD-10-CM: **R20.0** (Numbness)
ICD-9-CM: **782.0** (Numbness)
7. 95851 × 2 (both legs) (Range of Motion Test, Extremities or Trunk)
ICD-10-CM: **R27.8** (Incoordination, muscular)
ICD-9-CM: **781.3** (Incoordination, muscular)

Exercise 30-12

1. 96110 (Developmental Test Screening)
ICD-10-CM: **F91.1** (Disorder, conduct, childhood onset type)
ICD-9-CM: **312.81** (Disturbance, conduct, childhood onset type)

2. 96101-32 (MMPI)
   ICD-10-CM: **Z01.89** (Test, specified NEC)
   ICD-9-CM: **V72.85** (Test, specified type NEC)
3. 96116 (Cognitive Function Tests)
   ICD-10-CM: **R53.83** (Lethargy)
   ICD-9-CM: **780.79** (Lethargy)

Exercise 30-13

1. 96440 (Chemotherapy, Pleural Cavity)
   ICD-10-CM: **C34.90** (Neoplasm, lung, unspecified site, Malignant Primary)
   ICD-9-CM: **162.9** (Neoplasm, lung, Malignant, Primary)
2. 96521 (Chemotherapy, Pump Services, Portable)
   ICD-10-CM: **C18.9** (Neoplasm, intestine, large, colon, Malignant Primary)
   ICD-9-CM: **153.9** (Neoplasm, intestine, large, colon, Malignant, Primary)
3. 96401 (Chemotherapy, Subcutaneous)
   ICD-10-CM: **C43.59** (Melanoma, skin, chest wall)
   ICD-9-CM: **172.5** (Melanoma, skin, chest wall)
4. 96413 (Chemotherapy, Intravenous)
   ICD-10-CM: **C50.919** (Neoplasm, breast, Malignant Primary), **C79.51** (Neoplasm, bone, spine, Malignant Secondary)
   ICD-9-CM: **174.9** (Neoplasm, breast, Malignant, Primary), **198.5** (Neoplasm, bone, spine, Malignant, Secondary)
5. 96450 (Chemotherapy, CNS)
   ICD-10-CM: **C71.9** (Neoplasm, brain, Malignant Primary)
   ICD-9-CM: **191.9** (Neoplasm, brain, Malignant, Primary)
6. 96372 (Injection, Intramuscular, Therapeutic); J3420 (Vitamin B12)

Exercise 30-14

1. 99241-25 (Consultation, Office and/or Other Outpatient); 96900 (Ultraviolet Light Therapy, for Dermatology)
   ICD-10-CM: **L70.0** (Acne, vulgaris)
   ICD-9-CM: **706.1** (Acne)
2. 99244-25 (Consultation, Office and/or Other Outpatient); 96913 (Photochemotherapy)
   ICD-10-CM: **L13.9** (Dermatosis, bullous)
   ICD-9-CM: **694.0** (Dermatosis, bullous)

Exercise 30-15

1. 97010 (Physical Medicine/Therapy/Occupational Therapy, Modalities, Hot or Cold Pack)
2. 97761 × 2 (Physical Medicine/Therapy/Occupational Therapy, Prosthetic Training)
3. 97116 × 2 (Physical Medicine/Therapy/Occupational Therapy, Procedures, Gait Training)
   ICD-10-CM: **I69.398** (Sequelae, infarction, cerebral, specified effect NEC)
   ICD-9-CM: **438.89** (Late effect, Cerebrovascular disease, specified type NEC)
   (Note that the stand-alone code 97110 specifies "each 15 minutes.")

Exercise 30-16

1. 98940 (Chiropractic Treatment, Spinal, Extraspinal)
   ICD-10-CM: **M25.552** (Pain, joint, hip)
   ICD-9-CM: **719.45** (Pain, joint, hip)
2. 98925 (Osteopathic Manipulation)
   ICD-10-CM: **M54.5** (Pain, lumbar region)
   ICD-9-CM: **724.2** (Pain, lumbar region)

Exercise 30-17

1. 99050 (Special Services, After Hours Medical Services)
2. 99000 (Special Services, Specimen Handling)
3. 99070 (Special Services, Supply of Materials)

CHAPTER 31

Exercise 31-1

1. No answer required.
2. a. Pyelonephritis, acute
   b. ICD-10-CM: **N10**
      ICD-9-CM: **590.10**
   c. 590, Infections of Kidney
   d. no
   e. ICD-10-CM: **N10**
      ICD-9-CM: **590.10**
   f. because flank pain and hematuria are symptoms of pyelonephritis

Exercise 31-2

1. No answer required.
2. a. open fracture of the right humerus and right distal femur
   b. Fracture
   c. humerus
   d. (closed)
      ICD-10-CM: **S42.301B**
      ICD-9-CM: 812.30
   e. Yes, because the patient record did not specify the exact location of the fracture of the humerus, so the "unspecified part of the humerus, open" is as specific as you can get with the information that you have available.
   f. femur
   g. (closed)
   h. distal or distal end
   i. *see* Fracture, femur, lower end
   j. open
   k. ICD-10-CM: **S72.401B**
      ICD-9-CM: 821.30
   l. yes

Exercise 31-3

1. No answer necessary.
2. a. menorrhagia
   b. ICD-10-CM: **N92.0**
      ICD-9-CM: **626.2**
   c. anemia

d. ICD-10-CM: **D62**
ICD-9-CM: **285.1**

Exercise 31-4

1. No answer necessary.
2. a. Fracture
   b. *See also* Fracture, by site
   c. ICD-10-CM: **C79 .51**
      ICD-9-CM: **198.5**

Exercise 31-5

1. a. ICD-10-CM: **M25.569**
      ICD-9-CM: **719.46**
   b. ICD-10-CM: **M23.202**
      ICD-9-CM: **717.0**
   c. ICD-10-CM: **M23.40**
      ICD-9-CM: **717.6**

Exercise 31-6

1. a. ICD-10-CM: **K80.10** (Calculus, gallbladder, with, cholecystitis)
      ICD-9-CM: **574.10** (Cholelithiasis with cholecystitis)
   b. ICD-10-CM: **J18.9** (Pneumonia)
      ICD-9-CM: **486** (Pneumonia)
   c. Contraindicated
   d. ICD-10-CM: **Z53.09** (Procedure, not done, because of, contraindication)
      ICD-9-CM: **V64.1** (Surgery, not done because of, contraindication)
2. a. 2; sterilization and surgery not done
   b. ICD-10-CM: **Z30.2** (Encounter (for) sterilization)
      ICD-9-CM: **V25.2** (Admission for sterilization)
   c. ICD-10-CM: **Z53.29** (Refusal of, treatment [because of], patient's decision NEC)
      ICD-9-CM: **V64.2** (Surgery, not done, because of, patient's decision)

Exercise 31-7

1. a. Postoperative ileus
   b. ICD-10-CM: **K91.89** (Complication, following, gastrointestinal, postoperative, specified NEC)
      ICD-9-CM: **997.49** (Complication, postoperative, digestive system)
   c. yes
   d. ICD-10-CM: **K56.0** (Ileus, paralytic)
      ICD-9-CM: **560.1** (Ileus, paralytic)
   e. yes
      ICD-10-CM: **C18.9** (Neoplasm, colon, Malignant Primary), **Y83.2** (Reaction, anastomosis)
      ICD-9-CM: **153.9** (Neoplasm, malignant, colon, unspecified)
2. a. Malfunction insulin pump
      ICD-10-CM: **T85.614A** (Complication, insulin pump, mechanical, breakdown)
      ICD-9-CM: **996.57** (Complications, due to [presence of] any device, implant, or graft, insulin pump)

b. ICD-10-CM: **Z79.4** (Long–term [current] drug therapy [use of], insulin)
   ICD-9-CM: **V58.67** (Long–term [current] drug use, insulin)
c. ICD-10-CM: **E10.9** (Diabetes, type 1)
   ICD-9-CM: **250.01** (Diabetes); **E932.3** (Insulin, Therapeutic use)

Exercise 31-8

1. a. Probable aspiration pneumonia
   b. ICD-10-CM: **J69.0** (Pneumonia, aspiration)
      ICD-9-CM: **507.0** (Pneumonia, aspiration)
   c. yes
      ICD-10-CM: **I69.391** (Dysphagia, following, cerebral infarction), **I10** (Hypertension, unspecified)
      ICD-9-CM: **438.82** (Late effect, cerebrovascular disease); **787.20** (Dysphagia); **401.9** (Hypertension)
2. a. Suspected malignancy, right kidney
   b. ICD-10-CM: **C64.1** (Neoplasm, kidney [parenchymal], right, Malignant Primary)
      ICD-9-CM: **189.0** (Neoplasm, kidney [parenchymal], Malignant, Primary)
   c. yes
      ICD-10-CM: **R31.9** (Hematuria)
      ICD-9-CM: **599.70** (Hematuria)

Exercise 31-9

1. a. Postoperative atrial fibrillation
   b. ICD-10-CM: **I97.191** (Complication[s], postprocedural, cardiac functional disturbance, following other surgery)
      ICD-9-CM: **997.1** (Complications, surgical procedure, cardiac)
   c. ICD-10-CM: **I48.91** (Fibrillation, atrial or auricular [established]), **M32.14** (Lupus, nephritis)
      ICD-9-CM: **427.31** (Fibrillation, atrial); **710.0, 583.81** (Lupus, nephritis)
   d. yes, **55.23** (Biopsy, kidney, percutaneous [aspiration] [needle])
   e. ICD-10-CM: **Y84.8** (Complication [delayed] of or following [medical or surgical procedure], biopsy), **Y92.238** (External Cause Index: Place of occurrence, hospital, specified)
      ICD-9-CM: **E879.8** (Reaction, abnormal to or following [medical or surgical procedure], biopsy); **E849.7** (Accident, occuring [at] [in], hospital)

Exercise 31-10

1. History of hysterectomy
2. History of peptic ulcer disease
3. Remote history of appendectomy

Exercise 31-11

1. Yes
2. No

Exercise 31-12

1. F
2. 1
3. B
4. 0
5. D
6. 0

Exercise 31-13

1. 7
2. L
3. M
4. G
5. N
6. 1
7. R
8. 5
9. T
10. 8

Exercise 31-14

1. transfer
2. excision
3. inspection
4. transplantation
5. insertion
6. removal
7. fragmentation
8. occlusion
9. revision
10. release

Exercise 31-15

1. complete
2. expandable
3. multiaxial
4. standardized in terminology (in any order)
5. 7
6. alphanumeric
7. 34
8. O and I
9. procedure

Quick Check Answers

CHAPTER 1

Quick Check 1-1
1. a
2. b, c, d
3. a
4. d
5. b
6. b, c, d
7. a, b, c

CHAPTER 2

Quick Check 2-1
1. Y93.44

Quick Check 2-2
1. Q28.1
2. R10.0

Quick Check 2-3
1. 098.
2. J00-J22

CHAPTER 3

Quick Check 3-1
1. Z23
2. Z20
3. no

Quick Check 3-2
1. Z03.810
2. medical

CHAPTER 4

Quick Check 4-1
1. yes
2. no

Quick Check 4-2
1. K86.1
2. K85.0

CHAPTER 5

Quick Check 5-1
1. B95.62
2. vancomycin
3. *Staphylococcus*

Quick Check 5-2
1. C95, Z85.6
2. M84.5, neoplasm

CHAPTER 7

Quick Check 7-1
1. 14
2. 14, 28
3. 28

Quick Check 7-2
1. Z37.0
2. first
3. complicating

CHAPTER 8

Quick Check 8-1
1. a. 6
2. Notes instruct coder to "See listing at the beginning of the chapter for definitions" where a full list is included under each subclassification and "Knee joint" is listed under "6 lower leg."

Quick Check 8-2
1. *Official Guidelines for Coding and Reporting*
2. Footer of each page

CHAPTER 10

Quick Check 10-1
1. The presence and location of the *Official Guidelines for Coding and Reporting* may vary depending on the publisher of the ICD-9-CM manual, and some do not include them at all.

Quick Check 10-2
1. There is an instructional note to use an additional code to identify organism, such as *Staphylococcus* (041.1).
2. No, the fifth digit is missing.

CHAPTER 11

Quick Check 11-1
1. 229.9 (Neoplasm, unknown site or unspecified, Benign)

CHAPTER 12

Quick Check 12-1
d. All of the above

CHAPTER 13

Quick Check 13-1
1. True

Quick Check 13-2
1. unlisted

Quick Check 13-3
1. unlisted, III

Quick Check 13-4
1. Use, CPT

Quick Check 13-5
1. J0120-J9999
2. a. HCPCS

Quick Check 13-6
1. S
2. G
3. K
4. Q

Quick Check 13-7
1. c
2. b
3. a

Quick Check 13-8
1. True

CHAPTER 14

Quick Check 14-1
1. five

Quick Check 14-2
1. d. All of the above

Quick Check 14-3
1. ⊘ Symbol preceding a code indicates it is modifier -51 exempt.

Quick Check 14-4
1. No. Parenthetical notes following codes indicate modifier -63 is not reported with these codes.

CHAPTER 15

Quick Check 15-1
1. exceed, three

Quick Check 15-2
1. True

Quick Check 15-3
1. e. All of the above

Quick Check 15-4
1. Yes

Quick Check 15-5
1. outpatient

Quick Check 15-6
1. Time

Quick Check 15-7
1. Written or verbal request, written report

Quick Check 15-8
1. Yes

Quick Check 15-9
1. None
2. Yes

Quick Check 15-10
1. Any two of:
   - Interpretation of cardiac output measure (93561, 93562)
   - Chest x-rays (71010, 71015, 71020)
   - Pulse Oximetry (94760, 94761, 94762)
   - Blood gases and information data stored in computers (e.g., ECGs, blood pressures, hematologic data [99090])
   - Temporary transcutaneous pacing (92953)
   - Ventilator management (94002-94004, 94660, 94662)
   - Vascular access procedures (36000, 36410, 36415, 36591, 36600)

CHAPTER 16

Quick Check 16-1
1. In the CPT index, locate the main term "Injection," subterm "Spinal Cord," then subterm "Blood" for code 62273 OR main term "Spinal Cord," subterm "Injection," then subterm "Blood."

Quick Check 16-2
1. Anesthesia Guidelines

Quick Check 16-3
1. QX: Indicates medical direction of a CRNA by a physician and is appended to the CRNA portion of the charge. QY: Indicates medical direction by an anesthesiologist of one CRNA and is appended to the physician portion of the charge.

CHAPTER 17

Quick Check 17-1
1. True (The listing is found before each subsection of the Surgery section.)

Quick Check 17-2
1. III

Quick Check 17-3
1. False

CHAPTER 18

Quick Check 18-1
1. False

Quick Check 18-2
1. b
2. c
3. a

Quick Check 18-3
1. b. reported separately

CHAPTER 19

Quick Check 19-1
1. a. 27506

Quick Check 19-2
1. no

Quick Check 19-3
1. anatomic

Quick Check 19-4
1. -58

CHAPTER 20

Quick Check 20-1
1. open, intranasal

CHAPTER 21

Quick Check 21-1
1. The three main coronary arteries include: right coronary (RC), left anterior descending (LD), and left circumflex (LC).

Quick Check 21-2
1. CABG

Quick Check 21-3
1. Appendix L

Quick Check 21-4
1. c. saphenous vein graft

CHAPTER 22

Quick Check 22-1
1. True

Quick Check 22-2
1. -50

CHAPTER 23

Quick Check 23-1
1. cross

Quick Check 23-2
1. extent

Quick Check 23-3
1. Any two of the following: inguinal, lumbar, incisional (ventral), epigastric, umbilical, spigelian, diaphragmatic (hiatal).

   Hernia repairs using an abdominal approach are located in the Abdomen, Peritoneum, and Omentum subsection, Repair subheading (49491-49611). Laparoscopic hernia repairs are in the Laparoscopy subheading (49650-49659).

CHAPTER 24

Quick Check 24-1
1. False, they may not pass spontaneously

Quick Check 24-2
1. externally

Quick Check 24-3
1. nephrostomy, pyelostomy

Quick Check 24-4
1. 50945

Quick Check 24-5
1. 58240

Quick Check 24-6
1. cystoscopy, urethroscopy

Quick Check 24-7
1. Integumentary

Quick Check 24-8
1. 28

Quick Check 24-9
1. non-inflatable, inflatable

Quick Check 24-10
1. orchiopexy

Quick Check 24-11
1. 54700

Quick Check 24-12
1. abdomen, perineum

Quick Check 24-13
1. VLAP, ILCP

Quick Check 24-14
1. b
2. c
3. a

Quick Check 24-15
1. needle, punch

CHAPTER 25

Quick Check 25-1
1. 2

Quick Check 25-2
1. The weight of the uterus
2. b. approach, number, weight

Quick Check 25-3
1. Codes 58951, 58953, 58954, 58956

CHAPTER 26

Quick Check 26-1
1. anterior, posterior

Quick Check 26-2
1. 64400-64530
2. 64600-64681

CHAPTER 27

Quick Check 27-1
1. b
2. c
3. a

Quick Check 27-2
1. b
2. c
3. d
4. a

Quick Check 27-3
1. False

CHAPTER 28

Quick Check 28-1
1. 76810

Quick Check 28-2
1. False

CHAPTER 29

Quick Check 29-1
1. modifier -91

Quick Check 29-2
1. report separate entries

Quick Check 29-3
1. 88150-88154

CHAPTER 30

Quick Check 30-1
1. b

Quick Check 30-2
1. absence of the lens of the eye

Quick Check 30-3
1. d. EEG, EOG, EMG

EHR Screens

South Padre Medical Center						Melville, James Q	▢ ▢ ✕

| **Pt info** | Provider Info | Payer Info | Encounter Notes | Claim Info | Charge Capture | Admin Info | Emergency Contact | Exit |

Patient Name

Last [ ] First [ ] MI [ ] Suffix [ ]

Name Preference [ ] Patient ID [ ]

Patient Information

Address 1 [ ] DOB [MM] [DD] [YYYY] M/F/U [ ]

Address 2 [ ] Home Ph ([ ])- [ ] - [ ]

City [ ] Cell Ph ([ ])- [ ] - [ ]

State [ ] Zip [ ] – [ ] Work Ph ([ ])- [ ] - [ ]

Notes

Date Note

[MM] [DD] [YYYY] [ ]

[MM] [DD] [YYYY] [ ]

[MM] [DD] [YYYY] [ ]

FIGURE D–1 Sample EHR Screen, Patient Information

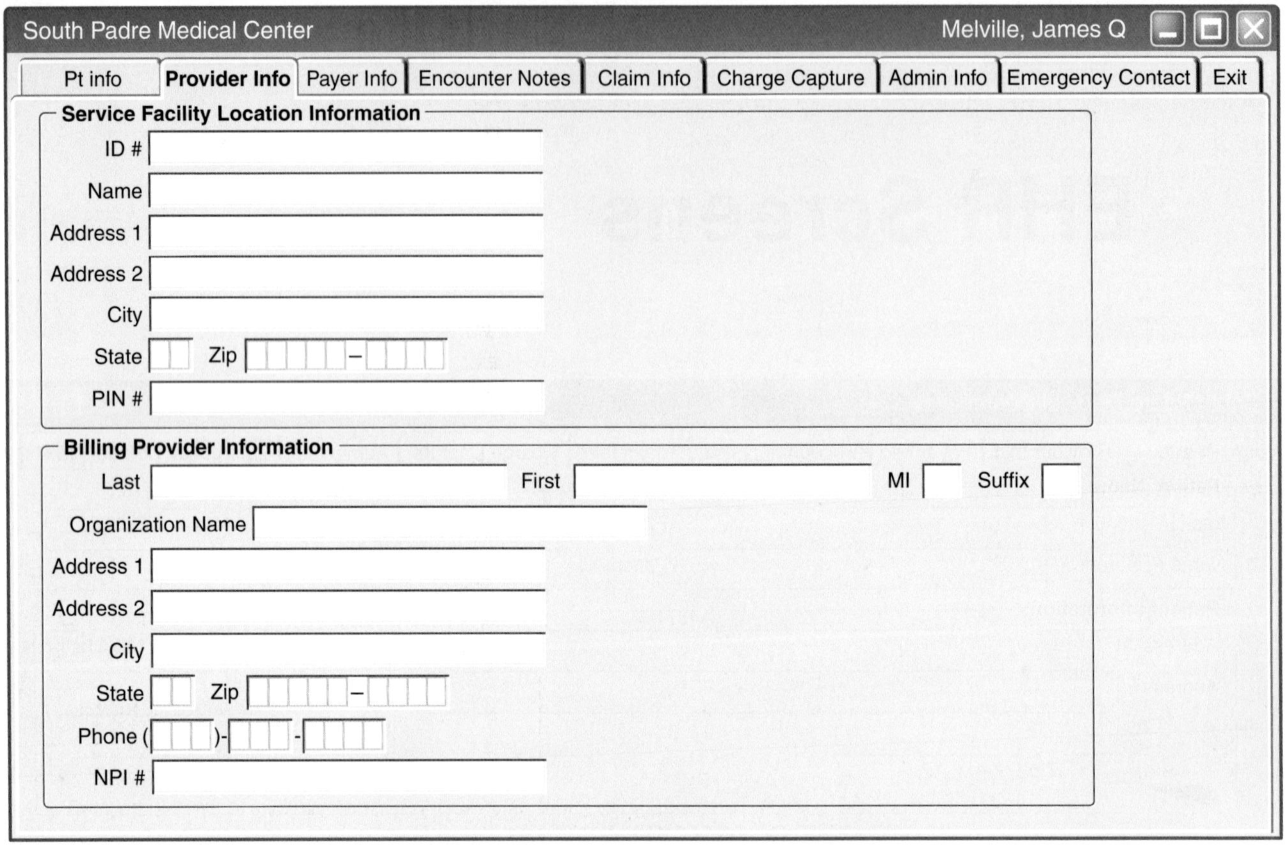

| South Padre Medical Center | | | | | | Melville, James Q | ▬ ☐ ✕ |

| Pt info | **Provider Info** | Payer Info | Encounter Notes | Claim Info | Charge Capture | Admin Info | Emergency Contact | Exit |

Service Facility Location Information

ID #

Name

Address 1

Address 2

City

State ☐☐   Zip ☐☐☐☐☐ – ☐☐☐☐

PIN #

Billing Provider Information

Last   First   MI ☐   Suffix ☐

Organization Name

Address 1

Address 2

City

State ☐☐   Zip ☐☐☐☐☐ – ☐☐☐☐

Phone (☐☐☐) - ☐☐☐ - ☐☐☐☐

NPI #

FIGURE D-2   Sample EHR Screen, Provider Information

South Padre Medical Center   Melville, James Q [_] [□] [X]

| Pt info | Provider Info | **Payer Info** | Encounter Notes | Claim Info | Charge Capture | Admin Info | Emergency Contact | Exit |

Payer Information

○ Primary   ○ Secondary   ○ Tertiary

Payer Name [_____ ▾]   Payer Identifier [_____]

Insured's Group # [_____]   Insured's ID # [_____]

Secondary ID [_____]   Qualifier [_____]   Prior Authorization [_____]

Payer Billing Address

Address 1 [_____]

Address 2 [_____]

City [_____]

State [__]   Zip [_____]–[____]

Phone ([___])-[___]-[____]

Insured's Name

Relation to insured

○ Self   ○ Spouse   ○ Dependent

Last [_____]   First [_____]   MI [__]   Suffix [__]

DOB [MM][DD][YYYY]   M/F/U [__]

Address 1 [_____]

Address 2 [_____]

City [_____]

State [__]   Zip [_____]–[____]

Phone ([___])-[___]-[____]

Employer name [_____]   School name [_____]

FIGURE D–3   Sample EHR Screen, Payer Information

South Padre Medical Center — Melville, James Q

| Pt info | Provider Info | Payer Info | **Encounter Notes** | Claim Info | Charge Capture | Admin Info | Emergency Contact | Exit |

Encounter Notes Opened by Dr. Morris Polson

Last: Melville First: James MI: Q Suffix: Age: 76 DOB: 01 12 1935 M/F/U:

HPI: James is here for a followup. Overall he has been doing well. His energy level has not changed much from the other time, but overall he is doing well. He does not have any acute complaints. When he saw Dr. Marcus, he was put on a new medication. Unfortunately, he does not recall the name. He seems to be tolerating it well.

REVIEW OF SYSTEMS: Today, it is negative for back pain and energy level is unchanged from last time, no nausea or vomiting, also lower leg edema is unchanged.

O: Blood pressure 118/60. Respirations 20. Pulse is 80. Temperature is 98.0. Weight is 214 lbs. In general, James is a very pleasant male in no acute distress. He is alert x3.

AP: Fatigue from before. At this time, I still think it could be related to the degree of his anemia and hypothyroidism. However, given the fact that he is currently followed by a nephrologist, rheumatologist, chronic pain physician, I have not much else to offer other than to be on standby for the time being. We are going to obtain the records from Dr. Marcus, but I would like to see him back in six months for a general followup, before that if needed.

Encounter Data
MM DD YYYY
1:15 PM

Lab Orders
Wellness panel
CBC

Rad Orders

Encounter Diagnoses

DX1	Pernicious anemia	DX5		DX9	
DX2	Hypothyroidism	DX6		DX10	
DX3	Fatigue	DX7		DX11	
DX4	Stage 2 CKD	DX8		DX12	

Signature of Physician

Signed ○ _____ Date MM DD YYYY

Federal Tax I.D. Number _____ ☐ SSN ☐ EIN

FIGURE D–4 Sample EHR Screen, Encounter Notes

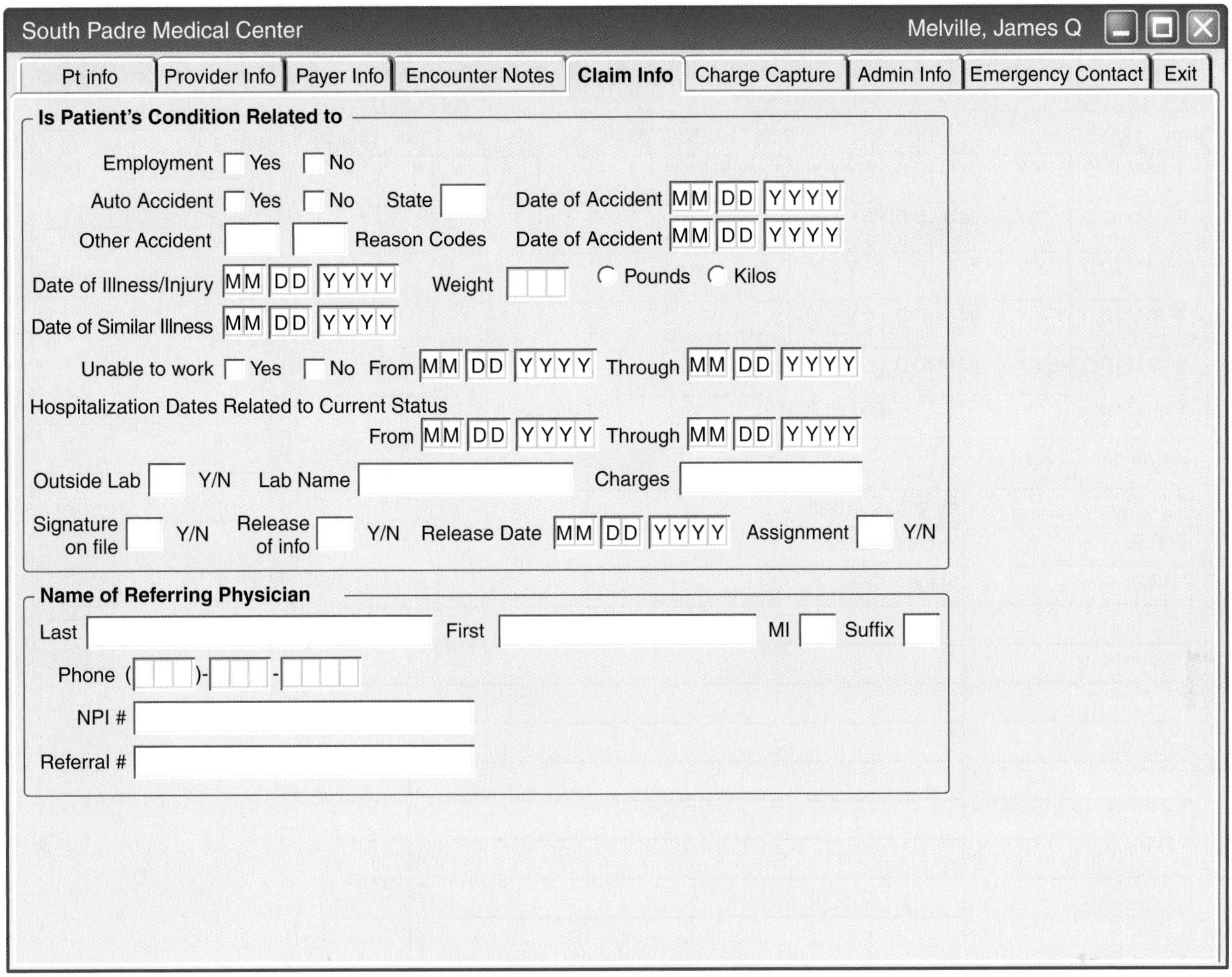

South Padre Medical Center   Melville, James Q   ⊟ ▣ ⊠

| Pt info | Provider Info | Payer Info | Encounter Notes | **Claim Info** | Charge Capture | Admin Info | Emergency Contact | Exit |

Is Patient's Condition Related to

Employment ☐ Yes ☐ No

Auto Accident ☐ Yes ☐ No   State ☐   Date of Accident MM DD YYYY

Other Accident ☐ ☐   Reason Codes   Date of Accident MM DD YYYY

Date of Illness/Injury MM DD YYYY   Weight ☐   ○ Pounds ○ Kilos

Date of Similar Illness MM DD YYYY

Unable to work ☐ Yes ☐ No From MM DD YYYY Through MM DD YYYY

Hospitalization Dates Related to Current Status

From MM DD YYYY Through MM DD YYYY

Outside Lab ☐ Y/N   Lab Name ☐   Charges ☐

Signature on file ☐ Y/N   Release of info ☐ Y/N   Release Date MM DD YYYY   Assignment ☐ Y/N

Name of Referring Physician

Last ☐   First ☐   MI ☐   Suffix ☐

Phone (☐)-☐-☐

NPI # ☐

Referral # ☐

FIGURE D-5 Sample EHR Screen, Claim Information

South Padre Medical Center — Melville, James Q

| Pt info | Provider Info | Payer Info | Encounter Notes | Claim Info | **Charge Capture** | Admin Info | Emergency Contact | Exit |

Item	DOS From	DOS To	POS	HCPCS	M1	M2	M3	M4	Units	Charge
1	MM DD YYYY	MM DD YYYY	11	99213					1	
2	MM DD YYYY	MM DD YYYY	11	99213						
3	MM DD YYYY	MM DD YYYY	11	99213						
4	MM DD YYYY	MM DD YYYY								
5	MM DD YYYY	MM DD YYYY								

Total Charge [ ]   Amount Paid [ ]   Balance Due [ ]

Recent Diagnoses
- E03.9
- D51.0
- R60.0
- M54.5
- M05.9
- N18.2
- K64.9

Diagnostic Codes

		Item
D51.0	Pernicious anemia	1
E03.9	Hypothyroidism	1
N18.2	Stage 2 CKD	1

FIGURE D–6   Sample EHR Screen, Charge Capture

South Padre Medical Center — Melville, James Q

| Pt info | Provider Info | Payer Info | Encounter Notes | Claim Info | Charge Capture | **Admin Info** | Emergency Contact | Exit |

HIPAA
Form on file? ✓ Yes ☐ No
Dated MM DD YYYY

Living Will
Copy on file? ✓ Yes ☐ No
Dated MM DD YYYY

Primary Physician
Name   Steven Poison, MD
Phone ( ) - -

FIGURE D–7   Sample EHR Screen, Administration Information

South Padre Medical Center   Melville, James Q

| Pt info | Provider Info | Payer Info | Encounter Notes | Claim Info | Charge Capture | Admin Info | **Emergency Contact** | Exit |

Emergency Contact

Name: Last _____   First _____   MI ____   Suffix ____

Relationship _____

Address 1 _____

Address 2 _____

City _____

State ____   Zip _____ – ____

Home (____)-____-____

Cell (____)-____-____

Work (____)-____-____

FIGURE D–8 Sample EHR Screen, Emergency Contact

Glossary

A-mode: one-dimensional ultrasonic display reflecting the time it takes a sound wave to reach a structure and reflect back; maps the structure's outline

ablation: removal by cutting or destruction

abortion: termination of pregnancy

abscess: localized collection of pus that will result in the disintegration of tissue over time

abuse: misuse of substance

acquired: not genetic

actinotherapy: treatment of acne using ultraviolet rays

acute: of sudden onset and short duration

addiction: dependence on a drug

admission: attention to an acute illness or injury resulting in admission to a hospital

adrenal: glands, located at the top of the kidneys, that produce steroid hormones

AHA: American Hospital Association

AHIMA: American Health Information Management Association

allogenic: a graft that is from the same species, but genetically different

allograft: tissue graft between individuals who are not of the same genotype

allotransplantation: transplantation between individuals who are not of the same genotype

amniocentesis: percutaneous aspiration of amniotic fluid

anastomosis: surgical connection of two tubular structures, such as two pieces of the intestine

aneurysm: is an abnormal weakening of a vessel wall with outpouching beyond the normal confines of the vessel

angiography: taking of x-ray films of vessels after injection of contrast material

angioplasty: surgical or percutaneous procedure in a vessel to dilate the vessel opening; used in the treatment of atherosclerotic disease

angioscopy: studying the capillaries of the eyes

anomaloscope: instrument used to test color vision

anomaly: abnormality

anoscopy: procedure that uses a scope to examine the anus

antepartum: before childbirth

anterior (ventral): in front of

anterior segment: those parts of the eye in the front of and including the lens, orbit, extraocular muscles, and eyelid

anterior synechiae: adhesions of the iris to the cornea

anteroposterior: from front to back

antrum: sinus

aortography: radiographic recording of the aorta

apexcardiography: noninvasive graphic recording of the movement of the chest wall from the cardiac pulsations from the region of the apex of the heart, usually of the left ventricle

APC (Ambulatory Payment Classification): a patient classification that provides a payment system for outpatients

aphakia: absence of the lens of the eye

apicectomy: excision of a portion of the temporal bone

Appendix A: located near the back of the CPT manual; lists all modifiers with complete explanations for use

Appendix B: located near the back of the CPT manual; contains a complete list of additions to, deletions from, and revisions of the previous edition

Appendix C: located near the back of the CPT manual; presents clinical examples of Evaluation and Management (E/M)

Appendix D: located near the back of the CPT manual; contains a list of the CPT add-on codes

Appendix E: located near the back of the CPT manual; contains a list of modifier -51 exempt codes

Appendix F: located near the back of the CPT manual; contains information about modifier -63, Procedures Performed on Infants less than 4-kg

Appendix G: located near the back of the CPT manual; contains CPT codes that include moderate (conscious) sedation

Appendix H: located near the back of the CPT manual; contains website to access information about performance measures of Category II codes

Appendix I: located near the back of the CPT manual; contains information about Genetic Testing Code Modifiers (deleted for 2013)

Appendix J: located near the back of the CPT manual; contains information on sensory, motor, and mixed nerves and the corresponding conduction study codes

Appendix K: located near the back of the CPT manual; contains the codes that are pending FDA (Food and Drug Administration) approval

Appendix L: located near the back of the CPT manual; contains the vascular families

Appendix M: located near the back of the CPT manual; contains deleted CPT codes

Appendix N: located near the back of the CPT manual; contains a summary of resequenced CPT codes

Appendix O: located near the back of the CPT manual; contains Multianalyte Assays with Algorithmic Analyses codes

arteriovenous fistula: direct communication (passage) between an artery and vein

artery: vessel that generally carries oxygenated blood from the heart to body tissues (pulmonary artery carries un-oxygenated blood)

arthrodesis: surgical immobilization of a joint

arthrography: radiographic recording of a joint

arthroplasty: reshaping or reconstruction of a joint

aspiration: use of a needle and a syringe to withdraw fluid

assignment: Medicare's payment for the service, which participating physicians agree to accept as payment in full

astigmatism: condition in which the refractive surfaces of the eye are unequal

asymptomatic: not showing any of the typical symptoms of a disease or condition

atrium: chamber in the upper part of the heart

attending physician: the physician with the primary responsibility for care of the patient

audi-: prefix meaning hearing

audiometry: hearing testing

aur-: prefix meaning ear

aural atresia: congenital absence of the external auditory canal

autogenous, autologous: from oneself

axillary nodes: lymph nodes located in the armpit

B-scan: two-dimensional display of tissues and organs

backbench work: special preparation of an organ before organ transplantation

bariatric surgery: gastric restrictive procedures that are used to treat morbid obesity and are accomplished by placing a restrictive device around the stomach to decrease its functional size

barium enema: radiographic contrast medium–enhanced examination of the colon

benign: not progressive

benign hypertension: hypertensive condition with a continuous, mild blood pressure elevation

bifocal: two focuses in eyeglasses, one usually for close work and the other for improvement of distance vision

bilateral: occurring on two sides

bilobectomy: surgical removal of two lobes of a lung

biofeedback: process of giving a person self-information

biometry: application of a statistical measure to a biologic fact

biopsy: removal of a small piece of living tissue for diagnostic purposes

blephar(o)-: prefix meaning eyelid

block: frozen piece of a sample

blood patch: a procedure in which a cerebrospinal fluid leak is closed by means of an injection of the patient's blood into the area used during spinal anesthesia

brachytherapy: therapy using radioactive sources that are placed inside the body

bronchography: radiographic recording of the lungs

bronchoplasty: surgical repair of the bronchi

bronchoscopy: inspection of the bronchial tree using a bronchoscope

bulbocavernosus: muscle that constricts the vagina in a female and the urethra in a male

bulbourethral gland: rounded mass of the urethra

bypass: to go around

calculus: concretion of mineral salts, also called a stone

calycoplasty: surgical reconstruction of a recess of the renal pelvis

calyx: recess of the renal pelvis

cannulation: insertion of a tube into a duct or cavity

carcinoma in situ: a cancerous tumor in its original place that has not invaded neighboring tissues

cardiopulmonary: refers to the heart and lungs

cardiopulmonary bypass: blood bypasses the heart through a heart-lung machine during open-heart surgery

cardioversion: electric shock to the heart to restore normal rhythm

cataract: opaque covering on or in the lens

Category I: CPT codes approved by the FDA and representing widely used services and procedures

Category II: Supplemental codes that can be used for performance measurements

Category III: Temporary CPT codes

catheter: tube placed into the body to put fluid in or take fluid out

caudal: away from the head, or the lower part of the body; same as inferior

cauterization: destruction of tissue by the use of cautery

cavernosa–corpus spongiosum shunt: creation of a connection between a cavity of the penis and the urethra

cavernosa–glans penis fistulization: creation of a connection between a cavity of the penis and the glans penis, which overlaps the penis cavity

cavernos–saphenous vein shunt: creation of a connection between the cavity of the penis and a vein

cavernosography: radiographic recording of a cavity, e.g., the pulmonary cavity or the main part of the penis

cavernosometry: measurement of the pressure in a cavity, e.g., the penis

-centesis: suffix meaning puncture of a cavity

central nervous system (CNS): brain and spinal cord

cervical: pertaining to the neck or to the cervix of the uterus

cervix uteri: rounded, cone-shaped neck of the uterus

cesarean: surgical opening through abdominal wall for delivery

CF (conversion factor): national dollar amount that is applied to all services paid on the Medicare Fee Schedule basis

cholangiography: radiographic recording of the bile ducts

cholangiopancreatography (ERCP): radiographic recording of the biliary system and pancreas

chole-: prefix meaning bile

cholecystectomy: surgical removal of the gallbladder

cholecystoenterostomy: creation of a connection between the gallbladder and intestine

cholecystography: radiographic recording of the gallbladder

chordee: condition resulting in the penis' being bent downward

chorionic villus sampling (CVS): biopsy of the outermost part of the placenta

chromotubation: surgical procedure to open obstructed fallopian tubes

chronic: of long duration

Clinical Documentation Improvement (CDI): programs used by medical providers to improve documentation keyed to the quality of coding, medical necessity, and denial standards

Cloquet's node: also called a gland; it is the highest of the deep groin lymph nodes

closed treatment: fracture site that is not surgically opened and visualized

CMS: Centers for Medicare and Medicaid Services, formerly HCFA, Health Care Financing Administration

colonoscopy: fiberscopic examination of the entire colon that may include part of the terminal ileum

colostomy: artificial opening between the colon and the abdominal wall

combination code: single ICD-10-CM/ICD-9-CM code used to classify two diagnoses

combination coding: a code from the Radiology section as well as a code from one of the other sections must be used to fully describe the procedure

communicable disease: disease that can be transmitted from one person to another or one species to another

comparative conditions: patient conditions that are documented as "either/or" in the medical record

component: part

component coding: a code from the Radiology section as well as a code from one of the other sections must be used to fully describe the procedure

computed axial tomography (CAT or CT): procedure by which selected planes of tissue are pinpointed through computer enhancement, and images may be reconstructed by analysis of variance in absorption of the tissue

concurrent care: the provision of similar services (e.g., hospital visits) to the same patient by more than one physician on the same day. Each physician provides services for a separate condition, not reasonably expected to be managed by the attending physician. When concurrent care is provided, the diagnosis must reflect the medical necessity of different specialties

congenital: existing from birth

conjunctiva: the lining of the eyelids and the covering of the sclerae

conscious sedation: a decreased level of consciousness in which the patient is not completely asleep

constitutional examination element: assessment of the patient's general condition and the recording of the vital signs

consultation: includes those services rendered by a physician whose opinion or advice is requested by another physician or agency concerning the evaluation and/or treatment of a patient; a consultant is not an attending physician

contralateral: the opposite side

contributory factors: counseling, coordination of care, nature of the presenting problem, and time of an E/M service

cordectomy: surgical removal of the vocal cord(s)

cordocentesis: procedure to obtain a fetal blood sample; also called a percutaneous umbilical blood sampling

corneosclera: cornea and sclera of the eye

corpora cavernosa: the two cavities of the penis

corpus uteri: uterus

counseling: a discussion with a patient and/or family concerning one or more of the following areas: diagnostic results, impressions, and/or recommended diagnostic studies; prognosis; risks and benefits of treatment;

instructions for treatment; importance of compliance with treatment; risk factor reduction; and patient and family education

CPT (Current Procedural Terminology): a coding system developed by the American Medical Association (AMA) to convert widely accepted, uniform descriptions of medical, surgical, and diagnostic services rendered by health care providers into five-digit codes

cranium: that part of the skeleton that encloses the brain

critical care: the care of critically ill patients in medical emergencies that requires the constant attendance of the physician (e.g., cardiac arrest, shock, bleeding, respiratory failure); critical care is usually, but not always, given in a critical care area, such as the coronary care unit (CCU) or the intensive care unit (ICU)

CRNA: certified registered nurse anesthetist

Crohn's disease: regional enteritis

cryosurgery: destruction of lesions using extreme cold

curettage: scraping of a cavity using a spoon-shaped instrument

cycl/o-: prefix meaning ciliary body or eye muscle

cyst: closed sac containing matter or fluid

cystic hygroma: congenital deformity or benign tumor of the lymphatic system

cystocele: herniation of the bladder into the vagina

cystography: radiographic recording of the urinary bladder

cystolithectomy: removal of a calculus (stone) from the urinary bladder

cystolithotomy: cystolithectomy

cystometrogram (CMG): measurement of the pressures and capacity of the urinary bladder

cystoplasty: surgical reconstruction of the bladder

cystorrhaphy: suture of the bladder

cystoscopy: use of a scope to view the bladder

cystostomy: surgical creation of an opening into the bladder

cystotomy: incision into the bladder

cystourethroplasty: surgical reconstruction of the bladder and urethra

cystourethroscopy: use of a scope to view the bladder and urethra

cytopathology: study of the diseases of cells

dacry/o-: prefix meaning tear or tear duct

dacryocyst/o-: prefix meaning pertaining to the lacrimal sac

dacryocystography: radiographic recording of the lacrimal sac or tear duct sac

debridement: cleansing of or removal of dead tissue from a wound

delivery: childbirth

Demerol: a narcotic analgesic

dermatoplasty: surgical repair of the skin

dermis: second layer of skin, holding blood vessels, nerve endings, sweat glands, and hair follicles

destruction: killing of tissue by means of electrocautery, laser, chemicals, or other means

DHHS: Department of Health and Human Services

diagnostic: that done to identify the cause, origin, or extent of a condition

diaphragm: muscular wall that separates the thoracic and abdominal cavities

diaphragmatic hernia: hernia of the diaphragm

dilation: expansion (of the cervix)

diskography: radiographic recording of an intervertebral joint

dislocation: placement in a location other than the original location

displacement therapy: procedure in which the physician flushes saline solution into the sinuses to remove mucus or pus

distal: farther from the point of attachment or origin

distinct procedure: one service or procedure that has no relationship to another service or procedure

Doppler: ultrasonic measure of blood movement

dosimetry: scientific calculation of radiation emitted from various radioactive sources

drainage: free flow or withdrawal of fluids from a wound or cavity

DRGs (Diagnosis Related Groups): a disease classification system that relates the type of inpatients a hospital treats (case mix) to the costs incurred by the hospital (now MS-DRGs)

dual-chamber pacemaker: electrodes of the pacemaker are placed in both the atria and the ventricle of the heart

duodenography: radiographic recording of the duodenum, or first part of the small intestine

E Codes: alphanumeric designations preceded by the letter "E," used to classify external causes in ICD-9-CM

ear, parts of the external: auricle, pinna, external acoustic, meatus, and tympanic membrane

ear, parts of the inner: vestibule, semicircular canals, and cochlea

ear, parts of the middle: malleus, incus, and stapes

ECG: *see* electrocardiogram

echocardiography: radiographic recording of the heart or heart walls or surrounding tissues

echoencephalography: ultrasound of the brain

echography: ultrasound procedure in which sound waves are bounced off an internal organ and the resulting image is recorded

-ectomy: suffix meaning removal of part or all of an organ of the body

ectopic: pregnancy outside the uterus (i.e., in the fallopian tube)

EEG: *see* electroencephalogram

electrocardiogram (ECG): written record of the electrical activity of the heart

electrocochleography: stimulation of the cochlea to measure electrical activity

electrode: lead attached to a generator that carries the electric current from the generator to the atria or ventricles

electrodesiccation: destruction of a lesion by the use of electric current radiated through a needle

electroencephalogram (EEG) (EKG): written record of the electrical activity of the brain

electrohydraulic fragmentation: use of a probe containing two electrodes that are applied, one on each side, of the calculus

electromyogram (EMG): written record of the electrical activity of the skeletal muscles

electromyography (EMG): recording of the electrical impulses of muscles

electro-oculogram (EOG): written record of the electrical activity of the eye

electrophysiology: the study of the electrical system of the heart, including the study of arrhythmias

embolectomy: removal of blockage (embolism) from vessels

embolism: blockage of a blood vessel by a blood clot or other matter that has moved from another area of the body through the circulatory system

emergency care services: services that are provided by the physician in the emergency department for unplanned patient encounters; no distinction is made between new and established patients who are seen in the emergency department

encephalography: radiographic recording of the subarachnoid space and ventricles of the brain

endarterectomy: incision into an artery to remove the inner lining so as to eliminate disease or blockage

endomyocardial: pertaining to the inner and middle layers of the heart

endopyelotomy: with the use of an endoscope, an incision is made to correct stenosis of the ureteropelvic junction

endoscopy: inspection of body organs or cavities using a lighted scope that may be inserted through an existing opening or through a small incision

endotracheal tube: can be inserted through the nose or mouth and passed into the trachea for ventilation

endovascular aneurysm repair (EVAR): an emerging technology that involves placing a stent graft, or a fabric tube, inside the affected area of the blood vessel by access through an artery

enterocystoplasty: surgical reconstruction of the small intestine after the removal of a cyst and usually including a bowel anastomosis

enucleation: removal of an organ or organs from a body cavity

epicardial: over the heart

epidermis: outer layer of skin

epididymectomy: surgical removal of the epididymis

epididymis: tube located at the top of the testes that stores sperm

epididymography: radiographic recording of the epididymis

epididymovasostomy: creation of a new connection between the vas deferens and epididymis

epidural anesthesia: injection of an anesthesia agent into the spaces between the vertebrae. Also known as peridural anesthesia, epidural, epidural block, and intraspinal anesthesia

epiglottidectomy: excision of the covering of the larynx

eponym: disease, structure, or procedure that is named after a person

ESRD: end-stage renal disease

established patient: a patient who has received professional services from the physician or another physician of the exact same specialty and subspeciality in the same group within the past 3 years

etiology: study of causes of diseases

eventration: protrusion of the bowel through the viscera of the abdomen

evisceration: pulling the viscera outside of the body through an incision

exacerbation: worsening or increase of severity of a condition or disease

excision: it is full-thickness removal of a lesion that may include simple closure

excisional: removal of an entire lesion for biopsy

Exclusive Provider Organization (EPO): similar to a Health Maintenance Organization except that the providers of the services are not prepaid, but rather are paid on a fee-for-service basis

exenteration: removal of an organ all in one piece

exostosis: bony growth

exstrophy: condition in which an organ is turned inside out

exteriorization: developing an artificial opening through the abdominal wall to take out a diseased portion of the intestine

External Cause Code: classification of health condition due to external cause

extirpation: taking or cutting out solid matter from a body part

false aneurysm: sac of clotted blood that has completely destroyed the vessel and is being contained by the tissue that surrounds the vessel

fascia lata grafts: a graft of fibrous tissue that is found beneath the skin

fasciectomy: excision of fascia

FDA (Food and Drug Administration): responsible for the safety of food and drugs in America; is an agency within the U.S. Public Health Service, which is part of the Department of Health and Human Services

Federal Register: official publication of all "Presidential Documents," "Rules and Regulations," "Proposed Rules," and "Notices"; government-instituted national changes are published in the *Federal Register*

fenestration: creation of a new opening in the inner wall of the middle ear

fimbrioplasty: surgical repair of the fringe of the uterine tube

first-listed diagnosis: outpatient diagnosis

Fiscal Intermediary (FI): handled administration of Medicare claims but was phased out by 2011 into MACs

fistula: abnormal opening from one area to another area or to the outside of the body

fluoroscopy: procedure for viewing the interior of the body using x-rays and projecting the image onto a television screen

forensic examination: a head to toe examination performed when an injury occurs that was not the result of natural causes; involves legal investigation

fracture: break in a bone

fulguration: use of electric current to destroy tissue

fundoplasty: repair of the bottom of an organ or muscle

gastro-: prefix meaning stomach

gastrointestinal: pertaining to the stomach and intestine

gastroplasty: operation on the stomach for repair or reconfiguration

gastrostomy: artificial opening between the stomach and the abdominal wall

general anesthesia: a state of unconsciousness produced by the administration of a drug; it can be administered by inhalation or intramuscularly, rectally, or intravenously

gloss(o)-: prefix meaning tongue

gonioscopy: use of a scope to gain a view of the iridocorneal angle, or the anatomical angle formed between the eye's cornea and iris

Group Practice Model: an organization of physicians who contract with a Health Maintenance Organization to provide services to the enrollees of the HMO

grouper: computer used to input the principal diagnosis and other critical information about a patient and then provide the correct MS-DRG code

Guidelines: provide specific instructions about coding for each section of the CPT manual; the Guidelines contain definitions of terms, applicable modifiers, explanation of notes, subsection information, unlisted services, special reports information, and clinical examples

HCFA: Health Care Financing Administration, now known as Centers for Medicare and Medicaid Services (CMS)

Health Maintenance Organization (HMO): a health care delivery system in which an enrollee is assigned a primary care physician who manages all the health care needs of the enrollee

hemodialysis: cleansing of the blood outside of the body

hepat(o)-: prefix meaning liver

hepatography: radiographic recording of the liver

hernia: organ or tissue protruding through the wall or cavity that usually contains it

histology: study of the minute structures, composition, and function of tissues

Hodgkin disease: malignant lymphoma

hydrocele: sac of fluid

hypertension, uncontrolled: untreated hypertension or hypertension that is not responding to the therapeutic regimen

hypertensive heart disease: secondary effects on the heart of prolonged, sustained systemic hypertension; the heart has to work against greatly increased resistance, causing increased blood pressure

hypogastric: lowest middle abdominal area

hyposensitization: decreased sensitivity

hypospadias: congenital deformity of the urethra in which the urethral opening is on the underside of the penis rather than at the end

hypotension: abnormally low blood pressure; sometimes induced during surgical procedures

hypothermia: low body temperature; sometimes induced during surgical procedures

hysterectomy: surgical removal of the uterus

hysterorrhaphy: suturing of the uterus

hysterosalpingography: radiographic recording of the uterine cavity and fallopian tubes

hysteroscopy: visualization of the canal of the uterine cervix and cavity of the uterus using a scope placed through the vagina

hysterotomy: incision into the uterus

ileostomy: artificial opening between the ileum and the abdominal wall

imbrication: overlapping

immunotherapy: therapy to increase immunity

implantable defibrillator: surgically placed device that directs an electric current shock to the heart to restore rhythm

incarcerated: regarding hernias, a constricted, irreducible hernia that may cause obstruction of an intestine

incision: surgically cutting into

incision and drainage: to cut and withdraw fluid

incisional: *see* incision

Individual Practice Association (IPA): an organization of physicians who provide services for a set fee; a Health Maintenance Organization will often contract with the IPA for services to their enrollees

infectious disease carrier: person who has a communicable disease but is symptom free despite having the disease

infectious disease contact: encounter with a person who has a disease that can be communicated or transmitted

inferior: away from the head or the lower part of the body; also known as caudal

inguinofemoral: referring to the groin and thigh

injection: introduction of fluid into a tissue, vessel, or cavity

inpatient: one who has been formally admitted to a health care facility

in situ: malignancy that is within the original site of development and has not invaded neighboring tissue

internal/external fixation: application of pins, wires, screws, and so on to immobilize a body part; they can be placed externally or internally

intracardiac: inside the heart

intramural: within the organ wall

intramuscular: into a muscle

intraoperative: period of time during which a surgical procedure is being performed

intravascular ultrasound: a test that uses sound waves to examine coronary vessels of the heart

intravenous: into a vein

intravenous pyelography (IVP): radiographic recording of the urinary system

introitus: opening or entrance to the vagina

intubation: insertion of a tube

invasive: entering the body, breaking the skin

iontophoresis: introduction of ions into the body

ischemia: deficient blood supply due to obstruction of the circulatory system

isthmus: connection of two regions or structures

isthmus, thyroid: tissue connection between right and left thyroid lobes

isthmusectomy: surgical removal of the isthmus

italicized code: an ICD-10-CM/ICD-9-CM code that can never be sequenced as the principal or primary diagnosis

jejunostomy: artificial opening between the jejunum and the abdominal wall

joint movement:

  abduction: movement of a limb away from the midline of the body

  adduction: movement of a limb toward the midline of the body

  circumduction: circular movement of a limb

  extension: movement by which two parts are drawn away from each other

  flexion: movement by which two parts are drawn toward each other

  hyperextension: excessive extension of a limb

  pronation: applied to the hand, the act of turning the palm down

  supination: applied to the hand, the act of turning the palm up

jugular nodes: lymph nodes located next to the large vein in the neck

kerat/o-: prefix meaning cornea

keratoplasty: surgical repair of the cornea

key components: the history, examination, and medical decision-making complexity of an E/M service

Kock pouch: surgical creation of a urinary bladder from a segment of the ileum

kyphosis: humpback, the abnormal curvature of the spine

labyrinth: inner connecting cavities, such as the internal ear

laminectomy: surgical excision of the lamina

laparoscopy: exploration of the abdomen and pelvic cavities using a scope placed through a small incision in the abdominal wall

laryngeal web: congenital abnormality of connective tissue between the vocal cords

laryngectomy: surgical removal of the larynx

laryngo-: prefix meaning larynx

laryngography: radiographic recording of the larynx

laryngoplasty: surgical repair of the larynx

laryngoscope: an endoscope used to view the inside of the larynx

laryngoscopy: viewing of the larynx using a fiberoptic scope

laryngotomy: incision into the larynx

late effect: residual effect (that a condition produced) after the acute phase of an illness or injury has terminated

lateral: away from the midline of the body (to the side)

lavage: washing out of an organ

lesion: abnormal or altered tissue, e.g., wound, cyst, abscess, or boil

ligament: a band of fibrous tissue that connects cartilage or bone and supports a joint

ligation: binding or tying off, as in constricting the bloodflow of a vessel or binding fallopian tubes for sterilization

litholapaxy: lithotripsy

lithotomy: incision into an organ or a duct for the purpose of removing a stone

lithotripsy: crushing of a gallbladder or urinary bladder stone followed by irrigation to wash the fragment out

lobectomy: surgical excision of a lobe of the lung

lymph node: station along the lymphatic system

lymphadenectomy: excision of a lymph node or nodes

lymphadenitis: inflammation of a lymph node

lymphangiography: radiographic recording of the lymphatic vessels and nodes

lymphangiotomy: incision into a lymphatic vessel

lysis: releasing

M-mode: one-dimensional display of movement of structures

MAAC (Maximum Actual Allowable Charge): limitation on the total amount that can be charged by physicians who are not participants in Medicare

MAC (Medicare Administrative Contractor): an entity that manages the process claims for CMS

magnetic resonance imaging (MRI): procedure that uses nonionizing radiation to view the body in a cross-sectional view

malignancy: used in reference to a cancerous tumor

malignant: used to describe a cancerous tumor that grows worse over time

malignant hypertension: accelerated, severe form of hypertension, manifested by headaches, blurred vision, dyspnea, and uremia; usually causes permanent organ damage

mammography: radiographic recording of the breasts

Managed Care Organization (MCO): a group that is responsible for the health care services offered to an enrolled group of persons

mandated service: a service required by an agency or organization to be performed for a patient; usually the agency or organization pays all or a portion of the patient's medical bills

manifestation: sign of a disease

manipulation or reduction: words used interchangeably to mean the attempted restoration of a fracture or joint dislocation to its normal anatomic position

marsupialization: surgical procedure that creates an exterior pouch from an internal abscess

mast-: prefix meaning breast

mastoid-: prefix meaning posterior temporal bone

MDC (Major Diagnostic Categories): the division of all principal diagnoses into 25 mutually exclusive principal diagnosis areas within the MS-DRG system

meatotomy: surgical enlargement of the opening of the urinary meatus

medial: toward the midline of the body

mediastinoscopy: use of an endoscope inserted through a small incision to view the mediastinum

mediastinotomy: cutting into the mediastinum

mediastinum: area between the lungs that contains the heart, aorta, trachea, lymph nodes, thymus gland, esophagus, and bronchial tubes

Medicare Administrative Contractor (MAC): handles the administration of Medicare claims

Medicare Risk HMO: a Medicare-funded alternative to the standard Medicare supplemental coverage

MEI (Medicare Economic Index): government-mandated index that ties increases in the Medicare prevailing charges to economic indicators

MeV: megaelectron volt

MFS (Medicare Fee Schedule): schedules that list the allowable charges for Medicare services

modality: treatment method

moderate (conscious) sedation: a decreased level of consciousness in which the patient is not completely asleep

modifiers: added to codes to supply more specific information about the services provided

monofocal: eyeglasses with one vision correction

morbidity: condition of being diseased or morbid

morphine: a narcotic analgesic

morphology: the science of the form and structure of organisms

mortality: death

MS-DRG (Medicare Severity Diagnosis Related Groups): a system of classifying patient groups by related diagnoses

MSLT: multiple sleep latency testing

multiple coding: use of more than one ICD-10-CM/ICD-9-CM code to identify both etiology and manifestation of a disease, to fully describe condition

muscle: fibrous structures that can contract and facilitate movement of the body. There are three types of muscles: smooth, skeletal, and cardiac

MVPS (Medical Volume Performance Standards): government's estimate of how much growth is appropriate for nationwide physician expenditures paid by the Part B Medicare program

myasthenia gravis: syndrome characterized by muscle weakness

myelography: radiographic recording of the subarachnoid space of the spine

myocardial infarction (MI): necrosis of the myocardium resulting from interrupted blood supply

myring-: prefix meaning eardrum

nasal button: a synthetic circular disk used to cover a hole in the nasal septum

nasopharyngoscopy: use of a scope to visualize the nose and pharynx

NCPAP: nasal continuous positive airway pressure

NEC: not elsewhere classifiable

neoplasm: new tumor growth that can be benign or malignant

nephrectomy, paraperitoneal: surgical removal of a kidney by a cut through the side along the twelfth rib

nephro-: prefix meaning kidney

nephrocutaneous fistula: a channel from the kidney to the skin

nephrolithotomy: removal of a kidney stone through an incision made into the kidney

nephrorrhaphy: suturing of the kidney

nephrostolithotomy: procedure to establish an artificial channel between the skin and the kidney to remove kidney stone

nephrostomy: creation of a channel into the renal pelvis of the kidney

nephrostomy, percutaneous: creation of a channel from the skin to the renal pelvis

nephrotomy: incision into the kidney

new patient: a patient who has not received professional services from the physician or another physician of the exact same specialty and subspeciality in the same group within the past 3 years

newborn care: the evaluation and determination of care management of a newly born infant

noninvasive: not entering the body, not breaking the skin

nonselective catheter placement: catheter or needle that is not manipulated and is placed directly into an artery or vein or is placed only into the aorta from any approach

NOS: not otherwise specified

nuclear cardiology: diagnostic specialty that uses radiopharmaceuticals to aid in the diagnosis of cardiologic conditions

nystagmus: rapid involuntary eye movements

objective information: findings observed by the physician during an examination

OBRA (Omnibus Budget Reconciliation Act of 1989): act that established new rules for Medicare reimbursement

ocul/o-: prefix meaning eye

ocular adnexa: orbit, extraocular muscles, and eyelid

office visit: a direct encounter between a physician and a patient in the physician's private office to allow for primary management of a patient's health care status

Official Guidelines for Coding and Reporting: rules of coding diagnosis codes (ICD-10-CM, ICD-9-CM) published by CMS and NCHS

omentum: peritoneal connection between the stomach and other internal organs

oophor-: prefix meaning ovary

oophorectomy: surgical removal of the ovary(ies)

opacification: area that has become opaque (milky)

open treatment: fracture site that is surgically opened and visualized

ophthalmodynamometry: test of the blood pressure of the eye

ophthalmology: body of knowledge regarding the eyes

optokinetic: movement of the eyes to objects moving in the visual field

orchiectomy: castration

orchiopexy: fixation or suturing of an undescended testicle to secure it in the scrotum

orthoptic: corrective; in the correct place

osteotomy: cutting into bone

ostomy: artificial opening

oto-: prefix meaning ear

-otomy: suffix meaning incision into

outpatient: a patient who receives services in an ambulatory health care facility and is currently not an inpatient

overdose: excessive dose

oviduct: fallopian tube

pacemaker: electrical device that controls the beating of the heart by electrical impulses

paraesophageal hiatal hernia: hernia that is near the esophagus

parathyroid: produces a hormone to mobilize calcium from the bones to the blood

paring: removal of thin layers of skin by peeling or scraping

Part A: Medicare's Hospital Insurance; covers hospital/facility care

Part B: Medicare's Supplemental Medical Insurance; covers physician services and durable medical equipment that are not paid for under Part A

Part C: Medicare Advantage is a set of health care options from which beneficiaries choose health care providers

Part D: Medicare's prescription drug program

participating provider program: Medicare providers who have agreed in advance to accept assignment on all Medicare claims; now termed QIO

pathologic fracture: fracture due to a bone disease or a change surrounding the bone tissue that makes the bone weak

patient-controlled analgesia (PCA): a system that allows the patient to self-administer an analgesic drug, such as morphine, to control pain. A hand-held device is attached to a pump holding the drug and the patient can depress a button to administer a dose of the drug. In this way, the patient can control the amount of the drug, frequency of administration, and manage postoperative pain. The system is used with patients with chronic pain.

pelviolithotomy: pyeloplasty

penoscrotal: referring to the penis and scrotum

percutaneous: through the skin

percutaneous skeletal fixation: considered neither open nor closed; the fracture is not visualized, but fixation is placed across the fracture site under x-ray imaging

pericardiocentesis: procedure in which a surgeon withdraws fluid from the pericardial space by means of a needle inserted percutaneously into the space

pericarditis: inflammation of the sac surrounding the first few centimeters of great vessels and the heart

pericardium: membranous sac enclosing the heart and the ends of the great vessels

perineal approach: surgical approach in the area between the thighs

perinephric cyst: cyst in the tissue around the kidney

perineum: area between the vulva and anus

peripheral nerves: 12 pairs of cranial nerves, 31 pairs of spinal nerves, and autonomic nervous system; connects peripheral receptors to the brain and spinal cord

perirenal: around the kidney

peritoneal: within the lining of the abdominal cavity

peritoneoscopy: visualization of the abdominal cavity using one scope placed through a small incision in the abdominal wall and another scope placed in the vagina

perivesical: around the bladder

perivisceral: around an organ

pharyngolaryngectomy: surgical removal of the pharynx and larynx

phlebotomy: cutting into a vein

phonocardiogram: recording of heart sounds

photochemotherapy: treatment by means of drugs that react to ultraviolet radiation or sunlight

physical status modifiers: modifying units in the Anesthesia section of the CPT manual that describe a patient's condition at the time anesthesia is administered

physician: legally qualified to practice medicine; CPT definition includes other qualified health care professional

physics: scientific study of energy

-plasty: suffix meaning technique involving molding or surgically forming

plethysmography: determining the changes in volume of an organ part or body

pleura: covering of the lungs and thoracic cavity that is moistened with serous fluid to reduce friction during respiratory movements of the lungs

pleurectomy: surgical excision of the pleura

pneumo-: prefix meaning lung or air

pneumonocentesis: surgical puncturing of a lung to withdraw fluid

pneumonolysis: surgical separation of the lung from the chest wall to allow the lung to collapse

pneumonostomy: surgical procedure in which the chest cavity is exposed and the lung is incised

pneumonotomy: incision of the lung

pneumoplethysmography: determining the changes in the volume of the lung

polyp: tumor on a pedicle that bleeds easily and may become malignant

polysomnography: measurement of the brain waves and various stages of sleep during sleep

posterior (dorsal): in back of

posterior segment: those parts of the eye behind the lens

posterior synechiae: adhesions of the iris to the lens of the eye

posteroanterior: from back to front

postoperative: period of time after a surgical procedure

postpartum: after childbirth

Preferred Provider Organization (PPO): a group of providers who form a network and who have agreed to provide services to enrollees at a discounted rate

preoperative: period of time prior to a surgical procedure

priapism: painful condition in which the penis is constantly erect

primary diagnosis: first-listed diagnosis, used in the outpatient setting to identify the reason for the encounter

primary site: site of origin or where the tumor originated

principal diagnosis: defined in the Uniform Hospital Discharge Data Set (UHDDS) as "that condition established after study to be chiefly responsible for occasioning the admission of the patient to the hospital for care"; the principal diagnosis is sequenced first

proctosigmoidoscopy: fiberscopic examination of the sigmoid colon and rectum

professional component: term used in describing physician's services in radiology or pathology

prognosis: probable outcome of an illness

prophylactic: substance or agent that offers some protection from disease

PROs (Peer Review Organizations): groups established to review hospital admission and care; now termed QIO

prostatotomy: incision into the prostate

PSRO (Professional Standards Review Organization): voluntary physicians' organization designed to monitor the necessity of hospital admissions, treatment costs, and medical records of hospitals

punch: use of a small hollow instrument to puncture a lesion

pyelo-: prefix meaning renal pelvis

pyelocutaneous: from the renal pelvis to the skin

pyelography: radiographic recording of the kidneys, renal pelvis, ureters, and bladder

pyelolithotomy: surgical removal of a kidney stone from the renal pelvis

pyeloplasty: surgical reconstruction of the renal pelvis

pyeloscopy: viewing of the renal pelvis using a fluoroscope after injection of contrast material

pyelostolithotomy: removal of a kidney stone and establishment of a stoma

pyelostomy: surgical creation of a temporary diversion around the ureter

pyelotomy: incision into the renal pelvis

pyloroplasty: incision and repair of the pyloric channel

QIO (Quality Improvement Organization): consists of a national network of 53 entities that work with consumers, physicians, hospitals, and caregivers to refine care delivery systems

qualifying circumstances: five-digit CPT codes that describe situations or conditions that affect the administration of anesthesia

qualitative: measuring the presence or absence of

quantitative: measuring the presence or absence of and the amount of

rad: radiation absorption dose, the energy deposited in patients' tissues

radiation oncology: branch of medicine concerned with the application of radiation to a tumor site for treatment (destruction) of cancerous tumors

radiograph: film on which an image is produced through exposure to x-radiation

radiologist: physician who specializes in the use of radioactive materials in the diagnosis and treatment of diseases and illnesses

radiology: branch of medicine concerned with the use of radioactive substances for diagnosis and therapy

RBRVS (Resource-Based Relative Value Scale): scale designed to decrease Medicare expenditures, redistribute physician payment, and ensure quality health care at reasonable rates

real time: two-dimensional display of both the structures and the motion of tissues and organs, with the length of time also recorded as part of the study

reanastomosis: reconnection of a previous connection between two places, organs, or spaces

rectocele: herniation of the rectal wall through the posterior wall of the vagina

reducible: able to be corrected or put back into a normal position

referral: the transfer of the total or a specific portion of care of a patient from one physician to another that does not constitute a consultation

regional anesthesia: the interruption of the sensory nerve conductivity in a region of the body, which is produced by field block (forming a wall of anesthesia around the site by means of local injections) or by nerve block (injection of the area close to the major sensory nerve supplying a field); also known as block anesthesia, block, or conduction anesthesia

Relative Value Guide®: comparison of anesthesia services; published by the American Society of Anesthesiologists (ASA)

renal pelvis: funnel-shaped sac in the kidney where urine is received

repair: to remedy, replace, or heal (in the Integumentary subsection pertains to suturing a wound)

residual: that which is left behind or remains

resource intensity: refers to the relative volume and type of diagnostic, therapeutic, and bed services used in the management of a particular illness

retrograde: moving backward or against the usual direction of flow

retroperitoneal: behind the sac holding the abdominal organs and viscera (peritoneum)

rhino-: prefix meaning nose

rhinoplasty: surgical repair of the nose

-rrhaphy: suffix meaning suturing

rubric: heading used as a direction or explanation as to what follows and the way in which the information is to be used. In ICD-10-CM coding, the rubric is the three-digit code that precedes the four to seven characters. In ICD-9-CM coding, the rubric is the three-digit code that precedes the four- and five-digit codes

rule of nines: rule used to estimate burned body surface area in burn patients

RUQ: right upper quadrant

RVU (Relative Value Unit): unit value that has been assigned for each service

salpingectomy: surgical removal of the uterine tube

salping(o)-: prefix meaning tube

salpingostomy: creation of a fistula into the uterine tube

scan: mapping of emissions of radioactive substances after they have been introduced into the body; the density can determine normal or abnormal conditions

sclera: the white, outer covering of the eye

scoliosis: abnormal lateral curvature of the spine

secondary site: place to which a malignant tumor has spread; metastatic site

section: slice of a frozen block

sections: the six major areas into which all CPT codes and descriptions are categorized

See: a cross-reference term within the index of the CPT manual used to direct the coder to another term or other terms. The *See* indicates that the correct code will be found elsewhere

segmentectomy: surgical removal of a portion of a lung

selective catheter placement: catheter must be moved, manipulated, or guided into part of the arterial system other than the aorta or the vessel punctured, generally under fluoroscopic guidance

seminal vesicle: gland that secretes fluid that ultimately becomes semen

sentinel node: the first lymph node to receive drainage from a tumor; used to determine whether there is a lymphatic metastasis in certain types of cancer

separate procedures: minor procedures that when done by themselves are coded as a procedure, but when performed at the same time as a major procedure are considered incidental and not coded separately

septoplasty: surgical repair of the nasal septum

sequela: a condition that follows an illness

severity of illness: refers to the levels of loss of function and mortality that may be experienced by patients with a particular disease

shaving: horizontal or transverse removal of dermal or epidermal lesions, without full-thickness excision

shunt: divert or make an artificial passage

sialography: radiographic recording of the salivary duct and branches

sigmoidoscopy: fiberscopic examination of the rectum and sigmoid colon that may include a portion of the descending colon

signal-averaged electrocardiography (SAECG): type of electrocardiography that can help physicians predict certain tendencies to abnormalities such as ventricular tachycardia

signal node: the first lymph node that may "signal" a malignant neoplasm's presence

single chamber pacemaker: the electrode of the pacemaker is placed only in the atrium or only in the ventricle, but not placed in both

sinography: radiographic recording of the sinus or sinus tract

sinus tract: a cyst or abscess inside the body with a tract (otherwise known as a fistula)

sinuses: cavities within the facial bones (maxillary, frontal, sphenoid, and ethmoid)

sinusotomy: surgical incision into a sinus

skin graft: transplantation of skin tissue

skull: entire skeletal framework of the head

slanted brackets: indicate that the ICD-10-CM/ICD-9-CM code can never be sequenced as the principal or primary diagnosis

soft tissue: tissues (fascia, connective tissue, muscle, and so forth)

somatic nerve: sensory or motor nerve that supplies a dermatome

special reports: detailed reports that include adequate definitions or descriptions of the nature, extent, and need for the procedure and the time, effort, and equipment necessary to provide the services

specimen: sample of tissue or fluid

spermatocele: cyst filled with spermatozoa

spirometry: measurement of breathing capacity

splenectomy: excision of the spleen

splenography: radiographic recording of the spleen

splenoportography: radiographic procedure to allow visualization of the splenic and portal veins of the spleen

spontaneous fracture: fracture due to a bone disease or a change surrounding the bone tissue that makes the bone weak

Staff Model: a Health Maintenance Organization that directly employs the physicians who provide services to enrollees

stem cell: immature blood cell

stent: mold that is surgically placed to reinforce or hold open an area

stereotaxis: method of identifying a specific area or point in the brain

strabismus: extraocular muscle deviation resulting in unequal visual axes

strangulated hernia: blood supply is cut off to hernia

subcutaneous: tissue below the dermis, primarily fat cells that insulate the body

subjective information: complaint or problem in the history portion of the encounter that is usually described by the patient

subsections: the further division of sections into smaller units, usually by body systems

superior: toward the head or the upper part of the body; also known as cephalic

supine: lying on the back

surgical package: bundling together of time, effort, and services for a specific procedure into one code instead of reporting each component separately

suture: to unite parts by stitching them together

Swan-Ganz catheter: central venous catheter

symbols: special guides that help the coder compare codes and descriptors with the previous edition. A bullet (●) is used to indicate a new procedure or service code added since the previous edition of the CPT manual. A solid triangle (▲) placed in front of a code number indicates that the code has been changed or modified since the last edition. A plus (+) is used to indicate an add-on code. A circle with a line through it (⊘) is used to identify a modifier -51 exempt code. Right and left triangles (▶◀) indicate the beginning and end of the text changes. A bullseye (⊙) indicates procedures that include moderate sedation.   A lightning bolt symbol (⚡) identifies codes that are being tracked by the AMA to monitor FDA status for approval of a drug.

sympathetic nerve: part of the peripheral nervous system that controls automatic body function and sympathetic nerves activated under stress

symphysiotomy: cutting of the pubic cartilage to help in birthing

systemic: affecting the entire body

tarsorrhaphy: suturing together of the eyelids

technical component: term used in describing the services provided by the facility

TEFRA (Tax Equity and Fiscal Responsibility Act): act that contains language to reward cost-conscious health care providers

tenodesis: suturing the end of a tendon to a bone

tenorrhaphy: suturing together two parts of a tendon

term location methods: service/procedure, anatomic site/ body organ, condition/disease, synonym, eponym, and abbreviation

thermogram: written record of temperature variation

thoracentesis: surgical puncture of the thoracic cavity, usually using a needle, to remove fluids

thoracic duct: collection and distribution point for lymph, and the largest lymph vessel located in the chest

thoracoplasty: surgical procedure that removes rib(s) to allow the collapse of a lung

thoracoscopy: use of a lighted endoscope to view the pleural spaces and thoracic cavity or perform surgical procedures

thoracostomy: surgical incision into the chest wall and insertion of a chest tube

thoracotomy: surgical incision into the chest wall

thrombosis: blood clot

thrombus: blood clot that occludes, or shuts off, a vessel

thymectomy: surgical removal of the thymus

thymus: gland that produces hormones important to the immune response

thyroglossal duct: a duct in the embryo between the thyroid primordium and the posterior tongue

thyroglossal duct cyst: a cyst of the neck caused by persistence of portions of or by the lack of closure of the primitive thyroglossal duct

thyroid: part of the endocrine system that produces hormones that regulate metabolism

thyroidectomy: surgical removal of the thyroid

thyroiditis: a thyroid gland inflammation

tissue transfer: piece of skin for grafting that is still partially attached to the original blood supply and is used to cover an adjacent wound area

tocolysis: repression of uterine contractions

tomography: procedure that allows viewing of a single plane of the body by blurring out all but that particular level

tonography: recording of changes in intraocular pressure in response to sustained pressure on the eyeball

tonometry: measurement of pressure or tension

total pneumonectomy: surgical removal of an entire lobe of a lung

tracheostomy: creation of an opening into the trachea

tracheotomy: incision into the trachea

traction: application of force to a limb

transabdominal: across the abdomen

transcutaneous: entering by way of the skin

transesophageal echocardiogram (TEE): echocardiogram performed by placing a probe down the esophagus and sending out sound waves to obtain images of the heart and its movement

transfer order: official document that transfers the care of a patient from one physician to another; often required by third-party payers to legally transfer the care of a patient

transglottic tracheoplasty: surgical repair of the vocal apparatus and trachea

transhepatic: across the liver

transmastoid antrostomy: called a simple mastoidectomy, it creates an opening in the mastoid for drainage

transplantation: grafting of tissue from one source to another

transseptal: through the septum

transthoracic: across the thorax

transtracheal: across the trachea

transureteroureterostomy: surgical connection of one ureter to the other ureter

transurethral resection, prostate: procedure performed through the urethra by means of a cystoscopy to remove part or all of the prostate

transvenous: across a vein

transverse: horizontal

transvesical ureterolithotomy: removal of a ureter stone (calculus) through the bladder

trocar needle: a sharp-pointed instrument equipped with a cannula, used to puncture the wall of a body cavity and withdraw fluid

tumescence: state of being swollen

tumor: swelling or enlargement; a spontaneous growth of tissue that forms an abnormal mass

tunica vaginalis: covering of the testes

tympanic neurectomy: excision of the tympanic nerve

tympanometry: procedure for evaluating middle ear disorders

UHDDS: Uniform Hospital Discharge Data Set

ultrasound: technique using sound waves to determine the density of the outline of tissue

unbundling: assigning multiple CPT codes when one CPT code would fully describe the service or procedure

uncertain behavior: refers to the behavior of a neoplasm as being neither malignant nor benign but having characteristics of both kinds of activity

uncertain diagnosis: diagnosis documented at the time of discharge as "probable," "suspected," "likely," "questionable," "possible," or "rule out"

unilateral: occurring on one side

unlisted procedures: procedures that are considered unusual, experimental, or new and do not have a specific code number assigned; unlisted procedure codes are located at the end of the subsections or subheadings and may be used to identify any procedure that lacks a specific code

unspecified hypertension: hypertensive condition that has not been specified as either benign or malignant hypertension

unspecified nature: when the behavior or histology of a neoplasm is not known or is not specified

uptake: absorption of a radioactive substance by body tissues; recorded for diagnostic purposes in conditions such as thyroid disease

urachal cyst: between the umbilicus and bladder dome, often diagnosed in young children when the cyst becomes infected

urachal sinus: congenital abnormality in which prenatal tissue remains, causes drainage to the umbilicus, and results in infection and umbilicus drainage

ureterectomy: surgical removal of a ureter, either totally or partially

ureterocolon: pertaining to the ureter and colon

ureterocutaneous fistula: the channel from the ureter to the exterior skin

ureteroenterostomy: creation of a connection between the intestine and the ureter

ureterolithotomy: removal of a stone from the ureter

ureterolysis: freeing of adhesions of the ureter

ureteroneocystostomy: surgical connection of the ureter to a new site on the bladder

ureteroplasty: surgical repair of the ureter

ureteropyelography: ureter and bladder radiography

ureteropyelonephrostomy: surgical connection of the ureter to a new site on the kidney

ureteropyelostomy: ureteropyelonephrostomy

ureterosigmoidostomy: surgical connection of the ureter into the sigmoid colon and out through a new opening in the skin

ureterotomy: incision into the ureter

ureterovisceral fistula: surgical formation of a connection between the ureter and the bladder

urethrocutaneous fistula: surgically created channel from the urethra to the skin surface

urethrocystography: radiography of the bladder and urethra

urethromeatoplasty: surgical repair of the urethra and meatus

urethroplasty: surgical repair of the urethra

urethrorrhaphy: suturing of the urethra

urethroscopy: use of a scope to view the urethra

urography: same as pyelography; radiographic recording of the kidneys, renal pelvis, ureters, and bladder

uveal: vascular tissue of the choroid, ciliary body, and iris

V codes: numeric designations in the ICD-9-CM preceded by the letter "V"; used to classify persons who are not currently sick when they encounter health services

vagina: canal from the external female genitalia to the uterus

vagotomy: surgical separation of the vagus nerve

Valium: a sedative

varicocele: swelling of a scrotal vein

vas deferens: tube that carries sperm from the epididymis to the urethra

vasogram: recording of the flow in the vas deferens

vasotomy: creation of an opening in the vas deferens

vasovasorrhaphy: suturing of the vas deferens

vasovasostomy: reversal of a vasectomy

VBAC: vaginal delivery after a previous cesarean delivery

vectorcardiogram (VCG): continuous recording of electrical direction and magnitude of the heart

vein: vessel that carries unoxygenated blood to the heart from body tissues; pulmonary veins carry oxygenated blood back to the heart

vena caval thrombectomy: removal of a blood clot from the blood vessel (inferior vena cava or superior vena cava)

venography: radiographic recording of the veins and tributaries

ventricle: chamber in the lower part of the heart

version: turning of the fetus from a presentation other than cephalic (head down) to cephalic for ease of birth

vesicostomy: surgical creation of a connection of the bladder mucosa to the skin

vesicovaginal fistula: creation of a tube between the vagina and the bladder

vesiculectomy: excision of the seminal vesicle

vesiculography: radiographic recording of the seminal vesicles

vesiculotomy: incision into the seminal vesicle

vitre/o-: prefix meaning pertaining to the vitreous body of the eye

vulva: external female genitalia including the labia majora, labia minora, clitoris, and vaginal opening

World Health Organization (WHO): group that deals with health care issues on a global basis

wound repair, complex: involves complicated wound closure, including revision, debridement, extensive undermining, and more than layered closure

wound repair, intermediate: requires closure of one or more subcutaneous tissues and superficial fascia, in addition to the skin closure

wound repair, simple: superficial wound repair, involving epidermis, dermis, and subcutaneous tissue, requiring only simple, one-layer suturing

xeroradiography: photoelectric process of radiographs

Z codes: numeric designations in the ICD-10-CM preceded by the letter "Z"; used to classify persons who are not currently sick when they encounter health services

Figure Credits

INTRODUCTION

Figure 1: Modified from Blackmer D: Salary Survey 2013: Coder Employment on the Rise, *Cutting Edge* 24[10]:39, 2013, American Academy of Professional Coders. 2: Modified from Blackmer D: Salary Survey 2013: Coder Employment on the Rise, *Cutting Edge* 24[10]:39, 2013, American Academy of Professional Coders. 3: Modified from Blackmer D: Salary Survey 2013: Coder Employment on the Rise, *Cutting Edge* 24[10]:39, 2013, American Academy of Professional Coders. 4, 5, 6: AHIMA 2012 Salary Survey, Courtesy of the American Health Information Management Association.

CHAPTER 1

Figures 1-1, 1-2: Modified from Centers for Medicare and Medicaid Services: *Medicare Administrative Contractor (MAC) Jurisdictions Fact Sheet* [website]: www.cms.gov/Medicare/Medicare-Contracting/Medicare-Administrative-Contractors/MACJurisdictions.html. Accessed February 21, 2014. 1-3: From *Federal Register,* January 2, 2014, Vol 79, No 1, Rules and Regulations.

CHAPTER 2

Figures 2-1: From American Academy of Professional Coders: *AAPC Code of Ethics* [website]: www.aapc.com/aboutus/code-of-ethics.aspx. Accessed July 7, 2014. 2-2, 2-3, 2-6*A*, 2-7, 2-8, 2-9: Courtesy U.S. Department of Health and Human Services, Centers for Disease Control and Prevention. 2-4, 2-5, 2-6*B*, 2-11, 2-12, 2-13, 2-14, 2-15, 2-16, 2-17, 2-18, 2-19, 2-20: Modified from Buck CJ: *2015 ICD-10-CM DRAFT,* St. Louis, 2015, Saunders. 2-10: Courtesy U.S. Department of Health and Human Services, Centers for Medicare and Medicaid Services.

CHAPTER 3

Figure 3-1: Modified from Buck CJ: *2015 ICD-10-CM DRAFT,* St. Louis, 2015, Saunders.

CHAPTER 4

Figures 4-1, 4-2, 4-3, 4-4, 4-5: Modified from Buck CJ: *2015 ICD-10-CM DRAFT,* St. Louis, 2015, Saunders.

CHAPTER 5

Figures 5-1, 5-2, 5-3, 5-4, 5-5, 5-6, 5-7, 5-8, 5-9, 5-10, 5-11, 5-12, 5-13, 5-14, 5-20, 5-22, 5-23, 5-24: Modified from Buck CJ: *2015 ICD-10-CM DRAFT,* St. Louis, 2015, Saunders. 5-18*A,* 5-19*A*: From Frazier MS, Drzymkowski JW: *Essentials of Human Diseases and Conditions,* ed 5, St. Louis, 2013, Saunders. 5-18*B*: From Seidel HM, Ball JW, Dains JE, Benedict GW, *Mosby's Guide to Physical Examination,* ed 6, St. Louis, 2006, Mosby Elsevier. 5-19*B*: From Ignatavicius DD, Workman ML: *Medical-Surgical Nursing: Critical Thinking for Collaborative Care,* ed 5, St. Louis, 2006, Saunders.

CHAPTER 6

Figures 6-1, 6-2, 6-4, 6-5, 6-6: Modified from Buck CJ: *2015 ICD-10-CM DRAFT,* St. Louis, 2015, Saunders.

CHAPTER 7

Figures 7-1, 7-3, 7-4, 7-5, 7-6, 7-7, 7-8, 7-9: Modified from Buck CJ: *2015 ICD-10-CM DRAFT,* St. Louis, 2015, Saunders. 7-2: From Damjanov I: *Pathology for the Health Professions,* ed 4, St. Louis, 2012, Saunders.

CHAPTER 8

Figure 8-1: From American Academy of Professional Coders: *AAPC Code of Ethics* [website]: www.aapc.com/aboutus/code-of-ethics.aspx. Accessed July 7, 2014. 8-2: Courtesy U.S. Department of Health and Human Services, Centers for Medicare and Medicaid Services. 8-3, 8-4, 8-5, 8-6, 8-7, 8-9, 8-10, 8-11, 8-12, 8-13, 8-14, 8-15, 8-16, 8-17, 8-18, 8-19, 8-20, 8-21: Modified from Buck CJ: *2015 ICD-9-CM for Hospitals, Volumes 1, 2, & 3, Professional Edition*, St. Louis, 2015, Saunders .

CHAPTER 10

Figure 10-1: *Modified from Buck CJ: 2015 ICD-9-CM for Hospitals, Volumes 1, 2, & 3, Professional Edition*, St. Louis, 2015, Saunders.

CHAPTER 11

Figures 11-1, 11-2, 11-3: Modified from Buck CJ: *2015 ICD-9-CM for Hospitals, Volumes 1, 2, & 3, Professional Edition*, St. Louis, 2015, Saunders.

CHAPTER 12

Figures 12-1, 12-2, 12-3, 12-4: Modified from Buck CJ: *2015 ICD-9-CM for Hospitals, Volumes 1, 2, & 3, Professional Edition*, St. Louis, 2015, Saunders.

CHAPTER 13

Figures 13-1, 13-30: Courtesy U.S. Department of Health and Human Services, Centers for Medicare and Medicaid Services. 13-21, 13-22, 13-23, 13-24, 13-25, 13-26, 13-27: Modified from Buck CJ: *2015 HCPCS Level II Professional Edition*, St. Louis, 2015, Saunders. 13-28, 13-29: Courtesy U.S. Department of Health and Human Services, Public Health Service, Centers for Medicare and Medicaid Services.

CHAPTER 14

Figure 14-2: Courtesy U.S. Department of Health and Human Services, Centers for Medicare and Medicaid Services.

CHAPTER 15

Figures 15-8, 15-9: Courtesy U.S. Department of Health and Human Services, Centers for Medicare and Medicaid Services.

CHAPTER 16

Figure 16-1B: From Stack RS, Roubin GS, O'Neill WW: *Interventional Cardiovascular Medicine: Principles and Practice*, ed 2, Philadelphia, 2002, Churchill Livingstone. 16-3: From Potter PA, Perry AG: *Basic Nursing: Essentials for Practice*, ed 6, St. Louis, 2007, Mosby. 16-6, 16-7, 16-10, 16-11: Excerpted from *2014 Relative Value Guide*®, © 2013 of the American Society of Anesthesiologists. All Rights Reserved. *Relative Value Guide* is a registered trademark of the American Society of Anesthesiologists. A copy of the full text can be obtained from ASA, 1061 American Lane, Schaumburg, Illinois, 60173-4973. 16-8: Courtesy U.S. Department of Health and Human Services, Centers for Medicare and Medicaid Services. 16-9A and B: Courtesy U.S. General Services Administration.

CHAPTER 17

Figure 17-9: From Forbes CD, Jackson WF: *Color Atlas and Text of Clinical Medicine*, ed 3, 2003, Mosby.

CHAPTER 18

Figure 18-1: From Forbes CD, Jackson WF: *Color Atlas and Text of Clinical Medicine*, ed 3, 2003, Mosby. 18-2: From Kumar V, Abbas AK, Fausto N, Aster JC: *Robbins and Cotran: Pathologic Basis of Disease*, ed 8, Philadelphia, 2010, Saunders. 18-5B: Courtesy Mary Garden. 18-6C: From Roberts JR, Hedges JR, editors: *Clinical Procedures in Emergency Medicine*, ed 4, Philadelphia, 2004, Saunders. 18-7, From Habif TP: *Clinical Dermatology: A Color Guide to Diagnosis and Therapy*, ed 4, Philadelphia, 2004, Mosby. 18-9: Courtesy U.S. Department of Health and Human Services, Centers for Medicare and Medicaid Services. 18-10A, 18-12: From Habif TP: *Clinical Dermatology: A Color Guide to Diagnosis and Therapy*, ed 5, Philadelphia, 2010, Mosby. 18-13: From Burkitt HG, Quick CRG: *Essential Surgery*, ed 3, 2002, Churchill Livingstone. 18-14: Modified from Buck CJ: *2015 HCPCS Level II Professional Edition*, St. Louis, 2015, Saunders. 18-15: From Rakel RE: *Saunders Manual of Medical Practice*, ed 2, Philadelphia, 2000, Saunders. 18-17B: From Henry MC, Stapleton ER: *EMT Prehospital Care-Revised Reprint*, ed 4, St. Louis, 2012, Mosby Jems. 18-7D: From Henry MC, Stapleton ER: *EMT Prehospital Care*, ed 3, St. Louis, 2004, MosbyJems. 18-17F and H: From McCance KL, Huether SE: *Pathophysiology: The Biologic Basis for Disease in Adults and Children*, ed 6, St. Louis, 2010, Mosby. 18-18: From deWit SC: *Fundamental Concepts and Skills for Nursing*, ed 4, St. Louis, 2014, Saunders. 18-19: From Robinson JK, Hanke CW, Siegel DM, Fratila A, editors: *Surgery of the Skin: Procedural Dermatology*, ed 2, Edinburgh, 2010, Mosby. 18-21A and B: From McCarthy, JG, ed: *Plastic Surgery*, vol 6, Philadelphia, 1990, WB Saunders. 18-21C and D: From Converse JM, ed: *Reconstructive Plastic Surgery: Principles and Procedures in Correction, Reconstruction and Transplantation*, vol 5, Philadelphia, 1964, WB Saunders. 18-23: From Achauer BM, et al, eds: *Plastic Surgery: Indications, Operations, and Outcomes,* vol 4, St. Louis, 2000, Mosby. 18-24: From Ignatavicius DD, Workman ML: *Medical-Surgical Nursing: Patient-Centered Collaborative Care,* ed 7, St. Louis, 2013, Saunders. 18-25, 18-26: From Gallico GG, O'Connor NE: Cultured epithelium as a skin substitute. *Clin Plast Surg* 12: 155, 1985. 18-27: From Bland KI, Copeland EM: *The Breast: Comprehensive Management of Benign and Malignant Disorders,* ed 3, St. Louis, 2004, Saunders. 18-28, 18-30: From Flint PW, Haughey BH, Lund VJ, Niparko JK, Richardson MA, Robbins KT, Thomas JR: *Cummings Otolaryngology-Head & Neck Surgery,* ed 5, Philadelphia, 2010, Mosby. 18-29: From James WD, Berger TG, Elston DM: *Andrew's Diseases of the Skin: Clinical Dermatology,* ed 10, London, 2000, WB Saunders. 18-31: From Regezi JA, Sciubba JJ, Jordan RCK: *Oral Pathology: Clinical Pathologic Correlations,* ed 5, St. Louis, 2008, Saunders. 18-33A: From Callen J, Greer K, Hood A, et al: *Color Atlas of Dermatology, Philadelphia,* 1993, Saunders. 18-37: From Converse JM, ed: *Reconstructive Plastic Surgery: Principles and Procedures in Correction, Reconstruction and Transplantation,* vol 1, Philadelphia, 1964, WB Saunders. 18-39: Modified from Bland Kl, Copeland EM, eds: *The Breast: Comprehensive Management of Benign and Malignant Disorders,* ed 3, St. Louis, 2004, Saunders. 18-40: Modified from Buck CJ: *2015 ICD-10-CM DRAFT,* St. Louis, 2015, Saunders.

CHAPTER 19

Figure 19-7: From *Dorland's Illustrated Medical Dictionary,* ed 32, Philadelphia, 2012, Saunders. 19-9: From Rakel RE: *Saunders Manual of Medical Practice,* ed 2, Philadelphia, 2000, Saunders. 19-10: From Swan KG, Swan RC: Principles of ballistics applicable to the treatment of gunshot wounds. *Surg Clin North Am* 71:221-239, 1991. 19-11: From Swan, KG, Swan RC: *Gunshot Wounds: Pathophysiology and Management,* ed 2, Chicago, Year Book Medical Publishers, Inc. 19-13B: from McCance KL, Huether SE: *Pathophysiology: The Biologic Basis for Disease in Adults and Children,* ed 6, St. Louis, 2010, Mosby. 19-14: From Canale ST, Beaty JH: *Campbell's Operative Orthopaedics,* ed 12, Philadelphia, 2013, Mosby. 19-16A: From Fillit HM, Rockwood K, Woodhouse K: *Brocklehurst's Textbook of Geriatric Medicine and Gerontology,* ed 7, Philadelphia, 2010, Saunders.

CHAPTER 20

Figure 20-3A: From Zitelli BJ, Davis HW: *Atlas of Pediatric Physical Diagnosis,* ed 5, Philadelphia, 2007, Mosby. 20-3B: From Monahan FD et al: *Phipps' Medical-Surgical Nursing: Health and Illness Perspectives,* ed 8, St. Louis, 2007, Mosby. 20-8: Modified from Netter FH: *Atlas of Human Anatomy,* ed 4, Philadelphia, 2006, Saunders. 20-9: Modified from Standring S, editor: *Gray's Anatomy:*

The Anatomical Basis of Clinical Practice, ed 40, Philadelphia, 2008, Churchill Livingstone.

CHAPTER 21

Figures 21-5, 21-24: From Forbes CD, Jackson WF: *Color Atlas and Text of Clinical Medicine,* ed 3, 2003, Mosby. 21-6: From Miller RD, editor: *Miller's Anesthesia,* ed 7, Philadelphia, 2010, Churchill Livingstone. 21-7B: From Lewis SL, Dirksen SR, Heitkemper MM, Bucher L, Camera IM: *Medical-Surgical Nursing: Assessment and Management of Clinical Problems,* ed 8, St. Louis, 2011, Mosby. 21-8B: From Damjanov I: *Pathology for the Health Professions,* ed 4, St. Louis, 2012, Saunders. 21-9: From Monahan FD, Neighbors M: *Medical-Surgical Nursing: Foundations for Clinical Practice,* ed 2, Philadelphia, 1998, Saunders. 21-14: From Roberts JR, Hedges JR, eds: *Clinical Procedures in Emergency Medicine,* ed 4, Philadelphia, 2004, Saunders. 21-22: From Young AP, Proctor DB: *Kinn's The Medical Assistant: An Applied Learning Approach,* ed 10, St. Louis, 2007, Saunders. 21-25A: From Proctor DB, Adams AP: *Kinn's The Medical Assistant: An Applied Learning Approach,* ed 12, St. Louis, 2014, Saunders. 21-29: From Zipes DP, editor: *Braunwald's Heart Disease,* ed 7, Philadelphia, 2005, Saunders. 21-32: From Bennett JC, Plum F: *Cecil Textbook of Medicine,* ed 20, Philadelphia, 1996, WB Saunders.

CHAPTER 22

Figure 22-2: Modified from Netter FH: *Atlas of Human Anatomy,* ed 4, Philadelphia, 2006, Saunders.

CHAPTER 23

Figure 23-2: Modified from Liebgott B: *The Anatomical Basis of Dentistry,* ed 3, St. Louis, 2011, Mosby, Inc. 23-3: From Kavanagh KT: Abbe-Estlander Flap for Lip Reconstruction in a Patient with Skin Cancer of the Lower Lip, Ear, Nose & Throat - U.S.A. (website): www.entusa. com/abbe_estlander.htm. Accessed February 21, 2014. 23-4A: Modified from Buck CJ: *2015 ICD-10-CM DRAFT,* St. Louis, 2015, Saunders. 23-4B: From Zitelli BJ, Davis HW: *Atlas of Pediatric Physical Diagnosis,* ed 5, Philadelphia, 2007, Mosby. 23-4C: Patton KT, Thibodeau GA: *Anatomy & Physiology,* ed 8, St. Louis, 2013, Mosby. 23-5: From Coran AG, Adzick NS, Krummel TM, Laberge J-M, Shamberger RC, Caldamone AA, et al, editors: *Pediatric Surgery,* ed 7, Philadelphia, 2012, Saunders. 23-6: From Liebgott B:*The Anatomical Basis of Dentistry,* ed 3, St. Louis, 2011, Mosby. 23-8: From Marx JA, Hockberger R, Walls R, editors: *Rosen's Emergency Medicine: Concepts and Clinical Practice,* ed 8, Philadelphia, 2014, Saunders. 23-13: From Feldman M, Friedman LS, Brandt LJ: *Sleisenger & Fordtran's Gastrointestinal and Liver Disease,* ed 8, Philadelphia, 2006, Saunders. 23-14B and C: From

Drake RL, Vogl W, Mitchell AWM: *Gray's Anatomy for Students,* ed 2, Philadelphia, 2010, Churchill Livingstone. 23-18: Courtesy U.S. National Cancer Institute, Surveillance, Epidemiology, and End Results (SEER) Program. 23-21: From Townsend CM, Beauchamp RD, Evers BM, Mattox KL: *Sabiston Textbook of Surgery,* ed 19, Philadelphia, 2012, Saunders. 23-22: From Roberts JR, Hedges JR, Chanmugam AS, Chudnofsky CR, Custalow CB, Dronen SC: *Clinical Procedures in Emergency Medicine,* ed 4, Philadelphia, 2004, Saunders. 23-23: From Roberts JR, Hedges JR, editors: *Clinical Procedures in Emergency Medicine,*ed 4, Philadelphia, 2004, Saunders.

CHAPTER 24

Figure 24-4: From White GM, Cox NH: *Diseases of the Skin: A Color Atlas and Text,* ed 2, Edinburgh, 2006, Mosby. 24-14: Modified from Wein AJ, editor: *Campbell-Walsh Urology,* ed 9, Philadelphia, 2007, Saunders.

CHAPTER 25

Figure 25-2: Modified from Townsend CM, Beauchamp RD, Evers BM, Mattox KL: *Sabiston Textbook of Surgery,* ed 19, Philadelphia, 2012, Saunders. 25-3: Modified from Sanfilippo JS, Muram D, Dewhurst J, Lee PA: *Pediatric and Adolescent Gynecology,* ed 2, Philadelphia, 2001, Saunders. 25-4: From DiSaia PJ, Creasman WT: *Clinical Gynecologic Oncology,* ed 7, St. Louis, 2007, Mosby. 25-5: Modified from Gabbe SG, Niebyl JR, Simpson JL, Landon MB, Galan H, Jauniaux ERM, Driscoll DA: *Obstetrics: Normal and Problem Pregnancies,* ed 6, Philadelphia, 2012, Saunders. 25-6: From Baggish MS: *Colposcopy of the Cervix, Vagina, and Vulva: A Comprehensive Textbook,* Philadelphia, 2003, Mosby. 25-9: From Katz VL, Lentz GM, Lobo RA, Gershenson DM: *Comprehensive Gynecology,* ed 5, Philadelphia, 2007, Mosby. 25-10: Modified from Goldman CC, Snyder TK: *Differential Diagnosis for Physical Therapists: Screening for Referral,* ed 5, St. Louis, 2013, Saunders. 25-13: From Roberts JR, Hedges JR, eds: *Clinical Procedures in Emergency Medicine,* ed 4, Philadelphia, 2004, Saunders. 25-14: From *Dorland's Illustrated Medical Dictionary,* ed 32, Philadelphia, 2012, Saunders. 25-15: From Damjanov I: *Pathology for the Health Professions,* ed 4, St. Louis, 2012, Saunders.

CHAPTER 26

Figure 26-2: Modified from Hall JE: *Guyton and Hall Textbook of Medical Physiology,* ed 12, Philadelphia, 2011, Saunders. 26-3: From Stoy WA, Platt TE, Lejeune DA: *Mosby's EMT-Basic Textbook,* ed 2, St. Louis, 2007, Mosby.

CHAPTER 27

Figure 27-7: From Rothrock JC: *Alexander's Care of the Patient in Surgery,* ed 15, St. Louis, 2015, Mosby. 27-8A, 27-9A: From Frazier MS, Drzymkowski JW: *Essentials of Human Diseases and Conditions,* ed 5, St. Louis, 2013, Saunders. 27-8B: From Ignatavicius DD, Workman ML: *Medical-Surgical Nursing: Critical Thinking for Collaborative Care,* ed 5, St. Louis, 2006, Saunders. 27-9B: From Seidel HM, Ball JW, Dains JE, Benedict GW: *Mosby's Guide to Physical Examination,* ed 6, St. Louis, 2006, Mosby Elsevier. 27-11: Modified from Drake RL, Vogl W, Mitchell AWM: *Gray's Anatomy for Students,* ed 2, Philadelphia, 2010, Churchill Livingstone. 27-13: From Microsurgery Instruments Inc.: *The Economic Operating Microscope* (website): www.microsurgeryusa.com/EOM. htm. Accessed February 21, 2014. 27-14: From Mopec: *AK100 Binocular Magnifying Loupe* (website): www. mopec.com/product/523/binocular_magnifying_loupe/. Accessed February 21, 2014.

CHAPTER 28

Figures 28-7, 28-14: From Goldman L, Schafer AI, editors: *Goldman's Cecil Medicine,* ed 24, Philadelphia, 2012, Saunders. 28-10A: From Drake RL, Vogl W, Mitchell AWM: *Gray's Anatomy for Students,* ed 2, Philadelphia, 2010, Churchill Livingstone. 28-10B, 28-13: From Stimac GK: *Introduction to Diagnostic Imaging,* Philadelphia, 1992, WB Saunders. 28-11: From Bragg DG, Rubin P, Hricak H: *Oncologic Imaging,* ed 2, Philadelphia, 2002, Saunders. 28-12: Modified from Bradley WG, Daroff RB, Fenichel GM, Jankovic J: *Neurology in Clinical Practice,* ed 5, Philadelphia, 2008, Butterworth-Heinemann. 28-15: From Tempkin BB: *Ultrasound Scanning: Principles and Protocols,* ed 3, St. Louis, 2009, Saunders. 28-16: From Crownover RL, ed: *Hematology/Oncology Clinics of North America,* Vol 13, Number 3, June 1999, p 645.

CHAPTER 29

Figure 29-1: From Young AP, Proctor DB: *Kinn's The Medical Assistant,* ed 10, St. Louis, 2007, Saunders. 29-2: Courtesy National Institute of Environmental Health Sciences—National Institutes of Health. 29-3: From Proctor DB, Adams AP: *Kinn's The Medical Assistant: An Applied Learning Approach,* ed 12, St. Louis, 2014, Saunders. 29-4: From Clinical Diagnostic Solutions, Inc.: *M-Series Hematology Analyzer CAP.* (website): www.cdsolinc.com/index. php?main_page=product_info&cPath=7_44&products_ id=97. Accessed February 21, 2014. 29-6: Courtesy United States Environmental Protection Agency.

CHAPTER 30

Figure 30-4: From Lewis SL, Dirksen SR, Heitkemper MM, Bucher L, Camera IM: *Medical-Surgical Nursing: Assessment and Management of Clinical Problems,* ed 8, St. Louis, 2011, Mosby. 30-5: From National Eye Institute, National Institutes of Health: *Ref#: EE69* (website): http://www.nei.nih.gov/photo/eye_exam/images/EE69_72.jpg. Accessed February 21, 2014. 30-8: From Gardenhire DS: *Rau's Respiratory Care Pharmacology,* ed 8, St. Louis, 2012, Mosby. 30-9: From deWit SC: *Fundamental Concepts and Skills for Nursing,* ed 4, St. Louis, 2014, Saunders. 30-10: From DeLee JC, Drez D: *DeLee & Drez's Orthopaedic Sports Medicine: Principles and Practice,* ed 2, Philadelphia, 2003, Saunders. 30-11: From Goldman L, Schafer AI, editors: *Goldman's Cecil Medicine,* ed 24, Philadelphia, 2012, Saunders. 30-13: Courtesy Argentum Medical, LLC. 30-14: From Townsend CM, Beauchamp RD, Evers BM, Mattox KL: *Sabiston Textbook of Surgery,* ed 19, Philadelphia, 2012, Saunders.

CHAPTER 31

Figures 31-1, 31-2, 31-3, 31-4, 31-5: Modified from Buck CJ: *2015 ICD-10-PCS DRAFT,* St. Louis, 2015, Saunders.

Coder's Index

References are to pages. Current Procedural Technology (CPT) codes begin on page 937, ICD-9-CM codes begin on page 944, ICD-10-CM codes begin on page 948, and HCPCS codes begin on page 952.

CPT CODES

00100:	369, 402	11300:	534	12057:	541	15783:	547
00142:	502t	11311:	893	13100:	541	15786:	547
00172:	892	11313:	534	13101:	893	15787:	547
00322:	892	11400:	534	13121:	893	15788:	547
00400:	504t	11401:	411	13131:	653	15793:	547
00635:	402	11402:	408	13132:	893	15819:	547–548
00740:	508	11406:	407	13153:	653	15820:	547–548
00756:	508	11420-11426:	717	13160:	534, 541	15823:	547–548
00810:	508	11423:	408	14000:	542	15824:	547–548
00914:	892	11440:	653	14040:	656, 893	15829:	547–548
01472:	892	11444:	653	14041:	893	15830:	547–548
01916:	494	11446:	653	14302:	656	15839:	547–548
01922:	494t	11450:	535	14350:	542	15840:	548
01925:	494t	11471:	534, 535	15002:	543–545, 893	15845:	548
01936:	494	11600:	535	15003:	893	15847:	547–548
01951:	494	11620-11626:	717	15004:	893	15850:	548
01953:	494, 498, 499	11640:	653	15005:	543	15852:	548
01958:	494	11644:	653	15040:	545	15876:	548
01961:	892	11646:	535, 653	15050:	544	15879:	547, 548
01968:	498	11719:	536	15100:	543, 551, 893	15900:	519
01969:	494, 498	11720:	536	15101:	543, 893	15920:	548
01990:	494	11730:	537	15110:	544	15946:	411
01996:	499, 749	11732:	537	15116:	544	15999:	548
01999:	369, 402, 494, 506, 892	11740:	537	15120:	543, 755–756, 762, 893	16000:	528, 551
10021:	369, 414, 512, 521, 709, 893	11750:	537	15121:	543, 755–756, 762	16020:	550, 551
10022:	521, 524, 594, 709, 893	11752:	537	15130:	544	16025:	893
10030:	419, 527	11765:	536	15136:	544	16030:	550, 551
10040:	527	11770:	538	15150:	544	16035:	551
10080:	519	11772:	538	15157:	544	16036:	528, 551
10081:	519	11900:	538	15260:	755–756	17000:	534, 552, 893
10160:	527	11920:	538	15261:	543, 545, 755–756	17003:	552, 893
10180:	527	11922:	538	15271:	544, 545	17004:	552
11000:	366, 528, 542	11950:	538	15272:	545	17110:	893
11001:	366, 528	11954:	538	15273:	545	17250:	534
11004:	528	11960:	538	15274:	545	17260:	535
11006:	528	11971:	538	15275:	545	17264:	412, 888
11042:	528	11976:	539	15276:	545	17274:	412, 888
11042-11047:	841	11980:	539	15277:	545	17286:	535, 552
11047:	528, 542	11981:	539	15278:	543–545, 551	17311:	552–553, 893
11055:	531	11983:	538	15501:	412	17311-17315:	755
11056:	893	12001:	539, 541	15570:	545	17315:	552–553
11057:	531	12002:	893	15732:	893	17999:	893
11100:	410, 553, 585	12004:	520, 520t, 521, 893	15738:	545	19000:	370, 554, 893
11101:	410, 553	12014:	520	15740:	545, 546	19081:	554
11200:	533, 893	12020:	520t	15750:	546	19086:	554
11201:	533	12021:	539	15777:	545	19100:	516–517, 521
		12031:	534, 541	15780:	547	19101:	521
		12032:	407, 893	15781:	547	19287:	893
		12042:	404	15782:	547	19288:	554

ICD-10-CM CODES

HCPCS CODES

Index

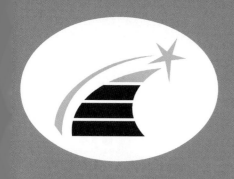
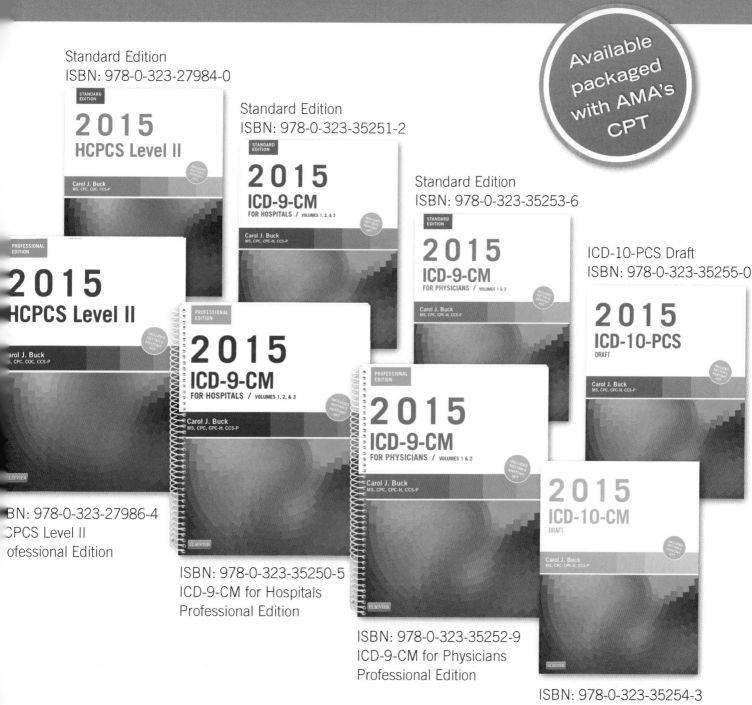

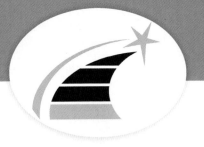
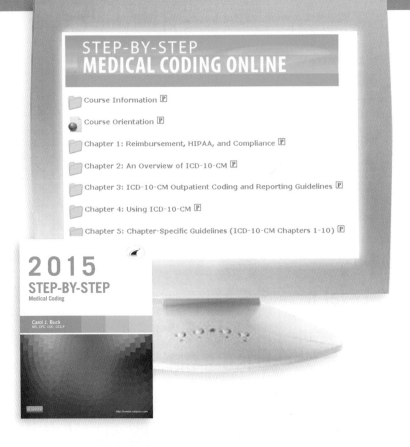
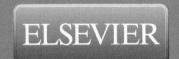

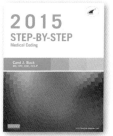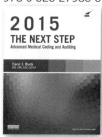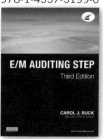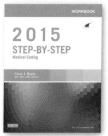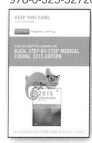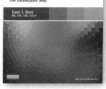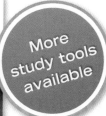
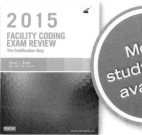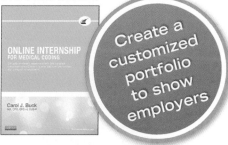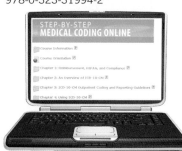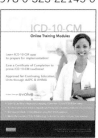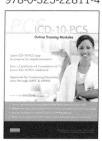
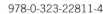

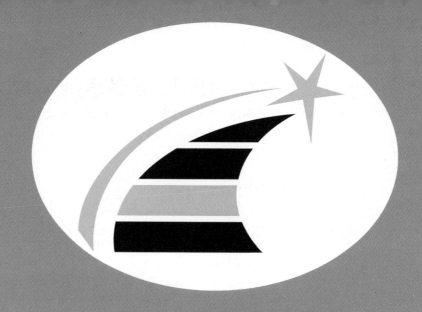

Step 2: Practice

"Before everything else, getting ready is the secret of success."

— Henry Ford

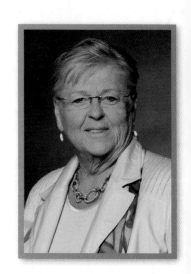

Thank you for pursuing excellence in your coding education! As coding becomes a more complex and specialized career, it is extremely important that we coders stay at the top of our coding game. That's why, as a lifelong coder and educator, I know that tools for more advanced learning and practice are crucial for today's top coders. ***Thank you for being committed to being one of the best and rising to the top in your career.***

— Carol J. Buck, MS, CPC, COC, CCS-P

Track your progress!

See the checklist in the back of this book to learn more about your next step toward coding success!